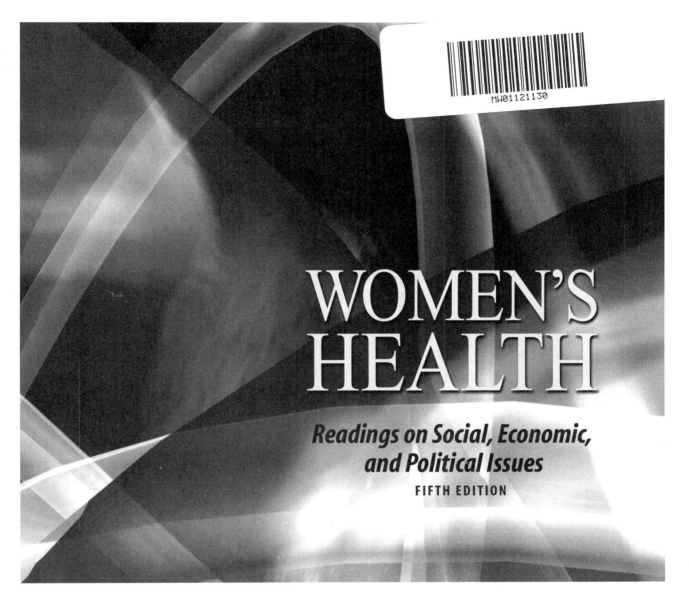

WOMEN'S HEALTH

Readings on Social, Economic, and Political Issues

FIFTH EDITION

edited by

NANCY WORCESTER • MARIAMNE H. WHATLEY

Department of Gender and Women's Studies

University of Wisconsin—Madison

KENDALL/HUNT PUBLISHING COMPANY
4050 Westmark Drive   P.O. Box 1840   Dubuque, Iowa 52004-1840

Book Team

Chairman and Chief Executive Officer   Mark C. Falb
President and Chief Operating Office   Chad M. Chandlee
Vice President, Higher Education   David L. Tart
Director of National Book Program   Paul B. Carty
Editorial Development Manager   Georgia Botsford
Developmental Editor   Denise LaBudda
Vice President, Operations   Timothy J. Beitzel
Assistant Vice President, Production Services   Christine E. O'Brien
Senior Production Editor   Charmayne McMurray
Permissions Editor   Renae Horstman
Cover Designer   Sandy Beck

Printed in the United States of America
10 9 8 7 6 5 4 3 2 1

CONTENTS

PREFACE

This fifth edition of this popular textbook builds on the success of the previous four editions and includes articles on the cutting edge issues, and responds to readers' comments to have an additional emphasis on consumer information for personal decision-making and activism.

This edition of the book:

- Includes more than eighty new articles, including a number of articles (not available elsewhere) written specifically for this book.

- Includes a totally new chapter on the medicalization and marketing of women's health.

- Provides a history of women's health movements, including "classic" articles on most topics, and updates and inspires people to be involved in *today's* issues and activism.

- Introduces readers to the organizations and publications that consistently provide scientifically accurate and personally empowering information. This edition of the book has a new emphasis on showcasing articles from the National Women's Health Network's *The Women's Health Activist.*

- Gives readers a feel for global women's health perspectives through overview articles, as well as a diversity of articles from Australian, British, and Canadian publications.

- Provides a guide to each chapter, highlighting why each article was included and how the articles fit together to build the chapter's themes.

- Provides worksheets to help teachers plan discussion or exam questions related to readings, and help students prepare for those discussions and exams.

- Inspires consumer literacy with a completely new directory of women's health web sites and how-to articles including "How to Read a Drug Ad" and "Finding Good Health Information on the Web."

ACKNOWLEDGMENTS

Each woman who has worked as a part of the Women's Studies 103 teaching team at the University of Wisconsin-Madison has made her own contributions to the course. This book reflects the input of all the women who have worked as Teaching Assistants for WS103 since the course was first taught in 1978. For the 5th edition, a special thanks goes to Sue Pastor (former WS103 TA and Lecturer), Ronna Popkin (former WS103 TA and Lecturer) and Stephanie Rytalahti (former WS103 student, now a WS103 TA) for writing original articles for this edition of the book and to Annie Kaatz (present WS103 TA) for working as our Project Assistant/Web Resources writer for this edition.

This book is dedicated to all the people who have been a part of Women's Health Movements. This book is about you, the way you have changed the world of health care and information for women, and the critical thinking and analysis you have put in place for future activists and leaders. And it is to all you future women's health activists that we give the biggest smile: we congratulate you for being a part of this most rewarding work to create a world that helps every woman, man, and child maximize on their mental and physical health.

A percentage of royalties from this book go to the National Women's Health Network (www.nwhn.org), as a thanks for being a leader in the women's health work movement work for more than thirty years. Readers will find that the many articles reprinted here from their newsletter, *The Women's Health Activist*, represent the cutting edge, social justice framework that the National Women's Health Network uses to combine sound scientific information and feminist critical thinking to affect policy and support consumer decision-making.

ABOUT THE AUTHORS

Nancy Worcester has a Ph.D. in Nutrition from the University of London. Her early life experiences included jobs in both the drug and food industries. She has been active in women's health movements in England and the USA for more than forty years. This work has included involvement in the Women and Science Group (London), The Politics of Health Group (England), the Women and Food Group (London), being a founding member of the National Women's Health Information Centre Collective (England), working as the state education coordinator for the Wisconsin Coalition Against Domestic Violence, and serving on Board of Directors for both the National (USA) Women's Health Network Board and the Society for Menstrual Cycle Research. Worcester also served as a Consumer Representative on the Food and Drug Administration's Endocrinological and Metabolic Drugs Advisory Panel. As UW-Madison's Women's Studies Outreach Coordinator, Worcester was the founder and key trainer for the WI Domestic Violence Training Project which trained more than 30,000 school and health professionals and she organized numerous local, state, and national women's health courses and conferences. Nancy led, organized or participated in health study tours to China (1978, 1983), Cuba (1981, 1994), Grenada (early 1983), and Nicaragua (1984.) Worcester is presently a Professor in Gender and Women's Studies at the University of Wisconsin-Madison where she teaches a science-based women's health course to 400 students each semester and coordinates the Women's Studies Internship Program.

Mariamne H. Whatley has been teaching women's health and biology of women at the University of Wisconsin-Madison since 1978, where she is a Professor of Gender and Women's Studies and Curriculum & Instruction, and Associate Dean in the School of Education. In addition to her work in women's health, she has written extensively on sexuality/health education, bringing a feminist analysis to textbooks and curricula. She teaches LGBTI health as part of the LGBT Studies Certificate Program. In an ongoing research collaboration with a folklorist, she co-authored, with Elissa Henken, *Did You Hear About the Girl Who . . .? Contemporary Legends, Folklore, and Human Sexuality*. She has served on the Board of the National Women's Health Network. Her undergraduate degree is in English from Radcliffe College and her PhD in Biological Sciences from Northwestern University.

Nancy Worcester and Mariamne Whatley were both members of the National Women's Health Network's Writing Group for several editions of *Taking Hormones and Women's Health and for The Truth About Hormone Replacement Therapy: How to Break Free from the Medical Myths of Menopause*.

INTRODUCTION

Women cannot have control over our lives until we have control over our bodies; thus, understanding and gaining control over our bodies and our health are essential to taking control of our lives. Consequently, activism around women's health issues has been a central part of struggles, by women and men, for improving the role of women in society.

The readings in this book are a representation of the exciting range of excellent resources now available on women's health issues. We intentionally include articles and chapters from the widest diversity of publications, to introduce readers to the amazing range of women's health writing and organizing being done throughout the world by individuals and groups actively striving for healthcare systems more appropriate to women's needs. Similarly, the lengthy list of websites gives readers a glimpse at the incredible number of good resources now available, and encourages teachers and students to follow up on topics covered here.

This collection of readings is designed specifically for use as a part of the women's health course, *Women's Studies 103: Women and Their Bodies in Health and Disease*, which is taught to 400 students each semester, in the Department of Gender and Women's Studies at the University of Wisconsin-Madison. (We are delighted to hear that the book is also being used in many other women's health courses throughout the country!) Readings and worksheets are particularly chosen or written to stimulate thought and analysis in preparation for discussion sections. Selections have been made to complement other materials used for the course: *Biology of Women* by Ethel Sloane, published by Wiley; *The Black Women's Health Book*, edited by Evelyn C. White, published by Seal Press; *Our Bodies, Ourselves: A New Edition for a New Era* by the Boston Women's Health Book Collective, published by Touchstone; and *Undivided Rights: Women of Color Organizing for Reproductive Justice* by Jael Silliman, Marlene Gerber Fried, Loretta Ross, and Elena R. Gutiérrez, published by South End Press.

This is the fifth edition of this book. Reflecting the rapidly changing area of women's health, the tremendous interest shown in women's health in recent years by both healthcare providers and consumers, and the new national debates, this book contains a very different range of articles than was available for the first four editions. In an effort to provide an historical context to the many present debates, we have deliberately included not only new articles but also those with an historical perspective, as well as older articles, which we mark as "classics." (We love the "classic" fist within a woman's symbol used to mark "classics" in this edition, as that graphic was such a part of our earliest women's health organizing. Mariamne even wore a large version of that symbol on the back of her gown at her college graduation!) A goal for this book is to have students learn to value and use women's health "classics" as a part of studying present-day issues and developing their own analyses. Often in the field of women's health, earliest articles written on a topic do an excellent job of identifying the crucial issues. Once that basic analysis has been written, other women's health writers are more likely to write an article updating the information, rather than writing an article very similar to the first one. When researching a women's health topic, students are encouraged to read both the "classics" and the most recent information to get the clearest overview of both the fundamental issues and which aspects of the area have and have not changed.

We have worked toward emphasizing an anti-racist, cross-cultural perspective on topics, and looked for articles that make the connections among social, economic, and political issues and women's mental and physical health. In many cases, there are still important articles to get written! We encourage readers to dig deeper in thinking about health ramifications related to poverty, ageism, racism, anti-semitism, heterosexism, fatphobia, and what it means to have a disability. **Then write your own articles or books or change the world. This project is now yours!**

WOMEN *and the* HEALTHCARE SYSTEM

The role of women in the health system and the priority given to work to maximize good mental and physical health for all women reflect much about the values of a society. Similarly, the priorities and visions each of us has for how to improve the healthcare system and women's health reflect much about our personal values, our goals, and our work for social change. Thus, studying the changing—and non-changing—roles of women in the health system and grassroots activism and professional organizing to improve women's health, becomes an effective lens for viewing societal changes of the last decades.

Since the late 1960s, modern women's health movements have critiqued curative medical systems based on the patriarchal values of the male medical establishment, organized for fundamental changes in the system, and worked for the empowerment of women, both as consumers and healthcare providers, to be more involved in healthcare decisions for themselves and the system.

Mary Halas's classic 1979 article, "Sexism in Women's Medical Care," sets the scene for the important ongoing discussion of how sexism in medical practice is rooted in the socialization of women to be passive patients, and the socialization of doctors (both men and women) to have a lack of respect for women and their right to information about their own bodies. Halas emphasized why it is essential for women to take a more involved role in their own health. The question of how much the sexism of the medical system has changed (or stayed the same) since 1979 will be a theme addressed throughout many specific topics in this book.

Andrea Irwin's article, "Diagnosing Gender Disparities in Healthcare," brings a contemporary perspective to some of the issues raised by Halas. Irwin's article begins, "Until I became a women's health advocate immersed in the nuances of Medicaid, health insurance, and other complicated policy issues, I never truly appreciated the numerous disparities that exist between the ways men and women access the healthcare system." She then lays out some of the many ways that health insurance policies—such as not covering contraceptives—work against good healthcare for women.

As reflected in the 1979 Halas article, much of the writing and debates of the 1970s and 1980s focused largely on why the health system was not adequately serving women and why women's health needed to be taken seriously. Today we can celebrate that women's health movements were extremely successful in many ways in convincing consumers, health practitioners, health systems and the federal government that women's health needed to be taken seriously. The next two classic articles, "PRO: Women's Health: Developing a New Interdisciplinary Specialty" and "CON: Women's Health as a Specialty: A Deceptive Solution," demonstrate how the debate increasingly changed from *why* women's health needed to be taken seriously to debates about *how* the health system should take women's health seriously. Both these articles, written by women doctors, describe key issues that the health system needed to address to better serve women. Centered around the specific debate about whether there should be a "women's health specialty" (more of a "hot" topic in the early 1990s than it is today), these "opposing" articles demonstrate that even when providers, consumers, or activists agree that there need to be fundamental changes in the health system for it to better serve women, we often do not agree on what strategies will be most effective.

The next five articles in this chapter represent a range of ways that women as consumers and healthcare practitioners have been working to help women individually and collectively be more informed, active patients, and to prepare the health system for consumers who expect a more respectful relationship with their healthcare providers. The classic, "How to tell Your Doctor a Thing or Two," published by Bread and Roses Women's Health Center (a feminist health center, *by* women, *for* women) is representative of how women's health movements have encouraged women to be a different kind of patient. In this article, Morton Hunt identifies changes in medical practices that had caused a deterioration in doctor-patient relationships, and proposes a seven-point program for becoming a more active patient.

From the other end of the speculum, Judy Schmidt's "The Gynecological Exam and the Training of Medical Students: An Opportunity for Health Education" gives an example of a training program that consciously aims to educate physicians to be "patient-orientated" so they can communicate appropriately with their patients. In a more theoretical approach to the same issues, Terri Kapsalis, in "Cadavers, Dolls, and Prostitutes: Medical Pedagogy and the Pelvic Rehearsal," explores how "the types of practice performances adopted reveal and promote specific ideas about female bodies and sexuality held by the medical institution." Next, Molly Kenefick, who had worked for a number of years as a "pelvic educator" at a medical school, presents her perspective about her experiences of doing this work, what she teaches the medical students, and why she sees this work as such an important role in changing the quality of healthcare for women.

The next article, by Megan Seely, changes the emphasis from improving the way healthcare practitioners give pelvic exams to encouraging women to learn more about their bodies through vaginal and cervical self-examination, an approach developed in the early 1970s that then faded away to a large extent. The instructions and illustrations provided by the Federation of Feminist Women's Health Centers make the process easy and accessible. Seely argues "that we gradually become disconnected from our bodies, particularly female bodies. And it is no wonder that we are disconnected—between the lack of adequate education and the widely endorsed negative attitudes about our bodies, our menstruation, and our sexuality—women learn early to ignore, underemphasize, or keep quiet about the functions of our bodies."

The years 1990/1991 are important "turning point" years for anyone studying the history of women's health movements. Decades of grassroots activism resulted in much visible organizing around women's health at the national level. Congressional hearings demonstrated that an embarrassingly small (13%) percentage of the national health research funding was earmarked for women's health; top-level policy-makers started seeing the need for increased attention to and funding of women's health issues. The Office of Research on Women's Health was established in 1990 and the U.S. Department of Health and Human Services' Office on Women's Health was established in 1991. Thus, it is fitting here to include the Office of Women's Health's own highlights of the women's health events of the twentieth century. Unfortunately, this list of highlights has not been updated to include the twenty-first century, so readers might decide to create their own lists.

Ruzek's and Becker's article, "The Women's Health Movement in the United States: From Grassroots Activism to Professional Agendas," is key to understanding the differences among groups that have worked to improve women's health. Identifying the early 1990s as "turning point" years for women's health activism, as discussed above, Ruzek and Becker contrast the work and philosophies of early grassroots organizations and newer (post-1990) "professionalized" women's health organizations on six important issues. Although these authors present organizational philosophies as "early organizing" versus "today's organizing," this textbook encourages readers to think about how crucial the philosophies of "early organizing" are to today's issues and how we can better incorporate more of those philosophies and activism into present-day organizing around women's health issues.

An excellent example that demonstrates that grassroots organizations are still alive, well, and extremely effective is the Boston Women's Health Book Collective (BWHBC), now known simply as *Our Bodies, Ourselves*. Their book, *Our Bodies, Ourselves (OBOS)*, continually updated since 1970, has been described as one of the most influential books ever published. "This book not only had a decisive impact on how generations of American women felt about their bodies, their sexuality and their health, but it was translated and adopted in 20 languages." [Quote from Kathy Davis in an excellent scholarly article on the BWHBC, "Feminist Body/Politics as World Traveler" published by *The European Journal of Women's Studies*, Volume 9 (3), 223–247, 2002.] The next four articles examine the impact that *OBOS* has had on women and healthcare throughout the U.S. and internationally. The first article, "Crossing Cultural Borders with *Our Bodies, Ourselves*" summarizes a gathering of grassroots feminists from 10 countries as they discussed the development and distribution of culturally appropriate versions of the classic women's health book for women in very different situations around the world; their conversations reflect, in many ways, the very different struggles facing women's health organizers around the world. The next two articles are by Kathy Davis, both from the book *The Making of Our Bodies, Ourselves: How Feminism Travels Across Borders*. The "Introduction" to Davis's book provides a short overview of the enormous popularity and impact of *OBOS* on generations of women. This is followed by Davis's chapter, "Transnational Knowledge, Transnational Politics," which examines *OBOS* from a contemporary feminist theoretical perspective, providing some important insights:

> . . . the politics of knowledge represented by *OBOS* not only allowed it to cross borders of class, race and ethnicity, sexual orientation, and generation within the United States, but it also enabled what was otherwise a local product—a typically U.S. book—to travel. One of the unique features of *OBOS* was that its content, form, and politics did not remain intact in the course of its border crossings. It invited women across the globe to rewrite the book, and ultimately, transform it in ways that would be accessible and relevant in their social, cultural, and geopolitical contexts.

To wrap up the *OBOS* section, Sheryl Ruzek also reviews some of the history and impact of the book, emphasizing the "critical role" *OBOS* played in "transforming patients from passive recipients of healthcare into active consumers. Today's concept of shared decision-making in healthcare is firmly rooted in the principles and practices of health communication set forth in *Our Bodies, Ourselves*."

The next two articles on women doctors provide perspectives on the question of whether increasing the number of women doctors is important in improving healthcare for women. Adriane Fugh-Berman's "Tales Out of Medical School" vividly describes some of the traumas facing women trying to become doctors, and reminds us that simply getting more women into medicine would do little to make the health system more appropriate for women (or men) unless the medical socialization of doctors during training were changed. We hope many of the problems identified in Fugh-Berman's 1992 article no longer exist, but whether the socialization of health practitioners is suitable for appropriately serving *all* patients remains an important question examined throughout this book.

Dr. Judith Lorber's answers to the question, "What Impact Have Women Physicians Had on Women's Health?" are both optimistic and realistic in recognizing the obstacles to, and potential for, women to have very positive influences on medicine when and if they are able to move into policy-making positions. (Readers may be interested in other articles on women physicians covered in *The Journal of the American Medical Women's Association*.)

The next group of articles focuses on healthcare reform, an unsolved problem in the U.S. While many in the U.S. know there is a need for major changes in the healthcare system, there are huge disagreements about how to proceed. Catherine DeLorey states, "Complicating this issue for women's health activists is the fact that—while women are often disproportionately affected by our healthcare system's problems—only fledgling efforts have been made to ensure that healthcare reform initiatives address women's concerns." She then lays out why women's health needs must be addressed in any healthcare reform.

Ahuva Segal, an Australian interning at the National Women's Health Network in Washington, D.C., describes her reaction to the U.S. healthcare system, having lived in a country where there is universal healthcare, and presents some suggestions to those who recognize that "now is the time to rally support for the U.S. adoption of universal healthcare." The article was written in 2004 and *now* is still the time to fight for this important right. Next, the short statement by the American Medical Student Association presents the case for a single-payer national health insurance system, stating that "everyone has a fundamental right to accessing healthcare."

The chapter concludes with "Scientific Terms Explained," from Adriane Fugh-Berman's excellent *Alternative Medicine: What Works*, a comprehensive pro-and-con easy-to-read review of the scientific literature. She demystifies many of the terms involved in describing scientific studies and helps the consumer become a more informed and critical reader of medical research, better able to judge which studies to take seriously.

Sexism in Women's Medical Care

by Mary A. Halas

A twenty-seven-year old woman complained that her health had taken a sudden unexplained change for the worse. She had a diffuse sense of not being well, with pains in various parts of her body, weakness, and fatigue. Her gynecologist gave her a physical exam and pronounced her fine. As the symptoms continued, she returned to her physician and also went to several other doctors—meeting reactions of disbelief and even ridicule with increasing frequency. Eventually one specialist recommended she see a counselor, because she obviously had no real physical problems.

That recommendation turned out to be a good one. After a few sessions the counselor concluded that the woman was in good mental health and concentrated on supporting her to continue seeking medical attention to evaluate the sudden change in her physical health.

Finally, months after her symptoms appeared and weeks after her last visit to her gynecologist, the woman had an appointment with a female physician who listened to an exhaustive list of her symptoms and concerns, and gave her an extremely thorough physical examination.

The results: the woman had a large lump in her left breast; after surgery two days later the lump was diagnosed as cancer. No one will ever know whether the lump was already there during her gynecologist's hurried and skeptical exam, but it is certain that the woman might have had a better chance of finding the lump herself if her doctor had ever taught her how to examine her own breasts. According to the woman's oncologist, there is a 70 percent chance that the cancer will recur, because of its type and size at the time of discovery.

Fortunately, the woman's counselor knew that sexism in the medical care system poses particular problems for women. Many physicians see women's physical complaints as trivial, neurotic disorders best treated with placebos or symptomatic therapy. A therapist who had conducted a prolonged analysis of the possible psychological causes of this woman's complaints or had considered the symptoms to be evidence of emotional disturbance would have put her life in even further jeopardy.

The medical needs of women and their problems in getting good healthcare are key issues. First, many women have psychosomatic illnesses, and counselors get many legitimate referrals from doctors who recognize that there needs to be a psychological as well as medical component to healing women's medical problems. Second, therapists get *too many* referrals from doctors, as the case of the woman with undetected breast cancer illustrates. Serious, treatable problems often progress to irreversible damage or death while a woman is trying to convince her doctor that her problems are not all in her head.

Before the advent of modern medical technology and the professionalization of medicine, women were the primary healers as "witches" and herbalists, and female midwives were the sole practitioners of physical care for women's special concerns—childbirth and gynecology. Now, however, the situation is radically reversed. Although women are the largest single group of healthcare consumers, 93 percent of all doctors are male, and 97 percent of all gynecologists are male.[1]

Women's experience in obtaining healthcare is different from men's in that women almost always are putting their bodies in the hands of someone of the opposite sex for medical care. In addition, women make 25 percent more visits to the doctors than men. They also take 50 percent more prescribed drugs than men and are admitted to hospitals more frequently.[2]

Sex-role stereotyping in the socialization of women has skewed the kind of medical care they seek. Women learn to identify themselves in terms of their reproductive potential, and the medical system reinforces this behavior. For example, a majority of women turn to the specialist obstetrician/gynecologist, not as a source of care for specialized problems, but as a first-line source for all medical care—rather than choosing a general practitioner or internist for routine care. A study which Helen Marieskind presented at a 1974 meeting of the American Association of Obstetricians and Gynecologists found that 86 percent of the women in the study saw no doctor other than an obstetrician/gynecologist on a regular, periodic basis.

Socialization of Women as Patients

The socialization of women to be passive recipients of medical care—especially from men—militates against their receiving adequate care. The attitude with which women seek medical care within the male-dominated system is one of subservient dependence on all-knowing authority. This dependence on all-powerful doctors and women's relinquishing of responsibility for their health to male doctors is the result of physician behavior that reduces the patient's sense of autonomy.

For example, a woman having a routine gynecological exam is ushered into the examining room without meeting the physician first in his office and is instructed to take off her clothes. Vulnerable, naked, and draped with a white sheet, she waits an indeterminate period for the doctor to enter. Once he arrives and her feet are in the examining table stirrups, she is literally helpless in his hands and feels this way—naked, supine, being manipulated with fingers and tools in her body by a male hidden behind a sheet. This dependence on male doctors works against women patients' interests. A patient's stereotyped respect for a doctor's wisdom and competence does not make a poor doctor into a good one.

Dependence on doctors also eliminates the woman's own desires and needs from decision-making about her care. Most medical care involves various levels of benefits and risks and choices about them, even when doctors do not allow patients to make those choices. Lack of information about their bodies, plus the dependent, fearful relationship with their physicians, make it difficult for women to find out what is really wrong with them physically and what methods of treatment are possible. In a study on doctor-patient communication, Barbara Korsch and Vida Negrete found that the use of medical jargon which is unintelligible to patients, plus doctors' frequent disregard for patients' concerns and perspectives, were obstacles to effective care.[3]

A logical result of this confusion and failure in doctor-patient communication is that only 42 percent of the women in this study carried out all the medical advice they received; 38 percent complied in part; and 11 percent did not follow instructions at all.

In gynecology and obstetrics the level of communication can be even poorer, because of an attitude generated by the fact that many of the visits are from healthy women. The attitude is that if there is nothing wrong, then there is nothing to tell. In 1970 hearings before the U.S. Senate, a physician who did research on oral contraceptives opposed labeling for these drugs which

would inform women of the risks. He said, "A misguided effort to inform such women leads only to anxiety on their part and loss of confidence in the physician. . . . They want him [the doctor] to tell them what to do, not to confuse them by asking them to make decisions beyond their comprehension. . . . The idea of informing such a woman is not possible."[4]

One would hope that this individual doctor's attitude represents an extreme case. However, in general many doctors neglect to give women information they do not ask for, and treat them as if they are not capable of understanding the basis of decisions and treatment. In the view of much of the medical profession, women cannot even be trusted with information about their own conditions or medication.

A graphic illustration of this point is the years-old controversy still raging over the government's proposal to require patient education leaflets on all prescription drugs. In response to tremendous pressure from Congressional advocates and the Food and Drug Administration, the major medical associations reluctantly have endorsed the abstract concept of such leaflets but continue to oppose specific applications.

The specter the medical associations raise in their congressional testimony on patient package inserts for drugs is that if patients are told all that can go wrong with a drug, a disease, or an operation, their hypochondriacal minds will ensure that all these things do go wrong. It is significant that it was a consumer group, the Center for Law and Social Policy, which sparked the government initiative on patient package inserts through a petition—and not the medical profession.

An example in which doctors have not given women information that can have life and death consequences for themselves and their children involves the hormone diethylstilbestrol (DES). During the 1950's many thousands of pregnant women received DES without being informed what the medication was. No one knew until fifteen years later that this drug greatly increased the risk of cancer in their children.

In October 1978, after years of press coverage of DES-caused cancer, the government issued a special letter and bulletin to the country's doctors because of the finding that some doctors were still prescribing DES for pregnant women and many others still were not informing their patients who had taken the drug of possible risks.[5]

Socialization of Doctors

Where do doctors get this lack of respect for a woman's right to information about healthcare and for her ability to participate intelligently in her medical care? Mary

Howell describes the process of professionalization of doctors in medical school—where they learn attitudes about work and patients—as strongly colored by a demeaning regard for women.[6] Medical schools teach discrimination against women as patients, Howell says, through lack of focus on diseases specific to women, in misogynic comparisons made between male and female patients with similar health problems, and in instructions regarding the appropriate behavior of doctors toward women patients.

In their classes, medical students learn both implicitly and explicitly that women patients have uninteresting illnesses, are unreliable historians of their health, and are beset by such emotionality that their symptoms are unlikely to reflect real disease.

Pauline Bart and Diana Scully reviewed twenty-seven gynecology textbooks published between 1943 and 1972 and found that at least half of the writers stated women are inherently frigid, have less sex drive than men, or are interested in sex only for procreation.[7] Two authors urged physicians to encourage women to simulate orgasm to please their husbands. The core of the female personality as described in these textbooks is narcissistic, masochistic, and passive.

Another much-used vehicle for the socialization of doctors in their attitudes toward women is drug advertisements in medical journals. Many of these ads serve to reinforce the prejudices against women. They teach doctors that women's physical complaints are trivial; their illnesses are irritating to others; and that women are emotional, have psychosomatic illnesses, and are bothersome to doctors.

Many ads for tranquilizers and antidepressants in particular suggest these products as treatment of choice before psychotherapy or social action for life situations and problems beyond the traditional concepts of illness and disease.

In a 1971 review of medical journals, Seidenberg found that misogynic statements in drug advertisements resonate with the bias of the intended observer—the male doctor. He targeted in particular advertisements that recommended doctors use drugs to adjust women to their lot when they are discontented with a humdrum environment. One caption accompanying a portrayal of a woman behind the bars of broom and mop handles read, "you can't set her free, but you can help her feel less anxious."[8]

In 1979 men are beginning to appear more frequently in drug advertisements as patients, but the difference in portrayal of men and women is still striking. Men on antidepressant medications are depicted as, "Alert on the job," and "functioning effectively in daily activities" (Pamelor). Women needing antidepressant medications,

however, appear in drug ads as helpless patients under a doctor's care because, "Everything I saw was negative" (Norpramin).

The insidious effects of the sexist bias doctors learn in medical school, the professional literature they read, and the drug advertising they are exposed to are broad-ranging. The bias affects decision-making about individual patients and perpetuates misinformation about women's psychic and physiological processes. Negative consequences of these medical myths about women include the justification of limited opportunities for education, employment, and participation in the political process.

The following three specific issues are examples of sexism in medical care. All pose particular threats to women's well-being and as such are illustrations of medical care delivery to women.

Contraceptive Methods   Every woman has a right to make a free and informed choice about birth control for herself. The information about methods and the freedom of choice are key, because there is no completely satisfactory method of birth control. Each method has a unique range of benefits and risks which will differ for women of various medical histories, personal preferences, income, and health habits.

There are widespread misunderstandings about the risks and failure rates of various methods of contraception.[9] Some of this is caused by unethical advertising by pharmaceutical firms. In addition, the biases of clinics or individual doctors frequently deprive women of complete information on which to base their choices. Planned Parenthood prides itself on giving women unbiased information so they can make choices, but many women have already made up their minds about a method before they come into the clinics. According to the Washington, D.C. Public Interest Research Group, the popularity of the Pill is based on its convenience, and fewer women would expose themselves to its many risks if they took these into account in making their choices. Much of the pro-Pill reasoning is fallacious, especially the comparison of risks of the Pill with risks of pregnancy. Such comparisons assume that women not taking oral contraceptives will become pregnant, whereas they could use other safer contraceptive methods; furthermore, many of the necessary studies on the Pill's long-term safety have not been done, and many complications are never reported, so that valid comparisons between the risks of pregnancy and oral contraceptives cannot be made.

Estrogen Use in Menopause   Uterine cancer used to be rare—about one in 1,000 postmenopausal women who had not had their uteruses surgically removed. Since 1970, however, the incidence of uterine cancer in women over fifty years of age increased dramatically—by 50 percent for invasive cancer and by 100 percent for localized cancer.[10] It is not a coincidence that in the last ten to fifteen years the use of estrogen has at least tripled, and recent studies have concluded that there is a causal connection, and that the major cause of the increasing rate of uterine cancer in the United States is estrogen therapy. The sharpest rise in uterine cancer rates is among white upper- and middle-class women, who are most likely to take estrogens. Fifty percent of all post-menopausal women have taken estrogens, and approximately half of these women have taken estrogen for more than ten years. The longer the estrogen treatment and the higher the dose, the higher the incidence of uterine cancer. There are strong social pressures causing the high use of estrogen. Unsupported claims that estrogen will retard the aging process, plus the sexism that devalues older women, combine to create strong consumer demand for the drug. This demand reinforces physicians' entrenched prescribing habits, despite new scientific findings.

Six million women are using estrogens, many of them in hopes that the drug will keep them "feminine forever." This attitude, created in large part by irresponsible drug company advertising, is not going to evaporate soon. Also resistant to change are the time-hallowed doctors' attitudes toward menopause as a disease rather than as a normal physiological process.

Psychoactive Drugs Use of legitimate psychoactive drugs among women is an important issue. An estimated one to two million people in the U.S. from all walks of life and social strata have abuse problems with prescription drugs, according to the National Institute of Drug Abuse's February and April 1978 *Capsules* press releases.

Almost twice as many women as men have had tranquilizers, sedatives, and stimulants prescribed for them. In many cases, there is no medical reason for use of the drugs, but they become a chemical support system to adjust a woman to a frustrating or unfulfilling marriage, divorce, lifestyle, or work situation. Psychoactive drugs become both a substitute and a barrier to use of counseling or other measures to combat or alter the distressing situation or the individual's response to it.

Chemical crutches for women are nothing new. In the 1800's it was common medical custom to prescribe then-legal opium for "female troubles."[11] A wide spread pattern of opium abuse grew among women—outnumbering male opium-eaters three to one in the late nineteenth and early twentieth centuries. In the drug pattern of the 1970's, general practitioners write most of the tranquilizer prescriptions for Valium alone; there were fifty-seven million prescriptions between May 1976 and April 1977.[12]

Doctors get their education about psychoactive drugs primarily from drug companies. A survey of seventy-two medical schools found that only 20 percent had any course in psychopharmacology, and the average time on the subject was seventeen hours in four years.[13] Medical advertising for drugs typically portrays women as frustrated, anxious, neurotic, and depressed.

Tranquilizers, sedatives, and stimulants are addictive, and in conjunction with alcohol they can be deadly. Persons who take excessive doses of either sedatives or certain tranquilizers for extended periods of time will experience dramatic withdrawal symptoms including convulsions, tremor, abdominal and muscle cramps, vomiting, and sweating.[14]

Alarming information that only recently has come to light is that some patients will experience withdrawal from such drugs as Librium and Valium when they have been taking normal therapeutic doses, with no abuse.[15] These symptoms include tremors, agitation, fear and anxiety, stomach cramps, and sweating. Since these symptoms of withdrawal so closely resemble the anxiety manifestations for which women in particular originally receive these drugs, and since so many millions of women are taking these drugs, they represent a complex problem for counselors.

Sexism in medical practice is rooted in the socialization of women to be passive recipients of care from authoritarian male doctors, plus doctors' socialization which trivializes women's medical problems and fosters attitudes that demean women patients. The results are that many women suffer needlessly from treatable organic problems labeled as psychogenic, experience irreparable damage or death because of ignored symptoms, or unwittingly fall into drug dependence due to doctors' attempts to "help" women adjust through drugs to an uncomfortable sex-typed role.

The implications are clear—it is vital for women to become informed partners in their own medical care. This will involve learning about key medical issues concerning women and developing skills to assert their rights in the sexist dynamics that pervade the healthcare of women. Useful tools in this task will be information sharing and assertiveness training to assist women in getting information on their own and getting responses they want from professionals. Some authors suggest limiting the practice of women's medicine (obstetrics/gynecology) to women practitioners. At some future date that may be thinkable or possible; at present, however, since 97 percent of all obstetrician/gynecologists are male, women are faced with the art of the possible in dealing with sexism in their medical care.

NOTES

1. Linda Bakiel, Susan Daily, and Carolyn Kott Washburne, ed., *Women in Transition: A Feminist Handbook on Separation and Divorce* (New York: Scribners, 1975), p. 392.

2. Boston Women's Health Collective, *Our Bodies Ourselves* (New York: Simon and Schuster, 1976), p. 337.

3. Barbara H. Korsch and Vida F. Negrete, "Doctor-Patient Communication." *Scientific American,* 227 (1972), 66–72.

4. Gena Corea, *The Hidden Malpractice* (New York:Marron Co., 1977), p. 77.

5. Food and Drug Administration, "Alert on DES," *FDA Drug Bulletin,* 8, (1978), p. 3.

6. Mary Howell, "What Medical Schools Teach About Women," *New England Journal of Medicine,* 291 (1974), 304–07.

7. Pauline Bart and Diana Scully, "A Funny Think Happened on the Way to the Orifice," *American Journal of Sociology,* 28 (1973), 1045–50.

8. R. Seidenberg, "Drug Advertising and Perceptions of Mental Illness," *Mental Hygiene,* 55 (1971), 21–31.

9. *Our Bodies Ourselves,* p. 185.

10. Food and Drug Administration, "Estrogens and Endometrial Cancer," *FDA Drug Bulletin,* 6 (1976), 2–3.

11. Annabel Hecht, "Women and Drugs," *FDA Consumer,* October 1978, pp. 7–12.

12. Jody Forman-Sher and Jonica Homiler, "An Overview of the Problem of Combined Drug/Alcohol Dependencies Among Women," paper presented at the International Conference on Alcoholism and Addictions, Zurich, Switzerland, June 1978.

13. Ann H. Clark, *National Consumers League Position on Minor Tranquilizers,* paper presented at the public hearing before the Food and Drug Administration, Rockville, Maryland, March 1978.

14. David Haskell, "Withdrawal of Diazepam," *Journal of the American Medical Association,* 233 (1975), 135.

15. Arthur Rifkin, Frederick Quitkin, and Donald Klein, "Withdrawal Reactions to Diazepam," *Journal of the American Medical Association,* 236 (1976), 2173.

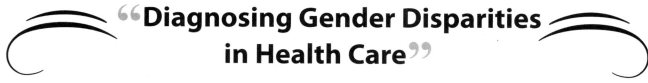

"Diagnosing Gender Disparities in Health Care"

by Andrea Irwin

Until I became a women's health advocate immersed in the nuances of Medicaid, health insurance, and other complicated policy issues, I never truly appreciated the numerous disparities that exist between the ways men and women access the healthcare system. Most of my female friends are now in their mid-to-late twenties and I am constantly amazed at the myriad medical concerns that are unique to the female anatomy. For starters, research shows that women's reproductive systems are just so much more complex than men's and women are more likely than men to need healthcare throughout their lifetimes. Our ovaries, uteruses, breasts, cervixes, and fallopian tubes are all subject to various cancers, infections and other complications making routine monitoring a necessity, in addition to women's overarching need for safe, effective and affordable birth control. Among my circle of friends we have experienced breast biopsies, vaginal ultrasounds, and colposcopies galore.

At a minimum, a young woman is advised to visit her gynecologist once a year to have a pelvic exam and Pap test, but she may require further and additional visits to receive contraception and STI/HIV testing, or to follow-up on any abnormalities discovered through these preventive screenings. For women with comprehensive health insurance, most of these preventive services are covered benefits—but, un-

"Young Feminists: Diagnosing Gender Disparities in Health Care," by Andrea Irwin, originally published in the *Women's Health Activist,* September/October 2007, pp. 8–9, the newsletter of the National Women's Health Network (NWHN). It is reprinted with the permission of the author and the NWHN.

fortunately, not all. Moreover, some of these services are not covered in a way that makes sense. For instance, I just learned that many insurance plans will not cover STI/HIV tests at a woman's annual physical visit, which forces a woman to make an additional appointment for these tests and adds an extra layer of stress and burden to an already anxiety-producing procedure. Luckily, my provider pointed this out to me, but most women are not likely to be aware of such hidden costs. Instead of creating disincentives for women to be smart, efficient consumers of healthcare, insurers should end this policy that may increase a woman's health expenses or lead her to avoid care altogether.

Even worse, some insurance plans do not cover contraceptives despite the fact that the plans usually cover other prescription drugs. And, even when plans do cover contraceptives, they may not cover Emergency Contraception (EC) now that it's sold over-the-counter. EC costs around $45, which impedes access for many young women. Some insurance plans (notably the federal government employees' plan) also refuse to pay for abortion services, despite the fact that abortion is a safe and legal procedure, and that plans cover all prenatal care and pregnancy-related services.[1] The typical first trimester abortion costs, on average, around $468, which is extremely expensive for many women, particularly young and low-income women.[1]

Beyond the reproductive health disparities between men and women in terms of needed services and covered benefits, young women are more likely than men to suffer from chronic conditions like rheumatoid arthritis, lupus, or asthma.[2] Over one-third (38%) of women suffer from chronic conditions that require ongoing treatment, compared with 30% of men.[2] I've seen my peers struggle with all of these illnesses first-hand, as well as with the on-going treatment and medications they necessitate.

Young women are also more prone to be diagnosed with anxiety, depression, eating disorders, and other mental health conditions that may require extensive therapy and/or medications, and which may also result in increased physical health problems if left untreated.[2] Twice as many women as men are diagnosed with certain mental health problems such as anxiety and depression.[2] Even for women who have health insurance, the costs of these services can add up and co-pays and deductibles can become very expensive.

Moreover, because most health insurance plans are not required to cover mental health services, many insurers refuse to cover treatment for some or all mental health conditions, or may set very low limits on the number of mental health visits an individual can receive.

These practices leave many young women with no ability to seek needed treatment. The high prevalence of violence against women—and the media's negative influences on women's body image that have largely shaped our generation's tormented relationships with our bodies (and driven us to seek out carcinogenic cigarettes to stay thin, and cancer-causing tanning beds to improve our appearance)—also exacerbate women's need for comprehensive healthcare.[3] We need to advocate for policies that reduce the powerful, negative, influence of these harmful external forces on our health and promote universal healthcare for all.

While these insurance practices are bad for women, more than one-third of all young women between the ages of 19 and 24 aren't insured at all.[4] For these women, the situation is far more dire because, without health insurance, women are more likely to avoid needed healthcare. Women in this age group are also more likely than men to have high medical debts or to experience bankruptcy because of medical expenses.[2] This is due to both women's lower incomes on average (thanks to the gender gap in pay) and their greater healthcare needs.[4] Proposals that expand healthcare coverage to more people—including individuals who work part-time, run their own businesses, or stay at home to raise families—are essential to ensuring women's autonomy and full equality with men.

One major lesson I've learned is that young women tend to underestimate the value of healthcare to our lives and well-being. We constantly sacrifice our mental and physical health so that we can nurture our careers, and build financial nest eggs for our futures. Like the importance of setting up a 401(k) at work or pursuing higher education to ensure access to better employment opportunities, accessing quality healthcare when we are young is an investment women must learn to make in order to ensure our health throughout our lives. Young women need to share our stories and encourage our peers to empower and educate themselves about the importance of preventive care. Most importantly, we must demand that lawmakers develop and implement healthcare reform proposals that meet young women's unique healthcare needs.

I am fortunate to have comprehensive health insurance through my employer. I was also raised by a strong feminist mother with more than 30 years of nursing experience who helps me to navigate the increasingly convoluted healthcare system. My hope is that my generation will continue to advocate for improved healthcare services and access for all so that everyone can enjoy a brighter, healthier future and better quality of life than our grandmothers experienced.

REFERENCES

1. National Network of Abortion Funds. *Policy Report—Abortion Funding: A Matter of Justice.* Amherst, MA: NNAF. 2005, 2, 6.

2. The Commonwealth Fund and The National Women's Law Center. *Issue Brief—Women and Health Coverage: The Affordability Gap.* Washington, DC: CF. April, 2007, p. 4.

3. Charlie Guild Melanoma Foundation (CGMF) Website. "10 Facts About Melanoma." Richmond, CA: CGMF. No date. Accessed June 6, 2007 from http://www.charlie.org/melanoma_facts.html.

4. The National Women's Law Center (NWLC). *Issue Brief—Women and Health Coverage: A Framework for Moving Forward.* Washington, DC: NWLC. April, 2007, p. 2.

PRO: Women's Health
Developing a New Interdisciplinary Specialty

by Karen Johnson, M.D.

Abstract   This paper argues that medicine is based on a male paradigm that does not permit high-quality comprehensive care for women within existing medical specialities. Suggestions are made to alleviate the shortcomings of the current paradigm by including women. A call for the development of a specialty in women's health is made. Types of resistance to this proposal, stemming from sexism, economics, and alliances to existing specialties, are also discussed. Finally, it is argued that bringing the study and practice of women's health to parity with the understanding and treatment of men must be achieved rapidly and comprehensively using an active and multifaceted approach.

Introduction

No existing medical specialty is devoted exclusively to the comprehensive care of women. Many of us providing healthcare for women in a variety of existing specialties believe that the absence of such a comprehensively trained specialist is a significant problem in the healthcare services offered to women. This problem could be solved through the development of an interdisciplinary specialty in women's health.

Medicine as a Paradigm Based upon Experiences with Men

With the exception of physicians in one surgical specialty, obstetrics-gynecology, physicians caring for women base the majority of their diagnoses and interventions on clinical trials and studies with men, often unknowingly. However benevolent the original intentions in excluding women from drug trials and clinical studies, their absence has led to unnecessary morbidity and premature mortality. For example, the Baltimore Longitudinal Study on Aging started in 1958 and did not include women for the first 20 years. This omission delayed the discovery of the link among osteoporosis, calcium, estrogen, and progesterone, resulting in the needless suffering and death of hundreds of thousands of women.

More recently the AIDS epidemic has highlighted the serious consequences of assuming that diseases in women manifest with exactly the same signs and symptoms as diseases in men. Until 1991 the Center for Disease Control (CDC) criteria for AIDS was based on men. HIV positive women presenting with cervical cancer, pelvic inflammatory disease, and vaginal thrush were diagnosed much later in the disease process. Not only did these uniquely female diagnoses delay treatment and thus shorten life expectancy compared with men, they often caused undue economic hardship because meeting the CDC criteria was a prerequisite to receiving public assistance available to patients with AIDS.

Other problems are created by the assumption that our experience with men is transferable to women. Although cardiovascular disease is the leading cause of death in women, we would hardly know it based on most of the research in this field. The initial study affirming that aspirin could be used as preventive therapy for coronary disease included more than 22,000 subjects, all male. The Mr. FIT study (Multiple Risk Factor Intervention Trials) identified coronary disease risk factors in 15,000 subjects, again all men. Even when women's risk of cardiovascular disease is assessed, clinical experience and interventions with men may not be applicable to women. Women may present with different symptoms in the office; they often arrive further in the progression of a myocardial infarction in the emergency room; they are more likely to die in the operating room.

Many diseases common in both men and women have a substantially higher incidence in women. It is not entirely clear why. Diseases of the gastrointestinal tract are just one example. Gallstones occur earlier in women and women continue to have a greater prevalence of them throughout their lives. Biliary dyskinesia occurs more often in women. Irritable bowel syndrome and gastroparesis are three times more common in women than men. Women are more susceptible to the hepatotoxic effects of alcohol than men. However, as is often the case in diseases that occur in both genders, clinical investigations have been carried out mostly in men. As a result in caring for women we cannot be confident that our diagnostic techniques and medical interventions are sound.

Health matters that occur exclusively (or primarily) in women such as menstruation, premenstrual symptoms, uterine fibroids, menopause, and breast cancer have received less attention than the patient population (52% of adults) would warrant. This has hindered our ability to offer advice with confidence.

Sometimes relying on the male paradigm is nothing short of ludicrous. Consider the study at Rockefeller University in which researchers were analyzing the effects of obesity on estrogen activity and the tendency to develop breast and uterine cancer. All the subjects were male. Although it is finally a widely held belief that women and men are equal, they are not the same—physiologically or psychologically. Using men as the medical standard from which women diverge is unpardonable.

Crossing Boundaries

Now that the consciousness of medicine has been raised, it has been suggested that improving women's healthcare can be achieved by making adjustments in the education of physicians within existing specialties. This plan on its own would not address the numerous health concerns experienced by women that do not easily fit into any existing specialty. Consider the woman whose abdominal pain is finally diagnosed as endometriosis. Lacking an interdisciplinary-trained women's health specialist, the recommended interventions are likely to be biased by the specialty training of her provider. A primary care physician may be inclined to prescribe analgesics for pain, whereas a gynecologist leans more toward hormonal or surgical interventions. A psychiatrist or other mental health provider may need to be included to assist with corollary emotional distress or sexual dysfunction. Two or more physicians are required to provide complete care, an inefficient and expensive process.

Many medical problems experienced by women present similar dilemmas. Two additional examples are premenstrual symptoms and domestic violence. Premenstrual symptoms are inadequately defined within the existing paradigm, but they are certainly experienced by many women. Lacking agreement about diagnosis and treatment, specialists tend to interpret symptoms through their own frame of reference. Domestic violence is a major health hazard for American women, but it is overlooked by many physicians. Untrained in a broader understanding of women's health, physicians' impressions are biased by the perspective of their own specialty. When presented with only a small part of the clinical problem, they often fail to piece together the larger diagnostic picture. A woman complaining of insomnia or suffering with a fracture may be treated in an emergency room or family practice center, but never asked directly about physical abuse. Although the lack of a unified approach to premenstrual symptoms can lead to discomfort and distress, the failure to accurately diagnose domestic violence can be life threatening. What is called for in these and many other situations experienced by women is an interdisciplinary approach.

Correcting the Paradigm

Most physicians until recently have been unaware that the practice of medicine is based on a male paradigm. Many of the problems that have arisen because of this have been identified. There is now relative agreement within the medical profession that these problems must be addressed, but we are by no means in agreement as to the method.

Some believe that we have crossed the barriers to the full inclusion of women's healthcare needs and that we can correct the existing medical paradigm by alterations within current specialties. This belief is at odds with the limited achievements women have made in other areas when analogous omissions were brought to light, as noted in Faludi's *Backlash*.

Representatives from at least three specialties—internal medicine, obstetrics-gynecology, and family practice—have argued that these specialties can adequately meet the comprehensive needs of women patients. I question their assertions. Unless practitioners of these specialties have taken it upon themselves to round out their standard residency training, few are qualified to call themselves women's health specialists in the manner I am arguing is required.

At present most internists have inadequate knowledge of women's reproductive health, extremely limited experience with the psychosocial aspects of women's healthcare, and a discipline that is built entirely on a male paradigm. Although obstetrics-gynecology training is based upon experiences with women, it is arguable whether it can genuinely be considered a primary care specialty. The training is fundamentally surgical, and the inclusion of a psychosocial perspective is also limited.

Family physicians argue that they are in the best position to offer high-quality comprehensive care for women. This is true within the context of the current medical paradigm. Their interdisciplinary training serves them well in approaching the multiplicity of women's healthcare concerns. However, the training and practice of family medicine require these physicians to divide their attention among women, men, and children.

Certainly family physicians treat the young as well as the elderly and more than other specialists gain a psychosocial perspective in their training. Nevertheless, this has not negated the need for the specialty of pediatrics or the subspecialty of geriatrics. Pediatricians' focused attention on children and geriatricians' focused attention on the elderly have led to improved healthcare for the youngest and the oldest of patients. Specialists in women's health will bring similar benefits to all our woman patients—no matter what specialty we practice.

I do agree with colleagues who caution that a specialty in women's health must not be viewed as alleviating the imperative that every existing medical specialty revise its content to include the accurate and respectful treatment of women. However, I do not believe that these efforts will be adequate. Nor do I think that these improvements and the development of a new interdisciplinary specialty are mutually exclusive. They would be complementary.

Placing Women's Health in the Larger Context

The idea of a specialty in women's health is a logical extension of the women's health movement that began in the 1960s. Physicians influenced by this movement began to articulate the need for a specialty in women's health by the 1980s. The recent increased interest in women's health at all levels is gratifying; however, attention to the concerns of women has been inconsistent during this century. It would be a mistake to assume the current flurry of activity in women's health will continue without formalizing the specialty.

Having a medical specialty in women's health could be viewed much like having a room of one's own. Just as departments of women's studies have been instrumental in assuring that women's experiences are accurately represented in the academic community, a specialty in women's health would serve a similar purpose in medicine.

Those who believe it will be sufficient to simply add women's health to existing specialties would be wise to study the history of science, the sociology of knowledge, and the role of values in science if the missed opportunities of other pioneers are to be avoided. Nineteenth century scientists argued that the rigors of a university education would drain energy from women's reproductive organs. These and other socially expedient biases were used to justify the exclusion of women from positions of authority and decision making. Unless health issues are approached from a solid interdisciplinary, pro-woman perspective, I am not confident that current or future physicians will serve women significantly better than their earlier counterparts. We have already seen a great deal of the money targeted for new research in women's health funneled into the existing "old boys" research network. This is worrisome and disappointing to those of us who had hoped for more adventuresome funding and innovative projects. Rest assured, the age-old debate of autonomy versus integration will wage on as we struggle with how to include women's health in medical training. Common sense and experience suggest that we must do both. It is from the power base of a residency in women's health that efforts to mainstream are most likely to be successful. Furthermore, women's health is a separate body of knowledge and deserves to be treated as a legitimate area of inquiry.

Positioning a Women's Health Specialty

There are several possible routes to specialization. Women's health could be a primary care specialty like pediatrics or subspeciality like geriatrics. Alternatively, much like toxicology, it could be a field of study. Entry from any number of specialties would be possible. The positioning of the specialty is less critical than its content. Women's health must be based on research and experience with women, not men.

Those of us interested in fostering the development of an interdisciplinary specialty in women's health have many resources to turn for valuable advice and information. Nursing, a female-dominated profession, has had training programs in women's health for over a decade. Feminist scholars in health psychology and women's studies also have much to offer.

There are already many interesting and active steps being taken within medicine to assure a better response to women's healthcare needs. Since 1982, hospital-affiliated multidisciplinary women's health centers have offered a closer approximation of an interdisciplinary approach than more conventional group practices. This summer Harvard Medical School held their fifth annual conference on women's health, combining internal medicine, obstetrics-gynecology, and psychiatry. The American Medical Women's Association is preparing a multidisciplinary postgraduate course on the healthcare needs of women. Fellowships in women's medicine have started to appear at several institutions, and a number of medical schools offer electives in women's health. Nevertheless, a growing number of medical students longing to specialize in women's health express frustration at the lack of a residency program anywhere in the United States. For now, highly motivated trainees are left to customize existing residencies to achieve their goal of specializing in women's health (D. Moran, personal communication).

Resistance

The resistance to this proposal has been intense and is no doubt determined by many factors. Change is almost always anxiety provoking. In this case the anxiety is fueled by forces as divergent as sexism, economics, and alliances to existing specialties.

Treating women with knowledge drawn from research on men is enough of a problem without being compounded by pervasive sexism. This is an issue in patient care that we have hardly begun to address. Sexist behavior ranges from simple patronizing to explicit harassment and abuse. One male obstetrician has suggested that unless male physicians correct their sexist attitudes and behavior, they should not be allowed to provide healthcare for women.

Unfortunately, sexism is not unique to male physicians. It is embedded in the professionalization of almost every medical student. How else can we interpret the disturbing revelation this year of a graduating medical student that in the anatomy lab female breasts were designated as "waste" and tossed in the trash without careful dissection and examination? This behavior is unconscionable when one in nine American women can expect to develop breast cancer within her lifetime.

Arguments that a specialty in women's health will lead to costly fragmentation and overspecialization do not make sense. It is the current arrangement that causes these problems. Divisions in medicine are arbitrary and based on any number of factors including physician interest, expanding scientific knowledge, and political agendas. Siphoning funds from other critical areas such as AIDS and cancer research will undoubtedly be used as economic scarecrows. At a less conscious level some will be concerned that specialists in women's health will compete more favorably for women patients. Women are the greatest users of healthcare. Yet another potential financial loss is hard to swallow when physicians are already feeling under siege.

Those of us specializing in the care of women have been cautioned against proposing the development of a new specialty just as medicine is being forced to tighten its belt. The proposal of a new specialty at this time may seem to burden a crumbling system. But it is in this climate that attending to the healthcare needs of women is even more urgent. Unless we are vigilant about the quality and availability of care for women, it is likely with any of the insurance reforms currently under consideration that healthcare services for women will be the first to suffer.

Even many well-meaning physicians are unconvinced that a specialty is needed. They believe that theirs is either providing perfectly adequate care for women or that with only modest efforts the quality of care can be raised to acceptable levels. Their identification with their own training interferes with an accurate understanding of the problem.

Framing the Solution

What most opponents fail to appreciate is that women's health is a unique body of knowledge and skills based upon experience with women that cross the boundaries of existing specialties. Women's healthcare needs are not being met, and cannot be met, within the existing medical paradigm.

The criterion of the American Board of Medical Specialists for a new specialty is that it must "represent a distinct and well-defined field of medical practice" such as "special concerns with problems of patients according to age, sex, organ systems or interaction between patients and their environment." With practice specialties ranging from addiction medicine to undersea medicine, I am hard pressed to understand why a specialty embracing 52% of the adult population is unreasonable or unnecessary.

Conclusion

When it comes to women's health, there are far more questions than answers. Specialists devoted to women's healthcare in a number of fields are beginning to provide some answers, but the information is fragmented and unknown to physicians who have no particular interest in the field.

It is not only discriminatory, but truly dangerous to fail to bring the study and practice of women's medicine to parity with the understanding and treatment of men rapidly and comprehensively. This can and must be achieved through an active and multifaceted approach. This includes physicians examining their practices and attitudes for social or cultural biases that affect medical care, funding medical research in women's health, and increasing the number of women in positions of authority in teaching, research, and the practice of medicine. The Women's Health Initiative, a multidisciplinary, multi-institute intervention study to address the major causes of death, disability, and frailty among middle-aged and older women, is an important step, as is the creation of the Office of Research on Women's Health. However, as valuable as these efforts are, they are insufficient. Women deserve no less than children who have specialists in pediatrics and the elderly who have specialists in geriatrics. A new interdisciplinary specialty in women's health is required.

REFERENCES
A list of references is available in the original source.

CON: Women's Health as a Specialty
A Deceptive Solution

by Michelle Harrison, M.D.

Abstract   A proposed call for a new specialty in women's health is an attempt to rectify current inadequacies in the care of women. This paper discusses nineteenth century origins of the current organization of medical specialties in which the male body is the norm and woman becomes "other." Nineteenth century attitudes toward women, with the belief in the biological inferiority of women due to their sexual organs, and the replacement of midwives by physicians, became the basis of this bifurcated system of care in which women require two physicians for their ongoing care. A reorganization of medical specialties is proposed in which: (1) Internal medicine incorporates the primary care aspect of gynecology, as does family medicine; (2) Obstetrics and gynecology remains the surgical and referral specialty that it is; (3) Interdisciplinary research addresses gaps in understanding the role of reproductive events, hormones, and cycles to normal and pathological functioning; (4) Medical students are taught to identify across gender lines; (5) All specialties are examined for the purpose of making them "user friendly" to women; and (6) The medical profession addresses and rectifies past inequities in the conceptual framework about women and their subsequent denial of leadership opportunities. The need for education in women's health is acknowledged, but with the goal of making that need obsolete. A new specialty has the potential to further isolate women's issues from mainstream medicine and to marginalize its practitioners.

The proposition that women's health become a separate specialty derives from the failure of the established medical system to address adequately the healthcare needs of women. These inadequacies exist in the social, medical, educational, and research aspects of women's health. Even though women consume proportionally more medical services than do men, the basic organization of medical specialization has been based upon a male standard to which woman is the eternal exception. Although the establishment of a separate specialty of women's health may initially seem appealing, it has the potential of further isolating the women's perspective in delivery of healthcare, while simultaneously marginalizing those practitioners who commit themselves to its practice.

This paper discusses the history of the development of the current system of medicine with its adaptation toward the male body and psyche. A model of healthcare in which women's bodies are the norm, not the exception, is developed.

Nineteenth Century Attitudes

The current treatment of women has its roots in the history of medicine in America, which in turn reflected the prevailing cultural attitudes toward women. Dr. Charles D. Meigs, Professor of Midwifery and the Diseases of Women and Children at Jefferson Medical College in Philadelphia, in 1838 translated the following from the French physician Velpeau:

> Puberty, or the marriageable age, is announced in girls, as it is in boys, by numerous changes. . . . The young girl becomes more timid and reserved; her form becomes more rounded. . . . Her eyes, which are at once brilliant and languishing, express commingled desires, fears, and tenderness; the sensations she experiences and the sense of her own weakness, are the causes why she no longer dares to approach the companions of her childhood but with a downcast look.

The biological transition from girl to young woman was seen as the causative factor in her change in personality. Biology was deemed destiny, and hers was to be one of fear and weakness.

The nineteenth century saw the development of a sizable population of women who, because of industrialization and urbanization, became part of a middle class in which women's employment outside the home was unnecessary. So, while the vast majority of women throughout the world toiled in fields and factories, bore child after child, then aged and died early, Western Europe and America were creating a new version of woman expressive of new political and economic times. The new version conveniently placed women out of competition with men and created a biological basis for that exclusion. Meigs, in an 1859 collection of his own lectures, wrote, "The sexuality of the woman does in its essence consist in the possession of that peculiar structure called

ovarian stroma—her heart, brain, lungs, all her viscera, all indeed that she is, would not make her a female without the primordial central essence—stroma." He continues, "She demands a treatment adapted to the very specialties of her own constitution, as a moral, a sexual, germiferous, gestative, or parturient creature." Women's sexuality then became the heart of the justification of difference, and difference invariably meant lesser.

Laqueur, in *Making Sex: Body and Gender from the Greeks to Freud,* describes the Greek model in which the genders were measured by metaphysical perfection in hierarchical relation to each other. This early model of "one sex" in various states of perfection and imperfection was replaced in the nineteenth century with a model of biological divergence based upon anatomical and physiological incommensurability. What had previously been a variation on a single human body became two distinct sexes, believed to be different in every aspect. The shift had been one of changing from comparing grades of apples to comparing apples and oranges, male and female.

Laqueur argues that the polarities of gender can be understood as polarities of power and that "the competition for power generates new ways of constituting the subject and the social realities within which humans dwell." As if to illustrate Laqueur's point, Dr. Alfred Stille in his presidential address to the American Medical Association in 1871 stated, "If, then, woman is unfitted by nature to become a physician, we should, when we oppose her pretensions, be acquitted of any malicious or even unkindly spirit." Woman had been discovered to be a new species, one conveniently unsuited to compete with men in the profession of medicine.

Nineteenth century medicine developed along two lines simultaneously. The body of medicine treated men and the nonreproductive aspects of women's health. Childbirth and common gynecologic problems were usually left to midwives, in part because of prohibitions against male physicians examining female sexual organs. Women's genitals began to be "observed" by physicians in the mid nineteenth century. With the development of gynecologic surgery, which established gynecology as a recognized field, and the successful effort on the part of medicine to define childbirth as a surgical procedure, female midwives were replaced by male obstetricians and gynecologists.

The lifting of cultural prohibitions against the gynecological examination of women by men opened the way for increasing male knowledge about female reproductive anatomy and physiology. If not for the pursuit of economic and professional power on the part of physicians, there might have been a partnership with the midwives, with benefit to both professions and especially to women as patients. Instead there was the destruction of midwifery and a loss of the ways in which women had for centuries attended to the needs of other women. The midwives' care of women exclusively meant that for midwifery, the female body was the standard, the normal, the regular. With the transfer of care to a male medical profession, in which the standard was the male body, the body without female parts, woman's body became "other." With the destruction of midwifery and the paucity of women physicians, the woman's body with its sexual organs was now a foreign body to the overwhelmingly male medical profession and the exclusively male gynecologic surgeons.

The stage was thus set for the current organization of medicine in which internal medicine attends to the non-reproductive aspects of women's health and the generative-related conditions are relegated to the obstetrician-gynecologist. The woman's body with its sexual and generative functions had been medicalized, even in those processes that can be viewed as normal functions. Because medicine was organized around a male body and because physicians were male, nothing about a woman's menstrual cycle or reproduction was "normal." It was all new. She had to be "managed," an approach to women that has not significantly changed.

Nineteenth century medicine attributed the state of women's mental health to the health of their ovaries. Mental illness (at times defined as the inability to accept culturally defined roles, with symptoms including a desire to run away from home, dislike of a husband, or a refusal to sleep with him) was attributed to the dysfunction of sexual organs. The reproductive organs became the seat of not just sexual passions but were seen as the cause of insanity. Clitoridectomy was the first operation performed to check woman's mental disorder. Proponents of castration described the benefits of removal of the ovaries: "the moral sense of the patient is elevated . . . she becomes tractable, orderly, industrious, and cleanly." There was apparently some recognition that castration could lead to postoperative insanity, in which case further surgery was recommended, namely removal of the uterus and Fallopian tubes. Clitoridectomy, castration, and hysterectomy were the nineteenth century treatment of uncontrolled female emotions. The operation was successful if the woman "was restored to a placid contentment with her domestic functions."

Normality was defined as male, with sanity therefore being closer to male function than to female function. Barker-Benfield suggests that the identification of female sexuality with madness was a result of the assumption that "man's madness" was the norm within the

society and therefore woman's was easier to cure. Female "madness" was also easier to see because to the extent it expressed resistance to stereotypic roles, it stood in sharp contrast to the social and political prohibitions of the society.

Such practices as the nineteenth century surgical treatments to return women to their acceptable "passivity" may seem shocking by contemporary standards. Less obvious are the current ways in which society accommodates male behavior and male "madness." For example, although the current diagnosis of postraumatic stress disorder describes the woman's reaction to rape, an adequate framework to describe the causative behavior on the part of the male aggressor is lacking. The psychological effects of sexual harassment on the part of the victim can be described, but the language and understanding of perpetrators is wanting.

The long delay in recognizing wife battering and marital rape may be traced to the nineteenth century when, "throughout much of the bourgeois century, all across the Western world, women remained virtual chattels in the hands of their fathers, and later, of their husbands." For the last two centuries it was the women victims of battering and marital rape who were brought for mental health services. Society's acceptance of, and possibly hopelessness about, male violence may prevent perception of these acts as deviant and destructive.

Sex role stereotyping within the mental health field was aptly described by Broverman et al., who described sex biases in interpretation of behavior by clinicians. In their 1970 study, a healthy adult (nonspecified sex) had attributes more like a healthy male than a healthy woman. They found that "clinicians are more likely to suggest that healthy women differ from healthy men by being more submissive, less independent, less adventurous, more easily influenced, less aggressive, less competitive, more excitable in minor crises. . . ."

These findings from 1970 are not unlike the descriptions of Velpeau (quoted above) in 1838 or those describing results of castration. In those intervening 130 years, a civil war was fought, women organized and fought for the right to vote, they organized against alcohol, they entered the professions of medicine and law against great odds, they joined the military for two world wars, and yet the stereotypes prove more resilient than reality. Women's sex and sexuality continued to be perceived as the basis for her inferiority. Physicians had, "turned the stereotype of feminine frailty into a medical principle."

The diagnosis of late luteal phase dysphoric disorder was added to the *Diagnostic and Statistical Manual* of the American Psychiatric Association in 1987. This diagnosis describes a mental disorder whose etiology is the menstrual cycle and whose language includes anger as a symptom of mental illness. Although few would dispute that the menstrual cycle may affect how some women feel, including anger, there is an important distinction between influencing and causing symptoms and behavior.

Men and women are influenced in mood by weather, light, diet, general health, and day of the week, but few would designate those as the determinants of mental illness. However, old beliefs persist, in practitioners and in women. When a contemporary woman visits her gynecologist because she is irritable with her children premenstrually, she is the "medical" expression of the nineteenth century view of women's mental state being controlled by her ovaries. Likewise, her gynecologist is supporting this premise when ovariectomy is the treatment recommended for the woman's mood or behavioral problems. Chemical and surgical castration remain accepted treatments for disorders of mood.

Educating for Women's Health

The establishment of training programs in women's health is a separate issue from the creation of a new specialty. There is an enormous job to be done in educating the medical profession and institutions. Ideally, this would be a task undertaken with the aim of eventual obsolescence. Fellowships are needed in order to teach and to create meaningful research. However, to create a new specialty, to certify those physicians trained to take care of women, would allow the rest of those in medicine to feel absolved of responsibility for addressing the needs of women, and more inclined to leave the sensitive care of women to those few practitioners who are now the "experts." In reality, only a very small percentage of women (and of a given social class) would have access to this care, and the vast majority of women would continue as they do now with their bifurcated care.

The Call for a Specialty

The problems in contemporary medicine that have brought forth the call for a new specialty in women's health are related to: (1) unexplored and unanswered questions in research and education related to women's health; (2) the ways in which women's health needs are not met; and (3) the bifurcation of routine medical care of women.

Given the shortcomings of the present medical system, the call for a separate specialty is understandable. It comes out of frustration, disappointment, and mistrust. The presence of increasing numbers of women physicians has led to a reassessment as to whether medicine could do a better job in addressing needs of women patients. However, there is no aspect of this new proposed specialty that should not be an integral part of the education and practice of every physician, male or female. Rather, the solutions lie in a reorganization of current medical specialization and a demand for the provision of services that more adequately address the needs of women patients.

Questions for Research and Education

Major gaps exist in the understanding of differences in female physiology and pathology, related, but not restricted, to the menstrual cycle. Because of the "foreign nature" of female bodies to a male medical profession, the menstrual cycle and its effects were for a long time ignored, stigmatized, or left strictly to gynecology. Were all males to menstruate, the interrelated effects of the menstrual cycle on other aspects of a person's health would have been considered essential, even fascinating, areas of study, worthy of the best research and funding. In fact, the vast majority of physicians have never experienced menstruation, looked at sanitary pads, handled tampons, or had cramps. Though it may not be necessary to experience illness in order to understand or treat them, the lack of understanding or familiarity with what is normal may result in a tendency to pathologize the entire process. That deficiency in personal experience may limit one's ability to be comfortable with integrating menstruation into a "normal" body.

On the other side, the fact that women are not defined by their menstrual cycles does not mean that this process is irrelevant. It is clear that many medications react differently over the course of the menstrual cycle, yet this area remains largely unexplored. Pharmacologic research has been done on males in part because the menstrual cycle becomes a confounding factor in analysis of results. However, the drugs are then used on women and those confounding effects become clinical effects—poorly understood because of a paucity of research. The research that is needed is not necessarily on the menstrual cycle itself, but rather interdisciplinary research that looks at the menstrual cycle in relation to heart disease, asthma, seizures, and lupus, areas where it is already clear that gender is relevant. Interdisciplinary and gender-conscious research is needed to look at osteoporosis in relation to nutrition, exercise, vitamins, *and* the menstrual cycle. Current research and understanding of substance abuse lacks any systematic or "systems" study of the effects of the menstrual cycle or of menopause.

The designation of obstetrics and gynecology as *the* women's specialty may have actually isolated the understanding of interrelations between menstruation, pregnancy, and other metabolic processes. And, because of the bifurcation in treatment and approach to women's health, the rest of medicine has tended to leave these questions to obstetrics and gynecology.

There is a consistency to the problems identified in the care of women. The common thread is the lack of integration of women's physiologic and metabolic processes into the body of medicine. As a result, the female body remains somewhat "foreign," something a bit more alien to (primarily male) physicians than a regular (male) body.

The Problem of Shortcomings in the System

The differential attention paid to male versus female patients has been documented. Armitage, Schneiderman and Bass, in a study of physician response to complaints in men and women, speculate that "they might be responding to current stereotypes that regard the male as typically stoic and the female as typically 'hypochondriacal!'" Recent literature has addressed differences in referral patterns for male and female cardiac patients and in their selection for coronary angiography and coronary revascularization. This research attempts to discriminate between bias in the care of women and their different needs because of different courses of specific illness. If there is bias in the care of women cardiac patients, it must be addressed, but it does not warrant the development of separate surgery based upon the "female" heart as opposed to a "male" heart. Whatever differences exist in severity of illness, circulation of coronary arteries, or innervation of conducting muscle, they are all within overlapping variations of both male and female hearts. With the exception of those organs involved in reproduction, the vast majority of human organs are truly androgynous.

The Bifurcation of Medical Care of Women

Internal medicine is founded on the model of a male body, with women as "other." That specialty attends to the medical illnesses of the entire male body and part of the female body, whereas obstetrics and gynecology treats those parts of the body related to reproductive health. The result is that most women during their reproductive years must go to two physicians to get their whole body attended to, or use one and forgo the services of the other.

The archaic nature of this arrangement is nowhere more evident than in the assessment of abdominal disorders. The partitioning of the abdominal cavity into the domain of two specialties reflects the dual origins of internists descending from the regular physicians and ob-

gyns replacing midwives. No clear anatomical distinction exists, however, between abdomen and pelvis in a female. The area is a continuous cavity divided by imaginary lines that delineate the boundaries of the specialist's territory rather than anatomical structures. The gastrointestinal tract passes through the pelvis and may adhere to the ovaries; endometrial tissue may migrate to the diaphragm, and yet the woman with abdominal pain must visit two doctors, each of whom only partially examines her and then communicates findings with the other by phone or written report, or through the patient. In a male it would be akin to having initial chest pain evaluated by two different doctors, one for the heart and one for the lungs. One doctor would only listen to heartbeats, the other only to breath sounds. Each would then write reports back to the other as to whether the shortness of breath and pain on deep inspiration were of cardiac or pulmonary origin. The need for two physicians to evaluate abdominal pain in a woman is equally absurd.

It is the organization of medical knowledge and practice that are the problem, not the female body. Whereas internal medicine and ob-gyn fall short of addressing the whole woman, family medicine takes care of the whole woman, but in the context of her family, a social role not a medical condition. The one specialty that teaches care of the whole woman also includes children and men. In other words, either a specialty treats only parts of the woman, or it treats all of her and her family.

Rather than the establishment of a new specialty based upon the care of more than half of all adult patients, the current system, in both its structure and content, must address the needs of women as an integral and legitimate aspect of the practice of medicine within every specialty. There simply is no special training for an orthopedist treating women or a radiologist reading women's films or a cardiologist listening to a woman's heart. There is rather the necessity for all orthopedists, all radiologists, and all cardiologists—indeed, all physicians—to look beyond bias and sex stereotyping, and to view being female as only one aspect of the biological, social, and psychological person.

If all human bodies were female and social structure was based upon some other factor than gender, the thorough knowledge of the body would be the medical standard. For instance, anatomically, the physician would examine the whole body because vaginas would not be alien anatomical parts but rather within the norm. If men had large breasts, they would be included in the routine examination of a person. The same physician who examines for spleens and prostrates would be expected to feel for breast lumps. The internist examining for abdominal pain would also do a pelvic exam as part of the assessment, and at the same time, would also do a Pap if needed. In other words, the female reproductive and sexual parts would be part of the everyday practice of an everyday physician.

Even though childbirth has become a surgical procedure, pregnancy remains a metabolic process with the major risk factors being related to the medical health of the woman. Hypertension and diabetes, normally the domain of internists, in pregnancy becomes the domain of the obstetrician-gynecologist, a highly trained surgeon. The major difficulties of the postpartum period are likewise not surgical. Bleeding may occasionally be a problem, but the physician is more likely to encounter thyroid disease, depression, and questions about medications that might pass into breast milk. These are areas more appropriately addressed by an internist or family physician than by a surgeon.

Marginalization of "Women's Health" Specialists

The entrance of women and minorities into male-dominated fields has more commonly led to what the anthropologists term "ritual contamination" of a field than to an increase in the prestige of the women who enter the profession. A field created for the nonsurgical routine care of women, whose practitioners would invariably be mostly female, would likely become a relatively low-paid, low-status field with little or no opportunities for advancement or access to power within universities or specialty societies. Just recently in this century women have entered into medicine in significant numbers. However, their continued inability to achieve positions of power makes it likely that "women's health" would become a marginalized area for a few dedicated (probably mostly female) physicians. Meanwhile, the rest of medicine would continue as it is, with both the male body and male psyche the standard of normality and health. And, as long as the standard is male, "other" invariably will mean less.

Women do not need special practitioners. Except for diseases of the male reproductive tract and some rare genetic diseases, there are no illnesses restricted to men only. The basic diseases of man are the diseases of woman. The surgical care of women's reproductive organs would rightfully remain the domain of the obstetrician/gynecologist. Although ob-gyns would like to be designated as the primary care physicians of women, it is more likely that internists or family physicians will retain expertise in pelvic exams rather than ob-gyns adding to their training the routine management of diabetes, hypertension, heart disease, gastric ulcers,

pneumonia, and all the other diseases encountered in the routine primary care of women.

Necessary Changes

The changes needed to rectify current shortcomings are broad in scope but necessary if anything except cosmetic changes are to be made. Hospital facilities can be dressed up in pink colors and new labeling, but unless the need for fundamental changes in the structure of medicine are acknowledged and implemented, health for the vast majority of women will go unaltered. The basic deficiencies and biases that exist in the conceptual framework of woman—as a biological, psychological, and social person—will continue to undermine any attempt to put women on an equal medical and professional footing with men. The changes needed are as follows.

1. The current specialty of internal medicine must incorporate the menstrual cycle and reproduction into its conceptual framework. The routine gynecologic care of women must be a part of the practice of internal medicine. Family medicine, while continuing to provide primary care for a woman, must recognize her individual existence separate from the family.

2. Obstetrics and gynecology should remain the specialty for referral of obstetric and gynecologic difficulties.

3. Interdisciplinary research must address gaps in the understanding of female functions and their relationship to normal and pathological conditions.

4. Medical students must be taught to identify with patients across gender lines.

5. All medical specialties must be examined for ways in which they are or are not "user friendly" to women.

6. Organized medicine, including medical schools and professional societies, must begin to actively address and rectify those unfounded assumptions about the biological inferiority of women that have been the basis for exclusion of women from medicine and from positions of leadership and power within medicine.

It is not clear what medicine would look like without the standard of the male body and the concomitant underlying assumptions of a biological basis for female passivity and weakness. However, we have the opportunity to find out. Women as patients and as professionals should not settle for a small corner of medicine as a women's health specialty, however appealing that might be. Women instead need to establish their rightful place and perspective within the body of medicine, a body that has been entirely too male in its conceptual framework as well as its membership. There is no medical imperative for a new specialty. Instead, there is an urgent social and economic imperative to restructure medical special-

ization and to create a nonadversarial body of knowledge and code of practice, in which gender may represent difference but not "other," and certainly not less.

REFERENCES
A list of references is available in the original source.

How to Tell Your Doctor a Thing or Two

by Morton Hunt

If you're like most Americans, you've lost a lot of faith in doctors in recent years. In 1966 the Louis Harris survey organization reported that 73 percent of Americans had a great deal of confidence in the medical profession: by 1977 the figure had dropped to 43 percent.

As a result a new kind of patient has appeared—a patient who is questioning and even argumentative, sometimes mistrustful, often balky. This patient goes doctor-shopping, files complaints with medical societies, sues for malpractice. She may join one of the hundreds of new medical-consumer (patient) organizations that defend patients against their own doctors. She—or he—no longer silently listens to the doctor with awe but speaks up, wants to be told everything and to be convinced, and reserves the right to reject the doctor's advice or to ask for a second opinion.

I've been talking to leaders of the medical profession and of medical-consumer groups, and both sides agree on one thing: Doctors throughout America are seeing the new kind of patient increasingly often in their offices. Although some doctors—including my own—look approvingly on patients of this new breed, the majority view them with disapproval and even hostility. By training, position and tradition, doctors tend to play the role of Wise Patriarch Whose Word is Law, and they expect their patients to be Good Children Who Obey Without Argument. They consider the new breed "difficult," "troublemakers" and—above all—"bad" patients.

But there is growing evidence that nowadays the "bad" patient is a better one, in terms of medical results, than the "good" patient. According to a number of recent research studies, the passive, uncomplaining, unquestioning patient is less likely to get well quickly than the new kind. Or as Eli Glogow, director of the graduate program in health administration at the University of Southern California, succinctly puts it, "the 'bad patient' gets better quicker."

Why? Not because the "bad" patient—whom I'll call the "active" patient— refuses to follow instructions. Indeed, medical journals report that the independent patient is apt to carry out doctors' orders faithfully, once he or she accepts them, while the passive patient is more likely to forget or quietly disobey.

But following instructions is only part of it. What gives the active patient better odds at regaining health quickly or staying healthy is a whole new concept of the patient's role. Essentially it consists of taking responsibility for one's own healthcare—becoming an adult rather than a child in the doctor-patient relationship. That means finding the best doctor available but getting another opinion if doubtful about a major recommendation; defending oneself against overmedication and unnecesary surgery; and in general acting as the doctor's partner, collaborator and equal.

It is out of necessity that such patients are becoming ever more numerous for there has been a revolution in the nature of medical practice. In recent years the doctor-patient relationship has become coldly impersonal, and

Reprinted with permission from Bread & Roses, Women's Health Center, Milwaukee, Wisconsin. (Specific date uncertain, probably late 1970s.)

not very reassuring to the patient. Here are some of the reasons:

- The number of drugs, tests and special technological procedures has vastly increased. As a result, patients spend more time with nurses and technicians, less time with the doctor himself. Diseases get treated but treatment becomes an assembly-line affair.

- The new technology makes for greater specialization. Specialization makes for higher fees—and so more doctors want to specialize (more than four out of five now do so). In consequence there are fewer general practitioners, and the patient has to wait longer and settle for less time with a G.P. than ever before.

- Specialization also means that the patient is sub-divided and parceled out among doctors—the gynecologist, the allergist, and so on—and is to each not a person but a symptom in some part of the body. Many patients get medical care from several doctors but have no one doctor who *cares*. There's the rub. Dr. W. Walter Menninger of the Menninger Foundation, a center of psychiatric research, says that most of the grievances patients have against doctors involve breakdown in the *caring* aspect of the physician-patient relationship, not in the quality of technical care.

  One young woman I know worried about menstrual spotting and went to a busy gynecologist who, with little explanation, did a suction extraction of the endometrium (the mucus lining of the uterus). Unprepared for the invasive and painful procedure, she left the office shaken and burst into tears on the sidewalk. Months later she said to him as casually as she could, "Doctor, that last visit was so unpleasant I thought I might never come back"—to which he replied just as casually, "If you ever feel that way again, I think you *shouldn't* come back." Caring? He'd sneer at the word.

- We Americans move about more than ever. We become separated from the doctor who knows us best, and what he or she knows about us is, in most cases, lost or forgotten. Yet you, the patient, have no legal right in most states to make the doctor turn over his records to you. (If you ask, he'll send them to another doctor—but few patients ask.)

- Group practice, growing by leaps and bounds, gives the busy doctor much-needed relief and free time and assures you that someone will be on hand when needed. But the substitute doctor rarely knows your medical history or has time to read through your folder. Unless you can fill in the gaps in this stranger's knowledge of you—and have the courage to do so—you may get indifferent or even hurtful treatment.

  One 30-year-old woman went to her medical group when a rash spread over her arms and chest. An overworked doctor who had never seen her before asked her a few questions and concluded—correctly—that it was an allergic reaction; summer sunshine and an antibiotic she'd been taking didn't go well together. He prescribed a form of cortisone to be taken by mouth, and a week later she was in the hospital with a bleeding ulcer. Buried in her folder and unread by the doctor had been notes about a tendency on her part toward ulcers: cortisone treatment brought the condition to an acute state.

- The profit motive has altered the patient-doctor relationship. Profitmaking is an old, respectable incentive to businessmen and professionals alike, but it can easily lead to exploitative and unfair practices. That's why watchdog agencies protect consumers from impersonal big business. But medicine, though it too is now impersonal and big business—doctors' fees total over $26 billion a year—remains virtually unregulated except by itself.

Exploitation by doctors takes many forms. In a study of one group of internists, researchers found that some of the doctors ordered patients to come back for follow-up visits twice as often as others did, even though all were treating the same kinds of patients. Three of four doctors polled by the American Medical Association this year admit that they now order anywhere from one to several extra tests per patient—not for the patient's benefit but for their own, as protection from potential malpractice suits. But it is the patient who pays—and who is exposed to extra risks.

The most serious conflict between the patient's best interest and the profit motive occurs when the doctor stands to gain the most. A surgeon who will earn many hundreds of dollars from performing an operation is likely to be less objective, when deciding whether to recommend it, than a surgeon who is not involved and therefore impartial. A recent Congressional study indicates that one of every six operations is unnecessary: that's more than 3 million needless operations per year, costing $4 billion and leading to nearly 12,000 postoperative deaths. In some specialties the figures are even higher; various research teams have termed anywhere from a quarter to a half of the 800,000 hysterectomies performed each year "unjustified" or "unnecessary."

Reaction to all this was inevitable. Liberal doctors and medical administrators drafted "bills of rights" for patients, and a few legislators tried to get some of them enacted into state law. Labor unions and veterans' organizations began to fight for "patients' advocates" in clinics and hospitals, to listen to patients' grievances and take their complaints to the authorities. Everywhere the new breed of patient began to appear.

And perhaps most important, medical-consumer organizations sprang up, most of them offshoots of the 1960s consumer movement. Public Citizen, the national organization headed by Ralph Nader, set up the Health Research Group in Washington, D.C. Headed by Sidney M. Wolfe, a dynamic young doctor, it gathers research data and uses them to lobby for stronger Government controls over drug advertising, prescription writing, the use of x-rays; for the patient's right to obtain personal medical records; and for controls over cost and quality of healthcare in general.

In recent years other medical-consumer groups have been started in many cities by churches, by campus organizations and by women's groups. Some of them, chiefly educational, publish pamphlets, newsletters or books on medical matters, or operate Tel-Med libraries. (You phone, ask to hear a tape on a medical matter that concerns you and get plugged in to a four-to-seven minute cassette at no charge.) Others also offer counseling and advice and make referrals to doctors or clinics. Still others, like Nader's health group, are interested chiefly in bringing pressure to bear on city and state officials to control medical costs and practices and in getting consumer-minded representatives onto the governing boards of hospitals, medical-insurance plans and relevant state agencies.

In the long run it will be these collective efforts that will rebuild the patient-doctor relationship in a new, democratic form. Meanwhile what can you, the individual, do for yourself? A good deal. From my conversations with medical-consumer leaders I have put together a seven-point program for the new-style patient:

1. **Care for yourself as far as possible.** Save the doctor's time and your own—and your money— by doing at home certain things you can learn through community-health projects and self-care courses taught by medical-consumer groups. You can learn to take and record your own blood pressure and that of your husband and children (these days *everyone's* blood pressure is considered important information; the equipment costs as little as $20). You can learn to adjust the dosage of your own or your children's medication, within limits set by the doctor. You can give yourself or others in your family regular injections (allergy shots, for instance), when needed. Professor Lowell S. Levin, of the Yale University School of Medicine, a specialist in public health, says that the time has come for the "rediscovery of the lay function in health," and maintains that the informed patient can become the most important practitioner in the medical-care system.

2. **Keep your own medical records.** Since in most states you can't gain access to doctors' records, ask your doctor for his findings every time you visit him—your pulse, blood pressure, hemoglobin and white-cell count—whatever he checks; and don't settle for "It's fine." You have a moral if not a legal right to precise information. So start a notebook. Keep track of whatever the doctor tells you, plus the dates of illnesses, their symptoms and duration, diagnoses, medications taken and their effects.

   Also ask your doctor for the results of all tests and lab reports. A few doctors already provide such information; others do not but will if you ask; and many others will refuse. If your doctor refuses, you can either accept defeat or look for another doctor. You also can ask any medical-consumer group what the law is in your state; it may support your claims, and if it does, tell the doctor so.

3. **Come to the doctor prepared.** Before your visit, jot down everything you want to tell the doctor. Include the questions you want to ask. It's amazing how things will slip your mind when you're talking to a hurried doctor or when you're spraddled out on an examination table with some unseen gadget making its way into you. Many feminist groups urge patients to take along a friend to hold the list of questions and remind you of things you forget. Most doctors will ask a third party to leave before an examination, but this is only custom: A.M.A. spokesmen and consumer-group leaders agree that doctors should, and for the most part will, allow a third party to remain if the patient asks them to.

4. **Exercise your right to choose and refuse.** Even with a doctor you believe in—and all the more with one who is new to you—you should take an active part in decisions affecting you. Ask for a detailed explanation of the possible side effects of any recommended drug or procedure. Ask if there

are alternate ways to treat your problem. Give due weight to the doctor's preference, but also to your own. It's your body and your life.

If the doctor calls for tests, ask how necessary they are; it's quite in order for you to say you'd like to keep costs down. And ask about risks; it's quite proper for you to say you'd like to avoid any x-rays that are of only marginal value, since it's not the individual exposure that endangers you but an excessive lifetime total of exposures. And it's also your right to say that you prefer to live with your medical problem—or even die of it—rather than submit to a painful, risky treatment if the outcome is highly uncertain.

But if you question the doctor's advice or decline to follow any of his recommendations, won't he be angered? It depends in part on how you put it—and on what kind of person he is. Says Dr. Wolfe, of the Health Research Group, "The doctor who gets huffy when you ask questions or express preferences is a doctor to stay away from. The doctor you should look for is the one who realizes that you have a right to ask questions and to decide what you want to do with your life."

Do you really have a right to refuse any of the doctor's orders? Medical-consumer leaders and A.M.A. officials agree that unless your disease endangers the public welfare, you do have such a right—but that if you exercise it, the doctor may exercise a corresponding right to stop treating you. If you're pregnant or seriously ill or worried, you may be afraid to risk it; you may choke back your questions or objections and play the part of the "good" patient.

But speaking up needn't mean confrontation. Denise Fuge, coordinator of the Women and Health Committee of the New York Chapter of NOW, says patients shouldn't *confront* the doctor, but should seek to *communicate* their fears, wishes and personal values openly and honestly. "Most doctors," she says, "don't know what women are thinking, and they'd like to. They'd respond to the patient much more sensitively if they did."

5. **Get a second opinion.** Before you agree to surgery or any other major procedure, or when some ailment isn't getting better under your doctor's management, tell him that you'd like a second opinion and that you feel sure he wouldn't mind your getting one. He probably will mind, but won't say so or threaten to stop treating you; publicly, most doctors are opposed only to mandatory

(legally required) second opinions. Privately, though, many of them feel like Dr. James Sammons, executive vice-president of the A.M.A., who is against them in general.

"I'm opposed to them," he told me, "because the patient's right of choice is lost—he tends to assume the second opinion is more intelligent than the first one." What Dr. Sammons ignores is that the second opinion, though not necessarily more intelligent than the first, is disinterested and hence less subject to unconscious bias. Not all doctors, incidentally, are against second opinions; one quarter of a sample of doctors polled by the magazine *Medical World News* favored them, and the trend is in that direction.

6. **Ask for enough time.** Don't let yourself be rushed. "You're paying for an expensive service," says Maryann Napoli, of New York's Center for Medical Consumers and Healthcare Information, "and consultation is part of it. It's important for your mental health as well as your physical health to have your questions fully answered and your doubts resolved."

   Denise Fuge, of NOW, recommends that you say something like, "Doctor, I came to you because I've been worried, and I need more time to talk to you. If you're too busy today, please tell me when you can spend more time with me and I'll come back." A women's medical-consumer group in New York, HealthRight, also suggests that you ask the nurse some of your unanswered questions; nurses are often sympathetic and less rushed than the doctor.

   But if your doctor regularly allows less time than normal—15 minutes is the national average duration of routine office visits—and doesn't respond to your request for more time, he may be the wrong doctor for you.

7. **Don't let yourself be treated as an inferior.** This is one of the trickiest points, and perhaps one of the most important. Many doctors treat you in ways that put you at a psychological disadvantage. Some gynecologists in particular address patients by their first names even when they scarcely know them; it makes the patient feel a little like a child. Many women resent this; a few fight back. When a gynecologist greeted one woman, whom he had seen only once before, with "What brings you here today, Lillian?" she said sweetly, "I've got galloping vaginitis again, Bernard." Bernard took the hint. Generally, though, a more formal

way of setting the matter straight will work better. For instance: "Doctor, I would much prefer to be called Ms. So-and-so," or, "I really don't like being addressed by my first name."

Similarly, it may make you feel inferior to be undressed and in a gown when you first meet the doctor. If so, tell the nurse you want to speak to him before you undress. This is a delicate matter; the doctor may have set office rules. But Dr. Menninger points out that when you come to exhibit some disease to the doctor, you are apt to feel shame and humiliation, and since such feelings tend to make you a docile patient rather than an active one, it is important to resist anything that intensifies them.

Things will never be what they once were. But the new doctor-patient relationship need not be one of antagonism; it can be one of equality and cooperation. This is what most of the medical-consumer groups, and most active patients are really seeking.

And within the ranks of doctors there are signs of evolution toward a new image of the good doctor—no longer the wise patriarch whose word is law, but a dedicated expert who is ready to give you the help you need and the kind of help you choose. Increasingly, medical journals carry articles advocating democratic ways of dealing with patients and favoring patient participation in the making of medical decisions.

Professor Julia Frank, of the Yale University School of Medicine, writing in the *New England Journal of Medicine,* urges doctors everywhere to make the patient "an equal member of the team." An editorial in a recent issue of the *Journal of the American Medical Association,* noting the spread of "participatory democracy" in our society, says, "It is simply no longer possible for the physician to make moral and value decisions for his patients." And Professor Levin, writing in *Public Health Reports,* sounds a call for massive self-reform by the health professions: "The high value placed on the compliant patient must be transferred to the active, even resistant, patient." He predicts the creation of a "new social contract between professionals and lay persons"—a contract from which the doctor will benefit, by sharing responsibility with those he treats.

And it is a contract from which the patient will benefit by gaining self-respect and a sense of control over her own life—and by getting better quicker.

The Gynecologic Exam and the Training of Medical Students
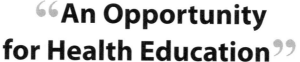
"An Opportunity for Health Education"

by Judith Schmidt

This article is a personal account written by a senior health education major about her experience as a teaching associate (TA) in training medical students for the gynecological examination. This method of using teaching associates who "teach on their own bodies" has evolved in medical schools across the country in recent years. It is an attempt to counter inadequate medical school preparation in this important area of women's health and to improve the physician-patient relationship in gynecological medicine. Lack of sensitivity to female patients has taken the form of high rates of malpractice litigation in gynecology, a situation which might well be reversed given the improved communication between physician and patient. Medical school teaching staff across the country have now widely accepted the use of teaching associates as the most effective teaching method for this part of the complete physical examination.

One of the ideas emphasized in this approach is that of the "activated patient." An activated patient is one who is fully and equally involved as a participant in the examination process. One projected outcome of this approach is greater personal responsibility for one's health such as doing self-breast exams. But the potential of using this approach goes beyond mere "disease prevention" of traditional medical care. It gives female patients a sense of control over what happens to them—both inside and out of a gynecologist's office—and enters a psychological and social health dimension that makes the concept known as "high-level wellness" accessible. In the context of medical intervention by physicians during the gynecological exam, the potential exists to take steps toward the goal of optimal wellness. This article attempts to explore that potential.

"What's it like doing that sort of thing?" curious and sometimes incredulous friends ask. I have just told them about my job. I am a teaching associate (TA) for the instruction of the gynecological examination to first and second-year medical students. As such, I am a "professional patient." I give feedback to these students about their technique and attitude, and most important, about the way they communicate with me as a patient during the gynecological exam.

I respond to my friends' questions by telling them my job is demanding. I experience the same feelings that any woman facing a breast and pelvic exam does, including anxiety and nervousness. But overall, I feel good about doing it. I feel that what I am doing is important.

The next question, "Does it pay well?" The implication is that the only reason for my engaging in such an occupation must be money. "Yes, it does," is my answer. "And well it should! My job takes a good deal of knowledge and ability." Not only does it require knowledge of female sexual and reproductive anatomy, but it means that I must be comfortable discussing my own anatomy with others. It requires good teaching and interpersonal skills, plus a lot of sensitivity about a topic that is emotionally loaded for students and patient alike.

"But money isn't the main reason I do it," I explain. My own experiences with gynecologists have for the most part not been satisfactory. The opportunity to improve this area of women's health through my input into the training of medical students appeals to me. Also, as a student majoring in health education at the same university, I see the potential for patient education and the role physicians might play in this process. As a TA, I feel I have some influence in this direction.

"Does your job take training?"

"Yes it does," I respond, as I visualize our initial training sessions. In these first sessions, we learn right along with the medical students. We all become part of a "learning team" which I can now see is beneficial for reducing anxiety and developing a comfortable working relationship with the students prior to the actual examination.

Just as the medical students do, we watch the Bates videotape, "Female Pelvic Examination." And just as they do, we practice inserting the speculum and examining internal anatomy manually on the plastic Gynny model. As I practice using the speculum on the Gynny model, the idea then seems less scary to me. I wonder, as a health educator, whether offering other women this experience on a Gynny model prior to a pelvic exam might lessen their anxiety, as it has mine.

In these initial training sessions my actual teaching role begins. I am called upon to recall my own feelings during the gynecological exam. The medical students are also encouraged to explore the kinds of feelings that they, as physicians, might experience. How should the physician, for example, handle a situation in the best interests of the patient and him or herself if sexually attracted to the patient prior to the examination? Issues such as these are dealt with in these sessions.

Emphasis in these training sessions is put on the importance of involving the patient during the process of the exam itself. An activated patient who is involved in such a way has some sense of control over what is happening to her during her exam. Again, as a teaching associate I am called upon to describe how being "activated" in this way as a patient allows me to feel less victimized during the gynecological exam.

Part of this initial discussion focuses on empathy. To learn to empathize with female patients, all the students are required to disrobe, drape, and get into the lithotomy position—or into the stirrups, as it is commonly called. Through this first-hand experience, medical students can vividly relate to the feelings of vulnerability shared by their female patients as they lie naked, legs suspended, waiting to be examined—covered only by a thin piece of paper that fails to intercept the cool flow of air over one's usually concealed private anatomy.

After these preliminary training sessions, my difficult work begins. I find that my anxiety soon disappears as I get actively involved in teaching. The students are much more nervous than I am so that relating to them in a calm and confident way has the effect of putting us both at ease.

The nature of the suggestions that I give during the actual examination stresses technique. I might suggest that a student flatten his or her hand while palpating my abdomen. I might help a student identify that fleeting moment when my ovaries roll past. But I do not emphasize the mechanics, as I know these will improve with practice.

The general feedback I give each student in turn afterward about how well he or she communicated with me and attended to my emotional needs is far more important. I begin by reinforcing those things which I like. This might include confirming that the student maintained eye contact with me and watched my face for nonverbal signals indicating discomfort. Or it might mean commending a student's effective use of firm and reassuring touch. Then, I follow with a suggestion for improvement. This might include suggesting to the student that he or she replace specialized medical jargon with common conversational language that the patient can more easily understand.

Occasionally, my job demands that I be assertive. For example, I had to tell a male student that I was uneasy having his groin against my knee, while having my breast examined—under ordinary circumstances a female patient might interpret this in a sexual way. We were both embarrassed, but he expressed appreciation for telling him this.

Only once did I find it necessary to tell a student about poor attitude. "I am uncomfortable with the way you treated me—as if I were a plastic model," I had to say. Fortunately, this is rare as most students are respectful and caring to the extreme.

I am proud of the student who is able to include me actively and equally as a participant. I keep a mental checklist during the exam of the various ways the student might accomplish this. Does the student remember to offer me a mirror? Does he or she offer it in such a way that is *not* just an off-hand question? ("Do you want a mirror?") But rather in a way so that *I,* as patient, understand that it is important and acceptable to know about my own female anatomy. "Would you like to hold a mirror while I examine your pelvic area? That way I can better explain to you what *I* see, and *you* can see everything for yourself?"

There are other check-offs on my mental list. Does the student offer me the option of having my head raised during the pelvic part of the examination to facilitate communication between us? Does the student actively solicit my verbal input; not just telling and explaining, but questioning and encouraging any questions *I,* as patient, might have regarding my anatomy or sexual functioning?

Finally, I consider certain non-verbal aspects of our communication exchange. I consider the student's attitude. Is it flippant or overbearing in any way? Does the student display appropriate respect and a willingness to share power in the interaction that goes on between us? What clues do I get from facial expression, body position and movement that support my assessment?

By assessing the answers to all these questions, I am able to evaluate how well I was activated as an involved and equal participant during the examination. When done effectively, this process allows me to feel in control—not as a passive bystander whose body is "being done to."

At this point, relating the notion of the activated patient to the idea of wellness begins. By actively engaging female patients in the gynecological exam itself, the physician can play an important role in aiding the female patient in knowing and being comfortable with her body. Not only might this have a spin-off effect of encouraging women to practice self-examination and prevention at home (I am an example of one who only began doing regular self-breast exams since beginning this job even though I had long known the appalling statistics about breast cancer), but it might help overcome those culturally programmed negative feelings that many women still have about their bodies and lead to a greater degree of sexual satisfaction.

At the end of the teaching session, it is my time for reinforcement. The students all express their gratitude. They are relieved that doing a procedure that had worried them has turned into a positive learning experience; they give me credit. I accept their thanks and express my hope that they will use what they have learned here to make the experience of the gynecological exam a better one for their patients.

One of my fears when I took this job was how the students would react when we would meet in public after the training sessions. I knew this was inevitable as I am a student on the same campus in a small city. Contrary to my worries, I have not felt the slightest embarrassment. Rather I sense a mutual respect between us resulting from the difficult task we shared together.

This feeling of mutual respect might not be something peculiar to my own particular experience. Perhaps it is a reflection of this kind of interaction between a patient-oriented physician and an activated, involved patient. It is an interaction that is designed to allow the patient to feel more in control and, in so doing, to enhance her self-esteem.

The positive effect of this interaction for the patient and its contribution to her overall health status should not be minimized. Replacing negative feelings that many women still have regarding their sexual-reproductive anatomy with positive ones can enhance a woman's sense of well-being and personal fulfillment. Satisfying such a psychological health need represents a step on that continuum toward that elusive concept known as high level wellness. Entering this psychological and social health dimension goes beyond the purely physical realm of traditional medical care.

Medical intervention by a physician which attempts to accomplish such a task is a concrete way to lessen the gap between disease prevention and that lofty goal of optimal wellness. It is an intervention mutually rewarding to patient and physician alike.

BIBLIOGRAPHY

1. DiMatteo R M, Friedman HS: *Social Psychology and Medicine.* Oelgeschlager, West Germany, Gum and Hain, Publishers, Inc., 1982.

2. Miller G D: The gynecological examination as a learning experience. *Journal of the American College Health Association* 1974; 23(2).

Cadavers, Dolls, and Prostitutes
"Medical Pedagogy and the Pelvic Rehearsal"
by Terri Kapsalis

My first question, as I suspect yours may be, was, "what *kind* of woman lets four or five novice medical students examine her?"—James G. Blythe, M.D.

Fearing the Unknown

In a paper entitled "The First Pelvic Examination: Helping Students Cope with Their Emotional Responses," printed in the *Journal of Medical Education* in 1979, Julius Buchwald, M.D., a psychiatrist, shares his findings after ten years of conducting seminars with medical students starting their training in OB/GYN. He locates six primary fears associated with a first pelvic examination: (1) "hurting the patient"; (2) "being judged inept"; (3) the "inability to recognize pathology"; (4) "sexual arousal"; (5) "finding the examination unpleasant"; and (6) the "disturbance of the doctor-patient relationship" (when a patient reminded them of somebody they knew, e.g., mother or sister).

Because the pelvic exam produces fear and anxiety in medical students, numerous methods have been used to offer them a pelvic exam "rehearsal." This practice performance is meant to help soothe or disavow student fears while allowing them to practice manual skills. The types of practice performances adopted reveal and promote specific ideas about female bodies and sexuality held by the medical institution. The use of gynecology teaching associates (GTAS), trained lay women who teach students using their own bodies, is a relatively new addition to pelvic exam pedagogy that will be examined at length. Previous to and contemporaneous with this practice, medical schools have cast a variety of characters as subjects of this pelvic exam rehearsal, including actual patients, cadavers, anesthetized women, prostitutes, and plastic manikins such as "Gynny," "Betsi," and "Eva". The ways medical students have been taught to perform pelvic exams illustrate the predicament of the gynecological scenario, a situation in which a practitioner must, by definition, examine women's genitals in a clinical and necessarily nonsexual manner. The array of pedagogical methods used to teach pelvic exams reveals how the medical institution views female bodies, female sexuality, and the treatment of women.

In pelvic exams, physicians-to-be are confronted with both female genital display and manipulation, two highly charged cultural acts. If students have previously engaged in gazing at or touching female genitals, most likely they have done so as a private sexual act (e.g., male students engaging in heterosexual activities and female students masturbating or engaging in lesbian activities). Occasionally there are male or female students who, for a variety of reasons, have had little or no exposure to naked female bodies, and their fears often revolve around a fear of the "unknown," which in the case of women's genitals takes the form of a particularly stigmatized mystery.

Students seem to find it very difficult to consider female genital display and manipulation in the medical context as entirely separate from sexual acts and their accompanying fears. Buchwald's list of fears makes explicit the perceived connection between a pelvic examination and a sexual act. "A fear of the inability to recognize pathology" also reflects a fear of contracting a sexually transmitted disease, an actual worry expressed by some of Buchwald's student doctors. Likewise, "a fear of sexual arousal" makes explicit the connection between the pelvic exam and various sexual acts. Buchwald notes that both men and women are subject to this fear of sexual arousal. "A fear of being judged inept" signals a kind of "performance anxiety," a feeling common in both inexperienced and experienced clinical and sexual performers. "A fear of the disturbance of the doctor-patient relationship" recognizes the existence of a type of "incest taboo" within the pelvic exam scenario. Buchwald shares anecdotes of students feeling sick or uncomfortable if the patient being examined reminded them of their mother or sister. Buchwald's work deviates from most publications dealing with the topic of medical students and pelvic exams. Largely, any acknowledgment of this precarious relationship between pelvic exams and sex acts is relatively private and informal, taking place in conversations between students, residents, and doctors, sometimes leaking into private patient interactions. For example, as a student in the 1960s, a male physician was told by the male OB/GYN resident in charge, "During your first 70 pelvic exams, the only anatomy you'll feel is your own." Cultural attitudes about women and their bodies are not checked at the hospital door. If women are largely marketed as sexualized objects of the gaze, why should a gynecological scenario necessarily produce different meanings?

Rehearsing Pelvics

Teaching medical practices is the act of constructing medical realities. In other words, the student is continuously learning by lecture and example what is right and acceptable and, conversely, what is wrong and unacceptable in medical practice. The intractability of medical teaching from medical practice is built into the very title of Foucault's *Birth of the Clinic*. The translator's note recognizes the importance of the choice of the word "clinic": "When Foucault speaks of *la clinique,* he is thinking of both clinical medicine and of the teaching hospital so if one wishes to retain the unity of the concept, one is obliged to use the rather odd-sounding clinic." Medical

pedagogy, including textbooks (the focus of the following chapter) and experiential learning, is symbiotic with medical practice; the two work together in the formation, transferal, and perpetuation of medical knowledge. With regard to pelvic exams, this medical knowledge has been acquired in a number of ways.

Many medical students have encountered their first performance of a pelvic exam on an actual patient. Oftentimes a group of students on rounds would repeat pelvic exams one after another on a chosen patient while the attending physician watched. If we consider that the pelvic exam is often sexualized by novice practitioners, this pedagogical situation resembles a "gang rape." Many times there is little communication with the woman being examined, nor is her explicit consent necessarily requested. Due to the intimidation of the medical institution, a woman may not resist repeated examination, even if she is adamantly against the use of her body for pedagogical purposes. This actual patient situation is one that Buchwald locates as anxiety provoking for the medical student (he fails to mention the anxiety this may cause the woman being examined). This situation adds to what Buchwald refers to as the student's "fear of being judged inept": "a frequent remark was, 'if the resident sees the way I'm going about it, he'll think I'm stupid.' In some respects what began to evolve was the image of the experienced, wise, worldly, and sexually competent adult (the resident or attending physician) sneering at the floundering explorations of an adolescent (the medical student) who is striving to become a 'man.'" Buchwald's reading of this situation is gendered inasmuch as he compares the pelvic exam to an adolescent male rite of passage. This gendered reading is telling. The medical apparatus, particularly this 1970s version, incorporates specifically gendered male positions of physician and medical student. Even though there are increasing numbers of women medical students, physicians, and medical educators, the structures of this apparatus, specifically the structures of medical pedagogy, are in many instances unchanged or slow in changing and require a female medical student to fit into this masculinized subject position. Her relationship to this ascribed subject position, particularly as a medical student, may be uncomfortable, as she may be split between identifying with the woman pelvic patient (as she herself has most likely undergone such exams) and with her newly forming role as masculinized spectator. As a medical educator, I frequently witness such a split in female medical students. As Laura Mulvey describes, "trans-sex identification is a *habit* that very easily becomes *second nature.* However, this Nature does not sit easily and shifts restlessly in its borrowed transvestite clothes." Although Mulvey is discussing female cinematic spectatorship, her words are applicable to female medical spectatorship as well. While the anxieties located and described by Buchwald as very "male" in nature may be the very same anxieties experienced by a female medical student, these anxieties take on different twists and meanings with female physicians-in-training.

Other than the attending physician, one person within the pelvic equation who might also judge the student as inept or whose presence might distract the student from performing a proper first exam and therefore cause the student anxiety, is the patient herself. Cadavers, anesthetized women, and anthropomorphic pelvic models like the plastic manikins "Gynny," "Betsi," and "Eva" are pelvic exam subjects who, for a variety of reasons, are rendered absent and therefore cannot talk back or have an opinion about the medical student's performance. These female models alleviate anxiety regarding inappropriate patient performance since they cannot possibly act out. The pedagogical use of these models may also have been developed in order to avert other student fears. If the woman's body is anesthetized, dead, or replaced altogether by a plastic model certainly there can be no fear of causing her pain. However, this logic is questionable in the case of the anesthetized patient: How might repeated pelvic exams under anesthetic affect how a woman "feels" both psychologically and physically when she wakens?

More importantly, the legality of this practice is extremely questionable. How many women would actually consent to this practice? Many women are anxious at the thought of a single pelvic exam, let alone multiple exams. Furthermore, the fear of a pelvic exam is often associated with feeling vulnerable and out of control; under anesthetic, a woman is particularly vulnerable and out of control. And yet teaching medical students how to do pelvic exams on anesthetized women appears to be widely practiced, although public discussion of this method outside (and inside) the medical community is relatively scarce. At a 1979 conference sponsored by the Women's Medical Associations of New York City and State, New Jersey, and Connecticut held at Cornell University Medical College, this issue was discussed and found its way into the *New York Times,* where the conference recommendation was quoted: "If examined in the operating room, patients must be told prior to anesthesia that they will be examined by the members of the operating team, including the medical student." Decades later this recommendation is often unheeded. For example, a surgical nurse I interviewed provided a common scenario: "While doing an exam on a woman who is sedated for a urological procedure, a physician may discover that she has a prolapsed uterus. The student or students observing the procedure will then be invited to perform a bi-manual exam on the woman [inserting two fingers in her vagina while pressing on her abdomen] in order to feel her uterus." I have overheard physicians at a prestigious Chicago medical school encouraging students to "get in surgery as much as possible to get pelvic exam practice." The assumption is that students will not be intimidated by an unconscious woman and that the patient will, in addition, have relaxed abdominal muscles, thus permitting easy palpation of her ovaries and uterus. Many physicians have not heard about such "practicing" and are outraged at the suggestion, maintaining that this is medically sanctioned sexual assault. Some physicians who are aware of the practice dodge the questionable issues, maintaining that for some students it is the only way they will learn.

But what *are* students learning in this scenario? By using anesthetized women, cadavers, or plastic models as pelvic exam subjects students are being taught that a model patient (or patient model) is one who is essentially unconscious or backstage to the performance of the pelvic exam; she should be numb to the exam, providing no feedback and offering no opinions. In the tradition of Sims's experiments, passive and powerless female patients are considered ideal "participants" in the learning process. In addition, students practicing on essentially silent and lifeless models are learning that the manual skills associated with completing a pelvic exam are more important than the fundamental skills needed to interact with the patient—skills that ideally would help the patient relax and participate in the exam.

Perhaps these rehearsal methods are used under the assumption that an anesthetized, dead, or plastic model is unerotic and will thus relieve students of Buchwald's fear #4, "a fear of sexual arousal." And yet the rendering of the object of manipulation or the gaze as passive simply heightens the power differential between examiner and examined that can in effect tap into an altogether different system of erotics. Necrophilia may be coded into a pelvic examination on a cadaver. Similarly, there have been noted cases of sexual abuse when patients are under anesthetic. Likewise, the anthropomorphically named pelvic manikins "Gynny," "Betsi," and "Eva," with their custom orifices for medical penetration, could be recognized as the medical correlates to inflatable sex dolls.

In the late 1970s, numerous medical pedagogues were reexamining what one physician referred to as "the time-honored methods" of pelvic exam pedagogy: students examining anesthetized women, conscious patients, cadavers, or plastic models. The problems with these methods were discussed in a number of articles. The authors of the 1977 article "Professional Patients: An Improved Method of Teaching Breast and Pelvic Examination" in the *Journal of Reproductive Medicine* found that training medical students on actual patients "has many disadvantages, including infringement of patients' rights, inadequate feedback and moral and ethical concerns. Another approach that is widely used is the anesthetized preoperative patient. Again, problems include informed consent, increased cost and/or risk and lack of an interpersonal exchange. The introduction of the 'Gynny' and 'Betsi' models has been an attempt at improvement, but not without drawbacks, which include a lack of personal communication, unreal exposure and difficulty with 'live' correlation." Where was the medical community to find these living models? Some went to what must have seemed a very natural source. In the early 1970s a number of schools, including the University of Washington Medical School and the University of Oklahoma Physician's Associate Program, hired prostitutes to serve as "patient simulators." What other women would accept payment for spreading their legs? Logically, these educators felt that a prostitute would be the most fitting *kind* of woman for the job. In a sense, the patriarchal medical establishment took the position of a rich uncle, paying for his nephew, the medical student, to have his first sexual experience with a prostitute. This gendered suggestion assumes that female medical students are structurally positioned as masculinized "nephew" subjects as well.

Although lip service has been paid to the supposed importance of desexualizing the pelvic patient, in choosing prostitute patient models, medical educators inadvertently situated the exam as a sexualized act. They must have thought that only a prostitute would voluntarily submit to exams repeatedly and for nondiagnostic purposes. Or perhaps the underlying assumption was that a lady *pays* to get examined whereas a whore *gets paid* for the same exam. It may have also been assumed that prostitutes are more accustomed to and have a higher tolerance for vaginal pain than other women and would thus be more fitting practice models for novice students. In choosing to hire prostitutes as patients the boundaries of pornographic and medical practice were collapsed. Within this scenario of a hired prostitute, the student physician was put in the position of a medicalized lover or "john." Certainly Buchwald's fear #3, "a fear of sexual arousal," was confirmed and even encouraged by hiring prostitutes. Buchwald notes that certain students "appeared to project their anxiety by asking, 'what should I do if the patient starts responding sexually?'" By hiring prostitutes as pelvic patients, the med-

ical establishment not only enforced the trope of the "seductive patient," but also paid for it. "Playing doctor" in this pelvic rehearsal cast with patient prostitutes threatened to translate the pelvic exam into an act of sexualized penetration and bodily consumption.

In many cases when prostitutes were hired, the medical student was led to believe that the woman being examined was a clinical outpatient rather than a prostitute. Thus the prostitute still had a relatively passive position in the training of medical students. In order to properly perform her role as clinical outpatient, she could offer the student little feedback. In addition, the working logic of the medical educators remained relatively opaque inasmuch as the student was not directly learning about the medical establishment's opinion of model patients. And yet these attitudes undoubtedly found their way into medical practice. Years later, students are still told by certain unaware medical faculty that GTAS are prostitutes. Today certain faculty still conclude that no other *kind* of woman would submit her body to multiple exams in exchange for a fee. This points to the importance of understanding the recent history of pelvic pedagogy. Those physicians trained in the 1970s are the same physicians practicing and educating today.

Some physicians found fault with the use of prostitutes as pelvic models. According to the authors of "Utilization of Simulated Patients to Teach the Routine Pelvic Examination," "the employment of prostitute patient simulators is not satisfactory. The prostitutes employed by the PA (Physician's Associate) program were not articulate enough to provide the quality of instructive feedback necessary for an optimal educational experience. Their employment was costly at $25 per hour, and that expense prohibited their extensive and long-term use. Also, and more importantly prostitutes had abnormal findings on examination prior to their utilization." Pathology was not desirable in these model patients: in the pelvic rehearsal, students were not to be distracted by abnormal findings. Rather, the patient simulator needed to be standardized as normal like the plastic model. In addition, the prostitute was expensive. She received market value for her bodily consumption, unlike the income-free corpse, indebted actual patient, and the cut-rate graduate students that the authors of the article hired at $10 per hour. And although prostitutes did offer some student critique (comments such as "poor introduction," "too serious," "too rough," and "forgot to warm the speculum") their language skills were not medically acceptable. What the medical establishment needed was a model who could engage in medicalese, was more cost efficient, and had normal, healthy anatomy. The GTA would be the answer.

The GTA Program

In 1968 at the University of Iowa Medical School's Department of Obstetrics and Gynecology, Dr. Robert Kretzschmar instituted a new method for teaching junior medical students how to perform the pelvic exam. For the pelvic model he used a "simulated patient," first defined in the medical literature as a "person who has been trained to completely simulate a patient or any aspect of a patient's illness depending upon the educational need." Many simulated patients were actresses and actors hired by the medical establishment to realistically portray a patient. Their critical feedback was not traditionally requested. They simply served as a warm body for the practicing student. This stage of Kretzschmar's program was not dissimilar to the other programs that hired prostitutes. Initially, Kretzschmar adhered to this simulated patient model. He hired a nurse for the role of patient. She agreed to repeated exams by medical students; "however, it was necessary to compromise open communication with her, as she was draped at her request in such a way as to remain anonymous." The curtain rose but the nurse's knowledge, thoughts, feelings, and face remained backstage. All that was revealed was the object of the exam: the woman's pelvic region. The logic behind draping the simulated patient presumed that if "only a whore gets paid" for a nondiagnostic exam, perhaps the nurse could avoid whore status by becoming faceless and silent.

In many gynecology textbooks, as will be examined in the following chapter, a similar logic prevails. Photographs picturing women are cropped so that faces are not shown or bands are placed across eyes to maintain the model's anonymity. If the woman's face and eyes are pictured, the photo could enter the realm of pornography; the woman imaged cannot be soliciting or meeting the medical practitioner's gaze, a potentially sexualized act. If the nurse who served as simulated patient was draped to maintain her anonymity she was in effect attempting to desexualize her body for the medical gaze. But is this an effective strategy for the desexualization of the exam? Is a faceless, vulnerable female body less erotic? In addition, although this professional patient model rehearsal did save actual patients from the task of performing the role of pelvic model, it did little to encourage communication between student and patient. Maintaining such anonymity taught the students that it was acceptable and even preferable for them to ignore the woman backstage behind the drape. They were also shown that a modest woman, unlike a prostitute, would need to disassociate her face from her body. And therefore, a modest woman preferred to be treated as though she were anonymous and invisible.

In 1972, Kretzschmar instituted a different program. The new simulated patient, now named the gynecology teaching associate (GTA), would serve as both patient and instructor, stressing the importance of communication skills in addition to teaching the manual skills required to perform a proper pelvic exam. Unlike the nurse clinician who was first hired as a simulated patient in 1968, the GTA would actively teach and offer feedback to medical students, forsaking any anonymity through draping. The GTAS first hired by Kretzschmar were women who were working on or had received advanced degrees in the behavioral sciences but who had no formal medical training. The women had normal, healthy anatomy and were willing to undergo multiple exams. They then received elaborate instruction in female anatomy and physiology, pelvic and breast examination, self-breast-examination and abdominal examination, with an emphasis on normal anatomy. They worked in pairs, one GTA serving as "patient" TA, one as "instructor" TA. They were assigned a small group of medical students and conducted the educational session in an exam room. The "patient" TA received the exam, role-playing as patient and co-instructor, while the "instructor" TA remained alongside the students, helping and instructing them during the exam. After receiving two exams the "patient" TA changed from gown to street clothes and became "instructor" TA, and the "instructor" TA changed from street clothes to gown to become the "patient" TA. The teaching session was then repeated with a new group of medical students, thus assuring that one TA of each pair would not receive all the exams.

Kretzschmar's GTA model provided a radically new way of teaching medical students how to do pelvic and breast exams. No longer was the simulated patient a teaching tool; now she was both teacher and patient. The women's movement undoubtedly influenced this model. In the 1960s and 70s women were demanding better healthcare and some took matters into their own hands by establishing self-help groups and feminist clinics. In fact, many early GTAS were directly associated with these groups and clinics and believed their new position within the medical establishment as GTA could allow them to bring their alternative knowledge to the heart of the beast.

Kretzschmar received a variety of critical responses from the medical community for his new GTA program. Some were positive, applauding him for his innovative method and his success in avoiding a "men's club" attitude by hiring women as teachers. Some, however, were skeptical at best. They were particularly cautious regarding the GTAS' motives for participating in such a perverse endeavor. The epigraph to this chapter—"What *kind* of woman lets four or five novice medical students examine her?"—was a question asked by many physicians, according to Kretzschmar. Some human subjects committee members who reviewed the GTA concept "felt that women who were willing to participate must be motivated by one or more of several questionable needs, such as desperate financial circumstances (in which case exploiting their need would be unethical). Others fear the women would be exhibitionists or that they would use the pelvic exam to serve some perverse internal sexual gratification (in which case portraying them as normal to medical students would be irresponsible)." Once again, the pelvic exam was compared to a sexual act by the medical establishment. Cultural fears regarding female sexuality and its perversions surface in these objections to the GTA program. Only a nymphomaniac would seek out multiple exams, enjoying repeated penetration with speculums and fingers. Also, poor women might lower themselves to such embodied work out of desperation, thereby aligning the GTA with the prostitute in an explanatory narrative. Furthermore, the committee questioned the psychological stability of the GTA, with the assumption "that women who are emotionally unstable might be attracted to the program, or that undergoing repeated examination might be psychologically harmful." These human subject committee members reveal their nineteenth-century ideas about (white) women: frail female psychological health and sexual health are seen as mutually dependent and delicate partners. If their equilibrium is tipped by the "pleasure" or pain incurred by the excessive sexualized act of multiple pelvic exams, then who knows what horrors will take place.

Unquestionably, teaching female genital display and manipulation has been the cause of a great deal of anxiety. These fears are much more reflective of the medical institution's constructions of the female psyche and female sexuality than of any actual threat to women posed by the role of GTA. One reason the role of GTA could seem threatening to these critics is that they were faced with a new and potentially powerful position for women in the predominantly male medical establishment. Their attempt at pathologizing the GTA could have been propelled by a desire to maintain the status quo: that *normal* women are passive, quiet, disembodied recipients of a hopelessly unpleasant but necessary pelvic exam. For them, perhaps this was the least threatening alternative.

Despite its early critics, Kretzschmar's model has become the pedagogical norm in the vast majority of institutions. Over 90 percent of North American medical schools employ this instructional method, recognized as "excellent" by the Association of Professors of Gynecology and Obstetrics Undergraduate Education Committee. Many GTA programs throughout the country maintain the same basic form as Kretzschmar's 1972 incarnation, though there is some variation. For example, some schools have GTAS working alone, rather than in pairs; a few schools still hire the more passive live pelvic model or "professional patient" to be used in conjunction with an instructing physician. The use of pelvic manikins, anesthetized women, cadavers, and actual patients continues to supplement some student learning.

Beginning in 1988, I was employed as a GTA by the University of Illinois at Chicago (UIC) medical school. Periodically, I also taught at two other Chicago-area medical schools and in one physician's assistant program. Excepting one institution, all my teaching experiences have followed Kretzschmar's GTA model. For the institution that had not adopted Kretzschmar's model, I worked as a "professional patient." A physician or nurse-midwife served as instructor, and I was hired primarily to model the exam for three students and the instructor. Whenever a clinician-instructor was unable to attend, I volunteered to work as both instructor and model, adopting a variation of Kretzschmar's model.

In discussing the GTA, I will collapse the roles of instructor and patient GTA into a single role. While this is reductive of the complexity of the partner relationship assumed by the instructor and patient GTAS, it may help clarify their common mission. And indeed many schools have collapsed the roles of the two GTAS into a single GTA who is paired with three or four students. After years of teaching, I find this to be a better model. It is impossible for students to position the instructor as silent patient if she is the only educator in the room. When there is a single teacher who also serves as "patient" students are faced with the jarring experience of examining a woman who knows more about gynecological exams than they do.

The Teaching Session

The students enter the exam room, where the GTA wears a patient gown. She is both their teacher and the object of their examination. The GTA explains the purpose of the teaching session. She is a healthy woman with normal anatomy who is there to help the students learn how to perform a proper breast and pelvic exam. Medical students, however, have been indoctrinated into a system that privileges pathology. They have learned that what is normal and healthy is not as interesting as what is abnormal and unhealthy. Some students seem disappointed when they are told that the GTA session is one part of their medical education in which they will not be presented with pathology.

The GTA explains that the patient, performed by herself, is there for a yearly exam. She has no complaints. Rather, they are there to have the experience of examining a normal, healthy woman and thus should offer the "patient" feedback after each part of the exam, letting her know that "everything appears healthy and normal." The GTA emphasizes that no woman can hear the phrase "healthy and normal" too much. For many medical students "healthy" and "normal" are new additions to their medical script. Often, these second- and third-year medical students admit that the GTA session is the first time they have been encouraged to use these words. In a moment that struck me as simultaneously encouraging and tragicomic, one student, upon hearing me discuss the phrase "healthy and normal," pulled a 3 × 5 notecard and pen out of his pocket. He then said, "Tell me those words again. I want to write them down so I can remember them." In medical pedagogy, pathology is the norm, and normalcy is often viewed as mundane or unremarkable. For a woman in need of her yearly pap smear, the clinician's preoccupation with pathology can have sad consequences, both adding to the woman's anxiety about the possibility of the clinician finding that something is wrong and leaving her with the feeling that something is wrong regardless of actual clinical findings.

During the GTA session, other aspects of the students' scripts are rewritten and relearned. They are taught to use words that are less sexually connotative or awkward. For example, "I am going to *examine* your breasts now" as opposed to "I'm going to *feel* your breasts now." A number of script adjustments are made: "insert" or "place" the speculum as opposed to "stick in"; "healthy and normal" as opposed to "looks great." Changes are encouraged with regard to tool names: "footrests" as opposed to "stirrups"; "bills" rather than "blades" of the speculum.

When I was working as a "professional patient" with a young white woman physician as instructor, she kept referring to the "blades" of the speculum while teaching the students. I explained to her that many people within the medical community were replacing the term "blades" with "bills" because of the obvious violent connotations of the term, especially given that it refers to that part of the speculum placed inside the woman's body. The physician replied, agitated, "Well, we don't say it to the *patient.*" Her assumption was that words that circulate within the medical community do not affect patient care or physician attitudes toward patients as long as those words do not reach the patient's ears. This is naive and faulty thinking, resistant to change, disabling the idea that language does indeed help structure attitudes and practice.

Furthermore, in that scenario *I* was the patient and the word "blade" was being used to refer to the part of an instrument that was to be placed inside *my* body. My thoughts were largely ignored even though I was hired to perform the role of patient. For the rest of the session, the physician begrudgingly used the word "bills," looking at me and punching the word each time she used it. Weeks later I worked at the same institution with a young white male physician whose language was considerate and carefully chosen and who continually encouraged my feedback and participation within the session. He consistently referred to the "bills" of the speculum of his own accord. By seeking out a patient's opinion and input within both a teaching situation and an actual exam, the clinician is relinquishing a portion of control and offering the patient more power within the exam scenario. As is evident in these two examples, gender does not necessarily determine a clinician's attitudes toward patients or the patient model.

The GTA offers many tips on how the clinician may help the patient feel more powerful and less frightened during an exam. "Talk before touch" is a technique used in the pelvic exam by which the clinician lets the patient know that she or he is about to examine the patient: with the phrase "You'll feel my hand now," the clinician applies the back of her or his hand to the more neutral space of the insides of a patient's thighs. Since the patient cannot *see* where the clinician's hands are, this technique offers her important information about where and when she will be touched.

Eye contact is another important and often ignored part of the pelvic exam. The GTA reminds the student to maintain eye contact with her throughout most parts of the exam. Many women complain that oftentimes clinicians have spoken at their genitals or breasts rather than to them. Eye contact not only offers the clinician another diagnostic tool, since discomfort and pain are often expressed in a patient's face, but it also makes the patient feel as though she is being treated as a person rather than as fragmented parts. In order to facilitate eye contact, the students are taught to raise the table to a 45-degree angle rather than leaving it flat. This has the added benefit of relaxing the woman's abdominal muscles. Specific draping techniques are taught so that the student-clinician cannot hide in front of the drape, ignoring the parts of the woman that reside backstage behind the curtain.

Given that the medical institution routinely segments and dissects bodies for examination, maintaining eye contact with the patient is often difficult for students. Considering the sexual overtones of this particular exam, many students (and practitioners) find it very difficult to meet their patient's gaze. Likewise, there are patients who will not look into their examiner's eyes due to shame or embarrassment or a desire to be "invisible." While this is always a possibility, the GTA asserts that the practitioner must initiate eye contact even if the patient declines the offer, so that the patient at least has a choice of whether to "look back" at the clinician.

Similarly, the GTA encourages students to continuously communicate with the patient, informing her as to what they are doing, how they are doing it, and why they are doing it. For example, the student must show the woman the speculum, holding it high enough so that she can see it (without aiming it at her like a gun), while explaining, "This is a speculum. I will insert this part, the bills, into your vagina, opening them so that I can see your cervix, the neck of your uterus. I do this so that I can take a pap smear, which is a screening test for cervical cancer." Many women have had dozens of pelvic exams without ever having had the opportunity to see a speculum. More often, they hear the clanking of metal as the speculum is snuck out of its drawer and into their vagina.

Clinicians should not use words that patients will not understand, nor should they patronize patients; rather, they should piggyback medical terms with simpler phrases. In addition, students are taught that women should be given verbal instruction when they need to move or undress. For example, the woman should not be handled like a limp doll as a clinician removes her gown for the breast exam; instead the woman should be asked to remove her own gown. This helps her feel a little more in control of her own body and space. Ideally, the pelvic exam can become an educational session and the patient a partner in her own exam.

Lilla Wallis, M.D., an OB/GYN professor at Cornell University Medical School and a strong advocate of the GTA program, promotes this idea of "the patient as partner in the pelvic exam," and in addition encourages the use of many techniques popular within the women's health movement. Wallis adopts what some institutions might consider radical techniques. For instance, she urges clinicians to offer patients a hand mirror so that they might see what is being done to them. The patient is encouraged to look at her own genitals and not feel as though this were a view limited to the practitioner. Wallis also questions the draping of the patient: "This separates the patient from her own body. It suggests that the genitals are a forbidden part of her body that she

should modestly ignore. It also isolates the doctor." Instead, she believes that patients should have the choice of whether to be draped or not. She refers to the use of GTAS as "a quiet revolution" in American medical schools, believing that GTA programs will lead to better, more thoughtful care by physicians.

Is the rehearsal with GTAS enough to change medical attitudes about women, female sexuality, and women's bodies? Can the use of GTAS actually affect these attitudes? While I was working as a "professional patient" or "model" at an esteemed Chicago-area medical school, an interesting sequence of events happened that pointed out to me the vast difference between teaching students as a GTA and serving as a "model." The physician I was to be working with was delayed at a meeting, so I started working with the four medical students. I stressed patient communication, helping the woman relax, "talk before touch," and educating the woman during the exam. The students were responsive, as the vast majority of students are, understanding my explanations for why these techniques were important and making an effort to adopt them as they made their way through the breast and pelvic exam.

I had finished teaching all four students how to do a breast exam and two students had completed pelvic exams, when the physician, a young white man, rushed in, apologizing for being late. He then proceeded to contradict much of what I had taught the students. I argued my points, but he insisted that many women were not interested in explanations or education but just "wanted it to be over with." He taught students a one-handed technique so that only one hand ever got "dirty," leaving the other hand free. He basically ignored my presence, so much so that at one point I had to dislodge his elbow, which was digging into my thigh as he leaned over, bracing himself on me, to see if my cervix was in view. The two remaining students were visibly more nervous than the students who had already had their turns. They were rushed and forgot "talk before touch" in an attempt to incorporate the shortcuts that the physician had taught them.

At the end of the session, he encouraged the students to get into surgery to examine as much pathology as possible: "I have an 18cm uterus I'll be working on. Come by." I pictured this enlarged uterus alone on a surgical table without it's woman-encasement. He assured the students, "The only way you're going to learn what is normal is to see a lot of pathology." I had emphasized the wide variety of what is normal, how vulvas were all different and that students would need to see a lot of normal anatomy to understand what was not normal. After this physician's intrusion, the lone female medical student in the group kept looking at me at each point the physician contradicted me. She smiled at me empathetically, understanding the severity of the emotional and political sabotage I must have been feeling as both an educator and a naked woman "patient." Before the students left, three of the four shook my hand, genuinely thanking me for helping them. The one student who had been resistant to some of the techniques I had taught them was more suspicious. He said to me sternly, "Can I ask you, what are your motivations for doing this?"

The View from the Table

Implicit in the role of the GTA is a fundamental contradiction. On the one hand, she is an educator, more knowledgeable than medical students about pelvic and breast exams although she holds no medical degree. In this sense she is in a position of power, disseminating various truths about the female body and its examination. On the other hand, the GTA is bound to a traditionally vulnerable and powerless lithotomy position: lying on her back, heels in footrests. Oftentimes, her body is viewed as the true learning tool, with her words taking a back seat to this "hands-on" educational experience. In an interview, one GTA expressed her frustration: "Sometimes I feel like it's strange being nice, being like an airline hostess of the body. For example [she points two fingers as stewardesses do at cabin exits], 'Now we're coming to the *mons pubis.*' You have to be nice. I've seen some GTAs who were strong and businesslike about it, and I don't feel comfortable doing that but it's a strain having to be nice." This is a beautiful metaphor for describing the GTA's predicament: She is there to make medical students comfortable as they journey across the female body. Comparing the GTA to an airline hostess highlights the pink-collar service role she performs: she is working for the medical school in a position that only women can fill and she is there to make the students feel less apprehensive and more knowledgeable. The fact that she needs to be "nice" while presenting her own body points to one of the performative aspects of the GTA's role as educator. Like the stewardess, the GTA is costumed with a smile, a well-defined script, and a uniform.

In her book *The Managed Heart: Commercialization of Human Feeling,* Arlie Russell Hochschild connects Marx's factory worker to the flight attendant; both must "mentally detach themselves—the factory worker from his own body and physical labor, and the flight attendant from her own feelings and emotional labor." The case of the GTA becomes an interesting blend of these two types of alienation. She is like the flight attendant in that she manages her own feelings, what the GTA above calls

"being nice." She must learn how to deal with the occasional hostile or overtly sexual medical student customer. She is there to make the student's trip through the female body comfortable, safe, and enjoyable. But it is her own body, not the meal tray or the fuselage of the airplane, that she is presenting to the paying customer. In this sense, the GTA is like Marx's factory laborer who uses his own body. She is getting paid for her body's use-value in the production of a trained medical student.

Structurally, with regard to physical labor and the management of feelings, the GTA resides in a position similar to that of a prostitute. Both GTAs and prostitutes sell the use of their body for what may be loosely termed "educational purposes." Both must manage their feelings, acting the part of willing recipient to probing instruments. Medical school history aside, GTAs and prostitutes have a good deal in common. This is perhaps why numerous GTAs have remarked on their husband's or partner's discomfort with their work. Certainly not all GTAs have partners who consider their teaching to be a sexual act and so object to or are threatened by it. But partner discontent is not uncommon. One GTA explains, "My boyfriend had problems with my teaching when I first moved in with him. It didn't bother him before I was living with him. I moved in only a couple of months before we got married and then he started voicing his complaints . . . I think they [significant others] are afraid it's sexual and I think the students are afraid it's sexual. They're afraid about how they're going to react, whether they're going to be aroused, but it's so clinical." Another GTA present at this interview said she had a similar problem in that her boyfriend was "concerned" and "uneasy": "I said to him if you're going to give me $150 to sit with you or have sex with you or whatever, fine, otherwise I'm going to make my money."

GTAs' partners are not the only ones who have been distressed by the GTA role. Some early women's health activists expressed a different kind of uneasiness as they quickly realized the pink-collar nature of the job. When the GTA program was first starting in the 1970S, these feminist health activists participating in the project sensed that they were still expected to mimic a patriarchal medical performance, employing language, techniques, and attitudes that reinforced the established power differential between pelvic exam clinician and female patient. These groups felt that working for a medical school did not allow them enough autonomy to teach what were, for them, important exam techniques. They believed that change within the medical establishment was virtually impossible and encouraged women not to participate in pelvic teaching within medical schools. Of these GTAs, some simply discontinued their work with medical students. Others continued teaching self-motivated medical students who would voluntarily visit feminist self-help clinics for continuing education. These feminist teachers regarded this new experience as highly valuable. As one activist notes: "The rapport experienced by the program participants and the [feminist teaching] nurses had been astounding . . . The result was an exploration with students of such topics as sexuality, abortion, contraception and ambivalent feelings regarding their roles." After refusing the medical institution's version of a proper pelvic exam rehearsal, these health activists composed their own.

In his article about medical students' six fears of pelvic exams, Buchwald accepted student fears without either questioning why young physicians-to-be would have such fears or searching for the cultural attitudes underlying them. Indeed, he might have been employing a Freudian psychoanalytic model that would entirely justify such fears: faced with the abject, castrated vulva, medical students *would* be terrified by the exam. These feminist teachers who rejected the GTA program, however, confronted and questioned student fears, realizing the importance of helping these future caregivers shed deep anxieties and ambivalences regarding female bodies. For years, medical pedagogues blatantly sidestepped these issues by employing teaching methods that would simply ignore or Band-aid student fears: hiring prostitutes would confirm student ideas regarding promiscuous female sexuality and its relationship to the pelvic exam; the use of plastic manikins would soothe student fears of touching real female genitals; while the use of anesthetized women and cadavers would present an unconscious "model" patient. Only with the use of GTAS have medical schools attempted to incorporate women patients' thoughts, feelings, and ideas into pelvic exam teaching. And yet, as these feminist teachers pointed out decades ago and as my experiences have occasionally confirmed, it may be impossible to educate students properly within the medical institution given unacknowledged cultural attitudes about female bodies and female sexuality.

• • •

The pelvic exam is in itself a pedagogical scenario. The woman receiving the exam, despite the political or philosophical orientation of the clinician, is taught attitudes about female bodies. In this respect, the physician is as much a pedagogue as a healer, if the two roles can be separated. In teaching medical students, one is therefore teaching teachers, transferring knowledge, methods, and attitudes to those practitioners who will in turn conduct private tutorials with individual women who

seek their care. Thus the methods used to teach medical students how to do pelvic exams significantly structure how these physicians-to-be will educate their future patients. The various ways medical students have been taught to do pelvic exams are intimately related to the medical institution's attitudes toward women and in turn structure how future practitioners perceive and treat their women patients.

The use of GTAS alters the normal pelvic scenario to some degree. Here the "doctor" is being educated by the "patient," a potentially powerful role for the GTA. As an educator, she may critique the student from the patient's perspective (e.g., "Use less pressure," "you're not palpating the ovary there"). One would think that the medical student would not argue with the woman who is experiencing the exam. And yet, because the GTA is not a physician, the student is sometimes skeptical of her expertise, doubting her advice even if it is based on her bodily experience. The very fact that her experience is bodily may serve to deny the importance of her role. Her embodiment of the exam makes her a curious and suspect educator in the eyes of many since she is being *paid* for the use of her body in addition to her teaching skills. Her role continually elicits questions about what *kind* of woman she must be to undergo multiple exams.

In the GTA's educational performance there is no hypothetical signified, no abstract female body; rather the GTA is a fleshy referent with her own shape, anatomical variation, and secretions. At the site of the GTA, medicine, pornography, and prostitution mingle, highlighting medical attitudes regarding female sexuality, vulvar display, and genital manipulation. The teaching session may be a "representation" of a "real" exam, but for the GTA, as well as the medical student, it is simultaneously representation *and* practice.

It is curious, but not surprising, that the medical institution has focused so much attention on the GTA's role. Instead of focusing on what *kind* of woman would allow multiple exams to be performed on her, physicians might be more justified in asking how the medical establishment perceives the proper pelvic model or model patient. Or to turn the question back onto the medical institution itself, one might ask what *kind* of man or woman will *give* multiple exams. Unless there is a continued investigation of the medical structures that construct and reflect attitudes about female bodies and sexuality, the answer to this question might indeed be something to really fear.

REFERENCES
A list of references is available in the original source.

"Spreading My Legs for Womankind"

by Molly Kenefick

Ever wonder how doctors learn to do pelvic exams? Well, I can answer that question for more than six hundred medical students: I taught them—on my body.

At some medical schools, students learn to do the exam on cadavers, women under anesthesia, or with "pelvic models" (women who function simply as bodies for professors to demonstrate on). Students on the campuses where I teach learn from "pelvic educators," women who instruct students in anatomy, physiology, palpation techniques, and various emotional and cultural issues that arise in a clinical setting.

When I first heard about the job, it sounded amazing. I'd already been working to overcome negative feelings about my body (the same body-image crap most women internalize growing up in our culture), and this seemed like a good next step. More important, I felt that teaching future doctors to do sensitive, thorough pelvic exams could positively impact the lives of many female patients down the line. I thought of Joan Rivers's joke that there should be a commemorative stamp of a woman on an examining table, feet in the footrests, to honor those who keep their annual appointments. I remember thinking at the time, *Joan is right: Many women do dread the exam. But it shouldn't* have *to be horrible.* Now, years later, I take pride in teaching my students the many details that can make an exam a positive, comforting experience.

I was scared at first. I'd take the hospital gown into the bathroom to change, and then climb onto the table, holding the johnny tight to make sure nothing extra was exposed. I felt shy about opening my legs to strangers (especially without any foreplay!), so as I did this, I avoided looking students in the eyes. I steeled myself by acting nonchalant and businesslike, and held onto the idea that this was important to women. Now, after six years, I simply turn my back to change (yes, in front of students), wrap a sheet around me, and casually hop onto the table.

Working with two to four students at a time, I first go over psychosocial issues. I tell them that though their patient may be an adult, it could be her first exam. I suggest they offer her a hand mirror so she can see what they are doing, and that they explain what they're doing as they do it. We discuss asking questions without making assumptions about a patient's sexual orientation or practices; looking for signs of sexual abuse, and, if they suspect it, how to handle it; words patients use to describe their anatomy; and culturally specific sexual customs.

Then it's time for the physical exam. I undress from the waist down and sit on the exam table, feet in the footrests ("Not stirrups; it's not a saddle"). I teach draping technique ("Expose only the area you will be examining"), the physician's first touch ("Put your hands by the outside of her knees, and ask her to bring her knees to meet your hands—that way she touches you first"), and subsequent touch techniques ("Clinical touch should feel as different from sexual touch as possible"). We start with the external exam, checking beneath the pubic hair for redness, lice, and scabies ("Don't mention lice and scabies unless she has them"). The external exam includes inspecting the vulva, perineum, and anus ("Always avoid touching the clitoris").

The internal exam is next. I teach them to insert an index finger to find my cervix and check my glands for infection and my vaginal walls for laxity. I demonstrate how to put in and open the speculum ("Warm it first, for patient comfort"). Then we view the cervix (a first sighting and a thrill for most students) and practice the Pap smear.

Next, the bimanual exam. With two fingers inside me, a student checks for cervical tenderness and feels for the uterus. The outside hand palpates the abdomen, pushing down toward the inside fingers. The most rewarding part for students is finding an ovary (yet another first), which feels like an almond hidden under layers of pastry dough ("The number of layers depends on how much pastry I've eaten"). Lastly, a student inserts one finger in my rectum, another in my vagina. They are often surprised at how much better they can feel my uterus from two angles.

In separate sessions with students, I also teach breast exams. The first time I did this, I looked at my 38-C breasts (heavy and pendulous: nipples soft, not pert) and wished they were perkier. Then I thought, *Who the hell looks like a centerfold in real life?* I'm a real woman, and this is what women look like. More important, this is what their patients will look like. My self pep talk ended with: *You're healthy. Get over it. Focus on the work.*

With up to eight students, we first practice on a silicone-filled model (with quite lumpy breasts). I show them the palpation technique: Fingers make circles of light, medium, and deep pressure as they move in a vertical stripe pattern (lawnmower versus zigzag). Then I take off my shirt and bra and we look for rashes, dimpling, and changes in the nipples (such as spontaneous discharge or inversion). I teach them to palpate my nodes along the clavicle and under the armpit ("No tickling!"). Then, one at a time, they practice the vertical stripe technique on my breast.

Most students have been a pleasure to teach. A few had terrible palpation skills (I can only hope they've gone into research). Two got noticeable erections (I sympathized, as they seemed mortified at this betrayal of their body). A couple were inappropriate (one kept asking if my parents and boyfriend knew I did this work), and one asked me out (though I thought, *Wouldn't this be a story to tell our grandkids?* I said *no*, of course). The majority of my students, however, have been respectful and grateful for the opportunity to learn from, and on, me.

I'm amazed by all the ways this job has impacted my life. As hoped (and as strange as it may sound), undressing in front of strangers has made me more comfortable with my body. Now, years into the job, I take off my shirt and bra, drop my pants, and often feel like a superhero. I'm not a "perfect 10," just a healthy, strong woman, unashamed of her body. I feel students' admiration and respect, and I deserve it because I am doing important work for women and women's health. In addition, I've become knowledgeable about my reproductive health. Knowing where my uterus is and what my cervix looks like makes me more in touch with being a woman. On the downside, as "party talk" goes, telling people I'm a pelvic educator can be a conversation starter—or stopper. And at times, no amount of kisses could summon my libido because it got lost earlier in the day during the third pelvic exam. In general, however, I've found this to be rewarding work, both because of the immediate positive changes I see in my students and because of the ripple effect I know my work will have on their future patients. Finally, a nice benefit is that every day when I go to work, I'm reminded that *Hey, I've got ovaries.*

 # "Take a Good Look"

by Megan Seely

We don't have to go very far back to find the origins of the modern feminist health movement. In 1971, the Feminist Women's Health Centers were founded by a group of Los Angeles women who wanted to know more about their bodies and their reproductive selves. At a time when pregnancy tests and yeast infection treatments were available only at physicians' offices and when libraries and bookstores were void of women's health books, the Feminist Women's Health Center provided a source of information and a place for women to gather to share experiences about their bodies, health, and lives.[4] They helped women across the country and around the world set up "self-help groups," where women came together to share information, learn from one another, and practice cervical self-exam. Yes, basically a group of women hangin' out and looking at their vaginas—despite the efforts of Eve Ensler to bring vaginas into fashion today, this still may sound a bit weird to people of my generation—but it was a real revelation to women then (and still is today!). The cervical self-exam was a way to gain control of one's body at a time when this domain belonged more to women's doctors and sexual partners. The practice continues to put women in touch with themselves and to assist in their awareness of their bodies—which returns our power to us. The Feminist Women's Health Centers' self-help is about understanding how our bodies work through our eyes; it is about making our bodily knowledge available and legitimate. Perhaps this is the first step in freeing ourselves from dependence on a medical system that does not value us. So, if you haven't done so, grab a mirror, and take a good look.

Vaginal and Cervical Self-Examination

Vaginal and cervical self-examination is one of the most useful health tools a woman can have. It enables us to see a vital part of our anatomy that is hidden from plain view—the vagina and cervix (the neck of the womb). By using a speculum, you can observe changes in your cervix and its secretions, the menstrual cycle, and indications of fertility; you can identify and treat common vaginal conditions such as yeast, trichomonas, or bacterial infections (which often cause itching or discharge); and you can learn what your cervix looks like day by day, rather than depending on a physician to look once a year to pronounce what is normal for you.

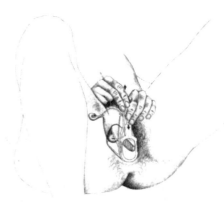

To insert a plastic speculum, spread the inner lips of the clitoris with two fingers of one hand, hold the bills of the speculum tightly together with the thumb and index finger of the other, and guide it into the vaginal canal. You can use a water-soluble jelly or just plain water to make insertion smoother. This woman is inserting her speculum with the handles upright, but some women prefer to insert it sideways initially. Inserting the speculum with the handles down is strictly for the doctor's convenience, and it requires that a woman put her feet into stirrups at the end of an exam table.

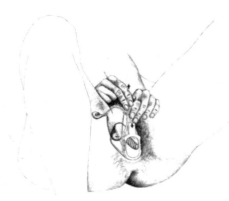

When the handles of the speculum are pinched together, they force the bills open, stretching the vaginal walls and revealing the cervix. With the handles held tightly together, the short handle slides down and the long handle slides up. When there is a sharp click the speculum is locked into place.

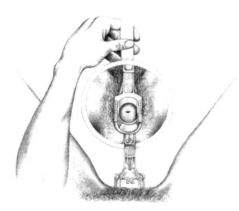

With the speculum locked, both hands are free to hold a mirror and a flashlight or gooseneck lamp. If a flashlight is used, shine the beam into the mirror, and it will, in turn, be reflected into the vagina, illuminating the vaginal walls and the cervix. The cervix won't always pop instantly into view. Sometimes you have to try several times. If it stubbornly refuses to appear, you can move around or jump up and down a few times. Sometimes it is also helpful to move to a firmer surface, like the floor or a tabletop. When the cervix is visible, you can see a rounded or flattened knob, between the size of a quarter and a fifty-cent piece, like a fat doughnut with a hole or slit in it. The hole, called the cervical os, is where the menstrual blood, other uterine secretions, and babies come out. Your cervix might be pink and smooth, or it might have a few reddish blemishes. It can also be uneven, rough, or splotchy. In any case, the only time to worry is when abnormal cells are found in a Pap smear.

*Material adapted from *A New View of A Woman's Body*, Federation of Feminist Women's Health Centers, Feminist Health Press, Los Angeles, CA. Suzann Gage created these beautiful illustrations, pp. 22–24. Reprinted with permission.

Beyond getting to know one's own vagina, a women-centered health agenda might also start at the beginning of our young lives and recognize the different ways that we are treated and taught to understand our own bodies. Little boys are often encouraged to be baseball players; little girls are encouraged to be fairy princesses. Little boys are encouraged to use their bodies in physical ways, whereas little girls are encouraged to dress their bodies in different clothes. When a little boy gets dirty, some say, "that's just a boy being a boy," but when a little girl does the same, she is a "tomboy" or "not acting like a nice little girl." While some of these tendencies may be biological, there is no doubting that society encourages these stereotypes. (Some might even say that this is how patriarchy continues itself.) Thankfully, there are now soccer leagues for both boys and girls, but there is still no doubting that there are many more athletic opportunities for boys than for girls and that, overall, boys are encouraged to be more physical and athletic than girls.

These bodily differences all but erupt at puberty. From the start, we are divided in gender-specific groups to see separate films about our changing bodies. Many of us struggle to pay attention during the coming-of-age video that highlights young girls that we barely recognize, while our curiosity wonders what the boys are learning about us—from someone else. We are both envious and fearful of the girls who begin menstruation before us—wanting to both be them and avoid the situation altogether. Very little if anything is shared ahead of time—as with most of our "education," we swap stories with our friends, trying to sort out this mess called *womanhood*. And then . . . the day—the day we see blood. We are indoctrinated into this new club, but usually with very little celebration. And our modern ritual begins—pads versus tampons, Midol versus heating pad—we learn the tortures of "the curse." We are bombarded with messages of fear—fear of someone knowing, fear of odor, fear of bloating, fear of leakage, fear of staining, fear of pain, fear, fear, fear. We are told that we need protection—but from what? Ourselves, our menstruating selves. The Solution: Deodorize, minimize, and hide the fact that we are women. Though this "secret" of womanhood is something that only women share as a rite of passage and though it may give us a certain sense of bonding (though the bonding over an "emergency" tampon gets you only so far), ultimately, this is a shameful secret to be kept, even from other women, in public.

Even if we may want to, it is no wonder that we don't embrace and celebrate our femaleness; the messages that we should be ashamed are too strong.

We usually learn that menstruation and our cyclic bodily functions are disgusting. Just as quickly, we learn to judge these bodies harshly, and from another's point of view. As Emily Martin writes in *The Woman in the Body: A Cultural Analysis of Reproduction*,

> [b]ut because women are aware that in our general cultural view menstruation is dirty, they are still stuck with the "hassle": most centrally no one must ever see you dealing with the mechanics of keeping up with the disgusting mess, and you must never fail to keep the disgusting mess from showing on your clothes, furniture, or the floor.[5]

As a result, I argue that we gradually become disconnected from our bodies, particularly female bodies. And it is also no wonder that we are so disconnected—between the lack of adequate education and the widely endorsed negative attitudes about our bodies, our menstruation, and our sexuality—women learn early on to ignore, underemphasize, or keep quiet about the functions of our bodies. As Martin writes, ultimately, women are taught to see bodily functions such as menstruation, birth, and menopause as happening to them; they become an object to be dealt with and manipulated by the medical field.[6]

If we are to create a women-centered health agenda, we must recognize and appreciate the differentness of our bodies, perhaps even celebrate our female bodies. In addition to the Feminist Women's Health Centers, organizations like the Boston Women's Health Collective and the National Women's Health Network advocate for women's health so that we may have research that represents us and information that is accessible and comprehensible. Organizations like Good Vibrations and Babes in Toyland offer women a positive image and support for our sexuality. Authors like Christiane Northrup, Inga Muscio, Laura Owen, Geneen Roth, Eve Ensler, Laura Fraser, and Marilyn Wann encourage us to embrace and celebrate our bodies. It is from each of these that we find resources and support for a women-centered approach to our health and wellness. Or, as Eve Ensler has said, "I love the word *vagina*."

REFERENCES
A list of references is available in the original source.

The Women's Health Movement in the United States "From Grass-Roots Activism to Professional Agendas"

by Sheryl Burt Ruzek and Julie Becker

The grass-roots women's health movement grew rapidly during the 1970s and 1980s, but contracted by the end of that decade. Surviving organizations must now negotiate roles and relationships with newer women's health organizations that burgeoned in the 1990s and that are typically professionalized and disease specific. They differ from grass-roots groups through: 1) their relationships to broader movements for social change; 2) leadership; 3) attitudes toward biomedicine; 4) relationships to corporate sponsors; 5) educational goals; and 6) lay versus professional authority. There is little overlap between women's health advocacy organizations identified by the National Women's Health Network and two Internet search engines. The proliferation of newer organizations dilutes the role of grass-roots groups as information brokers for women in the United States and raises questions about who will speak for women in the electronic age. (*JAMWA*. 1999;54:4–8)

Women's health activists have generated public debate and spearheaded social action in a number of waves throughout US history, waves that Carol Weisman views as part of a women's health "megamovement" that has spanned two centuries. The US women's health movement grew rapidly through the 1970s; broadened its base with women of color and others in the early 1980s; and contracted, was co-opted, and became institutionalized during the late 1980s and 1990s. Surviving grass-roots organizations are now negotiating roles and relationships with newer, more professional women's health support and advocacy organizations. While both older and newer women's health organizations seek improvements in women's healthcare, their focus and priorities vary.

In this article, we analyze the historical development of the grass-roots women's health movement in the United States, note key contributions, and differentiate surviving movement organizations from the newer, professionalized women's health advocacy groups. Distinguishing between grass-roots and more professional women's health groups becomes particularly important as we move into the global "information age." Because public trust of mainstream medical institutions is eroding, as evidenced by the growth of alternative and complementary medical practices and the increasing distrust of managed care organizations, both grass-roots and professionalized health advocacy groups are likely to play key roles in defining the quality and trustworthiness of health information. Growing calls for accountability and improved patient satisfaction create windows of opportunity for health advocates to use their influence and authority to shape how the quality of health information and services will be defined.

Social Movements and Social Change

The women's health movement's very success makes differentiating surviving grass-roots movement organizations from professionalized ones that are historically, ideologically, and strategically aligned with this episode of activism particularly challenging. For conceptual clarity, it is important to note that social scientists have long distinguished between general social movements and specific social movements. Theorists of social movements are particularly careful to differentiate between grass-roots movements and professionalized movements that emerge from within established institutions. General social movements affect the public's consciousness of many issues and bring about social change in many arenas. The general feminist movement of the 1960s and 1970s spawned dozens of specific movements and hundreds of movement organizations. As specific social movements gain momentum, they, like general social movements, shape public consciousness beyond the smaller world of movement organizations.

It is also crucial not to confuse formally constituted movement organizations with social movements themselves, although these groups represent the active components of a movement. As health activists differentiated themselves within the broader feminist movement and developed an identity as a specific grass-roots feminist movement, they founded organizations such as the Boston Women's Health Book Collective, the Federation of Feminist Women's Health Centers, DES Action, and the National Women's Health Network.

Rise and Development of the Women's Health Movement

More than three decades ago, when access to medical information was restricted almost exclusively to physicians (who were mostly men), laywomen's insistence on access to medical research was truly "revolutionary." Few books on women's health could be found in bookstores, except for books on childbirth. The assumption was simply that physicians were the experts and women were to do as instructed. Breaking open this closed system, laywomen asserted that personal, subjective knowledge of one's own body was a valid source of information and deserved recognition, not scorn.

The women's health movement grew rapidly through the leadership of several grass-roots groups with strong ties to other social change movements, particularly the abortion rights, prepared childbirth, and consumer health movements. As the general feminist movement of the 1960s and 1970s sought equal rights and the full participation of women in all public spheres, many believed that without control over reproduction, all other rights were in jeopardy. Thus in the early years, reproductive issues defined many branches of the movement and shaped group consciousness and social action. Reproductive rights remain central to feminist health agendas worldwide.

Feminist health writers such as Barbara Seaman, Barbara Ehrenreich and Deirdre English, Ellen Frankfort, Gena Corea, Claudia Dreifus, and columnists for prominent feminist newspapers galvanized women to explore their own health, providing critical momentum for the emerging grass-roots movement. The Boston Women's Health Book Collective produced the enormously popular *Our Bodies, Ourselves,* which has gone through numerous US and many other language editions world-

wide. The Federation of Feminist Women's Health Centers "invented" and championed gynecological self-help and woman-centered reproductive health services. The National Women's Health Network (NWHN) linked a wide array of local groups to provide a voice for women in Washington. Monitoring legislation, Food and Drug Administration actions, and informing the public about women's health issues continue to be central to this organization's mission. A few nationally prominent groups focused on specific diseases or conditions (eg, DES Action, the Endometriosis Association). Members of pivotal groups and other health activists traveled, spoke, and published widely, and used contacts with the media effectively, becoming spokespeople for the rapidly growing movement.

An important achievement of the women's health movement was transferring women's health from the domain of largely male experts to women themselves. Developing in parallel with self-help medical care movements, consciousness-raising and gynecological self-help became strategies for empowering women to define their own health and create alternative services. Local movement groups in all 50 states were providing gynecological self-help, women-controlled reproductive health clinics, clearinghouses for health information, and referral services and producing their own health educational materials. Advocacy ranged from accompanying individual women seeking medical care to advising and influencing state and local health departments. By the mid-1970s, more than 250 formally identifiable groups provided education, advocacy, and direct service in the United States. Nearly 2,000 informal self-help groups and projects provided additional momentum to the movement (B. Seaman, unpublished data, 1998). Although ideologically committed to being inclusive, the leadership of the women's health movement remained largely white and middle class in North America during the early years. Sterilization abuse mobilized women of color to seek government protection during the 1970s, and groups such as the Committee to End Sterilization Abuse (CESA) were founded.

The women's health movement grew increasingly visible globally, with groups such as ISIS in Geneva creating opportunities for worldwide feminist health activism. By the mid-1970s, there were more than 70 feminist health groups in Canada, Europe, and Australia. Today, there are growing efforts to make connections with feminist health activists worldwide, both in industrialized and developing countries.

As the women's health movement evolved in the United States, the distinct health needs of diverse women emerged, and women of color formed their own movement organizations such as the National Black Women's Health Project, the National Latina Women's Health Organization, the Native American Women's Health Education and Resource Center, and the National Asian Women's Health Organization. Women of color health organizations gained national recognition and developed agendas to protect women against racist sterilization and contraceptive practices; to widen access to medical care for low-income women, including abortions no longer covered by Medicaid; and to focus on diseases and conditions affecting women of color such as lupus, fetal alcohol syndrome, hypertension, obesity, drug addiction, and stress related to racism and poverty that were ignored or misunderstood by largely white movement groups. By the late 1980s, the National Black Women's Health Project had established local chapters with more than 150 self-help groups for African-American women.

Other women added distinct health agendas. Lesbians, rural women, and women with disabilities joined older women's groups and women with specific health concerns to direct attention to their particular needs. Groups such as the Dis-Abled Women's Network, the Older Women's League, and the Lesbian Health Agenda broadened constituencies and issues. With the rise of environmental health concerns, groups such as the Women's Environmental Development Organization (WEDO) built bridges between feminist health activism and other movements for social change.

Like other social movements, the women's health movement has gone through periods of emergence, rapid growth, decline, and institutionalization. Grass-roots feminist health organizations declined in the 1980s, apparently as a result of changes in movement adherents and the social context in which movement groups operated. For example, many founders of movement organizations returned to school, began families, or entered the paid labor force, as have the next generation of women who increasingly juggle careers and families, thus reducing the traditional volunteer labor pool. Much of organized feminism as it evolved both in media imagery and academe, came to be seen as distant or disconnected from ordinary women's lives. The success of single-issue groups, particularly acquired immune deficiency syndrome (AIDS) organizations, to secure funding for direct services, education, and research presented new models for health activism. And the discovery of mainstream health institutions that "marketing to women" could increase profits led to the designation of a wide array of clinical services as "women's health clinics." By the 1990s, women's health services were widespread, although most were now part of larger medical institutions. In a recent national survey of women's health ser-

vices, most centers founded in the 1960s and 1970s claimed a commitment to a feminist ideology; those founded later or sponsored by hospitals were significantly less likely to report this commitment.

By the end of the 1980s, most alternative feminist health clinics had ceased to exist, and the survivors had broadened their range of services and affiliated with larger health systems. Gynecological self-help has virtually disappeared. The surviving grass-roots movement advocacy and education groups such as the NWHN face declining support from both individuals and foundations as they compete with newer organizations for members and resources. Thus, grass-roots groups contracted internally as they were diluted externally by the growing prominence of both mainstream women's support groups (on a wide array of health issues ranging from alcohol problems to breast cancer) and disease-focused health advocacy groups whose efforts supported the growing federal initiatives for greater equity in women's health research (S.B. Ruzek, unpublished data, 1998).

From Grass-Roots Ideologies to Professional Institutional Agendas

The success of the women's health movement is reflected in the extent to which mainstream organizations and institutions, particularly federal agencies, have incorporated or adopted core ideas and created new opportunities for women's health advocates. By the 1990s, the reform wings of feminism had made significant claims for gender equity in all social institutions. With a growing number of women in Congress, in the biomedical professions, and in health advocacy communities, organizations that had pursued very different paths to improving women's health coalesced around the 1989 General Accounting Office (GAO) report showing that the National Institutes of Health (NIH) had failed to implement its policy of including women in study populations. The GAO report proved to be a catalyst for pressuring Congress and the NIH to take action, and by the end of 1990, the Women's Health Equity Act was passed, and the NIH established the Office of Research on Women's Health. In 1991, the NIH undertook the Women's Health Initiative, the largest project of its kind, seeking data on prevention and treatment of cancer, cardiovascular disease, and osteoporosis. Although grass-roots women's health groups have criticized many aspects of the research and have attempted to rectify perceived problems in consent procedures and inclusion criteria, they have largely supported greater federal funding of biomedical research into women's health. Thus the women's health movement critique of biomedicine and the call for demedicalizing women's healthcare was reframed into a bipartisan agenda for equity. Scientific and professional interest in women's health burgeoned in the early 1990s. Spurred by growing federal investment in women's health and by the "cold-war dividend" funding of women's research through the Department of Defense, health activists saw opportunities to collaborate with scientists and professionals who were eager to take advantage of these new research priorities.

To maximize the likelihood of obtaining federal funding for research on women's health, scientists and their consumer allies focused on specific diseases. This narrowing of focus was critical for navigating federal funding streams that are tied to specific diseases and organ systems. The new "disease-oriented" organizations reflect the interests of women who expect a high level of professionalism. Facing dual roles as workers outside the home and traditional caretakers inside the home, the highly educated women who support the new single-issue groups may find that their interests lie in organizations that dispense professionally endorsed information, solicit donations, and carry out advocacy efforts on behalf of women. Thus the success of women's entry into the labor force, changes in cultural ethos, and women's own commitment to specialization and professionalism may explain why the narrower, highly professionalized women's health equity organizations attract women who do not identify either with broader movements for social change or with feminism per se.

AIDS advocacy groups also raised a new standard of effectiveness for health activists. They not only successfully increased funding for education and research, but gained a voice in how these added appropriations from government and foundations would be spent. Thereafter, breast cancer advocates and others (ovarian cancer advocates, Parkinson patients and their families, etc.) adopted many of the AIDS organizations' strategies, albeit with a more professional and less confrontational style. A growing willingness to own illness and become "poster people" for cancer, as people with AIDS have done effectively, put a face on diseases that women privately and pervasively feared. Creating strong alliances between consumers, medical professionals, and researchers, breast cancer advocates rallied behind a specific cause that affected many of them directly or through family and friends. Many local support and advocacy organizations joined larger, well-funded organizations such as the National Breast Cancer Coalition, leaving behind older-style support groups and feminist health organizations with broader agendas.

Using well-established letter-writing and advocacy strategies, breast cancer activists testified at hearings, held press conferences, and took their case to the NIH. In collaboration with growing bipartisan support in Congress and the scientific community, advocates succeeded in increasing federal funding for breast cancer research from $84 million to more than $400 million in 1993. Breast cancer advocates also insisted that survivors be involved in shaping research agendas and educational efforts and aligned themselves more consistently and collaboratively with scientists than some AIDS activists or earlier grass-roots movement leaders had.

The success of breast cancer advocacy quickly created a "disease du jour" climate, where professionals rallied people directly or indirectly affected by particular diseases to lobby for increased funding. Ovarian cancer was the next women's disease to achieve national prominence. While this approach secures more resources for particular groups in the short run, it pits diseases against each other, turning research funding into a "popularity contest" or war of each against all—to be won by the group that can make the most noise or wield the greatest political pressure. A result may be overfunding some diseases without regard for their prevalence, contribution to overall population health, or likelihood of scientific value. In this environment, orphan diseases will join orphan drugs as the unfortunate, but unavoidable downsides of market-driven research and medicine.

Differences of Grass-Roots and Professionalized Women's Health Organizations

In a market-focused society, identifying differences is important for establishing a niche, and like other organizations, movement groups emphasize their unique features. Grass-roots women's health movement groups see themselves as different from what they perceive the more professional, mainstream organizations to be, although these differences are not always clearly articulated. After observing a wide range of groups for three decades, we have found that surviving grass-roots advocacy groups are differentiated from most professionalized, disease-focused groups in the following six ways.

Social Movement Orientation   The founders of many grass-roots feminist groups had ties to progressive or radical social movements that emphasized social justice and social change, to which many remain committed. In contrast, the newer professionalized support and advocacy organizations are typically more narrowly focused on a single disease or health issue, and except for environmentally focused groups such as WEDO, few are integral to broader social movements for social change (although some individual members may have such commitments).

Leadership Although some women physicians who were critical of medical education, training, and practice were leaders of the grass-roots women's health movement, lay leadership was the norm. The role of physicians relative to others remains a point of contention. In contrast, the professionalized support and advocacy groups formed in the 1990s had a growing pool of women physicians, scientists, and other highly trained professionals to turn to for leadership.

Attitude toward Biomedicine A recurring theme in the grass-roots women's health movement has been the demand for "evidence-based medicine," long before this term came into vogue. Major feminist advocacy groups aligned themselves with scientists and physicians who sought to put medical practice on a more scientific basis at a time when it was resisted by many clinicians. Grass-roots health activists were critical of the side effects of inadequately tested drugs and devices, particularly early high-dose oral contraceptives, diethylstilbestrol, and the intrauterine device. They also questioned the number of unnecessary hysterectomies and radical mastectomies performed. In short, consumer groups sought to protect women from unsafe or unnecessary biomedical interventions. The professionalized advocacy groups founded in the 1990s focus more on ensuring women an equitable share of biopsychosocial science and treatment. The growing number of women physicians and scientists also facilitates alliances with women consumers because perceived interests in safety and effectiveness make these relationships seem mutually beneficial.

Relationships with Corporate Sponsors Older grass-roots advocacy groups remain deeply concerned about the effects of drug and device manufacturers sponsoring journals and organizational activities. In fact, this issue is a pivotal source of strain between grass-roots groups and professionalized women's health organizations. While organizations of women physicians and professionalized advocacy groups rely heavily on corporate sponsorships, older grass-roots groups avoid such relationships on grounds that financial ties affect the willingness of groups to criticize sponsors, promote competitors' products, or address alternative or complementary therapies that might undermine conventional prescribing patterns. Refusing support from corporate sponsors remains a hallmark of grass-roots movement

groups, but they struggle financially as a result. Because professionalized groups accept corporate support, they have more resources for education and advocacy.

Goals of Education Both older and newer women's health organizations share the goal of educating women to improve their own health and make decisions about their own care. A central feature of grass-roots feminst groups, particularly through the 1970s was to demystify medicine and to encourage women to trust their subjective experience of their own health. Having access to larger numbers of women physicians may have reduced the perceived need to demystify medicine, and professionalized organizations appear largely concerned with making their highly educated constituencies aware of medical and scientific information.

Lay versus Professional Authority Grass-roots health groups remain committed to substantial lay control over health and healing and to expanding the roles of such nonphysician healers as midwives, nurses, and counseling professionals. They would involve consumers in all aspects of health policy making, not simply transfer legitimate authority from male to female physicians. In professionalized organizations, women physicians become the primary societal experts on women's health matters.

The grass-roots women's health movement organizations leave a legacy of making health an important social concern and educating women to take responsibility for their own health and healthcare decision making. The movement as a whole has made substantial efforts to influence powerful social institutions—organized medicine, the pharmaceutical industry, and regulatory agencies. In partnership with newer, professionalized equity organizations, health movement activists have taken up mainstream reform efforts that will become increasingly important as medical care is dominated by market forces. Thus the current episode of women's health activism overlaps with, but is, in many ways, different from the activism of the 1960s and 1970s. These distinct episodes of women's health activism need to be differentiated and understood in the specific historical contexts in which they emerged, recognizing the distinct roles that their history may lead them to play in the future.

The Next Challenge: Who Will Speak for Women in the Electronic Age?

The electronic communication technologies foster a climate in which researchers and consumers expect to find information instantaneously and effortlessly. The reliability of information in electronic media is often questionable, however. Until data can be transformed into usable knowledge that can shape human action, the information age will not fulfill its promise. Neither grass-roots women's health movement organizations nor newer professionalized disease agenda groups have adequately grappled with how to communicate with their constituencies effectively. Both types of groups as well as government and mainstream health organizations will have to assess, manage, and distribute what each sees as "reliable" health information. Organizational survival may depend increasingly on teaching both "customers" and staff how to use reliable information effectively.

Because of the role of advocacy groups in health policy making in the United States, how they present themselves and are perceived are important. As electronic media provide all-comers the opportunity to claim organizational status in an increasingly "virtual" world, and the number of groups claiming to speak for women increases, how will the public differentiate among them? As we navigate the uncharted "information age," the ability of the grass-roots women's health movement to remain viable appears somewhat precarious because the technology allows anyone with a computer and minimal skill to "create" an organization with worldwide visibility. Most movement organizations have not moved beyond hard copy resource centers and clearinghouses, in part because they have well-established communication networks that have served them well in the past (S.B. Ruzek, J. Becker, unpublished data, 1998). Newer professionalized advocacy groups are better funded and more attuned to technological advancements. As electronic communications gain prominence, those who position themselves in this media will be perceived as speaking for women. In an effort to address the complexity of electronic media, the Boston Women's Health Book Collective is including a section on how to assess the adequacy of electronic sources of information in the 1998 edition of *Our Bodies, Ourselves.*

To assess the complexity of the environment in which grass-roots activist groups find themselves at the close of this century, and to determine the array of groups that present themselves as speaking for women, we compared the number of national women's health advocacy organizations easily identified through two worldwide web search strategies with those identified by the National Women's Health Network in 1994 as meeting their criteria: national, women-controlled or a women-controlled

project of a larger organization, feminist outlook, mostly consumer controlled, and primarily advocacy, not just engaged in service or education. In an effort to identify organizations that might easily be identified by the public, Yahoo, a common Internet search engine, was used along with Healthfinders, the electronic database that the Department of Health and Human Services unveiled for public use in May 1997. Using the term "women's health organizations," 339 groups were located on the two Internet sources. After coding them for meeting two of the five NWHN criteria (being national and having an advocacy agenda beyond service or education), and removing duplications, 223 women's health advocacy organizations were identified, 46 by the NWHN, 53 by Healthfinders, and 124 by Yahoo.

When we cross-tabulated the data, it became clear that there is little overlap in the women's health advocacy organizations identified by these three sources. Only the Society for the Advancement of Women's Health Research was identified by all three. Six organizations were identified by both the NWHN and DHHS Healthfinders; 9 were identified by both DHHS and Yahoo; and 13 were identified by both NWHN and Yahoo. Thus, "who speaks for women's health" in the electronic age very much depends on where one looks—and how willing one is to sort through hundreds of self-characterized "women's health organizations." In this environment it is unclear how the women's health movement will continue to be perceived as a key information broker in an increasingly complex sea of women's health information.

Grass-roots health movement groups remain important forces for increasing awareness of women's health issues and are viewed as trustworthy sources of information by feminist groups in the United States and worldwide. Newer, professionalized equity organizations, too, face competition from a growing array of institutions that claim expertise in matters of women's health. The challenge for both types of women's health groups will be to differentiate themselves from others whose interests lie more in marketing than in meeting diverse women's health needs. Both types of groups need to be allies for widening access and equity in healthcare for all women, not just some women, in the next century.

REFERENCES
A list of references is available in the original source.

 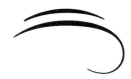

"Women's Health Events of the 20th Century"

by Office on Women's Health, U.S. Department of Health and Human Services

1906– The Food and Drug Administration Established: This agency is established by the Pure Food and Drug Act to regulate the safety of foods and medicines, giving women new support in protecting themselves and their families.

1908– Protecting Working Women and Children: The Supreme Court upholds the right of states to ensure the safety of working women and children who had not been included in labor union protection in *Muller vs. Oregon.*

1912– The Federal Children's Bureau Established: One of its first tasks was to write and distribute two public health pamphlets directed at women consumers: Prenatal Care and Infant Care. By century's end, women were able to access health information through thousands of self-help books, Internet web sites, and government publications.

1913– The First Public Discussion of the Word Cancer: A Ladies' Home Journal magazine article entitled "What Can We Do About Cancer?" was published. The American Society for the Control of Cancer was formed that same year.

1915– Radical Mastectomy Proven Effective for Breast Cancer: This disfiguring surgery, developed by Dr. William Halstead, became the standard of care for women with breast cancer.

1916– First Birth Control Clinic Opens: Margaret Sanger and her sister Ethyl Byrne opened a birth control clinic in Brooklyn, New York. The authorities shut it down ten days later under the Comstock Law. In those ten days, nearly 500 women came in for help and advice on contraception. The Comstock Law, passed in 1873, defined information on birth control and contraception as obscene and outlawed its distribution.

1921– The Sheppard-Towner Act: This law provided federal funding (with matching state funds) to reduce maternal and infant mortality. It was fiercely opposed by the American Medical Association (AMA), and some members of Congress as too socialistic. Some of the influential pediatricians in the AMA who were in favor of the bill broke off from the organization and created the American Academy of Pediatrics. The law was allowed to lapse in 1929.

1929– Selling Mrs. Consumer Published: This popular book was written by a female home economics and marketing expert, and highlighted women's roles as the primary household consumers.

1933– Sodium Pentathol Introduced as Anesthesia for Childbirth: This drug replaced opiates and other sedatives that had a longer lasting effect on mother and baby, and meant that more women could have pain relief during labor and delivery.

1935– Title V of the Social Security Act: This maternal and child health legislation authorized grants-in-aid to states to fund maternal, infant, and child health programs, including services for crippled children.

1935– Cure Found for "Childbed" Fever: Sulfanomides were introduced as a cure for puerperal fever,

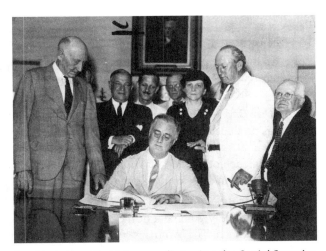

President Franklin D. Roosevelt signing the Social Security Act of 1935. Also shown from left to right: Representative Robert Doughton (D-NC); Senator Robert Wagner (D-NY); Representative John Dingell, Sr. (D-MI); Unknown man in bowtie; Secretary of Labor Frances Perkins; Senator Pat Harrison (D-MS); Congressman David L. Lewis (D-MD). Photo courtesy of the Library of Congress.

Source: *A Century of Women's Health: 1900–2000* by the U.S. Department of Health and Human Services, Office on Women's Health, 2002.

contracted from unsterile conditions during childbirth and a leading cause of maternal death.

1936– *U.S. vs. One Package:* Margaret Sanger and the National Committee for Federal Legislation on Birth Control won a judicial decision (*U.S. vs. One Package*) that exempted doctors from the Comstock Law restrictions on dissemination of contraceptive information.

1938– The Food and Drug Administration's Authority Broadened: The agency was given authority to regulate cosmetics and medical devices.

1942– Planned Parenthood Named: The American Birth Control League changed its name to Planned Parenthood, over the objections of its founder, Margaret Sanger. Planned Parenthood was believed to be a more acceptable name to mainstream America.

1943– Emergency Maternity and Infant Care Program: This program provided free and complete maternity care to the wives and infants of men serving in the four lowest grades of the military during World War II. The program ended in 1949.

1950– The American Cancer Society Begins Promotion of Breast Self-exam: There is still no scientific proof by century's end, that it actually improves breast cancer survival rate.

1953– The Kinsey Report Published: Sexual Behavior in the Human Female was published by researcher Michael Kinsey, as a companion to the 1948 Report, Sexual Behavior in the Human Male. More than 5,500 interviews with women showed that many enjoyed having a sexual life. This provoked widespread controversy, and altered the perception of women's sexuality. Later analyses have questioned much of Kinsey's methodology.

1956– La Leche League Formed: This group was started by seven mothers to promote breastfeeding after it fell out of fashion in the 1920s. It was not until the year 2001 that the U.S. Department of Health and Human Services released its first policy promoting breastfeeding, calling it the best source of infant nutrition.

1956– Dependents Medical Care Act: This program provided Government-sponsored health insurance (CHAMPUS) for the dependents of members of the Armed Forces.

1959– The Barbie Doll Created: This was the first popular doll to be shaped like a woman, with an impossible-to-attain figure. Little girls everywhere loved the doll, but critics claimed it encouraged girls to adopt unhealthy habits to stay unreasonably thin, and set an unrealistic standard of beauty for decades to come.

1960– The FDA Approves the Birth Control Pill: The Pill gave women unprecedented reproductive freedom. The controversy over its approval eventually led to the first package insert that explained the risks and benefits of a medication. By the year 2000, it was still one of the most popular forms of birth control.

1961– Worldwide Alert on Thalidomide: The efforts of a woman scientist, Frances Kelsey, M.D., Ph.D., led the FDA not to approve thalidomide for use in the U.S., saving countless numbers of babies from the severe deformities seen among babies in Europe. Worldwide alarm led to legislation in the United States in 1962 that gave the FDA new authority to require that drugs must be shown to be effective prior to approval, and also required manufacturers to report unexpected harm (adverse events).

1965– Birth Control Made Legal for Married Couples: In *Griswold vs. Connecticut,* the Supreme Court overturned one of the last state laws to prohibit the use of contraceptives by married couples.

1965– Medicaid and Medicare: Medicare was created as a national program to provide federal coverage for health services to individuals aged 65 and over, a population that was disproportionately female. Medicaid was passed as part of President Lyndon Johnson's War on Poverty and provided medical assistance to poor families with dependent children, low-income elderly, the blind, and people with disabilities. It was designed to be administered by each of the 50 states.

1965– Family Planning Funds: As part of the War on Poverty, the Office of Economic Opportunity made available federal funding for family planning for low-income women.

1970– *Our Bodies, Ourselves* Published: This popular book was produced by the Boston Women's Health Book Collective. It was written by women (not medically trained) to teach other women about their bodies, and it encouraged them to be critical healthcare consumers.

1970– Medical Schools Sued for Gender Discrimination: In 1965, only 7 percent of medical students in the U.S. were women. The Women's Equity Action League sued most medical schools in the nation to correct this inequity. By the late 1990's nearly half of medical students were women. Still, by the end of the century, only eight U.S. medical schools were headed by women deans.

1970– Title X Family Planning Funding: This law established a federally-funded program nationwide to provide family planning services to low-income women.

1971– The National Cancer Act Passed: This law, signed by President Richard M. Nixon, greatly expanded funding for cancer research.

1972– Title IX Revolutionizes Athletics for Women: Title IX of the Education Amendments of 1972 prohibited sex discrimination in all educational programs receiving federal funding.

1973– *Roe vs. Wade:* While a woman's right to abortion is not explicitly found in the Constitution, and while the practice of abortion was opposed by many Americans, the U.S. Supreme Court held in this landmark case that limiting a woman's right to terminate her pregnancy violated the Due Process clause of the 14th Amendment.

1974– The Food and Drug Administration Outlaws the Dalkon Shield: This brand of intrauterine device was ruled to be unsafe due to increased complications with pregnancies and a higher risk of pelvic inflammatory disease.

1975– National Women's Health Network: This organization was founded to give women a voice in the U.S. healthcare system.

1976– Hyde Amendment: This amendment banned the use of Medicaid funds for abortion services, unless a woman's life was in danger. The law was broadened in 1994 to allow Medicaid coverage for abortion in cases of rape or incest.

1978– Pregnancy Discrimination Act: This law prohibited sex discrimination in employment on the basis of pregnancy, childbirth, or related medical conditions.

1979– Patricia Harris, an African American, Is Appointed as the First Female Secretary of Health, Education, and Welfare: Later that year, Congress established a separate Department of Education and Harris' department became the Department of Health and Human Services. Harris was a professor at Howard University Law School and a businesswoman before her appointment.

1980– Surgeon General's Report on Women and Smoking: This report documented the growing number of women smokers and warned that if the trend was not reversed, smoking related diseases in women will reach epidemic proportions. By century's end, the prophecy was realized. A new Surgeon General's Report on Women and Smoking, written in 2000, revealed that since the release of the 1980 report, three million women had died prematurely from smoking related illnesses.

1981– National Black Women's Health Project: This organization was established by Byllye Avery to improve the health of Black women by providing wellness education and services, health information, and advocacy.

1981– Maternal and Child Health Services Block Grants: This law consolidated programs for maternal, infant, child, and adolescent health at the State level, and transferred funding directly to the states in a block-grant format.

1983– The Public Health Service's Task Force on Women's Health Established: This task force signified a new level of federal commitment to women's health issues.

1983– The Komen Race for the Cure Is Established: The Race for the Cure was established by Susan Goodman Komen to raise money for breast cancer research, education, screening and treatment programs. The five-kilometer race began as a single event in Dallas, Texas, and by century's end became a series of more than a hundred races in the U.S. and around the world, with 69,000 runners and walkers, raising three million dollars annually.

1983– Margaret Mary Heckler Is Named the First Secretary of the Department of Health and Human Services: She served 16 years in the United States House of Representatives as a Republican from Massachusetts. As Secretary, Heckler introduced a system of set rates for Medicare payments to hospitals. She also helped to win Congressional approval of a law that helped ensure payment of court-ordered child support.

1985– Lumpectomy Declared as Effective Breast Cancer Treatment: Studies were released that showed lump removal combined with radiation therapy was as effective a treatment as mastectomy for many breast cancers.

1986– New Policy on Women's Health Research: The National Institutes of Health established a policy to increase participation in women's health research, but in 1990, an Institute of Medicine Report said NIH was not moving quickly enough to implement this policy.

1987– Lung Cancer Surpasses Breast Cancer as the Leading Cause of Cancer Death in Women.

1989– Women's Health Equity Act: This law, introduced by the Congressional Caucus for Women's Issues, called for an increased focus on women's health through research, services, and prevention activities.

1990– Dr. Antonia Novello is Confirmed as the First Woman Surgeon General of the United States: She is also the first minority to be appointed to this position.

1990– Office of Research on Women's Health Is Established: This office was established at the National Institutes of Health to stimulate and serve as a focal point for women's health research. Public hearings and

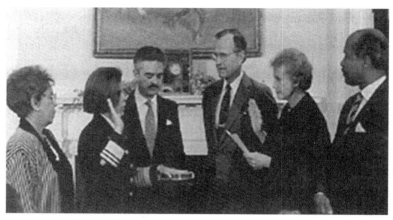

Antonia Coello Novello, M.D. (1944–), the first woman and the first minority to be appointed as Surgeon General of the United States. Pictured, Dr. Novello being sworn in by Justice Sandra Day O'Connor in a ceremony at the White House on March 9, 1990. Also in the photo, President George Bush (center right), Secretary of the Department of Health and Human Services Louis Sullivan (far right), and Dr. Novello's husband and mother. Photo courtesy of the U.S. Department of Health and Human Services, Washington, D.C.

a scientific workshop held at Hunt Valley, Maryland, produced the report "The National Institutes of Health: Opportunities for Research on Women's Health," which served as a blueprint for research at the NIH.

1990– Society for the Advancement of Women's Health Research Founded: This organization's mission was to improve the health of women through research.

1990– Breast and Cervical Cancer Mortality Prevention Act: This Congressional act provided mammograms and pap smears to underserved women (including low-income women, older women, and minority women).

1991– Office on Women's Health Established: The Office on Women's Health was established at the U.S. Department of Health and Human Services during the presidency of George H. W. Bush, to better coordinate women's health activities, programs, and research throughout the U.S. Public Health Service.

1992– Mammography Quality Standards Act: This law was designed to set national standards and a uniform system of quality control for mammography clinics across the country.

1992– Infertility Prevention Act: This Act provided additional funds to establish screening, treatment, counseling, and follow-up services for sexually transmitted diseases that could lead to infertility in women if left undiagnosed and/or untreated.

1993– NIH Revitalization Act: This law required the inclusion of women and members of racial and ethnic minority groups in all federally-funded population-based studies.

1993– Family and Medical Leave Act: This law provided employees with the right to take up to 12 weeks of unpaid leave during a 12-month period for family or medical reasons without the threat of having to leave their job permanently.

1993– National Action Plan on Breast Cancer (NAPBC) Established: This public-private partnership was established by President William J. Clinton in response to a national petition drive (2.6 million signatures) coordinated by the National Breast Cancer Coalition. Its goal was to establish a comprehensive national plan to address the breast cancer epidemic. After providing leadership and sparking interest on issues from genetic testing to public education and clinical trials, the work of the NAPBC was handed over to private groups and the National Cancer Institute in 2000.

1994– Violence against Women Act: This Act defined new federal crimes of violence against women and enhanced penalties to combat sexual assault and domestic violence.

1994– Offices of Women's Health Established at the Food and Drug Administration and the Centers for Disease Control and Prevention.

1994– BRCA1 and BRCA2 Identified: The DNA sequences of two genetic mutations linked to breast cancer were discovered, leading to the possibility of genetic testing for high risk women.

1994– Women of Childbearing Years Can Participate in Clinical Trials: The FDA issued guidance lifting the ban on inclusion of women with childbearing potential from early clinical studies (Phase 1 and early Phase 2). This ban (which had been in place since 1977) had been a significant barrier to women's participation in clinical trials.

1996– The Personal Responsibility and Work Opportunity Reconciliation Act of 1996: A provision of this bill, Support for Families Transitioning into Job, was designed to help more mothers move into jobs. The law also guaranteed that women on welfare would continue to receive health coverage for their families, including at least one year of transitional Medicaid when they leave welfare for work.

1996– National Centers of Excellence in Women's Health Designated: The DHHS Office on Women's Health designated the first six National Centers of Excellence (CoEs) at academic medical centers around the country. These were model "one-stop-shopping" health programs designed to integrate women's health research, clinical services and public education. By century's end, there were fifteen CoEs, and three National Community Centers of Excellence in Women's Health, with more planned for the future.

1996– Women's Health in the Medical School Curriculum Published: This first guideline for including women's health issues in medical school curriculum was published by the Office of Research on Women's Health, the Health Resources and Services Administration, and the DHHS Office on Women's Health.

1997– An Agenda for Research on Women's Health in the 21st Century: This document expanded the Hunt Valley vision for women's health research in the broader context of cultural and ethnic origins, geographic location, and socioeconomic strata.

1997– FDA Office of Women's Health Launches "Take Time to Care Campaign": This three year effort reached over 26 million Americans with the message "Use Medicines Wisely." Done in partnership with the National Association of Chain Drug Stores and more than 80 other participating organizations, this campaign targeted the issue of preventing adverse drug reactions and medication errors.

1998– Gender Differences in Susceptibility to Environmental Factors Published: This Institute of Medicine report encouraged more research into how certain factors, such as genetics and hormones, affect susceptibility to environmental influences in health status.

1998– The National Women's Health Information Center (NWHIC) Launched: The DHHS Office on Women's Health launched the first commercial-free combined Web site and toll-free phone number for women's health information. By century's end, NWHIC was receiving more than four million "hits" and several hundred thousand "user sessions" a month.

1999– Contraceptive Coverage in the Federal Employees Health Benefits Program: This law was attached to the 1999 Treasury, Postal Service, and General Government Appropriations Bill to offer contraceptive coverage to women insured through the Federal Employees Health Benefits Program.

1999– Women's Health in the Dental School Curriculum Published: The first women's health curriculum recommendations for dental schools were released by the NIH Office of Research on Women's Health and the Health Resources and Services Administration.

1999– Lesbian Health: Current Assessment and Directions for the Future: This Institute of Medicine report recommended more research into health issues that might be unique to lesbian women.

2000– The Breast and Cervical Cancer Prevention and Treatment Act: This Congressional Act is designed to enable states to provide treatment services to eligible women through the Medicaid program.

2000– Exploring the Biological Contributions to Human Health: Does Sex Matter?: This Institute of Medicine report was initiated in 2000. It concluded that "every cell has a sex" and that medical research should focus more on sex differences and determinants on the biological level.

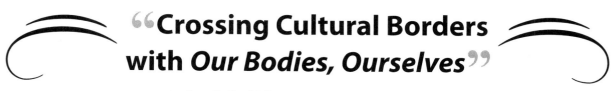

"Crossing Cultural Borders with *Our Bodies, Ourselves*"

by Sally Whelan and Jane Pincus

With just three weeks to go before the Utrecht meeting that would bring together groups from around the world that are translating/adapting *Our Bodies, Ourselves (OBOS)*, the last piece of funding came in, last minute requirements of embassies and visa offices were met, necessary documents produced, and the final hotel rooms booked. I (Sally) sat bolt upright in bed at 5 AM one morning, realizing that if I got on email immediately, I might be able to catch our colleague Codou Bop on-the-spot at her computer in Senegal, or Liana Galstyan in Armenia to find out if wired funds had gotten through. This instant messaging worked splendidly.

It was an honor to attend this exciting meeting; now, the events of the past two months have made us even more keenly aware of the essential need for this kind of global dialogue. The only other large gathering of groups working on translations/adaptations of *Our Bodies, Ourselves* was in 1995 at the Fourth World Conference on Women held in Beijing. This time we arranged to carve out our own time and place.

Kathy Davis, a feminist sociologist at the University of Utrecht, and Marlies Bosch, presently a facilitator of the Tibetan translation project, helped organize and facilitate the meeting. The Federation of Women's Self-help Centers, a coalition of groups funded by the Dutch government, graciously offered us a large, sunlit room. Chantal Soeters, one of Kathy's students, took notes. Seated at tables designed to come together in a comfortable ellipse, twenty-one participants from Japan, Armenia, Poland, Tibet, Senegal, Mexico, Bulgaria, Serbia, the Netherlands, and the U.S. put faces to the voices we had come to know through email and fax over the last several years. For the next three days, women described the dramatic challenges they faced in creating adaptations of *Our Bodies, Ourselves*.

Six New Books

Bulgaria
Kornelia Slavova and Tatyana Kotzeva

The Women's Health Initiative in Bulgaria took the risk of publishing their book in a culture where women's roles have been "re-traditionalized" in the transition from Communism to democracy, and where feminism is seen as a Western, anti-male, anti-family, and pro-lesbian ideology. The *collective* voice of *OBOS* reverberates cynically, as does the idea of *sisterhood*, conjuring up a leftist agenda that smacks of Marxism and Leninism. A straight translation would have been culturally inappropriate.

Over-medicalization is not an issue, as basic needs in healthcare are not yet met, nor are abortion rights an issue, particularly not a moral one, because abortion is the primary method of birth control. Pro-natalist attitudes make for an especially difficult and charged environment for women experiencing infertility.

Speaking to the societal antipathy towards feminism, the authors recast it within the perspective of gender justice, providing a special chapter about women's issues during the nineteenth and twentieth centuries. Throughout, they emphasized the rights of women in their roles as consumers, patients and citizens. They address their introduction to men as well as women.

After sometimes challenging negotiations, the book was published by a prestigious publisher, Colibri, and came out in July.

Serbia
Stanislava Otasevic and Bobana Macanovic

Much of the Serbian adaptation of *OBOS* was produced in war-torn Serbia. The coordinating group, The Autonomous Women's Center Against Sexual Violence supports and counsels women survivors of male violence.

A team composed of nine women from five groups, spent over a year translating and adapting *OBOS,* publishing it themselves. Stanislava and Bobana proudly brought copies—hot off the press!—to our meeting, with the cover photo of the first ever "Take Back the Night" march in 1995 in Belgrade. Each page contains just one column of text, leaving a lot of space for women to write in their own experiences, for they said "These books will have many owners."

This is the first book available in Serbia on the politics of women's health. In a country that conceals health statistics for military and economic purposes, documentation about women's health takes on a unique power. War has severely affected the healthcare situation, with long waiting lists, shortage of money and medicines, and general depression. Often Serbian women's bodies have literally been used as weapons for military and political purposes; thus, these women have experienced them as instruments of pain and suffering, not as a functional or pleasurable part of their lives. Material on sexuality takes on a special importance.

As the authors see it, living within a regime that abhorred diversity and had well developed 'mechanisms of hate,' it is essential to underscore the diversity of Serbian women, and they especially have attempted to give visibility to lesbians and women with disabilities.

Recent events have increased substance abuse and the use of anti-depressant drugs, discussed at length in the book. The authors dropped the 'Nutrition' chapter, for it seemed terrible to speak of food when people were starving; 'Women in Motion' was dropped too, for it also lacked relevance, pertinent only to affluent people.

The authors hope that their printer's comment, when they picked up the finished book in June, augurs well for a positive reception of the Serbian *OBOS.* He said: "This book should be given to each daughter by her father." It is a testament to their strength, courage and perseverance that there is any Serbian edition at all.

Armenia
Liana Galstyan

The Armenian adaptation of *OBOS* arrived last month in our mailbox, almost ten years after work on this book began. During the past decade, Armenia endured an earthquake, severe losses in electricity and heating fuel, and paper shortages—some photos from the project's first phase show the translators in a candlelit room wearing gloves. Faced with hardships and logistical problems, the project was stalled until Dr. Mary Khachikian met Judy Norsigian at the Armenian World Medical Congress in Boston during 1996 and agreed to assume

coordination of the project. After that point, the vision and dedication of Mary and her colleagues shaped a process and a product that is now beautiful to behold with its multi-colored cover filled with images of Armenian women of all ages.

With a declining birthrate and economic hardship causing serious emigration from the country, the book, with its extensive section on contraception, faced some resistance from some government officials and members of the media even before its actual publication. For some, the legacy of the Armenian genocide also contributes to a pro-natalist sentiment. Still, Liana reported, the authors managed to offer extensive information about birth control. They significantly adapted the infertility section of the book, as STDs cause infertility rates to be very high (28%). The book makes a special attempt to reach young women with chapters on body image and sexuality.

The coordinator of the Armenian Family Health Association plans to organize a series of awareness-raising workshops for women throughout Armenia, including educators, health providers and women in social service agencies. This edition holds special meaning for Judy Norsigian, who is also Armenian and visited Armenia for the first time last year to participate in an Armenian women's conference and to help with completion of the book project.

Senegal
Codou Bop

The present challenge for the authors of the "inspired" African-French edition of *OBOS, Notre Corps, Notre Santé* is to secure funding for printing and distribution of their already completed manuscript. The book will serve twenty-one francophone countries. With French (the language of colonization) as the necessary working language, it will be distributed for free to schools, health centers and women's groups, and translated into local dialects. The BWHBC is currently seeking donors who may wish to contribute to this endeavor.

Most Africans are being increasingly harmed by a new kind of re-colonization, among them the World Bank's structural adjustment policies, increased debts to the global North, devalued currencies and the privatization of health and education, which used to be free or cost very little.

Women have little or no access to healthcare, land, jobs, or schooling. False interpretations of the Koran increasingly stand in the way of women's health and rights. Young women rank low in the social hierarchy of power, with 56% married and mother of a baby by age seventeen. In general, women belong to fathers, husbands or uncles. Their role is to take care of others. Since they are not "allowed" to be ill, and there is no such thing as an "unhealthy" woman, women buy over-the-counter medications to ease symptoms enough to carry on with their work.

Some practices are oppressive and harmful: For instance, to be fat is desirable, since thinness is associated with poverty and AIDS. Thus, women are too often encouraged to eat high-fat diets and discouraged from exercising. Fifteen to nineteen year old women are most afflicted by HIV/AIDS (an insidious myth teaches that a man infected with AIDs need to have sex with a virgin to purify himself). Women use bleach to whiten their skin (a result of colonialism), causing skin cancer and kidney problems.

The book emphasizes the cultural, economic, political and religious contexts in which African women live. It empowers a woman by telling her she belongs to herself, and constantly encourages her not to feel guilty taking care of herself. One chapter describes pre-colonial matrilineal societies in which women did have a great deal of power.

Mexico

Ester Shapiro, Alan West, U.S., and Lourdes Ruiz

An extensive cultural adaptation of *OBOS* was produced by approximately twenty Latin American women's health groups spanning the Americas and the Caribbean in collaboration with a Boston-based editorial team of Latinas. Ester, coordinating editor of *NCNV,* discussed some of *NCNV's* departures from *OBOS,* the tasks faced in adapting a US feminist text (by emphasizing "mutual help" rather than "self-help" and eliminating some of the overtly ideological attitudes, for instance), and how the book's text became a living tool for lively networking and community organizing.

The audience for *NCNV* is huge and very varied. As women worked in coalition across lines of continent and nation, North and South, locally and regionally, they broadened the definition of social change work to emphasize working with men and other social change movements. The "Católicas por el Derecho a Decidir" (Catholics for a Free Choice) prolife/prochoice perspective on abortion within the framework of women's sacred responsibility for preserving life was tremendously important. *NCNV* embodies a participatory health education model, with an emphasis on community building and outreach.

As the only translation/adaptation project based at the BWHBC, *NCNV* has served in many ways as a bridge between *OBOS* and other projects worldwide. Important commonalities arise between *NCNV* and other books.

NCNV redefines feminism within a gender and social justice model, as in the Bulgarian edition. It places great emphasis throughout, as does the francophone African edition, on the need to balance the care of others with the care for one's self. And like the Arabic edition from Egypt, inspired by *OBOS,* but a new book altogether, *NCNV* acknowledges the importance of religion and spirituality in discussions of women's health.

Ester offered her extensive knowledge in networking, media outreach, and promotion and held special sessions with participants whose books are already published, and for whom promotion and community outreach are now a priority. Alan provided an analysis of cross-cultural translations, which always involve the implementation of power relationships via the language used. Translation consists of a constant historic, poetic interaction between the text itself, the language and the culture. Lourdes, developer of CIDHAL's impressive website, discussed the use of electronic media and encouraged us to think about how our books, or sections of books, can be brought into the electronic age.

Japan

Toyoko Nakanishi, Toshiko Honda, and Miho Ogino

Authors of the 1988 Japanese edition of *OBOS,* veterans of the translation/adaptation process, they brought to our circle at Utrecht invaluable experience and knowledge. They also brought, straight from the printer the day before their departure for Utrecht, the first-ever translation of *Sacrificing Ourselves for Love*—a book co-authored by deceased BWHBC founder Esther Rome and Jane Wegsheider Hyman. They chose this book to translate because it deals with dieting, eating disorders, cosmetic surgery, domestic violence, rape, STDs, and HIV/AIDS—all serious problems today in Japanese society. Research carried out in Osaka City reveals that 2 out of 3 women have experienced some kind of violence from their husbands or lovers. In May, 2001, Japan enacted a new law attempting to reduce this violence. The authors working on *SOFL* included information on shelters and counseling services for battered women.

The Japanese women did not face censorship in publishing *OBOS* in the late '80s, even when introducing subjects such as lesbians, masturbation, people with disabilities, or the sexuality of older women. However, the Japanese language itself was a challenge. For traditional characters, such as those for pubic hair ('shameful hair'), they substituted a new, positive language of sexuality.

It was useful to hear how a mostly direct translation of *OBOS* became specifically useful to Japanese women. The authors conducted their own research. They added the responses of over 200 clinics and hospitals to a survey designed to provide information on rates/policies on such things as episiotomy, labor positions, contraception, partners permitted at birth, and abortion services. They substituted information about the Japanese medical system, health insurance system, and Japanese law in pertinent places in the text, as well as the names of foods and drugs available in Japan.

OBOS inspired the formation of many groups that began to meet to discuss and conduct research on the birth control pill, endometriosis, menopause, reproductive technologies, sexual harassment, and domestic violence. Many new books have sprung up based on the information and experiences gathered. As a result of increased interest in and visibility of women's health issues, the atmosphere of shame and secrecy surrounding women's bodies and sexuality has been dispersed to a considerable degree.

Upcoming Projects
Poland
Malgorzata (Gosia) Tarasiewicz

Pending funding, the Network of East West Women—Polska will focus on reaching young women. They envision putting selected portions of *OBOS* on the internet, using popular stars. Already, three women singers have agreed to deliver messages about health and sexuality. The site will be interactive, with room for questions. Magazines will reach women in rural areas and a short story competition for young women will encourage them to talk about their bodies. In these ways they will collect Polish women's experiences for a booklet.

They anticipate attacks from the Catholic hierarchy and media that will cast them as "perverts." But given that in their country prenatal exams are forbidden, abortions illegal, homophobia extensive, and bribes often required for health services, they are determined to bring about some change. "In two years, when we meet again, we'll tell you our story," said Gosia.

Tibet
Lobsang Dechen with Marlies Bosch, the Netherlands

Five hundred Tibetan Buddhist nuns, their country occupied by the Chinese, live in exile in Dharamsala, India at the Tibetan Nun's Project. Lobsang Dechen, a co-director of the nunnery, attended the Utrecht meeting. Through body awareness workshops held last year, the nuns identified some of the topics most useful to them. In meetings held this fall at the nunnery with Marlies Bosch, co-facilitator of the project from the Netherlands, women selected content from *OBOS* to be used for booklets in Tibetan.

Because most of the nuns are young (seventeen to twenty-two years) and without previous exposure to health information, they may also use parts of Ruth Bell's *Changing Bodies, Changing Lives* (for teens) to enhance body awareness and teach basic health concepts. Dechen hopes that in the future they can make available to Tibetan women living in Tibet the information they have gathered.

The Last Day
Marlise Mensink of MAMA CASH, a women's foundation in the Netherlands

With fundraising a constant reality for all groups, we each spoke about how our groups had raised money for our book projects. Marlise stressed the collaborative aspects of the funder/recipient relationship—funders love to give their money away and 'ideals need money!'—and made amusing, practical suggestions about how raising money can be most effective.

Norma Swenson and Jane Pincus, BWHBC co-founders and *OBOS* co-authors

We presented a brief history of the first *OBOS*, BWHBC's early ideals and activities, and some history of the US Women's Health Movement. We mentioned the times of right-wing censorship of *OBOS*. In the post-meeting evaluations, participants said how important it was for them to hear BWHBC's story. Utrecht gave them a chance to:

> "listen to the extraordinary history of the book in the US; to learn stories and crucial moments in producing and publishing its different editions; I was impressed with the enthusiasm of the women who were struggling for the publication of *OBOS;* I was surprised to find that they faced inspection and religious restriction."

To complete the circle, Norma describes her reaction to the stories of these extraordinary women and their works:

> "As I listened to their stories of truly daunting conditions—war, political opposition, lack of funds, lack of time, inadequate and unreliable technology, and dozens of other obstacles—I was strongly moved. I felt there is really no comparison between what we have gone through to produce *OBOS* over the years, under conditions of peace and relative ease and prosperity, and what so many of them have been going through. What we all seem to have in common is the willingness to pour volunteer time, money and effort into producing these books if necessary and the determination to

get this vital information in accessible language into the hands of women who clearly need it. As I have felt many times over the years in many different places across the world, women can and do cross cultural borders powerfully with *OBOS,* and with us. I feel very privileged to have been there."

Upcoming Projects

The BWHBC plans to:

- provide ongoing technical assistance to groups in every stage of the translation/adaptation process;

- complete a translation/adaptation guidelines packet that identifies typical challenges faced by groups around the world and illustrates through first-hand accounts how coordinating groups have resolved problems;

- explore the establishment and coordination of a revolving loan fund program to support translation projects on a temporary basis, ensuring they can bring their projects to fruition and disseminate their books as widely as possible;

- and facilitate communication, through a listserv, among emergent and experienced groups producing *OBOS.*

A million thanks to all who participated in the meeting as well as those who contributed funds—the Global Fund for Women, the MacArthur Foundation, Conservation Food and Health Foundation, and an anonymous donor. Thanks also to Ester Shapiro, who coined the title of the meeting. We appreciate all who have joined with us in this critical global work.

Many thanks for the support we received this year from foundations not already mentioned in this newsletter: Ford Foundation, Packard Foundation, Rockefeller Foundation, Mellon Foundation, Pettus-Crowe Foundation, Educational Foundation of America, Dickler Family Foundation, Harvard Pilgrim Healthcare Foundation, and Tufts Health Plan.

The Making of *Our Bodies, Ourselves*

How Feminism Travels across Borders

by Kathy Davis

This is a book about a book: the feminist classic on women's health, *Our Bodies, Ourselves (OBOS),* and how it "traveled." The story begins in 1969. The country was in turmoil over the Vietnam War. Richard "Tricky Dick" Nixon had just been elected president after the riots at the Democratic National Convention in Chicago. Radical activism was everywhere: the civil rights movement and its offshoots—Black Power, La Raza, and the American Indian movement; antiwar demonstrations and draft resistance; radical student activism of the Marxist, socialist, or anarchist persuasion; hippies, yippies, and the "sexual revolution"; and, last but not least, a burgeoning women's movement. It was in this context that a small group of young women met at a workshop called Women and Their Bodies, held at one of the first feminist conferences in the United States, which took place in Boston. Some of the women had already been active in the civil rights movement or had helped draft resisters during the Vietnam War, but this was for many of them their first encounter with feminism. They talked about their sexuality (which was still, despite the sexual revolution, very much taboo), abortion (which was illegal—*Roe v. Wade* wasn't decided until 1973), their experiences with pregnancy and childbirth (several were young mothers), and their frustrations with physicians and healthcare. The group, which later evolved into the Boston Women's Health Book Collective (BWHBC), began to meet regularly. Its members collected information about health issues (which was, unlike today, scarce and hard to find) and wrote papers, which they discussed in meetings attended by increasing numbers of local women. These meetings were electrifying, leaving many of the participants irrevocably changed.

A year later the group assembled the discussion papers, and the first version of *OBOS* was born. Originally printed on newsprint by an underground publisher and selling for seventy-five cents, *OBOS* was a lively and accessible manual on women's bodies and health. It was full of personal experiences and contained useful information on issues ranging from masturbation (how to do it) to birth control (which methods were available and how to use them) to vaginal infections, pregnancy, and nursing. It combined a scathing critique of patriarchal medicine and the medicalization of women's bodies with an analysis of the political economics of the health and pharmaceutical industries. But, above all, *OBOS* validated women's embodied experiences as a resource for challenging medical dogmas about women's bodies and, consequently, as a strategy for personal and collective empowerment.

The book was an overnight success, and the group—to its surprise—found itself being wooed by commercial publishers. Since the first commercial edition was published in 1973, *OBOS* has sold over four million copies and gone through six major updates. The latest edition appeared in 2005. It occupied the *New York Times* best seller list for several years, was voted the best young adult book of 1976 by the American Library Association, and has received worldwide critical acclaim for its candid and accessible approach to women's health.

Often called the "bible of women's health," *OBOS* shaped how generations of women have felt about their bodies, their sexuality and relationships, and their reproduction and health. It has not only enjoyed a widespread popularity, unique for a feminist book, but has also transformed the provision of healthcare, helped shape healthcare policies, and stimulated research on women's health in the United States.[1] No family practice is complete without a copy of *OBOS* in the waiting room. Gynecological examinations have become more responsive to the patient's needs (e.g., by abandoning cold metal speculums in favor of more comfortable plastic ones), and hospitals have allowed women more control over the process of giving birth. As a result of *OBOS*, many women have been encouraged to enter medicine and midwives and nurse practitioners have been rehabilitated as respectable professionals in the U.S. healthcare system. The book has been a catalyst for myriad consumer and patient advocate organizations and campaigns for women's reproductive rights. It was instrumental in getting patient information inserts packaged with medications and has played an advocacy role in congressional hearings and scientific conferences on the safety of medications, medical devices, and procedures ranging from silicone breast implants to the injectable contraceptive Depo-Provera and the new genetic technologies. It has inspired research on women's health within the health sciences and medicine. Research protocols on—for example—heart disease no longer leave women out, and diseases that specifically effect women (such as breast cancer) have been given considerably more attention since the publication of *OBOS*. The recent study on the dangers of hormone replacement therapy (HRT), which exposed the negligence of the pharmaceutical industry and medical profession in indiscriminately promoting estrogen supplements for menopausal women, owes a debt to the pioneering work of *OBOS*.[2]

REFERENCES
A list of references is available in the original source.

The Making of *Our Bodies, Ourselves*

"Transnational Knowledge, Transnational Politics"

by Kathy Davis

While I was in the final stages of writing this book, I gave a presentation about *OBOS* and its travels to an audience of feminist scholars. Afterward one of these scholars, well known for her work in post-colonial feminist theory, approached me. "You know," she said, "I can't tell you how nice it is to hear a story like this. It's so . . ."— she seemed to be struggling to find the right word— "it's just so *hopeful*."

Her remark, I must admit, took me somewhat by surprise. I began this inquiry—as I set out in the introduction—with certain ambivalences, which were a reflection of my position as a feminist scholar. Within feminist scholarship, it is bon ton to situate oneself as a critic. Taking a critical and reflexive perspective is almost a kind of second nature, involving anything from debunking assumptions that are taken for granted in scientific discourse to exposing hidden inequalities and exclusions of power lurking within even seemingly benign practices and policies to being relentlessly vigilant concerning one's own blind spots and prejudices. While my experiences as a feminist health activist in the seventies made me embrace *OBOS*, my experiences as a feminist scholar in the nineties warned me to take a more cautious stance. Well versed in poststructuralist feminist theory, I was inclined to be suspicious of any text that glorified women's embodied experience as an unproblematic source of knowledge. Moreover, in the light of long-standing debates about "global feminism," I was disposed to be wary that any U.S. feminist export could exhibit imperialistic tendencies, which would obscure differences and hierarchies of power between U.S. feminists and feminists in non-Western contexts.

Throughout this inquiry, I have used these ambivalences as a resource for exploring the history and travels of *OBOS*, taking its trajectory within and outside the United States as an occasion to think critically about its politics of knowledge and its status as a transnational feminist project. As a result of my efforts to read *OBOS* through the critical lens of contemporary feminist schol-

arship, I find myself at the end of my own journey—much like the feminist scholar in my audience—left with an unfamiliar and yet unmistakably pleasant feeling that I can only describe as hopeful.

It is not my intention to romanticize *OBOS* as a feminist project, and, as I have shown throughout this book, it has produced its own problems and exclusions. Nevertheless, I will take the opportunity in this final chapter to explore some of the reasons for this strange and appealing sensation of hopefulness that the project has engendered, despite all its limitations. While I began this inquiry with the assumption that *OBOS* would have much to learn from contemporary feminist theory, in this chapter I will argue that it is contemporary feminist theory that may have just as much, if not more, to learn from *OBOS*. I will take the travels of *OBOS*—the scope and variety of its border crossings, the diversity of its multifaceted transformations, and the ways in which it has shaped encounters between feminists globally—as having implications for feminist scholarship and theory and, more specifically, for how we might begin to think about feminist history, feminist politics of knowledge, and transnational feminism.

Before I discuss these implications, however, I will return briefly to the questions that were raised at the outset of this inquiry: how a U.S. feminist book could resonate with women in such diverse social, cultural, and geographical locations; what happened to it as it traveled; and what these travels can tell us more generally about feminist knowledge and feminist politics in a transnational context.

Making *OBOS*

The present inquiry began with two somewhat unorthodox assumptions. The first was that *OBOS* should be regarded, first and foremost, as an *epistemological project* rather than a popular self-help book on women's health. Within feminist scholarship, the prevailing sentiment is that *OBOS* is historically important, practically useful, and undoubtedly well intentioned but has little of theoretical relevance to offer feminist scholarship. From the vantage point of postmodern feminist theory à la Donna Haraway, Joan Scott, Judith Butler, and many others, *OBOS* is regarded as theoretically naive and unsophisticated because it commits several cardinal theoretical sins: it naturalizes the biological female body, it valorizes women's experiences as authentic sources of the truth, and it glorifies the autonomous agency of individual women. Seen in this light, *OBOS* is at best old-fashioned and unsophisticated and at worst an object requiring critical deconstruction.

In the present inquiry, I have taken issue with this stance. I have argued that some of the assumptions made by postmodern feminist body theory, while helpful in deconstructing the problematic legacy of Western Enlightenment philosophy, have also become blinders, obscuring the analysis of *OBOS* as an epistemological project and, more generally, failing to engage seriously with feminist health activism. This theory gets in the way of exploring what has been the most distinctive feature of *OBOS*, namely, a politics of knowledge that invited individual women to use their own embodied experiences to engage critically with dominant practices of knowledge. This politics of knowledge was reflected in the book's distinctive format (accessible and accountable information, women's personal stories about their bodily experiences, and a critical framework situating women's health in a broader social, cultural, and political context). It was this politics of knowledge that enabled the readers of *OBOS* to become embodied, critical, epistemic agents.

The second assumption of the present inquiry was that in order to fully appreciate the impact and significance of *OBOS* as a feminist icon it would be necessary to connect the book's history *within* the United States with its travels *outside* the United States. This meant that I refrained from writing a straightforward history of *OBOS* as a U.S. feminist project. Instead I have taken the book's travels as a starting point for thinking critically about its impact during the past three decades, the myriad transformations it has undergone, and its worldwide significance as a transnational feminist knowledge project for transnational feminist health politics. This entailed situating the inquiry within contemporary theoretical debates about the politics of location. These debates explore how individuals use their material locations in the world as a resource for knowing what it means to be embodied as a particular kind of person in a particular social and cultural context. The politics of location is also a place from which to construct a critical subjectivity and political perspective for social change.

In the present inquiry, I have used the politics of location (social, cultural, and geographical) to understand how *OBOS* as a feminist knowledge project has been able to circulate internationally, thereby generating a transnational feminist politics of the body.

The combination of an approach that treats *OBOS* as an epistemological project and a perspective that decenters it as an exclusively U.S. feminist project has brought me to the following insights.

First, the politics of knowledge represented by *OBOS* was particularly suited to crossing borders of class, race and ethnicity, sexual orientation, and generation, allowing the book to speak to a wide diversity of women. The reason for its success in addressing different women was that it did not assume that women would automatically have identical experiences, needs, or interests simply by virtue of having a female body. Indeed, the book recognized differences in women's embodiment (experiences, social location, and circumstances), and this recognition had consequences for the process in which each new edition of *OBOS* was made. It assumed that this would not be a one-time affair but would require the ongoing critical interrogation of each new version of the book. Through the collaborative method of knowledge production, whereby different women were invited to "read against the grain" and to think critically about the text from their specific embodied location, *OBOS* was not only able to include a variety of perspectives on women's health, but it used these different perspectives to enable readers to think critically about their own embodied experiences, as well as become sensitized to the circumstances of women in social, cultural, and political locations different than their own.

Second, the politics of knowledge represented by *OBOS* not only allowed it to cross the borders of class, race and ethnicity, sexual orientation, and generation within the United States, but it also enabled what was otherwise a local product—a typically U.S. book—to travel. One of the unique features of *OBOS* was that its content, form, and politics did not remain intact in the course of its border crossings. It invited women across the globe to rewrite the book and, ultimately, transform it in ways that would make it accessible and relevant in their own social, cultural, and geopolitical contexts. This required something other than a straightforward translation; it required a feminist translation strategy of "friendly learning by taking a distance" (Spivak 2000). The translators of *OBOS* invariably participated in a collective process of contextualizing and critically reworking the U.S. text, whereby they creatively used differences between their own context and the U.S. context to open up controversial topics, celebrate local accomplishments, or suggest points for political coalitions. The same process of reading against the grain that had been instrumental to the widespread popularity of *OBOS within* the United States proved to be its most translatable feature *outside* the United States. In the course of translating *OBOS*, women from widely divergent locations were able to appropriate this collective, critical process of knowledge production, using *OBOS* as an occasion for developing their own brand of oppositional feminist politics of knowledge.

Third, the travels of *OBOS* have implications for how we think about the circulation of feminist knowledge and politics in a global context. One of the most notable features of the translations is that they were not simply transported from the "West to the rest" (Hall 1992) or imposed as a kind of feminist cultural imperialism. The international trajectory of *OBOS* suggests that the circulation of feminist knowledge is much more complicated and contradictory. When feminist knowledge moves from place to place, it is reworked and rearticulated, allowing new configurations of the original to emerge. Thus, while *OBOS* emerged initially in the United States, its flows were not unidirectional. The text not only moved from place to place, but its translations traveled as well, providing the basis for new translations or returning—literally—to the United States, where they were taken up and used by diasporic communities there. Thus, *OBOS* should be viewed less as a U.S. book with multiple translations than as an ongoing transnational feminist knowledge project.

Fourth, as a catalyst for transnational feminist politics, *OBOS* has created a global feminist imagined community. This community is not based on shared gender identity or common interests or even identical political goals. It has emerged through the engagement of women from different locations with *OBOS*, predicated on their willingness to engage in a shared politics of knowledge. Through the act of making, reading, or translating *OBOS*, women in different locations and at different points in time were able to participate vicariously in that first mythical discussion group "where it all began." The story of the first meeting in 1969 in Boston when a group of young women met to talk about their bodies not only became a foundational myth for U.S. feminism. This myth also traveled, capturing the minds and hearts of women across the globe, who imaginatively situated themselves within the mythical history of *OBOS*, making it their history, too. Thus, the very myth that created *OBOS* as a U.S. feminist success story has, through its travels, enabled *OBOS* not only to continue but to become much more than the original project. As transnational feminist project, *OBOS* has taken on a life of its

own, becoming a feminist icon for women across the globe.

Having looked at the making of *OBOS* and how it traveled, I will now turn to the implications of this transnational knowledge project for feminist scholarship—in particular, for feminist history, knowledge politics, and transnational practice.

Feminist History

The making of *OBOS* and the ways it has traveled have implications for how feminist history should be written. In recent years, U.S. feminist historians have devoted considerable attention to what has been called "second-wave feminism."[1]

Written against the backdrop of a widespread feminist backlash in the United States (Faludi 1992), these histories exude a sense of urgency—a desire to set the record straight before it is too late. There is a palpable sense that feminism has come and gone, leaving us with no other choice than to patiently await the next "wave"— a new generation that will pick up the torch and carry on where "we" left off. While many historians lament its passing, expressing an unmistakable nostalgia for the "good old days," others have been more critical, pointing to its mistakes and failings. However, in either case, feminism is treated very much as a U.S. phenomenon. Both its emergence and its demise seemed to occur without reference to what happened outside the United States. The implicit assumption is that what happens in the rest of the world is dependent on what happens to feminism in the United States. It is as if without U.S. feminism there would be no feminism at all.

The history of *OBOS* refutes the assumptions made by this particular brand of feminist historiography. It disrupts the notion that feminism is a thing of the past. While many of the projects of the so-called second wave of U.S. feminism may be over, *OBOS* is not only still around but feminism itself is very much alive and kicking in many different locations around the world. The longevity and the success of *OBOS* are inextricably linked to its capacity to transform itself so that it can speak across shifting lines of difference. Its resilience raises questions concerning the claim that feminism is dead or at least on its last legs. U.S. feminist history has been criticized for its "time-charged terminologies" (first wave, second wave, third wave), which marginalize the activism and worldviews of women of color.[2] Ironically, the very period that white feminist historians typically treat as the moment of decline is the time when women of color began to develop as a new political subject. From the point of view of multiracial feminism in the

United States, feminism gained momentum in the eighties and its best days are yet to come (Thompson 2002, 344).

But, even more powerfully, the transnational trajectory of *OBOS* demonstrates that feminism is not limited to the United States and, indeed, may presently play a more significant role outside the United States. U.S. feminism has often situated itself (and been situated by others) as the standard against which all women's struggles across the globe are to be measured. Ironically, even so-called international or comparative studies of feminism tend to treat the United States as the undisputed center of feminist history. Precedence is given to events and struggles occurring within the borders of the United States. A discourse of the Western Enlightenment is reproduced, whereby notions of progress and development are privileged so that what comes after is automatically better than what came before. This version of feminist history tends to leave non-Western women's movements "stuck" in an earlier and "less advanced" stage (Shih 2002, 98). The translations of *OBOS* demonstrate that, while notions about what might constitute a feminist politics of the body may differ, there is a broad interest among women's groups in widely divergent locations about issues of women's health. The international women's health movement is not only one of the most vibrant of the contemporary social movements, but it has become a force to be reckoned with in the terrain of international politics. The global interest in women's health, reproductive rights, and sexual integrity demonstrates that worries about the demise of feminism may be, in fact, little more than ethnocentric myopia, that is, the failure of U.S. feminism to look beyond its own backyard. A more accurate and politically viable vision of history would encompass the wide diversity of feminist histories and women's struggles across the globe.

The global dissemination of *OBOS* shows why—when it comes to the state of feminism in the world—there may be considerably more reason for optimism than despair. It provides a case in point for the importance of what Susan Stanford Friedman has called "thinking geographically" (2001), that is, for replacing the "overdeveloped historical contextualization" of U.S. feminist scholarship with a better-developed "spatial and geographical imagination" (16). This not only means acknowledging and learning about feminist histories of struggles in other parts of the world. At a time when the accelerating pace of globalization and transnational cultural traffic has made national borders increasingly porous, it also makes sense for contemporary feminist historiography to explore the ways in which the global is already implicated in local histories, as well as the diversity of feminist struggles across the globe.[3] By tracking the migratory and transcultural formations, feminism can become viewable as both more ubiquitous (global) and more historically specific (local), that is, as emerging in specific geographical locations and at specific historical moments.

Politics of Knowledge

The making of *OBOS* and its travels also have implications for how we should think about feminist knowledge and knowledge politics. Postmodern feminist scholarship, particularly under the influence of critical race and postcolonial theory, has devoted considerable attention to the production and dissemination of feminist knowledge in the context of global hierarchies of power. Many scholars have criticized the problematic legacy of Western Enlightenment philosophy, along with its humanistic conception of identity, its arrogant claims to universalist knowledge, and its notion of modernity, which locates progress and development squarely in the West, while the non-Western world remains mired in ignorance and tradition (Grewal and Kaplan 1994; Mohanty 2003). Attention has increasingly been paid to the unequal circulation of feminist knowledge, whereby feminist theory (with a capital *T*) is situated in the United States (or France) while non-Western women become the objects of that theory, the "subalterns" in whose name white, already emancipated, First World feminists may speak (Spivak 1988a).

While this critique has been extremely important in uncovering the relationship between power and knowledge in a transnational context, it has tended to focus—somewhat paradoxically—on feminist theory in the West.[4] Postcolonial feminist theorists have directed their critical energy inward, preferring to deconstruct the humanistic, modernist, or ethnocentric assumptions of Western feminist theory (John 1996). The unintended consequence of these critiques has been a centering (rather than a decentering) of feminist theory in the metropoles of the First World rather than an exploration of what actually happens when feminist knowledge and knowledge practices flow from the West to other parts of the globe and how "Western" feminism gets taken up outside the United States. It seems to be assumed that Western feminist conceptions and knowledge practices are automatically irrelevant for or even harmful to feminists in non-Western contexts. But, as Roy (2001) has noted, the assumption that universals are simply the outcome of First World hegemonies makes it difficult to imagine "careful and responsible modes of universalization" in feminist knowledge practices. In short, while sophisticated theoretical reflections on the feminist politics of knowledge in a global context abound, little attention has been paid to the vicisitudes of feminist knowledge practices on the ground and to how feminist knowledge travels and is transformed in ways that might make it oppositional in different locations.

One look at the international impact of *OBOS* as a feminist knowledge project belies the assumption that feminist knowledge that is relevant in the West will automatically be irrelevant for non-Western women. Aside from the fact that it is unclear why the modernization projects of other nations should not be subjected to the same critical scrutiny as the modernization projects of the West (Narayan 1998), the notions of modernity, humanism, and ethnocentrism are hardly limited to the West. The translations of *OBOS* suggest that a more complicated approach is needed. For example, the fact that discourses of equality originated in the West and many exclusions have since been enacted in their name does not mean that these discourses cannot be rearticulated outside the United States in ways that will make them oppositional. The notion of women's reproductive rights—which provides the undisputed ideological lynchpin of *OBOS*—obviously draws on Western notions of equality (with all their drawbacks). Nevertheless, the notion of reproductive rights has proved to be an effective rallying cry for feminist health activism internationally and has been strategic in empowering women in many contexts outside the United States (Petchesky 2003, 1995). It would be shortsighted to dismiss it with the "poison skull" label of ethnocentrism merely because it employs a modernist discourse and politics of rights, equality, and collective struggle (Pfeil 1994, 224).

In the present inquiry, I have shown how non-Western feminist scholars and activists from very different social, cultural, and geo-political locations have freely borrowed from the U.S. *OBOS*, including its concepts of individualism, choice, and informed consent. While these concepts were clearly modernist in origin, they could easily be used (albeit flexibly and strategically) to empower women in the context of their own (often very different) modernization projects. A case in point is the Bulgarian *OBOS*, which I discussed in chapter 6, in which the individualism of the U.S. book is embraced and rearticulated into a strategy for gendered citizenship and social change as an oppositional response to the postcommunist legacy of collectivist ideologies and state-imposed equality between the sexes. The Bulgarian case illustrates that rather than summarily dismissing Western feminism it makes more sense to explore how feminist concepts and practices associated with the West (e.g., the language and politics of rights, equality,

and collective solidarity) are taken up and rearticulated as potentially useful discourses within the contested terrain of oppositional feminist politics.

In other words, rather than viewing *OBOS* as just another typically U.S. feminist book about women's health, it should be regarded as a traveling theory par excellence. It is a prime example of how feminist knowledge and knowledge practices can travel in ways that both take up and reinscribe, but also transform and decenter, Western theory. By looking at how women in other contexts appropriated *OBOS*, a valuable site for theoretical exploration is opened up, offering an opportunity for analyzing how and why feminist knowledge can become oppositional at specific moments in time and in particular locations. Ironically, paying closer attention to the diverse sources and character of non-Western feminist knowledge practices might do more to revitalize Western feminist theory than the most "rigorously reflexive meta-theoretical ruminations" on its own intellectual practices (Stacey 2001, 102).[5]

As Edward Said (1983) argued in his seminal essay on traveling theory, what happens to a theory when it travels is at least as interesting as the "original" for what it can tell us about the limitations and problems, but also the possibilities, of the original. As traveling theory, *OBOS* has shown that it has a unique capacity to generate endless alternatives—a capacity that is, when all is said and done, what critical consciousness is all about (Said 1983, 247). For those theorists interested in decentering First World feminist theory, it may well be time to stop focusing on those theories that are most firmly embedded in the context that is being criticized (the U.S. academy and Western philosophy) and begin considering theories that have demonstrated that they are capable of movement and transformation. For anyone interested in the possibilities of a critical, nonimperialistic, feminist theory on a global scale, any theory with such a capacity clearly deserves our most serious attention.

Transnational Feminist Practice

Finally, the making of *OBOS* and its travels have implications for how transnational feminist practice should be theorized. This inquiry has critically engaged with the ideological commitment to internationalism that assumes that feminism can encompass all women regardless of nationality, uniting them against the masculine aberrations of fascism, imperialism, and war.[6] In its most recent incarnation, this dream of international feminist solidarity has come to be known as transnational feminism. This version of international feminist politics rejects binaries such as the West and the rest, global and local, and center and periphery, assuming instead that women are linked by globally structured relations of power that influence their lives at every level in ways that are both varied and historically specific (Grewal and Kaplan 1994, 13). Women are viewed as having different experiences, different needs, and different struggles depending on the particularities of their local circumstances, as well as their location within a global nexus of power. This conception of transnational feminism assumes that, while feminist alliances are necessary and desirable, they are also invariably infused with inequalities and hierarchies. It is essential, therefore, that feminists do not assume a natural affinity based on a shared gender identity but rather acknowledge their complicities in national histories of imperialism, colonialism, and slavery. Differences rather than similarities among women should be drawn on as an occasion for global dialogues about common issues and common struggles. That these alliances are complicated and often fraught with contradictions is illustrated by the recent emergence of feminist NGOS that adopt agendas inspired by the United Nations and engage in international coalitions aimed at helping Third World women. These coalitions can involve mainly urban, middle-class, white feminists ("globetrotting feminists") from different parts of the world who meet at international megaconferences to set feminist agendas, often to the detriment of the local activism of community-based women's groups (Alvarez 1998; Thayer 2000). While these transnational feminist alliances are undoubtedly undertaken out of a desire for international feminist solidarity, in practice they sometimes exacerbate inequalities among women at a local level and even deradicalize local feminist politics (Mendoza 2002). Thus, transnational feminism requires constant vigilance in order to ensure that global linkages between women remain mutually empowering (Mohanty 2003). However, by looking at how feminists actually work across lines of difference in the context of transnational alliances, some of the pessimism of this important critique can be tempered by a more realistic and simultaneously more hopeful perspective on transnational feminist politics.[7]

In the present inquiry, I have shown how the alliances generated in the course of translating *OBOS* bear many of the features of what might be called *good* transnational feminist practice—that is, practice based on the acknowledgment of differences among women, on an awareness of privilege and complicity in national histories of domination, and an attempt to discover common concerns and struggles.

As we have seen, *OBOS* went from an almost exclusively U.S. project to a transnational feminist project with offshoots across the globe. The "center" of *OBOS* gradually moved to the "periphery," whereby the translations increasingly became the raison d'être for the project as a whole. In the wake of waning sales and uncertainties concerning future editions of *OBOS* within the United States, the translation projects clearly were instrumental in the longevity and success of *OBOS* as feminist project. In this context, the U.S. collective increasingly took on a supportive role, facilitating the adaptation of the book in other contexts. The help provided was of the "no strings attached" variety, sometimes interventionist, sometimes "hands off," depending on the needs of the local groups doing the translations. Members of the U.S. collective was consistently mindful of their status, using their financial and organizational resources, international status, expertise, and substantial international network to help local women's groups do what they wanted to do. Moreover, the groups involved in translating and disseminating *OBOS* did not passively adopt the agenda set out by their U.S. "sisters" but rather used the project in ways that fit their own needs and political agendas, sometimes explicitly in opposition to the U.S. project. Thus, *OBOS* provides a promising example of how U.S. feminism can be decentered while maintaining an awareness of and responsibility toward the unequal division in resources (financial, institutional, and informational) between First and Third World feminists. It shows how feminist political practice can recognize and (re)dress global power hierarchies while remaining mutually beneficial for all parties concerned.

However, *OBOS* is not simply an illustration of how transnational feminism works in practice. It also suggests some directions in which contemporary scholarship on transnational feminist politics should be elaborated. While postcolonial feminist scholarship tends to highlight difference as the sine qua non of any feminist alliance across national borders, the transnational alliances around *OBOS* indicate that the similarities or commonalities among women may be equally important.[8] Despite its commitment to the struggles of non-Western women, postcolonial feminist scholarship has not paid sufficient attention to the actual practices of activists from the First and Third Worlds who are already working across lines of difference. As a result, the lessons that these practices might teach us have been foreclosed in advance by a perspective that commits itself to "unbridgeable distance between differently constituted individuals or groups" (Pfeil 1994, 226).

Ultimately, a political perspective of "unity in difference," a determination to remain "full of hope," may be just as—or even more—important for a transnational feminist politics than the recognition of the many differences and conflicts that divide us (Pfeil 1994, 227). The efforts of feminist activists already working across borders to create workable coalitions attest to an awareness of conflict but also to a belief in the possibility of solidarity. As we have seen, this unity in difference does not have to be of the "common world of women" variety that has been so perceptively criticized by Mohanty (2003) and others. Nor does it require a shared identity, a common experience of oppression, or even a collective political ideology. As the translation projects have shown, community can be constructed imaginatively as a common history that begins with a small group of Boston women meeting in 1970 to talk about their bodies and continues through space and time to include Serbian activists, Japanese feminist scholars, Armenian physicians, and even Tibetan nuns. Incommensurable differences in personal history, social and cultural contexts, and geopolitical circumstances are not forgotten but momentarily transcended in order to create a liminal unity. The global feminist imagined community that is generated through working together on *OBOS* is a shared political project—a project aimed at developing empowering knowledge practices concerning women's bodies, sexuality, and health.

On a Hopeful Note

Up until now, I have dealt with the reasons for a hopeful assessment of *OBOS* and its travels. It's unlikely that *OBOS* could have emerged at a different time or in a different place than during the exuberant activism of the sixties in the United States. Nor could it have happened without a group of women (the "founders") with the vision and motivation to launch such a project and the stamina to persevere through several more decades. It required a mass audience eager to read and be inspired by what the book had to say. But the success and longevity of *OBOS* cannot be attributed to these historically specific conditions alone. Processes of globalization have enabled knowledge and information to circulate around the globe. People are on the move (willingly or unwillingly), making the borders between nations and cultures more permeable and creating opportunities for cross-cultural exchange. Information and communication technologies make global connections possible across time and space. The global expansion of capital has done much to increase disparities between the postindustrial nations of the First and the Third Worlds. However, while the threatening cloud of globalization has given us ample reason for pessimism, it has also provided cause for optimism, particularly because it has enabled what Appadurai (2000) has called "grassroots globalization" or "globalization from below."

It is my contention that the global dissemination of *OBOS*—its seemingly unstoppable ability to cross borders—is just such an example of grassroots globalization. Despite its limitations, it has—through its myriad transformations—invariably provided opportunities for dialogue among differently embodied and differently located women. While these dialogues are hardly a sinecure for the global empowerment of women, they offer the possibility of understanding points of divergence and intersection among women across multiple borders, whether personal, cultural, national, or political.

Throughout this inquiry, I have been puzzled over the willingness of many feminist groups to undergo enormous hardship in order to get a mere book translated. I have wondered at the equanimity with which they struggled to finish the book only to have their publishers balk at giving it proper distribution. And I have observed with growing despair how foundations are more than willing to finance translation projects under the banner of international feminism and yet have no interest in the less sexy and more mundane task of keeping these projects afloat once the book has come out. And yet, despite all odds, those women involved in *OBOS*, both within and outside the United States, seem prepared to carry on, taking difficulties in stride in order to produce new editions of the book. It is, ultimately, the process of collaboration rather than the outcome that justifies the enormous expenditure of time and effort and makes the project worth doing.

The process of transforming *OBOS*, whether updating it for a new generation of readers or translating it for another audience, involves getting women together and discussing the book against the backdrop of their specific experiences. It involves finding ways to make the book interrogate and speak across lines of difference shaped by class, race, ethnicity, sexual orientation, and more. This process invariably entails introducing feminist discourses and initiating collective forms of political activity that can make sense in specific locations. This project of cultural translation—in the broadest sense of the word—is an occasion for what can become a transnational, cross-cultural dialogue among women loosely united under the banner of a shared, but differently conceived, feminist political project. Such encounters inevitably provide an opportunity for what Lugones (1990) has called "world traveling"—the delight and pain of entering another's world, in learning "what it is to be them and what it is to be ourselves in their eyes" (401).

It is, of course, an open question whether such encounters will provide the kind of dialogue necessary for mutually empowering and reflexive transnational feminism. It may not always be possible for future editions of *OBOS* to maintain a commitment to the critical politics of knowledge that made it oppositional and translatable to other contexts: its commitment to women's embodied experience as critical resource; its critical engagement with dominant forms of knowledge; and its

conviction that all knowledge is situated and partial, requiring ongoing reflection and critique. However, based on the present inquiry into the making of *OBOS* and its travels as an epistemological project, my inclination is to end this book on a note of optimism and an appreciation for the hopeful glimpse that this particular feminist project provides of what might someday become a better world.

REFERENCES
A list of references is available in the original source.

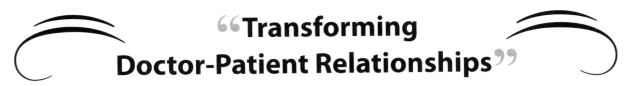

"Transforming Doctor-Patient Relationships"

by Sheryl Ruzek

Historians often ponder how books change history. *Our Bodies, Ourselves*, the enormously popular and influential work, will long be studied for igniting and sustaining a worldwide women's health movement. It should also be studied for how it transformed doctor-patient relationships and why it is such a trusted source of health information.

The book began in a small discussion group on 'women and their bodies' at a Boston women's conference in 1969. It grew into a course on women and their bodies and finally into a book with global appeal.[1] Between 1973 and 2005, the Collective published seven English language and two Spanish language editions in the USA and over 20 foreign language editions. Within five years of its first publication it was a bestseller, and by 1999 had sold over four million copies.

In her history of the women's health movement, Morgan argues that it would be difficult to exaggerate the impact of *Our Bodies, Ourselves*. It filled the void where there existed few popular books on women's health. Many colleges, universities and medical schools adopted it as a text.[2] It was unique in that it gave voice to women's own experiences of reproductive health and body issues. Elevating and validating women's experiential knowledge, the Collective broke new ground in medical com-

munication. The authors urged women to demand answers and explanations and to insist on enough information to negotiate the healthcare system. They envisioned creating a new type of partnership between patient and doctor that bore almost no resemblance to the model that existed. In the new model, it was envisioned that doctors and patients would have different responsibilities with the latter having ultimate control.

Our Bodies, Ourselves evolved through a dialogue whereby ordinary readers communicated with the Collective to get information, lodge concerns and complaints, and suggest revisions to the book. The Collective was urged to add information relevant to an ever-growing array of 'people like me'. As they corresponded with their readers, they enhanced coverage for women with disabilities and women of colour, weathered tumultuous storms over how to address lesbian health issues, and expanded the scope and coverage of a growing array of issues. Kline's research on letters from women to members of the Collective during the 1970s and 1980s details how critical a role readers played in the evolution of this work.[3]

Finding ways to include many voices and yet retaining control over the final product posed many challenges. Invited contributors and people who corresponded

"Transforming Doctor-Patient Relationships," by Sheryl Ruzek, reproduced from *Journal of Health Services Research & Policy* 2007; vol. 12: pp. 181–182, with permission from Royal Society of Medicine Pess, London.

sometimes had conflicting views on what was important. Keeping the book affordable was always at odds with expanding coverage. Editorial effort increased exponentially. For the 2005 edition, editors Judy Norsigian, Heather Stephenson and Kiki Zeldes managed and coordinated the work of 102 contributors and hundreds of 'voices' with the help of a 'tone and voice editor' and a photo editor.

The evolution of *Our Bodies, Ourselves* is visible in the front matter of each edition. For example, the preface to the 25th Anniversary Edition, written by feminist luminaries Byllye Avery, Helen Rodriguez-Trias and Gloria Steinem anchored the volume in a continuation of second wave feminism.[4] The current edition takes a very different approach. Reaching out to a new generation of women for whom second wave feminism is history, not lived experience, the front matter includes only a brief 'Introduction'. A short letter from the founders tells readers that the history of the book is available on the web.

How has the content evolved? The 1973 edition focused-heavily on women's changing sense of self in response to the second wave of feminism. It encouraged women to change internalized sexist volume covered the anatomy and physiology of reproduction and sexuality, the social and cultural aspects of sexuality and relationships, and included a controversial chapter written by a Boston gay collective that was replaced in later editions. Short chapters on nutrition, exercise, rape, self-defence, venereal disease, birth control, abortion, deciding about having children and childbearing were followed by a limited discussion of the menopause. A well-formulated critique of the American healthcare system rounded out the 275-page paperback that sold for $2.98, but with substantial discounts to clinics and women's groups.

The 2005 edition, an 832-page encyclopedic version, opens with chapters on body image, eating well, drugs, exercise, complementary health practices, emotional wellbeing, environmental and occupational health, and violence and abuse against women. Expanded sections address relationships and sexuality, sexual health, reproductive choices and childbearing, and over 170 pages are devoted to growing older and to medical problems and procedures. The companion website provides breaking health news, as well as the history of the book.[5] For women living under conditions of censorship, web-based information supplements that can be published or promoted locally.

The organization itself has changed. The book is no longer produced by a collective but by an incorporated entity with a board and a unionized staff. What has not changed is a commitment to validating women's personal experience and organizing for change. The accolades continue to pour in. Bylle Avery, founder of the National Black Women's Health Project, has called it the 'bible for women's health' and the *Journal of the American Medical Association* has hailed it as 'A mother lode of information and resources for the client/consumer and the physician'.

How did it come to be such a trusted source? Bell's account of how editions were painstakingly updated to translate scientific information into health information for women shows how committed the Collective was to producing evidence-based information.[6] But the success of the book really lies in the powerful combination of presenting solid evidence framed in terms of self-determination, patients' rights and social justice through women's own voices. Women's experience, not professional opinion, made this groundbreaking volume so powerful. While its appeal has always been its usefulness as a source of personal health information, it continues to confront the politics of women's health. By producing a personal health manual that doubles as an organizing tool, it has been able to retain its core values and feminist principles even as it became institutionalized.

The organization's global impact continues to grow from working collaboratively with women's groups worldwide to developing local editions that are far more than translations.[7] Twenty-one adaptations have been nurtured around the globe, each reflecting the social and cultural conditions of women in different countries. It has inspired groups in Tibet, Senegal, India, Denmark, South Africa and Egypt to develop similar types of books that put health knowledge directly into the hands of women.

The Collective, along with other self-help health and consumer groups that emerged in the late 1960s, played a critical role in transforming patients from passive recipients of healthcare into active consumers. Today's concept of shared decision-making in healthcare is firmly rooted in the principles and practices of health communication set forth in *Our Bodies, Ourselves*. Scholars now debate which patients prefer being active decision-makers and even ask if passive patients should be urged to take more active roles in decision-making. These controversies reflect the diffusion of models of doctor-patient communication and relationships that the book set out to create over three decades ago.

As healthcare in the USA has changed, *Our Bodies, Ourselves* has attempted to suggest how to manage those changes. For example, because primary care visits are largely limited to 15 minutes, with insufficient time to resolve many of women's most pressing issues, the book suggests that women improve doctor visits by bringing in their own information or even an advocate. A new ideal model of the doctor-patient relationship is also evolving. A woman's voice in the current edition tells readers, 'Friends now marvel at my close relationship with my current doctor and my ability to talk back, question, and disagree with him and his colleagues. He respects me and trusts me to tell him what is going on, and I, in turn, trust him to listen, make suggestions, and consult with me before any action is taken'. As elusive as this type of relationship may be to many, if not most women, its inclusion suggests an evolving model of health communication that was unimaginable when the book first appeared.

Looking back over 35 years, it has retained its core strategy of providing the best available evidence accompanied by women's own voices. It has also earned the distinction of being a trusted source of information. That trust is deeply embedded in the organization's steadfast refusal to accept funding from the pharmaceutical industry or other sources that would create conflicts of interest. This sets it apart from many of the newer, highly professionalized women's health advocacy groups that have flourished from such infusions of resources.[8] As one of a small number of women's health organizations that has survived beyond the active phase of the second wave of feminism,[9] *Our Bodies, Ourselves* continues to be a source of trustworthy health information for women. As such, it is well worth another look.

REFERENCES
A list of references is available in the original source.

Tales Out of Medical School

by Adriane Fugh-Berman

With the growth of the women's health movement and the influx of women into medical school, there has been abundant talk of a new enlightenment among physicians. Last summer, many Americans were shocked when Frances Conley, a neurosurgeon on the faculty of Stanford University's medical school, resigned her position, citing "pervasive sexism." Conley's is a particularly elite and male-dominated subspecialty, but her story is not an isolated one. I graduated from the Georgetown University School of Medicine in 1988, and while medical training is a sexist process anywhere, Georgetown built disrespect for women into its curriculum.

A Jesuit school, most recently in the news as the alma mater of William Kennedy Smith, Georgetown has an overwhelmingly white, male and conservative faculty. At a time when women made up one-third of all medical students in the United States, and as many as one-half at some schools, my class was 73 percent male and more than 90 percent white.

The prevailing attitude toward women was demonstrated on the first day of classes by my anatomy instructor, who remarked that our elderly cadaver "must have been a Playboy bunny" before instructing us to cut off her large breasts and toss them into the thirty-gallon trash can marked "cadaver waste." Barely hours into our training, we were already being taught that there was nothing to be learned from examining breasts. Given the fact that one out of nine American women will develop breast cancer in her lifetime, to treat breasts as extraneous tissue seemed an appalling waste of an educational opportunity, as well as a not-so-subtle message about the relative importance of body parts. How many of my classmates now in practice, I wonder, regularly examine the breasts of their female patients?

My classmates learned their lesson of disrespect well. Later in the year one carved a tick-tack-toe on a female cadaver and challenged others to play. Another gave a languorous sigh after dissecting female genitalia, as if he had just had sex. "Guess I should have a cigarette now," he said.

Ghoulish humor is often regarded as a means by which med students overcome fear and anxiety. But it serves a darker purpose as well: Depersonalizing our cadaver was good preparation for depersonalizing our patients later. Further on in my training an ophthalmologist would yell at me when I hesitated to place a small instrument meant to measure eye pressure on a fellow student's cornea because I was afraid it would hurt. "You have to learn to treat patients as lab animals," he snarled at me.

On the first day of an emergency medicine rotation in our senior year, students were asked who had had experience placing a central line (an intravenous line placed into a major vein under the clavicle or in the neck). Most of the male students raised their hands. None of the women did. For me, it was graphic proof of inequity in teaching; the men had had the procedure taught to them, but the women had not. Teaching rounds were often, for women, a spectator sport. One friend told me how she craned her neck to watch a physician teach a minor surgical procedure to a male student; when they were done the physician handed her his dirty gloves to discard. I have seen a male attending physician demonstrate an exam on a patient and then wade through several female medical students to drag forth a male in order to teach it to him. This sort of discrimination was common and quite unconscious: The women just didn't register as medical students to some of the doctors. Female students, for their part, tended (like male ones) to gloss over issues that might divert attention, energy or focus from the all-important goal of getting through their training. "Oh, they're just of the old school," a female classmate remarked to me as if being ignored by our teachers was really rather charming, like having one's hand kissed.

A woman resident was giving a radiology presentation and I felt mesmerized. Why did I feel so connected and involved? It suddenly occurred to me that the female physician was regularly meeting my eyes; most of the male residents and attendings made eye contact only with the men.

"Why are women's brains smaller than men's?" asked a surgeon of a group of male medical students in the doctors' lounge (I was in the room as well, but was apparently invisible). "Because they're missing logic!" Guffaws all around.

Such instances of casual sexism are hardly unique to Georgetown, or indeed to medical schools. But at Georgetown female students also had to contend with outright discrimination of a sort most Americans probably think no longer exists in education. There was one course women were not allowed to take. The elective in sexually transmitted diseases required an interview with the head of the urology department, who was teaching the course. Those applicants with the appropriate genitalia competed for invitations to join the course (a computer was supposed to assign us electives, which we had ranked in order of preference, but that process had been circumvented for this course). Three women who requested an interview were told that the predominantly gay male clinic where the elective was held did not allow women to work there. This was news to the clinic's executive director, who stated that women were employed in all capacities.

The women who wanted to take the course repeatedly tried to meet with the urologist, but he did not return our phone calls. (I had not applied for the course, but became involved as an advocate for the women who wanted to take it.) We figured out his schedule, waylaid him in the hall and insisted that a meeting be set up.

At this meeting, clinic representatives disclosed that a survey had been circulated years before to the clientele in order to ascertain whether women workers would be accepted; 95 percent of the clients voted to welcome women. They were also asked whether it was acceptable to have medical students working at the clinic; more than 90 percent approved. We were then told that these results could not be construed to indicate that clients did not mind women medical students; the clients would naturally have assumed that "medical student" meant "male medical student." Even if that were true, we asked, if 90 percent of clients did not mind medical students and 95 percent did not mind women, couldn't a reasonable person assume that female medical students would be acceptable? No, we were informed. Another study would have to be done.

We raised formal objections to the school. Meanwhile, however, the entire elective process had been postponed by the dispute, and the blame for the delay and confusion was placed on us. The hardest part of the struggle, indeed, was dealing with the indifference of most of our classmates—out of 206, maybe a dozen actively supported us—and with the intense anger of the ten men who had been promised places in the course.

"Just because you can't take this course," one of the men said to me, "why do you want to ruin it for the rest of us?" It seemed incredible to me that I had to argue that women should be allowed to take the same courses as men. The second or third time someone asked me the same question, I suggested that if women were not allowed to participate in the same curriculum as the men, then in the interest of fairness we should get a 50 percent break on our $22,500 annual tuition. My colleague thought that highly unreasonable.

Eventually someone in administration realized that not only were we going to sue the school for discrimination but that we had an open-and-shut case. The elective in sexually transmitted diseases was canceled, and from its ashes arose a new course, taught by the same man, titled "Introduction to Urology." Two women were admitted. When the urologist invited students to take turns working with him in his office, he scheduled the two female students for the same day—one on which only women patients were to be seen (a nifty feat in a urology practice).

The same professor who so valiantly tried to prevent women from learning anything unseemly about sexually transmitted diseases was also in charge of the required course in human sexuality (or, as I liked to call it, he-man sexuality). Only two of the eleven lectures focused on women; of the two lectures on homosexuality, neither mentioned lesbians. The psychiatrist who co-taught the class treated us to one lecture that amounted to an apology for rape: Aggression, even hostility, is normal in sexual relations between a man and a woman, he said, and inhibition of aggression in men can lead to impotence.

We were taught that women do not need orgasms for a satisfactory sex life, although men, of course, do; and that inability to reach orgasm is only a problem for women with "unrealistic expectations." I had heard that particular lecture before in the backseat of a car during high school. The urologist told us of couples who came to him for sex counseling because the woman was not having orgasms; he would reassure them that this is normal and the couple would be relieved. (I would gamble that the female half of the couple was anything but relieved.) We learned that oral sex is primarily a homosexual practice, and that sexual dysfunction in women is often caused by "working." In the women-as-idiots department, we learned that when impotent men are implanted with permanently rigid penile prostheses, four out of five wives can't tell that their husbands have had the surgery.

When dealing with sexually transmitted diseases in which both partners must be treated, we were advised to vary our notification strategy according to marital status. If the patient is a single man, the doctor should write the diagnosis down on a prescription for his partner to bring to her doctor. If the patient is a married man, how-

ever, the doctor should contact the wife's gynecologist and arrange to have her treated without knowledge of what she is being treated for. How to notify the male partner of a female patient, married or single, was never revealed.

To be fair, women were not the only subjects of outmoded concepts of sexuality. We also received anachronistic information about men. Premature ejaculation, defined as fewer than ten thrusts(!) was to be treated by having the man think about something unpleasant, or by having the woman painfully squeeze, prick or pinch the penis. Aversive therapies such as these have long been discredited.

Misinformation about sexuality and women's health peppered almost every course (I can't recall any egregious wrongs in biochemistry). Although vasectomy and abortion are among the safest of all surgical procedures, in our lectures vasectomy was presented as fraught with long-term complications and abortion was never mentioned without the words "peritonitis" and "death" in the same sentence. These distortions represented Georgetown's Catholic bent at its worst. (We were not allowed to perform, or even watch abortion procedures in our affiliated hospitals.) On a lighter note, one obstetrician assisting us in the anatomy lab told us that women shouldn't lift heavy weights because their pelvic organs will fall out between their legs.

In our second year, several women in our class started a women's group, which held potlucks and offered presentations and performances: A former midwife talked about her profession, a student demonstrated belly dancing, another discussed dance therapy and one sang selections from *A Chorus Line*. This heavy radical feminist activity created great hostility among our male classmates. Announcements of our meetings were defaced and women in the group began receiving threatening calls at home from someone who claimed to be watching the listener and who would then accurately describe what she was wearing. One woman received obscene notes in her school mailbox, including one that contained a rape threat. I received insulting cards in typed envelopes at my home address; my mother received similar cards at hers.

We took the matter to the dean of student affairs, who told us it was "probably a dental student" and suggested we buy loud whistles to blow into the phone when we received unwanted calls. We demanded that the school attempt to find the perpetrator and expel him. We were told that the school would not expel the student but that counseling would be advised.

The women's group spread the word that we were collecting our own information on possible suspects and that any information on bizarre, aggressive, antisocial or misogynous behavior among the male medical students should be reported to our designated representative. She was inundated with a list of classmates who fit the bill. Finally, angered at the school's indifference, we solicited the help of a prominent woman faculty member. Although she shamed the dean into installing a hidden camera across from the school mailboxes to monitor unusual behavior, no one was ever apprehended.

Georgetown University School of Medicine churns out about 200 physicians a year. Some become good doctors despite their training, but many will pass on the misinformation and demeaning attitudes handed down to them. It is a shame that Georgetown chooses to perpetuate stereotypes and reinforce prejudices rather than help students acquire the up-to-date information and sensitivity that are vital in dealing with AIDS, breast cancer, teen pregnancy and other contemporary epidemics. Female medical students go through an ordeal, but at least it ends with graduation. It is the patients who ultimately suffer the effects of sexist medical education.

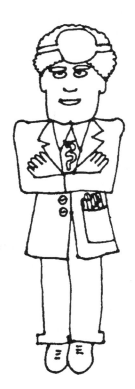

Is Medical School the right choice for *you?*
A SELF-EVALUATION TEST FOR THE PRE-MEDICAL STUDENT
Answer true or false

T   F

☐   ☐   1. Mothers often overreact to the most trivial symptoms in their children.

☐   ☐   2. Mothers are often guilty of denial followed by neglect in not bringing a symptomatic child to the doctor.

☐   ☐   3. Women often imagine breast lumps.

☐   ☐   4. Women should examine their breasts often enough, but not too often.*

☐   ☐   5. Informing patients of the side effects of the drugs prescribed for them will cause the patients to experience these side effects in their most virulent form.

☐   ☐   6. Women are sexually excited by gynecological examinations.

☐   ☐   7. Patients never ask the really interesting questions.

☐   ☐   8. A certain amount of physical discomfort is to be expected in anyone over 35, and old people should keep their symptoms to themselves.

☐   ☐   9. No doctor can ever really be guilty of malpractice.

☐   ☐   10. Most people when asked to describe your personality would say, "He's not real warm."

Too often if the lump disappears in a few months; *not often* enough if the lump turns out to be malignant.

ANSWERS: You know who you are.

"What Impact Have Women Physicians Had on Women's Health?"

by Judith Lorber

The proportion of women in medicine in the United States is approaching that of men, but women physicians are still the minority in positions of power. Research has shown that women physicians order more preventive tests for women patients, are more attuned to patients' psychosocial needs, and have developed more patient-oriented communication styles than men physicians. Recent organized efforts of women physicians have brought attention to many gender gaps in medical research and practice. If more women move into policy-making positions, especially in education and research, their gender-sensitive perspective could permanently influence the profession as a whole.

Women have been entering medical schools in the United States in greater numbers since the 1960s. In the last decade, women have even outnumbered men in some medical school classes, including at Harvard. As in other countries where the proportion of women physicians is growing, it may be time to assess the impact women physicians have had on US medicine. Has their presence made a difference in women's healthcare, or have they assimilated men's biases and perspectives? What effect have women physicians' organizations had? What is the future role of women in American medicine?

Is Medicine Turning into Women's Work?

The changing structure of medical practice in countries with medical systems once dominated by men has led to an influx of women into medicine. In the United States before World War II, physicians were usually solo, fee-for-service practitioners with sole authority over their patients. Since 1945, medicine has been subject to more regulation and has been paid for by governments and an expanding insurance industry. As doctors' authority has been diluted and their income decreased, fewer white men have applied to medical school, leaving an occupational niche for women and nonwhite men, similar to what has happened in other desegregating occupations. Despite their increasing numbers, however, women physicians are not equitably represented in medical leadership. They are not usually mentored by senior men physicians for positions of authority in medical schools and research centers, and their rate of promotion in medical schools tends to be slower than that of men.

The structure of work and family life has not allowed women physicians with family responsibilities to add extensive administrative responsibilities or committee work to the time they spend with patients. Women physicians who remain single or enter into childless dual-career marriages could be formidable competitors for men with homemaker wives, but there is still a glass ceiling on how far women can rise in positions of authority.

As a result, the top positions in large medical centers, medical schools, and research centers are still predominantly held by men. These institutions develop medical knowledge, decide what medical students are taught, and determine practice standards for diagnosis and treatment. Because women are underrepresented in high-level positions as chiefs of service in hospitals, deans of medical schools, or directors of large research centers, they have yet to make much impact on the production and dissemination of medical knowledge and standards of practice. I believe that where they themselves are in control—in their own practices—they have made a difference for women patients.

Are Women Physicians Better for Women Patients?

Referral rates for breast and cervical cancer screening seem to depend on the gender of the doctor. Studies including thousands of patients in the United States have found large, statistically significant differences in the rate at which women and men physicians recommend these tests.

Even though coronary heart disease is the major cause of death for women in the United States, they are less likely than men to be routinely tested for cardiovascular symptoms and more likely to suffer unrecognized heart attacks. Women with severe symptoms are not as likely as men with lesser symptoms to be given coronary arteriography, catheterization, or bypass surgery. As a result, they are more likely to die of myocardial infarction than men of the same age, and the postoperative mortality rate for coronary artery bypass surgery has been found to be significantly higher in women than men.

In order to address problems like these, Bernadine Healy, MD, as director of the National Institutes of Health, established an Office of Research on Women's Health and began the Women's Health Initiative. The WHI not only studies the illnesses that affect women alone, but also looks at previously neglected gender differences in illnesses that affect women and men, such as acquired immune deficiency syndrome (AIDS).

Do Women Physicians Have More Caring Practice Styles?

Today, men and women physicians both say they have to understand their patients' daily lives, work and family roles, and emotional needs to adequately treat them for physical illness, but patients claim that women physicians are more "humane." Women physicians may act differently toward patients, or patients may feel they are less intimidating and so can be asked more questions and argued with. Women physicians tend to encourage patients to participate by asking what they expect and think—and by listening to their answers. They talk more to their patients, but, more important, allow patients to talk more as well, especially about personal and family issues. A study that found little difference in verbal communication between men and women physicians also found that women physicians' nonverbal communication styles were more supportive than those of men physicians. In comparing patients' behavior, they found that both men and women patients spoke more to women physicians, and that women patients offered more medical information to women than to men physicians. The women physicians encouraged their women patients' narratives with supportive statements, "uh-huhs," and nodding. In contrast, the women physicians' interactions with men patients, who were usually older than they were, showed evidence of tension and role strain.

In another study, 45 lesbians, half of whom were women of color, were more likely to evaluate men physicians negatively than they were women physicians. These patients wanted knowledge that would enable them to promote and maintain their own health and wellbeing, and they also appreciated being involved in the diagnosis and decisions about treatment.

The overall thrust of these studies of doctor-patient relationships in the United States, where seeing a woman doctor is a relatively new phenomenon for older patients, is that women physicians present themselves to patients as warm and supportive, which may be at odds with the expected image of authority and competence.

Because so many women physicians are in primary care, patients come to them with all their problems—major and minor illnesses, physical and emotional symptoms. There is a danger, then, that women will become "the de facto psychosocial experts in the care of patients and increasingly assume responsibility for the management of emotionally distressed patients." This expertise can have a backlash; patients may be more dissatisfied with their care if a woman doctor does not live up to their expectations.

Physicians of either gender in office practice generally prefer patients who allow them to carry out their work with a minimum of fuss and who are cooperative, trusting, appreciative, and responsive to treatment. In one study, however, more women than men physicians said they liked their patients. The differences patients perceive between men and women physicians may be a self-fulfilling prophecy. If patients think women physicians are more empathic, the women may cultivate an expressive style to meet patients' expectations. Women physicians may or may not be more attuned to the "whole patient" because they are women, but if patients think they are, they may prefer a woman physician, especially for primary care. Doctors in group practice or clinic settings, however, have a fixed time to spend with patients. They are usually not in a position to structure their delivery of healthcare to be sensitive to patients unless they are in their own solo or small group practices.

In sum, where they are in control of their work, women physicians have had a positive impact on women's healthcare through more extensive screening for life-threatening illnesses and through practice styles that are sensitive to patients' social and psychological problems.

Have Women Physicians Transformed Medicine?

In the 1970s in the United States, activists in the feminist health movement established client-run clinics for women patients that stressed education in health matters, gynecological self-examination, and alternative therapies. Their goal was to take the control of women's bodies out of what they saw as an oppressive medical system. The problem women patients faced, according to the ideas of the feminist health movement, was twofold: men physicians who allowed patients very little control over their own care, and medical research and practices that ignored many of women's needs.

Although the directors of feminist clinics preferred women physicians for their legally required medical backup, they were not trusted any more than men physicians because both had been trained in the masculinist medical curriculum. The activists in the feminist health movement thought that by educating women patients to be more assertive and knowledgeable health consumers, they would put pressure on the medical system to modify the way physicians were taught to practice. The feminist health movement, the influx of women physicians into obstetrics/gynecology, and the presence of mid-wives in hospital settings did change how pelvic examinations were done and made childbirth more participatory and family-oriented. But medicine in general continued to be insensitive to gender issues.

Much of the feminist health movement's critical thrust had been abandoned by the 1990s, but it left a heritage of clinics and managed care centers that offer woman-centered family practices and obstetrics/gynecology, often provided by women physicians. The consumer movement in healthcare has also enormously strengthened all patients' rights to question their care.

Have these individual assets coalesced into an impact on medicine as a whole?

The greater number of women physicians has tilted the gender balance; women are no longer a minority vulnerable to stereotyping and informal discrimination, but a visible, vocal, and increasingly powerful group. Numbers alone have not made the difference, however. Organizing *as* women professionals and *for* women patients has been equally important. The arguments over whether women physicians should form a separate "interest bloc" and whether women's health should be a separate spe-

cialty seem to have evolved into a strategy of wide-ranging woman-centered medicine.

In the last few years, women physicians in the United States have promoted research and held conferences on women's medical needs and insisted that trials of new drugs include women. A workshop held in 1997 called for participatory research based on "women's experience, both of their physiology and of their psychosocial, home, and work environments." Women physicians have called attention to the particular needs of lesbians and women with AIDS and disabilities, and to such human rights issues as female genital mutilation and politically motivated rape.

If women physicians are to make a transformative impact, their specialized knowledge of women's medical needs has to become part of medical school curricula, and their patient-oriented perspective has to be routinely incorporated into teaching and training. In addition, the gender-sensitive perspective developed in women's healthcare conferences and journals needs to become part of mainstream medical thinking and include men's gender-based risks and traumas as well. Making such an impact takes the authority, prestige, and resources held only by heads of medical institutions. When women are equal to men in these positions as well as in clinical practice, I predict that the differences women have made in their own practices, through their own medical organizations, and in their research and publications will be seen throughout the profession.

REFERENCES
A list of references is available in the original source.

Healthcare Reform
"A Woman's Issue"
by Catherine DeLorey

Dissatisfaction with the cost and quality of the healthcare available in the United States is increasing. With the Democratic take-over of Congress in the November elections, there is new interest in changing the healthcare system, but little agreement on the best alternative for improving access to healthcare.

Complicating this issue for women's health activists is the fact that—while women are often disproportionately affected by our healthcare system's problems—only fledgling efforts have been made to ensure that healthcare reform initiatives address women's concerns. It is important that current proposals consider women's

"Healthcare Reform—A Woman's Issue," by Catherine DeLorey, D.Ph., originally published in the *Women's Health Activist*, March/April 2007, pp. 4–5, the newsletter of the National Women's Health Network (NWHN). It is reprinted with the permission of the author and the NWHN.

healthcare needs, and for activists and advocates to support efforts that prioritize and recognize women's issues.

Access to Healthcare Is a Women's Issue

The failures of our current healthcare system greatly affect women, especially women of color. Women constitute more than 52 percent of the U.S. population, and are the major consumers of health services, as well as the traditional caretakers of their families' health. Women have greater annual healthcare expenses than men ($2,453 vs. $2,316) and pay a greater proportion of their healthcare expenses out-of-pocket (19 percent vs. 16 percent).[1] Women make 58 percent more visits per year to primary care physicians, and are more likely than men to take at least one prescription drug on a daily basis.[1]

Because women are disproportionately represented among low-wage workers and/or work in industries that do not offer benefits, they are more likely to be uninsured or under-insured than men. In fact, women work in jobs that are 15 percent less likely to offer healthcare and, because of their low incomes and high healthcare costs, women are 20 percent more likely than uninsured men to have trouble obtaining healthcare.[1] Women are also more likely to be dependent on spouses for coverage: they are more than twice as likely as men to receive employer-based health coverage as "dependents" through their spouses' insurance (26 percent vs. 11 percent).

This dependent status makes women vulnerable to losing their coverage as a result of being divorced or widowed.[2] The predominance of employer-based insurance also hampers lesbians from accessing health coverage through their partners, since many companies do not recognize domestic partners and, of course, with limited exceptions, gay and lesbians cannot get married.

Although American women tend to live longer than men, this is not the case for uninsured women, compared to uninsured men. Women who are uninsured tend to forgo getting healthcare, especially preventive services, and they are more likely not to fill prescriptions than are women with insurance coverage. Of the 17 million uninsured women in America, more than 67 percent did not seek healthcare because they could not afford it. The direct result of the way our healthcare system is structured is that women are more likely than men to be sick and to find health services unattainable.

Biological and physiological issues are not the only factors that influence women's concerns in health and healthcare. Other influences include women's social/cultural roles, and how we both use and are treated by the healthcare system. These other influences include inequities in healthcare that result in women traditionally not being included in clinical research studies on drugs and medical procedures; and not receiving the same rigorous care and treatment for cardiac problems as men do. In addition, important aspects of women's lives (such as pregnancy or menopause) are treated as medical conditions or diseases, rather than life experiences.

These problems—particularly access to healthcare—are magnified for women of color. Thirty-eight percent of Latinas and 23 percent of African American women are uninsured, compared to just 13 percent of White women.[3] Difficulties accessing healthcare are compounded for immigrant women who face both linguistic and cultural barriers to their receipt of healthcare. For undocumented women, the problems in accessing healthcare are compounded by State and Federal restrictions on their ability to use public health services.

Because women are more likely to be employed in industries that do not provide health insurance, and because they spend more time out of the workforce as caregivers and mothers, women are less likely to have adequate health insurance and more likely to face barriers in accessing care and other services. For these reasons, the fight for universal healthcare is a fight for equality and justice for all women. Only a system that guarantees access to affordable, comprehensive healthcares for everyone will resolve the healthcare disparities that women experience.

What Should Be Included in Women's Healthcare?

There can be no health security for women without protection of the full range of women's reproductive needs that include, but are not limited to, abortion services. Comprehensive reproductive healthcare supports a woman's right to information and services that both prevent pregnancy and help her to become pregnant when she wants to; that support her during a healthy pregnancy; and promote healthy outcomes for pregnancy.

In addition to comprehensive reproductive rights, the following principles are central to health system change that meets women's needs:

- Universal access to quality healthcare;
- Comprehensive health benefits for all women, employed or not;
- Access to health services from a variety of providers;
- Access to health services provided in a variety of settings;
- Systems accountable to women and other consumers; and
- Complete information for women to use to make own healthcare decisions.

Making Women's Needs a Central Priority

The only way to achieve an adequate health system for women is for women to work together to have our voices heard. It is critical that women's health advocates come together to support initiatives that prioritize women's healthcare needs. The following organizations are among the many that are working on healthcare reform:

- The Avery Institute for Social Change (www .averyinstitute.org), MergerWatch (www .mergerwatch.org), and the National Women's Health Network (www.nwhn.org) are working together on an effort called "Women Lead on Healthcare Reform". This effort mobilizes and unites advocates who are committed to achieving universal healthcare that meets women's comprehensive reproductive healthcare needs and works to ensure that any new system will meet women's comprehensive reproductive healthcare needs. More information is available on the organizational web sites.

- Women's Universal Health Initiative (www.wuhi .org) is a national organization dedicated to building diverse communities of women and work for

healthcare reform. In addition, the organization publishes a quarterly electronic newsletter on women and healthcare reform.

These initiatives are a start, but we must ensure that our voices are heard by those who are making decisions about the future of healthcare in the U.S. Those of us who are working in health reform organizations must raise awareness of women's needs, and keep advocates focused on the issue of comprehensive reproductive rights. Those of us in professional organizations need to speak out and make sure health reform and women's needs are included in all of our efforts. And, in our own communities, we all need to communicate about the importance of healthcare reform, and inform others about efforts to enhance women's health.

REFERENCES

1. Lambrew, J, *Diagnosing Disparities in Health Insurance for Women: A Prescription for Change*. NY: Commonwealth Fund, Aug. 2001.

2. Sered, S. "Seven Reasons Why Healthcare Coverage is a Women's Issue." Boston: Center for Women's Health and Human Rights, Suffolk University, 2006.

3. Salganicoff A, Ranji U, Wyn R. *Report: Women and Healthcare: A National Profile*. Kaiser Family Foundation: Menlo Park, CA, Summer, 2005.

 # "Worlds Apart"

by Ahuva Segal

I had left the Australian summer to intern with NWHN and spend time with my sister, and from the minute I stepped off the plane I found myself constantly (and unconsciously) comparing everything. Food portions? Very big! Cars? Even bigger! Houses? Bigger yet! But another subject that I found myself comparing was universal healthcare—something Australia has and the United States desperately needs.

Shortly after my arrival, another NWHN intern told me she had been feeling under the weather for several weeks. I encouraged her to visit a doctor and follow it up, since benign symptoms such as tiredness could mask a

more serious situation. She replied that she had no health insurance, and that seeing a doctor for such a "trivial" matter would cost her more than she could afford, especially if the doctor sent her for blood tests or other diagnostic examinations. I soon learned her story was familiar to millions of Americans. "How could this be," I asked myself "how could someone from a middle-class family, with a degree from a good university and a part-time job, not have any insurance?"

As my internship progressed, I became more grateful every day to be an Australian with benefits such as public health insurance. Australia's universal healthcare

"Young Feminists: Worlds Apart," by Ahuva Segal, originally published in the *Women's Health Activist*, March/April 2004, pp. 4–5, the newsletter of the National Women's Health Network (NWHN). It is reprinted with the permission of the author and the NWHN.

system (Medicare) is based on several guiding principles whose ultimate goal is to provide affordable treatment to all Australian citizens and permanent residents. The first principle is universality: the system should serve the needs of all Australians, independent of race, sex or income. The second principle is that access to care is dependent on the user's health needs, not his or her ability to pay for the services. Third, funding is based on general public taxation and income taxes, resulting in little or no cost to the patient at the point of service. Finally, the system is efficient and simple to use, with low overheads and consumer-friendly claims-processing.[1] The government also heavily subsidizes more than 1,350 prescription drugs under the Pharmaceutical Benefits Scheme.[2]

The Australian Medicare system has its share of critics. Many rail against long waiting lines for "elective" surgery in public hospitals, understaffed and underfunded public hospitals, and a lack of doctors who "bulk bill"—that is, bill Medicare directly for services, requiring no out-of-pocket fees from patients. The majority of Australian doctors still require full payment from patients, who then must file for a Medicare rebate capped at 85 percent.

Nevertheless, Medicare is a great improvement on the United States' so called "two-tiered" health system, which is actually three-tiered, as so many Americans are underinsured or uninsured but do not qualify for Medicaid. In fact, where Australia spends only 8.4 percent of its gross domestic product on universal healthcare, the United States spends more than 14 percent of its GDP on all health insurance—private and public alike.[3] Despite this, 14.6 percent of the U.S. population had no health insurance whatsoever in 2001.[4] Even employment does not guarantee health insurance; in 2002, 75 percent of uninsured people had jobs.[5]

Research shows the uninsured are less likely to access healthcare when needed, less likely to receive early diagnoses and early treatment for curable diseases, and more likely to die young.[6]

What Can We Do?

In January, the National Academy of Sciences released results from a study recommending that "universal insurance coverage is an important and achievable goal for the country."[7] Intended to put universal healthcare back on the national agenda, the report came at a fortuitous time, since politicians tend to pander to public demands during election years. Clearly, now is the time to rally support for the U.S. adoption of universal healthcare. Here are some suggestions to that end:

- Organize events to bring attention to the issue. Events can be as small as inviting lunch-time speakers to local schools or workplaces, or as large as weeklong health-awareness campaigns in the community.

- Organize a letter-writing campaign to your member of Congress. Encourage her or him to propose a bill that supports universal healthcare. Or encourage media interest by writing to local and national newspapers and TV stations and/or calling in to radio stations.

- Organize a coalition of like-minded individuals and businesses to join your fight for universal healthcare coverage.

REFERENCES

1. Defend Medicare, www.defendmedicare.info.
2. Medibank Private, www.medibank.com.au/productandservices/overseas/students/aushealth.asp.
3. "Medicare has served us well." *The Age* Newspaper 1998: December 23.
4. National Coalition on Health Care, www.nchc.org/facts/coverage.shtml.
5. Ibid.
6. *The High Cost of Being Poor*, www.vakids.org/FES/Health.pdf.
7. Pear R. "Academy of Sciences Calls for Universal Health Care by 2010." *New York Times* 2004: January 15.

amsa®

Cover Me NOW Campaign

Achieving Quality Healthcare for ALL

The American Medical Student Association supports a
Single-Payer National Health Insurance System
to achieve affordable, quality healthcare for all.

As physicians-in-training, we believe that **everyone has a fundamental right to accessing healthcare** and receiving both acute and preventive care to avoid illness and all the associated heartaches and costs.

What's the deal with our system:
- We have the most expensive per capita system in the entire industrialized world
- 46 million uninsured and millions more underinsured
- half of all personal bankruptcies in America are caused by healthcare bills—three-fourths of these are with people who *had* insurance at the onset of their illness
- 18,000 people DIE every year from lack of health insurance
- Our health outcomes are mediocre at best when compared to other rich nations

In the clinics and in the wards, AMSA members see every day the effect of a profit-driven healthcare system.
- Patients don't get better because they can't afford their medicines
- Our teaching hospitals are compromised financially because of the burden of uncompensated care
- When we decide how to treat a patient, we not only think of what is medically best for the patient, but whether the patient's insurance will cover the treatment.
- Insured patients decide not to follow-up on their care because they can't afford the deductibles and co-pays.

Private insurance companies value profit, not the public's health. Every cent they pay out in care is a cent less in profit. They deny care and avoid covering those who are sick or frail. We believe that the only way to ensure that everyone gets the care they need is to develop a system where profit is no longer the primary incentive. Our system has to value comprehensiveness and universality if we hope to improve the health of the American public.

Please visit www.amsa.org/uhc and www.sickocure.org for more information on our healthcare system and what you can do for real healthcare reform.

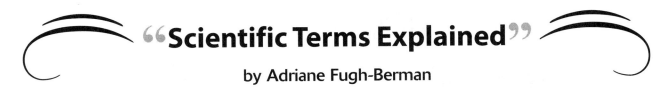

"Scientific Terms Explained"

by Adriane Fugh-Berman

Some of the terms you'll come across repeatedly in this book may be unfamiliar to you. It's worth learning them, since they're universally used to explain the results of scientific experiments. and knowing them will not only help you read this book but will stand you in good stead when you read about scientific experiments elsewhere.

Fortunately, scientific terminology isn't hard to learn. That doesn't mean you're going to remember every single term after reading this chapter once. Just let whatever sticks in your mind stick, and ignore the rest. Then, when you encounter a term you're not sure about, refer back to this chapter, or look it up in the index. (I've boldfaced the terms where they're defined in this chapter, to make them easy to find.)

Study is a very broad term that covers almost everything that's looked at objectively. A human participant in a study—that is, one of the people whose responses, reactions or whatever are being studied—is called a **subject.**

A **case study** is a report on one unusual subject by a doctor. Both case studies and stories patients report themselves are called **anecdotal evidence.** Doctors joke that if we see two cases, we say we're seeing something "time after time," and if we see three cases, we call it a **case series.** Joking aside, a case series should consist of at least five cases. Case series are useful for indicating that something interesting is going on that may merit more formal study.

A **survey** is a kind of study that reports the results of interviewing people on whom no **intervention** is done. (Compare *trial,* below.) Since nothing new—no new drug, procedure, dietary restriction or whatever—is given to them or done to them, we say surveys are **observational.** Like the three studies cited in the *Introduction,* surveys simply try to discover how common a disease, treatment. condition or behavior is—or what **correlations,** or **associations,** there may be between various diseases, behaviors, etc. (There's a subtle distinction between a *correlation* and an *association* that isn't worth going into here.)

A **positive correlation** means that the more you have of A, the more you have of B. A **negative** (or **inverse**) **correlation** means that the more you have of A, the *less*

you have of B. So, for example, there's a positive correlation between a high-fat diet and heart disease (the more fat you eat, the greater your chance of getting heart disease), and a negative correlation between eating broccoli and getting certain cancers (the more broccoli you eat, the smaller your chance of getting these cancers).

Correlations can't prove anything absolutely. For example, just because an increased number of storks in an area coincides with an increased number of births, that doesn't prove that storks bring babies.

How many people have a given condition at a given point in time is called its **prevalence** (for example, the number of color-blind people per 100,000 in the US today, or the number of people who were carrying tuberculosis bacteria on January 1, 1900). How many new cases of a condition occur over a given period of time is called its **incidence** (for example, the number of babies born in a given year who are color-blind, or the number of new TB cases in the last month). The study of prevalence and incidence falls into the field of **epidemiology,** which looks at patterns of disease and the factors that influence those patterns.

A **retrospective study** looks to the past for clues—you start with the disease and try to find out what caused it. For example, retrospective studies found that the prevalence of cigarette smoking among patients with lung cancer was higher than the prevalence of cigarette smoking among people without lung cancer. (Since you can't intervene in the past, all retrospective studies are observational.)

Retrospective studies can be large or small. To improve their quality, the **case-control** method is often used. This means that, when comparing a group with the disease to a group without it, the two groups are matched as closely as possible with regard to factors like age, sex, geographic location or any other variable that might affect the likelihood of getting the disease. The perfect case-control study would be of a group of identical twins where one twin in each pair developed a disease and the other twin in each pair didn't.

A **prospective study** is one in which subjects are followed forward in time instead of backward. Unlike retrospective studies, prospective studies can be either observational or interventional. Two famous prospective trials are the Nurses' Health Study, in which about 100,000 nurses have been answering annual questionnaires since 1976, and the Health Professionals Follow-up Study, in which about 50,000 physicians and other health professionals have been answering annual questionnaires since 1986.

By analyzing their responses, many associations have been discovered, including the positive correlation between hormone replacement therapy and breast cancer (that is, hormone replacement tends to increase one's risk of getting breast cancer) and the negative correlation between vitamin E intake and cardiovascular disease (that is, taking E tends to decrease heart disease risk).

Unlike a survey, a **trial** is a study in which the subjects receive an experimental intervention. Since you can only intervene in the present, not in the past, trials are always prospective. A **clinical trial** is one in which the subjects are human—as opposed to **preclinical trials** that use animals, bacteria, cells, etc.

In a **controlled trial,** at least two groups are compared. The **treated,** or **experimental** group receives the intervention, while the other—called the **control group** or simply the **control**—doesn't. Or different groups may receive different interventions. The groups studied in a trial are also called **arms.**

In a **placebo-controlled** trial, an inactive pill or procedure—the **placebo**—is given to the control group. *Placebo* is Latin for *I will please [you];* placebos got that name because any intervention, including simple attention, tends to make people feel better. Certain conditions, such as headaches, arthritis and hot flashes, are particularly responsive to placebos—as are some individuals.

Overall, the average **placebo effect** is an astonishing 33% (although it can range from much lower to much higher). In other words, an average of a third of the subjects in clinical trials will report significant improvement simply from being given a sugar pill (or some other placebo). So to demonstrate that a treatment works, you have to show that it does significantly better than the placebo that's given to the control group.

A **randomized** trial is one in which subjects are assigned to different groups as randomly as possible—by flipping a coin, or using a random number generator. If the researcher decides which subjects go into which group, or if the subjects assign themselves, intentional or unintentional **bias** can creep in and the groups may no longer be comparable (all the sicker patients might end up in one group, for example).

A **crossover** trial is one in which each patient is in each group at different times. For example, group A starts on drug X, and group B starts on the placebo; then, midway through the trial, the subjects are crossed over to the other arm (group A starts taking the placebo and group B starts taking the drug).

Blinding (sometimes, but less frequently, called **masking**) means that the researchers and/or the subjects don't know which group each subject is in. In a **single-blind** study, the subjects don't know but the researchers do (theoretically, it could also mean that the subjects know and the researchers don't, but there wouldn't be much point to that). Most nonsurgical studies are at least single-blind, since subjects' knowing whether they're getting an experimental treatment or a placebo is obviously likely to affect their responses.

In a **double-blind** study, neither the researchers nor the subjects know which group the subjects are in; all information is coded, and the code isn't broken until the end of the trial. (An exception is made when the difference between the two groups is so pronounced—everyone in the control group is dying, say, and everyone in the treated group is getting well—that it would be unethical to continue to deny the treatment to the controls.)

Double-blinding is important because researchers can give subtle, unconscious cues that can change subjects' responses quite independently of the treatment being tested. If the researchers don't know who's getting the treatment and who's getting the placebo, they can't put out those signals.

Saying that a treatment worked in 50% of the subjects tested obviously means a lot more if you're talking about 2000 subjects than if you're talking about two. So a good researcher involves statisticians before a trial begins in order to determine the **sample size** (the number of subjects) that will be necessary to show that the results are **statistically significant**—that is, unlikely to be due to chance.

Statistical significance isn't black and white; it's a matter of degree—what are the *odds* that this result was due to chance? It's measured by something called the **p value** (the *p* stands for *probability*). P values look like this: $<.1$, $<.05$, $<.01$, etc. ($<$ means *less than*). To translate a p value into English, move the decimal point two spaces to the right and say "percent."

A p value of $<.01$ means that the probability that the results occurred by chance is less than 1%. That's a good study. A p value of $<.1$ means that the probability that the results occurred by chance is less than 10%. That isn't so great, since it means that there's almost one chance in ten that the results are meaningless. In general, a p value of $<.05$ is considered statistically significant.

A large sample size helps to control for **confounding variables** (also called **confounding factors** or simply

confounders). For example, a small trial on cardiovascular disease might happen to have a larger number of smokers in one group than the other. In this case, smoking would be a confounding variable, since it's known to cause cardiovascular disease.

If the sample size is large enough, however, one can assume that known—and unknown—confounders will be evenly distributed between the groups. To see why this is, imagine flipping a coin. If you flip it ten times, there's a reasonable chance it will come up heads 70% of the time (7 heads, 3 tails). If you flip it a thousand times, there's almost no chance it will come up heads 70% of the time (700 heads, 300 tails).

To put all this together—the gold standard for medical research is a prospective, randomized, double-blind, placebo-controlled trial with a sample size large enough to produce a p value of <.05 or lower. Many of the studies in this book don't achieve that standard—but then neither do most of the studies behind conventional medical therapies. If I limited the studies cited here to ones that meet that standard, this wouldn't be a book but an article . . . a short article.

Still, it's useful to know what the gold standard is, because everything—including trials of conventional medical therapies—should be held up to it. (Studies that don't meet the standard aren't necessarily wrong, but they're not proof. Future trials should adhere to the gold standard as much as possible.)

There are just a few more terms you should know. A **meta-analysis** is a relatively new kind of study in which you combine the results from a number of selected trials in order to come to some general conclusions. Meta-analyses are usually done when a number of small trials give ambiguous, conflicting or statistically insignificant results. When all of the decent trials are combined, there may be enough subjects in the combined treatment group to reach a statistically significant conclusion.

Let's say we're doing a survey of weights in a tiny village that has just eleven inhabitants. There are five children, who weigh 40, 50, 65, 65 and 65 lbs (the last three are triplets); three women, who weigh 105, 110 and 125 lbs; and three men, who weigh 150, 160 and 840 lbs (this last guy has a hormonal disorder).

If we add up all the weights, we get 1780 lbs; if we divide that by 11, we get 162 lbs. This is the **mean**—it's

what we're talking about when we use the word *average* in everyday speech. But it would be very misleading to say that the average person in this village weighs 162 lbs, since all but one of the inhabitants weigh less than that. To deal with situations like this, statisticians have come up with two other kinds of averages—the median and the mode.

The **median** is the value in the middle of the distribution—the one halfway between the bottom and the top. In this particular example, the median—105 lbs—gives a much better idea of the average weight than the mean does.

The **mode** is the value that occurs most frequently; in this example, it would be 65 lbs (the triplets). In some distributions, the mode is a better indication of what's representative than either the mean or the median.

The **FDA** (the Food and Drug Administration, a regulatory agency of the federal government) requires specific kinds of trials on human subjects before it will approve new drugs. (Animal studies and the like have typically been done before these trials take place.) A **Phase I** trial simply tests for safety; it's usually done on healthy volunteers, without a control group.

In a **Phase II** trial, the drug is given to people with the condition or disease to be treated; it supplies some preliminary data on whether the treatment works, and supplements the safety data of the Phase I trial. Phase II trials may or may not use a control group.

A **Phase III** trial assesses efficacy, safety and dosage, compared with standard treatments or a placebo. Phase III trials are usually randomized and controlled.

Phase I, II, and III trials are usually performed as part of an **IND** (an *investigational new drug* application to the FDA). After the Phase III trial is completed, the manufacturer can submit an **NDA** (a *new drug application*) which requests permission to market the drug.

Not routinely required, **Phase IV** studies are done after drugs are approved by the FDA and can be sold to the public. They're randomized trials or surveys that attempt to evaluate longterm benefits and risks.

Finally, **in vitro** (literally, "in glass") refers to studies done in artificial environments like test tubes, and **in vivo** to studies done in living organisms.

WORKSHEET—CHAPTER 1

Women and the Healthcare System

1. The 1979 classic article "Sexism in Women's Medical Care" sets the scene for discussions on how sexism impacts women's health and the field of medicine. Using this article, identify at least two things that you feel have improved significantly since 1979 and identify two things that you feel still need to be improved:

   have improved since 1979   still need to improve

2. Describe your "best" and "worst" healthcare experiences. Briefly, identify the behaviors (or other characteristics) that were different for you and the health providers in the two situations. Referring to "How to Tell Your Doctor a Thing or Two," identify ways that you were or were not an "active patient" in the two situations.

3. Building on information in several articles, describe how the gynecological exam is symbolic of the consumer-health practitioner relationship, and identify things every woman should be able to expect as a part of a good gynecological exam.

4. Outline both sides of the debate on the question, "Will increasing the number of women doctors increase the quality of care which women receive as healthcare consumers?"

   yes

   no

5. *Our Bodies, Ourselves,* even though it was originally written in the U.S., has been successfully adapted in many parts of the world. Discuss a few examples of ways in which transforming *OBOS* into a different cultural and societal context involves much more than just translating it into another language.

6. List at least three reasons why women's health issues must be considered in any movement toward health-care reform.

7. The Ruzek and Becker article, "The Women's Health Movement in the US," identifies different philosophies and priorities of grass-roots and professionalized women's health organizations. Briefly summarize information from the articles on the chart below and identify your own values/visions on each topic.

Topic	Grass-roots Organizations	Professionalized Organizations	My View
1. Social Movement Orientation			
2. Leadership			
3. Attitude toward Biomedicine			
4. Relationship with Corporate Sponsors			
5. Goal of Education			
6. Lay versus Professional Authority			

INEQUALITIES
and HEALTH

Acore part of developing an analysis of women's health issues is working toward an understanding of why "some women have a better chance of being healthy than other women." This involves learning how racism, anti-semitism, poverty, homophobia, ageism, attitudes toward disabilities, fatphobia, and other forms of oppression multiply the effects of sexism, impact on women's mental and physical health, affect access to the determinants of health (such as good nutrition, pollution-free environment, housing, education, rewards for employment), influence or determine one's access to the health system, impact the cultural appropriateness of the health system if one has access to it, and affect whether or not one is appropriately and respectfully represented in research on women's health issues.

Articles in this chapter are chosen to stimulate dialogue on this complex topic and help us work towards a better understanding of how oppressions impact on health, so that working against oppressions and our own ways of perpetuating oppressions can be an ongoing part of our work toward a healthcare system more appropriate for *all* women (and men). This book is planned to complement, rather than overlap with, *The Black Women's Health Book*. As African-American women, and the National Black Women's Health Project specifically, have played a leadership role in the activism and writing on how racism has impacted women's health, much of the most ground-breaking work on this topic is covered or reflected in *The Black Women's Health Book*. Readers are also encouraged to study *Undivided Rights: Women of Color Organize for Reproductive Justice,* by Jael Silliman, Marlene Gerber Fried, Loretta Ross, and Elena R. Gutiêrrez. Chapters in *Undivided Rights* give detailed information and powerful examples of organizing related to the unique women's health issues faced by specific groups of women of color.

The first articles in this chapter set the tone for how we have tried to work on anti-oppression issues in this book. Audre Lorde's classics, "Age, Race, Class, and Sex: Women Redefining Difference" and "There is No Hierarchy of Oppressions," look at the intersection of *all* forms of oppression and how a basic understanding of power and control issues (who benefits from the inequalities in society and what strategies are used to keep the status quo/the inequalities in place) is fundamental to understanding any and all forms of oppression. (It is important to note that while Audre Lorde's life was devoted to educating us about the widest range of oppressions and strongly encouraging us to look at their intersections rather than looking at a hierarchy of oppressions; Lorde also emphasized that in a racist society, racism plays a dominating role in maintaining power differentials.)

In "Racism," Megan Seely (from her *Fight Like a Girl: How to Be a Fearless Feminist)* shares her commitment as a white "third wave" feminist to discover "How did racism infiltrate itself into a movement (the women's movement) determined to fight for equality?" and what can she/we do to unlearn racism and build more inclusive movements. We think readers will be particularly inspired by the gems of wisdom she shares from bell hooks' *Feminism is for Everyone*, Peggy McIntosh's "White Privilege: Unpacking the Invisible Knapsack" (reprinted in the 4th edition of this Worcester/Whatley book), and Paul Kivel's *Uprooting Racism: How White People Can Work for Racial Justice.*

Ricky Sherover-Marcuse's "Unlearning Racism" captures some of the essence of the powerful, life-changing Unlearning Racism Workshops, which she facilitated around the country, encouraging each of us to take responsibility for starting to unlearn oppressive misinformation, which we have learned as a part of our socialization in a racist society. Perhaps her most inspiring work was to stimulate everyone committed to anti-oppression work to look at how we could consciously work at being *allies* for each other and for "each other's issues."

The next articles present overviews and "big picture" analyses to encourage critical thinking, discussions, and work related to oppressions-as-health issues. Additionally, the excellent book *Unequal Health: How Inequality Contributes to Health or Illness,* by Grace Budrys (Rowman and Littlefield, 2003) is highly recommended.

"Does Racism Harm Health?" specifically addresses connections between racism and health, though frameworks introduced will also be useful for making connections between other forms of oppression and health. As stated in the abstract, this article explores: (1) links between racism, biology, and health; (2) methodological issues related to studying racism's impact on health; and (3) the roles of both racism and class in racial/ethnic inequalities.

"What Are Health Disparities?" and "Why Do Health Disparities Exist?" from the American Medical Student Association (AMSA) website give a number of facts related to the problem of health disparities and move on to identify reasons for disparities. Articles and websites like these are positive examples of important action being taken to confront inequalities and improve the healthcare system. As AMSA represents the future of medicine, it is promising to read, "As the future doctors of America, AMSA believes that all physicians-in-training must take a pro-active role in eliminating health disparities."

"Cultural Humility versus Cultural Competence" introduces a profoundly useful and realistic way to think of anti-oppression work. The article, specifically addressing physician training outcomes for multi-cultural education, helps us think through what will be necessary to meet the above-stated AMSA goals that all physicians-in-training actively eliminate inequalities in health. However, the analysis offered is just as relevant to *all* readers of this book studying and working to improve women's health. Slightly paraphrasing Tervalon and Murray-García:

> Cultural humility is proposed as a suitable approach for our anti-oppression work. Cultural humility incorporates a life-long commitment to self-evaluation and self-critique, to redressing power imbalances wherever they occur, and to developing mutually beneficial and non-paternalistic partnerships whenever and wherever possible on behalf of individuals and defined populations.

Serving as an introductory overview to focusing attention on specific issues for particular groups, the "umbrella" article, "Health at the Margins," draws attention to commonalities and unique issues of being distanced from the center of power and privilege experienced by women of color, lesbians, women with disabilities, women in poverty, rural women, and women living in the Global South. In order to recognize the ways that racism and other forms of oppression impact on every health issue, we have tried to include articles by a diverse group of people in many chapters of this book. The next articles in this chapter are intended to highlight, rather than isolate, a few of the many specific issues, which are related to racism, anti-semitism, class, and disability issues.

Vanessa Gamble's "Under the Shadow of Tuskegee: African Americans and Healthcare" examines the long history of racism, including more recent examples of the ways racist medicine has hurt Black people, which results in the fact that many African Americans do not trust the health system.

In "Health and Indigenous people," Michael Bird, former President of the American Public Health Association, highlights both the health problems (worst health status of any group in this country, including high infant mortality and low life expectancy) and contributions of indigenous people. Drawing attention to the urgency of improving the health of indigenous people, Bird also emphasizes that indigenous people have much to offer, including "the importance of the spiritual essence of all people, and our relationships to each other and the environment."

"Reclaiming Choice, Broadening the Movement" looks at unique issues for Asian-Pacific Islander women. For example, because over 40 percent of U.S. nail technicians are Asian Pacific Americans, the cancer, birth defects, and spontaneous abortion risks associated with phthalates in nail chemicals are an urgent problem for this population. (For more information, see "The High Price of Beauty" in Chapter 8.) This article reminds us of why *all* groups of women need to be studied, and the disservice it does for a group with much internal diversity to be lumped together when there are specific subpopulation needs to be recognized. Health consequences discussed in relation to the "model minority" stereotype are an important addition to other anti-oppression issues discussed in this book.

In "On Being a Jewish Feminist Valley Girl," Tobin Belzer takes both a personal and political view of the damages done by stereotypes, living up to them, learning to critique them, and learning to live with one's own contradictions. After identifying the power of the "Valley Girl"/"Jewish American Princess" stereotype as "the most recent permutation of the age-old condemnation of Jews," Belzer describes:

> As a Jewish feminist Valley Girl, I am trying to honor my multiple selves while acknowledging the contradictions inherent in doing so. . . . Embracing my Jewish feminist Valley Girl identity allowed me to honor all sides of myself. As a Valley Girl, I had paid meticulous attention to altering my appearance. When I became a feminist, I decided to learn to love and honor my body, rather than investing all of my energy in trying to improve it. Instead, I set out to change the world.

"Immigrant Women's Health a Casualty in the Immigration Policy War" demonstrates how our broken immigration system breaks women. Immigrant women are "more likely than U.S.-born women to live in poverty, be unemployed, and lack insurance." Instead of improving the dire situation, recent legislation has made it much more difficult for immigrants to access public benefit programs, and has drastically increased barriers to healthcare.

"Trans Health Crisis: For Us It's Life or Death" is also a powerful reminder of how inequalities are literally a matter of life and death if people do not have access to the health system, or if health practitioners are not educated and committed to serving all patients. In raising awareness about the health crisis for the trans population, Leslie Feinberg's personal story painfully demonstrates how health practitioners' ignorance and prejudice are dangerous and life-threatening for their trans patients:

> After the physician who examined me discovered I am female-bodied, he ordered me out of the emergency room despite the fact that my temperature was above 104D F.
>
> (Later hospitalized for the same undiagnosed bacterial endocarditis . . .) They place transsexual women who have completed sex-reassignment surgery in the male wards. Putting me in a female ward created a furor. I awoke in the night to find staff standing around my bed ridiculing my body and referring to me as a "Martian". The next day the staff refused to work unless "it" was removed from the floor. These and other expressions of hatred forced me to leave. Had I died from this illness, the real pathogen would have been bigotry.

A major gap in this book is that it is still nearly impossible to find useful data on how class impacts health in the USA. Class analysis, building on officially published figures (always open to criticism, such as why is a woman's class defined by her husband's occupation?) is core to women's health writing in many other countries, but "the U.S., unlike most industrialized nations, does not regularly collect or publish mortality statistics or other health information by class" ("The Class Gap" by Vincente Navarro in *The Nation*, April 8, 1991, pp. 436-437). Is that a reason for, or a reflection of, Americans' confusion about the role of class in our lives? Class differs from other forms of oppression in a very fundamental way. For other issues, a goal is to celebrate and value our differences and to eliminate *the oppression* related to the issue. With poverty, the goal is to *eliminate* that form of difference.

While understanding that poverty is certainly correlated with ill health, it is also important to look at how financial problems are *caused* by lack of universal healthcare or health insurance. In "Financially Vulnerable," an article written specifically for this book, Stephanie Rytilahti, a women's health teaching assistant, combines her analysis as a Women's Studies graduate student with her years of experience in banking. With unique insight, she describes "the financially vulnerable situation many Americans find themselves in when trips to the hospital are either uninsured or only partially covered by health insurance."

"Rural Health Care" identifies the unique challenges of accessing healthcare faced by the one-quarter of Americans who live in rural areas. These include "Lack of insurance, limited economic opportunities, . . . inadequate funding for targeted public health interventions, . . . healthcare provider shortages and geographic isolation."

"Disability and the Medical System" gives us an overview of some of the health and medical issues for women with disabilities. This article again reminds us that people who most need a good health system are often exactly the people least likely to be served by a profit-driven system that caters to a "mythical norm." Through illustrations, "Simply Friend or Foe?" offers (temporarily?) able-bodied people ideas for how to be allies to people with disabilities. "Letting Justice Flow" relates how, as a non-disabled woman, Alison Kafer, "saw myself as a political activist only when involved in a demonstration or a protest" but now, as a woman with disabilities, she recognizes:

I understand my very body as a site of resistance. Every single time I leave my house, people stare. Their eyes linger on my scars, my half-legs, and my wheelchair as they try to understand what happened and why I look the way I do. Their stereotypes about disability are written in their expressions of confusion and fear as they watch me pass. I am powerfully aware that merely by living life in a wheelchair, I challenge their stereotypes about what bodies look like and what bodies do. I feel like an activist just by rolling out my front door.

She describes how a full bladder and her activism around the right to pee resulted in more disability-awareness of her classmates—and eventually, an accessible bathroom.

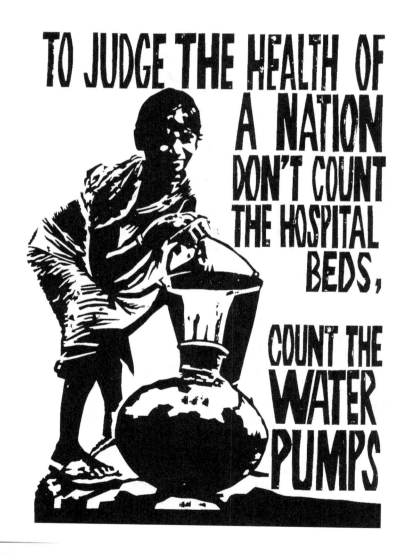

From the graphic "To Judge the Health of a Nation Don't Count the Hospital Beds, Count the Water Pumps" is reproduced with permission of Oxfam GB, Oxfam House, John Smith Drive, Cowley, Oxford OX4 2JY, UK, www.oxfam.org.uk. Oxfam GB does not necessarily endorse any text or activities that accompany the materials.

Age, Race, Class, and Sex
Women Redefining Difference *

by Audre Lorde

Much of western European history conditions us to see human differences in simplistic opposition to each other: dominant/subordinate, good/bad, up/down, superior/inferior. In a society where the good is defined in terms of profit rather than in terms of human need, there must always be some group of people who, through systematized oppression, can be made to feel surplus, to occupy the place of the dehumanized inferior. Within this society, that group is made up of Black and Third World people, working-class people, older people, and women.

As a forty-nine-year-old Black lesbian feminist socialist mother of two, including one boy, and a member of an interracial couple, I usually find myself a part of some group defined as other, deviant, inferior, or just plain wrong. Traditionally, in American society, it is the members of oppressed, objectified groups who are expected to stretch out and bridge the gap between the actualities of our lives and the consciousness of our oppressor. For in order to survive, those of us for whom oppression is as American as apple pie have always had to be watchers, to become familiar with the language and manners of the oppressor, even sometimes adopting them for some illusion of protection. Whenever the need for some pretense of communication arises, those who profit from our oppression call upon us to share our knowledge with them. In other words, it is the responsibility of the oppressed to teach the oppressors their mistakes. I am responsible for educating teachers who dismiss my children's culture in school. Black and Third World people are expected to educate white people as to our humanity. Women are expected to educate men. Lesbians and gay men are expected to educate the heterosexual world. The oppressors maintain their position and evade responsibility for their own actions. There is a constant drain of energy which might be better used in redefining ourselves and devising realistic scenarios for altering the present and constructing the future.

Institutionalized rejection of difference is an absolute necessity in a profit economy which needs outsiders as surplus people. As members of such an economy, we have *all* been programmed to respond to the human differences between us with fear and loathing and to handle that difference in one of three ways: ignore it, and if that is not possible, copy it if we think it is dominant, or destroy it if we think it is subordinate. But we have no patterns for relating across our human differences as equals. As a result, those differences have been misnamed and misused in the service of separation and confusion.

Certainly there are very real differences between us of race, age, and sex. But it is not those differences between us that are separating us. It is rather our refusal to recognize those differences, and to examine the distortions which result from our misnaming them and their effects upon human behavior and expectation.

Racism, the belief in the inherent superiority of one race over all others and thereby the right to dominance. Sexism, the belief in the inherent superiority of one sex over the other and thereby the right to dominance. Ageism. Heterosexism. Elitism, Classism.

It is a lifetime pursuit for each one of us to extract these distortions from our living at the same time as we recognize, reclaim, and define those differences upon which they are imposed. For we have all been raised in a society where those distortions were endemic within our living. Too often, we pour the energy needed for recognizing and exploring difference into pretending those differences are insurmountable barriers, or that they do not exist at all. This results in a voluntary isolation, or false and treacherous connections. Either way, we do not develop tools for using human difference as a springboard for creative change within our lives. We speak not of human difference, but of human deviance.

Somewhere, on the edge of consciousness, there is what I call a *mythical norm,* which each one of us within our hearts knows "that is not me." In america, this norm is usually defined as white, thin, male, young, heterosexual, christian, and financially secure. It is with this mythical norm that the trappings of power reside within this

---

society. Those of us who stand outside that power often identify one way in which we are different, and we assume that to be the primary cause of all oppression, forgetting other distortions around difference, some of which we ourselves may be practicing. By and large within the women's movement today, white women focus upon their oppression as women and ignore differences of race, sexual preference, class, and age. There is a pretense to a homogeneity of experience covered by the word *sisterhood* that does not in fact exist.

Unacknowledged class differences rob women of each others' energy and creative insight. Recently a women's magazine collective made the decision for one issue to print only prose, saying poetry was a less "rigorous" or "serious" art form. Yet even the form our creativity takes is often a class issue. Of all the art forms, poetry is the most economical. It is the one which is the most secret, which requires the least physical labor, the least material, and the one which can be done between shifts, in the hospital pantry, on the subway, and on scraps of surplus paper. Over the last few years, writing a novel on tight finances, I came to appreciate the enormous differences in the material demands between poetry and prose. As we reclaim our literature, poetry has been the major voice of poor, working class, and Colored women. A room of one's own may be a necessity for writing prose, but so are reams of paper, a typewriter, and plenty of time. The actual requirements to produce the visual arts also help determine, along class lines, whose art is whose. In this day of inflated prices for material, who are our sculptors, our painters, our photographers? When we speak of a broadly based women's culture, we need to be aware of the effect of class and economic differences on the supplies available for producing art.

As we move toward creating a society within which we can each flourish, ageism is another distortion of relationship which interferes without vision. By ignoring the past, we are encouraged to repeat its mistakes. The "generation gap" is an important social tool for any repressive society. If the younger members of a community view the older members as contemptible or suspect or excess, they will never be able to join hands and examine the living memories of the community, nor ask the all important question, "Why?" This gives rise to a historical amnesia that keeps us working to invent the wheel every time we have to go to the store for bread.

We find ourselves having to repeat and relearn the same old lessons over and over that our mothers did because we do not pass on what we have learned, or because we are unable to listen. For instance, how many times has this all been said before? For another, who would have believed that once again our daughters are allowing their bodies to be hampered and purgatoried by girdles and high heels and hobble skirts?

Ignoring the differences of race between women and the implications of those differences presents the most serious threat to the mobilization of women's joint power.

As white women ignore their built-in privilege of whiteness and define *woman* in terms of their own experience alone, then women of Color become "other," the outsider whose experience and tradition is too "alien" to comprehend. An example of this is the signal absence of the experience of women of Color as a resource for women's studies courses. The literature of women of Color is seldom included in women's literature courses and almost never in other literature courses, nor in women's studies as a whole. All too often, the excuse given is that the literatures of women of Color can only be taught by Colored women, or that they are too difficult to understand, or that classes cannot "get into" them because they come out of experiences that are "too different." I have heard this argument presented by white women of otherwise quite clear intelligence, women who seem to have no trouble at all teaching and reviewing work that comes out of the vastly different experiences of Shakespeare, Molière, Dostoyefsky, and Aristophanes. Surely there must be some other explanation.

This is a very complex question, but I believe one of the reasons white women have such difficulty reading Black women's work is because of their reluctance to see Black women as women and different from themselves. To examine Black women's literature effectively requires that we be seen as whole people in our actual complexities—as individuals, as women, as human—rather than as one of those problematic but familiar stereotypes provided in this society in place of genuine images of Black women. And I believe this holds true for the literatures of other women of Color who are not Black.

The literatures of all women of Color recreate the textures of our lives, and many white women are heavily invested in ignoring the real differences. For as long as any difference between us means one of us must be inferior, then the recognition of any difference must be fraught with guilt. To allow women of Color to step out of stereotypes is too guilt provoking, for it threatens the complacency of those women who view oppression only in terms of sex.

Refusing to recognize difference makes it impossible to see the different problems and pitfalls facing us as women.

Thus, in a patriarchal power system where white-skin privilege is a major prop, the entrapments used to neutralize Black women and white women are not the same. For example, it is easy for Black women to be used by the power structure against Black men, not because they are men, but because they are Black. Therefore, for Black women, it is necessary at all times to separate the needs of the oppressor from our own legitimate conflicts within our communities. This same problem does not exist for white women. Black women and men have shared racist oppression and still share it, although in different ways. Out of that shared oppression we have developed joint defenses and joint vulnerabilities to each other that are not duplicated in the white community, with the exception of the relationship between Jewish women and Jewish men.

On the other hand, white women face the pitfall of being seduced into joining the oppressor under the pretense of sharing power. This possibility does not exist in the same way for women of Color. The tokenism that is sometimes extended to us is not an invitation to join power; our racial "otherness" is a visible reality that makes that quite clear. For white women there is a wider range of pretended choices and rewards for identifying with patriarchal power and its tools.

Today, with the defeat of ERA, the tightening economy, and increased conservatism, it is easier once again for white women to believe the dangerous fantasy that if you are good enough, pretty enough, sweet enough, quiet enough, teach the children to behave, hate the right people, and marry the right men, then you will be allowed to co-exist with patriarchy in relative peace, at least until a man needs your job or the neighborhood rapist happens along. And true, unless one lives and loves in the trenches it is difficult to remember that the war against dehumanization is ceaseless.

But Black women and our children know the fabric of our lives is stitched with violence and with hatred, that there is no rest. We do not deal with it only on the picket lines, or in dark midnight alleys, or in the places where we dare to verbalize our resistance. For us, increasingly, violence weaves through the daily tissues of our living—in the supermarket, in the classroom, in the elevator, in the clinic and the schoolyard, from the plumber, the baker, the saleswoman, the bus driver, the bank teller, the waitress who does not serve us.

Some problems we share as women, some we do not. You fear your children will grow up to join the patriarchy and testify against you, we fear our children will be dragged from a car and shot down in the street, and you will turn your backs upon the reasons they are dying.

The threat of difference has been no less blinding to people of Color. Those of us who are Black must see

that the reality of our lives and our struggle does not make us immune to the errors of ignoring and misnaming difference. Within Black communities where racism is a living reality, differences among us often seem dangerous and suspect. The need for unity is often misnamed as a need for homogeneity, and a Black feminist vision mistaken for betrayal of our common interests as a people. Because of the continuous battle against racial erasure that Black women and Black men share, some Black women still refuse to recognize that we are also oppressed as women, and that sexual hostility against Black women is practiced not only by the white racist society, but implemented within our Black communities as well. It is a disease striking the heart of Black nationhood, and silence will not make it disappear. Exacerbated by racism and the pressures of powerlessness, violence against Black women and children often becomes a standard within our communities, one by which manliness can be measured. But these women-hating acts are rarely discussed as crimes against Black women.

As a group, women of Color are the lowest paid wage earners in America. We are the primary targets of abortion and sterilization abuse, here and abroad. In certain parts of Africa, small girls are still being sewed shut between their legs to keep them docile and for men's pleasure. This is known as female circumcision, and it is not a cultural affair as the late Jomo Kenyatta insisted, it is a crime against Black women.

Black women's literature is full of the pain of frequent assault, not only by a racist patriarchy, but also by Black men. Yet the necessity for and history of shared battle have made us, Black women, particularly vulnerable to the false accusation that anti-sexist is anti-Black. Meanwhile, womanhating as a recourse of the powerless is sapping strength from Black communities, and our very lives. Rape is on the increase, reported and unreported, and rape is not aggressive sexuality, it is sexualized aggression. As Kalamu ya Salaam, a Black male writer points out, "As long as male domination exists, rape will exist. Only women revolting and men made conscious of their responsibility to fight sexism can collectively stop rape."[1]

Differences between ourselves as Black women are also being misnamed and used to separate us from one another. As a Black lesbian feminist comfortable with the many different ingredients of my identity, and a woman committed to racial and sexual freedom from oppression, I find I am constantly being encouraged to pluck out some one aspect of myself and present this as the meaningful whole, eclipsing or denying the other parts of self. But this is a destructive and fragmenting way to live. My fullest concentration of energy is available to me only when I integrate all the parts of who I am, openly, allowing power from particular sources of my living to flow back and forth freely through all my different selves, without the restrictions of externally imposed definition. Only then can I bring myself and my energies as a whole to the service of those struggles which I embrace as part of my living.

A fear of lesbians, or of being accused of being a lesbian, has led many Black women into testifying against themselves. It has led some of us into destructive alliances, and others into despair and isolation. In the white women's communities, heterosexism is sometimes a result of identifying with the white patriarchy, a rejection of that interdependence between women-identified women which allows the self to be, rather than to be used in the service of men. Sometimes it reflects a diehard belief in the protective coloration of heterosexual relationships, sometimes a self-hate which all women have to fight against, taught us from birth.

Although elements of these attitudes exist for all women, there are particular resonances of heterosexism and homophobia among Black women. Despite the fact that woman-bonding has a long and honorable history in the African and African-American communities, and despite the knowledge and accomplishments of many strong and creative women-identified Black women in the political, social and cultural fields, heterosexual Black women often tend to ignore or discount the existence and work of Black lesbians. Part of this attitude has come from an understandable terror of Black male attack within the close confines of Black society, where the punishment for any female self-assertion is still to be accused of being a lesbian and therefore unworthy of the attention or support of the scarce Black male. But part of this need to misname and ignore Black lesbians comes from a very real fear that openly women-identified Black women who are no longer dependent upon men for their self-definition may well reorder our whole concept of social relationships.

Black women who once insisted that lesbianism was a white woman's problem now insist that Black lesbians are a threat to Black nationhood, are consorting with the enemy, are basically un-Black. These accusations, coming from the very women to whom we look for deep and real understanding, have served to keep many Black lesbians in hiding, caught between the racism of white women and the homophobia of their sisters. Often, their work has been ignored, trivialized, or misnamed, as with the work of Angelina Grimke, Alice Dunbar-Nelson, Lorraine Hansberry. Yet women-bonded women have always been some part of the power of Black communities, from our unmarried aunts to the amazons of Dahomey.

And it is certainly not Black lesbians who are assaulting women and raping children and grandmothers on the streets of our communities.

Across this country, as in Boston during the spring of 1979 following the unsolved murders of twelve Black women, Black lesbians are spearheading movements against violence against Black women.

What are the particular details within each of our lives that can be scrutinized and altered to help bring about change? How do we redefine difference for all women? It is not our differences which separate women, but our reluctance to recognize those differences and to deal effectively with the distortions which have resulted from the ignoring and misnaming of those differences.

As a tool of social control, women have been encouraged to recognize only one area of human difference as legitimate, those differences which exist between women and men. And we have learned to deal across those differences with the urgency of all oppressed subordinates. All of us have had to learn to live or work or coexist with men, from our fathers on. We have recognized and negotiated these differences, even when this recognition only continued the old dominant/subordinate mode of human relationship, where the oppressed must recognize the masters' difference in order to survive.

But our future survival is predicated upon our ability to relate within equality. As women, we must root out internalized patterns of oppression within ourselves if we are to move beyond the most superficial aspects of social change. Now we must recognize differences among women who are our equals, neither inferior nor superior, and devise ways to use each others' difference to enrich our visions and our joint struggles.

The future of our earth may depend upon the ability of all women to identify and develop new definitions of power and new patterns of relating across difference. The old definitions have not served us, nor the earth that supports us. The old patterns, no matter how cleverly rearranged to imitate progress, still condemn us to cosmetically altered repetitions of the same old exchanges, the same old guilt, hatred, recrimination, lamentation, and suspicion.

For we have, built into all of us, old blueprints of expectation and response, old structures of oppression, and these must be altered at the same time as we alter the living conditions which are a result of those structures. For the master's tools will never dismantle the master's house.

As Paulo Freire shows so well in *The Pedagogy of the Oppressed,*[2] the true focus of revolutionary change is never merely the oppressive situations which we seek to escape, but that piece of the oppressor which is planted deep within each of us, and which knows only the oppressors' tactics, the oppressors' relationships.

Change means growth, and growth can be painful. But we sharpen self-definition by exposing the self in work and struggle together with those whom we define as different from ourselves, although sharing the same goals. For Black and white, old and young, lesbian and heterosexual women alike, this can mean new paths to our survival.

We have chosen each other
and the edge of each other battles
the war is the same

if we lose
someday women's blood will congeal
upon a dead planet
if we win
there is no telling
we seek beyond history
for a new and more possible meeting.[3]

NOTES

1. From "Rape: A Radical Analysis, An African-American Perspective" by Kalamu ya Salaam in *Black Books Bulletin*, vol. 6, no. 4 (1980).

2. Seabury Press, New York, 1970.

3. From "Outlines," unpublished poem.

There Is No Hierarchy of Oppression

by Audre Lorde

I was born Black, and a woman. I am trying to become the strongest person I can become to live the life I have been given and to help effect change toward a liveable future for this earth and for my children. As a Black, lesbian, feminist, socialist, poet, mother of two including one boy and a member of an interracial couple, I usually find myself part of some group in which the majority defines me as deviant, difficult, inferior, or just plain "wrong."

From my membership in all of these groups I have learned that oppression and the intolerance of difference come in all shapes and sizes and colors and sexualities; and that among those of us who share the goals of liberation and a workable future for our children, there can be no hierarchies of oppression. I have learned that sexism (a belief in the inherent superiority of one sex over all others and thereby its right to dominance) and heterosexism (a belief in the inherent superiority of one pattern of loving over all others and thereby its right to dominance) both arise from the same source as racism—a belief in the inherent superiority of one race over all others and thereby its right to dominance.

"Oh," says a voice from the Black community, "but being Black is NORMAL!" Well, I and many Black people of my age can remember grimly the days when it didn't used to be!

I simply do not believe that one aspect of myself can possibly profit from the oppression of any other part of my identity. I know that my people cannot possibly profit from the oppression of any other group which seeks the right to peaceful existence. Rather, we diminish ourselves by denying to others what we have shed blood to obtain for our children. And those children need to learn that they do not have to become like each other in order to work together for a future they will all share.

The increasing attacks upon lesbians and gay men are only an introduction to the increasing attacks upon all Black people, for wherever oppression manifests itself in this country, Black people are potential victims. And it

---

Reprinted with permission from *Council on Interracial Books for Children Bulletin*, vol. 14, No. 3–4, 1983. (1841 Broadway, Rm. 500, New York, N.Y. 10023)

is a standard of right-wing cynicism to encourage members of oppressed groups to act against each other, and so long as we are divided because of our particular identities we cannot join together in effective political action.

Within the lesbian community I am Black, and within the Black community I am a lesbian. Any attack against Black people is a lesbian and gay issue, because I and thousands of other Black women are part of the lesbian community. Any attack against lesbians and gays is a Black issue, because thousands of lesbians and gay men are Black. There is no hierarchy of oppression.

It is not accidental that the Family Protection Act, which is virulently anti-woman and anti-Black, is also anti-gay. As a Black person I know who my enemies are, and when the Ku Klux Klan goes to court in Detroit to try and force the Board of Education to remove books the Klan believes "hint at homosexuality," then I know I cannot afford the luxury of fighting one form of oppression only. I cannot afford to believe that freedom from intolerance is the right of only one particular group. And I cannot afford to choose between the fronts upon which I must battle these forces of discrimination, wherever they appear to destroy me. And when they appear to destroy me, it will not be long before they appear to destroy you.

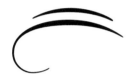
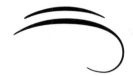

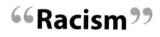"Racism"

by Megan Seely

Of the criticisms of feminism and the women's movement, the most poignant is that of racism. It is a myth that women of color are not involved in the women's movement. They are and always have been. Unfortunately, a division formed that served to separate women of color from white women. As a third waver, I have many questions about this division—did white women honor the perspectives of women of color? Were women of color incorporated into the leadership of the movement? Whose issues were of primary focus? How did racism infiltrate itself into a movement determined to fight for equality? I feel as if I have inherited much of this strain and daily confront the past when mobilizing for change today. But, as a white girl, it is a challenge to talk about race. What do I know about being "of color" in this culture? How can I speak to the issue of racism, not having lived it myself? I used to want to be colorblind, not to see race, but then I realized that this was essentially ignoring the role of race in a society that is far from colorblind. I realize that to try not to see color in this culture is to ignore the challenges of race and ethnicity, to undervalue the struggle that has been waged to end racial discrimination, and to distance myself from the ongoing fight to end racism. To do so also ignores the importance of celebrating our differences as a means of expanding our individual and collective knowledge.

I recognize the power of growing up white in a racist society. And, in that, I recognize that I say and do prejudicial things without fully knowing the impact of my actions or words. While I work every day to unlearn racism, to listen without prejudice, to hear the realities of my sisters, I also recognize that in a global culture with such tense race relations, I am seen first as a white woman. The assumption by some, I believe, is that I have no greater commitment to diversity than that assumed by my foremothers. So, how do we break through this? How do we create a venue to get real with each other? To have a dialogue that understands that, while we may not say the right words, while we may not fully understand the realities of living with racism, we come into the conversation with honest intentions? How do we have a dialogue about the multitude of oppressions we face without valuing one over the other? How do we get to a respectful understanding that, while a person of color knows racism in a way that a white woman can only imagine, the oppression of sexism is also real? I believe that we need to come to a place of understanding that no longer asks people to define narrowly who they are primarily—a person of color *or* a woman *or* a lesbian *or* a gay man *or* a person with a disability—but that recognizes our diversity and the importance of eradicating all discrimination and oppression. I own the fact that because I grew up white in a racist society, on some level I will have prejudice, and, though without the intent to offend, I sometimes say or do things that are offensive. In my quest for better understanding, better communication, better partnership, I unknowingly tokenize—not because I believe that one person can speak for her group but because I want the conversation to occur.

I want there to be a place where we can all sit down and really talk it all out, where we come to the conversation with honest intentions. I want us to give one another the benefit of the doubt, understanding that fear of offending has kept us from meaningful interaction. I am not talking about truly, overt racist people who hate on the basis of skin color and think they are right in doing so—they are a whole other, more obvious, problem. I am talking about the people who care about equality, who are conscious of racism but who largely are ignorant of the implications of their own words and actions and their impact, or the people who spend so much energy searching for the right words that they say nothing. I realize that just sitting down together is not the solution, but it is an important step.

One of the greatest moments in my activist life occurred at the 1996 San Francisco "Fight the Right" March. As Californians, we were fighting two horrible propositions—Prop. 209, the "civil rights initiative" that proposed the elimination of affirmative action in the state, and Prop. 187, which proposed cutting health and social services (including public education) for immigrant populations in California. For the first time, at this march, I saw all the "groups" come together to fight discrimination. The women's movement, the civil rights movement, the labor movement, the immigration movement, the GLBT movement—six hundred different organizations were represented, and approximately fifty thousand participants were at the march. In that moment, we were powerful—instead of focusing on our differences and debating who had more at stake, we recognized that we were all oppressed by the power structure. Because we are female or gay or a person of color or an immigrant, we are denied access to full participation in society—we are denied housing, jobs, promotions, and free movement. We are disenfranchised, ignored, targeted, or denied basic rights because of characteristics inherent to who we are. We are divided and pitted against one another, fighting over a small piece of the social pie, while all the while the power structure takes the bulk of the pie. I believe that there is a conscious effort to divide our groups. But, if we can begin to recognize our commonalities rather than believe in the lines that divide us, we can share the struggle, unite forces, and emerge stronger. The power structure fears this most—fears an organizing of the oppressed who can rise up collectively and change the distribution of the proverbial pie. Unfortunately, in the end, both propositions were approved. The movements are still fractured. Today, we continue with the struggle to see the importance of our diversity and to share leadership across the board.

I have seen racism within the women's movement. I have heard the frustrations of women of color who come to the table only to be shut out by white reality. I have seen white women negate the importance of religion and faith to women of color who often hold these as central to who they are. I have seen many well-intentioned white women make racist remarks. But I have also seen women from all ethnic backgrounds sit together in a room and discuss the challenges to women today and collectively work toward a solution. I have seen the bridging of our lives, the raising of consciousness and the commitment to band together. And it is a powerful sight.

The second wave's approach of consciousness raising is regaining momentum as young feminists are reviving the tradition and practice. And it is not just young people who need this consciousness raising, I see everyday examples of racial tensions among people of all ages and across all ethnicities. The reality is that we live in a multicultural, multiracial society. But, despite this diversity, when it comes to the debate about race, we tend to see and talk only in black and white. Certainly, historical and current tensions are significant between African Americans and whites, but these are not the only racial tensions that exist. Racism occurs between white people and every people of every other ethnicity, but it also exists among other ethnic groups. The idea of valuing one's skin color over another is not unique to white people. As JeeYeun Lee writes in her article, "Beyond Bean Counting," "Issues of exclusion are not the sole province of white feminists."[1] We categorize and discriminate in all areas of race, creating a hierarchy of value within and among varying ethnicities. At the core are issues of power—getting it, having it, and keeping it. And, indeed, historically, white people have systematically held the most power. This is, of course, still true today. However, not all white people have power. Class, age, gender, physical and mental ability, and sexual orientation all come into play when determining power. But skin color alone does afford benefits for whites. Whiteness itself provides an unearned privilege for those who carry the pigmentation. In her book *Feminism Is for Everyone*, bell hooks writes:

> No intervention changed the face of American feminism more than the demand that feminist thinkers acknowledge the reality of race and racism. All white women in this nation know that their status is different from that of black/women of color. They know this from the time they are little girls watching television and seeing only their images, and looking at magazines and seeing only their images. They know that the only reason nonwhites are absent/invisible is because they are not white. All white women in this nation know that whiteness is a privileged category. The fact that white females may choose to repress or deny this knowledge does not mean they are ignorant: it means that they are in denial.[2]

I believe that white women must confront this denial and deconstruct our role in racism. In her writings on white privilege, Peggy McIntosh encourages looking beyond individual acts of racism to invisible systems of privilege and dominance of whites. She writes, "as a white person, I realized I had been taught about racism as something that puts others at a disadvantage, but had been taught not to see one of its corollary aspects, white privilege, which puts me at an advantage."[3] White women must begin (and continue) to deconstruct and understand this privilege if we are to be true allies in ending racism and the discrimination that accompanies it. If you are white, consider these statements when evaluating your benefits as a white person:[4]

> I live in a school district where more money is spent on schools that white children go to than on those that children of color attend.
>
> I went to a school where the textbooks reflected my race as heroes and builders of the United States, and there was little mention of contributions of people of color.
>
> I work in a job, career, or profession where there are few people of color.
>
> I can always vote for candidates that reflect my race.
>
> My race needn't be a factor in where I choose to live or where I send my children to school.
>
> I don't need to think about racism every day.

For a white person, examining these statements is the start to unlearning racism and beginning to look critically at the tensions we keep at arm's length—because we are certain (and often loudly proclaim) that we are not racist. In meeting after meeting of "progressive-minded" activists, I hear white women argue against concerns brought forward by women of color. Perhaps this happens because progressive white women have a lot invested in being politically correct. Perhaps it happens because there is a lot of guilt about being white among those whites who fight for equality. But fear of being accused of being racist gets in the way of *hearing* the points and views of women of color. And, instead of building a bridge, we deepen the divide.

White people need to get beyond their feelings of guilt and understand that guilt for being white (or male or straight) is self-indulgent and paralyzing. This isn't about you. It is about the structure of society and your actions within it. Feel guilty if you are not contributing to the solution, but not over something over which you have no control. Energy is much better spent working to be allies of people of color in ending racial discrimination. In his book *Uprooting Racism: How White People Can Work for Racial Justice*, Paul Kivel sets forth some important guidelines for being a white ally to people of color:

1. Assume racism is everywhere, every day.
2. Notice who is the center of attention and who is the center of power.
3. Notice how racism is denied, minimized, and justified.
4. Understand and learn from the history of whiteness and racism.
5. Understand the connections between racism, economic issues, sexism and other forms of injustice.
6. Take a stand against injustice.
7. Be strategic. Decide what is important to challenge and what's not.
8. Don't confuse a battle with the war.
9. Don't call names or be personally abusive.
10. Support the leadership of people of color.
11. Learn something about the history of white people who have worked for racial justice.
12. Don't do it alone.
13. Talk with your children and other young people about racism.[5]

As a white woman, let me add another guideline: Don't look to people of color to educate you on racism. It is not the job of people of color to take care of white folks. It is the job of white folks to raise their consciousness, to reach out and partner with people of color, to consult, include, and take the lead from people of color on the issues of racism . . . and on other issues of social justice, as well. As McIntosh asks, "having described [white privilege], what will I do to lessen or end it?" White people need to share positions of power, support and encourage the leadership of people of color in organizations and in the larger society.

Racism and the Feminist Movement

What about the feminist movement? Does it truly represent all women? As a third waver, I have learned the history of exclusion and the politics between white women and women of color. I have heard the arguments that white women focused on issues about their lives—for example, fighting for the rights to abortion—while women of color were fighting for their rights to have children; white women have neglected to embrace and support the issues of women of color. I have seen conflict arise when white women focus solely on their gender as their oppression, putting gender above all else. All the while, women of color fight to be recognized as such and resist being forced to choose their ethnicity over their gender or vice versa. I have seen the fighting between women, and, more tragical, I have seen women give up and move further away from one another. The conflict for third wavers is in knowing this past and respecting the feelings and opinions that came from that time, while living our commitment to a more inclusive movement, doing this work every day and confronting and changing this heritage. The third wave is acutely aware of the reality of racism and the history of exclusion of women of color by so-called mainstream organizations—it has been taught to us through women's studies and is present in our day-to-day interactions, our writings, our dialogues, and our activism. The discussion of race is integral to all that the third wave does, as are gender politics, class, sexuality, and disability. And, while we certainly don't have everything figured out, we have had the benefit of learning from the women who came before us, and, as a result, we recognize and appreciate the inadequacy of valuing gender as the only oppression.

White women need to recognize and respect that women of color have always been involved in social justice movements—for suffrage, women's rights, civil rights, GLBTQQI rights, disability rights, and so on. There is a misconception that women of color are not interested in the feminist movement; quite the contrary, they are leaders and visionaries working for change every day. This, of course, is not news to women of color, but it just might be news to those who know of the feminist movement only what they see on TV or read in history books. In fact, this movement is multifaceted—from nationally based mainstream organizations to local, grass-roots efforts, we all contribute to this fight for equality. We need to come together to define feminism, to define our work, and to commit to working together. Collectively, we can reclaim and redefine the image of feminism and women's rights—so that all women, all experiences, and all perspectives are represented. We are in this together, not in spite of but because of our differences and because of our commitment to justice. We must ensure that this is the foundation upon which we build and that the images of the movement reflect all women.

One of our greatest contributions as third wavers can be to close the gap across ethnicities, to build upon the failures and successes of this movement, and to live a politics that is about, and represents, all women. In order to do this, we need to be willing to join together, to be honest with one another, to build and share a dream together. And we need to tell the true story of feminism, one that is not controlled by the media, does not put forth one leader but rather reflects the contributions, the perspectives, and the lives of us all. I see today's feminists attempting to do this work everyday, choosing not to inherit this divide but to learn from our foremothers and change the course of this movement. We need to be able to call one another on our misconceptions and inaccuracies, to hold each other accountable, to listen and hear one another—each of us, across all ethnic and racial lines. It is difficult, it is confusing, it is sensitive, it is raw, but it is also vital.

What Can You Do?

Listen. Read. Support. Advocate. Join multicultural efforts to address issues as defined by those affected. Hold your own organizations, friends, school, and family accountable for racism, exclusion, and ignorance. Get honest with yourself and about your actions. It is not enough to believe that you are not racist; you must also deconstruct racism within our culture, your role, and how you benefit from it. We need to question the structure of society and the hierarchy of race. We must raise our racial consciousness. We need to get honest about this, about who benefits and who does not—even when this system is not what we wish for or consciously support. We *all* need to do this. I do hold the feminist movement to a higher standard, as I do all social justice movements, but I believe that we must also recognize that racism is a challenge throughout our culture, that there is not an answer out there that the feminist movement is choosing to ignore. Which means that we—the multiracial, multicultural, multigendered, progressive masses—need to lead the way in finding the solutions.

Unlearning Racism

by Ricky Sherover-Marcuse

Because racism is both institutional and attitudinal, effective strategies against it must recognize this dual character. The *undoing* of institutionalized racism must be accompanied by the *unlearning* of racist attitudes and beliefs, and the *unlearning* of racist patterns of thought and action must guide the practice of political and social change.

Institutionalized racism can be defined as the systematic mistreatment of people of color (Third World people). Defining racism in this way highlights the fact that racism is not a genetic disease which is inherent in white people, but that it is a form of social oppression which is the result of the institutionalized inequalities in the structure of a given society.

Attitudinal racism can be defined as the set of assumptions, feelings, beliefs, and attitudes about people of color and their cultures which are a mixture of *misinformation* and ignorance. By "misinformation" I mean any assumption or attitude which in any way implies that people of color are less than fully human. Defining attitudinal racism as misinformation about people of color which has been imposed upon white people means that racism is not a moral defect which some (bad) white individuals have, but a social poison which has been given to all of us, albeit in many different forms.

Attitudinal racism and institutional racism feed off each other. The systematic mistreatment of any group of people generates misinformation about them which in turn becomes "explanation" of or justification for their continued mistreatment. As a result, misinformation about the victims of social oppression becomes socially empowered or *socially sanctioned misinformation*. This is what differentiates this sort of misinformation from prejudice. Socially sanctioned misinformation gets recycled through the society as a form of conditioning which becomes part of our "ordinary" assumptions, and as a result social oppression is viewed either as "natural" or as the fault of the victims themselves.

For example, the misinformation that people of color are stupid or indifferent to the value of human life becomes the "explanation" as to why there is a higher rate of infant mortality among certain groups in the populations. This "explanation" then justifies the attitude that there is really nothing one can do about infant mortality since this problem is basically due to the character or personality structure of the ethnic group involved.

For the past five years I have been doing workshops with groups of white people on "Unlearning Racism". The purpose of these workshops is to help whites to become aware that we have a personal stake in overcoming and unlearning the racist conditioning that was imposed upon us. Having racist beliefs and attitudes is like having a clamp on one's mind. *Unlearning* racism is partly a process of *relearning* how to get accurate information from and about people of color. This involves *relearning* how to really listen to people of color without making judgments or assumptions about what we think they are going to tell us.

When white people become aware of the ways in which *our lives* have been limited and restricted by racism, we become aware of *our interest* in ending this oppression. The most effective action that white people can take against racism will be action which springs not from a sense of guilt or pity, but from our own *knowledge* that in working against racism we are moving towards our own human liberation.

Does Racism Harm Health? Did Child Abuse Exist Before 1962? On Explicit Questions, Critical Science, and Current Controversies
"An Ecosocial Perspective"

by Nancy Krieger

Research on racism as a harmful determinant of population health is in its infancy. Explicitly naming a long-standing problem long recognized by those affected, this work has the potential to galvanize inquiry and action, much as the 1962 publication of the Kempe et al. scientific article on the "battered child syndrome" dramatically increased attention to—and prompted new research on—the myriad consequences of child abuse, a known yet neglected social phenomenon. To further work on connections between racism and health, the author addresses 3 interrelated issues: (1) links between racism, biology, and health; (2) methodological controversies over how to study the impact of racism on health; and (3) debates over whether racism or class underlies racial/ethnic disparities in health. (Am J Public Health. 2003;93:194-199)

Did child abuse exist before 1962, when C. Henry Kempe and coauthors published the now classic article "The Battered-Child Syndrome"? Certainly. Did it harm health? Yes, if current research is any guide. Before the Kempe et al. article catapulted the issue onto the mainstream US medical and public health agenda, had anyone previously raised concerns about child abuse? Absolutely. Since the early 1800s, numerous individuals and organizations—many in fields that came to be known as public health, medicine, social work, philanthropy, and criminal justice—had attempted to investigate, raise public awareness about, and ameliorate problems of family violence. Public and scientific attention to the issue, however, waxed and waned in concert with broader societal concerns.

Kempe's article in a prominent scientific journal nevertheless was and remains enormously influential. Why? In part, because it explicitly named—and simultaneously highlighted the health consequences of—a volatile societal problem then hidden from view by dominant beliefs about the sanctity of family life. The unnamable problem, once named, became less nebulous and more tangible, something that could be more rigorously documented, monitored, and analyzed, bolstered by the belief that—with adequate will and resources—it could ultimately be rectified.

Forty years later, in 2002, we are reaching a similar juncture: the unnamable is again becoming named, and explicit investigation of racism as a harmful determinant of population health is gaining entry into mainstream public health and medical discourse. At issue are the myriad ways in which racism—and other forms of social inequality and discrimination—can adversely affect health across the life course via varied, intertwined economic, environmental, psychosocial, and iatrogenic pathways. The scientific question "Does racism harm health?" prompts a plenitude of hypotheses, each meriting serious scientific attention and resources.

Is it, however, novel to posit that racial/ethnic disparities in health arise from inequitable race relations? Surely not. Are we the first to suggest that health is harmed not only by heinous crimes against humanity, such as slavery, lynching, and genocide, but also by the grinding economic and social realities of what Essed has aptly termed "everyday racism"? Once again, no. In the mid-1800s, leading US abolitionists and physicians, Black and White alike, challenged convention by arguing that the poorer health of the Black relative to the White population resulted not from innate inferiority but rather White privilege, enforced via slavery in the South and legal racial discrimination in the North.

The Choctaw and Cherokee nations, forcibly evicted from their homelands after the U.S. Congress passed the Indian Removal Act in 1830, likewise understood that their health was being decimated by not only territorial but also cultural dispossession, justified in the name of

White supremacy. Concerns about health consequences of racism clearly are not new; to suggest otherwise is to misstate the historical record. Rather, reflecting the historical impact of racial inequality on not only health but also health sciences, the stark reality is that, despite long-standing awareness of the problem, the serious scientific study of racism as a determinant of population health remains in its infancy.

One way to move to the next stage is to consider current conceptual issues in the field, given that scientific knowledge is more often spurred by clarification of our thinking than by technological breakthroughs. In this spirit, I address 3 interrelated issues from the vantage of an epidemiologist guided by an ecosocial perspective: (1) links between racism, biology, and health, including recognition of biological expression of race relations and racialized expressions of biology; (2) methodological controversies over how to study the impact of racism on health; and (3) debates over whether racism or class underlies racial/ethnic disparities in health.

Racism, Biology, and Health

Clarity of terminology is critical for any science. A first step for analyzing the contribution of racism to racial/ethnic disparities in health is being explicit about definitions of racism, race/ethnicity, and the link between these concepts. In essence, both are interdependent expressions of inequitable and institutionalized societal race relations. More specifically, *racism* refers to institutional and individual practices that create and reinforce oppressive systems of race relations whereby people and institutions engaging in discrimination adversely restrict, by judgment and action, the lives of those against whom they discriminate.

Race/ethnicity, in turn, is a social rather than a biological category, referring to social groups, often sharing cultural heritage and ancestry, that are forged by oppressive systems of race relations justified by ideology. One group benefits from dominating other groups and defines itself and others through this domination and the possession of selective and arbitrary physical characteristics (e.g., skin color). Although once trumpeted as scientific "fact," the notion that "race" is a valid, biologically meaningful a priori category has long been—and continues to be—refuted by work in population genetics, anthropology, and sociology. The fact that we know what "race" we are says more about our society than it does our biology.

Why do these sorts of explicit definitions matter? Because they provide a conceptual foundation for integrating thinking about racism *and* biology as a means of understanding and investigating the impact of racism on health. Both matter. Two diametrically opposed constructs are at issue, constructs that nevertheless are routinely conflated in the scientific literature. The first is *biological expressions of race relations;* the second is *racialized expressions of biology.* The former draws attention to how harmful physical and psychosocial exposures due to racism adversely affect our biology, in ways that ultimately are embodied and manifested in racial/ethnic disparities in health. The latter refers to how arbitrary biological traits are erroneously construed as markers of innate "racial" distinctions.

Consider skin color. The biology of pigmentation and its direct relationship to certain skin-related disorders is real. Whether or not racism existed, people with lighter vs darker skin (i.e., less vs more dispersed melanosomes) would be at higher risk of malignant melanoma, given sufficient exposure to sunlight (and especially bad sunburns before puberty). By contrast, damage resulting from adverse use of skin lightening products, as prompted by the ideology that lighter is better, would constitute a biological expression of race relations.

Skin color, in turn, would become a racialized expression of biology if, absent any evidence, it were treated as a valid marker for other unspecified genetic traits, reflecting a presumption that the biology of "race" equals the biology of gene frequencies. This was the logic of the flawed research agenda egregiously exemplified by the Tuskegee syphilis study, unnaturally intended to determine whether the "natural history" of untreated syphilis in Blacks was the same as that previously observed in Whites, in light of hypothesized differences in their nervous systems.

As Cruickshank has recently pointed out, however, drawing on lessons from the Human Genome Project and systems biology, it is a logical and biological fallacy to assume that gene expression is equivalent to gene frequency. Consider the recent, rapid secular changes in obesity, hypertension, and diabetes among populations of West African descent living in the United Kingdom, the Caribbean, and the United States, as well as in West Africa, to use but one diasporic example. Only changes in gene expression, not gene frequency, can explain the speed of these trends. Even so, myriad epidemiological studies continue to treat "race" as a purely biological (i.e., genetic) variable or seek to explain racial/ethnic disparities in health absent consideration of the effects of racism on health.

By clearly distinguishing between and emphasizing the importance of taking into account both racism and biology, these 2 constructs make clear that we can never study human biology—or behavior—in the abstract. Exemplifying that we instead study people in context is Sapolsky's cautionary tale: If adrenal glands are studied only among cadavers of the poor, long since hypertrophied as a result of excess excretion of cortisol, then—as occurred in the early 20th century—the wealthy will be diagnosed with adrenal deficiency disorder. Simplistic divisions of the social and biological will not suffice. The interpretations we offer of observed average differences in health status across socially delimited groups reflect our theoretical frameworks, not ineluctable facts of nature.

Methodological Controversies

How then, methodologically, can we test the hypothesis that racism harms health? Addressing this scientific question raises several critical questions and controversies. At issue is the need for—and strengths and limitations of—studies that directly and indirectly assess the impact of racism on health, whether employing quantitative or qualitative methods. By direct, I mean health studies explicitly obtaining information on people's self-reported experiences of—and observing people's physiological and psychological responses to—real-life or experimental situations involving racial discrimination. By indirect, I mean studies that investigate racial/ethnic disparities in distributions of deleterious exposures or health outcomes and explicitly infer that racism underlies these disparities. Each approach has its flaws, and both are necessary, addressing questions the other cannot.

Highlighting why both direct and indirect approaches are necessary are 5 key pathways through which racism can harm health, by shaping exposure and vulnerability to the following: (1) economic and social deprivation; (2) toxic substances and hazardous conditions; (3) socially inflicted trauma (mental, physical, and sexual, directly experienced or witnessed, from verbal threats to violent acts); (4) targeted marketing of commodities that can harm health, such as junk food and psychoactive substances (alcohol, tobacco, and other licit and illicit drugs); and (5) inadequate or degrading medical care. Also relevant are health consequences of people's responses to discrimination. These responses—each with its own set of potential health impacts—can range from internalized oppression and harmful use of psychoactive substances to reflective coping, active resistance, and community organizing to end discrimination and promote human rights and social justice.

From this perspective, the direct approach is necessary for investigating pathways pertaining to socially inflicted trauma. There is no substitute. The caveat, well recognized in the enormous body of literature on "stress" and health, is that such research must reckon with not only exposures but perceptions of these exposures, as well as

cognitive issues pertaining to memory and disclosure. The scientific task is therefore to understand how various threats to validity can affect investigations relying on self-report data. Potential solutions include the following: research on what constitutes valid self-report measures of racial discrimination; experimental studies (as conducted in the areas of housing and job discrimination) that employ "testers" of the same age, gender, and physical size, equipped with identical resumes but differing in terms of their race/ethnicity; or psychological and criminal justice studies investigating differences in perception of and responses to designated scenarios.

Notably, conduct of such studies requires appraisal of participants' racial/ethnic identity. Recent suggestions, however well intentioned, to "abandon" use of racial/ethnic categories in public health research, on grounds that "race" is not a valid scientific concept, err on 2 accounts. First, such an argument implies that only biological, and not social, variables are "real" and can be studied scientifically. Second, it presumes that the race/ethnicity of persons reporting experiences of racial discrimination is irrelevant, thereby rendering it impossible to distinguish between—or evaluate the health effects of—racial discrimination reported by people of color and that reported by White people.

The indirect approach, in turn, is necessary for most of the other pathways listed, precisely because they involve exposures that extend beyond individual perception. Knowledge of racial discrimination in wages, for example, can be obtained only if one knows what others are paid. Similarly, knowledge of racial inequality in the provision of medical care, above and beyond disrespectful interpersonal interactions, can be obtained only by comparing the types of treatment offered to groups that exhibit equivalent morbidity rates but differ in regard to their race/ethnicity.

Herein lies the rub. A claim recently advanced by some social epidemiologists, notably Cooper and Kaufman, is that we cannot make causal inferences based on studies comparing health outcomes across different racial/ethnic groups. Why? Because, they argue, such studies violate the counterfactual criterion of exchangeability. That is, people who are "exposed" should, in principle, be capable of being "unexposed." Using this logic, their debatable example is that smokers differ from nonsmokers only because they smoke; in principle, the "treatment" of smoking could be randomized.

By contrast, according to Cooper and Kaufman, there is no way a White person could ever be or become a Black person or have the lifetime set of related experiences contingent upon being Black. The exposure of "race" is thus nonexchangeable and also, in their examples, uniform. Because commonly used statistical tests presume exchangeability, they assert that parameter estimates for racial/ethnic contrasts have no valid causal interpretation, including in relation to racial discrimination.

The fallacy of their argument is contained within their counterfactual propositions. Cooper and Kaufman in effect relegate "race" to an intrinsic trait. They confuse the fact that people cannot simply "choose" their race/ethnicity, in that it is conditioned by the racial/ethnic relations of the society into which they are born, with the consequences of experiencing differential—and variable—treatment by virtue of inequitable race relations. The appropriate counterfactual is thus as follows: What would happen if people were randomized to discriminatory treatment, as occurs with racial discrimination? As is often the case in epidemiology, we cannot perform such an experiment to test this hypothesis regarding racial/ethnic disparities in health across the life course and instead must rely on observational studies.

More broadly, the counterfactual contrast is of a world with and without racism. In the latter, people with darker vs lighter skin would in fact be "exchangeable"—as human beings—and thus equally at risk for all ailments other than those directly involving skin color (e.g., melanoma, vitiligo). This contrast, premised upon a common humanity, underlies the "tester" studies alluded to earlier regarding housing and job discrimination. It also underlies inferences made comparing health outcomes across birth cohorts; obviously, someone born in 1910 cannot be "exchanged" with or have the same set of experiences as a person born in 1940 or in 1970. Birth cohort comparisons of both rates of disease and exposures, however, are critical for assessing whether cross-sectional associations—even those derived from randomized clinical trials—can in fact explain secular changes in health.

As with any scientific research, poorly specified counterfactuals are what threaten causal interpretation, and all observational studies—not only those concerned with social determinants of health—must consider carefully their motivating counterfactuals. Even the smokers and nonsmokers of Cooper and Kaufman's example would, after all, violate a strict "exchangeability" criterion, because the fact and process of being a smoker brings with it an array of other correlated exposures and life histories.

Racism or Social Class: The Limits of "Either/Or" Logic

The third and final conceptual controversy builds on the first and second. It is the debate over whether "racism" or "social class" explains racial/ethnic disparities in

health and, relatedly, which is causally prior. Typically argued with reference to the Euro-American legacy of colonization and the slave trade, the logical and historical fallacy is to frame this debate as "either/or" rather than as "both/and." As attested to by reams of sociological and historical research, class and race relations are in fact intertwined. Since the global expansion of European power and economies in the mid-15th century and contingent territorial conquest and intercontinental slave trade, people have lived in a world of racialized class relations and class-contingent race relations. It logically follows that racial/ethnic inequalities are shaped and fostered by class inequalities, and vice versa.

The same holds for other types of discrimination that render people socially and economically vulnerable (e.g., discrimination based on gender or sexuality). Translated to health research, it is therefore an empirical question, not a philosophical principle, whether pathways involving economic deprivation and/or non-economic manifestations of racial discrimination contribute to racial/ethnic disparities in health. Or, put simply, the answer to the crude question "Which matters—race or class?" can be one, the other, neither, or both. This is why we need scientific research: to test competing hypotheses.

Being Explicit about Racism: A Scientific Necessity

In conclusion, recalling the example of child abuse, the point of explicitly naming and scientifically investigating racism as a determinant of population health is to generate valid knowledge to guide actions designed to improve public health. It is not to imply that racism is solely a public health or medical problem or that solutions will come primarily from public health or medical initiatives. Nor is health research required to "prove" that racism is "bad"; it is, by definition, and in many instances it is illegal as well. Rather, the point is that neglecting study of the health impact of racism means that explanations for and interventions to alter population distributions of health, disease, and well-being will be incomplete and potentially misleading, if not outright harmful. Of course, work in this field will, inevitably, be fraught with controversy, because the exposure raises important themes of accountability, agency, and human rights.

That there are legal, political, and economic consequences of attributing disparities in health status to racial discrimination is, however, no more or less germane than it is for research on any other determinant of societal health, whether child abuse, ambient air pollution, tobacco, or food. The canard that research on health consequences of racism is "political" rather than "scientific" is blatantly incorrect: it is in fact political and unscientific to exclude the topic from the domain of legitimate scientific inquiry and discourse. Nor is this insight new: James McCune Smith and John Rock, 2 of the first credentialed African American physicians in the United States, said as much a century and a half ago. Rather, the task at hand is to bring the knowledge and methods available in our generation to the pressing public health problem of persistent racial/ethnic disparities in health.

REFERENCES
A list of references is available in the original source.

"What Are Health Disparities?"

by American Medical Student Asociation

The existence of racial and ethnic disparities in healthcare represents a failure of the healthcare system to provide equal, high quality healthcare to all individuals, regardless of ethnicity, race and other factors. The publication of Healthy People 2010 in 2000 advanced a goal for the elimination of all health disparities in the United States, and acknowledged that a comprehensive strategy incorporating research, education, policy changes, and community partnerships is fundamental to accomplishing this goal. Medical education is an important component of an overall strategy to eliminate health disparities. As the United States becomes increasingly diverse, the next generation of physicians is challenged to expand their knowledge of the different racial and ethnic populations and healthcare inequities facing the U.S. and develop new skills to take care of these patients effectively with cultural competency. As Unequal Treatment suggests, students must learn the underlying causes of health disparities to prepare themselves to care for diverse patient populations. These causes include disparities in healthcare access, resources, treatment, outcomes, and health status for racial and ethnic minority patients; the patient-physician relationship; the healthcare delivery system; language problems; understanding of cultural and folk illnesses; patient beliefs; provider biases; and stereotyping. In addition, students must appreciate the relationship between psychosocial issues and health disparities in order to become culturally competent physicians.

Access: Minorities are less likely than non-minorities to have access to regular medical care and to have health insurance

- Low-income Americans run the highest risk of being uninsured. In 2003, 45 million people lacked health insurance, and the numbers have increased since. Among minority groups, Hispanics are the least likely to have health insurance (32.7% uninsured), followed by American Indians and Alaska Natives (22.7% uninsured) based on a 2-year average (2002–2003). Compare this to 19.6% of Blacks, 18.8% of Asians and Pacific Islanders, and 11.1% of white non-Hispanics who lack health insurance.

Treatment: Minorities are more likely to receive inappropriate or insufficient care than non-minorities

- Numerous studies over the past two decades have documented racial and ethnic differences in care for heart conditions. The strongest studies provide credible evidence that African Americans are less likely than whites to receive diagnostic procedures, revascularization procedures and thrombolytic therapy. Eighty-four percent of studies (done from 1984–2001) investigating this idea found racial/ethnic differences in cardiac care for at least one of the minority groups under study.

Source: *Racial/Ethnic Differences in Cardiac Care, The Weight of the Evidence*, October 2002.

- HIV infection is now the leading cause of death among African Americans between the ages of 25 and 44 and the second leading cause of death among Latinos in this age group. The most telling data regarding adequacy of treatment for minorities come from the HIV Cost and Services Utilization Study that looked at the use of triple drug antiretroviral therapy, a treatment regimen that is very effective in delaying disability and prolonging the life of persons with HIV. African Americans were more than twice as likely as whites to not receive combination drug therapy and 1.5 times more likely to not get preventive treatment for pneumocystic carinii pneumonia (a common, but preventable, infection in people with HIV) than whites. Latinos were 1.5 times more likely than whites to not get combination drug therapy.

Outcomes: Minorities are more likely to have worse health outcomes than non-minorities

- Heart disease is the leading cause of death for all racial and ethnic groups in the United States. In 1999, rates of death from cardiovascular disease were about 30% higher among African American adults than among white adults.

    Source: *HHS Fact Sheet, U.S. Dept of Health and Human Services,* Sept. 2002

Health status

- The incidence of diabetes among American Indians and Alaska Natives is more than twice that of the total population, and the Pima Indians of Arizona have the highest known prevalence of diabetes in the world. The prevalence of diabetes is 70% higher among African Americans and nearly 100% higher among Hispanics than among Caucasian individuals.

    Source: *HHS Fact Sheet, U.S. Dept of Health and Human Services,* Sept. 2002

- As recently as 2000, African Americans and Hispanics accounted for roughly 75% of all adult AIDS cases, although they only comprise 25% of the U.S. population. African American and Hispanics also make up 81% of all pediatric AIDS cases.

    Source: *HHS Fact Sheet, U.S. Dept of Health and Human Services,* Sept. 2002

- In women, racial and ethnic minority groups are more likely to be overweight or obese than non-Hispanic whites. The same holds true for Mexican-American men vs. non-Hispanic men. This risk factor contributes to the fact that 8.2% of all Hispanic Americans have diabetes.

    Source: HHS Fact Sheet, U.S. Dept. of Health and Human Services, Sept. 2004, Health Gap Datastats, OMHRC

A disparity is an inequality. In the United States, we believe that healthcare should not differ by race, ethnicity, socioeconomic status, or geographic location. When these differences do exist, they are referred to as disparities. We see this when racial and ethnic minorities receive lower quality healthcare than whites. It is important to understand that differences in race and ethnicity (among other things) will always exist; it is wrong, however, when these differences lead to unequal care.

 **"Why Do Health Disparities Exist?"**

by American Medical Student Asociation

There are many factors that may contribute to racial and ethnic disparities in healthcare. Among the better-controlled studies performed to assess these factors, the vast majority indicated that minorities are less likely than whites to receive needed services, including clinically necessary procedures. Let's look at some of the reasons for this:

- **Healthcare delivery systems and access to healthcare.** In examining healthcare access issues, one must also consider the legal and regulatory climate in which healthcare systems operate, including factors such as **cultural or linguistic barriers** (e.g. the lack of interpretation services for patients with limited English speaking skills), **fragmentation of healthcare systems** (which could include the possibility that minorities are disproportionately enrolled in lower-cost health plans that put greater per-patient limits on healthcare spending and available services), and **incentives to physicians to limit services.** Where minority patients tend to receive care is also important to consider, as they are less likely to access care in a private physician's office, even when insured at the same level as whites. When asked why the healthcare system treats people unfairly based on race or ethnic background, 58% of physicians cite as a major reason the simple fact that many people from minority groups live in medically underserved areas where there are fewer doctors or other health providers.

- **Physician biases and patient perceptions.** Medical school does an excellent job of teaching the diagnosis and treatment of clinical disease but fails to prepare future physicians to incorporate psychosocial and cultural factors and overcome personal biases in the care of patients. It is reasonable to assume that the majority of healthcare providers find prejudice morally wrong and at odds with their professional values, but healthcare providers, like other members of society, may not recognize manifestations of prejudice in their own behavior. A study based on actual clinical encounters done by van Ryn and Burke (2000) found that doctors rated black patients as less intelligent, less educated, more likely to abuse drugs and alcohol, more likely to fail to comply with medical advice, more likely to lack social support, and less likely to participate in cardiac rehabilitation than white patients, even after patients' income, education, and personality characteristics were taken into account. These findings suggest that while the relationship between race or ethnicity and treatment decisions is complex, providers' perceptions and attitudes toward patients are often influenced in subtle ways by patient race or ethnicity

- **Greater clinical uncertainty when interacting with minority patients.** Any degree of uncertainty a physician may have relative to the condition of a patient can contribute to disparities in treatment. In order to make a diagnosis, a doctor must depend on inferences about severity based on what they can see about the illness and on what they observe about the patient (including race, age, gender, and sometimes socioeconomic status). If the information related to the illness is lacking or deemed to be inaccurate, the doctor tends to rely on his observations of the patient (which may include unfair assumptions) to make diagnostic decisions. The consequence is that treatment decisions and patients' needs are potentially less well matched.

Sources: The National Healthcare Disparities Report, Agency for Healthcare Research and Quality (AHRQ) and U.S. Dept. of Health and Human Services (July 2003) (accessed December 9, 2004); *The Right to Equal Treatment Report, Physicians for Human Rights*, (September 2003) (accessed December 9, 2004); and "*Racial and Ethnic Disparities in Access to Health Insurance and Health Care*," UCLA Center for Health Policy Research and The Henry J. Kaiser Family Foundation (April 2000) (accessed December 9, 2004)

Cultural Humility versus Cultural Competence: "A Critical Distinction in Defining Physician Training Outcomes in Multicultural Education"

by Melanie Tervalon and Jann Murray-García

Abstract   Researchers and program developers in medical education presently face the challenge of implementing and evaluating curricula that teach medical students and house staff how to effectively and respectfully deliver healthcare to the increasingly diverse populations of the United States. Inherent in this challenge is clearly defining educational and training outcomes consistent with this imperative. The traditional notion of competence in clinical training as a detached mastery of a theoretically finite body of knowledge may not be appropriate for this area of physician education. Cultural humility is proposed as a more suitable goal in multicultural medical education. Cultural humility incorporates a lifelong commitment to self-evaluation and self-critique, to redressing the power imbalances in the patient-physician dynamic, and to developing mutually beneficial and nonpaternalistic clinical and advocacy partnerships with communities on behalf of individuals and defined populations.

The increasing cultural, racial, and ethnic diversity of the United States compels medical educators to train physicians who will skillfully and respectfully negotiate the implications of this diversity in their clinical practice. Simultaneously, increasing attention is being paid to nonfinancial barriers that operate at the level of the physician/patient dynamic. This dynamic is often compromised by various sociocultural mismatches between patients and providers, including providers' lack of knowledge regarding patients' health beliefs and life experiences, and providers' unintentional and intentional processes of racism, classism, homophobia, and sexism.

Several recent national mandates calling for innovative approaches to multicultural training of physicians have emerged from various sources. The Pew Health Professions Commission, specifically seeking to give direction to health professions education for the twenty-first century, stated that "cultural sensitivity must be a part of the educational experiences that touches the life of every student." The Institute of Medicine defines *optimal primary care* as including "an understanding of the cul-tural, nutritional and belief systems of patients and communities that may assist or hinder effective healthcare delivery."

The necessity for multicultural medical education provides researchers and program developers with the challenge of defining and measuring training outcomes and proving that chosen instructional strategies do indeed produce these outcomes. However, in the laudable urgency to implement and evaluate programs that aim to produce cultural competence, one dimension to be avoided is the pitfall of narrowly defining competence in medical training and practice in its traditional sense: an easily demonstrable mastery of a finite body of knowledge, an endpoint evidenced largely by comparative quantitative assessments (i.e., MCATs, pre- and post-exams, board certification exams).

Rather, cultural competence in clinical practice is best defined not by a discrete endpoint but as a commitment and active engagement in a lifelong process that individuals enter into on an ongoing basis with patients, communities, colleagues, and with themselves

"Cultural Humility versus Cultural Competence: A Critical Distinction in Defining Physician Training Outcomes in Multicultural Education," by Melanie Tervalon and Jann Murray-Garcia, *Journal of Health Care for the Poor & Underserved*, 9:2 (1998), 117–125. Reprinted by permission of The Johns Hopkins University Press.

(L. Brown, MPH, Oakland health advocate, personal communication, March 18, 1994). This training outcome, perhaps better described as cultural humility versus cultural competence, actually dovetails several educational initiatives in U.S. physician workforce training as we approach the twenty-first century. It is a process that requires humility as individuals continually engage in self-reflection and self-critique as lifelong learners and reflective practitioners. It is a process that requires humility in how physicians bring into check the power imbalances that exist in the dynamics of physician-patient communication by using patient-focused interviewing and care. And it is a process that requires humility to develop and maintain mutually respectful and dynamic partnerships with communities on behalf of individual patients and communities in the context of community-based clinical and advocacy training models.

Self-reflection and the Lifelong Learner Model

Increasing trainees' knowledge of health beliefs and practices is critically important. For instance, the Cambodian child who comes in with the linear marks of "coining," a Southeast Asian healing practice, should not be mistaken for the victim of parental child abuse.

To be avoided, however, is the false sense of security in one's training evidenced by the following actual case from our experience: An African American nurse is caring for a middle-aged Latina woman several hours after the patient had undergone surgery. A Latino physician on a consult service approached the bedside and, noting the moaning patient, commented to the nurse that the patient appeared to be in a great deal of postoperative pain. The nurse summarily dismissed his perception, informing him that she took a course in nursing school in cross-cultural medicine and "knew" that Hispanic patients overexpress "the pain they are feeling." The Latino physician had a difficult time influencing the perspective of this nurse, who focused on her self-proclaimed cultural expertise.

This nurse's notion of her own expertise actually stereotyped the patient's experience, ignored clues (the moaning) to the patient's present reality, and disregarded the potential resource of a colleague who might (albeit not necessarily) be able to contribute some relevant cultural insight. The equating of cultural competence with simply having completed a past series of training sessions is an inadequate and potentially harmful model of professional development, as evidenced by this case.

In no way are we discounting the value of knowing as much as possible about the healthcare practices of the communities we serve. Rather, it is imperative that there be a simultaneous process of self-reflection (realistic and ongoing self-appraisal) and commitment to a lifelong learning process. In this way, trainees are ideally flexible and humble enough to let go of the false sense of security that stereotyping brings. They are flexible and humble enough to assess anew the cultural dimensions of the experiences of each patient. And finally, they are flexible and humble enough *to say that they do not know when they truly do not know* and to search for and access resources that might enhance immeasurably the care of the patient as well as their future clinical practice.

In a related manner, an isolated increase in knowledge without a consequent change in attitude and behavior is of questionable value. In fact, existing literature documenting a lack of cultural competence in clinical practice most reflects not a lack of knowledge but rather the need for a change in practitioners' self-awareness and a change in their attitudes toward diverse patients. These data indicate that the prescription of clinical resources from prevention services to potentially life-saving procedures is often differential, dependent on the race or ethnicity of the patient. For example, a study in a university emergency department showed that Latinos were half as likely as white patients to receive analgesia for the same, usually very painful, long-bone fractures, regardless of the linguistic capability or insurance status of the patient. A follow-up study in the same institution showed no difference in physicians' assessment of the level of pain experienced by white and Latino patients experiencing the same, isolated injury. Another study showed that while African Americans are twice as likely to go blind from progressive ophthalmologic diseases such as glaucoma, they are half as likely to receive sight-saving procedures. Such disturbing evidence from the medical profession is a sobering reflection of the parallel reality and tragic costs of racism that persist in American society and that potentially influence every physician.

Clearly, program developers and researchers cannot, in our cultural competency training, simply stimulate a detached, intellectual practice of describing "the other" in the tradition of descriptive medical anthropology. At the heart of this education process should be the provision of intellectual and practical leadership that engages physician trainees in an ongoing, courageous, and honest process of self-critique and self-awareness. Guiding trainees to identify and examine their own patterns of unintentional and intentional racism, classism, and homophobia is essential.

One way to initiate such a constructive process is to have trainees think consciously about their own, often ill-defined and multidimensional cultural identities and backgrounds. In leading trainees into this process of cultivating self-awareness and awareness of the perspectives of others, trainers and program planners have used the following pedagogical approaches with success: small-group discussions; personal journals; availability of constructive professional role models from cultural groups and from the trainee's groups; and videotaping and feedback, including directed introspection of residents' interactions with patients. Recognition and respect for others' cultural priorities and practices is facilitated by such initial and ongoing processes that engender self-knowledge.

At the same time and by the same process of self-reflection, awakening trainees to the incredible position of power physicians potentially hold over all patients, particularly the poor, is critical. Especially in the context of race, ethnicity, class, linguistic capability, and sexual orientation, physicians must be taught to repeatedly identify and remedy the inappropriate exploitation of this power imbalance in the establishment of treatment priorities and health promotion activities.

Again, humility, and not so much the discrete mastery traditionally implied by the static notion of competence, captures most accurately what researchers need to model and hold programs accountable for evaluating in trainees under the broad scope of multicultural training in medical education.

Patient-focused Interviewing and Care

Embodied in the physician who practices cultural humility is the patient-focused or language-focused interviewing process. Studies of patient-physician communication have shown a strong bias on the part of physicians against patient-initiated questions and agendas, with physicians in one study initiating over 90 percent of the questions. Another study demonstrated that although poor and minority patients wanted as much information regarding their conditions as did other patients, they received less information regarding their conditions, less positive or reinforcing speech, and less talk overall.

Patient-focused interviewing uses a less controlling, less authoritative style that signals to the patient that the practitioner values what the patient's agenda and perspectives are, both biomedical and nonbiomedical. With these communication skills, perhaps along with other specifically cross-cultural interaction techniques, physicians potentially create an atmosphere that enables and does not obstruct the patient's telling of his or her own illness or wellness story. This eliminates the need for a complete mastery of every group's health beliefs and other concerns because the patient in the ideal scenario is encouraged to communicate how little or how much culture has to do with that particular clinical encounter.

For example, Ridley describes the uniqueness of a patient by detailing the patient's "conjoint membership in eight cultural roles:" as a Mexican American, male, father, husband, Catholic, mechanic, night-school student, and resident of East Los Angeles. Only the patient is uniquely qualified to help the physician understand the intersection of race, ethnicity, religion, class, and so on in forming his (the patient's) identity and to clarify the relevance and impact of this intersection on the present illness or wellness experience. Relevant and effective prevention, health promotion, and therapeutic strategies can then be developed that take into account the patient's life priorities, health beliefs, and life stressors. Humility is a prerequisite in this process, as the physician relinquishes the role of *expert* to the patient, becoming the *student* of the patient with a conviction and explicit expression of the patient's potential to be a capable and full partner in the therapeutic alliance.

Community-based Care and Advocacy

There is increasing consensus that a substantial portion of physicians' clinical training needs to occur in community sites. It is argued that training needs to happen in arenas where most physicians will eventually practice, away from the university-based, largely tertiary medical center. Part of this training directive includes a population-based approach to health promotion and disease prevention that works toward the optimal health of communities; that is, health in its broadest sense of physical, mental, and social well-being. Evans states that "surely a small part of each physician's responsibility should extend beyond the care of individual patients to the advocacy for changes in the community's policies and practices that influence determinants of health, causes of disease, and the effectiveness of health services."

Competency in advocacy is actually mandated by the American Academy of Pediatrics as a skill to be acquired during pediatric residency. This professional skill is to be taught by way of "structured educational experiences that prepare residents for their future role as advocates for the health of all children . . . with particular attention to underserved populations."

It is hoped that community-based care and advocacy training would go beyond working with community physicians and even beyond training in legislative advocacy to include systematically and methodically immersing trainees in mutually beneficial, nonpaternalistic, and respectful working relationships with community members and organizations. Experiencing with the community the factors at play in defining health priorities, research activities, and community-informed advocacy activities requires that the physician trainee recognize that foci of expertise with regard to health can indeed reside outside of the academic medical center and even outside of the practice of Western medicine. Competence, thus, again becomes best illustrated by humility, as physician trainees learn to identify, believe in, and build on the assets and adaptive strengths of communities and their often disenfranchised members. Requiring ongoing self-reflection and a parallel notion of patient- (community-) focused interactions, the possibility then exists for planning, practice, and advocacy in community health work in which physicians and physician trainees are both effective students of and partners with the community.

Institutional Consistency

The same processes expected to affect change in physician trainees should simultaneously exist in the institutions whose agenda is to develop cultural competence through educational programs. Self-reflection and self-critique at the institutional level is required, encompassing honest, thorough, and ongoing responses to the following questions: What is the demographic profile of the faculty? Is the faculty composition inclusive of members from diverse cultural, racial, ethnic, and sexual orientation backgrounds? Are faculty members required to undergo multicultural training as are the youngest students of the profession? Does the institutional ethos support inclusion and respectful, substantive discussions of the clinical implications of difference? What institutional processes contradict or obstruct the lessons taught and learned in a multicultural curriculum (i.e., if it is taught that practitioners should not use children or other family members as translators, does the institution provide an accessible alternative?)? What is the history of the healthcare institution with the surrounding community? And what present model of relationship between the institution and the community is seen by trainees?

Time-limited and explicit educational goals are one dimension of demonstrated institutional cultural competence. For instance, developing a written plan of faculty recruit-

ment and/or curricular development to be in place by a designated date could be a point to which the community and/or other external entities hold the institution publicly accountable with regard to issues of race, ethnicity, language, culture, sexual orientation, and class in healthcare.

Summary of the Challenge to Medical Education Researchers

The emphasis on demonstration of process as opposed to endpoint is not meant to imply that training outcomes in cultural competence programs cannot be measured or monitored. Capturing the characteristic of cultural humility in individuals and institutions is possible, especially with mixed methodologies that use qualitative methods (including participant observation, key informant interviews, trainees' journals, and mechanisms for community feedback) and action research models to complement traditional quantitative assessments (pre- and postknowledge tests, patient and trainee surveys) of program effectiveness. A potentially valuable measure is the documentation of an active, ongoing institutional process that includes training, established recruitment and retention processes, identifiable and funded personnel to facilitate the meeting of program goals, and dynamic feedback loops between the institution and its employees and between the institution and patients and/or other members from the surrounding community.

This is not to say that the measurement of individuals' or institutions' cultural competence is a well-developed area of research. Witness this present discussion on defining training outcomes. Indeed, the definition and measurement of program effectiveness in producing cultural competence is a relatively new arena of inquiry in need of careful and attentive intellectual leadership. Nonetheless, acknowledging the necessity for creativity in a program's development and evaluation stages will help avoid the pitfall of adopting the status quo in documenting clinical competence.

Conclusion

In this critically important dialogue of defining training outcomes, it is proposed that the notion of cultural humility be distinguished from that of cultural competence. Cultural humility incorporates a lifelong commitment to self-evaluation and critique, to redressing the power imbalances in the physician-patient dynamic, and to developing mutually beneficial and non-paternalistic partnerships with communities on behalf of individuals and defined populations.

Acknowledgments

This work was supported by grants from the California Wellness Foundation, the Federal Office of Minority Health (DHHS), the East Bay Neonatology Foundation, and the Bay Area Physicians for Human Rights.

REFERENCES

A list of references is available in the original source.

"Health at the Margins"

by Gabrie'l J. Atchison

In this issue, we are asking how different forms of discrimination affect the quality of healthcare that women receive. What are the barriers to women's health? We include information about women of color, lesbians, women with disabilities, women living in poverty, rural women, and women living in the Global South. This article is a brief overview of information about women in different groups, which shows that there are some interesting similarities from group to group. Marginalized women in general seem more likely to die from preventable diseases and health conditions, because they reach professionals too late. They experience higher levels of stress and have less leisure time, which contributes to unique health problems. There is not enough research about the health needs of women at the margins, so healthcare providers cannot help them adequately. Violence is a major health risk in the lives of marginalized women. Poverty and racism are also especially linked to high incidences of HIV infection and AIDS deaths.

Women of Color
African American Women

Black women face stereotyping and discrimination in their healthcare. They are less likely to have health insurance, more likely to face great financial barriers to adequate healthcare, less likely to have information about symptoms, and less likely to have healthcare facilities in their neighborhoods. Due to high levels of stress, African American women are disproportionately represented among the obese in this country and have high rates of hypertension, heart disease, and stroke,

three other stress-related conditions. African American women have the highest death rate due to HIV of any racial/ethnic group. There is no research explaining why this is so. AIDS is the leading cause of death for African American women between the ages of 25 and 44. Homicide and violence is the fourth leading cause of death in this group. Maternal mortality is four times higher for African American women than white women, and African Americans have the highest infant mortality rate of any racial group. Native American women and African American women experience and witness violence more often than other groups of women.

Latinas

Latino families have the highest rates of poverty in the United States; almost 30 percent of Latinas live in poverty. Their healthcare problems are compounded by language barriers, racism, and lack of access to healthcare facilities. Like African American women, Latinas are often diagnosed when it is too late for proper treatment, especially with breast cancer. For undocumented Latinas, there is an additional fear of being reported and deported, so many women do not have access to healthcare at all for themselves or their children. Latinas experience high levels of severe depression, and have the highest prevalence of lifetime depression. For Latinas, the leading causes of death are heart disease, diabetes, and stroke. Diabetes is the second highest cause of death for Latinas between the ages of 55 and 74. Latinas have the second highest death rate due to HIV.

Asian American Women

Like Latinas, the Asian American community is diverse in language, culture, and geographic location. There is not enough information about this diversity, so more research is needed. According to the information that is available, Asian Americans who live in poverty face similar racial discrimination in healthcare, combined with the added burden of language and cultural differences and undocumented immigration status among some communities. Some of the research suggests that Asian American women do not have adequate access to reproductive healthcare providers. Many Asian American women work in factories or in small, family-owned businesses and do not have any access to healthcare. Unsafe and unhealthy work environments also contribute to their health problems.

Native American Women

Native American women face logistic and cultural barriers to obtaining healthcare services. Many Native American women live in rural communities and have limited access to transportation, and there is only a small number of healthcare facilities available to them. In some Native communities, women have traditionally been the healers for other women, so Native American women find going to male doctors uncomfortable. Many women do not seek preventative services. There are high rates of smoking and alcohol and drug addiction in these communities and very few culturally specific recovery programs. Accidents and violence are the most common causes of death among this group of women. Almost one quarter of all Native American women live in poverty. They experience racial discrimination, high unemployment, environmental racism, and poor quality housing; and they often live near toxic waste or other forms of environmental hazards and lack access to safe water.

Immigrant Women of Color

Ten percent of the United States population are immigrants. Of that group, more than half are from Latin America and one quarter is from Asia. Women in these populations experience racism as well as language and cultural barriers to receiving healthcare. The Personal Responsibility Work Opportunity and Reconciliation Act of 1996 restricted immigrant women's access to healthcare services and insurance by allowing states to deny Medicaid benefits to immigrant families. Many immigrants live in poverty and have no access to healthcare.

Lesbians

Little attention is paid to the special health needs of lesbians. There should be more research which takes into account the diversity of lesbian women. Lesbians experience job discrimination and because of this may end up in low-paying jobs or feel forced to stay in the closet about their sexuality. Most lesbians are not covered by their partners' insurance. Lesbians also face a great deal of discrimination trying to receive healthcare, most of which stems from the assumption of heterosexuality by providers. Lack of legal recognition can prevent lesbians from getting financial support when a partner becomes ill or dies. Typically lesbians cannot benefit from life insurance, family leave, workers' compensation, or hospital visitation rights. Lesbian women are also susceptible to hate crimes and violence. Since lesbians are less likely to use contraceptives and may be reluctant to discuss their sexual lives with providers they fear will discriminate against them, they may not have regular gynecological checkups, including preventative services like cervical and breast cancer screenings. There is a lack of information about the health habits of lesbians outside of their sexual behaviors. The issue of domestic violence in lesbian communities is a major health concern. A disproportionate number of youth suicides are young lesbians who cannot find acceptance or approval. Because of ageism and homophobia, the special health needs of the older lesbian community are invisible. There can be safety problems in nursing homes because of homophobia among attendants and other personnel. Healthcare providers are urged to challenge their own assumptions of heterosexuality and those of their colleagues to make healthcare more inclusive of lesbians. Simply using language like "partner" as opposed to "boyfriend" or "husband" would make a difference. Physicians could also change office registration forms, questionnaires, and informational brochures to include information about lesbians.

Women with Disabilities

Women with disabilities face a multitude of barriers to proper healthcare. Some of these barriers include physical inaccessibility of medical offices, limited availability of information, inaccessible public transportation, and inadequate treatment or outright refusals of treatment by healthcare providers. Health maintenance organizations place strict limits on therapeutic, supportive, and home services, which severely limit disabled women's ability to live independently. There are also problems because women are not able to use specialists as primary care providers, and alternative therapies are often not covered. There is a lack of research on disabled women and health, but some of the special concerns for this group are violence and barriers to adequate mental and reproductive healthcare. Disabled women are at high risk for depression and eating disorders, and are often either denied medication or are oversedated. They experience forced sterilization, coerced abortions, and unauthorized hysterectomies. Disabled women and girls are very vulnerable to emotional, physical, and sexual abuse by partners, family members, and care givers, and since they are often not believed when they report this abuse many of these crimes go unreported. Girls with disabilities are almost twice as likely as other girls to be sexually abused and assaulted.

Caring for a Disabled Child

Taking care of a child with a disability demands a great deal of time and can cause a lot of stress. When a woman lives in poverty, having a disabled child can be completely overwhelming. Visits with doctors and specialists can be an all-day event, especially if one had to spend a long time on public transportation. This often means missing days from work. Working low-income women most often receive no sympathy from employers for these absences. Low-income women who have to work to provide for the care of their children are often accused by their children's care providers of not loving or attending to their children enough. For developmentally disabled children, the quality of attention they receive in their early years affects the quality of life they will have as adults.

Women Living in Poverty

In the United States and globally, women are disproportionately represented among the people living in poverty. In the United States, health is a commodity, and things like gym memberships, medication, and vacations and leisure time are all too expensive for women living in poverty. Without an adequate income, women cannot afford healthcare, health insurance, safe housing, or nutritious food. Serious illness of a parent or child can result in economic ruin for many poor families. Many of the women and girls in prison are there because they sold drugs or did sex work to support themselves and their children. The lack of public transportation in poor communities makes travel to healthcare facilities difficult. Violence is a major cause of death among poor women and many advocacy groups are pressuring politicians

for gun control laws to reduce the level of deaths and serious injuries to women caused by gunshots.

Rural Women

Rural Women are almost non-existent in psychological literature, but we know that rural women experience barriers to healthcare because of isolation, fewer resources, lack of transportation, and lack of access to medical and mental health services, which are often concentrated in cities. Rural women have a higher incidence of anxiety and depression. Often, the only providers in rural areas are from the public health centers. Rural women have to travel far for healthcare, only to see a doctor with less training. Because rural women have less contact with doctors, they have lower levels of preventive care.

Women in the Global South

"The Global South" is a phrase used to describe countries commonly referred to as "developing countries"—the term is meant to bring attention to the relationship between the colonizer and the colonized and to economic privilege and control. The phrase incorporates many different countries and relationships between countries. Women are overrepresented among the poor in the Global South, and women's poverty is destructive to women and children's health in these countries. Women and girls are often the last to eat and thus are often malnourished. Their health problems are considered less important than men's problems. For example, the number of women with HIV in Africa is considerably higher than that of men with the disease, yet men are receiving more care and treatment. Adolescent girls are particularly vulnerable because of lack of information about reproductive health, lack of power in sexual relations, scarcity of reproductive health services, and susceptibility to sexual abuse and violence. It is estimated that women in the Global South work twice as many hours as men. They also work in dangerous, unhealthy environments like sweatshops, the informal economy, and the sex industry. Many women work at paid jobs and still have to provide care for children, men, and the elderly. Poverty combined with high levels of stress exacerbate health problems faced by women.

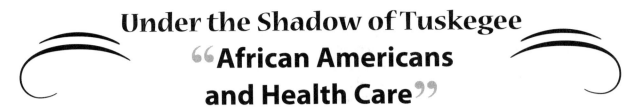

Under the Shadow of Tuskegee
"African Americans and Health Care"

by Vanessa Northington Gamble

Abstract   The Tuskegee Syphilis Study continues to cast its long shadow on the contemporary relationship between African Americans and the biomedical community. Numerous reports have argued that the Tuskegee Syphilis Study is the most important reason why many African Americans distrust the institutions of medicine and public health. Such an interpretation neglects a critical historical point: the mistrust predated public revelations about the Tuskegee study. This paper places the syphilis study within a broader historical and social context to demonstrate that several factors have influenced—and continue to influence—African Americans' attitudes toward the biomedical community. (*Am J Public Health*. 1997;87:1773–1778)

Introduction

On May 16, 1997, in a White House ceremony, President Bill Clinton apologized for the Tuskegee Syphilis Study, the 40-year government study (1932 to 1972) in which 399 Black men from Macon County, Alabama, were deliberately denied effective treatment for syphilis in order to document the natural history of the disease. "The legacy of the study at Tuskegee," the president remarked, "has reached far and deep, in ways that hurt our progress and divide our nation. We cannot be one America when a whole segment of our nation has no trust in America." The president's comments underscore that in the 25 years since its public disclosure, the study has moved from being a singular historical event to a powerful metaphor. It has come to symbolize racism in medicine, misconduct in human research, the arrogance of physicians, and government abuse of Black people.

The continuing shadow cast by the Tuskegee Syphilis Study on efforts to improve the health status of Black Americans provided an impetus for the campaign for a presidential apology. Numerous articles, in both the professional and popular press, have pointed out that the study predisposed many African Americans to distrust medical and public health authorities and has led to critically low Black participation in clinical trials and organ donation.

The specter of Tuskegee has also been raised with respect to HIV/AIDS prevention and treatment programs. Health education researchers Dr Stephen B. Thomas and Dr Sandra Crouse Quinn have written extensively on the impact of the Tuskegee Syphilis Study on these programs. They argue that "the legacy of this experiment, with its failure to educate the study participants and treat them adequately, laid the foundation for today's pervasive sense of black distrust of public health authorities." The syphilis study has also been used to explain why many African Americans oppose needle exchange programs. Needle exchange programs provoke the image of the syphilis study and Black fears about genocide. These programs are not viewed as mechanisms to stop the spread of HIV/AIDS but rather as fodder for the drug epidemic that has devastated so many Black neighborhoods. Fears that they will be used as guinea pigs like the men in the syphilis study have also led some African Americans with AIDS to refuse treatment with protease inhibitors.

The Tuskegee Syphilis Study is frequently described as the singular reason behind African-American distrust of the institutions of medicine and public health. Such an interpretation neglects a critic historical point: the mistrust predated public revelations about the Tuskegee study. Furthermore, the narrowness of such a representation places emphasis on a single historical event to explain deeply entrenched and complex attitudes within the Black community. An examination of the syphilis study within a broader historical and social context makes plain that several factors have influenced, and continue to influence, African Americans' attitudes toward the biomedical community.

Black Americans' fears about exploitation by the medical profession date back to the antebellum period and the use of slaves and free Black people as subjects for dissection and medical experimentation. Although physicians also used poor Whites as subjects, they used Black people far more often. During an 1835 trip to the United States, French visitor Harriet Martineau found that Black people lacked the power even to protect the graves of their dead. "In Baltimore the bodies of coloured people exclusively are taken for dissection," she remarked, "because the Whites do not like it, and the coloured people cannot resist." Four years later, abolitionist Theodore Dwight Weld echoed Martineau's sentiment. "Public opinion," he wrote, "would tolerate surgical experiments, operations, processes, performed upon them [slaves], which it would execrate if performed upon their master or other whites." Slaves found themselves as subjects of medical experiments because physicians needed bodies and because the state considered them property and denied them the legal right to refuse to participate.

Two antebellum experiments, one carried out in Georgia and the other in Alabama, illustrate the abuse that some slaves encountered at the hands of physicians. In the first, Georgia physician Thomas Hamilton conducted a series of brutal experiments on a slave to test remedies for heatstroke. The subject of these investigations, Fed, had been loaned to Hamilton as repayment for a debt owed by his owner. Hamilton forced Fed to sit naked on a stool placed on a platform in a pit that had been heated to a high temperature. Only the man's head was above ground. Over a period of 2 to 3 weeks, Hamilton placed Fed in the pit five or six times and gave him various medications to determine which enabled him best to withstand the heat. Each ordeal ended when Fed fainted and had to be revived. But note that Fed was not the only victim in this experiment; its whole purpose was to make it possible for masters to force slaves to work still longer hours on the hottest of days.

In the second experiment, Dr J. Marion Sims, the so-called father of modern gynecology, used three Alabama slave women to develop an operation to repair vesico-vaginal fistulas. Between 1845 and 1849, the three slave women on whom Sims operated each underwent up to 30 painful operations. The physician himself described the agony associated with some of the experiments: "The first patient I operated on was Lucy. . . . That was before the days of anesthetics, and the poor girl, on her knees, bore the operation with great heroism and bravery." This operation was not successful, and Sims later attempted to repair the defect by placing a sponge in the bladder. This experiment, too, ended in failure. He noted:

> The whole urethra and the neck of the bladder were in a high state of inflammation, which came from

the foreign substance. It had to come away, and there was nothing to do but to pull it away by main force. Lucy's agony was extreme. She was much prostrated, and I thought that she was going to die; but by irrigating the parts of the bladder she recovered with great rapidity.

Sims finally did perfect his technique and ultimately repaired the fistulas. Only after his experimentation with the slave women proved successful did the physician attempt the procedure, with anesthesia, on White women volunteers.

Exploitation after the Civil War

It is not known to what extent African Americans continued to be used as unwilling subjects for experimentation and dissection in the years after emancipation. However, an examination of African-American folklore at the turn of the century makes it clear that Black people believed that such practices persisted. Folktales are replete with references to night doctors, also called student doctors and Ku Klux doctors. In her book, *Night Riders in Black Folk History,* anthropologist Gladys-Marie Fry writes, "The term 'night doctor' (derived from the fact that victims were sought only at night) applies both to students of medicine, who supposedly stole cadavers from which to learn about body processes, and [to] professional thieves, who sold stolen bodies—living and dead—to physicians for medical research." According to folk belief, these sinister characters would kidnap Black people, usually at night and in urban areas, and take them to hospitals to be killed and used in experiments. An 1889 *Boston Herald* article vividly captured the fears that African Americans in South Carolina had of night doctors. The report read, in part:

> The negroes of Clarendon, Williamsburg, and Sumter counties have for several weeks past been in a state of fear and trembling. They claim that there is a white man, a doctor, who at will can make himself invisible and who then approaches some unsuspecting darkey, and having rendered him or her insensible with chloroform, proceeds to fill up a bucket with the victim's blood, for the purpose of making medicine. After having drained the last drop of blood from the victim, the body is dumped into some secret place where it is impossible for any person to find it. The colored women are so worked up over this phantom that they will not venture out at night, or in the daytime in any sequestered place.

Fry did not find any documented evidence of the existence of night riders. However, she demonstrated through extensive interviews that many African Americans expressed genuine fears that they would be kidnapped by night doctors and used for medical experimentation. Fry concludes that two factors explain this paradox. She argues that Whites, especially those in the rural South, deliberately spread rumors about night doctors in order to maintain psychological control over Blacks and to discourage their migration to the North so as to maintain a source of cheap labor. In addition, Fry asserts that the experiences of many African Americans as victims of medical experiments during slavery fostered their belief in the existence of night doctors. It should also be added that, given the nation's racial and political climate, Black people recognized their inability to refuse to participate in medical experiments.

Reports about the medical exploitation of Black people in the name of medicine after the end of the Civil War were not restricted to the realm of folklore. Until it was exposed in 1882, a grave robbing ring operated in Philadelphia and provided bodies for the city's medical schools by plundering the graves at a Black cemetery. According to historian David C. Humphrey, southern grave robbers regularly sent bodies of southern Blacks to northern medical schools for use as anatomy cadavers.

During the early 20th century, African-American medical leaders protested the abuse of Black people by the White-dominated medical profession and used their concerns about experimentation to press for the establishment of Black controlled hospitals. Dr Daniel Hale Williams, the founder of Chicago's Provident Hospital (1891), the nation's first Black-controlled hospital, contended that White physicians, especially in the South, frequently used Black patients as guinea pigs. Dr Nathan Francis Mossell, the founder of Philadelphia's Frederick Douglass Memorial Hospital (1895), described the "fears and prejudices" of Black people, especially those from the South, as "almost proverbial." He attributed such attitudes to southern medicine practices in which Black people, "when forced to accept hospital attention, got only the poorest care, being placed in inferior wards set apart for them, suffering the brunt of all that is experimental in treatment, and all this is the sequence of their race variety and abject helplessness." The founders of Black hospitals claimed that only Black physicians possessed the skills required to treat Black patients optimally and that Black hospitals provided these patients with the best possible care.

Fears about the exploitation of African Americans by White physicians played a role in the establishment of a Black veterans hospital in Tuskegee, Ala. In 1923, 9 years before the initiation of the Tuskegee Syphilis Study, racial tensions had erupted in the town over con-

trol of the hospital. The federal government had pledged that the facility, an institution designed exclusively for Black patients, would be run by a Black professional staff. But many Whites in the area, including members of the Ku Klux Klan, did not want a Black-operated federal facility in the heart of Dixie, even though it would serve only Black people.

Black Americans sought control of the veterans hospital, in part because they believed that the ex-soldiers would receive the best possible care from Black physicians and nurses, who would be more caring and sympathetic to the veterans' needs. Some Black newspapers even warned that White southerners wanted command of the hospital as part of a racist plot to kill and sterilize African-American men and to establish an "experiment station" for mediocre White physicians. Black physicians did eventually gain the right to operate the hospital, yet this did not stop the hospital from becoming an experiment station for Black men. The veterans hospital was one of the facilities used by the United States Public Health Service in the syphilis study.

During the 1920s and 1930s, Black physicians pushed for additional measures that would battle medical racism and advance their professional needs. Dr Charles Garvin, a prominent Cleveland physician and a member of the editorial board of the Black medical publication *The Journal of the National Medical Association,* urged his colleagues to engage in research in order to protect Black patients. He called for more research on diseases such as tuberculosis and pellagra that allegedly affected African Americans disproportionately or idiosyncratically. Garvin insisted that Black physicians investigate these racial diseases because "heretofore in literature, as in medicine, the Negro has been written about, exploited and experimented upon sometimes not to his physical betterment or to the advancement of science, but the advancement of the Nordic investigator." Moreover, he charged that "in the past, men of other races have for the large part interpreted our diseases, often tinctured with inborn prejudices."

Fears of Genocide

These historical examples clearly demonstrate that African Americans' distrust of the medical profession has a longer history than the public revelations of the Tuskegee Syphilis Study. There is a collective memory among African Americans about their exploitation by the medical establishment. The Tuskegee Syphilis Study has emerged as the most prominent example of medical racism because it confirms, if not authenticates, long-held and deeply entrenched beliefs within the Black community. To be sure, the Tuskegee Syphilis Study does cast a long shadow. After the study had been exposed, charges surfaced that the experiment was part of a governmental plot to exterminate Black people. Many Black people agreed with the charge that the study represented "nothing less than an official, premeditated policy of genocide." Furthermore, this was not the first or last time that allegations of genocide have been launched against the government and the medical profession. The sickle cell anemia screening programs of the l970s and birth control programs have also provoked such allegations.

In recent years, links have been made between Tuskegee, AIDS, and genocide. In September 1990, the article "AIDS: Is It Genocide?" appeared in *Essence,* a Black woman's magazine. The author noted "As an increasing number of African-Americans continue to sicken and die and as no cure for AIDS has been found some of us are beginning to think the unthinkable: Could AIDS be a virus that was manufactured to erase large numbers of us? Are they trying to kill us with this disease?" In other words, some members of the Black community see AIDS as part of a conspiracy to exterminate African Americans.

Beliefs about the connection between AIDS and the purposeful destruction of African Americans should not be cavalierly dismissed as bizarre and paranoid. They are held by a significant number of Black people. For example, a 1990 survey conducted by the Southern Christian Leadership Conference found that 35% of the 1056 Black church members who responded believed that AIDS was a form of genocide. A *New York Times*/WCBS TV News poll conducted the same year found that 10% of Black Americans thought that the AIDS virus had been created in a laboratory in order to infect Black people. Another 20% believed that it could be true.

African Americans frequently point to the Tuskegee Syphilis Study as evidence to support their views about genocide, perhaps, in part, because many believe that the men in the study were actually injected with syphilis. Harlon Dalton, a Yale Law School professor and a former member of the National Commission on AIDS, wrote, in a 1989 article titled, "AIDS in Black Face," that "the government [had] purposefully exposed Black men to syphilis." Six years later, Dr Eleanor Walker, a Detroit radiation oncologist, offered an explanation as to why few African Americans become bone marrow donors. "The biggest fear, she claimed, is that they will become victims of some misfeasance, like the Tuskegee incident where Black men were infected with syphilis and left untreated to die from the disease." The January 25, 1996, episode of *New York Undercover,* a Fox Network police drama that is one of the top shows in Black households, also reinforced the rumor that the U.S. Public Health Ser-

vice physicians injected the men with syphilis. The myth about deliberate infection is not limited to the Black community. On April 8, 1997, news anchor Tom Brokaw, on "NBC Nightly News," announced that the men had been infected by the government.

Folklorist Patricia A. Turner, in her book *I Heard It through the Grapevine: Rumor and Resistance in African-American Culture,* underscores why it is important not to ridicule but to pay attention to these strongly held theories about genocide. She argues that these rumors reveal much about what African Americans believe to be the state of their lives in this country. She contends that such views reflect Black beliefs that White Americans have historically been, and continue to be, ambivalent and perhaps hostile to the existence of Black people. Consequently, African-American attitudes toward biomedical research are not influenced solely by the Tuskegee Syphilis Study. African Americans' opinions about the value White society has attached to their lives should not be discounted. As Reverend Floyd Tompkins of Stanford University Memorial Church has said, "There is a sense in our community, and I think it shall be proved out, that if you are poor or you're a person of color, you were the guinea pig, and you continue to be the guinea pigs, and there is the fundamental belief that Black life is not valued like White life or like any other life in America."

Not Just Paranoia

Lorene Cary, in a cogent essay in *Newsweek,* expands on Reverend Tompkins' point. In an essay titled "Why It's Not Just Paranoia," she writes:

> We Americans continue to value the lives and humanity of some groups more than the lives and humanity of others. That is not paranoia. It is our historical legacy and a present fact; it influences domestic and foreign policy and the daily interaction of millions of Americans. It influences the way we spend our public money and explains how we can read the staggering statistics on Black Americans' infant mortality, youth mortality, mortality in middle and old age, and not be moved to action.

African Americans' beliefs that their lives are devalued by White society also influence their relationships with the medical profession. They perceive, at times correctly, that they are treated differently in the healthcare system solely because of their race, and such perceptions fuel mistrust of the medical profession. For example, a national telephone survey conducted in 1986 revealed that African Americans were more likely than Whites to report that their physicians did not inquire sufficiently about their pain, did not tell them how long it would take for prescribed medicine to work, did not explain the seriousness of their illness or injury, and did not discuss test and examination findings. A 1994 study published in the *American Journal of Public Health* found that physicians were less likely to give pregnant Black women information about the hazards of smoking and drinking during pregnancy.

The powerful legacy of the Tuskegee Syphilis Study endures, in part, because the racism and disrespect for Black lives that it entailed mirror Black people's contemporary experiences with the medical profession. The anger and frustration that many African Americans feel when they encounter the healthcare system can be heard in the words of Alicia Georges, a professor of nursing at Lehman College and a former president of the National Black Nurses Association, as she recalled an emergency room experience. "Back a few years ago, I was having excruciating abdominal pain, and I wound up at a hospital in my area," she recalled. "The first thing that they began to ask me was how many sexual partners I'd had. I was married and owned my own house. But immediately, in looking at me, they said, 'Oh, she just has pelvic inflammatory disease.'" Perhaps because of her nursing background, Georges recognized the implications of the questioning. She had come face to face with the stereotype of Black women as sexually promiscuous. Similarly, the following story from the *Los Angeles Times* shows how racism can affect the practice of medicine:

> When Althea Alexander broke her arm, the attending resident at Los Angeles County-USC Medical Center told her to "hold your arm like you usually hold your can of beer on Saturday night." Alexander who is Black, exploded. "What are you talking about? Do you think I'm a welfare mother?" The White resident shrugged: "Well aren't you?" Turned out she was an administrator at USC medical school.

This example graphically illustrates that healthcare providers are not immune to the beliefs and misconceptions of the wider community. They carry with them stereotypes about various groups of people.

Beyond Tuskegee

There is also a growing body of medical research that vividly illustrates why discussions of the relationship of African Americans and the medical profession must go beyond the Tuskegee Syphilis Study. These studies demonstrate racial inequities in access to particular technologies and raise critical questions about the role of racism in medical decision making. For example, in 1989 *The Journal of the American Medical Association* published a report that demonstrated racial inequities in the treatment of heart

disease. In this study, White and Black patients had similar rates of hospitalization for chest pain, but the White patients were one third more likely to undergo coronary angiography and more than twice as likely to be treated with bypass surgery or angioplasty. The racial disparities persisted even after adjustments were made for differences in income. Three years later, another study appearing in that journal reinforced these findings. It revealed that older Black patients on Medicare received coronary artery bypass grafts only about a fourth as often as comparable White patients. Disparities were greatest in the rural South, where White patients had the surgery seven times as often as Black patients. Medical factors did not fully explain the differences. This study suggests that an already-existing national health insurance program does not solve the access problems of African Americans. Additional studies have confirmed the persistence of such inequities.

Why the racial disparities? Possible explanations include health problems that precluded the use of procedures, patient unwillingness to accept medical advice or to undergo surgery, and differences in severity of illness. However, the role of racial bias cannot be discounted, as the American Medical Association's Council on Ethical and Judicial Affairs has recognized. In a 1990 report on Black-White disparities in healthcare, the council asserted:

> Because racial disparities may be occurring despite the lack of any intent or purposeful efforts to treat patients differently on the basis of race, physicians should examine their own practices to ensure that inappropriate considerations do not affect their clinical judgment. In addition, the profession should help increase the awareness of its members of racial disparities in medical treatment decisions by engaging in open and broad discussions about the issue. Such discussions should take place as part of the medical school curriculum, in medical journals, at professional conferences, and as part of professional peer review activities.

The council's recommendation is a strong acknowledgment that racism can influence the practice of medicine.

After the public disclosures of the Tuskegee Syphilis Study, Congress passed the National Research Act of 1974. This act, established to protect subjects in human experimentation, mandates institutional review board approval of all federally funded research with human subjects. However, recent revelations about a measles vaccine study financed by the Centers for Disease Control and Prevention (CDC) demonstrate the inadequacies of these safeguards and illustrate why African Americans' historically based fears of medical research persist. In 1989, in the midst of a measles epidemic in Los Angeles, the CDC, in collaboration with Kaiser Permanente and the Los Angeles County Health Department, began a study to test whether the experimental Edmonston-Zagreb vaccine could be used to immunize children too young for the standard Moraten vaccine. By 1991, approximately 900 infants, mostly Black and Latino, had received the vaccine without difficulties. (Apparently, one infant died for reasons not related to the inoculations.) But the infants' parents had not been informed that the vaccine was not licensed in the United States or that it had been associated with an increase in death rates in Africa. The 1996 disclosure of the study prompted charges of medical racism and of the continued exploitation of minority communities by medical professionals.

The Tuskegee Syphilis Study continues to cast its shadow over the lives of African Americans. For many Black people, it has come to represent the racism that pervades American institutions and the disdain in which Black lives are often held. But despite its significance, it cannot be the only prism we use to examine the relationship of African Americans with the medical and public health communities. The problem we must face is not just the shadow of Tuskegee but the shadow of racism that so profoundly affects the lives and beliefs of all people in this country.

REFERENCES

A list of references is available in the original source.

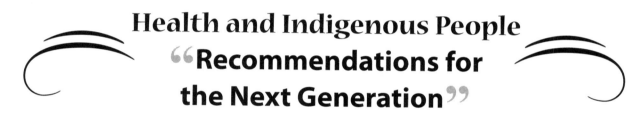

Health and Indigenous People "Recommendations for the Next Generation"

by Michael E. Bird

We are the first people of this land. . . . We are Indigenous peoples throughout this land and all over the planet we call Mother Earth.

For American Indians, the reality is that the founding fathers of the United States (none of them Indians), in order to establish a more perfect union that provided them with life, liberty, and the pursuit of happiness, displaced a people who had occupied this continent for thousands of years and denied those people their lives, liberty, and happiness. It is a fact.

Disparity, Dispossession, and Health Inequalities

In 1970, President Richard Nixon delivered the following statement in a message to Congress:

The first Americans—the Indians—are the most deprived and most isolated minority group in our nation. On virtually every scale of measurement—

employment, income, education, health—the condition of the Indian people ranks at the bottom. This condition is the heritage of centuries of injustice. From the time of their first contact with European settlers, the American Indians have been oppressed and brutalized, deprived of their ancestral lands, and denied the opportunity to control their own destiny.[1]

Last year at the 129th annual meeting of the American Public Health Association, we created a plenary session on indigenous health. This session provided an opportunity for indigenous people to speak to the issues that affect the health of the native peoples of Hawaii, Central America, Canada, Alaska, and the continental United States. We shared our experiences as individuals and as indigenous people from a variety of settings. We learned

From *The American Journal of Public Health,* Vol. 92, No. 9, September by Michael E. Bird. Copyright © 2002 by American Public Health Association. Reprinted by permission.

more about our similarities and differences. And what we gained was a sense of network, of a community brought closer by the threat of the power of ignorance and hate, and by the unacceptability of despair and disparity.

In my mind, disparity and dispossession go hand in hand. The massive dispossession that removed native people from their ancestral lands—not to mention the genocide and cultural eradication that followed—can hardly be imagined by most people. This story is not unique to American Indians. It is all too familiar for Native Hawaiians, Australian Aborigines, the Maori of New Zealand, and tribes throughout Central and South America. It may even apply to the Irish of Northern Ireland.

Wherever there has been dispossession, we see in the dispossessed populations significant damage in health, in educational levels, and in social well-being. And dispossession of one's land is not the only form of dispossession. Native peoples have been dispossessed of their labor, language, culture, and religious beliefs as well. We are only beginning to comprehend the consequences of what occurred long ago and still continues throughout the world. What is most important, though, is that we raise the collective awareness in this country to the level of undeniable truth: dispossession is at the root of health disparities.

Indian Health Services data show that American Indians and Alaska Natives have the worst health status of any group in this country. In 1993, their infant mortality rates were higher and life expectancy lower than those of the general population. American Indian and Alaska Native people are dying at younger ages than the rest of the nation. The leading causes of death among American Indians and Alaska Natives are heart disease and cancer, but in the area of behavioral health, these peoples' death rates are significantly higher as well: death from alcoholism, 579% higher; unintentional injury, 21% higher; suicide, 70% higher; and homicide, 41% higher. The diabetes mortality rate is 231% higher among American Indians and Alaska Natives than in the US population as a whole. Unfortunately, some of the highest rates of diabetes in the world are found in American Indian communities.

United We Stand

The most interesting result of the 2001 plenary session on indigenous health was how remarkably similar the historical experience has been for all indigenous populations. Another similarity was the description across the board of the relatively healthy nature of indigenous populations prior to contact, and the healthy living conditions that are universally described by historians and the first explorers. Clearly, the stories and the statistics bear witness to a certain pathology.

Indigenous peoples have given so much of themselves. And they offer the world even more at a time when the United States is struggling: The importance of the spiritual essence of all people, and our relationships to each other and the environment. Respect for all living things, and for human beings' place in the web of life. The importance and recognition of the role of spirituality in health. The concept of the well-being of all vs the benefit of few. The value of family and family wellness. The importance of balance in one's life and life choices. The village concept. The concept of mind, body, and spirit, and the importance of this concept to the health of individuals and communities. Generosity and reciprocity. An indigenous world view that predates the "alternative" Western view that has yet to prove its long-term sustainability and viability.

Indigenous people know the meaning of personal responsibility—but in a different, non-Western context. The concept is much broader, more humane and functional. If I am responsible only to myself, that kind of personal responsibility can be selfish and self-serving. It does not recognize the symbiotic nature of relationships that are important on this shrinking planet. Personal responsibility for indigenous people recognizes relationships and connections to others (family, tribe, community, world community). If I am to do well, then others must also do well. I am not isolated in thought, deed, or action. All are related and interconnected. I am personally responsible; I am my brother's keeper!

Improving the Health of Indigenous Peoples

Improving the health of indigenous peoples will require an effort beyond the indigenous community, from all individuals and institutions in public health. Our task is to reach and educate those people and organizations, and all branches of the federal, state, and local governments. We must help them understand who we are and how we have been affected. We must assume that this is a doable task, to bring together the data and the political process with wisdom and heart.

As a means to that end, we can put our energy into supporting and encouraging students from indigenous communities to enter the field of public health. Scholarship programs do exist, but many, many more could be established. Mentoring programs that create helpful relationships between students and those of us already in the field will ensure that the next generation continues to explore developments in healthcare while at the same time honoring traditional values and beliefs.

And we must maintain our commitments within our indigenous communities to be supportive of each other. Together, we are strong and capable. We are not the sum of our disparities. We will enter the broad arena as brothers and sisters on our way to building positive health and greater visibility for all of us.

But if justice on this earth can be imagined, so can a practical way to achieve it. Provided, that is, we are willing to reconcile ourselves to achieve it. Provided, that is, we are willing to reconcile ourselves to each other, and to historical truth.[2]

REFERENCES

1. Message from the President of the United States transmitting recommendations for Indian policy 91st Cong. 2nd sess (July 8, 1970; H Doc 91-363).

2. Bothwell ARX. We live on their land: implications of long-ago takings of Native American Indian property. Annual Survey of International and Comparative Law (Golden Gate University School of Law). 2000:6:175.

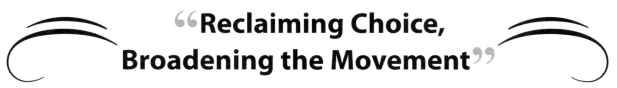

"Reclaiming Choice, Broadening the Movement"

by Courtney Chappell

Abortion, teenage pregnancy, and comprehensive sexuality education are the primary topics that guide the national dialogue about reproductive rights in America. Yet, the intersection of reproductive rights and other critical factors that influence sexual health is often missing from the debate. Many of these issues—including immigration, healthcare, welfare reform, and environmental justice—intimately impact the reproductive and sexual health of women, including women of color like Asian Pacific Americans.

The Asian Pacific American (APA) population includes individuals whose heritage or origins derive from Asia or the Pacific Islands, a region stretching from Hawaii to India, and from China to Australia. (See text box.) The APA population is extremely diverse, and is comprised of more than 30 ethnic subpopulations that speak over 200 languages and dialects. Asian Americans and Pacific Islanders represent over 4 percent of the total U.S. population, or nearly 12 million people; by 2050, that figure is expected to double to 8 percent of the population (a projected 33.4 million people). Four percent of women in the U.S. are Asian Pacific Americans (139 million women), of whom 50 percent are of reproductive age.

Despite the millions of APA women who need sexual and reproductive care, a very small number of studies specifically document trends and needs among APA women and girls. Only two percent of all published reproductive and sexual healthcare articles include APA women, the lowest percentage for all racial/ethnic groups. Even fewer studies disaggregate APA data by ethnic subpopulations, such as Hmong, Chinese, Vietnamese, or Native Hawaiian groups. APAs are either overlooked in research studies, or lumped together despite the broad differences that exist among subpopulations. This insufficient and inadequate research on APAs prevent both the public and healthcare providers from understanding sexual and reproductive healthcare issues that shape APA women's lives.

Moreover, the 'model minority' stereotype (by which Asians are viewed as trouble-free and successfully assimilating to mainstream American culture) inhibits recognition of APAs as individuals facing very real challenges and reproductive healthcare needs. In reality, the few studies that include APA populations present a very different and alarming picture of these women's overall health risks and outcomes. For example:

"Reclaiming Choice, Broadening the Movement," by Courtney Chappell, originally published in the *Women's Health Activist*, May/June 2006, pp. 6, 7, 10, the newsletter of the National Women's Health Network (NWHN). It is reprinted with the permission of the author and the NWHN.

- The incidence of cancer is steadily increasing among particular APA ethnic subpopulations. The rate of cervical cancer among Vietnamese American women is five times higher than White women's, and is the highest rate among all racial and ethnic groups.

- Between 1994–2000, abortion rates fell for all groups except APA women; over one-third (35 percent) of APA pregnancies end in abortion, the second highest percentage for all racial/ethnic groups.

- Laotian American teenagers have the highest teenage birth rate in California; almost 19 percent of California's teen births were to Laotian American teens, compared to 12 percent for White teens.

- Although less than one percent of reported U.S. HIV cases are among APAs, the number is steadily increasing, particularly among Filipino Americans and Native Hawaiians.

- Prolonged exposure to phthalates (chemicals used in many cosmetics and highly concentrated in nail polish) is a serious occupational hazard that has been linked to cancer, birth defects, and spontaneous abortions. Over 40 percent of U.S. nail technicians are APAs; in California, 80 percent of the industry workers are Vietnamese immigrant women.

Why do APA women have poor health outcomes and suffer health disparities compared to other women in the U.S? One of the primary reasons is their lack of access to healthcare services and insurance coverage. Legal restrictions on providing healthcare services to undocumented workers, the high cost of obtaining private health insurance, and the lack of employment-based health benefits are among the primary reasons that APAs are uninsured. Currently, 36 percent of all APA women under age 65 are uninsured; 12 percent of school-age APA children are uninsured (compared to 7 percent of White children). Over half of APA men (52 percent) have not met the minimum standard of adequate doctor visits, as defined by the American Medical Association. Korean Americans are the least likely of all racial and ethnic groups to be insured.

Moreover, even APA women who are covered and have access to healthcare services face barriers to obtaining appropriate care. Language differences create enormous challenges to receiving high-quality and effective care. Approximately 60 percent of APAs are foreign-born (APAs make up a quarter of the U.S. foreign-born pop-

Asian American refers to Chinese, Filipinos, Japanese, Koreans, South Asians (individuals whose heritage or origins derive from Bangladesh, Bhutan, Myanmar, India, and Maldive Islands, Nepal, Pakistan, and Sri Lanka), and Southeast Asians (Individuals from Cambodia, Indonesia, Laos, Malaysia, Thailand, and Vietnam.)

Pacific Islander refers to individuals from the thousands of islands in the Pacific Ocean that are classified as Micronesian (Marshal Islands, Kiribati, Guam), Melanesian (Fiji, Papua New Guinea, Vanuatu), and Polynesian (Hawaiians, Tongans, Samoans.)

ulation). The U.S. Census Bureau has found that 79 percent of APAs speak a language other than English at home; 40 percent of APAs are limited in English proficiency, or speak English less than "very well." It can be intimidating, if not impossible, for women to discuss their sexual and reproductive health when they do not share a common language with their provider, or when either a family member or stranger are the only available interpreters.

Further, studies have found that the cultural stigmatization of disease (including cancer) and lack of culturally competent healthcare prevent many APA women from seeking preventive reproductive healthcare services. For instance, one survey found that Vietnamese American women reported lower rates of preventive cervical cancer care because they fear a positive diagnosis and/or have misconceptions about the Pap test. Another focus group with South Asian American women revealed that many were uncomfortable asking South Asian health providers for sexual or reproductive health guidance or services, because they feared the doctors would bring cultural biases to their practices or violate confidentiality.

Inspired by women of color organizations that have long mobilized around reproductive justice, the National Asian Pacific American Women's Forum (NAPAWF) has developed a national action agenda on APA women's sexual and reproductive healthcare issues. This action agenda outlines eight legislative priorities for national and grassroots advocacy, and offers recommendations for policymakers, advocates, allied organizations, and community leaders.

NAPAWF's eight priorities include: providing access to healthcare for all APAs; promoting linguistic and cultural competence in health and human services;

demanding the collection of community-relevant sexual and reproductive health data and research; protecting and expanding sexual and reproductive rights; eliminating all forms of violence against women; increasing comprehensive sexuality education; linking women's reproductive health to environmental justice; and ending gender discrimination and the promotion of sex selection technologies.

By promoting this broad sexual and reproductive justice framework, NAPAWF seeks to broaden the pro-choice framework beyond the constitutional right to access abortion and provide APA women with real choices in their sexual and reproductive healthcare decisions. What is "choice" if a woman can't talk to her doctor confidentially, understand her provider's recommendations, access preventive care because of immigration restrictions, or ensure that her workplace is safe and healthy? NAPAWF hopes to work with other national and grassroots organizations to create change so that every woman and girl's life, including Asian Pacific Americans', is lived in dignity and equality.

⁶⁶On Being a Jewish Feminist Valley Girl⁹⁹

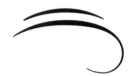

by Tobin Belzer

I was one of six Jewish teens in my high school to return from summer vacation with a new nose. On the first day of school, we gathered in the hallway to examine one another's profile, compare costs and enjoy our post-operative popularity. A surgically modified nose was a source of pride amid the white, upper middle-class Jewish students at my high school in the San Fernando Valley. It was my first American Jewish rite of passage.

It was the mid-1980s. Middle-class Americans were prospering in the booming Reagan-era economy, and conspicuous consumption was heralded as the nation's favorite pastime. Financial prosperity was the only economic climate I'd ever known. Until the emergence of the Valley Girl and Jewish American Princess (JAP) stereotypes, I thought everyone shared my aspirations: to be thin and rich. I didn't know that Valley Girl was only the first of many identities I would eventually embrace. I had never heard of women's studies and I'd never met a feminist. I could barely imagine myself in college, much less as a doctoral candidate in sociology. And I never dreamed that I would eventually leave L.A.

At fifteen, I had become almost completely acculturated to Valley Girl life. In the San Fernando Valley—often referred to as simply "the Valley"—having a perfect body was an achievement. I listened to advice from Hollywood and advertising agencies; I believed I would be lovable if I bought the right products. Taking control of my appearance felt empowering, so I shopped and shopped and *shopped*. In my quest for self-improvement, I waxed, painted and polished every inch of my body, changing every part of my self that I could. Cosmetic surgery was my ultimate acquiescence to societal norms about beauty.

Like many of my friends, I contended with Eastern European genes: I was hairy. And since the portrait of ideal womanhood had no discernible body hair, I felt doomed. Remaking myself required a tremendous amount of time, money and effort. I spent countless hours every week removing hair from my body and face, waxing my legs and upper lip, shaving my underarms and trimming my nose hair. My eyebrows were arched and my eyelashes tinted. I had the hairs on my chin permanently removed through electrolysis. And I bought expensive products to cleanse, moisturize and style the kinky Jewish hair on my head.

Grooming was so central to the daily life of a Valley Girl that it evolved into a social event. Once a week, I met my friends at a salon after school to socialize while our nails were manicured. When one of us got our hair cut, the others accompanied her. We did each other's makeup and traded clothes. We attended Weight Watchers meetings and encouraged each other to stick to our diets. We cared for one another by cooperatively improving our appearances.

My friends and I hung out at the mall in packs. We educated each other about the importance of wearing the right clothes and owning the right accessories. As Valley Girls, we luxuriated in our weekly grooming sessions, which we affectionately called "girl bonding time." When I later discovered a feminist community, I was already accustomed to women-centered spheres. Shopping, grooming and dieting are, after all, female-dominated activities.

In my family, Judaism was our ethnicity, but our religion was dieting. We had our own version of keeping kosher: At home, we ate only low-calorie food, but outside the house, we ate anything we wanted. While my peers went to Hebrew school, I went to a nutritionist; I knew that I was learning the more valuable dietary laws. Like everyone I knew, I attempted to transform my body into that of the ideal Anglo woman. I believed that if I were able to fit into the right clothes, I would be popular and happy. I weighed myself twice a day.

Everything around me encouraged and promoted my behavior. In 1982, radio stations played Moon Unit Zappa's parody, "Valley Girl," nonstop; the song title gave a name to the culture I had already internalized. Girls my age made the 1983 movie *Valley Girl* a smash hit. For a brief moment in American history, the Valley Girl became a cultural icon. The Valley was no longer just a place to live; it was a way to be. Bolstered by the media's frenzy, Valley Girl culture saturated mainstream culture. Valley Girl slang became a national fad. The sound bite "Oh, my, gawd!" was heard around the country.

The media hype surrounding Valley Girl culture simultaneously celebrated and mocked us. We were sold products to accentuate our Valley Girl identities while we were ridiculed for our excessive consumerism. Our enthusiastic engagement in mall culture made us famous, but we were disparaged because Valley Girl life was void of the trappings of high culture. Both class- and race-based anxieties were embedded in the criticism of Valley Girls' lack of refinement. The Valley Girl was born in L.A.'s largest suburban Jewish community; Valley Girls were daughters of the Jewish nouveau riche. The stereotype was the most recent permutation of the age-old condemnation of Jews for being crass and money-grubbing.

On the East Coast, the anti-Semitic nature of the insult was less thinly veiled. Girls with our characteristics were called Jewish American Princesses (JAPs); the labels gained popularity simultaneously. Like the Valley Girl, the JAP moniker began as a fairly mild stereotype depicting the over-indulged daughter of newly prosperous parents. A JAP wanted to date the right guy and dress according to magazine styles; she drove an expensive car and used multiple credit cards. Like Valley Girls, JAPs had a dialect that included the exclamation "Oh my gawd!"

JAP Jokes were everywhere. (Q: How many JAPs does it take to change a light bulb? A: Two. One to get the Diet Coke and one to call Daddy.) The jokes evolved into JAP-bashing, which erupted on college campuses. Jewish girls were maligned, held up as warnings of what becomes of those who try to acquire social status through consumerism.

On the more tolerant West Coast, we Valley Girls escaped the overt prejudice that accompanied the JAP label; the geography-based nature of the Valley Girl label made the anti-Semitism embedded in the stereotype less obvious. Since the anti-Jewish sentiment remained unnamed, identifying the malice in the stereotype was more difficult.

I was not able to recognize the extent of the psychic damage that I incurred because of this until I left the Valley at age twenty-three. By then I had realized that I would never be thin enough or rich enough, so I decided to leave L.A. altogether. I enrolled in graduate school at Brandeis University in Massachusetts because I was eager to discover another way of life.

Everything I knew about the East Coast I had learned in movies, so I was unprepared for the extent of the cultural differences I would encounter in Boston. I felt like a foreign exchange student. My peers did not wear makeup or openly obsess about their weight. They did not exchange Hollywood gossip, and they detested the mall. I learned that people from the East Coast proudly despised everything about L.A. In order to fit in, I believed I had to disavow the city of my birth, so I enthusiastically colluded with East Coast natives who were eager to delineate the depravity of Los Angeles. I stopped wearing lipstick and I rarely visited the mall.

In some ways, Valley Girl culture had prepared me for the world of East Coast academia. As a Valley Girl, complaining was one of my fundamental methods of communication. As a feminist, I'm empowered to complain. I'm as comfortable now naming a social injustice as I was sending a salad back when the dressing was not "on the side."

The constant criticism of one's self and peers was fundamental to both Jewish and Valley Girl cultures. So even before I became a feminist sociologist, I acquired substantial training in the art of social critique. Acquiring a feminist consciousness and a sociological awareness in graduate school enabled me to turn my critical voice outward, and use that ability to better understand the social world. I began to examine my world through the lenses of race, class and gender. I learned to analyze behavior by looking at social context as well as an individual's actions. In my research as a Jewish feminist sociologist, I aim to dispel stereotypes and correct the misconceptions about young Jewish women.

My stories about L.A. never fail to shock my friends from the East Coast. And my stories about the East Coast are similarly received by my friends from the Valley. When I told my graduate student friends about a new pubic hair waxing fad that was popular in L.A., they were horrified. And when I showed my West Coast friends the alternative menstrual product I bought at a co-op in Cambridge, they thought I was kidding. I feel like an intermediary between two foreign lands. I am simultaneously at home in, and alien to, each world I inhabit.

As a Jewish feminist Valley Girl, I am trying to honor my multiple selves while acknowledging the contradictions inherent in doing so. This can be tricky. My conflicting reactions to the Lewinsky/Clinton scandal are particularly illustrative. My response developed as an internal battle between my differing selves. I was fascinated by the fact that a voluptuous, sassy Jewish girl from L.A. was the focus of international news. I was also excited: the President of the United States was attracted to a girl who was practically my peer. If Bill was attracted to Monica, I reasoned, that meant that the ruler of the free world could be attracted to me!

At the same time, as a young Jewish woman from L.A., I felt embarrassed to be represented by Monica. In the media's eyes, she embodied everything disgusting about being Jewish, wealthy and female. She was depicted as a spoiled-rotten princess whose father (a Jewish doctor) gave her everything. Her appearance, as well as her behavior, was critiqued. She was charged with using her father's influence to forward her career, but she was also accused of sleeping her way to the top. She was described as young, naive and stupid, but was also seen as a manipulative temptress. I regarded the scandal as a reminder that a woman's most potent power is her ability to be sexually objectified (but when she uses that power, she will be vilified).

Even though Monica grew up in Beverly Hills, she was often referred to as a Valley Girl by the press. She was never called a Jewish American Princess. While the two terms are practically synonymous, the use of JAP is no longer socially acceptable. During the late 1980s, Jewish feminists condemned the JAP stereotype as anti-Semitic and sexist. In 1987, *Lilith* magazine devoted its fall issue to analyses of the problem.

After much deliberation, the organized Jewish community made a systematic effort to publicly condemn the image. Jews were called upon to abandon the stereotype, and by the 1990s, JAP T-shirts, buttons, humor books and the like had largely disappeared. The media was cautious when referring to any aspect of Monica's Jewish background. "Valley Girl" was used to evoke the same anti-Semitic sentiment of the JAP epithet without the political or social consequences of using that term directly.

When Monica finally agreed to an exclusive interview with Barbara Walters, I realized, with a moment of pride, that two Jewish women would be the focus of the world's attention. I waited enthusiastically, both to hear Monica's voice and to see what she would be wearing. It was the first time I would learn about her experience from her perspective.

Monica had obviously had a makeover in preparation for the interview. She wore a pink sweater and pink lipstick, and I wondered, from my feminist perspective, if she had been advised to look as feminine and innocent as possible. Yet at the same time, I found myself admiring how meticulously her eyebrows had been manicured, and I wondered which Beverly Hills salon she had visited. I also speculated about where I could purchase that fabulous lipstick. From my friends in L.A., I learned that I was not the only one; after the broadcast, that shade was impossible to find. During the interview, Monica seemed young and insecure. But when she described her sexual experiences with President Clinton, her eyes lit up and her body language became animated. Her nervousness turned to mania. It was clear that she derived a great deal of self-esteem from her sexual prowess. I felt sorry for her, remembering a time in my life when I, too, believed that my self-worth depended on my sexual attractiveness to men. I realized that she was simply adhering to the same lessons I had learned as a girl growing up in L.A.

During my East Coast experience, I acquired a feminist consciousness and met a wonderful therapist. During Monica's East Coast experiences, she acquired a stained blue dress and the negative attention of the nation. Instead of learning to love her body, she made a million-dollar deal with Jenny Craig. I felt grateful for our differing experiences, but saddened by the fact that Monica did not fare as well as I had.

Embracing my Jewish feminist Valley Girl identity has allowed me to honor all sides of my self. As a Valley

Girl, I had paid meticulous attention to altering my appearance. When I became a feminist, I decided to learn to love and honor my body, rather than investing all of my energy in trying to improve it. Instead, I set out to change the world. My Valley Girl identity enables me to feel entitled to complain, while my feminist identity compels me to acknowledge the class- and race-based privilege behind that entitlement. As a Jewish feminist, I acknowledge the importance of community and the significance of history while working to critique and correct the myopic attitudes that pervade American Jewish culture.

I have challenged myself to accept the positive aspects from each of my cultures and to leave behind the qualities that are not useful. I now know that critiquing my identities does not necessarily mean rejecting them completely. I listen to National Public Radio as religiously as I read *People* magazine. I critique pop culture through a feminist lens and regard fashion with a Valley Girl sensibility. I am a lipstick enthusiast who detests the beauty industry. And I am a young Jewish leader whose Jewish nose has been altered.

I am one of scores of young Jewish women who use our privilege to make the world a better place. We have defiantly refused to be hindered by stereotypes. In doing so, we are learning to honor the inevitable contradictory realities that come from occupying multiple identities. I wear my contradictions proudly: in my heart, in my mind and on my face.

"Immigrant Women's Health a Casualty in the Immigration Policy War"

by Aishia Glasford and Priscilla Huang

As the immigration policy battles rage in legislatures and presidential primaries and state elections throughout the country, there's been little attention to a serious casualty in these skirmishes: immigrant women's health. Immigrant women are facing serious threats to their health, and in the most dire cases, have even lost their lives as a result of problems in this broken system. Rosa Isela Contreras-Dominguez and Victoria Arrellano died in Federal custody awaiting deportation to Mexico; Contreras-Dominguez was 38 and pregnant at the time of her death, and Arrellano who had AIDS, deteriorated steadily in a San Pedro, California prison, eventually dying there at the age of 23.[1] In another tragic loss, Jiang Zhen Xing, pregnant with twins miscarried when Immigration and Customs Enforcement officials tried to forcibly deport her.[2] Among the estimated 37.5 million foreign-born people living in the United States, there are probably tens of thousands more women experiencing serious health and reproductive health problems that are being made worse by the violence, discrimination, and hurdles that U.S. immigration policy perpetuates.

The National Coalition for Immigrant Women's Rights (NCIWR) was formed in 2006 to bring a gender perspective to the immigration debate and to advocate for a truly comprehensive reform of the broken immigration system that is devastating the lives of women like Contreras-Dominguez, Arrellano, and Jiang and their families. One of NCIWR's goals is to bring to light the harm being done to immigrant women

"Immigrant Women's Health a Casualty in the Immigration Policy War," by Aishia Glasford and Priscilla Huang, originally published in the *Women's Health Activist*, March/April 2008, pp. 1, 3, 6, the newsletter of the National Women's Health Network (NWHN). It is reprinted with the permission of the author and the NWHN.

and their children's health as they attempt to secure the most basic rights, such as access to healthcare and reproductive health services.

Welfare, Immigration Reform and Immigrant Women's Healthcare

In 2006, approximately 12.5 percent of the total U.S. population was foreign-born.[3] (The term "foreign-born" describes anyone who is a naturalized citizen, legal permanent resident, or undocumented immigrant.[4]) About 53 percent of the U.S. foreign-born population immigrated from Latin America, 25 percent from Asia, and 14 percent from Europe.[5] Foreign-born women, who represent five percent of the total U.S. population, are twice as likely as their male counterparts to be widowed, divorced, or separated.[6] They are also more likely than U.S.-born women to live in poverty, be unemployed, and lack health insurance. Approximately 42 percent of immigrant women are of reproductive age (between 25-44 years of age), compared to 26 percent of native-born women.[6]

U.S. immigration laws and policies have restricted the mobility, status, and livelihood of immigrant women since the country began regulating its borders. In fact, the United States' first immigration law, the 1875 Page Law, targeted Asian women, particularly Chinese women. While the law specifically prohibited the entry of Chinese prostitutes, in practice it was intended to prevent wives and prospective brides of Chinese laborers from joining their husbands in the U.S. (Notably, many immigration scholars cite the 1882 Chinese Exclusion Act as the nation's first U.S. immigration law, however, the Page Law pre-dated this Act.)

Until the mid-1990's, immigrants were generally eligible for public benefit programs, such as Medicaid, on the same basis as their native-born counterparts. In 1996, however, the Welfare Reform Act (formally called the "Personal Responsibility and Work Opportunity Reconciliation Act of 1996," P.L. 104-193) and Illegal Immigration Reform and Immigrant Responsibility Act (IIRIRA) both made it increasingly difficult for immigrant women to flourish in their new homeland by creating barriers to accessing social services such as healthcare.

One of the Welfare Reform Act's most onerous provisions narrowed Medicaid eligibility criteria by imposing a "five-year bar" to access on most new immigrants. Thus, immigrant women who enter the country after August 22, 1996 must continuously reside in the U.S. for five years before becoming eligible for Federally funded health programs. Consequently, State and local governments which value the importance of a social net of services for both immigrant and U.S.-born residents must now use their own funds to extend public health programs to new immigrants. In addition, IIRIRA made it more difficult for immigrants to establish their income eligibility for Medicaid, even after reaching the five-year barrier. The law requires new immigrants with sponsors to include (or "deem") their sponsors' income when applying for Federal benefits. Thus, deeming and sponsor liability rules often render many immigrant women ineligible for services even after they have been in the U.S. for the required five years.

Both Acts restrict newly arriving, low-income immigrant women from accessing Federal benefits, and compound the financial strain and hardship that many immigrant families face when they first enter the country. (It is important to specify that neither welfare nor immigration "reform" laws changed the eligibility requirements for undocumented immigrants, who have always been ineligible for Medicaid and most other entitlement benefits.)

Impact on Immigrant Women

In 1996, when immigrants and native-born citizens had similar eligibility for public benefit programs, immigrants represented just 9 percent of the U.S. population and 15 percent of all welfare recipients.[7] By 1999, the number of immigrant welfare recipients dropped to 12 percent.[7] The number of low-income, immigrant children and parents receiving Medicaid fell by 7-8 percent between 1995–2000, while the same population experienced a 6-7 percent increase in un-insurance rates during the same period.[7]

The decline in welfare and Medicaid utilization by immigrant women was partly due to the increased restrictions imposed by the 1996 reforms. In addition, these policies created a chilling effect that discouraged Medicaid use even by immigrants who were eligible for, and needed, such services. As a result, thousands of eligible immigrant women and children have not accessed public programs and services for which they are eligible—including Medicaid and the State Children's Health Insurance Program (SCHIP)—and must either pay out-of-pocket for care or go without it altogether.[8]

The situation is far worse for undocumented immigrants. These individuals are eligible for services under Emergency Medicaid, but treatment is limited to serious health emergencies such as labor and childbirth. Therefore, most undocumented women forgo routine healthcare, including prenatal care and other preventive reproductive health services.

The Impact of Immigration Status, Economic Injustice, and Violence on Immigrant Women

Many immigrant women who wish to obtain a viable path of entry and citizenship to the U.S. face bleak prospects. Many U.S. citizens do not realize that obtaining a visa for entry to this country is a far more complicated and lengthy process than obtaining a passport or a driver's license. Applicants are routinely denied visas to travel to the U.S. Immigration procedures for both entry to the U.S. and citizenship are long, arduous, and extremely expensive. It takes many months of paperwork, large administrative and legal fees (up to thousands of dollars), and intense interviews with foreign consulate and immigration officers before one can get a visa or become a legal permanent resident (the first step to becoming a citizen). This process requires immigrant women to navigate a system that many trained immigration attorneys have difficulty fully understanding. The system's challenges mean that many immigrant women enter the U.S. without immigration documents (e.g., a visa).

Many other immigrant women enter the U.S. with some form of immigration status, such as a student, work, or tourist visa. Yet, they can easily lose this immigration status and become undocumented when their visa expires. This is common, because the U.S. immigration system is slow to notify visa holders and citizenship applicants of changes in their immigration status and/or relevant immigration rules.

For many immigrant women, the lack of documented immigration status and/or confusion over their status is a huge obstacle to accessing care, because access to publicly funded programs is now usually contingent upon one's immigration status. Moreover, lacking (or losing) immigration status endangers immigrant women because it makes them vulnerable to manipulation, coercion, and exploitation at the hands of employers, traffickers, smugglers, or intimate partners. Women who lack (or are unsure they have) immigration status are often forced to accept low-paying jobs where they are easily exploited. Domestic service, child care, agricultural work, nail salons, sweatshops, and forced sex work are a few industries in which exploitation can occur.

Immigrant women's working conditions are often deplorable and sometimes illegal, and may expose them to toxic chemicals, pesticides, poor ventilation, and dangerous equipment. Many immigrant women work long hours for little pay, without health benefits, and with no job security. For example, in 2001, 41 percent of immigrant women did not have health insurance.[9]

In 2000, 85 percent of migrant and seasonal farm worker women were uninsured,[10] of whom only 42 percent accessed prenatal care during their first trimester of pregnancy, compared to 76 percent of pregnant women nationally.[11] Exploitative working conditions are a covert form of violence, as these workers are exploited precisely because they tend to be undocumented. Immigrant women also experience overt violence including physical, emotional, and/or sexual abuse by their employers, traffickers, and/or intimate partners. Immigrant women may be raped or harassed by those who have power over them. Women may also be forced to remain in abusive relationships or employment when their undocumented status is used to intimidate them from reporting abuse to the authorities.

The Lack of Information on Immigrant Women's Reproductive Health Disparities

Compared to native-born women, immigrant women are more likely to have lower incomes, educational attainment, and acculturation levels; they are more likely to be uninsured and to lack awareness about preventative care and physician referrals. In addition, approximately 30 percent of immigrant households are linguistically isolated (defined by the U.S. Census Bureau as "a household in which all members 14 years old and over speak a non-English language and also have difficulty speaking English")[12] Linguistic isolation creates significant barriers to accessing reproductive and maternal health services. Studies have found that linguistically isolated individuals receive far fewer preventative services than English-speakers (including Pap tests, mammograms, and prenatal care).[13] These factors play important roles in if, how, and when immigrant women access healthcare.

While the consequence of the broken immigration system, economic exploitation, and violence is a multitude of reproductive health disparities for immigrant women, these negative outcomes remain hard to see because they are not adequately captured by current research. Statistical data on reproductive health disparities are not disaggregated by race, ethnicity and immigration status; thus, existing data are likely to be skewed and to underreport immigrant women's health problems. This means that an Afro-Latina immigrant woman may be categorized as African-American rather than as an immigrant or as Latina. The lack of specific information about foreign-born women is important because, as noted, immigrant women experience different constraints than native-born women, (including native born women of color) and require different strategies to increase their access to preventive and reproductive healthcare. Without such strategies we will continue to see in States, for example, with large Latina immigrant populations, disparities in access to services such as prenatal care: in 2002, 87.2 percent of White women in Arizona began prenatal care in the first trimester, compared to just 66.7 percent of Latinas who did so.[14]

The paucity of data on foreign-born women's health outcomes makes it hard to assess either the number of women who receive appropriate reproductive health services or strategies to improve their access to needed care. This problem is compounded by the fact that policymakers have failed to support funding and opportunities to study immigrant women's health in order to identify and address these disparities. Without such research, it is impossible to develop policies and programs that provide immigrant women with the care needed to protect their own and their children's health.

Policy Recommendations

In order to address the legal and reproductive health needs of immigrant women and their children, NCIWR advocates several policy recommendations:

- Comprehensive immigration reform must include legal and safe immigration options for undocumented men, women, and children; and a path to citizenship that allows immigrant women to obtain work permits, travel internationally, and access higher education and Federal financial aid.

- Reproductive healthcare coverage that is financed through public funds must be provided to all immigrant women regardless of their legal or economic status.

- Equitable access must be guaranteed to confidential and non-coercive family planning services; and to linguistically, culturally competent, and medically accurate reproductive healthcare services.

- Funding must be provided to research specific data on the reproductive health disparities, needs, and services for immigrant women, as well as for outreach to engage immigrant women and their children in care.

- Federal policy should impose a moratorium on immigration raids, and ensure better access to medical and legal services for immigrant women held in detention centers.

The National Coalition for Immigrant Women's Rights is working to eradicate discriminatory practices in public policies that impact the reproductive health and well-being of immigrant women. As part of the Coalition's principles of defending and protecting the well-being of immigrant women, their children, and their communities, NCIWR will tackle immigration reform, reproductive health and wellness, and labor policies and practices. NCIWR seeks to highlight not only immigrant women's lives but also U.S. policies and practices that impact these women's lives. In doing so, the NCIWR will also confront a society that has, for too long, contributed to the violence perpetrated against immigrant women, and advocate for enforcement policies and a judicial system that treats immigrant women with respect and dignity.

For further information about the NCIWR, please contact Aishia Glasford at Aishia@latinainstitute.org, or Priscilla Huang at phuang@napawf.org.

REFERENCES

1. Fears D, "Three Jailed Immigrants Die in a Month," The *Washington Post*, August 15, 2007, page A02. Retrieved September 10, 2007 from http://www.washingtonpost.com/wp-dyn/content/article/2007/08/14/AR2007081401690.html

2. Huang P, "Which Babies Are Real Americans?" TomPaine.com, February 20, 2007. Retrieved September 10, 2007 from http://www.tompaine.com/articles/2007/02/20/which_babies_are_real_americans.php.

3. U.S. Census Bureau, 2006 American Community Survey Data Profile Highlights, Washington, DC: US Census Bureau, 2006. Retrieved September 12, 2007 from http://factfinder.census.gov/servlet/ACSSAFFFacts?_event=&geo_id=01000US&_geoContext=01000US&_street=&_county=&_cityTown=&_state=&_zip=&_lang=en&_sse=on&ActiveGeoDiv=&_useEV=&pctxt=fph&pgsl=010&_submenuId=factsheet_1&ds_name=DEC_2000_SAFF&_ci_nbr=107&qr_name=DEC_2000_SAFF_R1010®=DEC_2000_SAFF_R1010%3A107&_keyword=&_industry=.

4. U.S. Census Bureau, The Foreign-Born Population in the United States: 2003, Washington DC: US Census Bureau, August 2004, page 1. Retrieved February 6, 2008 from http://www.census.gov/prod/2004pubs/p20-551.pdf.

5. U.S. Census Bureau, 2006 American Community Survey Origins and Language, Washington, DC: U.S. Census Bureau, 2006. Retrieved September 12, 2007 from http://factfinder.census.gov/servlet/ACSSAFFPeople?_event=&geo_id=01000US&_geoContext=01000US&_street=&_county=&_cityTown=&_state=&_zip=&_lang=en&_sse=on&ActiveGeoDiv=&_useEV=&pctxt=fph&pgsl=010&_submenuId=people_8&ds_name=null&_ci_nbr=107&qr_name=DEC_2000_SAFF_R1010®=DEC_2000_SAFF_R1010%3A107&_keyword=&_industry=

6. Greico E, U.S. in Focus: Immigrant Women, Washington DC: Migration Policy Institute, May 2002. Retrieved January 6, 2008 from http://www.migrationinformation.org/USFocus/display.cfm?ID=2.

7. Levinson A, U.S. in Focus: Immigrants and Welfare Use, Washington DC: Migration Policy Institute, August 2002. Retrieved January 6, 2008 from http://www.migrationinformation.org/USfocus/display.cfm?ID=45.

8. SCHIP is a Federal public health program that provides health coverage for many documented immigrant children and pregnant women. States have the option to use SCHIP funds to cover prenatal services for undocumented immigrant women, an option implemented in 2002 to provide much-needed services for pregnant immigrant women in several states. Yet, the added coverage comes at the cost of reproductive freedom: in order to receive prenatal care, the Centers for Medicare and Medicaid Services (CMS), which administers SCHIP, defines the undocumented pregnant woman's fetus as a "child," and therefore extends healthcare coverage by giving personhood status to the fetus. Ensuring that undocumented immigrant women receive prenatal care coverage is a step in the right direction, but the change should not have come at the cost of taking away women's ability to make autonomous reproductive health decisions.

9. Maternal and Child Health Bureau (MCHB), Women's Health USA 2003, Rockville, MD: MCHB, 2003, page 58. Accessed September 20, 2007 from http://mchb.hrsa.gov/pages/page_58.htm.

10. National Latina Institute for Reproductive Health (NLIRH), Fact Sheet: The Reproductive Health of Migrant and Seasonal Farm Worker Women, New York, NY: NLIRH, December 2005, page 1. Accessed February 5, 2008 from http://www.latinainstitute.org/pdf/MgrntFrmwkrs-4.pdf.

11. Rosenbaum S and P Shin, Migrant and Seasonal Farm Workers: Health Insurance Coverage and Access to Care, Washington, DC: Kaiser Commission on Medicaid and the Uninsured, April 2005, page 2. Accessed on February 5, 2008 from http://www.kff.org/uninsured/upload/Migrant-and-Seasonal-Farmworkers-Health-Insurance-Coverage-and-Access-to-Care-Report.pdf

12. U.S. Census Bureau, Summary File 3: 2000 Census on Population and Housing, Technical Documentation, Washington, DC: Census Bureau, 1997, Appendix (B-32). Accessed January 28, 2008 from http://www.census.gov/prod/cen2000/doc/sf3.pdf.

13. Leighton Ku, Reducing Disparities in Health Coverage for Legal Immigrant Children and Pregnant Women, Washington, DC: Center on Budget and Policy Priorities (CBPP), April 2007, page 3. Accessed February 5, 2008 from: http://www.cbpp.org/4-20-07health2.htm#_ftn3.

14. NLIRH, Policy Brief: Prenatal Care Access Among Latina Immigrant Latinas, New York, NY: NLIRH, December 2005, page 1. Accessed February 6, 2005 from http://www.latinainstitute.org/publications/index.html.

Trans Health Crisis
"For Us It's Life or Death"
by Leslie Feinberg

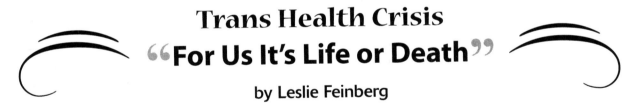

'm sitting in a cardiologist's waiting room filling out my intake forms. The tip of my pen hovers above the ubiquitous binary boxes. Female or male? I was born female-bodied and I identify as female—as a lesbian butch. However, some people see me as a feminine male. And whether they guess male or female, I am always perceived as "queer" because my gender expression is very fluid and complex. I am transgender. Which box do I check to get the medical attention I need so badly right now?

I sit here recalling recent studies showing that females my age are more likely than males to die from heart attacks. The symptoms of females are not necessarily the same as those of men. Distorted through the lens of sexism, these symptoms are often not recognized or taken seriously enough. I consider all this and decide to check the "F" box, hoping the doctor will take my birth sex into account in listening to my cardiac symptoms.

One of the 2 women at the front desk takes the clipboard and flashes me a generous smile. "Have a seat, sir." Minutes later she calls out, "Miss Feinberg, do you have insurance?" I stand up; she looks bewildered. To her credit, she recovers quickly. She goes out of her way to be warm to me.

I sit back down and leaf through a magazine. The other woman at the front desk explodes in derisive laughter.

She comments out loud about a patient's records: "Do you know what's on this *man's* chart? This man had a *breast* biopsy!" She snorts and snickers in a mean-spirited way. Everyone in the waiting room can hear her.

You may be appalled at that breach of patient confidentiality. But as a transgender patient, I have another take on it. I hear her backwardness about sex and gender variance, and I hear her intolerance. I feel more fearful about this appointment today. My reluctance isn't just because of how I might be treated by the front office staff. I dread seeing a physician because of a lifetime of experiences.

Five years ago, while battling an undiagnosed case of bacterial endocarditis, I was refused care at a Jersey City emergency room. After the physician who examined me discovered that I am female-bodied, he ordered me out of the emergency room despite the fact that my temperature was above 104° F (40° C). He said I had a fever "because you are a very troubled person."

Weeks later I was hospitalized with the same illness in New York City in a Catholic hospital where management insists patients be put in wards on the basis of birth sex. They place transsexual women who have completed sex-reassignment surgery in male wards. Putting me in a female ward created a furor. I awoke in the night to find staff standing around my bed ridiculing my body and referring to me as a "Martian." The next day the staff refused to work unless "it" was removed from the floor. These and other expressions of hatred forced me to leave.

Had I died from this illness, the real pathogen would have been bigotry.

I could recount many terrible incidents that illustrate the various ways hostility to trans patients is conveyed. This is not my individual problem; it is a widespread social crisis. You may have heard of Billy Tipton, a well-known white jazz musician who died of a bleeding ulcer in 1989 rather than see a doctor. After his death, lurid headlines revealed that he had been born female-bodied.

In 1995, African American hairdresser Tyra Hunter was in a car accident in Washington, DC. Eyewitnesses reported that rescue medics suspended treatment and made ridiculing remarks after they cut open her pants to treat her and discovered she had male genitals. On-lookers shouted at the medics until they took her to the emergency room, where she died. Hunter's mother won a wrongful-death lawsuit against the District, in which the jury also ruled against the emergency room physician for failing to diagnose Tyra's injuries and for not following nationally accepted standards of care.

Everyone who is living in a sex other than the one assigned to them by a stranger at birth, or who is born on the anatomical spectrum between female and male, or who cross-dresses, or who is perceived as a feminine male or masculine female, or who is gender-ambiguous or gender-contradictory, can most likely recount similar horror stories. As a result, many of us fear contact with health professionals.

Too many of us have already died unnecessarily, have been turned away from a doctor's office or a hospital, or have delayed pursuing preventive or emergency care because of previous mistreatment. And many individuals who are socially identifiable as transsexual or gender-variant are so marginalized by oppression—specifically, in the workforce—that we lack health insurance and a primary care physician. Those who do have insurance often cannot afford healthcare plans that allow us to choose our own doctors. Then, trans patients hesitate to go to HMOs and start over each time with a new physician who might be hostile.

There are also many people in this society who may not identify as trans but who have been humiliated because of some perceived difference in their secondary sexual characteristics or because their mode of self-expression is not considered "man" enough or "woman" enough. All of this shaming drives people underground. As a result, there is no way of knowing how large a segment of the population avoids seeking healthcare because they have been wounded by sex and gender oppression.

Beyond Pink or Blue

How the term "trans" is defined, and by whom, will shape the approach of public health to our population. Many communities—representing a spectrum of sexualities and a wide range of individual identities—march under the banner of trans liberation. And transsexual, transgender, and intersexual people can be found in every economic class, nationality, ethnicity, and region.

Broad generalizations about gender and sex will oversimplify this manifold segment of the population. A female who is considered feminine in her rural community may find herself harassed on urban streets for being too masculine. A Latina drag queen who has lived homeless on the streets of Manhattan since she was 10 years old does not experience the world in the same way as does a white heterosexual male who owns a corporation and cross-dresses several times a year at private parties.

I would recommend that public health professionals put aside definitions for now. They can be conceptually self-limiting.

The crisis for trans patients won't be solved by creating 2 more boxes: female-to-male and male-to-female. While that would create greater recognition of transsexual patients, it does not take into account that a diverse segment of the human population is reluctant to seek healthcare because of current social and medical models of what is "natural."

Sex is best viewed as a continuum. That truth is being articulated by courageous intersexual adults—those who were born on the anatomical sweep between female and male. Intersexual people have been surgically and hormonally shoehorned to fit into the either–or categories of female or male. Intersexual activists are speaking out publicly about their rights to self-determination and to make informed decisions about their own bodies. And birth biology is not the sole determinant of what it means to be a woman or a man. That is demonstrated by the bravery of transsexuals, who live in the sex that feels like home.

Gender expression is also represented most accurately by a continuum. Those pink and blue birth caps in delivery rooms are knitted with inaccurate assumptions that girls will grow up to be feminine and boys to be masculine. Trying to talk about gender articulation using only the terms widely used in English today—feminine, masculine, androgynous—is as ludicrous as trying to make yourself understood in a language composed of 3 words.

Even in this society, in which departures from the Ozzie-and-Harriet paradigms of gender are cruelly punished, I still see uniqueness and complexity, contradiction and ambiguity—what each individual has fashioned out of the social cloth they were issued. And if we are going to defend this full spectrum of self-expression, we must be prepared to defend its poles: masculinity is not rewarded in females, and femininity in a misogynist society is not a privileged gender expression in females or males.

To impose rigid social binaries on this range of human self-expression is to deny what actually exists. Evidence reveals the prevalence and acceptance of gender variance, sex reassignment, and intersexuality in societies on every continent since the earliest oral and recorded history. Historically, laws that partitioned the sexes and punished individuals who bridged or blurred the divide arose with the creation of patriarchal class divisions. The paradigm of 2 genders based on 2 biological sexes began to prevail in Western dominant culture only in the early 18th century.

This historical overview needs to be factored into any discussion about trans healthcare, especially because bigots use a vulgarization of the modern biological model of sex and gender to denounce any variation as "unnatural."

Experts on Our Own Oppression

For many decades, trans people have been told that the way to change the system is to talk to medical students about our bodies and identities, and even about some of the problems we've faced in accessing healthcare. But those individual patient narratives, introduced and framed by non-trans professionals, have not solved the problems.

The degree to which we as trans people are committed to helping change institutional patterns can be understood when I say that for us to describe to an audience what we have suffered as patients is oftentimes as painful as it is to recount a rape—a metaphor I do not use lightly. There are incidents that I have endured in healthcare settings that I still will not talk about.

I have spoken to classes of medical students about my overall experiences for more than 30 years. Sometimes students would later approach me on the street or in a supermarket to tell me how moved they were by my account. But in the course of those 3 decades I was not able to get a Pap test or find a primary care physician. And even the individuals who were sympathetic lacked the tools to change the systems they worked in.

Education is important. But attitudinal change is not the same as institutional change. If education is not tied to transforming systems of healthcare delivery, then it's as effective as putting out a forest fire with teacups full of water. Sensitivity and diversity training has to be linked to a commitment to institutional change and mechanisms for compliance.

Our standing before medical audiences to tell personal stories as patients has not been effective in ushering in change. Now we as an emerging political movement of trans communities are speaking out with a collective voice to say that we are experts on our own lives and what we need as patients.

Imagine that you discovered that male researchers and physicians—no matter how well-meaning—had written the entire body of medical literature on women's health needs, and that these articles narrowly defined "woman" and made sweeping, often erroneous, generalizations about women's psychology, experiences, and health needs. What if, as the basis for their "expertise," these men cited that they had seen some female patients and had read some books by women? Would this literature be problematic because more female patient narratives were needed? Or could this problem be solved only by the organized intervention of women?

Equal Partners in Problem Solving

Now here is a moment of truth for you. I want to talk to you as an equal partner in problem solving about how to remove institutionalized obstacles for trans people. If this is controversial, I welcome that controversy. I believe that this kind of debate will motivate the most progressive, self-confident, and compassionate members of the healthcare community—many of you battling your own oppression—to insist that we as trans people must be part of any dialogue or any plan about how to solve what is an urgent crisis for us.

This participation must include the most downtrodden and disenfranchised of the sex- and gender-oppressed populations, including people of color, street youths, the homeless, and prisoners. As trans grassroots organizers, we can also enlist the organizational networks established by intersexuals, cross-dressers, and trans men and women.

Will our insistence that we be included as peers create a struggle among divergent currents in the healthcare community? You bet! But as Frederick Douglass wisely and succinctly explained, "Power concedes nothing without a struggle."

So let me begin with a few concrete ideas that would make a big difference for us as trans people.

We need immediate changes in treatment-based situations, because those are often the most life threatening for us. We urgently need a centralized listing of trans-friendly healthcare providers and facilities. Those individuals and institutions need ongoing educational information and training about what constitutes sensitive care.

Some of the solutions are so easy, really. Refer to patients by their first and last names, not Mr. or Ms., sir or ma'am. Remove sex-specific signs and stick-figure symbols from single-occupancy restrooms. Provide unisex equipment, such as wide-mouth urinary devices.

We need healthcare providers to understand why it is so important not to ask us to remove our clothing unless it is absolutely necessary, and if it is necessary, to explain why. You may not realize how many times we have been told to strip and have suffered genital examinations and prurient questions when we were seeking treatment for strep throat or removal of a mole on the upper body.

We need written institutional standards establishing the minimum of good care for trans patients. We need healthcare worker competencies. We need on-site patient advocates to help us redress our grievances.

These and other actions will send up a signal flare to trans people that a transformation is taking place in healthcare. This signal will help us reach trans populations that are currently underground in order to do needs assessments.

Trans research should be community-based because of our specific sensitivities, understanding, experience, and consciousness. How will research be conceptualized and formulated? How will teams locate the most oppressed segments of the population? How will the results of research be interpreted? How will the findings be distributed—not only to the public health community, but also to trans communities that need that information? The quality and success of trans research will depend on how you answer these questions.

But trans needs assessment cannot be determined by community-based research alone. We also need to look at how misunderstandings or prejudices in the non-trans healthcare community affect needs assessment. For example, are very masculine females less likely than others to do breast self-examinations? Or are healthcare providers less likely to educate them about the need to do breast examinations?

We need profound changes to show the trans population that it is safe to seek care. Imagine if a prestigious group of public health educators, researchers, administrators, doctors, nurses, and healthcare unions issued a statement saying that sex and gender are much more complex than the currently accepted paradigm, that expressions of sex and gender are much more accurately represented by Kinsey-type continua than by either–or boxes. Suppose these medical professionals said they were going to work with sex- and gender-variant people to create models that more accurately reflect the range of human bodies and self-expression. That would have a stunning impact on social consciousness as a whole, not just the healthcare community.

I believe that our trans movement will find strong allies in public healthcare. More than any other area of medicine, public healthcare has always factored in social, economic, and political impacts—specifically oppression and poverty—on community wellness.

I have brought you just a few of the ideas that I, and other trans activists, have about our health crisis. We want to hear your thoughts about how the barriers to trans healthcare can be removed. Now we arrive at another moment of truth: When and where will our dialogue continue?

REFERENCES
List of references is available in the original source.

 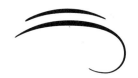

"Financially Vulnerable"

by Stephanie Rytilahti

This article places the reader in the position of a young woman I will call "Helena." Helena is a fictitious representation of the many clients I met with during my career in the financial industry. Although her story is untrue, her situation accurately reflects the financially vulnerable situation many Americans find themselves in when trips to the hospital are either uninsured or only partially covered by health insurance companies. In this narrative, I will optimistically guide Helena through a variety of options for dealing with her medical collections. None of these options will be without compromises, but, unlike many of the clients I assisted, she will have options. Her tale will be complicated by the same institutional hurdles many of my clients faced: gender, race, class, ethnicity, sexual orientation, parenthood, and limited educational and financial resources.

In a country where hospitals, financial institutions, and employment-based insurance are inextricably linked, many Americans face overwhelming and invisible obstacles on a daily basis. Helena largely represents the mythical norm. She is 25 years old, white, college-educated, and healthy. She works three different jobs to cover her expenses. None of her employers offers health insurance. She looks into a few different options after graduating from college, but the monthly premiums are beyond her financial resources. Thus far, she has avoided the need for major medical care. She knows her situation is risky, and eventually hopes to move into a position with full benefits. Unfortunately, a few months elapse and Helena is injured in a biking accident. The injuries are relatively minor, but without insurance she ends up owing the hospital over $1200. She sets up a payment plan to begin paying down the debt, but over the course of the next year she calls upon the healthcare system three additional times for strep throat, an ear infection, and a burn injury.

Two more years elapse, and Helena eventually finds a job that offers health insurance. She is delighted to have this aspect of her health covered. She has taken a total of seven trips to urgent care over the last two years, and knows there are still quite a few outstanding charges to pay. Her first priority is a new vehicle. Her new job is over thirty minutes from her apartment, and she walks a portion of the way every night in the dark because public transportation does not go directly to her office. It is not the safest part of town, and she is beginning to dread the walk each evening. She makes an appointment at her financial institution to apply for a loan, and the loan officer she meets with asks a few general questions about her employment, rent, and marital status. She lets Helena know it will take a few minutes to pull her credit report and determine her eligibility. Helena breathes a sigh of relief. She worked very hard, even during the months when illness kept her out of work, to keep up with her student loan payments and a small credit card bill. Thus, she is surprised when the loan officer begins to ask her about her outstanding collections. The names of the companies she owes money to do not make sense to her, and the loan officer explains that doctors regularly turn unpaid bills over to collection agencies for repayment, even if a patient has insurance and it is simply taking too long for bills to be reconciled. This strategy puts the pressure on the patient to cover unpaid expenses instead of hospitals arbitrating with insurance companies for past due bills.[1]

Now the intimidating calls from unknown collections agencies begin to make sense to Helena, but she is also relieved it is only medical collections appearing on her credit report. A friend told her a few years ago that these cannot hamper her ability to receive credit. Unfortunately, the loan officer goes on to explain that when a hospital chooses to turn over an unpaid medical bill to a collection agency, it has the same impact as any other unpaid debt. This situation is the same for those who lack insurance entirely, or when an insurance company makes a mistake and neglects to cover a bill. The overall effect can be devastating for a credit score. She indicates that advocacy groups have attempted to change the impact of medical collections in the past, but collection agencies are very lucrative businesses and have fought changes impeding debt collection.[2] She informs Helena that with twelve outstanding collections totaling over $8500.00, her request for a vehicle loan cannot be met. She hands Helena a copy of her credit report and the overwhelming number of unpaid medical bills jump off the page. The loan officer circles them in red, and Helena is suddenly very embarrassed. Her score is a 457, and she is kindly told that other lenders may work with consumers possessing "colorful" credit, but usually at a very high rate of interest. This makes the payments much higher and more difficult to manage monthly.

Similar to Helena, many of my clients never understood the ramifications of unpaid medical bills until a life event prompted a need for a vehicle loan, credit card, or mortgage loan. Most healthcare facilities will continue to send clients a bill for unpaid services, but after a period of time elapses; (in most states 45 days)[3] the debt is transferred to a state collection agency for repayment. Helena does not realize that medical collections will impact her credit score. She, like many others, has heard anecdotally that debts relating to medical services have little to no impact on her credit report. Although this is accurate in the initial stages of the billing process, when the medical establishment sells the debt to a collection agency it has the same devastating impact as any other outstanding bill. The 2003 Fair Credit Reporting Act allows for some consumer protections, but the reporting of any unpaid debt by a collection agency leaves the consumer in a financially precarious situation.[4]

Research relating to credit bureau reporting has found that over 50 percent of reportable collections are due to unpaid medical bills.[5] The conversation Helena has with her loan officer is very similar to others I had with clients in her situation. To obtain a loan with a reasonable interest rate, most lenders will require the consumer to have paid all or most of her collections.[6] Many consumers do not know where to start, because they did not receive or because they lost information from collection agencies stating an identification number for their unpaid account or even the appropriate number to call. Some financial institutions or debt counseling services will assist with this process, but the consumer can spend hours on the phone attempting to unravel years of financial history to no avail.

Based on my experience in the financial industry, it is safe to assume that Helena's situation will end in one of three ways. Faced with the inability to quickly conquer such a large amount of debt, she will simply go without a vehicle. This will decrease her physical safety during late hours, and also impact her mental health as she worries about walking alone to the bus stop at night. If she is a single parent, transporting children to and from school or daycare, purchasing groceries for a family, or dealing with unexpected trips to the hospital, it will be more difficult without her own vehicle. The stress of having no vehicle or "getting by" with something undependable is another unforeseen side effect of unpaid medical bills. Collections will stay on a credit report for seven years after they have been reported.[7] Thus, strep throat from five years ago could also impact Helena's ability to purchase her own home in the future. Many clients I worked with had no choice but to go without a credit card, new vehicle, or their own home because of unpaid medical debts.

Let's assume that going without a car is unthinkable to Helena. She is not willing to compromise her safety any longer, and her boss has intimated that she may be in line for some upcoming travel to other business sites. She investigates other options, and is pre-approved for a $20,000 vehicle loan! Helena is thrilled. This will allow her to buy a brand new vehicle, and not face the embarrassment of admitting to her employer that she is unable to get a car loan. When she sees the monthly payment amount of $618.00, she quickly understands how much her medical collections are costing her. Due to her credit problems, the alternative lender offers her a rate of 15.99% for her vehicle. The standard interest rate for new vehicles in her area is only 5.99%, and this would make monthly payments for the same vehicle only $490.00. However, due to her three years without insurance, Helena feels she has no choice but to accept the higher payments. Over the next few years, she will struggle greatly with this monthly requirement, and worry continually about her future financial picture.

Many of my clients would come to me after receiving these types of unfavorable loan terms, and hope to refinance the debt and escape unmanageable payments. Even if they were successfully making payments at the higher amount, it was often impossible to assist them if medical bills were still unpaid or lowering a score. In this tale, Helena begrudgingly accepts and understands the relationship between healthcare and affordable credit in the United States. This allows her to rationalize a tough financial decision. Many of my clients in same-sex relationships lamented the unfairness of a system that provides joint medical coverage for heterosexual couples, but requires same sex partners to individually find their own forms of insurance. Additionally, many of my clients struggled with language barriers or were new to the United States. As I attempted to bridge both cultural and linguistic divides, it was sometimes nearly impossible to explain that a broken arm from three years ago prohibited a client from receiving an auto loan today. The client may have understood what I was saying, but the logic behind my explanation struck many as blatantly absurd and unimaginable. My office served a sizable

Hispanic population, and the connection between access to healthcare and reasonable credit terms was often a tough lesson for newly arrived workers and their families.

Returning to Helena's final compromise, she may choose to pay down her collections based on her other available resources. She may have a modest sum in her savings account earmarked for unplanned expenses and a down payment on a house. Paying off her medical debt will significantly reduce her access to funds in an emergency, and delay home ownership by several years, but will make it easier for her to get more favorable loan terms in the present. If Helena were a few years older, she might have the option to withdraw funds from a retirement account to cover past medical debts. She will be required to pay a large penalty on the pre-retirement age withdrawal,[8] and she will be less prepared for the staggering costs of prescription drugs, co-pays, and other expenses in her retirement years, but $8500.00 is a lot of debt to pay off without making other sacrifices. Helena may hedge her bets that she won't the miss the money in her retirement years, and finally pay off the sums for minor medical treatment from over six years ago. Although Medicare provides assistance to retirement age citizens, supplemental insurance and other long-term care policies are often needed to cover gaps. If this long-term planning was not conducted or was not financially viable, medical collections can also hamper the financial stability of ageing populations.

Overall, Helena's situation with her medical collections is not only inconvenient but also leaves her physically and mentally vulnerable. Based on my ability as a writer to manipulate her scenario to fit a variety of possible outcomes, I attempted to illustrate some of the compromises I witnessed clients making to overcome the repercussions of medical collections. Each option is not without its short and long-term consequences, and can impact one's access to safe housing and transportation. I only illustrated briefly the acute anguish medical collections can impart on one's mental health, and the guilt and humiliation that can result from needing to depend on family members for assistance, admit past debts to a partner, or deal with collection agencies on the phone. Helena was embarrassed to have her situation revealed to the lending officer and did not want her supervisor to find out about her situation. Her past indebtedness to the medical establishment probably also created stress-related issues that impacted her mental and physical well-being, job performance, and personal relationships.

In my lending experience, struggles relating to unpaid medical collections were significantly more common with non-Caucasian groups. According to a 2003 study conducted by the Office of Human Development, 45 million Americans lack health insurance. As a group, 13% of white Americans are without coverage. Hispanic Americans are more than twice as likely to be uninsured, at a rate of 34%, and 21% of black Americans are without insurance.[9] Similar work undertaken by the Office of Minority Health and Health Disparities found that black Americans, Hispanics, American Indians, Alaska Natives, Native Hawaiians, and other Pacific Islanders all experienced additional barriers to receiving appropriate medical care based on a variety of factors, including insurance coverage.[10] As a lender in Madison, Wisconsin, I began to understand the disparate racial impact this has on credit reports. Credit scores remain low because past and present medical debts go unpaid. This closes the door on affordable loans, and those loans granted tend to be under highly unfavorable terms, which can lead to additional delinquencies on unreasonable payments. As the above data supports, minority groups suffer disproportionately from this adverse situation, and, as a result, access to fair credit remains elusive.

The unfairness and inequities I witnessed in the financial industry prompted me to become an advocate for change. Lack of access, inadequate coverage, and discrimination-based barriers will continue to plague Americans seeking reliable healthcare unless more voices join the calls for reform. Listed below are steps you can take to protect your own health and financial future. Inaction and acceptance will only result in additional unpaid elbow fractures and fewer affordable car loans.

1. Learn more about the health insurance industry and how it impacts your physical, mental, and financial health. Visit the nearest locally owned feminist bookstore or library for books covering this topic.

2. Follow current political debates regarding healthcare coverage in the newspaper.

3. Use on-line networking connections and personal contacts to inform others about the health insurance industry and its link to financial wellness.

4. Write to your local and national representatives and let them know you care about this issue.

5. Track the voting record of your elected representatives on issues relating to affordable healthcare, and volunteer to support fundraisers, networking events, and other campaigns in support of candidates mobilizing for change.

6. Join or create a local organization to raise awareness and fight for a change in the current health insurance and/or financial industry.

REFERENCES

1. McDonald, Jay. "Medical Bills Can Make Your Credit Sick." *Bank Rate*. 7 July 2003. 17 July 2008. <http://www.bankrate.com/brm/news/insur/20020828a.asp>

2. Ulzheimer, John. "Medical Collections . . . Oh, What Trouble They Cause." *Credit.Com*. n.d. 16 July 2008. <http://www.credit.com/rs/vol20.jsp>

3. McDonald, Jay.

4. Hendricks, Evan. "Credit Scores and Credit Reports." *Veracity*. 2005. 17 July 2008. <http://www.veracitycredit.com/credit-scores-and-credit-reports-c-001.html>

5. Hendricks, Evan.

6. Hendricks, Evan.

7. Fair Isaac Corporation. "Managing Your Credit in Turbulent Financial Times." *My Fico Credit Education Center*. n.d. 22 July 2008. < http://www.myfico.com>

8. Orszag, Peter. "Penalties on Early IRAs and 401(k)s." *Tax Policy Center: Urban Institute and Brookings Institution*. 2007. 21 July 2008. <http://www.taxpolicycenter.org/publications/url.cfm?ID=1000812>

9. Rowland Diane, and Catherine Hoffman. "The Impact of Health Insurance Coverage on Health Disparities in the United States." *Human Development Reports*. 2005. 17 July 2008. <http://hdr.undp.org/en/reports/global/hdr2005/papers/hdr2005_rowland_diane_and_catherine_hoffman_34.pdf>

10. Centers for Disease and Control Prevention. "About Minority Health." *Office of Minority Health and Health Disparities*. 6 June 2007. 17 July 2008. < http://www.cdc.gov/omhd/AMH/AMH.htm>

Rural Health Care
"A Report from Montana and Beyond"

by Nicole Winbush and Renee Crichlow

America's small towns and rural areas are facing a mounting healthcare crisis. Most of the nation's healthcare infrastructure is located in metropolitan areas, at some distance from America's more isolated areas. In these communities, limited economic opportunities and social isolation can combine to create seemingly insurmountable obstacles to accessible and high-quality healthcare. The result is a growing gap between the health of rural and urban Americans.

While definitions constantly change, most recent definitions describe rural areas as those with "open country and settlements with fewer than 2500 residents."[1] Beyond rural communities is the "frontier": areas with fewer than 6 people per square mile.[1] In Montana, our home, almost half of the population lives in frontier areas.[2] We live in Red Lodge, a town of 2,200 located in south-central Montana. In Red Lodge, many people work in ranching, agriculture, and service industries supported by the local tourist economy. Many do not have health insurance as part of their jobs and have to decide if it's "worth it" to have insurance—whether the freedom from worry justifies the expense of insurance.

Jen Nelson and her partner, Piney Hardiman, live in Red Lodge and waitress at a local restaurant. Their employer does not offer healthcare benefits, so Jen and Piney have purchased outside coverage with a $10,000 deductible. While it covers any serious injuries, the couple knows that smaller injuries or illnesses will require sacrifices in order for them to cover the deductible. Jen says, in a worst-case scenario if serious illness strikes, they can turn to "some savings, credit cards and family members."

"Rural Health Care: A Report from Montana and Beyond," by Nicole Winbush, M.D. & Renee Crichlow, M.D., originally published in the *Women's Health Activist*, March/April 2005, pp. 13–14, the newsletter of the National Women's Health Network (NWHN). It is reprinted with the permission of the author and the NWHN.

Last summer, Jen injured her foot, an experience that brought home the realities of her uncertain healthcare coverage. She comments, "I had to process all of the what ifs . . . It was very stressful. I knew I couldn't wait tables with a broken foot." In the end, she had a speedy recovery and was able to return to work sooner than expected, to her great relief.

Insurance and Opportunities Are Lacking in Rural and Frontier Areas

Nationally, 20 percent of the 41 million Americans who lack health insurance live in rural areas. In Montana, the figure is much higher: fully 70 percent of the state's uninsured live in a rural community.[3] Many are self-employed or work for small companies with non-existent or limited health insurance benefits. In addition, rural Americans are often employed in so-called "high-poverty jobs"—jobs where the likelihood that the worker will remain in poverty is high, despite the worker's employment.

Even workers who are insured are likely to have sub-optimal coverage and large deductibles. Premiums are higher in rural areas than in urban areas, and incomes are lower; thus, rural residents spend a larger proportion of their income for health insurance than non-rural Americans do.[4] Gay and lesbian couples face additional obstacles. While marriage and common law statutes often extend health insurance benefits to heterosexual spouses, same-sex partners are unlikely to be able to access insurance through their partner's coverage. In Montana, for example, no health insurance provider offers domestic partner benefits for same sex-partners.[5]

A lack of educational opportunities also disadvantages rural residents when it comes to protecting their health. Educational levels directly effect both an individual's and their children's health, partly because education is linked with increased employment opportunities that bring with them better benefits, including insurance.[6,7] In rural areas, significantly more people of all ethnicities fail to finish high school, compared to their urban-dwelling peers. The percentage of rural women living in poverty is higher than that of rural men; the average salary of a rural woman with less than a high school education is $213 per week, barely enough to survive, let alone purchase health insurance.[8]

Health Disparities and Lack of Access

A growing disparity in the number of healthcare providers in rural versus urban areas is taking its toll on the health status of rural residents. While one-quarter of the U.S. population lives in rural areas, only 10 percent of physicians practice in these communities.[9] Often, the physicians who remain do so at the cost of excessive work hours and staggering patient populations.

Dr. Heather Diaz is a family practice physician in Chelan, a town of 3,000 in eastern Washington. After her residency, she took a job in the small town. She expected to join a small clinic and work with another physician partner. When she arrived, however, Dr. Diaz found that the other physician had left. She spent the majority of the next year on call 24 hours a day, seven days a week. Of practicing in a small town, Diaz says, "There is no reprieve. I am not the kind of person who is good at saying no . . . [so] there is no downtime and it is starting to get to me." There is another clinic in Chelan, but its doctors are older and some are nearing retirement. Diaz comments, "I just do not know what these women will do when the doctors here retire . . . they will have to drive [for prenatal care]." Although Dr. Diaz has great fondness for her patients and town, she had reached the point where she thought she might have to leave. Just as things were looking most bleak, however, she may have found another physician to join her practice.

Over the past 25 years, 470 rural hospitals have closed, forcing individuals to travel further to receive in-patient care. In addition, physician shortages and lack of insurance mean that rural residents are 10-20 percent less likely than urban residents to receive preventive screenings and regular medical check-ups.[3] Rural women are 10 percent less likely to receive a Pap test every three years, and 20 percent less likely to receive an annual mammogram, than women who live in suburban or rural areas. This is increasingly significant, since rural populations are usually older.

Limited access is often most apparent in the provision of reproductive services. In some rural areas there are counties where women cannot obtain Emergency Contraception even with a doctor's prescription, because pharmacies refuse to stock the medication. At the same time, the number of abortion providers continues to decline nationally—dramatically so outside metropolitan areas. In 1978, 47 percent of metropolitan counties lacked an abortion provider; today, 61 percent of counties lack a provider. In the same period, the number of non-metropolitan counties without an abortion provider climbed from 85 to 97 percent.[11]

Targeted Solutions Can Enhance Health in Rural Communities

What can be done to improve access to healthcare in rural areas and improve rural residents' health status? Solving this problem will necessitate increasing the number of rural healthcare providers at all levels—nurses, physician assistants, physicians and public health workers—and supporting healthcare workers so they can remain in their communities.

Attempts to expand the number of rural providers through loan forgiveness and recruiting foreign medical graduates have had some success. Studies show, however, that individuals who have ties to a rural community are most likely to stay and practice in a rural environment.[12] Minnesota's Rural Physicians Associate Program (RPAP) draws on just such connections. The RPAP has been very successful in identifying and training individuals committed to rural medical practice: over 65 percent of RPAP graduates now practice in rural sites.[13] In addition to gaining healthcare services, these communities also benefit from increasing the number of well-paying local jobs and preserving local services.

The role of public health service delivery also must be addressed. Small towns and rural communities often lack large public health infrastructures. Yet, many of the disparities in rural versus urban/suburban health can be impacted by targeted public health services (i.e. alcohol-related motor vehicle injuries/fatalities, smoking, domestic violence, etc). Small towns and communities need access to funding, technical assistance and the financial discretion to create public health initiatives that appropriately address their community's needs. Organizations like the Rural Women's Health Project (RWHP), in Gainesville, FL, help communities develop and implement educational and outreach programs. RWHP can serve as a model and resource for communities seeking to develop public health campaigns and materials in collaboration with local agencies.

Finally, technology means even the most remote communities can access medical specialties that were previously unavailable. Through "telemedicine," telecommunications technology is being used to expand access to medical care and connect patients with health professionals. Using telemedicine, a patient can go to a clinic in her own community and meet with a distant physician by using high-resolution cameras and monitors. Mental health services are one of the least available in rural communities. Thus, telemedicine is most frequently used for psychiatry, followed by dermatology.

Conclusion

Rural and frontier Americans face many of the same challenges as their urban and suburban counterparts in accessing health insurance and care, including: lack of insurance, limited economic opportunities, and inadequate funding for targeted public health interventions. In addition, rural Americans face many unique challenges including healthcare provider shortages and geographic isolation.

To ensure that all Americans have health services and education, we must continue to fight for meaningful healthcare reform. Furthermore, we must not neglect the needs of rural Americans. We must direct resources to expanding the services and information available throughout rural areas, as well as to identifying, training, and supporting workers who can help meet the needs of America's rural communities and reduce disparities in rural health.

REFERENCES
Available from editor@nwhn.org

"Disability and the Medical System"

by the Boston Women's Health Book Collective

Women with disabilities constantly struggle to find healthcare workers who are sensitive to their needs. For nondisabled women, experiences such as childbirth tend to raise awareness of abuses in the medical system. But women with disabilities, particularly those raised with a disability or with very severe medical difficulties, constantly encounter patronizing attitudes and ignorance by healthcare practitioners, damaging their sense of independence and well-being, and seriously reducing the quality of care.

The overlap of sexism with discrimination against people with disabilities restricts employment, education, and participation in the community for the approximately 30 million U.S. women with disabilities, who are among the most frequent consumers of medical services. Wile not all disabled people need medical treatment, such non-medical services as Social Security benefits, wheelchair transportation, and personal care attendant benefits require "certification as disabled" by a doctor.

Yet physicians get little, if any, training about or exposure to people with disabilities. A woman with cerebral palsy reported going to the doctor for an ear infection; he told her he'd never met a person with CP and spent 20 minutes asking her probing questions unrelated to her ear. When another woman visited a dermatologist because of a blister from her brace, he became visibly alarmed to find a woman in a wheelchair in the examining room. On the other hand, some doctors only meet disabled people who are in medical crisis, and disability is viewed solely as a dysfunction; medical schools offer virtually no training in the social and political issues of disability, let alone the impact of sexism, racism, or homophobia on women with disabilities.

The recent passage of the Americans with Disabilities Act of 1990, which has sweeping provisions for accessibility of facilities and services, signals the growing political strength of disabled people. But the medical system lags behind in recognizing disabled women as adults, capable of independent, self-directed lives. For example, if a disabled woman questions a doctor's recommendation, the response is often brutal; a blind diabetic woman who questioned her doctor's prescription was told, "You are hardly in a position to decide. If you'd

Preventing Doctor Abuse

1. Remember: you are in charge of your care; regard the doctor and other health workers as consultants who are employed by you.
2. Don't accept inappropriate or hurtful interaction. If confronting your doctor is hard, role playing first with friends may help you assert yourself.
3. Take a friend with you to take notes and provide support. Make sure the doctor knows that the friend or interpreter, if you use one, is not your guardian and that all communication should be directed to you.
4. To find a good doctor, ask women you trust; avoid the phone book or other listings. Call first to ask if the doctor has experience with your disability; ask about wheelchair or other accessibility.
5. Ask your general practitioner to find out about a specialist's experience with disabled people before referring you for an appointment.
6. Get a new doctor if you feel frightened, threatened, abused, or not respected as a capable adult; if your friend isn't allowed in the examination room without an acceptable reason; if the doctor isn't understandable and willing to learn from you about disabled people.
7. If you like your physician, tell her or him why. Refer others to that doctor.—M.S.

From *Ms. Magazine,* Sept./Oct. 1991, pp. 36–37. Copyright © 1991 by *Ms. Magazine.* Reprinted by permission.
Marsha Saxton, a disability rights and women's health activist, herself disabled with spina bifida, is director of the Project on Women and Disability, a program sponsored by the Boston Women's Health Book Collective.

followed your doctor's advice, you probably wouldn't be blind."

Disabled women, often displayed with little or no clothing in front of groups of medical students, are beginning to communicate their feelings of violation and humiliation. Doctors justify this kind of objectification—bordering on abuse—as necessary to teach students; they are baffled that disabled women have begun to protest.

One of the most pervasive myths is that disabled women are not sexual beings capable of sexual relationships and motherhood. A woman with spina bifida asked her gynecologist for birth control and was asked, "What for? What would you do with it?" The medical system has lagged in addressing the reproductive health needs of women with various kinds of disabilities. By far, most of the medical research on the topic focuses on male reproduction and sexual function.

Medical benefits are another quagmire of inequity. Women with disabilities must fight harder than men to justify their need for benefits since women may not have "worked" in the Social Security system enough to qualify for Medicare. Often only the most sophisticated self-advocates who have access to legal advice can obtain their rights in the system. Others become discouraged by the vast bureaucratic requirements and give up.

With the increasing competition and privatization in the healthcare industry, hospitals are under pressure to be profitable. Screening technologies such as genetic testing, and extensive investigation into family medical histories, are being used increasingly to identify patients who may be poor financial risks. This strategy, called "skimming," often used by insurance companies to disqualify policyholders, hits women the hardest.

Another area of concern is personal care attendant services, which would allow severely disabled people to live in the community outside of institutions; obtaining such services is the new priority of the Denver-based activist organization Americans with Disabilities for Attendant Programs Today (ADAPT), which led the successful fight for wheelchair-accessible transportation.

Women with disabilities have few resources to challenge abuses; many are just now gaining the confidence to speak out, and their organizations have only begun to identify the nature of the mistreatment. As a group, disabled women tend to be poor, unemployed, and unlikely to pursue malpractice litigation; pro bono legal services are needed to support the legal rights of this emerging constituency.

We must assist disabled women in becoming more assertive, understanding their legal rights, and exploring medical alternatives, so that all of us can function as informed consumers of medical services.

"Simply . . . Friend or Foe?"

from New Internationalist

The able-bodied can be allies of disabled people—or they can be patronizing oppressors. Here are a few ways in which non-disabled readers can be friends instead of foes.

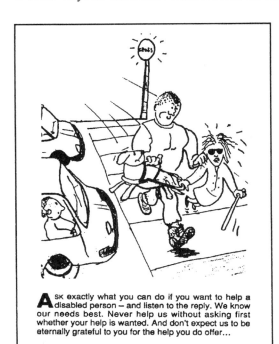

ASK exactly what you can do if you want to help a disabled person – and listen to the reply. We know our needs best. Never help us without asking first whether your help is wanted. And don't expect us to be eternally grateful to you for the help you do offer...

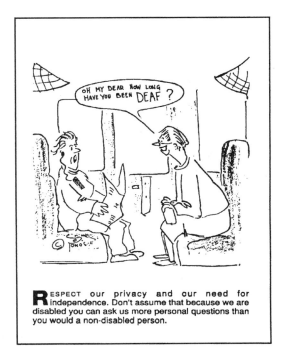

RESPECT our privacy and our need for independence. Don't assume that because we are disabled you can ask us more personal questions than you would a non-disabled person.

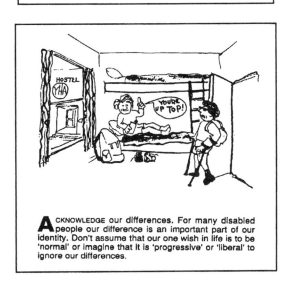

ACKNOWLEDGE our differences. For many disabled people our difference is an important part of our identity. Don't assume that our one wish in life is to be 'normal' or imagine that it is 'progressive' or 'liberal' to ignore our differences.

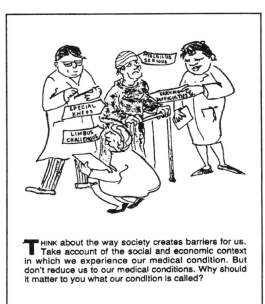

THINK about the way society creates barriers for us. Take account of the social and economic context in which we experience our medical condition. But don't reduce us to our medical conditions. Why should it matter to you what our condition is called?

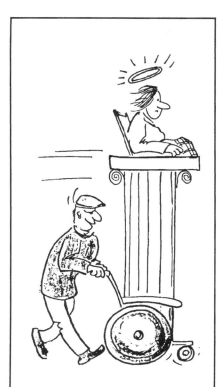

Challenge patronizing attitudes towards us. We want your empathy not your pity. Putting us on a pedestal or telling us how 'wonderful' and 'heroic' we are does not help. This attitude often conceals the judgment that having an impairment is intolerabale — which is very undermining for us.

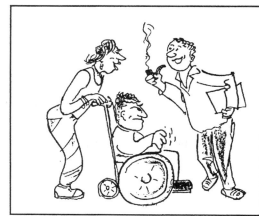

RECOGNIZE our existence. A gaze can express recognition and warmth. Talk to us directly. Neither stare at us — nor immediately look away either. And never talk about us as if we weren't there.

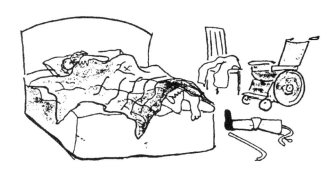

REALIZE that we are sexual beings, with the same wishes, needs and desire for fulfilling relationships as non-disabled people. Don't assume that we will never have children. And if a disabled person has a non-disabled lover don't jump to the conclusion that the latter is either a saint or has an ulterior motive.

APPRECIATE the contribution that we make to society in the fields of work, politics and culture. We engage in these activities for the same reasons as you do — but we may have some different insights to offer. Don't assume that we are passive — or that our activities are a form of 'therapy' to take our mind off our disability. Most disabled people are financially hard up and so we may have a greater need to earn a living than you.

This section is inspired by *Pride Against Prejudice* by Jenny Morris and produced in conjunction with Claire King and Beverly Ashton. The cartoons are by Tony Meredith.

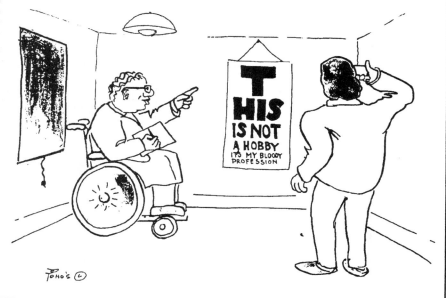

"Letting Justice Flow"

by Alison Kafer

I have no legs.

One night, six years ago, I fell asleep an active, able-bodied young woman. Months later I woke up, my arms, belly, and back covered in burn scars. The legs that had carried me for years were missing, amputated above the knees as a result of my burns. The last few years have been a continual process of learning how to move and understand myself in this new, and yet old, body.

Before my disability, I saw myself as a political activist only when involved in a demonstration or protest. Now, however, I understand my very body as a site of resistance. Every single time I leave my house, people stare. Their eyes linger on my scars, my half-legs, and my wheelchair as they try to understand what happened and why I look the way I do. Their stereotypes about disability are written in their expressions of confusion and fear as they watch me pass. I am powerfully aware that merely by living life in a wheelchair, I challenge their stereotypes about what bodies look like and what bodies do. I feel like an activist just by rolling out my front door.

Sometimes, however, simply rolling outdoors isn't enough of a statement. Sometimes you have to pee outdoors, too.

Three years ago, during my first semester of graduate school, I took an exchange class at a local seminary. A month into the course, I was assigned to give a presentation on the week's readings. Halfway through class we took a break, after which I was to give my talk. I desperately had to pee, and I rolled over to the library, sure I'd find accessible toilets there. I was met only with a wall of narrow stalls—too narrow to slide my wheels into.

I dashed about campus, rolling from one building to another, hoping to find a wide stall door, muttering to myself, "There *has* to be an accessible can somewhere on this damn campus." After checking every bathroom in every building, I realized I was wrong.

What the hell was I going to do?

Going home wasn't possible because I would never make it back to school in time to give my presentation. "Holding it" also wasn't possible because . . . well, when a girl's gotta go, a girl's gotta go. I exercised my only remaining option: I went outside, searched for a dark and secluded part of campus, hiked up my skirt, leaned my body over the edge of my wheelchair, and pissed in the grass.

It just so happened that the dark, secluded place I'd found was the Bible meditation garden.

I went back to class angry. With mild embarrassment, I told the professor what had happened. I felt validated when she stopped the class to tell everyone the seminary president's name so they could write letters demanding an accessible bathroom at the school.

The next day, I, too, wrote a letter to the president informing him of both my accessibility problem and my solution. "Odds are," I wrote, "I will need a bathroom again. And I am doubtful that my 'christening' of the Bible garden is a practice you would like me to continue." In closing, I mentioned the Bible verse I'd found emblazoned on the garden wall (the one I'd practically peed on), and hoped its irony would not escape him. "Let justice roll down like waters," the words proclaimed, "and righteousness like an everlasting stream." Never before had the Bible seemed so relevant to me!?

Within forty-eight hours, I had an appointment with the school president. He ushered me into his office and sat down across from me. "Before we discuss possible construction," he said, "I just want to give you a moment to share your pain."

I paused, thinking his comment a rather condescending way to begin a meeting. "I'm not in any pain," I said curtly, "I just want a place to go to the bathroom."

Our conversation could only go downhill from there.

The president informed me that although he wanted to provide me with an accessible bathroom, the school could not currently afford such construction. When I suggested that removing a forty-year-old skanky couch from one of the women's rooms would free up space for an accessible stall, he responded with a sentiment as old as the couch: "Well, I'm reluctant to remove the sofa because some of the lady students like to rest there *during their time*."

Right. I'd forgotten how much we lady students, brains overtaxed by academia, liked to rest, bleeding, on musty couches in dank bathrooms. What a traitor to my sisters

I must have been to suggest that my need to pee was more important than a couch that hadn't seen human contact since 1973.

Not surprisingly, that meeting did not result in an accessible toilet. So, as threatened, I continued to piss in the garden and complain in the halls. What had started out as a necessity became an interesting combination of necessity *and* protest—a pee protest. Word got around, and to my delight most students supported me. Petitions were signed in a number of classes. One student even proposed a documentary on *The Bathroom Debates* to her film class, showing them a short teaser clip she'd made. I became a bit of a celebrity, known in the halls as "the bathroom girl."

About a month after the first incident, I fired off another letter to the president informing him of my continued use of the Bible meditation site. This time I meant business. I told him I was ready to expose his total disregard of the needs of disabled Americans by going to the press with my story. Bingo. Construction began on the most beautiful accessible bathroom you ever did see.

Justice and righteousness were rolling down at last. They had just needed a little boost from a girl, her wheelchair, and a full bladder.

WORKSHEET—CHAPTER 2

Inequalities and Health

Although this chart of oppressions deserves much discussion and different people may choose to express this differently, this chart may be useful in answering questions on this worksheet.

Mythical norm (Non-target)	Oppressions	Targets
White people	Racism	People of color
Men	Sexism	Women
Young (not too young)	Ageism	Old/very young
Heterosexual	Homophobia, Heterosexism	Gays, lesbians, bisexuals
Fits gender binaries	Transphobia	Transgender or Gender Queer
Able-bodied	Ableism	People with disabilities
Christian	Anti-Semitism (Religious Narrowness)	Jews Other religious groups
Thin	Fatphobia	Fat people
Middle class	Classism	Poor people

The term "mythical norm" comes from Audre Lorde's writings, particularly in *Sister Outsider*. Ricky Sherover-Marcuse used the terms "non-target" and "target" groups in her Unlearning Racism Workshops.

1. Identify two ways that you think that your sex, race, or family income has influenced your interactions with healthcare providers or your access to the healthcare system.

2. Based on the oppressions chart above, identify one "mythical norm" (or non-target) group you are in. Describe the age and situation in which you first became aware that you had certain privileges or power because you belonged to this group.

3. "Racism" by Megan Seeley lists several examples of white privilege. If you are a white person, add to that list by specifically identifying ways that white privilege is *presently* a part of your life. Whether you are a person of color or a white person, make a list identifying ways you experience privilege because of your education. Make lists for any ways you experience privilege because of your class, sexual identity, age, or because you do not have a disability.

4. Based on the oppressions chart on top of page 143, identify one "target" group to which you belong. Identify ways in which you think belonging to this target group is similar and different from belonging to another target group. (Be specific about which two target groups you are comparing.)

5. Having identified a target group you are in, describe ways in which you feel you may have internalized society's negative messages about this group.

6. List ways that in your daily life you could or do interrupt sexist, racist, anti-Semitic, ageist, or homophobic incidents or behaviors.

7. You are helping plan a women's health course. Choose two different women's health topics. Suggest specific ideas of how you could plan to make sure that anti-oppression issues are central to the material covered for these topics.

SEX, GENDER, ROLES, *and* HEALTH

Most introductory women's studies courses devote some class time to a discussion of gender roles. Many of the inequalities in our society are reinforced through the perpetuation of gender roles and through the arguments that these roles are somehow biologically determined and inevitable. (We use the term *gender* roles to emphasize that these roles are socially and culturally constructed, not biologically determined sex roles.) Gender role stereotyping plays a part in every issue discussed in this book, and has an impact on women's roles as healthcare consumers and providers. This chapter brings together a number of themes related to the health ramifications of narrowly defined gender roles and narrow definitions of "males" or "females" as absolutes and binaries.

Leslie Doyal's classic "Hazards of Hearth and Home" gives an excellent global overview of women's health issues in the context of women's roles in different societies, exploring, among other issues, both the physical and psychological hazards of housework, the stress of caretaking and "emotional housework," and the impact of economic inequalities on women's health.

There are health issues that many might think of as not affected by gender. For example, both women and men smoke cigarettes and use alcohol, so it might be easy for someone to think that alcohol and tobacco are gender-neutral issues. Nothing could be further from the truth. In fact, issues related to smoking and alcohol consumption or abuse are sufficiently different for women and men that the topics of tobacco and alcohol can serve as teaching tools to help students learn why a gender analysis is essential for almost all health issues and how to develop a gender analysis.

To develop a gender analysis of tobacco and alcohol issues, we would want to ask questions about the widest range of ways that physiological sex differences, "acceptable" social roles for women and men, and institutional responses to women and men might influence tobacco and alcohol use, misuse, and the consequences. Here are some of the questions we might want to explore: How do sex role stereotypes have an impact on women's and men's use or non-use of tobacco and alcohol? How does the physiology of women's and men's bodies affect how tobacco and alcohol are used and metabolized, and what are the consequences? How do hormonal changes associated with contraception, pregnancy, lactation, and menopause affect tobacco and alcohol metabolism and consequences? How do sociocultural roles make cigarette and alcohol use or dependency/addiction different issues for women and men? How do issues of pregnancy, breast feeding, and women as care givers affect the issues of substance use, dangers of use, and stigma of use? What are health practitioners' attitudes towards women's and men's use and abuse of tobacco and alcohol? Is the health system equally effective at diagnosing and helping women and men who are abusing, dependent on, or addicted to tobacco or alcohol?

Lorraine Greave's thought-provoking work on theories of women's smoking demonstrates how societies benefit from women's smoking:

> When smoking reduces or erases women's demands, emotions, or challenges, women can be seen as compliant and less troublesome. The true scope of women's feelings, particularly anger, remains invisible. Women smokers describe "sucking back anger" with each drag on a cigarette. If women smokers continue to internalize the tensions of interpersonal and societal relations, the responsibility of others in their lives to deal with legitimate emotions is lifted. . . .

Women smokers are using a socially acceptable (among some cultures) form of self-medication. Unlike alcohol and most other drugs, tobacco does not render a woman incapable of carrying out her more traditional nurturing and caretaking social roles. In fact, as we have seen, it often helps women carry out numerous social roles that are unequal and unsatisfying.

It is important to recognize variations in gender roles cross-culturally, yet often discussions of this topic do not take into account cultural and societal differences in gender roles, and, therefore, how gender expectations that are seen by some as oppressive are seen by others as freeing. In "Veiled Intentions," Maysan Haydar, a Muslim feminist, discusses her feelings about veiling:

As an adult, I embrace the veil's modesty, which allows me to be seen as a whole person instead of a twenty-piece chicken dinner. In spite of the seeming contradictions of my life—I'm married to a white man who was raised Catholic, I love heavy metal, I consider myself a feminist, and I sport a few well-disguised piercings—I follow my religion's standard of modesty and appearance.

Later in the article, she compares some gender roles in the U.S. with her own comfort being veiled, "Ironically, the population that spends millions on beauty products, plastic surgery and self-help guides is the same one that takes pity on me for being so 'helpless' and 'oppressed.'"

In discussing gender, it is also crucial to discuss the role of sex—what are biological factors (genetic, hormonal, anatomical) and how do the biological and sociocultural interact? "Male and Female Hormones Revisited" critiques the common use of the terms "male hormones" and "female hormones" and how this terminology reflects and perpetuates misunderstandings about the role of hormones versus socialization in determining male and female similarities and differences. Many people find it liberating, or at least interesting, to learn that women and men are much more alike biologically than most of us have been led to believe and that many differences between girls and boys, women and men, are more socially constructed than biologically determined. Of course, in a society where females and males were equally valued, it would not particularly matter what was biological or social/cultural in origin. However, in a society in which what is identified as "masculine" is valued/rewarded more than what is labeled "feminine" (for example, see "If Men Could Menstruate" in Chapter 5 and "Women and Mental Health" in Chapter 6), demystifying biological vs. societal roles of sex/gender differences is an important political issue. Biological determinism (the attempt to explain complex human behaviors by simplistic biological explanations), which has been used as a very powerful tool to maintain the status quo and inequalities, needs to be examined and critiqued.

Feminists and others working for social change have certainly questioned rigid sex role socialization. Similarly, transsexuals and transgender people have questioned our narrow definitions of "male" and "female" as absolute binaries and moved (some of) us toward thinking about what more fluid definitions of sex and gender would mean. Julia Serano, in a chapter from her book, *Whipping Girl: A Transsexual Woman on Sexism and the Scapegoating of Femininity*, discusses language and terminology related to sex and gender, particularly to those who identify as transsexual or transgender. This is not an attempt to enforce language that some people might (inaccurately and inappropriately) call "politically correct." Instead it is her exploration of why she and others choose to use terms that can explain much about how some transgender or transsexual people understand their own relationship to sex and gender. She uses the term *cissexual*, meaning "the people who have only ever experienced their subconscious sex and physical sex as being aligned," that is, *not* transsexual. The use of this term may have an impact on those who never questioned their identity in terms of sex, similar to the impact on heterosexuals who never thought of themselves as having a sexual orientation or whites who never thought of themselves as having a "race." (See Leslie Feinberg's article in Chapter 2 for some of the healthcare experiences of transgender people.)

Continuing the discussion of transgender and transsexual topics is a chapter from Cris Beam's book, *Transparent: Love, Family, and Living the T with Transgender Teenagers*. Beam's insights and stories drawn from her close work and friendships with trans young people, help us to see the diversity of their experiences, the impact that race/ethnicity and economic issues have on their lives, and how central and varied the appearance of the body is to the need to be able to express gender identity:

> Everything in our culture pushes us to be "completely" male or female. It's in the language: a transsexual is either "pre-op" or "post-op"—the "operative" being presumed and non-negotiable. But contrary to mainstream imagination, there isn't one way to be transsexual—there isn't a fixed trail of body modifications you undergo, leading to genital surgery. Rather, there's a range of physical alterations you can make, depending on your financial situation, how permanent or temporary you want the change to be, your patience with a lengthy process, your tolerance for risk, and what you want to look like at the end.

Reading Beam's work can help those who fall into the cis rather than the trans category to understand the intensity of the search to have physical appearance and gender expression be congruent with internal identity. It also should come as no surprise, given that we live in a society in which many people who already feel their appearance and identity are congruent go through costly and sometimes risky body modification to achieve gender ideals of appearance, including breast augmentation, a range of other plastic surgeries, electrolysis to remove unwanted hair, and hormone use. As with several articles in this chapter, we could have placed this in Chapter 8 under the topic of "Body Modification." However, we placed these articles here to emphasize the relationship between the cultural construction of gender and the extent to which individuals choose to or have chosen for them body modifications that may include serious health risks and long term consequences because of gender expectations in their society.

"Intersexuals: Exploding the Binary Sex System" looks at how one group of people, at least 17 of every 1,000 births (depending on which source you read), would benefit from living in a society in which the definitions of "male" vs. "female" were less rigid and where the medical establishment was not given the power to mutilate the bodies of children who do not easily fit into the male/female sex system. This article introduces us to the Intersex Society of North America (ISNA) and the issues they are raising about the routine practice of doctors' performing major surgery on young children who are labeled as intersex. (Note: The older term "intersexuals" is found in a number of places in these articles but has been replaced more recently by the term "intersex" to recognize that the issue is not about *sexuality* but about biological *sex.*) But more than that, it raises much more fundamental questions about whether we can even envision a society in which new parents could be told, "You have a healthy child who is intersex, in other words, neither a boy nor a girl. There are resources available to help you raise your child in a healthy way. Go home and love your child as you would any other." (For a discussion of the challenges for trans and intersexuals to live safely, read "Trans and Intersex Survivors of Domestic Violence" in Chapter 6.)

Anne Fausto-Sterling, a developmental biologist, published an article titled "The Five Sexes" in 1993; in it she proposed that the two-sex system was not sufficient and should be replaced by five sexes. In the next article in this chapter she revisits that work, describing how much visibility and activism of intersex people and their allies have grown and how far the medical establishment has come in revising old approaches to intersex infants.

In another article on the same topic, Cheryl Chase, a founder of the ISNA interviewed for "Intersexuals: Exploding the Binary Sex System" and a key player in Fausto-Sterling's article, becomes the author challenging feminists and the medical system to recognize our double standards in ignoring or encouraging the issue of intersex genital mutilation in the U.S. but critiquing female genital mutilation in Africa. In her thought-provoking chapter, "'Cultural Practice' or 'Reconstructive Surgery'? U.S. Genital Cutting, the Intersex Movement, and Medical Double Standards" from the excellent book *Genital Cutting and Transnational Sisterhood*, edited by Stanlie M. James and Claire C. Robertson, Cheryl Chase states that:

> Examining the way that first-world feminists and mainstream media treat African practices and comparing that treatment with their response to intersex genital mutilation (IGM) in North America exposes some of the complex interactions between ideologies of race,

gender, colonialism, and science that effectively silence and render invisible intersex experience in first-world contexts.

She concludes,

> I suggest that intersex people have had such difficulty generating mainstream feminist support not only because of the racist and colonialist frameworks . . . but also because intersexuality undermines the stability of the category "woman" that undergirds much first-world feminist discourse.

We might also note the irony that many intersex people have experienced extensive genital surgery without consent, while many trans people have been denied the genital surgery they sought as consenting adults.

The chapter ends with two articles continuing the discussion of genital surgery. "Made-to-Order Vaginas" discusses the marketing of expensive vaginal surgery that will allegedly "enhance sexual gratification," though it has been shown to have no benefits and does have risks. The author states that "promoting surgery as a solution to bad sex or poor self-image is dangerous and perpetuates myths about women's psycho-social health and sexuality."

As Cheryl Chase pointed out in her article, U.S. feminists have been quick to critique female genital mutilation (FGM) in other nations but had not looked at the experiences of intersex children in the U.S. (such as having the clitoris removed or shortened—because it was "too big" to be a clitoris and "too small" to be a penis—causing loss of sexual response, scarring, and pain). This chapter ends with an interview with Waris Dirie, a Somalian woman who is now a well-known model in London. Because of her own experience of FGM, she told her story publicly and became a leader in activism against FGM. Her words carry the message that western feminists should listen to the voices of women from the societies that practice FGM and follow their lead as to how to work to support ending FGM in ways that work within specific cultures and societies. At the same time, it is important to examine our own societies and work against destructive practices at home.

FOR EVERY GIRL WHO IS TIRED OF ACTING WEAK WHEN SHE IS STRONG, THERE IS A BOY TIRED OF APPEARING STRONG WHEN HE FEELS VULNERABLE. FOR EVERY BOY WHO IS BURDENED WITH THE CONSTANT EXPECTATION OF KNOWING EVERYTHING, THERE IS A GIRL TIRED OF PEOPLE NOT TRUSTING HER INTELLIGENCE. FOR EVERY GIRL WHO IS TIRED OF BEING CALLED OVER-SENSITIVE, THERE IS A BOY WHO FEARS TO BE GENTLE, TO WEEP. FOR EVERY BOY FOR WHOM COMPETITION IS THE ONLY WAY TO PROVE HIS MASCULINITY, THERE IS A GIRL WHO IS CALLED UNFEMININE WHEN SHE COMPETES. FOR EVERY GIRL WHO THROWS OUT HER E-Z-BAKE OVEN, THERE IS A BOY WHO WISHES TO FIND ONE. FOR EVERY BOY STRUGGLING NOT TO LET ADVERTISING DICTATE HIS DESIRES, THERE IS A GIRL FACING THE AD INDUSTRY'S ATTACKS ON HER SELF-ESTEEM. FOR EVERY GIRL WHO TAKES A STEP TOWARD HER LIBERATION, THERE IS A BOY WHO FINDS THE WAY TO FREEDOM A LITTLE EASIER.

CrimethInc. Adapted from a poem by Nancy R. Smith. **CrimethInc. Gender Subversion Kit #69-B.** Copies of this poster are availble individually and in bulk quantities from CrimethInc. Genders Anonymous / PO Box 1963 / Olympia WA 98507 or if waiting ain't your thing, go to **www.crimethinc.com**.

Hazards of Hearth and Home

by Lesley Doyal

Synopsis   Women's health cannot be understood simply in terms of their biological characteristics. Improved theoretical analysis and more effective political action both require an exploration of the causal links between women's daily lives and their experiences of health, illness and disability. Recent research relating to these issues is explored in two linked articles: "The Hazards of Hearth and Home" and "Waged Work and Women's Well Being" (Vol. 13 No. 6).

Domestic work varies around the world but it universally involves low status, lack of economic power, and extensive social and emotional responsibilities. The implications of this labour for women's health are explored in this first article through an examination of the physical and psychological hazards of housework, the impact of caring on women's well-being, the stresses of emotional housework, inequalities in the allocation of household resources, the social and economic context of the ageing process in women, and the effects of domestic violence. These issues are placed in the context of the feminisation of poverty and differences between women in the developed countries and the Third World are explored.

Introduction

Women's health has traditionally been understood in terms of their reproductive systems. Thus, doctors locate women's problems in the specialist areas of gynaecology and obstetrics and assume that this takes care of those health problems peculiar to the female sex. Even women's overrepresentation among those diagnosed as suffering from certain types of mental illness is frequently explained by reference to some ill-defined biological nature, related, however obscurely, to their reproductive characteristics.

The reductionist model of health and illness that lies behind these practices has come under increasing attack in recent years. Research has shown that social and economic factors such as class, race, and country of residence are crucially important in mediating the biological processes underlying disease, death, and disability in both sexes. People do not become sick or remain healthy simply because of their genetic inheritance and their accidental contact with disease causing agents. The causal processes involved are much broader, encompassing living and working conditions, access to basic necessities, power and autonomy, and the quality of human relationships.

Feminists have taken this analysis a step further, using these ideas to explore the particular health problems experienced by women. While most women have a longer life expectancy than men from the same social group as themselves, they report more ill health and distress than men, use primary care and hospital services more than men, and suffer more long-term disability. The nature and severity of women's health problems obviously vary according to race, class, and economic status, but this overall gender difference remains remarkably constant. Researchers are now beginning to explore the reasons for this, linking women's patterns of morbidity and mortality to the nature of gender divisions in society and particularly to the continuing inequalities between the sexes. Findings from this new research are used to explore the links between women's health and two main areas of activity in their lives—domestic labour and waged work.

Domestic Labour in a Global Context

Women have traditionally been responsible for most of the work done in the domestic sphere. However, very little is known officially about the nature of household work or the conditions under which it is performed. While there have been periodic panics about women's capacity to look after their families'—and therefore the nation's—health, the impact of their domestic work on women's own well-being has rarely been a cause for concern. Indeed the role(s) of housewife and mother have generally been seen as healthy, despite considerable evidence to the contrary. So what is the nature of this work that most women spend so much of their time performing?

Their domestic responsibilities involve women in a complex web of activities that are often difficult to disentangle. For most, the central threads consist of care of a husband (or male partner), care of children and other dependents, and housework. Although the balance of these responsibilities will vary during the life cycle, these basic jobs form the core of women's domestic work in most societies. Not surprisingly, the nature and volume of this labour and the circumstances under which it is carried out have profound effects on women's physical and mental health.

In the developed countries, the common stereotype of the housewife is of a consumer who does a relatively small amount of low status, unskilled work, much of which involves spending money earned by a man. The reality, however, is very different. In the first place, most domestic work is done not by full-time housewives, but by women who are also engaged in some combination of paid and unpaid work outside the home. This pattern now applies in the majority of countries around the world—rich and poor, socialist and capitalist. In the second place, domestic work involves many (often unrecognized) skills and much effort. Indeed, most women with children (with the exception of the very affluent) spend their lives in continuous activity, putting together what the Italian feminist Laura Balbo has called "survival strategies" for themselves and their families (Balbo, 1987, p. 45).

But despite its obvious social utility, women's domestic work is unpaid—a fact which demeans it, and sets it apart from most other work done by adults. This inevitably has psychological significance for women, lowering their self-esteem and minimizing their sense of their own worth. It also affects them in more material ways, by reinforcing their economic dependence on others. Although many mothers with young children are now in paid employment, few can earn enough to support themselves and their families while continuing to do unpaid domestic work. Hence, most are forced, along with full-time housewives, into economic dependence on a male wage earner. Others have to rely not on an individual man but on the state to provide for their basic needs. In either case, economic dependence seriously limits women's autonomy and inhibits their control over their own lives and their health.

At the same time, women also have to take responsibility for those who are dependent on them for emotional and physical sustenance. Most of their daily work involves women in the servicing of others (Kickbusch, 1981). Put in more romantic terms, women's work consists of care of their "loved ones." This care can range from washing a partner's clothes through cooking a child's dinner to comforting a teenager worried about spots or cleaning up after the dog has been sick. It is distinguished from the same work in a laundry, cafe, or health centre because it is done for love rather than money. That is to say, women are expected to care *about* other people as well as caring *for* them (Graham, 1984). Thus, many women bear the double burden of their own economic dependence on a man or the state along with the dependency of their families on them for physical and psychological survival.

So far we have been talking in general terms about the elements of domestic work as it is performed by women in most countries around the world. The recognition of these basic similarities is important in reminding us that whatever the circumstances, patriarchal societies give women ultimate responsibility for the well-being of their families, often at considerable cost to their own health. However, this responsibility will have different implications according to the socioeconomic circumstances in which it has to be fulfilled. This point is most clearly illustrated through contrasting the lot of the majority of women in the industrialized countries with those in the Third World.

Housework and childcare are not the same in Birmingham, England or Birmingham, Alabama, as they are in the slums of Sao Paolo or the rural wastes of the Sahel. The most obvious difference is the level of material resources to which a woman has access to meet her family's needs. As we shall see, poverty itself is a major factor influencing the impact that a woman's domestic work has on her health, and most Third World women are very poor by comparison with those in Britain or the United States. But taking the analysis one stage further, we also need to recognize that the nature of domestic work itself is very different in the Third World.

Women in the rich countries work out their survival strategies through their own and often a partner's negotiations with the labour market and/or the state. This will often be difficult, time-consuming and exhausting, and the impact on the health of poor women should not be underestimated as they cobble together wages, benefits, subsidies, or rebates to underwrite the purchase of their necessities. However, even these options are not available to millions of women in the Third World. They have little or no money to spend in the cash economy and welfare services are not available to fill the gap. As a result, they have to weave their patchwork of survival through the direct production of their own and their family's needs. Many are engaged in subsistence agriculture, growing and then processing the food they are not rich enough to buy. Fuel is collected in the form of firewood rather than purchased from a gas or electricity supply company and water is collected from a local source rather than flowing to the house through pipes. Thus, the physical burdens of their domestic labour are very much greater and this is clearly reflected in their experiences of morbidity and mortality. These international variations will be explored in more detail as we look at the different aspects of women's domestic work and its impact on their health.

The Hazards of Housework

Throughout the world, women perform many millions of hours of housework every day—most of it unacknowledged and barely visible. In the developed countries it is widely assumed that technological innovation has led to a reduction in the hours spent on housework. However, there is little evidence to support this belief. The introduction of basic services, such as running water and gas and electricity, along with the later development of vacuum cleaners, washing machines, and other domestic appliances certainly ameliorated the hard physical labour that characterized the lives of so many workingclass women in the 19th and early 20th centuries (Oren, 1974; Pember Reeves, 1980; Llewellyn Davies, 1978; Spring Rice, 1981). However, there was little reduction in the number of hours worked (Vanek, 1974; Meissner et al., 1988). Nor is there evidence that women's greater participation in waged work has led to a more equal division of domestic labour. Instead, women have retained the moral responsibility for ensuring that all domestic work is done, whether they are employed outside the home or not. They must organize it and worry about it, even if they do not do everything themselves, with inevitable effects on their health.

Despite (or sometimes because of) the development of modern technology, housework can still be physically and mentally exhausting, especially when conditions are difficult. Domestic accidents are a common hazard, especially for older women, and are more likely to happen when the fabric of the home is substandard. An old and dilapidated house will be more difficult to keep clean and will often threaten the safety of women and children. Since they have to spend more time than men indoors, women are more affected by defects, such as condensation and dampness which can aggravate respiratory disorders, as well as increasing the physical burden of housework. Looking after a home and its in-

habitants can also bring the worker into contact with a wide range of toxic chemicals that are largely unregulated and have often been inadequately tested (Dowie et al., 1982; Rosenberg, 1984). Most of these are domestic products of various kinds such as cleaning fluids, bleaches, detergents, insecticides, and pesticides that are commonly used in the home and garden. It has been estimated that the average household in the United States contains some 250 chemicals that could send a child to hospital (Rosenberg, 1984).

There is also growing evidence that in the course of their housework women may be put at risk by hazardous chemicals encountered by their partners at their place of work. Research has shown that they can be endangered by asbestos fibers and radiation brought home on their husband's clothes or on his person. It also seems likely that some cases of cervical cancer may be caused by substances to which the man is occupationally exposed, which are then passed on to the women during intercourse (Robinson, 1981). Thus, the domestic workplace is not necessarily free from the chemical hazards of the industrial setting. Toxic substances do not become safe simply because they cross the threshold of the home and more research is needed to identify these dangers, as well as more effective regulation to control them.

However, it is the psychological hazards of housework which have attracted most attention, at least in the developed countries. To understand the reasons for this we need to look more closely at the nature of the work itself, at its social and economic status, and at the conditions under which it is performed. We can then explore the effects these have on women's sense of themselves, their control over their lives, and their potential for growth.

In Ann Oakley's study of full-time British housewives, most saw the main advantage of their job as the negative one of freedom from the constraints of employment (Oakley 1974). Few were positively happy with their work, with 70% expressing themselves 'dissatisfied' overall (Oakley, 1974). The women described most of their household tasks as monotonous, boring, and repetitive. Interestingly, it is these very characteristics of unskilled labour that occupational psychologists have shown to be most stressful in the context of male waged work. Although they are not formally controlled by a boss, most women doing housework experience very powerful pressures, both from other people and from inside their own heads. Ann Oakley asked one of the women in her study whether she found housework monotonous. Sally Jordan replied:

> Well, I suppose I do really, because it's the same thing every day. You can't sort of say, "I'm not going to do it," because you've got to do it. Take prepar-

ing a meal: it's got to be done, because if you didn't do it, the children wouldn't eat. I suppose you get so used to it, you do it automatically. When I'm doing housework, half the time I don't know what I'm thinking about. I'm sort of there, and I'm not there. Like when I'm doing the washing—I'm at the sink with my hands in water, and I drift off. I daydream when I'm doing anything really—I'm always going off in a trance, I don't hear people when they talk to me. (Oakley, 1976, p. 147)

Thus, women are able to get little job satisfaction from routine housework and this is exacerbated by their lack of social and economic status (Berk, 1980). Most adults are paid for their work, and lack of such rewards limits self-esteem and gives a sense of worthlessness. Moreover, housework tends to be noticed only when it has *not* been done, giving women little opportunity for positive reinforcement, even of a nonmaterial kind.

These negative feelings are reinforced by the circumstances under which domestic labour is carried out. Housework is paradoxical in that it is usually done at home in isolation from most other adults, but when combined with childcare it also offers little opportunity for solitude. Despite widespread social and economic change, women continue to do almost all their household tasks in individual nuclear family units, with modern architectural styles often reinforcing this separation. However, the housewife may also find that her time is not her own. She will have to respond to the needs of others, may find very little time or energy to do things for herself, and rarely has physical space of her own. Under these circumstances, the demands on women are often high, and the real possibilities for control are low—again a situation clearly identified as stressful in the context of waged work (Karasek, 1979).

An additional feature of domestic work which can pose a threat to women's health is its open-endedness. Just as there are no absolute goals or standards, so there is no obvious end to the working day. For men and older children, home is perceived as a place of rest and recovery from the stresses and strains of real work done in the world outside. However, for most women the home is also a workplace and remains so for most of their waking hours. Many find it difficult to separate work and leisure; indeed those with young children are never really off duty, and their working hours can even extend to periods of sleep.

Not surprisingly, surveys in the developed countries have shown that women indulge in fewer leisure activities than men. The hobbies and pastimes they do mention tend to be domestic or home-based (listening to records or tapes, watching TV, reading, needlework and knitting, crafts and cooking) and they are frequently combined with ironing or child care (Deem, 1986). Relatively few are able to have outside interests, and active participation in sport is rare indeed. The reasons for this are closely related to women's family situation: lack of material resources, reluctance of men to allow them out alone, and the difficulty of getting someone else to look after the children, as well as the male-domination of many leisure and sporting facilities. This lack of leisure in general, and sport in particular, has obvious implications for women's physical and mental health:

> . . . the notion of "wellbeing" is closely tied up with opportunities for leisure. The fewer opportunities women have for leisure, the less the chance that they will see themselves as enjoying such wellbeing, which includes more than feeling healthy and/or fit and implies a sense of confidence about and enjoyment of life in general, which is difficult if that life consists mainly of being stressed, overworked, tense and continually feeling tired as well as having a poor body image. (Deem, 1986, p. 425)

Ultimately, the most damaging aspect of housework for women's mental health may be the lack of opportunity it offers for personal development. Some women do get a great deal of satisfaction from tasks done in and for their households, and develop considerable skills in the process. However, the structure of the job offers no opportunity for growth or advancement and few chances of wider social recognition for achievement. Of course, women do learn to deal creatively with challenges and crises throughout their lives. Indeed many individuals and families would not have survived without their tenacity, problem-solving abilities, and sheer hard work. However, those tasks are rarely of their own choosing and may offer little in the way of increased personal autonomy.

Why then do so many women go on doing housework under these conditions with so little complaint? One reason is their early socialisation which means that many have extreme difficulty in expressing any dissatisfaction they may have with housework. To do so may be to threaten their identity as a good wife and loving mother.

The power of this repression is reflected in what Jessie Bernard has called the "paradox of the happy marriage." During her classic investigation of male and female perceptions of marriage, men expressed a considerable degree of dissatisfaction, but appeared to have relatively good mental health as measured by a questionnaire. Women, on the other hand, were more likely to say they were happily married but exhibited much poorer mental health (Bernard, 1972). This contradiction was especially acute among full-time housewives, many of whom simultaneously expressed high levels of satisfaction with marriage, as well as serious psychiatric symptoms. Indeed Bernard describes what she calls the "housewife syndrome" consisting of nervousness, fainting, insomnia, trembling hands, nightmares, dizziness, heart palpitations, and other anxiety symptoms. She concluded that "the housewife syndrome is far from a figment of anyone's imagination" (p. 47) and that "being a housewife makes women sick" (p. 48).

But it is depression above all, that seems to be an occupational hazard among fulltime housewives, especially those with young children. Both clinical experience and community research have shown that many women staying at home experience intense frustration, which is usually expressed in feelings of emptiness, sadness and worthlessness (Brown & Harris, 1978; Nairne & Smith, 1984). Too often these feelings go unacknowledged; women are said to be "like that" and the front door closes on a great deal of misery and distress. George Brown and Tirril Harris working in South London found that one-third of a random sample of workingclass women with children under six who were full-time caregivers were suffering from what could be classified as "clinical depression." However, few had sought medical help. When women do take emotional problems to their doctors they are usually offered a chemical solution. In reality, however, it is the nature of women's domestic labour, their relationships with other people and their dependent status that makes them more likely than any other group to experience depression and anxiety, but less likely to confront the real reasons for their frustrations and dissatisfactions.

Who Cares for the Caregivers?

As well as doing the housework the majority of women also care for dependents. The intensity of this work varies over the lifecycle and some women never do it at all. However the vast majority become mothers at least once in their lives—in Britain the figure is now about 80%. This can be immensely rewarding and for many women motherhood is the most important and creative aspect of their lives. However, the reality of day to day childcare can also be both physically and emotionally demanding, especially under difficult circumstances (Graham & McKee, 1980; Richman, 1976; Boulton, 1983). For first-time mothers in particular, the responsibility of a tiny baby can be very onerous and nights without sleep exhausting and demoralizing.

Despite the lip service paid to motherhood as a social duty and a valued activity, few researchers have explored the reality of childcare from a woman's perspective. In an attempt to fill this gap, the British sociologist Mary

Boulton recently carried out a series of in-depth interviews with young mothers (Boulton, 1983). Her intention was to disentangle women's feelings about the daily labour of childcare from their love for their children or their response to the status of motherhood itself. Almost two-thirds of women in the study experienced a strong sense of meaning, value, and significance in looking after their children. This is clearly important because a purpose in life is central to a feeling of well-being. However over one third did not feel this way (Boulton, 1983). Moreover, some 60% of her middle-class respondents and 44% of those who were working class found looking after children to be predominantly an irritating experience. Thus, the majority did not find childcare "naturally rewarding." Yet this was their fulltime work.

Many of the women referred to stress in their lives and identified a number of factors contributing to it. The lack of boundaries to their role meant that they were always trying to create structures and find themselves physical and mental space. They complained that childcare interfered with other activities, especially housework, and that children often undid what had just been achieved. For some women, childcare was isolating and limited them to relationships with other women in a similar position. Many also pointed out that children greatly curtailed their freedom of action because there was so much effort and anxiety involved in taking them out.

Overall, about 50% of Mary Boulton's sample said they were wholly content with their lives as mothers, about one-fifth were wholly discontented, while about one-quarter were in between. That is to say they accepted the situation, but wished it could be different. Significantly however, many of those who reported themselves satisfied also stated that their experiences of childcare were negative. This suggests that, as we saw in the context of housework, many women may simply accept situations over which they have no control, living much of their lives vicariously through others, with inevitable effects on their own well-being.

As well as caring for healthy children, women also look after dependent adults and chronically sick children. Again, precise information is difficult to obtain because this domesticated nursing is one of the most invisible of all forms of labour. In the British context, estimates suggest that at least 1.4 million people (out of a total population of just over 60 million) act as principal caregivers to adults and children with disabilities severe enough to warrant support in daily living tasks (Green, 1988). The vast majority of these are women. Some 15% of all British women of working age care for dependents over and above their normal family duties and many of them are also in paid employment (Martin & Roberts, 1984). Moreover, the need for such care is rising as the number of elderly and disabled people in the population increases. Indeed, the community care policies now fashionable in much of the industrialized world are based on the implicit assumption that women will continue with these unpaid labours (Osterbusch et al., 1987; Finch, 1984; Finch & Groves, 1983). Yet there is evidence that they may not be conducive to the promotion of women's own well-being.

The daily grind of caring has been well documented in a number of research studies (Equal Opportunities Commission, 1982; Finch & Groves, 1983; Briggs & Oliver, 1985). Caring for adults can be especially demanding both physically and psychologically. Much of the strain comes from the nature of the job itself—long hours, nightly disturbances and sometimes the trying behaviour of the person being cared for or the inability to hold a serious conversation. Stress is also caused by the conditions of caring, particularly the isolation that often results when the person cannot be taken out and no substitute care is available. Above all, caring for adults can cause emotional problems that do not arise in caring for normal children. The daughter who cares for a parent and the wife who cares for a husband may have to negotiate new relationships under difficult circumstances, often with very little support. One British woman looking after her husband has described her experiences in the following terms:

> The tiredness associated with looking after someone disabled was the hardest thing for me to adjust to . . . the tiredness is, of course, due to different causes for each caregiver, but the exhaustive effect is the same—for me, the tiredness comes from the physical exertion of caring for someone with severe multiple sclerosis, and from the mental stress of seeing the person you love best in the world suffering from such a disease. (Briggs & Oliver, 1985, p. 39)

Under these circumstances, women's own health will often suffer. This is especially true for women on what has been called the caring tricycle—the lifetime of responsibility which begins with care of children, continues into middle age with care of an aging parent, and ends with responsibility for a frail partner.

Doing Emotional Housework

Some of the more subtle aspects of women's domestic labour can be summarized as emotional housework. This is the least visible part of their work and consists of activities designed to ensure the happiness and emotional wellbeing of other family members—managing social relationships within the home to keep the old man happy and the kids quiet. While this labour is rarely perceived as such by women or their families, it is often a major burden. Arlie Hochschild has vividly described the processes involved:

> The emotion work of enhancing the status and wellbeing of others is a form of what Ivan Illich has called "shadow labour": an unseen effort which, like housework, does not quite count as labour but is nevertheless crucial in getting things done. As with doing housework the trick is to erase any evidence of effort, to offer only the clean house and the welcoming smile. (Hochschild, 1983)

But who is looking after women's needs while they smile for others? Sadly, the answer for many is no one. The traditional division of labour in the family means that women frequently do not receive the emotional sustenance they might have expected from their nearest and dearest. While adult daughters may provide support, this is rarely true of grown-up sons and male partners.

Luise Eichenbaum and Susie Orbach have written extensively on this problem from their experiences as feminist psychotherapists (Orbach & Eichenbaum, 1984; Eichenbaum & Orbach, 1985). They make the important point that the social stereotype of the clinging, passive female leaning on a strong and independent man is usually the reverse of the truth. Most men, they say, are looked after by women all their lives, from their mothers and other female relatives through female teachers to their wives or female partners in adulthood. A girl, on the other hand, is brought up to assume that she will marry a man and provide nurturance, care, and emotional support for him and his children. While she is expected to *appear* "dependent, incompetent and somewhat fragile," the internal reality is rather different:

> . . . behind this outward facade is someone who, whatever the inner state, will have to deal with the emotional problems met in family relationships, a person who knows that others will expect to rely and lean on her, a person who fears that she will never really be able to depend on others or never feels content about her dependency. (Eichenbaum & Orbach, 1985, p. 21)

Thus, many adult women cannot fulfill their own basic need for nurturance and emotional fulfillment, despite—or because of—their position at the hub of what is widely regarded as the most caring institution in modern society.

These insights derived from the psychoanalytic tradition are consonant with women's own accounts of their situation, as reported in a number of recent studies. Agnes Miles, a British sociologist, recently carried out in-depth interviews with some 65 women and men diagnosed as suffering from depression. About half of the women blamed their depression on an unhappy marriage, whereas most men referred to work and health problems (Miles, 1988). When asked about the support they had received, only 24 out of 65 women named their male partner as their main confidante and not all of these were satisfied with the quality of the relationship:

> (Iris, 24, no children). "There is only my husband. I wish there was someone else. Mostly I keep my thoughts to myself. I hoard my thoughts, then I get upset and tell my husband because there is nobody else. I usually regret it afterwards. He is part of the trouble, but who else can I talk to?"
>
> (Bridget, 29, two children 4 and 7). "I wish I had more people, I wish I had a woman friend. My husband is there but he doesn't want to talk, not like women talk to each other. He doesn't understand. He just says, don't bother me with nonsense." (Miles, 1988, pp. 94–95)

Many of the women in Miles' sample also expressed their fear of putting too much of a burden on other people. They were afraid that what little help was available would be withdrawn and, even more fundamentally, saw themselves as unworthy of support. Interestingly, the men in Miles' sample did not report the same problems in getting support from their wives. As Miles expressed it, "both took for granted that this was the natural order of things" (p. 113).

Susannah Ginsberg and George Brown uncovered a similar pattern in their study of women in the North London suburb of Islington. Again they were interviewing women who would be clinically diagnosed as a case of depression, in an attempt to see how relatives, friends, and doctors responded to their problems. This research repeated the now-common finding that signs of depression in women (such as inexplicable crying) are often given little attention since they are regarded as normal for women, especially when they are young mothers or menopausal (Ginsberg & Brown, 1982). Three quarters of those interviewed (27/37) who were living with their husbands felt that he had given little or no support. Mrs. Thomas, for instance, commented as follows:

> "I told my husband how depressed I've been feeling. He just sits in silence. If he could just talk things out and suggest something—but he doesn't."
>
> "Has he suggested you should go to the doctor?"
>
> "No, he doesn't realize anything is wrong. He doesn't notice that I haven't been getting on with things." (Ginsberg & Brown, 1982, p. 93)

Three quarters of the women (34/45) also felt they received little or no support from their mother or other relatives such as sister, or friends. The majority (32/37) who were living with their husbands said they did try to talk about their depression but most were unsuccessful. The majority of husbands apparently responded with such comments as "You're imagining it all," "Stop being silly," or "You mustn't talk like that, there's the baby" (Ginsberg & Brown, 1982, p. 95).

It seems, then, that women's domestic labour, especially their role in caring for others, is not always conducive to their own good health. Their mental well-being in particular will often be put at risk, and adequate support is not available when they are in need. As we shall see, this is especially true in the context of material poverty.

The Feminisation of Poverty

Women have always been overrepresented among the world's poor and recent years have seen a worsening of their situation (Scott, 1984). Although impoverished women are to be found in all countries, the majority live in underdeveloped parts of the world and it is here that the rigours of domestic work are at their most severe (Buvinic, Lycette, & McGreavey, 1983). Of course, men in the Third World are also poor, but it is women who must manage the consequences of poverty for the whole family. This often means performing physically heavier work and working longer hours than men (Dankelman & Davidson, 1988; Momsen & Townsend, 1987; Sen & Grown, 1988). In Tanzania, for instance, a recent study showed that women work an average of 3069 hours a year compared with 1829 hours for men (Taylor, 1985). Similarly, women in the Gambia spend 159 days a year on farmwork compared to men's 103 days (Mair, 1984). Moving to Asia, a study conducted in several rural villages in Kaunataka showed that the labour of women and children together contributed almost 70% of the total human energy expended on village work, even when strictly domestic tasks such as sweeping, washing clothes and childcare were excluded (Kishwar & Vanita, 1984).

Thus, women in the Third World bear a heavy weight of domestic responsibilities. Moreover, their material poverty and, for many, the exhaustion of frequent childbearing, add to their burdens. While climate, culture, and conditions vary between countries, these women are united by their poverty and the harshness of the social, economic, and physical environment in which they carry out their labours. As we shall see, this daily struggle is reflected in their general state of health and well-being.

In the richer parts of the world, most housewives can take for granted the existence of a constant supply of clean water. However, there are millions of women from rural areas of Bangladesh to the crowded barrios of Latin America who must face the daily task of acquiring enough water to meet the needs of their families. This is a physically demanding job which in rural areas will often mean a lengthy journey, but it is very rarely done by men.

Water is needed not just for drinking, but for sanitation and waste disposal, washing, childcare, vegetable growing, and food processing and also for economic uses such as keeping animals, irrigating crops, and brewing beer (Dankelman & Davidson, 1988). All this has to be fetched by women—usually on their heads because few have access to a vehicle of any kind or even a donkey (Wijk-Sijbesma, 1983). Many walk miles every day to a stream, well, or pond for a few pots of water. In urban areas, women depend on public taps which will usually mean long waits and no privacy for bathing. In many slums even public taps are not available, so that women face a long journey or the payment of a high price to a street vendor for water of dubious quality (Dankelman & Davidson, 1988).

Under these circumstances, water will have to be consumed sparingly, making other domestic tasks more difficult. Moreover, insufficient or polluted water will often result in illness, adding to the woman's burden. It is generally assumed that some 80% of all diseases in Third World countries are water-related. Diarrhoea, for instance, is a major cause of death among young children and is closely correlated with the absence of a clean water supply. Women themselves suffer additional problems caused by lack of adequate sanitation because religious and moral prohibitions mean they often have to wait until dark to avoid being seen in the act of defecation. This can lead to constipation and strain on the bladder and also exposes them to the risk of assault (Dietrich, 1986).

As well as supplying water, many Third World women are also responsible for ensuring an adequate amount of fuel for cooking, boiling water, and heating and lighting the house. Again, this very arduous task is rarely done by men and is a significant factor in the endemic exhaustion of many rural women. Throughout the world women are carrying loads of up to 35 kilograms, distances as much as 10 kilometers from home. This weight exceeds the legal allowance for women carrying heavy loads in an industrial setting in many countries. The distance women have to travel varies depending on where they live, and the time taken can be as much as three or four hours per day. In some areas including the Sahel, Gambia, and parts of India, the journeys can be even

longer and deforestation means that they are increasing (Agarwal, 1986). As supplies of firewood diminish, women and children are having to spend even more time on collection. In parts of Bihar, for instance, where seven to eight years ago poor women could get enough wood at 1.5 to 2 kilometers, they now have to trek 8 to 10 kilometers every day (Agarwal, 1986).

This growing shortage of fuel has meant that cooking has now become more labour-intensive and traditional methods have to be adapted to conserve energy. In some places the traditional wood fuel has been replaced by substances, such as cattle dung and crop residues. These biomass fuels are less convenient for cooking; the fire has to be stoked continuously and the smoke is even more dangerous than woodsmoke (WHO, 1984). Emissions from biomass fuels are major sources of air pollution in the home, and studies have shown that cooks inhale more smoke and pollutants than the inhabitants of the dirtiest cities. In one study quoted by WHO, a female cook was said to inhale an amount of benzopyrene (a known carcinogen) equivalent to 20 packs of cigarettes a day. Chronic carbon monoxide poisoning has also been reported (Dankelman & Davidson, 1988). Pollution of this kind has been identified as a causal factor in the high level of respiratory and eye disease found among Third World women. It can also cause acute bronchitis and pneumonia, as well as nasopharyngeal cancer among those exposed from early infancy (WHO, 1984).

As well as ensuring supplies of water and fuel, many Third World women are also directly involved in the production of food for their families (Dixon-Mueller, 1985). They grow a variety of crops either for immediate consumption or to be sold or bartered in the village or local market, and raise poultry or small animals. When food is scarce or there is a drought, they may have to scour the countryside for edible matter such as the roots and leaves of plants. This raw food then has to be processed, often by laborious and lengthy methods. These processes will vary between cultures and climates, but Madhu Kishwar's account of Indian peasant women gives some indication of the quantity of work involved:

> Grain or pulses to be consumed have to be hardcleaned, little pebbles or pieces of dirt hand-sifted or painstakingly removed, one by one before the cooking of every meal. Many women have to handpound the paddy or grind the wheat two or three days a week in order to make it consumable. The paddy first has to be boiled and dried in the sun before it is husked. To husk 20 pounds of paddy, two women can easily spend two to three hours, and it takes much

longer if a woman has to do it alone. . . . Thus, cooking even the most simple and basic foods commonly used in the diet of ordinary families is very exhausting. (Kishwar & Vanita, 1984, p. 4)

These accounts make it clear that the domestic labour of most Third World women is extremely hard. The work is physically strenuous and the hours are long, leaving many millions exhausted, undernourished, and vulnerable to premature death. Moreover, most are involved in frequent childbearing, resulting in levels of debility which can only be guessed at, since morbidity data for rural women are rare, and mortality data crude and uninformative.

While some of the worst living and working conditions are suffered by women in the Third World, this should not blind us to the fact that there are also many women in the developed countries who suffer the ill effects of both absolute and relative poverty on their health (Gelpi, Hartsock, Novack, & Strober, 1983; Glendinning & Millar, 1987; Scott, 1984). In the United States, the richest country in the world, almost two-thirds of impoverished adults are women. This overrepresentation of women among the poor must be explained by reference to the sexual division of labour in the wider society. Women are confined to a secondary status in the labour market, yet their work in the home is not financially rewarded. State welfare benefits mirror this low earning capacity, thus perpetuating a lifetime of economic dependence and poverty for many working-class women. In Britain, for instance, working women make up over two-thirds of the 8 million people whose wages are below the poverty line. Similarly, some two-thirds of all elderly people live in poverty and six million of this nine million are women. Female-headed families, too, represent a significant group in poverty. Thus, many women in rich as well as poor countries suffer the ill-effects of poverty.

The ill health women experience as a result of deprivation is often compounded by the allocation of resources within the family. Research has shown that even in households where the aggregate income is above the poverty line, women may not have enough to meet their own needs. This is because the division of income and wealth between individuals is often unequal (Glendinning & Millar, 1987; Land, 1983; Pahl, 1980). Women tend to get (or take) less both because of their economic dependence and lack of power, but also because of their concern for other family members. Thus, women are more likely than men to be poor when living alone, they may be poor members in nonpoor households, or they may be the poorest in a poor household. In all cases, their health will be at risk.

Bread for the Breadwinner?

We can illustrate these inequalities in the allocation of household resources by looking at gender differences in nutrition. Although women are usually responsible for the purchase and preparation of food and often its production too, many do not have the power to determine distribution between family members, and their own health may suffer as a consequence. Adequate nutrition is a basic human need which cannot always be met for the entire household in conditions of poverty. Research in many countries around the world has shown that when the family income is too low, it is women who are especially prone to nutritional deficiency. Under these circumstances, food is often the only item of expenditure that can be manipulated to make ends meet and it is usually women who go short to ensure that the needs of the children and the breadwinner are met (Oren, 1974).

Yet women themselves have particular nutritional needs, which often go unrecognized or ignored. Menstruation, pregnancy, and lactation all increase women's need for protein and iron. This is difficult to measure precisely, but it has been estimated that pregnant women need 350 extra Calories per day, while those feeding their babies need another 550 Calories, as well as three times the normal intake of calcium and double the amount of vitamin A (Protein-Calorie Advisory Group, 1977). Research in both the developed countries and the Third World has shown that many women do not get enough of the right food to meet these needs.

A study carried out by the London-based Maternity Alliance in 1984 showed that despite the existence of the British welfare state some women are still not able to feed themselves adequately during pregnancy. The average cost of the diet recommended for pregnant women by the Department of Health in 1988 was £15.88. This represented nearly half the weekly benefit payable to a single person and a third of that for a couple (Durward, 1988). As a result, the many pregnant women on supplementary benefit could not afford to eat what was officially defined as necessary to sustain their own health and that of their unborn children.

In the Third World, the nutritional problems of poor women are, of course, much greater. The combination of lack of food and, in some countries, severe discrimination against women, results in serious undernutrition for many mothers and daughters (World Health Organization, 1986). According to the Protein-Calorie Advisory Group of the United Nations (PAG), there are definite indications of maldistribution of food at the family level in many parts of Africa with women getting the least even in pregnancy (Protein-Calorie Advisory Group,

1977). In some cultures, it is common for boys to be breastfed considerably longer than girls and for girl children to be fed less well than boys, thus reducing their chances of surviving infancy. Adult men often sit down to eat before their women and children, who get what remains (Leghorn & Roodkowsky, 1977; Carloni, 1981; Maher, 1981). Thus, food which is itself in scarce supply is distributed according to the prestige of family members rather than their nutritional needs. As a result, many women become anemic, especially during pregnancy, due to a lack of basic nutrients. Estimates suggest that in the Third World as many as half of nonpregnant women and two-thirds of pregnant women are anemic due to iron deficiency and folate and vitamin B12 deficiency combined with parasitic infections (WHO, 1979).

The authors of a recent study in Bangladesh set out to determine whether or not the very poor health record of women in that country could be explained by inequalities in the allocation of food and medical care (Chen, Huq, & d'Souza, 1981). The results were startling. Fourteen and four-tenths percent of female children in the sample were found to be severely malnourished, compared with 5.1% of males. This appeared to be directly related to food intake because dietary surveys showed that per capita male food intake considerably exceeded that of females at all ages. Overall, males averaged 1,927 calories per capita compared with 1,599 calories for females. The male excess was as high as 29% during the childbearing years of 15 to 44. These differences remained even when the data were adjusted for body weight, pregnancy, lactation, and activity levels, indicating that they must be seen as a relevant factor in explaining women's excess mortality.

In concluding, the authors of the study make the important point that these gender inequalities in life and death should not be seen as merely the response to scarcity. Indeed, they were found in rich as well as poor families, reflecting the fundamental inferiority of women's position in a profoundly patriarchal society. Of course, the reasons for male preference are a complicated mixture of the material as well as the ideological— girls cannot earn as much to help the family budget, have to be given a dowry, and are not able to support their parents during old age. But all too often the end result is serious damage to the health of girls, with many of those who survive to adulthood passing on their debility to future generations.

Older Women: The Invisible Majority

So far we have talked mainly about the impact of domestic tasks on the health of women in their childbearing years. However, in the developed countries, at least, it is older women who are most often confined to the home and who form the largest single group living in poverty. Even those who are not materially deprived frequently face serious health problems, yet these go largely unnoticed in societies that prioritize youth, vitality, and innovation. A combination of ageism and sexism means that older women are all too often marginalised sexually, socially, and economically in ways that threaten their well-being.

Older women are now the fastest growing group in poverty in the United States and Britain. In the United States, one-fifth of women aged 65 and over are below the poverty line, and women are twice as likely as men to experience poverty in old age. The single elderly are poorest of all and are predominantly female—three-fifths of women over 65 are alone compared with only a quarter of men. This reflects both the age difference of most couples at marriage and women's longer life expectancy. Older women from ethnic minorities suffer disproportionately from the effects of poverty. Forty-two percent of aged black women are in absolute poverty and a staggering 82% in near poverty, according to the 1980 U.S. Census. A similar situation prevails in Britain, with two-fifths of elderly women (38%) living on or below the poverty line, compared with 25% of men; two-thirds of all older British women are on the margins of poverty (Walker, 1987).

The poverty of older women stems directly from their lifelong economic dependency on men, the nature of their domestic responsibilities, and the existence of a dual labour market. Those women who do not engage in waged work are never able to earn state benefit in their own right. Hence, dependency in their early and middle years is carried over into old age. Even those who do work outside the home are often unable to build up a reasonable income for themselves in retirement. Many worked in low paid jobs without pension provision. Moreover, their working lives are usually disrupted by childrearing and sometimes caring for elderly parents, giving them little opportunity to build up a reasonable contributions record. Most, therefore, remain dependent on men, who usually die first, leaving them with only a minimal state pension to rely on. As a result, many experience health problems either caused or exacerbated by inadequate living conditions, insufficient heating, and lack of a nutritionally balanced diet.

Of course, not all the health problems older women face can be related directly to poverty. Many also suffer the psychological problems associated with retirement from work. Almost no research has been carried out on this topic because it has generally been assumed either that women do not work outside the home or that they are not deeply attached to their jobs (Fennell, Phillipson, & Evers, 1988). Thus, women appear only as shadowy wives in studies of men's retirement problems. Yet the few accounts we have from older women themselves suggest that the tensions are very similar for both sexes, and are likely to result in similar health problems (Ford & Sinclair, 1987). Most older women also have to cope with the denial of their sexuality at the same time as the physical and psychological distancing of their children.

Very few studies have investigated the health problems of older women, and routine medical statistics tell us little about their well-being. However, we know that in both the United Kingdom and the United States, elderly women are much more likely than men to be disabled. Twice as many British women in the over-65 age group are severely or very severely disabled compared with men of the same age, while the figure is five times greater in the 75-plus age group (Harris, Cox, & Smith, 1971). Women suffer three times as much arthritis as men and osteoporosis is also a significant cause of reduced female mobility. Mental health problems are even more difficult to identify and measure, but older women appear to continue the excess identified in younger age groups, with higher rates of depression and dementia than their male counterparts. Alan Walker comments on the basis of British data that older women are "more likely than men to suffer from psychological problems such as loneliness or anxiety and to have lower levels of morale and life satisfaction" (Walker, 1987).

Overall, women seem to suffer longer periods of chronic ill health than men, but their deaths are rarely caused by the same disease(s) that disabled them in life. Men, on the other hand, tend to have shorter periods of disability and to die from the problems that have bothered them while they are alive (Verbrugge, 1985). Interestingly many older women seem to play down their ill health, either because of low expectations—"You can't expect much at my age"—or shame at being unable to manage any more (Fennell et al., 1988, p. 109). However, others seem to welcome illness as liberating them from a lifetime of caring for others, especially when their dependents are no longer alive (Herzlich, 1973). In any case, too many remain behind closed doors, struggling to look after themselves with little material or emotional support.

The situation of older women in underdeveloped countries is obviously different in several ways. In the first place, relatively few survive to old age at all, and those who do are often severely debilitated by frequent childbearing and hard physical labour. Second, they are more likely than women in the developed countries to be supported and looked after within the extended family. Indeed in many societies older women occupy important social roles—grandmother, mother, or mother in law,

performer of religious or magical rites, senior wife—which offer more status than those of younger men. Those societies where women are required to be attached to a male adult usually have mechanisms to ensure that widows are not left alone. In India, for instance, remarriage is not encouraged among high-caste Hindu women and a son will be expected to support his mother while in some African societies, a widow is inherited by her husband's brother. Thus, older women in many parts of the Third World are less likely to suffer the isolation and invisibility of those in the developed countries, and in some cultures their status is even enhanced.

However, this is by no means always the case. Childless widows in particular often find themselves without social or financial security. Moreover, there is growing evidence that in many countries the breakdown of the traditional family-support system with industrialization and urbanization is increasing the vulnerability of divorced and widowed women (Youssef & Hetler, 1983). In parts of India, the expectation that a widowed daughter-in-law will be absorbed into her husband's family is no longer always adhered to. Instead, widows often return to their own families or set up (often very poor) households. Similar findings of lack of support for widows have been reported from Africa, from Upper Volta, Morocco, Zambia, and Swaziland (Youssef & Hetler, 1983). Thus, the problems of older women in the industrialized countries are increasingly being felt by those in the Third World as modernization removes their traditional sources of emotional and material sustenance, and therefore their access to reasonable health.

The Home as Haven?

Despite the dangers discussed above, it is a common myth that the home is a haven, offering protection from the dangers of the world outside. Indeed, many women are afraid to go out at night, staying behind closed doors to ensure their safety. The reality, however, is very different, as I explore in this final section.

It is clear that both the fear and the reality of domestic violence constitute a major threat to women's health. The use of physical force in the home is relatively common and most of it is inflicted on women by men (Dobash & Dobash, 1980). Precise estimates are difficult to achieve because so many victims are reluctant to reveal their private suffering. Indeed, the authors of a major British study suggest that only 2% of such assaults are reported to the police (Dobash & Dobash 1980). However, a number of studies designed to reveal the extent of this hidden violence have given broadly similar findings for the United States and Britain. A large-scale national study carried out by Murray Straus and his colleagues in the United States reported that over 12% of the married women interviewed had suffered severe violence at some point in their marriage, while a total of 28% had experienced physical violence of some kind (Straus et al., 1980). A British study involved interviews with all the women living in seven neighbouring streets in inner Leeds. About one-fifth of those interviewed had been the victims of violent attacks in their homes during the previous year (Hanmer & Saunders, 1984).

There is evidence of domestic violence in most countries around the world. In India, in particular, the uncovering of this abuse and its elimination has been a major focus of the new feminist movement (Mies, 1986). Urban and rural women, working class and middle class are all potential victims of domestic violence and Mies argues that their suffering has increased as the process of modernization gets under way. The most dramatic and widely publicized cases include the so-called dowry murders, in which women have been abused and eventually murdered because their husband and often his family are not satisfied with the money and goods she brought to the marriage. Many are deliberately burnt to death, but a cooking accident is blamed. Others commit suicide because the pressures on them are too great (Mies, 1986; Kishwar & Vanita, 1984).

Thus, the evidence demonstrates that a significant proportion of the women who live with men have the quality of their lives diminished by domestic violence. Moreover, this experience is shared by those in different social groups and societies, uniting women across class and racial divides. All women are potentially at risk from male violence, but paradoxically it is wives or cohabitees who get the worst treatment. Moreover, it is often their domestic work that provides the immediate excuse for a battering—a meal not ready on the table, a shirt not ironed, the house not clean enough, too much money spent on food, or a bout of "nagging." The physical damage caused is often severe, necessitating medical treatment or hospitalization. In the Dobashes' study of the survivors of violence, nearly 80% reported visiting the doctor at least once during their marriage for injuries inflicted by their husbands. Nearly 40% said they had sought medical care on five or more occasions and many felt their husbands had prevented them from getting medical help when they needed it. Another study of women in British refuges found that 73% had put up with violence for three or more years. Thirty percent had suffered life threatening attacks or had been hospitalized for serious injuries such as fractured bones (Binney, Harkell, & Nixon, 1981).

As well as the physical damage, it is clear that domestic violence is a major cause of psychological stress and trauma. Sixty-eight percent of the British women in refuges said that mental cruelty was one of the reasons they left home (Binney et al., 1981). Many victims are emotionally debilitated by anxiety about the next attack and feel shocked, upset, angry, and bitter at what is happening to them. Sadly, many feel guilty and blame themselves:

> I actually thought if I only learned to cook better or keep a cleaner house everything would be OK. . . . It took me five years to get over the shame and embarrassment of being beaten. I figured there had to be something wrong with me. (Dobash & Dobash, 1980, p. 119)

The authors of a recent study in North London found that women who had been battered were twice as likely to be depressed and had lower self-esteem than those who had not received such treatment (Andrews & Brown, 1988). Years of violence often leave women in a situation where alternatives are difficult to visualize. The socially constructed dependencies that they already experience are exacerbated by physical intimidation and violence. Moreover, attempts to get help from social workers, police, and other authorities too often lead to further humiliation and rejection (Stark, Flitcraft, & Frazier, 1979).

Thus, women become double victims of the batterer and the social agencies who too often assign the blame to women and resist any intervention in the private lives of man and wife. Indeed, one American writer has used the term *learned helplessness* to describe the condition in which so many battered women find themselves (Walker, 1979). Constrained by lack of confidence, isolation, fear, and lack of money, too many are forced to remain for lengthy periods in relationships that threaten their health and sometimes even their lives.

Conclusion

Thus, research findings accord with some women's own subjective experience in associating many of their health problems with their domestic responsibilities. Women's traditional duties are not always good for their health, given the circumstances of inequality and sometimes deprivation under which they often have to be carried out. Not surprisingly perhaps, there is growing evidence that despite their subordination in the labour market, women sometimes improve their health by working outside the home. I explore the implications of this in Part Two.

REFERENCES
A list of references is available in the original source.

"What Is a Theory of Women's Smoking? *and* How Do Societies Benefit?"

by Lorraine Greaves

The analysis expressed in the first part of this chapter forms a useful starting point from which to develop a more thorough explanation of women's smoking:

> Smoking may be an important means through which women control and adapt to both internal and external realities. It mediates between the world of emotions and outside circumstances. It is both a means of reacting to and/or acting upon social reality, and a significant route to self-definition.

This view reflects the words of the women in this book. A consciousness and self-analysis is revealed by the women smokers, showing awareness of the discrepancies between emotional states and cultural and social expectations. Smoking mediates between these two fields. Women smokers use cigarettes to assist with their taking responsibility for social relationships and the maintenance of emotional equilibrium in their social groups.

Each cigarette serves as a temporary answer to these women's search for meaning. But as each one is stubbed out, the limitations of the answer it provided likely becomes clear. Not only do unpleasant aspects of life reenter consciousness, but the guilt. contradiction and tension associated with smoking also re-emerge.

Smoking a pack of cigarettes per day may offer repeated "meditations." It protects against full engagement with reality, allowing those realities to continue unabated. This is how smoking benefits the social order surrounding women. Not simply a lucrative and desirable aspect of commerce, fashion or femininity, smoking is also a way of perpetuating unsatisfying and unequal social relations.

The question remains whether women's smoking is a passive or active response to the world. Women can be either "passive victims" of or "active resisters" to patriarchal domination or possibly both, depending on their cultural or subcultural milieu. In some instances, women are victims and are limited to reacting. Other times, we have the energy and opportunity to be proactive in defining the self and negotiating social life. Depending on time, place and personal circumstance, women can use smoking to absorb inequality or resist it.

It is facile to assume that all women are victims. Seen this way, women smokers would be understood to be either completely duped by the culture or driven to smoke as a direct result of their treatment in the world. Neither of these is true. But it is equally facile to assume that a clear sense of self can be forged in a world that largely excludes the female experience in defining female identity. Smoking seems to assist in the assertion of the self in such circumstances.

Women across the social spectrum experience the failure of the ideal, but specific experiences such as abuse help expose the range of ways in which smoking can serve women. These interviews suggest that cigarettes are shock absorbers for abused women; smoking mediates between reality and ideal and eases the rawness of women's pain and life. Not surprisingly, suppressing negative emotions and using cigarettes as comfort were both more common in the testimony of abused women smokers. Many abused women know that directly expressing emotions could be perceived as aggressive and, as such, could potentially further endanger them.

The feminist smokers interviewed consciously analyze their reality. Their conflict centres on the discrepancy between their experience (as feminists and smokers) and their own and others' definitions of feminists and smokers. Is smoking liberating or did they just buy the advertising line? Is their continuing to smoke evidence of disempowerment? Is there a way to analyze this that fits with a feminist critique of the world? Tensions surround the personal and the political are the source of self-punishment and guilt. The politics of empowerment clash with the fact that these women are being controlled to varying degrees by their need to smoke. But throughout, smoking is useful in negotiating life circumstances.

How *Do* Societies Benefit?

In industrial countries when women use smoking to mediate existence, whether taking the edge off their emotional reactions, giving themselves space and time away from pressures or even staying thin and looking sophisticated, there is often a tangible benefit to others in their society.

Culturally and economically, women's smoking is approved of (in some cultures) in advertising, movies and fashion and as a weight control method. Women's image, size and superficial beauty is treated as a commodity. Generally, when a fashion magazine shows a thin model with a cigarette or a film shows an independent woman defiantly smoking, smoking is seen as positive in the industrial world. Several industries, includ-ing the tobacco industry, will benefit directly. Naomi Wolf describes the Western patriarchal definitions of women's beauty and the lucrative industries and practices that support these definitions. She argues that women who smoke to control their weight are actually reflecting the logic of the (North American) culture where women's external body image is valued far more than their internal health. She says women should not be blamed for making the decision to smoke as there is no real social or economic reward for choosing otherwise, nor is there any particular reward for women who live longer (1990, 229–30).

When smoking reduces or erases women's demands, emotions or challenges, women can be seen as compliant and less troublesome. The true scope of women's feelings, particularly anger, remains invisible. Women smokers describe "sucking back anger" with each drag on a cigarette. If women smokers continue to internalize the tensions of interpersonal and social relations, the responsibility of others in their lives to deal with legitimate emotions is lifted.

Some women describe quit attempts that appear to be sabotaged by partners or family members. Sometimes cigarettes will be presented to a woman struggling to quit simply because she is being too irritable or difficult. In fact, this pattern indicates the strength and impact of emotions concealed by smoking.

When women depend on cigarettes instead of a partner or friend in cultures which approve of women's smoking, the pressure and collective responsibility to offer comfort and care is often relieved. The intensity of feelings toward cigarettes as friends and the grief connected to giving them up is a key indicator of some women's security needs that go unfulfilled by others.

Both individual and collective responsibility for providing comfort and consistency to women may be abrogated. Recognizing and countering this situation is critical to effective and ethical cessation programming for women. If women are being asked to give up smoking, what can be offered to replace it?

Women smokers are using a socially acceptable (among some cultures) form of self-medication. Unlike alcohol and most other drugs, tobacco does not render a woman incapable of carrying out her more traditional nurturing and caretaking social roles. In fact, as we have seen, it often helps women carry out numerous social roles that are unequal and unsatisfying.

The women in this study generally have few legitimate avenues for expression of negative emotion and angst. While smoking is profoundly self-destructive for a woman, it does not undermine the patriarchal family. Indeed, as long as it does not interfere with child bearing, childrearing and the maintenance of heterosexuality, women's smoking can be regarded as useful by advocates of the status quo to both the woman and her society.

On the other hand, women who get drunk or stoned are unable to care for children or continue working. This is one explanation why women's use of alcohol and drugs is much less acceptable from a Western societal point of view, despite the fact that alcohol consumption and drug use cause much less death and disease than does smoking. Several of the women interviewed, especially the First Nations women, were particularly clear about this. Smoking is most similar to the use of legal drugs—the traditionally overprescribed tranquilizers and sedatives—which have also been used in the service of pacifying women. In this sense, tobacco is a preferred drug, a socially acceptable form of medication.

There are rare exceptions to this. Pregnant women who smoke are the subject of a great deal of attention regarding women and smoking. Indeed, for many years in industrial countries the only form of attention paid to women smokers focused on smoking in pregnancy. Even now, there is an overemphasis on pregnant smokers. Not discounting the serious health problems created by smoking during pregnancy, the best intervention would be respectfully focused on women, not the fetus, long before and long after pregnancy.

A related, more recent concern among anti-smoking activists is the effect of women's smoking on children they are looking after. The issue of children being exposed to smoke, while very important, arouses passions in anti-smoking activists far in excess of the concern invested in women's health. In many instances involving children, societal reaction and attention from the international tobacco control movement has been, and continues to be, swift, sexist and woman-blaming (see Jacobson 1986, 124–26). There is a widespread and strong motivation to intervene in these circumstances.

How can we specify the benefits of women's smoking to a society? The cultural meaning of women's smoking changes rapidly over time and from place to place. These shifts often affect the development of women's identity and pressure it to fit with new prevailing values and political realities. Over time, this has led to many social meanings being applied to women's smoking. Cultural meanings have demarcated occupations and class groups and evoked images, qualities and aspirations. In contemporary industrialized societies, smoking serves as a socially useful and legal method of self-medication for some women. In Third World countries, or countries where women's smoking rates are low it may still be a

mark of resistance, the emblem of the "bad girl." In either case, smoking is a form of social control.

What would industrial societies do if women did not suppress emotions through smoking? What would happen if women refused to overwork instead of coping through smoking? What would happen if women took control and stopped adapting? Even anti-tobacco activists in the West fail to consider these questions! Could it be that women's health is so undervalued that the benefits to industrial societies of women's smoking will likely be perpetuated and the negative effects of smoking on women will not arouse a great deal of effective concern?

REFERENCES
A list of references is available in the original source.

Veiled Intentions
"Don't Judge a Muslim Girl by Her Covering"

by Maysan Haydar

O Prophet! Tell thy wives and daughters and the believing women that they should cast their outer garments over their persons. That is most convenient that they should be known and not be molested.

—The Quran, Chapter 33, Verse 59

And say to the believing women that they should lower their gaze and guard their modesty: that they should not display their beauty and ornaments except what ordinarily appears thereof; that they should draw their veils over their bosoms and not display their beauty . . .

—The Quran, Chapter 24, Verse 30–31

I have a confession to make.

I've been covering my hair, as is prescribed for Muslim women, since I was twelve years old. And while there are many good reasons for doing so, I wasn't motivated by a desire to be different, to honor tradition or to make a political statement.

I wanted the board game Girl Talk.

When girls from our small, Midwestern Muslim community donned their first *hijab* (headscarf), their families rewarded them with parties and monetary gifts. At

twelve, I wasn't nearly as physically developed as a Muslim girl is supposed to be when she starts covering, but I desperately wanted Girl Talk. I knew that if I announced my intention to begin veiling in the board game aisle at Kmart, I could ask for anything and receive it.

My choice of Girl Talk as reward for taking on a religious responsibility is amusing to me now, because it's so antithetical to what veiling is supposed to represent. Girl Talk was the ultimate slumber party game, where players performed gags or revealed embarrassing secrets, then got to choose from four kinds of fortune cards as a prize. My favorite cards hooked me up with the class president, the football captain or a hunky lifeguard who saved me from drowning. And I still have a sheet of "zit stickers," which were meant to punish gamers who failed to share their dirt.

Now that I'm twenty-five and have worn a veil for more than half my life, I can admit to this shallow beginning, which is so far from my reason for veiling today. As an adult, I embrace the veil's modesty, which allows me to be seen as a whole person instead of a twenty-piece chicken dinner. In spite of the seeming contradictions of my life—I'm married to a white man who was raised Catholic, I love heavy metal, I consider myself a feminist, and I sport a few well-disguised piercings—I follow my religion's standard of modesty and appearance. It's only now, after comparing my turbulent teen experiences with those of other women, that I can fully appreciate how much of a saving grace this small piece of cloth was.

Much to my chagrin, many Americans see veiling as an oppressive tool forced on Muslim women by the men in our culture. Yet, the practice of covering hair and body is a choice for many women—and it is not specific to Islam. All the monotheistic religions (Christianity, Judaism and Islam) advocate modesty in dress, though the interpretation of "modesty" varies greatly. Ironically, the population that spends millions on beauty products, plastic surgery and self-help guides is the same one that takes pity on me for being so "helpless" and "oppressed." On a New York City bus a couple weeks ago, I sat with another woman, also veiled, but wearing a traditional *jilbab* (a cloak that women wear over their clothing). A girl two seats over remarked to her friend, while flipping her hair for effect, that she couldn't understand how we could dress this way. "Me, I got to be *free*."

To my eyes, her idea of freedom involved a complicated hairstyle, loads of makeup and jeans she probably had to sew herself into. If anything, I would find that ensemble more caging, more oppressive and more painful than clothes that allow me to walk in front of construction sites confidently, with minimal risk of harassment. (Construction workers may feel obligated to say something to every passing woman, but I often get things like "I like your skirt!" or "Girl, I would marry you!"—harmless compared to the degradation I've heard many women complain about.)

As for freedom, my parents have a healthy understanding of Islam, especially the Quranic verse "Let there be no compulsion in religion" (2:256). Having been raised in religiously different homes themselves (Mom: very liberal, European-minded, not so religious; Dad: religious, culturally structured gender roles and

expectations), they only practiced traditions that they understood, accepted and believed. Thus, my mother knew the best way to introduce veiling to me was to emphasize its feminist, forward-thinking reasons: Covering removes that first level of being judged, of being assessed based on my measurements, and it absolves me of the need or desire to be wanted solely for my looks. My choice of Girl Talk didn't showcase a deep understanding of that idea. But reflecting back, I see that wearing a scarf greatly influenced how people viewed me and my goals, before I could ever appreciate that it was having that effect.

In high school, my interactions with the opposite sex were different than the norm. If I hadn't yet been inclined to deal with boys in an unpressured, ungiggly, unmade-up way, the scarf shoved me in that direction. So, without being given handbooks or informative flyers about how they should curb their posturing and come-ons, guys sensed that they should treat me with respect.

I didn't watch boys and girls learn about each other from the sidelines. I have many rich friendships with men, and over the years a good number of them have made a go at becoming "more than friends." I didn't participate in dating games, but I was flattered by the attention, especially since I knew I was being liked for who I was beyond my body. What made me attractive was my ability to relate to everyone in a very natural way, without all the confusing sexual pressure. The weirdness that normally clouds boy-girl interactions was lifted, because most guys automatically assumed I wasn't available for dating. Of course, girls deserve to be treated with respect no matter what they wear. But since we live in a world of mixed messages, I got to bypass a lot of damaging experiences.

The veil bestowed other experiences upon me that I wouldn't quite classify as negative, but definitely educational. Like anyone else who's visibly different from the norm, I encountered ridiculous ideas about what a covered person should be, do and enjoy. If someone overheard me talking about my interests, which included karate and skateboarding, I grew to enjoy their disbelief and shock. I didn't pick my hobbies to prove that stereotypes are often false, but it was nice to make people reconsider their notions of a Muslim girl.

Moving to New York City right after college and living alone was the most affirming thing I've done to solidify my resolve and truly understand what veiling means. Here, for the first time, people believed that I was wearing a scarf because I wanted to, not because my family coerced me into it. On the other hand, New York exemplifies what's wrong with our image-obsessed society. I worked for a couple of magazines and saw the way women acted out to draw attention to themselves. It was especially apparent at my anything-goes dot-com job, where women showed up to work in backless halter tops and were fawned over by male coworkers.

And now, as I write this, I can watch women subjugate themselves on reality dating shows. On a show about aspiring models I heard a woman say that her greatest goal would be to appear in *Stuff* magazine. I can't imagine centering my life on something as fleeting and meaningless as being admired simply for my body.

You might assume that because Muslim women traditionally don't display our bodies, we don't hold them as important or feel connected to them—or that we don't value ourselves as sexual beings. Guess again. While our degree of modesty is high, the value Muslim women place on the bodies underneath our veils is higher. In Sunday school, girls are taught that our bodies are beautiful ("God is beautiful and loves beauty" is a *hadith*, or saying, of the prophet Muhammad) and that they're so valuable that they're only meant to be shared in an intimate relationship: husband and wife, mother and baby, among women and in clinical or safe spaces (for example, with your doctor, among family members). Historically, the most severe-looking coverings used to be limited to the richest women in Arab society; being swathed in so much cloth was regarded as a sign of status.

People who have written about being in the secluded quarters of Arab homes or at their parties often express surprise at the degree to which these cloaked women maintain themselves via fitness, style and decadent rituals. (Let's not even get started on the body hair-removal process in the Middle East.) I'm not one for creams and blushes, but I understand that there are women who enjoy the beauty process, and I see no harm in indulging it for the right reasons. Feminist author Geraldine Brooks, in her book *Nine Parts of Desire*, quotes women across the Middle East who extol the virtues of prettying up for their loved ones. To me, this demonstrates that Western priorities are out of line: American women spend hours getting ready for strangers to see them but don't give the same effort to those who see them in intimate settings.

As for the variation in Muslim women's dress, it demonstrates the wide-ranging interpretations of modesty. I often get asked what the most "right" version is: the Afghani *burqah*, the Iranian *chador*, the Pakistani *salwar kameez*, the Arab *jilbab* or a sweatshirt and jeans. The short answer is that the recommendations for modesty are to be interpreted and applied at the discretion of the woman picking her clothes.

All through high school, I wore a *jilbab* exclusively, because I didn't have to spend any effort worrying about what was in season or what I would be expected to wear to fit in. I now cover my hair, but generally wear jeans and a long-sleeved shirt. My once-strict interpretation of modesty has been adapted to my urban lifestyle. Is wearing an *abaya* (the head-to-toe gown that completely covers the wearer) and a face veil a good idea in New York City? Probably not, since the abaya would likely get stuck in a subway door or pick up the dust off any floor you glide across. But not wearing an *abaya* in Saudi Arabia would probably make getting around very difficult for a woman.

It's utopic and ridiculous to assert that looks don't matter and that by veiling I'm avoiding the messiness—particularly after September 11th. Now some people hold their breath a bit longer, assuming I'm a fundamentalist or wondering if I'm there to cause them harm. I sense people studying me on the trains, reading the cover of the book in my hand and trying to gauge if I'm one of "us" or one of "them." I grapple with the frustration that I can't reassure everyone individually that my goals have everything to do with social justice and nothing to do with holy war. But I have seen suspicions fade in the eyes of the pregnant woman to whom I've given my subway seat, or the Hasidic man whose elbow I've taken to help him up the stairs.

Though many of the stereotypes and incorrect assumptions people had while I was growing up still prevail (that Muslim equals backwards/oppressed/fundamentalist/terrorist), current events have pedestrians describing their secondhand "expertise" of Islam—the history of Wahhabi Islam, the export of Sayyid Qutb and the Muslim Brotherhood's ideas—or trying to argue that the Quranic requirements for modesty don't include veiling. It's much harder to explain why I cover to those who think they have a full understanding of the culture and the faith than those whose "knowledge" of the Middle East is limited to *Aladdin* and *hummus*.

I do appreciate the status Islam and the Middle East have in the news these days—the interest has generated new scholarship on Arabia's history and anthropology and on Islamic law, all of which I'm interested in and am relieved is being researched. This research includes a pool of female scholars reexamining Islamic texts with a feminist lens, and separating actual religious commands from their long-held, culturally laden interpretations, which often smack of patriarchy.

Forcing women to veil or unveil usually has the opposite effect. When I attended elementary school in Saudi Arabia and flew home to Michigan each summer, a parade of women swathed in black *abayas* would head to the airplane bathrooms once we were safely in the air and emerge wearing short, tight ensembles. Conversely, banning the veil in Syria and Turkey sparked a resurgence in its popularity.

The question of veiling comes up once someone finds out that I've married into a family that celebrates Christmas, with my full participation. "If you have a daughter, what will she wear?" they ask. I haven't yet cracked a pregnancy or parenting book, but I hope that my policy will be similar to the egalitarian way I was raised. If she wants to, she can; if she doesn't want to, then she won't.

It's far more important for her to respect herself, her body and her life.

At the heart of my veiling is personal freedom. I dress this way because it has made it easier to get through adolescent phases and New York City streets with no self-loathing, body hang-ups or sexual harassment. I wish more women emerged unscathed; no one should suffer for what they look like or what they wear.

"Male and Female Hormones Revisited"

by Mariamne H. Whatley

In 1985 a chapter I wrote, "Male and Female Hormones: Misinterpretations of Biology in School Health and Sex Education," in which I examined in detail problems with both content and language in health and sexuality texts, was published in *Women, Biology, and Public Policy* (edited by Virginia Sapiro, Sage Yearbooks in Public Policy Studies, vol 10). Since then there have been a lot of changes in health education, sexuality education, and general knowledge about women's health and biology. However, when I reread the chapter to see how out-of-date it was, I was interested to find that the main points I made then are still very relevant.

One of central examples I presented was of the common use of the terms "male hormones" and "female hormones" to refer to androgens and estrogens respectively. By using this terminology, educators imply that men and women have two very different sets of hormones, which naturally could be seen as affecting development, behavior, and abilities, and could serve as the basis for believing incorrectly that there are biologically-determined sex roles, rather than culturally and socially influenced gender roles. In fact, men and women share the same hormones, but they appear in varying amounts. The average man will have higher levels of androgens than the average woman and the average woman will have higher levels of estrogen than the average man. However, just by looking at hormone levels a scientist could not determine

with certainty whether an individual were male or female, because there is so much variation across individuals, across the lifespan, at different parts of the menstrual cycle for women, and even at different times of the day (Men's levels of androgens may vary more in a day than a woman's estrogen levels do over a month). There are a number of reasons, therefore, why it is scientifically inaccurate to refer to male hormones and female hormones:

1. Both males and females produce both androgens and estrogens.

2. The adrenal glands and the gonads (ovaries, testes) produce both hormones in both sexes.

3. Both males and females need both androgens and estrogens for normal development.

4. Both hormones increase in both males and females at puberty.

5. Androgens and estrogens are steroids which are very similar in structure and can be interconverted (changed from one to the other) in our bodies.

6. Knowing hormone levels alone is not enough to determine whether an individual is biologically male or female.

In spite of these facts, much sexuality and puberty education material still refers to estrogens and androgens

Printed by permission of the author, 1999.

as very distinctly female or male. For example, in discussing female puberty, only estrogen will be discussed as a factor in changes in development, leaving out the fact that androgens do play a role in the development of girls, as well as of boys, in such changes as muscle growth, hair distribution, acne, and libido (sex drive). If androgen is presented as only a *male* hormone, then muscle development in girls is seen as abnormal. Boys on the other hand also normally produce estrogen, which sometimes reaches high levels at puberty, causing changes that may be seen as "female," such as temporary breast enlargement (gynecomastia) or more fat distribution on the hips. A boy with gynecomastia will undoubtedly feel uncomfortable no matter how sensitively the topic is handled, but it certainly won't help if he and his peers have all learned that breast enlargement is caused by estrogen, the *female* hormone. On the other hand, if the message is that all boys and men produce estrogens but that the levels can fluctuate, especially during puberty, and cause temporary breast enlargement, that boy might at least have some assurance that he is "normal."

At the other end of the reproductive cycle, there are often discussions of hormones in relationship to aging. Information on menopause may present postmenopausal women as becoming more "male" as their estrogen decreases and androgen becomes proportionately higher. Such changes may have to do with loss of breast size and density, growth of facial hair, and redistribution of body fat, so there is less on hips and thighs and more in the abdomen. Because her whole life, a woman has been told that she has "female hormones," the menopause literature which presents menopause as a total lack of estrogen or an "estrogen deficiency disease" is giving the message that the factor that makes her female is gone. She is, therefore, not really female any longer. When Robert Wilson wrote the book *Feminine Forever,* which extolled the virtues of exogenous estrogen to counter the effects of menopause, much of his focus was on the loss of estrogen as causing a loss in femininity and sexuality. While there has been much criticism of his work and, in recent years, there has been a decrease in the negative descriptions of menopause, these views do still persist. Discussing the fact that estrogen does not disappear after menopause and that androgens are actually converted to estrogens in fat and muscle cells can help give women a clearer view of what the real hormonal changes are. Also recognizing that their whole lives, they have gone through changing balances of hormones

places menopause more in the context of ongoing biological processes rather than a new, completely different stage. Before puberty, girls and boys have very similar levels of hormones and the low estrogen in girls is certainly not considered an "estrogen deficiency disease" that needs to be treated with "estrogen replacement."

There are other implications of viewing estrogens and androgens as distinct hormones not shared by the sexes. If hormones are believed to have certain effects on behavior or abilities, then the association of a hormone with only one sex will imply biological limitations. For example, some scientists believe that androgen levels cause changes in aggression. There has been a long debate about this which includes such key opposing arguments as: the fact that behavior and environment can themselves alter hormone levels, so a high level of androgen may be a *result* of being in an aggressive position rather than a *cause* of it; the definition of aggression as very loose, ranging from rough and tumble play in primates to success in business and politics. If it were accepted that androgen levels cause aggression and aggression were loosely defined as meaning being able to compete in a highly competitive field, such as business or politics, then women would be seen as unable to compete in these areas. And, of course, women who are as aggressive (or assertive) as men may be seen as not really normal women. While we hope most people have discarded these outdated views, the basic misunderstanding of biology seeps into many discussions of women's abilities in general and in discussions of specific women. When someone refers to a woman as "ballsy," it may be seen as a compliment for her being a gutsy woman ready to take on challenges, but is also a backhanded compliment because it also implies she is not fully a woman, figuratively possessing testes—the major producer of androgens.

A discussion of changing the language which is used to describe hormones may seem trivial, as did attention to changing the generic male (e.g., mankind). However, a view of the world underlies choices we make in language and a change in language—however small—can cause a shift in perception. Just as we now refer to firefighters and police officers rather than firemen and policemen, to represent more accurately the status of women in the workforce, so must we also clean up our scientific language to reflect scientific reality, which is so often distorted and misrepresented.

"Coming to Terms with Transgenderism and Transsexuality"

by Julia Serano

Most non-trans people are unfamiliar with the words that we in the transgender community use to describe ourselves, our experiences, and our most pressing issues. Books and websites that discuss transgenderism and transsexuality often include some kind of glossary, where these terms are laid out and defined in a nice, orderly, alphabetical fashion. However, a potential problem with the glossary approach is that it gives the impression that all of these transgender-related words and phrases are somehow written in stone, indelibly passed down from generation to generation. This is most certainly not the case. Many of the terms used these days to describe transgender people did not exist a decade ago. Conversely, many of the terms that were commonly used a decade ago are now considered to be out of fashion, outdated, or even offensive to many people in the transgender community. Even the terms that are used frequently today are regularly disputed, as individual transgender people may define words in a slightly different manner or have aesthetic or political preferences for certain words over others. So in lieu of a glossary, I will use this chapter to define many of the transgender-specific terms used throughout the book and to explain why I chose these particular words and phrases rather than others.

It is difficult to talk about people who are trans*sexual* or trans*gender* without first defining the words "sex" and "gender." "Sex" commonly refers to whether a person is physically female and/or male. Because the physical traits that we most often take into account when describing "sex" are biological in origin (e.g., sex chromosomes, hormones, reproductive systems, genitals, and so forth), there is a tendency to see sex as being a "natural" aspect of gender. However, this is not quite the case. Cultural expectations and assumptions play a large role in shaping how we determine and consider sex. For example, in our culture, such assumptions are very genital-centric: A person's sex is assigned at birth based on the presence or absence of a penis. Thus, our genitals play a far more important role in determining our legal sex than do our chromosomes (which in most cases are never actually examined) or our reproductive capacity. After all, a woman can have a hysterectomy, or a man can have a vasectomy, without changing or nullifying their legal sex. Indeed, the fact that we even have a "legal" sex demonstrates that society greatly shapes our understanding of sex. Thus, throughout this book, I will use the word "sex" primarily to refer to a person's physical femaleness and/or maleness, but I will also sometimes use it to refer to the social and legal classes that are associated with one's physical sex.

The word "gender" is regularly used in a number of ways. Most commonly, it's used in a manner that's indistinguishable from "sex" (i.e., to describe whether a person is physically, socially, and legally male and/or female). Other people use the word "gender" to describe a person's gender identity (whether they identify as female, male, both, or neither), their gender expression and gender roles (whether they act feminine, masculine, both, or neither), or the privileges, assumptions, expectations, and restrictions they face due to the sex others perceive them to be. Because of the many meanings infused into it, I will use the word "gender" in a broad way to refer to various aspects of a person's physical or social sex, their sex-related behaviors, the sex-based class system they are situated within, or (in most cases) some combination thereof.

Now that we understand "sex" and "gender," we can begin to consider the word *transgender*, which is perhaps one of the most confusing and misunderstood words in the English language. While the word originally had a more narrow definition, since the 1990s it has been used primarily as an umbrella term to describe those who defy societal expectations and assumptions regarding femaleness and maleness; this includes people who are transsexual (those who live as members of the sex other than the one they were assigned at birth), intersex (those who are born with a reproductive or sexual anatomy that does not fit the typical definitions of female or male), and genderqueer (those who identity outside of the male/female binary), as well as those whose gender expression differs from their anatomical or perceived sex (including crossdressers, drag performers, masculine women, feminine men, and so on). I will also sometimes use the synonymous term *gender-variant* to describe all people who are considered by others to deviate from societal norms of femaleness and maleness.

The far-reaching inclusiveness of the word "transgender" was purposely designed to accommodate the many gender and sexual minorities who were excluded from the previous feminist and gay rights movements. At the same time, its broadness can be highly problematic in that it often blurs or erases the distinctiveness of its constituents. For example, while male crossdressers and transsexual men are both male-identified transgender people, these groups face a very different set of issues with regards to managing their gender difference. Similarly, drag queens and transsexual women generally have very different experiences and perspectives regarding gender, despite the fact that they are often confused with one another by mainstream society.

Thus, the best way to reconcile the nebulous nature of the word is to recognize that it is primarily a political term, one that brings together disparate classes of people to fight for the common goal of ending all discrimination based on sex/gender variance. While useful politically, *transgender* is too vague of a word to imply much commonality between individual people's identities, life experiences, or understanding of gender.

Another point that is often overlooked in discussions about transgenderism is that many individuals who fall under the transgender umbrella choose not to identify with the term. For example, many intersex people reject the term because their condition is about physical sex (not gender) and the primary issues they face (e.g., non-consensual "normalizing" medical procedures during infancy or childhood) differ greatly from those of the greater transgender community.[1] Similarly, many transsexuals disavow the term because of its anti-transsexual roots or because they feel that the transgender movement tends to privilege those identities, actions, and appearances that most visibly "transgress" gender norms.[2] This tendency renders invisible the fact that many of us struggle more with issues related to our physical femaleness or maleness than we do with our expressions of femininity or masculinity. Throughout this book, I will use the word *trans* to refer to people who (to varying degrees) struggle with a subconscious understanding or intuition that there is something "wrong" with the sex

they were assigned at birth and/or who feel that they should have been born as or wish they could be the other sex. (It should be noted that some people use the word "trans" differently, as a synonym or abbreviation for the word *transgender*). For many trans people, the fact that their appearances or behaviors may fall outside of societal gender norms is a very real issue, but one that is often seen as secondary to the cognitive dissonance that arises from the fact that their *subconscious sex* does not match their physical sex. This *gender dissonance* is usually experienced as a kind of emotional pain or sadness that grows more intense over time, sometimes reaching a point where it can become debilitating.

There are many different strategies that trans people may use to ease their gender dissonance. Perhaps the most common one is trying to suppress or deny one's subconscious sex. Others may allow their subconscious sex to come to the surface occasionally, for example through either crossdressing or role-playing. Still others may come to see themselves as *bigendered* (having a mixture of both femininity and masculinity and/or femaleness and maleness), *gender-fluid* (moving freely between genders), or *genderqueer* (identifying outside of the male/female gender binary). And those of us who make the choice to live as the sex other than the one we were assigned at birth are commonly called *transsexuals*.

Perhaps the most underacknowledged issue with regard to the transgender community—and one that is a continuing source of both confusion and contention—is the fact that many of the above strategies and identities that trans people gravitate toward in order to relieve their gender dissonance are also shared by people who do not experience any discomfort with regards to their subconscious and physical sex. For example, some male-bodied crossdressers spend much of their lives wishing they were actually female, while others see their crossdressing as simply a way to express a feminine side of their personalities. While many drag artists view themselves primarily as entertainers or enjoy performing and parodying gender stereotypes, some trans people gravitate toward drag because it provides them with a rare opportunity to express aspects of their subconscious sex in a socially sanctioned setting. And while many trans people identify as genderqueer because it helps them make sense of their own experiences of living in a world where their understanding of themselves differs so greatly from the way they are perceived by society, other people identify as genderqueer because, on a purely intellectual level, they question the validity of the binary gender system.

Thus, not only do transgender people vary in their perspectives and experiences, but individuals within the same transgender subcategory (whether it be crossdresser, drag artist, genderqueer, etc.) may also differ greatly in what drives them to embrace that identity. And while this book primarily focuses on transsexuality, and more specifically on trans women (as that is my experience and perspective), it is not because I believe that transgender people who are not transsexual are any less important or legitimate; their expressions of gender are just as valid as mine and the discrimination they may face as a result of those expressions is just as real. It is also crucial for us to recognize that it is equally valid for a trans person to decide to transition and live as the other sex as it is for them to instead choose to blur gender boundaries and identify themselves outside the gender binary. There is no one right way to be trans. Each of us simply needs to figure out what works best for us and what allows us to best express who we feel we are.

When discussing transsexuals, it is often necessary to distinguish between those who transition from male to female—who are commonly referred to as *trans women*—and those who transition from female to male—who are called *trans men*. I prefer these terms over others because they acknowledge the lived and self-identified gender of the trans person (i.e., woman or man), while adding the adjective "trans" as a way to describe one particular aspect of that person's life experience. In other words, "trans woman" and "trans man" function in a way similar to the phrases "Catholic woman" or "Asian man." Because many trans people choose to relieve their gender dissonance in ways other than transitioning, I will often use the phrases *male-to-female (MTF) spectrum* and *female-to-male (FTM) spectrum* to describe all trans people (regardless of whether they are genderqueer, transsexual, crossdresser, etc.) who experience their gender as being different from or more complex than the gender they were assigned at birth.

Sometimes people have a tendency to dismiss or delegitimize trans women's and trans men's gender identities and lived experiences by relegating us to our own unique categories that are separate from "woman" or "man." This strategy is often adopted by non-trans folks who wish to discuss trans people without ever bringing into question their own assumptions and beliefs about maleness and femaleness. An obvious example of this phenomenon is the prevalence of the terms "she-males," "he-shes," and "chicks with dicks" in reference to trans women. Sometimes attempts to *third-sex* or *third-gender* trans people are more subtle or subconscious than that, such as when people merge the phrase "trans woman" to make one word, "transwoman," or use the adjectives MTF and FTM as nouns (for example, "Julia Serano is an MTF."). I do not identify as a "male-to-female"—I identify as a woman. These attempts to relegate trans people to "third sex" categories not only disregard the profoundly felt gender identity of the transsexual in

question, but also ignore the very real experiences that trans person has had being treated as a member of the sex that they have transitioned to.

When discussing transsexuals' lives, it is important to find words that accurately describe their gendered experiences in both the past and present. Many trans people say they understood themselves to be female or male for most of their lives despite the fact that it wasn't the sex they were assigned at birth. Therefore, when a trans person transitions, their subconscious sex or gender identity essentially stays the same—rather, it is their physical sex that changes (hence the term trans*sexual*). With regards to the trans person's original sex, I will often use the somewhat clunky phrase *the sex (or gender) they were assigned at birth* to emphasize the nonconsensual nature of how we are raised, socialized, and treated by society on the basis of our physical sex. For convenience, I may also refer to it as their *assigned gender/sex* or (to a lesser extent) their *birth sex*. I may refer to the sex that the trans person has transitioned to as their *preferred sex*, their *identified sex* (to emphasize the fact that it agrees with their gender identity), or their *lived sex* (to emphasize the fact that they now live and experience the world as a member of that sex).

It is common for people to assume that being or becoming a transsexual involves some kind of "sex change operation." However, this is not necessarily the case. While some transsexuals undergo numerous medical procedures as part of their physical transitions, others either cannot afford or choose not to undergo such procedures. Indeed, attempts to limit the word "transsexual" to only those who physically transition is not only classist (because of the affordability issue), but objectifying, as it reduces all trans people to the medical procedures that have been carried out on their bodies. For these reasons, I will use the word *transsexual* to describe anyone who is currently, or is working toward, living as a member of the sex other than the one they were assigned at birth, regardless of what procedures they may have had. Further, because there are so many different paths that a transsexual person may take toward living in their identified sex, I will use the word *transition* to describe the process of changing one's lived sex, rather than in reference to any specific medical procedure.

The most common medical procedure for transsexuals to seek out is *hormone replacement therapy*, which involves taking testosterone in the case of trans men, or taking estrogen (and sometimes progesterone) in the case of trans women. These are the same sex hormones that kick in during puberty in all people and they produce many of the same bodily changes in adult transsexuals as they do in adolescents: Some effects are changes in skin complexion and muscle/fat distribution, breast growth in trans women, and deepened voices and facial hair growth in trans men. These hormone-produced body changes are often referred to as *secondary sex characteristics* (to distinguish them from so-called *primary sex characteristics* such as reproductive organs and genitals). Secondary sex characteristics are the cues that we most often use when we classify adults as being either women or men, which explains why hormone replacement therapy is often sufficient to allow trans people to live unnoticed in their identified sex.

While there are a number of possible surgeries that a trans person may undertake, the one that seems to most capture public imagination is *sex reassignment surgery (SRS)*, which involves reconstruction of the genitals to better match that of the transsexual's identified sex. Some trans people object to the term *SRS* and instead prefer alternatives such as *genital reassignment surgery*, *gender confirmation surgery*, or *bottom surgery* (to contrast it with *top surgery*: the removal or enhancement of breasts). Personally, I am not bothered by the technical name of the surgery so much as I am by the fact that it gets so much attention in the media and the general public. After all, as someone who is not a cardiologist nor has ever had a heart condition, I really don't feel any compelling need to know all of the technical names or hear play-by-play accounts of heart surgeries. Nor do I need to know all of the specific names and doses of chemotherapies in order to be touched by the story of someone who has survived cancer. For this reason, I am rather disturbed by the fact that so many people—who are neither medical professionals nor trans themselves—would want to hear all of the gory details regarding transsexual physical transformations, or would feel that they have any right to ask us about the state of our genitals. It is offensive that so many people feel that it is okay to publicly refer to transsexuals as being "pre-op" or "post-op" when it would so clearly be degrading and demeaning to regularly describe all boys and men as being either "circumcised" or "uncircumcised."

While the specific details of transsexual-related medical procedures should be readily available for those contemplating sex reassignment, such information is neither relevant nor necessary for one to understand the experiences and perspectives of trans people. After all, while my physical transition occurred primarily over a period of a year and a half—a mere fraction of my life—what has remained constant and pervasive (both pre-, during, and post-transition) has been the resistance and prejudice that I have faced from those who are not transgender, those who become irrationally uncomfortable or disturbed by my gender expression and/or female identity, and those who presume that their identified gender is more natural

or valid than my own. For this reason, I believe that one cannot begin to fully understand transsexuality without thoroughly examining and critiquing the prejudices and presumptions of the non-transsexual majority. So although I will be discussing transsexuals throughout this book, I will also be spending a great deal of time discussing the beliefs and attitudes common among cissexuals—that is, people who have only ever experienced their subconscious sex and physical sex as being aligned. Similarly, people who are not transgender may be described as being *cisgender* (although I will be using this term less often, since the focus of this book is on transsexual women rather than the transgender population as a whole). I prefer these terms, but I occasionally use the synonymous terms *non-transsexual* and *non-transgender*.

Some might feel that all of these trans- and gender-related terms I've introduced are overwhelming or confusing. And others, particularly those in the fields of gender and queer studies, might dismiss much of this language as contributing to a "reverse discourse"—that is, by describing myself as a transsexual and creating trans-specific terms to describe my experiences, I am simply reinforcing the same distinction between transsexuals and cissexuals that has marginalized me in the first place. My response to both of these arguments is the same: I do not believe that transsexuals and cissexuals are inherently different from one another. But the vastly different ways in which we are perceived and treated by others, and the way those differences impact our unique physical and social experiences, lead many transsexuals to see and understand gender very differently than our cissexual counterparts. And while transsexuals are extremely familiar with cissexual perspectives of gender (as they dominate in our culture), most cissexuals remain largely unfamiliar with trans perspectives. Using only words that cissexuals are familiar with in order to describe my gendered experiences would be similar to a musician only choosing words that nonmusicians understand when describing music. It can be done, but something crucial would surely be lost in the translation. Just as musicians cannot fully explain their reaction to a particular song without bringing up concepts such as "minor key" or "time signature," there are certain trans-specific words and ideas that will appear throughout this book that are crucial for me to use in order to precisely convey my thoughts and experiences regarding gender. To have an illuminating and nuanced discussion about my experiences and perspectives as a trans woman, we must begin to think in terms of words and ideas that accurately describe that experience.

REFERENCES
A list of references is available in the original source.

"Body"

by Cris Beam

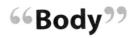

When I started meeting regularly with Christina and therefore talking about her to non-transsexual friends, they would often ask, "So has she had the surgery?" This is a very personal question and not my place to answer—as I don't make it my business to talk about anyone's genitalia without permission. Still, it's an understandable question. Everything in our culture pushes us to be "completely" male or female. It's in the language: a transsexual is either "pre-op" or "post-op"—the "operative" being presumed and non-negotiable. But contrary to mainstream imagination, there isn't one way to be a transsexual—there isn't a fixed trail of body modifications you undergo, leading to the genital surgery. Rather, there's a range of physical alterations you can make, depending on your financial situation, how permanent or temporary you want the change to be, your patience with a lengthy process, your tolerance for risk, and what you want to look like in the end.

For a few months, I ran a weekly transgender youth group for transgender girls at the Jeff Griffith Center, on Santa Monica Boulevard. At these meetings were the regular suspects—Foxx, Ariel, and Christina—but there were also Lu, Miguel, and Joelle, and occasionally other stragglers. They talked a lot about their bodies and what they wanted to do with them, and their visions and plans were varied.

"I want to have implants, I want to be hormoned out, I want to be extremely beautiful, and I want my own hair to grow," said Joelle, a seventeen-year-old girl in an olive skirt and a floppy fisherman's hat on her head who perpetually whined like an exasperated mother. "And I want to wake up in the morning and be thankful and not all horrible and sad."

Lu, the girl with the Xena obsession, only wanted to gain weight and wasn't thinking about hormones or implants or any other surgery: she felt her lack of hips was what got her clocked. "I'm tired of shopping in the children's department," Lu said. "I mean, I know it's cheaper, but it's embarrassing."

Ariel also wasn't interested in any body modification beyond shaving her head so it would be smooth under a wig. Ariel's wigs are her most prized possessions. She keeps them on stands and combs and styles them regularly; when she puts on her hair, she feels most at home in herself. I once went wig shopping with Ariel in Compton; she was looking for an auburn bob that was angled close to the chin, but she spent four hours in the shop trying on almost every style, gazing at herself in the mirror and making small, nearly inaudible cooing and clucking sounds at herself like a bird.

In the group, Ariel told the story of getting her hair snatched twice—by other transgirls. When girls are envious or mad, the first thing they go after in a fight is another girl's hair.

"Our hair is where we keep our power," Foxx said. Foxx's fashion at the time was all about dime-sized confetti glitter, glued to her eyelids and cheeks. She paired this with a baseball cap, which she was wearing to practice traveling undercover, because that's what she figured she would have to do when she became famous. Foxx was growing out her hair and weaving in extensions.

Ironically, while the girls can choose to do a lot or a little to their bodies, they're all expected to look a certain way—at least by one another, at least in Hollywood. "We might say, 'Miss Thing's a brick—she's bricking it up,'" Foxx said, and all the kids went "*mmmhmmm*" in agreement. "Brick" means a man in a dress, and on the street the girls will clock one another, calling out the ones who don't look feminine enough, especially if she's perceived as a nuisance or a bitch. "We're too shady toward each other."

Ariel leaned in. "Yeah. Sometimes your friends won't want to walk down the street with you because they think you look like a man."

In part to combat this, Foxx and Joelle were taking hormones, and Christina was considering them. Lu just wanted weight. Joelle would have surgeries; Foxx wasn't sure. That left Miguel.

Miguel was someone I had never met before, and he identified as a "plainclothes transgender." He looked undeniably male in a nondescript pair of jeans and an oversize T-shirt, but his eyes were soulful and soft. Plainclothes transgenders, Miguel explained, don't change the exteriors of their bodies at all; they move about in the world as their birth sex, demanding only that their lovers and most intimate friends use the opposite-gender pronouns.

Miguel had grown up a parentless "glue sniffer" in the roving child gangs of Tijuana, but crossed the border when he was sixteen. After landing in an American group home, Miguel recognized a long-sleeping need to become Alison. He folded his broad shoulders into modest, knee-length dresses and bought cheap wigs that he clasped into buns at his neck. "I looked like a librarian," Miguel told me. It was the look of a virginal Mexican Catholic girl, which earned him taunts on the slicker streets of Los Angeles. Miguel couldn't stand the teasing, so he went back to living as a boy but believed—and told anyone he got close to—that he was really a woman.

"That's not what it's all about, transgender," Miguel said, clearly translating his sentences from the Spanish in his head. "It's not about how you look. Being fierce is about being happy with yourself."

I would say Miguel is a rarity; for most people, being happy includes being recognized for who you feel you are. And that means altering your physical appearance to align with your inner self.

Christina's best friend, Domineque, wanted estrogen the first time she heard about it. She "caught T" about black-market hormones from her drag mother Juliana and from Shavonne—my student who choreographed the weight room dance from juvenile hall. Juliana and Shavonne were together when they started on street hormones, when they were fifteen.

"I asked Shavonne what hormones do, and she said basically it softens your skin, it doesn't prevent but it slows the growth of facial hair, and it makes you grow breasts," Domineque told me. At the time she decided to go for it, she was sixteen and Juliana and Shavonne were walking Domineque down Santa Monica Boulevard pointing out the girls who were, and were not, on hormones. "When she said it makes you grow breasts, I was like, 'Okay! I want to!'"

Unlike surgeries, which target a single spot, hormones are systemic and can change your overall appearance, and even mood and sensibility. When Juliana and Shavonne got their hormones, they believed the medicines were a race against puberty, and in a way they are: if you can start a regular estrogen protocol before, say, the onset of full facial hair, you can halt its growth—though a beard will sputter forth again if you stop the pills. But once the beard is there, it will never disappear without electrolysis, though it will thin out on hormones. If your voice has already dropped into the male register, there's also no going back (except by surgically tightening the vocal cords, and that often tweaks voices into

a Mickey Mouse falsetto). Estrogen, or a combination of estrogen and progesterone administered through pills or shots, will make existing facial and leg hair thinner and wispier, promote breast growth, and redistribute body fat in a more feminine manner—away from the belly and onto the hips, butt, and thighs. On hormones, transgirls become softer and rounder and, depending on how much they're taking, moodier. For some girls, libido drops considerably, and they often can't get erections when they're taking high doses—which means they can't have orgasms. This complicates an already-complicated relationship to sex: many girls are ashamed of what they consider their unfeminine genitalia, and losing interest in sex psychologically distances them even further from that part of their body. All of these effects, save for the extra breast tissue that will forever flap down in a thin fold, are completely reversible if the hormones are discontinued.

And some do go back. For instance, Juliana, who decided to return home to her estranged and religious mother in Texas and live as a boy again. The kids who kept in touch with her last heard she had graduated from high school and was still living as a boy, so it's a good thing her robust testosterone system had only been temporarily repressed.

Still, Juliana is the exception. Most of the kids I met have known for so long that their biological gender didn't match their internal knowledge of self that they stay the course. Many save their money to buy their estrogen from a swap meet in East Hollywood, where a long-standing black market does a brisk underground business in liquid hormones and syringes smuggled up from Tijuana.

The swap meets in L.A. are giant warehouse—type affairs, where vendors rent space and set up tables or racks or crates of goods. Some are fancy, with mannequins and pop-up changing rooms, and some are little more than tarps on the ground with piles of Beefy-T's or knockoff Nikes in plastic wrap. Sometimes the hormones are sold out of a swap meet stall that sells "botanica" and Santeria supplies—candles and soaps that bring about love or cast off curses—and sometimes one that sells CDs, racks of Shakira and Paula Rubio glistening behind their shrink wrap. The locales shift temporarily if someone hears that a cop has been tipped off, but that doesn't happen very often. Still, the sales exchange stays the same. It goes like this: A transgender girl walks up to the stall and, instead of looking at music, she just stands there. A salesperson asks if she can help her. The girl responds, vaguely, with something like, "Um, I was hoping someone could sell me something." As with narcotics, if nobody says the word, nobody gets busted. The vendor usually goes to get another person who handles the medicines, and the transaction will continue like this:

Salesperson: "Are you?"

Customer: "Uh-huh . . ."

Salesperson: "But you don't even look—!" (Flattery makes a buck in every business.)

Customer: "Thank you."

Salesperson: "Forty-five."

Customer: "That's so much! For Gravidinona?" Here, the customer is the first to say the drug name. Gravidinona is a regulated combination of progesterone and estradiol, marketed to menopausal women, generally in a single dose with its own syringe. It can be more expensive than estrogen by itself. The salesperson shrugs; she doesn't have to bargain with these drugs, and she wants to be quick.

Customer: "Prema?" Premarin—or plain estrogen.

Salesperson: "Twenty. Two dollars for the syringe."

At this, money and a small brown bag are exchanged, and the customer walks away. The whole thing takes less than two minutes, and the salesperson is back to hawking Shakira.

The rate of breast growth depends on how much testosterone the estrogen has to knock out, and every body naturally starts with different amounts. In general, a girl will feel a tingling or sensitivity in the nipples within a couple of weeks; in a month or two, the nipple will swell to a bulgy, raised marble with skin that prickles and aches against every brush of fabric. After three or four months, there may be a slight curve to the breast, a little tissue growing beneath the skin, and after that, the breasts continue to develop to their genetic destiny; a teenager on hormones will often end up with a cup size roughly the same as her mother's. Essentially, transgirls on hormones have to go through a second puberty, with all the emotions and pimples and weird breast shapes that genetic girls endure.

As with genetic girls, the whole messy prospect of puberty generally takes about two years to complete. Even though kids like Domineque or Juliana can rush things by shooting copious amounts of street hormones, their bodies still won't settle into a final shape until they've been at it for a few years. By this time, their hips and buttocks will have filled out, and their cheeks and chins will be less angled and bearded. Their skin everywhere will be plumper and softer, and, some say, the hair on their head will be more lustrous too, though this may come from increased investments in hair products. But the real payoff is the breasts; this is often the main drive behind the cost and the emotional instability and the inconvenience of hormones. It certainly was for Domineque.

It only took Domineque a few months to get breasts, but this is unusual. Her social worker, Andrea Biffle, said Domineque was growing breasts on her own even before the drugs, though this may have been due to the way she wore her clothes or held her shoulders. Domineque is just naturally fleshy, and her body seems to want to ripen somehow into roundness. At the time she bought her first shot, Domineque was living with her brother Tadeo and a foster dad named Johnny. The situation was decent; Domineque claimed Johnny was gay and was understanding about Domineque's boyfriend. He also was willing to foster siblings, which is not always available to DCFS wards, especially to teenagers. Domineque was getting to the age where she was likely to be put in group homes; private families are often saved for younger children. Plus, Johnny was kind enough, and he promoted homework and chores and other basic values that made Domineque and Tad feel homey and loved. Domineque was only dressing as a girl with her drag mother Juliana and with Shavonne; she hadn't yet shown that self to Johnny. She decided to talk to him about the hormones.

Domineque said Johnny panicked. He wasn't comfortable with transsexuality, and if Domineque—then Javier—were to become a girl, she would have to leave. He would keep Tad. According to Andrea, the issue was more complicated: Domineque was a troubled teenager and was acting out in other ways (like running away), and Johnny was upset by the misbehavior overall. In any case, Domineque certainly didn't want to leave Tad, the one steady element in her flail-about life and the brother she believed she protected. Still, the hormone idea was worming deeper into her brain. She decided to buy the hormones and hide them from Johnny.

It took Domineque five months from the day of her purchase to inject the estrogen-progesterone mix, though she wanted to so badly, her body ached. Then, the first time she tried, it was a disaster.

"I didn't know how to open the vial; I didn't know you're supposed to flick the top until it pops off, so I hit it against the wall and it cracked open," Domineque said, indicating with her hands that it spilled everywhere. She filled the needle as best she could with the small liquid puddle on the floor. The best place to inject is the buttocks because you want to shoot into muscle rather than veins, so Domineque dropped her pants. "I tried to get the needle in, but it wouldn't go in and I got scared, so I pulled it out and I was like, 'I can't do this,' and I threw the needle away. Finally I just asked Shavonne for some of her pills."

Hormones in tablet form are also sold on the street, and prescribed by doctors in special clinics or in private practice. Because transgender culture is unfortunately invisible to much of the larger medical world, many doctors are not specifically trained in gender care at all. Instead, they learn about it on the fly, usually when a patient of theirs complains of conflicting gender feelings or specifically requests hormones or surgical treatment. When this happens, the doctor will discover that there are no codified rules or laws governing how to treat transsexual patients, but rather a list of suggested guidelines, known collectively as the Harry Benjamin "Standards of Care," or SOC.

Harry Benjamin, the man, was born in 1885 and is credited with bringing much of the German knowledge of transsexuality and its accompanying treatments and surgeries to the United States. Before the Nazis shut it down, the bulk of radical sex and gender research in the world was happening in Germany at an institute called the Institute for Sexual Science, launched by the sexologist Magnus Hirschfeld in 1919. At the institute Hirschfeld studied sexual biology, pathology, sociology, and ethnology, and he also oversaw some of the first experimental sex reassignment surgeries. In 1933 the Nazis burned the institute's library, including 20,000 books, 35,000 photographs, and 40,000 confessions and biographical letters. Benjamin, who had been forced to relocate to New York in 1915 but returned many times to Berlin, studied with Hirschfeld. He went on to write the landmark book on transsexuality, *The Transsexual Phenomenon*, in 1966.

The Harry Benjamin International Gender Dysphoria Association was started in 1979 as a renamed assemblage of another group that was launched a decade earlier, which held talks and conferences on surgeries and therapies or treatments for transsexuals, attended by medical professionals. Harry Benjamin, the organization, was designed to establish guidelines for the increasing number of medical personnel who were coming into contact with transsexuals and didn't know what to do with them. Now the association hosts a major international conference every other year, and its committees dispense ethical guidelines for psychiatrists, endocrinologists, surgeons, sexologists, counselors, sociologists, and lawyers.

The "Standards of Care" was originally written in 1979 by six men—five medical doctors and one Ph.D.—and then approved by the attendees of the Harry Benjamin Symposium. The current incarnation was created by a committee more than three times that size—some women, some men, some transgender, some not, all with a variety of pedigrees—and the result is a twenty-two-page document that outlines what has become the generally accepted transition process from diagnosis to hormones to surgery. The "overarching treatment goal," as defined in the SOC, is "psychotherapeutic, endocrine, or surgical therapy" to create "lasting personal comfort with the gendered self in order to maximize overall psychological well-being and self-fulfillment." Most doctors who work with the transgender population follow association guidelines.

The resulting document is both impressive in terms of the scope of people it addresses and somewhat cautious—likely because it has to cover such a range. The authors recognize that not all transpeople want surgery or any other uniform body modifications, for instance, and they address this. They also recognize that young transpeople reach psychological maturity at different ages, so, I'm guessing, in order to be as safe and general as possible, the "Standards of Care" mostly mandates against treatment for minors, especially without parental involvement. To start hormones, it says, patients should be at least sixteen, with parental consent and a minimum of six months of therapy. On surgeries it's unequivocal: eighteen is the starting line.

One of the most exciting and, some would say, radical doctors treating transgender youth in California—and probably in the whole country, actually—is a man named Marvin Belzer. Dr. Belzer runs a clinic called the Division of Adolescent Medicine in Childrens Hospital Los Angeles (CHLA). Out of a standard-looking medical office with fluorescent lighting and construction-papered bulletin boards, a place with scuffed chairs and big windows, Dr. Belzer prescribes hormones to minors. He has patients as young as thirteen and a waiting list up to six months long.

Because estrogen is a menopause drug and prescribed widely, it's not federally monitored, the way something like Xanax or Vicodin is. It's easy to obtain and, because it's so common, Medi-Cal, the insurance agency for the poor in California, doesn't question the prescriptions for children with male names. (Belzer said that Medi-Cal recently started recognizing transgender care, so the hormone coverage may no longer be an oversight.) In any case, in practical terms Belzer's job is straightforward and legal. But in philosophical ones, it's more complicated. At first glance, one might say it's reckless to give adolescents hormones; teenagers are known for changing their minds and could suffer physically and psychologically if they wanted to revert back to their biological sex in adulthood. But for Belzer, age isn't the most important consideration. Dr. Belzer follows a "harm reduction" model. Essentially, he explained, if kids are prostituting for hormones, if kids are living on the street rather than in foster care to earn enough money to buy hormones, if kids are risking their lives and HIV status for hormones, then for goodness' sake, give them hormones. The equation, for him, is obvious.

In my universe Belzer was something of a hero. He had taken a community of kids with little money and excess baggage and stepped in to help them. His work didn't even start in the hospital; because several of his patients were wards of the state, Belzer had to get permission from a bevy of judges and social workers and sometimes probation officers before he could even treat them. In the process he was curbing the kids' HIV rates, and because he mandated counseling along with his meds, he provided a template for long-term psychological care; many kids would go on with therapy long after Belzer's program. While he started the program in 1991 for the very high-risk kids, he now sees the low-risk cases too, modeling what he calls the "human right to access healthcare." Simply, and perhaps most profoundly, Belzer showed kids that someone with authority really saw them and then cared.

The day of my first interview with Belzer, amazingly, the movie *Mrs. Doubtfire* was playing on the television in his lobby, and I watched Robin Williams totter around in a dress as I waited for him. His office was dominated by paper piles; three- and four-inch heaps on every available surface made the furniture feel secondary to the journal articles, the printed e-mails, the various studies and grants, which were all quietly demanding to be read or completed. Belzer wore green jeans and a business shirt and tie; he's white and was in his midforties, with thick boyish brown hair and a wandering right eye. With his good eye, he looks at you thoughtfully and listens closely, and all those papers fade away; I understood immediately why the kids liked him. He listens as much as he talks.

"Clinically, we see about fifty adolescents per year, aged thirteen to twenty-four," Dr. Belzer said, though if they had more funding, they could see more. There's always a waiting list. Of these fifty, he said, only about seven are female-to-male, not necessarily because there aren't as many, but because they're so much harder to fund. The male-to-female kids have an identifiable, well-documented HIV risk, and Belzer has traditionally gotten his major grants by citing his HIV-reduction work. But the transboys aren't involved in prostitution or drug use at the same levels, so Belzer can't justify their funding. Men are the prostitutes' buyers, and they don't want the female-to-males. (They're not a common fantasy on the porn racks either.) These FTMs aren't using drugs in the same volume either, perhaps because they aren't generally trafficking in sex work. What Belzer really needs, he said, is someone to simply care about the physical and psychological health of transboys, regardless of

their HIV status or risk, and subsidize them too. So far this hasn't happened.

It was through HIV work actually that Dr. Belzer discovered the young transgender community. He was treating HIV-positive patients when one who happened to be transgender mentioned that she was getting her hormones on the streets. Belzer reasoned that he may as well prescribe her hormones, so she could use her money to take care of herself in other ways. Then several more patients requested this service. Soon they were asking him to help out their HIV-negative friends, and "that just released the floodgates," Belzer said, adding that he quickly applied for grants to meet the growing need. "Word filtered down, and we went from seeing everyone from the really high-risk to the fourteen-year-olds with the intact families."

Even now, with the program's popularity, nobody who walks in off the street gets turned away. She'll get an initial appointment with a case manager who'll explain how the program works. "She'll learn what we offer and what our requirements are—we are a program that requires counseling—and if it's a good match for her, then she'll go on the wait list," Belzer explained. The Harry Benjamin standards require that a sixteen-year-old undergo a half year of counseling before being prescribed hormones, but because Belzer's patients are an at-risk population, each case is considered individually. Some of his patients are bruised from familial abuse or time on the street, and some are young and really do need to sort out their gender orientation before they're given shots or pills. Everyone, he reasons, can benefit from therapy, and some of his patients come to CHLA specifically because they want the free talk.

"I would say 90 percent of the time it's clear after the first visit that this person needs hormones. But then there's the 10 percent who go through therapy and they realize they're an effeminate gay male or they're transgender, but they can't cope with the transition process. They may say, 'I know I'm transgender, but it's just too hard. I'm going to live with my body the way it is for now because there's too much prejudice, and I need to be successful at school or at a job or my family's not supportive or whatever,'" Belzer said. For the 90 percent, the therapy can last anywhere from a week to six months before they start hormones, depending upon a child's psychological stability, emotional maturity, and mental flexibility.

On the streets, where Belzer and CHLA are widely known, this translates to "You gotta go through three months of therapy to get hormones at Childrens." This common perception, Foxxjazell said, means a number of kids who might benefit from the free counseling, regular medical checkups, and HIV-prevention education don't even ride the elevator up the four flights to Belzer's waiting room. Like most teenagers, when they want something, they want it now, and they hate to have an adult slow them down.

Foxx herself went to one of the free clinics that would prescribe her hormones right away. The clinics won't treat minors (likely because of the "Standards of Care" requirements and parental consent laws), and patients still have to pay for the hormones out of pocket unless they have insurance—both hurdles that Foxx could leap because she was nineteen and had a job. "I got a prescription for Premarin, the little purple pills, and I was just so happy. I really wanted to swallow the whole bottle," Foxx remembered.

She continued: "A lot of girls are very desperate and can't wait for Dr. Belzer; a lot of us will do whatever it takes to become women, even if it means stealing hormones." She shook her purse so I could hear the faint rattle of pills within. She said that once when she let some young girl who was new to Los Angeles crash at her place, that girl stole a whole bottle of Premarin from her. At that time if you didn't have insurance, a legal bottle cost about $180. Street hormones are now around $50, depending on what you get. Foxx now carries her hormones around with her all the time. "A lot of girls think, 'If I know I'm a girl, why do I have to confirm that with you? Why do I have to sit through therapy for three months, then go through medical exams, then wait for pills to come in, when I can just get street hormones?'"

Belzer is well acquainted with this attitude and can respond with some degree of flexibility when he thinks it's appropriate. "If a kid comes to us and she's been on hormones for weeks or months or years and she's already feminized, then we usually try to bridge that gap; we have a much more expedited way of doing things," Belzer said, explaining that this patient will still receive free psychotherapy but will likely get hormone prescriptions right away to parallel a regimen she's already been on.

The three-month therapy guideline comes from the "Standards of Care," which recommends even adults cross-live or get therapy for three months before they're given any body-altering medication. While this formula might sound reasonable, many critics say the cross-living concept can be dangerous; they're exposed to too much violence walking around as a "man in a dress." Adult transwomen often prefer to take hormones and get electrolysis for several months while still presenting themselves to the outside world as men, until their bodies and features have shifted enough to make the change. Others see the therapy as patronizing; they say it's taken

tremendous courage and generally years of internal preparation to make it to a psychiatrist's chair—they don't need to endure more months of mandated talk therapy to get the hormones they already know they need.

Another problem with the SOC's hallmark approach of "safe" and "general" is that it doesn't resonate with teenagers. "The principles are very good, but they're rigid," Belzer said. "You can follow all the guidelines, and you won't take any chances of messing anything up—or you can say, 'Where is this kid at? What are the dangers of starting hormones? What are the dangers of *not* starting hormones?'"

Even when he does start the hormones, Belzer explained, his team of psychologists has to spend extensive appointment time managing expectations. A lot of kids project their visions of Madonna or Britney or Marilyn onto their initial pill or injection and are devastated when their first sign of female puberty is a pimple on the chin.

"Hormones can do a lot for the girls, but just like a relationship, they take time," Foxx said. "You have to be faithful and patient with hormones, and a lot of girls aren't that."

So they'll shoot up and shoot up and shoot up, on top of what they get at Childrens—sometimes as many as four doses in one week. While you can't technically overdose on estrogen or Depo-Provera, you can get intensely moody (like PMS on overdrive)—and for the many kids who already suffer from depression, this can be dangerous. But the real risk is one that's not fully understood, and won't be until these young people are in their thirties or forties or fifties: breast cancer.

"That's the thing that just scares me to death," Dr. Belzer said, leaning forward in his chair. "There's more and more evidence that estrogen has a small but real risk associated with breast cancer, and we are not giving them physiologic doses, but pharmacologic doses. We're not trying to just give them enough estrogen; we're trying to *overcome* their testosterone. And there are no long-term, studies on the effects."

What this means is this: Genetic women have between 20 and 80 nanograms of testosterone per deciliter in their bodies; normal males have around 600. Belzer uses the estrogen to push the testosterone levels down to the lowest reaches of a normal female. The few articles in the medical literature suggest staying in the higher female realms, but few kids are satisfied with these effects, and Belzer wants to mimic what they can get on the streets to keep them in his program. A much safer way to bring down the testosterone, Belzer feels, would be to prescribe something that works as an anti-androgen, which blocks the production or effects of testosterone, something like the cancer drug Lupron. Then he could just use estrogen, in much smaller doses, for breast growth and other feminization, much like MTFs with more discretionary income will do. But most antiandrogens are prohibitively expensive, and insurance plans would require a cancer diagnosis to cover the cost.

It's possible, too, that the hormone regime isn't a terrible threat for transwomen. "When you give progesterone and estrogen together, you're converting a patient's risk factor from that of a male to that of a female, so probably overall you're lowering risk [of death]," he said, nothing that a person can die of more than cancer. He said that men, in general, have higher cholesterol and higher risk of heart disease, so the hormones he's providing could be protective against some illnesses while boosting risk for others. Belzer has seen girls on staggering levels of street hormones, and he said he's never seen the kinds of troubles that a Women's Health Initiative study of genetic women on estrogen and progestin found, such as strokes or blood clots, but that may be because his patients are so much younger than the postmenopausal subjects in the study. "There are not a lot of people who have been on hormones for thirty years, and there haven't been a lot of reports," Belzer said, but after another few decades, we'll know more about how patients on high levels of hormones fare over the long term. "The guidelines say, 'Be conservative,' but if I'm too conservative, the kids do the hormones on their own and avoid us, so there's a balance."

Belzer said he gets regular calls and e-mails from general practitioners or endocrinologists around the country who suddenly have a transgender teenager in their office seeking help and don't know what to do with her. "I get about an e-mail a month from a doctor saying, 'I was never trained for this, and I don't want to do anything dangerous,'" said Belzer, who will direct people to the Harry Benjamin Web site and to the primer books of Dr. Sheila Kirk, a transsexual surgeon who writes about feminizing hormonal therapy. "There's an amazing willingness on the part of the physicians [to treat these kids].

"I don't think anybody had a youth program before us," Belzer told me modestly. Chicago has a multifaceted adolescent program at the Howard Brown Health Center with case management, support groups, and medical services for up to a hundred trans youth. Unfortunately, Illinois laws make it difficult to provide hormones to people under eighteen, unless they have parental consent. Dr. Rob Garofalo, the director of youth services at Howard Brown, said judges won't generally allow doctors to prescribe hormones to, for instance, homeless minors. Garofalo also started a transgender youth program in Boston, where, he said, laws are similar. Still,

programs like Garofalo's are growing, as are the cities around the country with free clinics that offer hormones to teenagers in the mix of their adult offerings. San Francisco, for instance, has this.

And if a teenager has known since early childhood that she needed to change her gender, how early should a hormone regimen be implemented? "As early as possible," Belzer said. "Before they develop depression, before they develop substance abuse, before they run away from home because their parents are abusive and then get involved in sex work or get HIV without getting educated about their risk for HIV from sex."

When I first met Christina, she swore she would never take hormones. Even though she had struggled with far more dangerous drugs, weeping through monthlong spells of crack and crystal meth use here and there, she worried about altering her physiological chemistry with estrogen. She also worried about getting clocked. She knew she was a girl inside, but she'd had enough pain as a child; she didn't want to willingly sign up for more harassment and abuse as an adult. "I would have backed up any minute if I was embarrassing myself; it would have not been worth it to go on hormones if I looked too manly," Christina said, meaning that if her own natural puberty had masculinized her too much, she wouldn't have even tried to live full-time as a woman. She carefully watched the distress of all the transgirls who didn't easily pass. "I wanted to wait and see what my body would look like without hormones."

Christina's father didn't give her much, but he passed along convenient genes. Just after her eighteenth birthday, Christina was still only five foot five, right around the average height for an American woman, with no Adam's apple, and only eight or ten thin hairs teasing her upper lip, which she plucked ferociously, checking for stubble in a compact mirror several times a day. Puberty seemed to only graze her, whereas it throttled other kids, leaving them hairy and pock-marked from acne, thick necked, and broad. Christina was naturally thin with a full face, and since she was really only clocked when she was in Hollywood and people knew to scrutinize details like hand width or shoe size, she decided she was ready for hormones.

Christina signed up for Childrens but couldn't wait: she took her first shot illegally with Luisa, a main supplier for the community who goes to Tijuana several times a year to buy hormones and syringes to shoot up the girls who are too squeamish or simply don't want to do it themselves. Luisa is Mexicana and in her fifties, of average height and average looks. She wears stretch pants and embroidered sweatshirts and mules that clack when she walks, and if you saw her on the streets, you'd never suspect her of doing anything undercover. I first saw Luisa working at a community meeting for transgender women. As the agenda was being read and grievances aired, women one by one got up and strolled to the corner, sometimes still tossing comments over their shoulders as they went. Then they faced the wall and dropped the top corner of their pants or skirt. Luisa swabbed them in the upper quadrant of their behinds and injected them. They handed her a twenty and went back to the meeting, never stopping their train of talk. It seemed a clean operation, and Luisa always used new needles.

Luisa also makes house calls and works at the nightclubs. People like her because she's discreet and respectful and gentle, and, as Christina said, her hormones are strong. Christina said, in general, the shots seem to work most on skin softening and overall appearance, and pills seem to work on bust size. Belzer explained that shots and pills serve the same function and produce the same result, but a body will utilize and tolerate higher doses via syringe because the hormones don't get broken down by the liver or cause nausea as frequently. That first day Christina had the shot, she didn't know the details of where the hormones would go or what they would do; she just felt a generalized joy. She was with an older friend who was transitioning from female to male; he held her hand, and she didn't even flinch when the needle went in.

A few months after that first Luisa shot, Christina was accepted into the program at Childrens. She didn't mind the psychotherapy and believes people need it whether they'll admit it or not. "I think the therapy should be mandatory, because living the trans life, you need ways of coping," she said to me after she'd been taking hormones—both street and prescription—for a while. "Plus hormones can lead to some serious depression for a few days."

The mood swings don't stop kids from experimenting. Foxx, just shy of her twenty-first birthday, was also augmenting her prescription with shots. "My mother has big breasts, and my breasts will be close to my closest female relative—but I'm a size A now, and I wanted something hanging down," said Foxx. "So far they [the shots] have been working wonders. They've made my breasts bigger, my skin softer, and made my face more clear and round."

But other teenagers don't have the patience to still be a size A after nearly two years (though some, like Domineque, can be a B or C) and, if they can afford it, will opt for implants. A $4,000 or $6,000 surgery is no option, so another black-market business has developed, with much more dangerous consequences than the hormones: pumping, or shooting loose silicone directly into the body where you want it to be larger or fleshier. There are cliques of women who pump and those who don't, and they often don't socialize together, as pumping is perceived as a dangerous or sometimes even "trashy" thing to do.

Silicone is considered biologically inert, and because people inject it with immediate and visually impressive results, the girls who do it can think it's reasonably safe. In the medical literature, it's a less reassuring picture. Depending upon where it's injected, the most common sites being the hips and breasts, the silicone can become a mass of infected tissue that can slide into the lower legs or scrotum or cause real trouble if it travels to the lungs. Transwomen have had long latency periods, where their silicone behaved appropriately for up to seventeen years, and then it has suddenly caused a deformity or infection. In the lungs silicone has led to respiratory difficulty, chemical pneumonia, and even heart failure. It has killed several transsexuals over the past few years. In 2004 a few pumping deaths made the AP newswire, though the victims were referred to as men, or the community as transvestites. Even in the medical literature, it's difficult to get a real grasp on how widespread the practice is or how much silicone it takes to cause a problem; the evidence is all anecdotal, and the writing has a startled "Hey, guys, look what stumbled into my office—isn't this weird?" quality to it. What seems apparent is that some women are pumping excessively; in autopsies women have been described as having silicone deposits in their lymph nodes, spleens, livers, and adrenal glands. One was so full that when incisions were made in her body, a clear, brownish liquid flowed out.

Silicone came into vogue post-World War II when Japanese prostitutes found they could inject the substance into their breasts and boost business. It caught on in the States shortly thereafter, primarily among topless dancers but also in alternative circles, and by the mid-sixties, the silicone breast implant was being medically marketed and surgically inserted. The implant, as opposed to the purely liquid injection, was not supposed to leak, but it did (even through the sacs and foams that contained it), and Dow Corning, a producer of the implants, settled a class-action lawsuit in 1998 for $3.2 billion. Women who have implants do not commonly experience the more serious side effects as injectors (though they can get hardening and shifting and lumps), in all likelihood because they aren't taking in the same quantities. Now silicone implants are banned in the United States, and women have saline implants instead. Silicone has gone underground for transwomen who can't afford other options.

I first heard about pumping parties when I was a teacher and my students would get buzzed up about a "surgeon's wife" coming to town, which happened about twice a year. It was important that she was married to a doctor, the kids said, because she had access to medical-grade (as opposed to industrial-grade) silicone and because she had watched her husband perform surgeries. She knew how to handle needles and was very safe and clean. This mysterious woman flew in from Florida and rented a house in San Fernando Valley, the way porn directors do (at least in my imagination). I was told that eighty to a hundred transwomen would pay her a few hundred for each breast, several hundred for the buttocks or hips, and then extra for the face: cheeks, foreheads, and lips. Some even got shots in their knees to look less bony, little squirts of perfection here and there. The doctor's wife would work from early morning into the late night and sometimes into the next day, and then she'd be gone, off to another city, clearing a cool couple hundred grand or more.

When the "doctor's wife" or someone like her isn't around, many kids, being young and poor and reckless in other areas of their lives, will use industrial-grade silicone found in sealants and adhesives sold in hardware stores. Usually, some member of the community will rise up as a pumping expert, knowing how deep to place the needle, and how much to inject for the desired effect and so on, and the girls will pay her, but sometimes they'll even pump themselves. The silicone is always injected subcutaneously, in the tissue just below the skin, to the place where you can feel the tissue tearing away from the muscle. If it's too shallow, the skin will discolor.

On transgender websites and chat rooms, there are all kinds of warnings about pumping. Some are blanket admonitions, talking about fatal pulmonary embolisms, and displaying monstrous photographs of women whose breasts were so laden with granulomatous lumps that they had to be scraped of silicone, leaving them with a concave, watermelon-sized scar. Other sites are more moderate, simply claiming that if you are going to pump, you're less likely to die if you do it in small amounts; even though it's cheaper and more exciting to jump three breast sizes in one sitting, it's safer to go for several treatments. Plus, they say, no hot baths right after an injection; the silicone could ooze from the syringe holes. And then after a few days, go back to the hot baths: they're good for massaging the "silicone bubbles" out. After injections some women feel little knots or lumps that must be massaged and smoothed so as not to permanently harden. This, according to one site, "hurts like a mother."

Foxx finally gave up on the hormones working all alone and went to her first pumping party in 2002. She doesn't know if she got industrial-grade or medical-grade silicone. She didn't know to ask.

"I went to this girl named Michele—she eventually died of gangrene in her foot—who came from another state and went from state to state pumping the girls," Foxx said, adding that she paid $200 for each breast, which took about fifteen minutes each to complete. To make the breasts keep their shape, Foxx had to wear a firm training bra for two months, even while she slept. Afterward Foxx's breasts were a cup size larger, and she was hooked. She now goes to a clinic in Tijuana, where the process is publicly available. Over three sessions she's had her breasts, hips, and cheeks pumped. She now wants to do the backs of her thighs and butt area to look, as she said, thicker.

"I want to master that thickness that a lot of beautiful black women have; I want to look bottom heavy. If my hips come out more, then my shoulders will look smaller," Foxx said, dropping her pants and pushing on her hips to show me what she would look like if her figure were more hourglass. What about the risks, I asked, noting that her shoulders were already pretty small. Here, Foxx's normally safety-conscious attitude took a backseat to her vision of perfection. "I'm mostly worried about the hardness and the lumps," she said. "You've got to bust any lumps and break the silicone down for the rest of your life."

Foxx is driving toward a vision of an idealized feminine form, but she's not driving toward what many people believe is the end goal for all transsexuals—the genital surgery. This is the arena of body modification that's separate from the others: there are the procedures you do for everyone to see (things for your breasts, face, body shape, and so on), and then there's the "bottom surgery," concealed from view. Some need to change their entire bodies; some don't.

I find it interesting that the unadorned penis is, for Foxx and some others, a holdout for identity politics. I think most people would say that the soul resides in the inside of their bodies rather than on the outside, in the unseeable, unknowable blood and organs and cells that keep them alive, simply because they cannot imagine the soul as invisible, antimatter, ether. So there is the physical person that people see, and there is the "real me," that's "on the inside," literally, with the brains or intestines or heart. The genitals are, in a way, messengers from this interior world; like the mouth or nose, they bring forth inside things for us to examine, a litmus for inner health. Like wounds or secrets, we keep genitals covered most of the time, exposing them only to clean them or to show to doctors or lovers. So I understand the reluctance to change them. Breasts, clothing, hairstyle, walk, and voice are the external cues that convince the outside world that transwomen are women, the cues that make that world a comfortable place for her to move around in; a penis is something that's just between a woman and her partners—and if all interested parties are fine with it, then why change it?

Of course, many transsexuals are sure they want the SRS (sex reassignment surgery), and when they are, they enter an even more complicated relationship with the medical industry. Domineque is one person who has known she wanted it since she was a child, which is part of the reason she stayed with the program at Childrens Hospital. She'll ultimately need proof of her long-term care, as all surgeons require letters from patients' primary doctors and therapists saying they've been on hormones and in counseling for "gender identity disorder," or GID. In a way, the requisite diagnosis puts Domineque in the double bind of being both sane and sick at the same time. This is the law, as set by the Harry Benjamin "Standards of Care," which most every surgeon follows. Gender identity disorder is a mental illness in the American Psychiatric Association's fourth edition of the *Diagnostic and Statistical Manual of Mental Disorders*, the manual all physicians use to diagnose and treat mental disorders of all stripes. (Homosexuality was also "on the books" as a psychological sickness until 1973, when the APA voted to remove it. Such choices are largely more social and political than medical.) To have GID (previously called "transsexualism"), a person must have "the desire to live and be accepted as a member of the opposite sex, usually accompanied by the desire to make his or her body as congruent as possible with the preferred sex through surgery and hormone treatment." In addition, according to the *DSM-IV*, these feelings have to have been present for at least two years, and the "disorder" cannot be a "symptom of another mental disorder or a chromosomal abnormality."

For Domineque, who's felt like a girl since she was two, she'd get a check mark next to all three criteria. That's the "sick" part; SRS is not a cosmetic surgery— it's a medical necessity. The surgery is the treatment, and a patient needs a letter to her surgeon saying she's got this mental ailment that can only be cured through physical intervention. The letter also has to say that the illness is a physical one—that while GID is technically a mental disorder, the patient is of a sound-enough mind to be able to make such a decision. It's her body that just doesn't fit, the letter will say; that's the "sane" part. In other words, to get such a surgery, a patient can't just ask for it; she needs at least two psychological professionals (one with a Ph.D., the SOC demands) saying she deserves it.

The first American to undergo sex reassignment surgery was a transwoman named Christine Jorgensen in 1952. Because the procedure wasn't yet available in the States, Christine traveled to Denmark for the operation, and her transition made international news—in some ways, perhaps, making her responsible for the contemporary mainstream notion that the end goal for all transpeople is surgery. Christine was a quiet person and a former GI, and some accounts say she wanted to transition in private, while others say she relished being in the spotlight. In any case, when Christine returned to the United States, she was mobbed by reporters, and headlines across the country shouted, "EX-GI BECOMES BLONDE BOMBSHELL!" Christine stories ranked number one for 1953 in the *New York Daily News*, and she became so famous that letters addressed to "Christine Jorgensen, U.S.A.," would reach their destination.

In a book called *How Sex Changed: A History of Transsexuality in the United States*, author Joanne Meyerowitz theorizes that part of the reason Jorgensen enflamed the American imagination was her timing: the postwar era was one fixated on gender roles and whether the war-worker women could be coaxed happily back into their homes. It was also the atomic age, and Jorgensen tapped right into the issue of whether science could and even should win out over nature. Her case literally made "sex change" a household phrase. Before Jorgensen, a person's physical sex, psychological "gender," and sexuality were one fused thing determined by a doctor's quick glance in a delivery room; Jorgensen (or what she represented) ripped them apart.

Jorgensen ultimately used her fame to make a living, as she developed a stage act singing and telling jokes, and appealing to her audience's sympathies. She aligned herself with the American ideal of the lonely dreamer who strives to reach her goals despite the odds. Her beauty throughout her life was deemed sophisticated and understated, earning her comparisons to stars like Eve Arden and Lauren Bacall. (Still, Christine wasn't "American" enough to be allowed to perform in Boston, where lawmakers called her tame act "risqué," nor woman enough to get married, as she was denied a license in the state of New York in 1959.) She lived off and on with her Danish immigrant parents in New York and on her own in California until she died of bladder cancer in 1989.

Fifty years after that first operation, there are still only a handful of surgeons in the United States providing transgender genital surgery, which costs anywhere from $20,000 to $100,000 depending on what you get, how far you travel, and so on. It's odd to me that so few doctors do it, because just as with plastic surgery, your patients come willingly and leave ecstatic that you cut them open and sewed them up again. The surgeries are relatively low risk, there are a lot of ways to creatively approach each operation and implement improvements, and there's a certain aesthetic art to them. Also, because insurance won't pay for the job, you can be assured money up front. In fact, there'll likely be a waiting list for your services.

The young people I know can't afford the surgery, though they regularly talk and argue about wanting it—or never wanting it. Often these discussions are in the context of men and whether having the SRS would make their relationship prospects better. Some, like Domineque, don't care about the men at all; she wants the surgery to feel at peace within her own skin. Some, like Ariel, are still struggling with passing in a dress in daylight; talking about surgery with Ariel is akin to discussing college with a preschooler. But most play with the idea of what they would look like with a vagina, what they would feel like, how it would be to dress every day without tucking (wherein they tuck their penis up between their buttocks so as not to show a bulge), what it would be like to date and not be worried. It's a distant dream, they realize. Some talk of putting $2 or $5 a week toward the plan, but few do. If they do save up, perhaps later when they're older or more stable, they may well go to a surgeon named Dr. Toby Meltzer.

Dr. Meltzer runs his practice out of a hospital in Scottsdale, where he has twenty-one inpatient beds with views of the mountains and a staff of eleven—sizable, for one surgeon. Two-thirds of his surgeries every year are SRS; the rest are just standard cosmetic surgeries—liposuction, breast augmentations, and the like. Most transgender patients hear of Dr. Meltzer through word of mouth and, if they can afford it, will visit him in Scottsdale to talk about their surgical options. But several times a year, Dr. Meltzer also makes presentations at gay and transgender community centers, to show slides of his work and speak to potential patients, who line up with questions about tracheal shaves or feminizing nose jobs. Some cry with relief just to meet him. One Saturday afternoon on a chilly fall day, I went to see Dr. Meltzer make such a presentation in New York City.

Forty adults hunched into folding chairs and stared, rapt, at slide after slide of spread-leg genitalia, whispering to their friends and pointing with pencils at particular regions, nodding happily. This was not porn. This was salvation. In the "after" pictures of both men and women, the women looked better; it's easier to construct a vagina from a penis than the other way around. Meltzer explained that there are a few ways to do it, but that the most common is something called "penile inversion." What this means, in lay terms, is that the penis is basically turned inside out and pushed inside the body to form a vagina. "I don't get rid of much," Meltzer said to

the group that day. "It's all still there; it's just in a different location."

For the patient, there are several steps to the process. Before she even sees Dr. Meltzer, she has to have several treatments of electrolysis on her testicles so no hair ultimately ends up where it shouldn't. Then, she undergoes the first surgery to construct the basic vulva and vagina. Dr. Meltzer can't do what's called the "labiaplasty," which is constructing the labia minora and a clitoral hood, until a second surgery, because he needs to let the area heal. Some women stop at this first stage, but many don't; the aesthetics can be noticeably off-kilter.

When everything is completely healed after several weeks, a transwoman will be able to have a healthy sex life, with genitalia that's usually indistinguishable from a genetic woman, except for lubrication. Her vagina will have a depth of five and a half to six and a half inches and, because she has a clitoris constructed from the former glans of her penis, she can orgasm.

There's a saying that goes: "FTMs pass on the streets and MTFs pass in the sheets." There's a reason. Transmen, on hormones, look amazing. Even children under five, famous for loudly noting people's differences, don't clock them. Beards, baldness, deep voices, thick necks, everything. But get them to drop their pants, and you'll have a tough time finding a man-made penis that looks quite like the genetic version. They're either terribly small or large enough but the wrong color, or else they're a funny shape and weight because they're filled with tissue that's heavier than a genetic male's penis. And none of the reconstructed versions can get erect without a pump. The science just isn't there yet.

Fetuses are sexually undifferentiated until eight weeks of age, at which point girls begin to get ovaries and males get testes, boys get penises, girls get clitorises, and so on. The body parts parallel one another, so it actually makes intuitive sense to turn a transman's clitoris into a penis, in a procedure called a "metoidioplasty." After Meltzer's patients have had a hysterectomy, oophorectomy (to remove the ovaries), and a vaginectomy (to close the vagina) with some other doctor—because these aren't cosmetic procedures—he sets about constructing a penis. Essentially, this means removing the skin around the clitoris so it can extend from the pubic region and rotating the labia majora to the midline to form the scrotum. He puts expanders into the scrotum, which are later replaced with a prosthesis.

The average-length metoidioplasty penis is under three inches. It looks like a penis, but there's no chance that a date won't notice its smaller size. So the other option is penile reconstruction, which, in general, is slightly more dangerous, often more ugly, and sometimes less sensate. What you've got with penile reconstruction is—*big*.

Meltzer mostly sends patients who want penile reconstruction to Belgium, where surgeons specialize in the practice. To make a penis, you need skin, and you can take it from a few different areas: the thigh, the belly, or the forearm. With all three, a patient will have a brutal scar at least a foot long and several inches wide, and all three have their downsides. Leg skin is good because it's the same color and you can make a big penis, but the skin is insensitive, it's a less reliable blood supply during the operation, it requires multiple operations, and the urethral lengthening is precarious. If you go with the belly, the skin will be a different color. The forearm is sensitive skin and often makes the best-looking penis in the end, but the surgery is technically difficult and there are complications; a good 40 percent have a narrowing of the urethra and have to have it tracked back to their perineum. Plus the scarring on the arm is the worst of all three, and it's the most visible; even several years after healing, it's a shiny mass of pink and white noodles and suture marks.

In the States, average metoidioplasty costs can range from $2,000 to $18,000 (for clitoral release all the way up to urethral extension and testicular implants); penile reconstruction costs anywhere from $50,000 to more than $100,000. Add to that the cost of a hysterectomy, oophorectomy, vaginectomy, and a double mastectomy, and the price tag jumps another $30,000. And the time off work for surgery, bed rest, and the costs for traveling to the handful of surgeons who do the work. This is why relatively few transmen have the bottom surgery at all. For transwomen, a vaginoplasty in the States will cost from $12,000 to $20,000, and labiaplasty can cost an extra $3,000 to $5,000. A typical breast augmentation can cost a few to several thousand dollars, in addition to the hormones. But those are just fundamentals: some women feel they need a tracheal shave (to remove the Adam's apple), which costs around $3,000, or a jaw feminization, nose job, chin reduction, cheekbone augmentation, or forehead contouring, which can obviously add tens to hundreds of thousands of dollars to the total price tag. And while transsexuals are considered medically, mentally ill in the *DSM-IV* and have to be diagnosed as such to even be considered for the most basic of surgeries, no insurance will cover the cost.

Foxx went back and forth about wanting SRS. Almost twenty-one, she still had not had a boyfriend, not ever, and she attributed that tragedy to mere inches of skin and tissue. It didn't have to do with her face or her body; men in cars and malls who hooted or pressed phone numbers into her palms told her that. It didn't have to do with her personality or her voice, which could charm both sexes into buying extra long-distance services or registering for a trip to Hawaii; her countless telemarketing jobs proved that. Foxx passed everywhere but the bedroom. Still, she couldn't decide what was more important: the intense and personal love from one boyfriend (whom she felt would be easier to snag if she had the surgery) or the diffuse love from countless music fans whom she could encourage to respect themselves and the bodies they were born with.

"It changes from month to month. Some months it's like I want a pussy; other months I want to be a transsexual with a big old—"Foxx paused. She looked at her hands. "More and more I want to feel comfortable with what I have, with my own uniqueness, and I'm scared that once I have SRS, I'll no longer truthfully be transsexual in a way. I'll be categorized the way every other woman is, in the way that a lot more men will feel comfortable with."

Here Foxx grew more adamant. "But I don't want SRS because my boyfriend is going to like it or because people in society will finally accept me. I want it because I want it—and if I have it, I feel I won't be the same role model."

One cold January morning I was over at Foxx's place, and she was cooking grits and bacon for me and a twenty-year-old friend of hers named Keandra who had had implants. On impulse Foxx took off her shirt and asked me to feel the bumps in her breasts. They were small, she said, but they were worrisome. She didn't want them to harden any more or grow into anything unusual. I probed around where she told me and felt the normal, sinewy "rice and peas" that any gynecologist tells a woman to feel for during her monthly self-exams. Foxx's breasts hung down with a satisfying weight, heavier at the base, tiny stretch marks shining along their sides.

"Feel mine too!" Keandra said, and implants bounced out of her terrycloth bathrobe. Keandra's breasts were round like globes, the nipples pointing toward her chin, the skin unnaturally taut. Keandra had never felt a genetic woman's breasts before, so I took off my shirt too, and suddenly we were all at a sixth-grade slumber party, comparing size and lift and nipple shape and then lying on the floor to see how they flopped to the side, as the grits burned in the pan.

"Foxx, yours feel just like Cris's!" Keandra said, and she was right. This only made Foxx more sure about her decision to get more work done. I asked if Foxx remembered how she used to teach her daughters about the dangers of pumping and to have patience with the hormones. "I remember," she said. "But my patience wore out! It's like that Janet Jackson song, 'Let's Wait Awhile.' It's like, 'How long you want me to wait? Till I'm thirty-six and still singing that song?'"

Intersexuals
 ## "Exploding the Binary Sex System"

by Kim Klausner

I sat in a restaurant in the Castro section of San Francisco waiting to meet Cheryl Chase, founder of the Intersex Society of North America (ISNA). A lone woman entered the eatery and it soon became clear that this was the person I was waiting for. After settling ourselves at a table I did my best with innocuous small talk, hoping to find a connection with this person I would soon be interviewing. "So, you were born in New York City?" I ventured. Cheryl looked at me oddly and replied, "No, why?" I scratched my head and mentioned that I had seen a reference to her being operated on as an infant at a prestigious New York City hospital. She matter-of-factly said, "I wasn't born in New York; I was mutilated there."

Cheryl's response took my breath away, and well it should have. I gazed at this courageous woman and saw someone who was determined to transform an intensely personal experience into far reaching political action. As we ate, she willingly revealed intimate details about her life and body to me, a stranger, with the hope that I would join her effort to change oppressive medical practices and the assumptions behind them. Her particular experience is important to know only insofar as it can be used to illustrate larger social relations. During our lunch I was alternately struck by two processes that seemed to underlie all that Cheryl talked about: (1) that the personal is the political and (2) that the medical profession embodies the prevailing cultural assumptions about sex, biology, and gender and uses its authority to enforce particular power relations.

Before I get too far along with *my* thoughts, however, let me share a little about what ISNA is, mostly in the words of the organization itself. ISNA is "a peer support, education, and advocacy group founded and operated by and for intersexuals, individuals born with anatomy or physiology which differs from cultural ideals of male and female." Intersexuals, sometimes called hermaphrodites, are a physically diverse group of people, with bodies that are not easily categorized in our either/or male/female sex system. According to doctors, intersexuals are females born with clitorises that the doctors consider too long and males born with penises that are deemed too short. In a certain sense, the medical establishment hardly recognizes the integrity of the category "intersexual," preferring to dismiss intersexuals as deficient males or females. One of ISNA's first goals is to redefine the terms of their very existence.

The concept of intersexuality confronts the dominant cultural conception of "sex anatomy as a dichotomy: humans come in two sexes, conceived of as so different as to be nearly different species." ISNA challenges this view with the assertion that "anatomic sex differentiation occurs on a male/female continuum with several dimensions."

(If your eyes glaze over at the mention of chromosomes and you can't quite remember, or never knew, what gonads are, feel free to skip the next two paragraphs.) ISNA continues its explanation of intersexuality with, "Genetic sex, or the organization of the 'sex chromosomes,'

Author's note: If you want to know more about inersexuality or ISNA, contact the organization by e-mail (info@isna.org or cchase@isna.org), at their web site (http://www.isna.org), or by snailmail at P.O. Box 31791, San Francisco, CA 94131.

is commonly thought to be isomorphic to some idea of 'true sex.' However, something like 1/500 of the population have a karyotype [that is, chromosomal arrangement] other than XX (most females) or XY (most males)." As an example, ISNA points to women athletes subject to genetic testing. In recent years, women Olympic athletes have had to undergo genetic tests, and as a result a number of them have been disqualified as 'not women,' after winning. These women, of course are not men—they, like many other intersexuals, have atypical karotypes (though one gave birth to a healthy child after having been barred from competition).

The genitals of intersexual people vary along the male-female continuum. As is pointed out in ISNA literature:

Intersexual genitals may look nearly female, with a large clitoris, or with some degree of posterior labial fusion. They may look nearly male, with a small penis, or with hypospadias [a condition where the urethra opens on the under surface of the penis]. They may be truly "right in the middle," with a phallus that can be considered either a large clitoris or a small penis, with a structure that might be a split, empty scrotum, or outer labia, and with a small vagina that opens into the urethra rather than into the perineum.

Internal reproductive organs may be partially developed or discordant with external genitals. For instance, there are people whose genitals have the same appearance as most females, but inside have testes and no uterus or ovaries. Some people have combined gonads, that is, ovo-testes. Some people who have male-appearing genitals have a uterus, ovaries, and tubes.

To summarize, ISNA asserts that medical science has effectively promoted the "objective fact" that there are but two sexes, male and female, and that people are either one or the other. If truth be told, and it is, thanks to ISNA, people can be virtually all male, all female, or some of both (though, the popular concept of two sets of genitals—male and female—is not possible). It should be noted that we're just talking biology here; this doesn't even attempt to address questions about the social construction of gender or how children are raised to be boys or girls.

ISNA wants the immediate end to practices that arise from the medical model established in the 1950s that asserts that "children with visibly intersexual anatomy cannot develop into healthy adults." They want to stop emergency sex assignment and reinforcement of sex assignment with early genital surgery, which often causes serious sexual dysfunction. They also want an end to the dishonesty of healthcare providers who, in their discus-sions with parents and intersexuals, cover up the true status of the intersex child. ISNA does not, however, oppose using medical technology when it is necessary. "For instance," Chase explains, "some children are born with ambiguous genitals because of adrenal hyperplasia, which can be life threatening. Doctors should treat those aspects of this condition that affect the health and comfort of the child, such as preventing him or her from going into salt shock."

When an infant is born with genitals that don't conform to our idea of either male or female, ISNA wants doctors to be honest and not say, as they currently do, "Well, we can't determine what sex your child is by looking at it, but we can perform tests that will tell us, and then we can alter its genitals so it looks more like the sex it is." Rather, they'd prefer that new parents be told, "Your child is intersexual, in other words, neither a boy nor a girl. There are resources available to help you raise your child in a healthy way. Go home and love this child as you would any other." Chase succinctly sums it up with "we want an end to harmful and medically unnecessary cosmetic surgery, secrecy, and lying."

Obviously, this approach requires a radical rearrangement of our society. At the least, we need some new pronouns since "it" hardly describes a new baby. What ISNA is advocating is so profoundly disorienting that I've even had feminist friends roll their eyes at me and say, "So what, these people want to dismantle our society's concept of the male-female dichotomy? Good luck!" Or "How many people does this affect anyway? I mean, shouldn't we be dealing with issues like racism or poverty, things that affect much larger groups of people?" The number of people born intersexual is not huge, although it is probably greater than you imagine (1 out of every 2,000 births).

Accepting ISNA's claims means recovering the authority we have given to the medical establishment to assign and enforce sex roles. Most people hardly give the concept that sexes are assigned by society a thought. It is something that is determined by biology; if an infant has a penis, then it is a boy. It sounds simple enough. But transgendered people, who don't fit neatly into male or female categories, know that the medical establishment closely guards its prerogative to enforce sex roles. In most parts of the United States, transpeople have to feign a mental disorder to obtain an operation that is forced on intersexual children. In both cases the medical profession assumes the role of sex judge. Doctors tell the parents of the intersexual infant, "Based on the evidence, this is a girl, even though part of her anatomy looks almost male," while telling the person who wants to take hormones in the hopes of uncovering a body that more closely resembles their identity, "I will not prescribe these drugs unless you prove to me that you think you're really a (wo)man (and straight, too)."

If we are to honor the experience of many transsexuals, we must admit it is possible to be a female born with a penis or a male born with a vagina. We feel compelled to identify newborns as male or female, but maybe we should wait and let the kid decide whether s/he is male, female, or both. Chase points out that it's only been in the past 50 years or so that the medical profession has arbitrated these questions. For centuries, intersexuals navigated without the "help" of the sex judges. In some cultures, intersexuals were ignored, in some they were accorded high status, and in others they were reviled.

Feminists have long advocated that gender is culturally constructed. Well, why not sex? Somehow, the material nature of genitals, internal organs, and even hormones coursing through our bloodstreams lends credence to the medically or biologically based construction of sex. You cannot be fooled by something you can actually see or touch. Intersexuals and transpeople are starting to tell us otherwise. Sex cannot always be easily articulated in morphological terms and the diversity of anatomical differences among humans arrays us along a sex spectrum, not into two mutually exclusive categories.

The argument that sex is not biologically determined challenges decades of feminist theory and practice. If it is no longer clear that there are two distinct sexes, a theory resting on these two categories of existence becomes unstable. How can men oppress women if the boundaries between each group are permeable? Or if we no longer know who fits in each category? For these reasons, some feminists have found transpeople and intersexuals threatening. But do intersexuals alter the paradigm?

Unfortunately, oppressive relations can flourish without immutable, biologically based categories. The existence of mixed-race people has not brought an end to racism. While some Black civil rights organizations may fear that the institutionalization of mixed-race categories on the census will dilute their political power, I doubt that any of them think that the disappearance of mixed-race people from their statistical ranks will cause racism to crumble. And a person with parents of different races still faces racist prejudice and discrimination as s/he walks through life. In the case of men and women, perhaps imagining a sex continuum makes gender more important than sex. And this raises the question of the connection between gender and sex. The more I think about it, the more unsure I am that things are as they seem. But of course, many queer people have known this with their bodies and minds since they were young children.

Having the medical establishment (aided and abetted by the legal system) in charge of defining what the sexes are and how individual people fit into this schema provides reassurance—at least to those who have faith in the medical-judicial system—that sex assignment is not done on an arbitrary or capricious basis. It is, after all, scientifically proven. But what happens when people's experiences deviate from the accepted medical facts? Intersexual bodies are mutilated to maintain the current paradigm, just as gay people are institutionalized, women are called hysterical, and transpeople are thwarted in their efforts to realize themselves.

Here you might ask, "Why wouldn't a parent want to take advantage of the amazing medical techniques we have available to help her newborn child adjust to the world as it is? Wouldn't it be cruel to the child to force it to lead a life of being different?" The intersexuals connected with ISNA are saying simply and clearly they would rather be "different" than mutilated. Further, they want to help change our conception of normal so they won't have to feel out of place. Since an intersexual person knows, at some level, that s/he is different, the only thing surgical alteration seems to accomplish is the mental well-being of doctors, parents, and others who are more concerned with the intersexual's body than their mental well-being. In fact, the doctor's or parents' peace of mind is sometimes obtained at a monumental price: intersexuals report both sexual dysfunction and profound feelings of being unacceptable.

(It is certainly possible that some intersexuals are happy that they were altered. But they are the only ones who know. There have been no long-term studies on the effects of surgery on intersexual infants. The medical profession seems remarkably uninterested in knowing about the lives of intersexual adults. Perhaps if you are in this situation you will share your feelings with other *Sojourner* readers.)

This professionally sanctioned violation of a human body not only causes physical trauma but is also accompanied by a tremendous sense of shame about one's body. When an intersexual is born, a life of secrecy begins. It starts in the labor and delivery room. One can feel the palpable discomfort of the medical staff when they are unable to quickly answer the question, "is it a girl or a boy?" The intersexual teen is generally not told the truth about what has been done to his/her body, which magnifies an already difficult period of transition. And many intersexual people eventually carry the secret themselves as they hide their status from lovers.

When Cheryl Chase was born, the doctors told her parents that their child was a boy. When their son was a year old, a medical expert informed them, "This child is not really a boy. We will fix the problem by removing what looks like a penis but we suggest that you move to another city and start over again, telling people you have a daughter." Her parents renamed her Cheryl and did exactly that. Does the shame and secrecy sound similar to that experienced by the child of alcoholics or one who is sexually abused?

At 40, Cheryl still feels the painful reverberations of how the medical profession and her family treated her as someone born intersexual. Of this experience, she says simply, "It destroyed my whole family; we are scattered to the winds." From her mother who was given tranquilizers in response to her concerns about her infant's body, to her father who lay on his deathbed telling Cheryl that she was "bad from the day you were born," to her sisters who do not want biological children of their own, to her aunt who was unable to support Cheryl in her quest for the truth out of "loyalty" to her sister, there have been no winners here.

ISNA provides ample material from which to analyze power relations, particularly the way that science, as it is embedded in our particular culture, helps maintain a sexist hierarchy. For me, as someone who fits quite easily into a binary sex system, intersexual liberation is somewhat of an intellectual issue, removed from my day-to-day identity experience. At the same time, I recognize that this movement is led by people whose very core identities and bodies are at stake. As a political activist, I am incredibly rejuvenated by being a witness to this movement. There is something very powerful about a group of people who fuse the intensely personal with the theoretical to create change. I can take this concentrated sense of mission to other political work I do.

The process by which ISNA formed echoes the women's movement of the late '60s. A severe emotional breakdown provoked Chase to start asking questions about how her body came to be. In the course of her investigation, she found other people who had had similar experiences. Last summer, a group of ten intersexual people met for a weekend in Northern California. I happened to meet two of these people shortly after

their gathering. They shared a small pile of photographs taken during the weekend. The photos show a bunch of people hanging out in a nice place, nothing remarkable at all. The photos, though, stimulated these two women to recount parts of the weekend, and it soon became clear how potent it had been. The simple act of coming together to share experiences was what they needed to name an oppressive force. Speaking the unspoken is at once both personal and political. In this case, collective action arises from the recognition that one's individual life is not an isolated experience. Cheryl says of her work with ISNA, "If I wasn't doing this, I'd be dead now." Cheryl and other ISNA members are providing an opportunity for other intersexuals, who may be confused or despairing, to continue their healing among those who know the pain from first hand experience. And in doing so, they will change the world.

I am a lesbian parent of two sons. (Or at least I'm assuming they're male, until they tell me otherwise.) When my oldest child was born eight years ago, a lot of people thought that it was unfair to bring a child into the world to face the anticipated harassment he would receive as the son of lesbians. As a parent, it is painful to think that my children will face prejudice (and they will never face discrimination based on their skin color, language learned at home, or income level). I didn't send my son to be raised by a straight couple; instead, I've tried to do what I can to reduce negative attitudes about lesbians. I am lucky that I live in a community that supports me in doing this. It certainly would have been harder and more isolating to take this approach in other parts of the country (even 50 miles from here). But not impossible. Some people are willing to take risks in the hopes that oppressive attitudes or power structures will change. As feminists, what can we do to help parents of intersexual children accept their children as they are and fight to change a world that says they should be changed?

❝**The Five Sexes, Revisited**❞

by Anne Fausto-Sterling

As Cheryl Chase stepped to the front of the packed meeting room in the Sheraton Boston Hotel, nervous coughs made the tension audible. Chase, an activist for intersexual rights, had been invited to address the May 2000 meeting of the Lawson Wilkins Pediatric Endocrine Society (LWPES), the largest organization in the United States for specialists in children's hormones. Her talk would be the grand finale to a four-hour symposium on the treatment of genital ambiguity in newborns, infants born with a mixture of both male and female anatomy, or genitals that appear to differ from their chromosomal sex. The topic was hardly a novel one to the assembled physicians.

Yet Chase's appearance before the group was remarkable. Three and a half years earlier, the American Academy of Pediatrics had refused her request for a chance to present the patients' viewpoint on the treatment of genital ambiguity, dismissing Chase and her supporters as "zealots." About two dozen intersex people had responded by throwing up a picket line. The Intersex Society of North America (ISNA) even issued a press release: "Hermaphrodites Target Kiddie Docs."

It had done my 1960s street-activist heart good. In the short run, I said to Chase at the time, the picketing would make people angry. But eventually, I assured her, the doors then closed would open. Now, as Chase began to address the physicians at their own convention, that prediction was coming true. Her talk, titled "Sexual Ambiguity: The Patient-Centered Approach," was a measured critique of the near-universal practice of performing immediate, "corrective" surgery on thousands of infants born each year with ambiguous genitalia. Chase herself lives with the consequences of such surgery. Yet her audience, the very endocrinologists and surgeons Chase was accusing of reacting with "surgery and shame," received her with respect. Even more remarkably, many of the speakers who preceded her at the session had already spoken of the need to scrap current practices in favor of treatments more centered on psychological counseling.

What led to such a dramatic reversal of fortune? Certainly, Chase's talk at the LWPES symposium was a vindication of her persistence in seeking attention for her cause. But her invitation to speak was also a watershed in the evolving discussion about how to treat children with ambiguous genitalia. And that discussion, in turn, is the tip of a biocultural iceberg—the gender iceberg—that continues to rock both medicine and our culture at large.

Chase made her first national appearance in 1993, in these very pages, announcing the formation of ISNA in a letter responding to an essay I had written for *The Sciences*, titled "The Five Sexes" [March/April 1993]. In that article I argued that the two-sex system embedded in our society is not adequate to encompass the full spectrum of human sexuality. In its place, I suggested a five-sex system. In addition to males and females, I included "herms" (named after true hermaphrodites, people born with both a testis and an ovary); "merms" (male pseudo-hermaphrodites, who are born with testes and some aspect of female genitalia); and "ferms" (female pseudo-hermaphrodites, who have ovaries combined with some aspect of male genitalia).

I had intended to be provocative, but I had also written with tongue firmly in cheek. So I was surprised by the extent of the controversy the article unleashed. Right-wing Christians were outraged, and connected my idea of five sexes with the United Nations—sponsored Fourth World Conference on Women, held in Beijing in September 1995. At the same time, the article delighted others who felt constrained by the current sex and gender system.

Clearly, I had struck a nerve. The fact that so many people could get riled up by my proposal to revamp our sex and gender system suggested that change—as well as resistance to it—might be in the offing. Indeed, a lot has changed since 1993, and I like to think that my article was an important stimulus. As if from nowhere, intersexuals are materializing before our very eyes. Like Chase, many have become political organizers, who lobby physicians and politicians to change current treatment practices. But more generally, though perhaps no less provocatively, the boundaries separating masculine and feminine seem harder than ever to define.

Some find the changes under way deeply disturbing. Others find them liberating.

"The Five Sexes, Revisited," by Anne Fausto-Sterling, *The Sciences*, July/August 2000, Volume 40, pp. 18–24. Reprinted by permission of The New York Academy of Sciences.

Who is an intersexual—and how many intersexuals are there? The concept of intersexuality is rooted in the very ideas of male and female. In the idealized, Platonic, biological world, human beings are divided into two kinds: a perfectly dimorphic species. Males have an X and a Y chromosome, testes, a penis and all of the appropriate internal plumbing for delivering urine and semen to the outside world. They also have well-known secondary sexual characteristics, including a muscular build and facial hair. Women have two X chromosomes, ovaries, all of the internal plumbing to transport urine and ova to the outside world, a system to support pregnancy and fetal development, as well as a variety of recognizable secondary sexual characteristics.

That idealized story papers over many obvious caveats: some women have facial hair, some men have none; some women speak with deep voices, some men veritably squeak. Less well known is the fact that, on close inspection, absolute dimorphism disintegrates even at the level of basic biology. Chromosomes, hormones, the internal sex structures, the gonads and the external genitalia all vary more than most people realize. Those born outside of the Platonic dimorphic mold are called intersexuals.

In "The Five Sexes" I reported an estimate by a psychologist expert in the treatment of intersexuals, suggesting that some 4 percent of all live births are intersexual. Then, together with a group of Brown University undergraduates, I set out to conduct the first systematic assessment of the available data on intersexual birthrates. We scoured the medical literature for estimates of the frequency of various categories of intersexuality, from additional chromosomes to mixed gonads, hormones and genitalia. For some conditions we could find only anecdotal evidence; for most, however, numbers exist. On the basis of that evidence, we calculated that for every 1,000 children born, seventeen are intersexual in some form. That number—1.7 percent—is a ballpark estimate, not a precise count, though we believe it is more accurate than the 4 percent I reported.

Our figure represents all chromosomal, anatomical and hormonal exceptions to the dimorphic ideal; the number of intersexuals who might, potentially, be subject to surgery as infants is smaller—probably between one in 1,000 and one in 2,000 live births. Furthermore, because some populations possess the relevant genes at high frequency, the intersexual birthrate is not uniform throughout the world.

Consider, for instance, the gene for congenital adrenal hyperplasia (CAH). When the CAH gene is inherited from both parents, it leads to a baby with masculinized external genitalia who possesses two X chromosomes and the internal reproductive organs of a potentially fertile woman. The frequency of the gene varies widely around the world: in New Zealand it occurs in only forty-three children per million; among the Yupik Eskimo of southwestern Alaska, its frequency is 3,500 per million.

Intersexuality has always been to some extent a matter of definition. And in the past century physicians have been the ones who defined children as intersexual—and provided the remedies. When only the chromosomes are unusual, but the external genitalia and gonads clearly indicate either a male or a female, physicians do not advocate intervention. Indeed, it is not clear what kind of intervention could be advocated in such cases. But the story is quite different when infants are born with mixed genitalia, or with external genitals that seem at odds with the baby's gonads.

Most clinics now specializing in the treatment of intersex babies rely on case-management principles developed in the 1950s by the psychologist John Money and the psychiatrists Joan G. Hampson and John L. Hampson, all of Johns Hopkins University in Baltimore, Maryland. Money believed that gender identity is completely malleable for about eighteen months after birth. Thus, he argued, when a treatment team is presented with an infant who has ambiguous genitalia, the team could make a gender assignment solely on the basis of what made the best surgical sense. The physicians could then simply encourage the parents to raise the child according to the surgically assigned gender. Following that course, most physicians maintained, would eliminate psychological distress for both the patient and the parents. Indeed, treatment teams were never to use such words as "intersex" or "hermaphrodite"; instead, they were to tell parents that nature intended the baby to be the boy or the girl that the physicians had determined it was. Through surgery, the physicians were merely completing nature's intention.

Although Money and the Hampsons published detailed case studies of intersex children who they said had adjusted well to their gender assignments, Money thought one case in particular proved his theory. It was a dramatic example, inasmuch as it did not involve intersexuality at all: one of a pair of identical twin boys lost his penis as a result of a circumcision accident. Money recommended that "John" (as he came to be known in a later case study) be surgically turned into "Joan" and raised as a girl. In time, Joan grew to love wearing dresses and having her hair done. Money proudly proclaimed the sex reassignment a success.

But as recently chronicled by John Colapinto, in his book *As Nature Made Him*, Joan—now known to be an adult male named David Reimer—eventually rejected his female assignment. Even without a functioning penis and testes (which had been removed as part of the reassignment) John/Joan sought masculinizing medication, and married a woman with children (whom he adopted).

Since the full conclusion to the John/Joan story came to light, other individuals who were reassigned as males or females shortly after birth but who later rejected their early assignments have come forward. So, too, have cases in which the reassignment has worked—at least into the subject's mid-twenties. But even then the aftermath of the surgery can be problematic. Genital surgery often leaves scars that reduce sexual sensitivity. Chase herself had a complete clitoridectomy, a procedure that is less frequently performed on intersexuals today. But the newer surgeries, which reduce the size of the clitoral shaft, still greatly reduce sensitivity.

The revelation of cases of failed reassignments and the emergence of intersex activism have led an increasing number of pediatric endocrinologists, urologists and psychologists to reexamine the wisdom of early genital surgery. For example, in a talk that preceded Chase's at the LWPES meeting, the medical ethicist Laurence B. McCullough of the Center for Medical Ethics and Health Policy at Baylor College of Medicine in Houston, Texas, introduced an ethical framework for the treatment of children with ambiguous genitalia. Because sex phenotype (the manifestation of genetically and embryologically determined sexual characteristics) and gender presentation (the sex role projected by the individual in society) are highly variable, McCullough argues, the various forms of intersexuality should be defined as normal. All of them fall within the statistically expected variability of sex and gender. Furthermore, though certain disease states may accompany some forms of intersexuality, and may require medical intervention, intersexual conditions are not themselves diseases.

McCullough also contends that in the process of assigning gender, physicians should minimize what he calls irreversible assignments: taking steps such as the surgical removal or modification of gonads or genitalia that the patient may one day want to have reversed. Finally, McCullough urges physicians to abandon their practice of treating the birth of a child with genital ambiguity as a medical or social emergency. Instead, they should take the time to perform a thorough medical workup and should disclose everything to the parents, including the uncertainties about the final outcome. The treatment mantra, in other words, should be therapy, not surgery.

I believe a new treatment protocol for intersex infants, similar to the one outlined by McCullough, is close at hand. Treatment should combine some basic medical and ethical principles with a practical but less drastic approach to the birth of a mixed-sex child. As a first step, surgery on infants should be performed only to save the child's life or to substantially improve the child's physical well-being. Physicians may assign a sex—male or female—to an intersex infant on the basis of the probability that the child's particular condition will lead to the formation of a particular gender identity. At the same time, though, practitioners ought to be humble enough to recognize that as the child grows, he or she may reject the assignment—and they should be wise enough to listen to what the child has to say. Most important, parents should have access to the full range of information and options available to them.

Sex assignments made shortly after birth are only the beginning of a long journey. Consider, for instance, the life of Max Beck: Born intersexual, Max was surgically assigned as a female and consistently raised as such. Had her medical team followed her into her early twenties, they would have deemed her assignment a success because she was married to a man. (It should be noted that success in gender assignment has traditionally been defined as living in that gender as a heterosexual.) Within a few years, however, Beck had come out as a butch lesbian; now in her mid-thirties, Beck has become a man and married his lesbian partner, who (through the miracles of modern reproductive technology) recently gave birth to a girl.

Transsexuals, people who have an emotional gender at odds with their physical sex, once described themselves in terms of dimorphic absolutes—males trapped in female bodies, or vice versa. As such, they sought psychological relief through surgery. Although many still do, some so-called transgendered people today are content to inhabit a more ambiguous zone. A male-to-female transsexual, for instance, may come out as a lesbian. Jane, born a physiological male, is now in her late thirties and living with her wife, whom she married when her name was still John. Jane takes hormones to feminize herself, but they have not yet interfered with her ability to engage in intercourse as a man. In her mind Jane has a lesbian relationship with her wife, though she views their intimate moments as a cross between lesbian and heterosexual sex.

It might seem natural to regard intersexuals and transgendered people as living midway between the poles of male and female. But male and female, masculine and feminine, cannot be parsed as some kind of continuum. Rather, sex and gender are best conceptualized as points in a multidimensional space. For some time, experts on gender development have distinguished between sex at the genetic level and at the cellular level (sex-specific gene expression, X and Y chromosomes); at the hormonal level (in the fetus, during childhood and after puberty); and at the anatomical level (genitals and secondary sexual characteristics). Gender identity presumably emerges from all of those corporeal aspects via some poorly understood interaction with environment and experience. What has become increasingly clear is that one can find levels of masculinity and femininity in almost every possible permutation. A chromosomal, hormonal and genital male (or female) may emerge with a female (or male) gender identity. Or a chromosomal female with male fetal hormones and masculinized genitalia—but with female pubertal hormones—may develop a female gender identity.

The medical and scientific communities have yet to adopt a language that is capable of describing such diversity. In her book *Hermaphrodites and the Medical Invention of Sex*, the historian and medical ethicist Alice Domurat Dreger of Michigan State University in East Lansing documents the emergence of current medical systems for classifying gender ambiguity. The current usage remains rooted in the Victorian approach to sex. The logical structure of the commonly used terms "true hermaphrodite," "male pseudohermaphrodite" and "female pseudohermaphrodite" indicates that only the so-called true hermaphrodite is a genuine mix of male and female. The others, no matter how confusing their body parts, are really hidden males or females. Because true hermaphrodites are rare—possibly only one in 100,000—such a classification system supports the idea that human beings are an absolutely dimorphic species.

At the dawn of the twenty-first century, when the variability of gender seems so visible, such a position is hard to maintain. And here, too, the old medical consensus has begun to crumble. Last fall the pediatric urologist Ian A. Aaronson of the Medical University of South Carolina in Charleston organized the North American Task Force on Intersexuality (NATFI) to review the clinical responses to genital ambiguity in infants. Key medical associations, such as the American Academy of Pediatrics, have endorsed NATFI. Specialists in surgery, endocrinology, psychology, ethics, psychiatry, genetics and public health, as well as intersex patient-advocate groups, have joined its ranks.

One of the goals of NATFI is to establish a new sex nomenclature. One proposal under consideration replaces the current system with emotionally neutral terminology that emphasizes developmental processes rather than preconceived gender categories. For example, Type I intersexes develop out of anomalous viriliz-

ing influences; Type II result from some interruption of virilization; and in Type III intersexes the gonads themselves may not have developed in the expected fashion.

What is clear that since 1993, modern society has moved beyond five sexes to a recognition that gender variation is normal and, for some people, an arena for playful exploration. Discussing my "five sexes" proposal in her book *Lessons from the Intersexed*, the psychologist Suzanne J. Kessler of the State University of New York at Purchase drives this point home with great effect:

> The limitation with Fausto-Sterling's proposal is that . . . [it] still gives genitals . . . primary signifying status and ignores the fact that in the everyday world gender attributions are made without access to genital inspection. . . . What has primacy in everyday life is the gender that is performed, regardless of the flesh's configuration under the clothes.

I now agree with Kessler's assessment. It would be better for intersexuals and their supporters to turn everyone's focus away from genitals. Instead, as she suggests, one should acknowledge that people come in an even wider assortment of sexual identities and characteristics than mere genitals can distinguish. Some women may have "large clitorises or fused labia," whereas some men may have "small penises or misshapen scrota," as Kessler puts it, "phenotypes with no particular clinical or identity meaning."

As clearheaded as Kessler's program is—and despite the progress made in the 1990s—our society is still far from that ideal. The intersexual or transgendered person who projects a social gender—what Kessler calls "cultural genitals"—that conflicts with his or her physical genitals still may die for the transgression. Hence legal protection for people whose cultural and physical genitals do not match is needed during the current transition to a more gender-diverse world. One easy step would be to eliminate the category of "gender" from official documents, such as driver's licenses and passports. Surely attributes both more visible (such as height, build and eye color) and less visible (fingerprints and genetic profiles) would be more expedient.

A more far-ranging agenda is presented in the International Bill of Gender Rights, adopted in 1995 at the fourth annual International Conference on Transgender Law and Employment Policy in Houston, Texas. It lists ten "gender rights," including the right to define one's own gender, the right to change one's physical gender if one so chooses and the right to marry whomever one wishes. The legal bases for such rights are being hammered out in the courts as I write and, most recently, through the establishment, in the state of Vermont, of legal same-sex domestic partnerships.

No one could have foreseen such changes in 1993. And the idea that I played some role, however small, in reducing the pressure—from the medical community as well as from society at large—to flatten the diversity of human sexes into two diametrically opposed camps gives me pleasure.

Sometimes people suggest to me, with not a little horror, that I am arguing for a pastel world in which androgyny reigns and men and women are boringly the same. In my vision, however, strong colors coexist with pastels. There are and will continue to be highly masculine people out there; it's just that some of them are women. And some of the most feminine people I know happen to be men.

"Cultural Practice" or "Reconstructive Surgery"? "U.S. Genital Cutting, the Intersex Movement, and Medical Double Standards"

by Cheryl Chase

One of the forms of power that maintains gender boundaries in the United States is the surgical "correction" of infants whose genitals are deemed by medical professionals to be socially unacceptable. Media and scholarly discourses on "female genital mutilation," however, have not engaged these surgeries, instead serving up only representations of African women. These discourses continue a long tradition of making Africans into the "others," suggesting that ethnocentrism is a key factor in the sometimes purposeful maintenance of ignorance about contemporary U.S. genital surgeries. This essay will describe how Americans participate in the production of normatively sexed bodies from those born intersexed, the consequences of such genital surgeries for those subjected to them, the efforts of intersex people to organize to eliminate pediatric genital surgeries and how those efforts have been treated by many feminists, and the double standard regarding representations of genital cutting, depending upon who is cutting and where in the world the cutting is done.

"New Law Bans Genital Cutting in United States" read the headline on the front page of the *New York Times*. The law seems clear enough: "Whoever knowingly circumcises, excises, or infibulates the whole or any part of the labia majora or labia minor or clitoris of another person who has not attained the age of eighteen years shall be fined under this title or imprisoned not more than five years, or both." Yet this law was not intended and has not been interpreted to protect the approximately five children per day in the United States who are subjected to excision of part or all of their clitoris and inner labia simply because doctors believe their clitoris is too big.

Sexual anatomies, genitals in particular, come in many sizes and shapes. U.S. doctors label children whose sexual anatomies differ significantly from the cultural ideal "intersexuals" or "hermaphrodites" (a misleading term because these children are born with intermediate genitals, not two sets). Medical practice today holds that possession of a large clitoris, or a small penis, or a penis that has the urethra placed other than at its tip is a "psychosocial emergency." The child would not be accepted by the mother, would be teased by peers, and would not be able to develop into an emotionally healthy adult. The medical solution to this psychosocial problem is surgery—before the child reaches three months of age or even before the newborn is discharged from the hospital. Although parental emotional distress and rejection of the child and peer harassment are cited as the primary justifications for cosmetic genital surgery, there has never been an investigation of nonsurgical means—such as professional counseling or peer support—to address these issues.

The federal Law to Ban Female Genital Mutilation notwithstanding, girls born with large clitorises are today routinely "normalized" by excising parts of the clitoris and burying the remainder deep within the genital region. And boys with small penises? Current medical practice holds that intersex children "can be raised successfully as members of either sex if the process begins before 2½ years." Because surgeons cannot create a large penis from a small one, the policy is to remove testes and raise these children as girls. This is accomplished by "carv[ing] a large phallus down into a clitoris, creat[ing] a vagina using a piece of [the child's] colon," marveled a science writer who spoke only to physicians and parents, not to any of the intersex people subjected to this miracle technology. Efforts to create or extend a penile urethra in boys whose urethra exits other than at the tip of the penis—a condition called hypospadias—frequently lead to multiple surgeries, each compounding the harm. Heart-rending stories of physical and emotional carnage are related by victims of these surgeries in "Growing up in the Surgical Maelstrom" and, with black humor, in "Take Charge: A Guide to Home Catheterization."

"Reconstructive" surgeries for intersex infant genitals first came into wide-spread practice in the 1950s. Because intersexuality was treated as shameful and physicians actively discouraged open discussion by their patients—indeed, recommended lying to parents and to adult intersex patients—until recently most victims of these interventions suffered alone in shame and silence.

By 1993 the accomplishments of a progression of social justice movements—civil rights, feminism, gay and lesbian, bisexual and transgender—helped make it possible for intersex people to speak out. Initially, physicians scoffed at their assertions that intersexuality was not shameful and that medically unnecessary genital surgeries were mutilating and should be halted. One surgeon from Johns Hopkins, the institution primarily responsible for developing the current medical model, dismissed intersex patient-advocates as "zealots." Others cited the technological imperative. Doctors "don't really have a choice" about whether or not to perform surgery insists George Szasz.

By 1997 the intersex movement had gathered enough strength to visit Congress and ask that the Law to Ban Female Genital Mutilation be enforced to protect children not only against practices imported from other cultures but also against this uniquely American medicalized form of mutilation. Their work won coverage in the *New York Times* and on *Dateline NBC,* and by the following year the *Urology Times* was reporting a small but growing "new tidal wave of opinion" from physicians and sex researchers supporting the activists. Sad to report, the struggle of intersex activists against American medicalized genital mutilation has yet to attract significant support or even notice from feminists and journalists who express outrage over African genital cutting.

Hermaphrodites: Medical Authority and Cultural Invisibility

Many people familiar with the ideas that gender is a phenomenon not adequately described by male/female dimorphism and that the interpretation of physical sex differences is culturally constructed remain surprised to learn how variable sexual anatomy is. Although the male/female binary is constructed as natural and therefore presumably immutable, the phenomenon of intersexuality offers clear evidence that physical sex is not binary. Intersexuality therefore furnishes an opportunity to deploy "the natural" strategically as a means for disrupting heteronormative systems of sex/gender/sexuality. The concept of bodily sex, in popular usage, refers to multiple characteristics, including karyotype (organization of sex chromosomes); gonadal differentiation (e.g., ovarian or testicular); genital morphology; configuration of internal reproductive organs; and pubertal sex characteristics such as breasts and facial hair. These characteristics are assumed and expected to be concordant in each individual—either all-male or all-female.

Because medicine intervenes quickly in intersex births to change the infant's body, the phenomenon of intersexuality has been, until recently, largely unknown outside specialized medical practices. General public awareness of intersex bodies slowly vanished in modern Western European societies as medicine gradually appropriated to itself the authority to interpret—and eventually manage—the much older category of "hermaphroditism." Victorian medical taxonomy began to efface hermaphroditism as a legitimated status by settling on gonadal histology as the arbiter of "true sex." The Victorian taxonomy (still in use by medical specialists) required both ovarian and testicular tissue types, microscopically confirmed, to be present in a "true hermaphrodite." Conveniently, given the limitations of Victorian surgery and anesthesia, such confirmation was impossible in a living patient. All other anomalies were reclassified as "pseudo-hermaphroditisms" masking a "true sex" determined by the gonads.

With advances in anesthesia, surgery, embryology, and endocrinology, however, twentieth-century medicine moved from merely labeling intersexed bodies to the far more invasive practice of "fixing" them—altering their physical appearance to conform with a diagnosed true sex. The techniques and protocols for physically transforming intersexed bodies were developed primarily at Johns Hopkins University in Baltimore during the 1920s and 1930s under the guidance of urologist Hugh Hampton Young. "Only during the last few years," Young enthused in the preface to his pioneering textbook *Genital Abnormalities,* have we begun "to get somewhere near the explanation of the marvels of anatomic abnormality that may be portrayed by these amazing individuals. But the surgery of the hermaphrodite has remained a terra incognito." The "sad state of these unfortunates" prompted Young to devise "a great variety of surgical procedures" by which he attempted to normalize the their bodily appearances to the greatest extent possible.

Quite a few of Young's patients resisted his efforts. Emma T., a "'snappy' young negro woman with a good figure" and a large clitoris, had married a man but found her passion only with women. Emma refused surgery to "be made into a man" because removal of her vagina would mean the loss of her "meal ticket" (i.e., her husband). By the 1950s, the principle of rapid postnatal detection and intervention for intersex infants had been developed at Johns Hopkins, with the stated goal of completing surgery early enough so the child would have no memory of it. One wonders whether the insistence on early intervention was not at least partly motivated by the resistance offered by adult intersex people to "normalization" through surgery. Frightened parents of ambiguously sexed infants were much more open to suggestions of normalizing surgery than were intersex adults, and the infants themselves could, of course, offer no resistance whatsoever.

Most of the theoretical foundations justifying these interventions are attributable to psychologist John Money, a sex researcher invited to Johns Hopkins by Lawson Wilkins, founder of pediatric endocrinology. Wilkins's numerous students subsequently carried these protocols from Hopkins to hospitals throughout the United States and abroad. In 1998 Suzanne Kessler noted that Money's ideas enjoyed a "consensus of approval rarely encountered in science." But the revelation in 2000 that Money had grossly misrepresented and mishandled the famous "John/Joan" case (in which an infant was castrated and raised as a girl after his penis was destroyed in a circumcision accident) sent Money's stock into a steep decline.

In keeping with the Hopkins model, the birth of an intersex infant is today deemed a "psychosocial emergency" that propels a multi-disciplinary team of intersex specialists into action. Significantly, they are surgeons and endocrinologists rather than psychologists, bioethicists, intersex peer support organizations, or parents of intersex children. The team examines the infant and chooses either male or female as a "sex of assignment," then informs the parents that this is the child's *true* sex. Medical technology, including surgery and hormones, is then used to make the child's body conform as closely as possible to the assigned sex.

Current protocols for choosing a sex are based on phallus size: to qualify for male assignment the child must posses a penis at least one inch long; clitorises may not exceed three-eighths inch. Infants with genital appendages in the forbidden zone of three-eighths to one inch are assigned female and the phallus trimmed to an acceptable size. The only exception to this sorting rule is that even a hypothetical possibility of female fertility must be preserved by assigning the infant as female, disregarding masculine genitals and a phallus longer than one inch.

The sort of deviation from sex norms exhibited by intersex people is so highly stigmatized that emotional harm due to likely parental rejection and community stigmatization of the intersex child provides physicians with their most compelling argument to justify medically unnecessary surgical interventions. Intersex status is considered to be so incompatible with emotional health that misrepresentation, concealment of facts, and outright lying (both to parents and later to the intersex person) are unabashedly advocated in professional medical literature.

The Impact of "Reconstructive" Surgeries

The insistence on two clearly distinguished sexes has calamitous personal consequences for the many individuals who arrive in the world with sexual anatomy that fails to be easily distinguished as male or female, who are labeled "intersexuals" or "hermaphrodites" by modern medical discourse. About one in one hundred births exhibits some anomaly in sex differentiation, and about one in two thousand is different enough to render problematic the question, Is it a boy or a girl? Since the early 1960s, nearly every medium-sized or larger city in the United States has had at least one hospital with a standing team of medical experts who intervene in these cases to "assign"—through drastic surgical means—a male or female status to intersex infants. The fact that this system for enforcing the boundaries of the categories "male" and "female" existed for so long without drawing criticism or scrutiny from any quarters is an indication of the extreme discomfort that sexual ambiguity excites in our culture. Pediatric genital surgeries literalize what many might otherwise consider a purely theoretical operation—the attempted production of normatively sexed bodies and gendered subjects through constitutive acts of violence. Since the early 1990s, however, intersex people have begun to politicize intersex subjectivity, thus transforming intensely personal experiences of violation into collective opposition to the medical regulation of bodies that queers the foundations of heteronormative gender identifications and sexual orientations.

This system of hushing up the fact of intersex births and using technology to normalize intersex bodies has caused profound emotional and physical harm to intersex people and their families. The harm begins when the birth is treated as a medical crisis, and the consequences of that initial treatment ripple out ever afterward. The emotional impact of this treatment is so devastating that until the middle of the 1990s people whose lives have been touched by intersexuality maintained silence about their ordeal. As recently as 1993, no one publicly disputed surgeon Milton Edgerton when he wrote that in forty years of clitoral surgery on children "*not one has complained of loss of sensation, even when the entire clitoris was removed*" (emphasis in the original).

The tragic irony in all this is that while intersexual anatomy occasionally indicates an underlying medical problem such as adrenal disorder, ambiguous genitals are, in and of themselves, neither painful nor harmful to health. The often debilitating pediatric genital surgeries are entirely cosmetic in function. Surgery is essentially a destructive process. It can remove tissue and to a limited extent relocate it, but it cannot create new structures. This technical limitation, taken together with the framing of the feminine as a condition of lack, leads physicians to assign 90 percent of anatomically ambiguous infants as female by excising genital tissue. Surgeons justify female assignment because "you can make a hole, but you can't build a pole." Heroic efforts shore up a tenuous masculine status for the one-tenth assigned male, who are subjected to multiple operations—twenty-two in one case—with the goal of straightening the penis and constructing a urethra to enable standing urinary posture. For some, the surgeries end only when the child grows old enough to resist.

Children assigned female are subjected to surgery that removes the troubling hypertrophic (i.e., large) clitoris. This is the same tissue that would have been a troubling micropenis (i.e., small penis) had the child been assigned male. Through the 1960s, feminizing pediatric genital surgery was openly labeled "clitoridectomy" and was compared favorably to the African practices that have now become the focus of such intense scrutiny. As three Harvard surgeons noted, "Evidence that the clitoris is not essential for normal coitus may be gained from certain sociological data. For instance, it is the custom of a

number of African tribes to excise the clitoris and other parts of the external genitals. Yet normal sexual function is observed in these females." Authors Robert E. Gross, Judson Randolph, and John F. Crigler apparently understand normal female sexual function only as passive penetration and fertility. A modified operation that removes most of the clitoris and relocates a bit of its tip is variously (and euphemistically) called clitoroplasty, clitoral reduction, or clitoral recession and described as a simple cosmetic procedure in order to differentiate it from the now-infamous clitoridectomy. The operation, however, is far from benign.

Johns Hopkins surgeons Joseph E. Oesterling, John P. Gearhart, and Robert D. Jeffs have described their technique. They make an incision around the clitoris, at the corona, then dissect the skin away from its underside. Next they dissect the skin away from the upper side and remove as much of the clitoral shaft as necessary to create an "appropriate size clitoris." Then they place stitches from the pubic area along both sides of the entire length of what remains of the clitoris; when they tighten these stitches, the tissue folds, like pleats in a skirt, and recesses into a concealed position behind the pubic mound. If they think the result still "too large," they further reduce the tip of the clitoris by cutting away a pie-shaped wedge.

For many intersex people, this sort of arcane, dehumanized medical literature, illustrated with close-ups of genital surgery and naked children with blacked-out eyes, is the only available version of *Our Bodies, Ourselves*. Thus, even as fierce arguments over gender identity, gender role development, and social construction of gender rage in psychology, feminism, and queer theory, we have literally delegated to medicine the authority to police the boundaries of male and female, leaving intersex people to recover as best they can, alone and silent, from violent normalization.

My own case, as it turns out, was not unusual. I was born with ambiguous genitals. A doctor specializing in intersexuality deliberated for three days—and sedated my mother each time she asked what was wrong with her baby—before concluding that I was male, with micropenis, complete hypospadias, undescended testes, and a strange extra opening behind the urethra. A male birth certificate was completed for me, and my parents began raising me as a boy. When I was a year and a half old, my parents consulted a different set of intersex experts, who admitted me to a hospital for "sex determination." "Determine" is a remarkably apt word in this context, meaning both to *ascertain* by investigation and to *cause* to come to a resolution. It perfectly describes the two-level process whereby science produces through a series of masked operations what it claims merely to observe. Doctors told my parents that a thorough medical investigation, including exploratory surgery, would be necessary to determine (that is, ascertain) what my "true sex" was. They judged my genital appendage to be inadequate as a penis: too short to effectively mark masculine status or to penetrate females. As a female, however, I would be penetrable and potentially fertile. My anatomy having now been re-labeled as vagina, urethra, labia, and outsized clitoris, my sex was next determined (in the second sense) by amputating my genital appendage—clitoridectomy. Following doctors' orders, my parents then changed my name; combed their house to eliminate all traces of my existence as a boy (photographs, birthday cards, etc.); engaged a lawyer to change my birth certificate; moved to a different town; instructed extended family members to no longer refer to me as a boy; and never told anyone else—including me—just what had happened. My intersexuality and change of sex were the family's dirty little secrets.

At age eight, I was returned to the hospital for abdominal surgery that trimmed away the testicular portion of my gonads, each of which was partly ovarian and partly testicular in character. No explanation was given to me then for the long hospital stay or the abdominal surgery, nor for the regular hospital visits afterward in which doctors photographed my genitals and inserted fingers and instruments into my vagina and anus. These visits ceased as soon as I began to menstruate. At the time of the sex change, doctors had assured my parents that their once-son/now-daughter would grow into a woman who could have a normal sex life and babies. With the confirmation of menstruation, my parents apparently concluded that that prediction had borne out and their ordeal was behind them. For me, the worst part of the nightmare was just beginning.

As an adolescent, I became aware that I had no clitoris or inner labia and was unable to experience orgasm. By the end of my teens, I began to research in medical libraries, trying to discover what might have happened to me. When I finally determined to obtain my personal medical records, it took three years to overcome the obstruction of the doctors whom I asked for help. When I did obtain a scant three pages from my medical files, I learned for the first time that I was a "true hermaphrodite" who had been my parents' son for a year and a half, with a name that was unfamiliar to me. The records also documented my clitoridectomy. This was the middle 1970s, when I was in my early twenties. I had come to identify myself as lesbian at a time when lesbianism and a biologically based gender essentialism were virtually syn-

onymous. Men were rapists who caused war and environmental destruction; women were loving beings who would heal the earth; lesbians were a superior form of being uncontaminated by "men's energy." In such a world, how could I tell anyone that I had actually possessed the dreaded "phallus"? I was an impostor, not really a woman but rather a monstrous and mythical creature. And because my hermaphroditism and long-buried boyhood were the history that underlay the clitoridectomy, I could never speak openly about that either, or about my consequent inability to orgasm. I was so traumatized by discovering the circumstances that produced my embodiment that I could not speak of these matters with anyone.

Nearly fifteen years later, in my middle thirties, I suffered an emotional meltdown. In the eyes of the world I was a highly successful businesswoman, a principal in an international high-tech company. To myself, I was a freak, incapable of loving or being loved, filled with shame about my status as a hermaphrodite, about the imagined appearance of my genitals before surgery (I thought "true hermaphrodite" meant that I had been born with a penis), and about my sexual dysfunction. Unable to make peace with these facts about myself, I finally sought help from a professional therapist, only to find my experience denied. She reacted to each revelation about my history and predicament with some version of "no it's not" or "so what?" I'd say, "I'm not really a woman." She would say, "Of course you are. You look female." I'd say, "My complete withdrawal from sexuality has destroyed every relationship I've ever entered." She would say, "Everybody has their ups and downs." I tried another therapist and met with a similar response. Increasingly desperate, I confided my story to several friends who shrank away in embarrassed silence. I was in emotional agony and found myself utterly alone, with no possible way out. I decided to kill myself.

Confronting suicide as a real possibility proved to be my personal epiphany. In contemplating my own death, I fantasized killing myself quite messily and dramatically in the office of the surgeon who had sliced out my clitoris, forcibly confronting him with the horror he had imposed on my life. But in acknowledging that desire to put my pain to some use, not to waste my life completely, I turned a crucial corner, finding a way to direct my rage productively out into the world rather than aim it destructively at myself. My breakdown became my breakthrough, and I vowed that, whatever it took, I would heal myself. Still, I had no conceptual framework for developing a more positive self-consciousness. I knew only that I felt mutilated, not fully woman, less than fully human even, but I was determined to heal. I struggled for weeks in emotional chaos, unable to eat or sleep or work. I could not accept my image of a hermaphroditic body any more than I could accept the butchered one left me by the surgeons. Thoughts of myself as a Frankenstein patchwork alternated with longings for escape by death, only to be followed by outrage, anger, and determination to survive. I could not accept that it was just or right or good to treat any person as I had been treated—my sex changed, my genitals cut up, my experience silenced and rendered invisible. I bore a private hell within me, wretchedly alone in my condition without even my tormentors for company. Finally, I began to envision myself standing in a driving rain storm but with clear skies and a rainbow visible in the distance. I was still in agony, still alone, but I was beginning to see the painful process in which I was caught up in terms of revitalization and rebirth, a means of investing my life with a new sense of authenticity possessing vast potentials for further transformation. Since then I have seen this experience described by other intersex and transsexual activists.

I slowly developed a newly politicized and critically aware form of self-understanding. I had been the kind of lesbian who at times had a girlfriend but who had never really participated in the life of a lesbian community. I felt almost completely isolated from gay politics, feminism, and queer and gender theory. I did possess the rudimentary knowledge that the gay civil rights movement had gathered momentum only when it could effectively deny that homosexuality was sick or inferior and assert to the contrary that "gay is good." As impossible as it then seemed, I pledged similarly to affirm that "intersex is good" and that the body I was born with was not sick or shameful, only different. I vowed to embrace the sense of being "not a woman" that I had initially been so terrified to discover.

I began a search for community that brought me to San Francisco in the fall of 1992 on the theory that people living in the "queer Mecca" would have the most conceptually sophisticated, socially tolerant, and politically astute analysis of sexed and gendered embodiment. I found what I was looking for, in part because my arrival in the Bay Area corresponded with the rather sudden emergence of an energetic transgender political movement. At the same time, a vigorous new wave of gender scholarship had emerged in the academy. In this context, Morgan Holmes could analyze her own clitoridectomy for her master's thesis and have her study taken seriously as academic work. Openly transsexual scholars, including Susan Stryker and Sandy Stone, were visible in responsible academic positions at major universities.

Into this heady atmosphere, I brought my own experience. I started telling my story to everyone I met. Before long I learned of six other intersex people—including two who had been fortunate enough to escape medical attention. Realizing that intersexuality, rather than being extremely rare, must be relatively common, I decided to create a support network. Soon I was receiving several letters per week from intersex people throughout the United States and Canada and a few from further afield. Although details varied, the letters gave a remarkably coherent picture of the emotional consequences of medical intervention:

> All the things my body might have grown to do, all the possibilities, went down the hall with my amputated clitoris to the pathology department. The rest of me went to the recovery room—I'm still recovering.
>
> —Morgan Holmes

> I am horrified by what has been done to me and by the conspiracy of silence and lies. I am filled with grief and rage, but also relief finally to believe that maybe I am not the only one.
>
> —Angela Moreno

> As soon as I saw the title *Hermaphrodites with Attitude* I cried aloud for sheer joy. . . . Finally I can say, 'I'm hermaphrodite, I'm intersex, I'm transgender, I'm queer and damn proud,' as tears of joy and belonging stream down my face.
>
> —Lee

> Doctors never consulted me. . . . [T]he idea of asking for my opinion about having my penis surgically altered apparently never occurred to them. . . . Far too many people allow social stigma to cloud their judgment. It's OK to be different.
>
> —Randy

> I pray that I will have the means to repay, in some measure, the American Urological Association for all that it has done for my benefit. I am having some trouble, though, in connecting the timing mechanism to the fuse.
>
> —Thomas

Toward Social Justice

The peer support network that I formed grew into the Intersex Society of North America (ISNA). ISNA's long-term and fundamental goal is to change the way intersex infants are treated. We advocate that surgery not be performed on children born with ambiguous genitals unless there is a medical reason (to prevent physical pain or illness) and that parents be given the conceptual tools and emotional support to accept their children's physical differences. We also advocate that children be raised either as boys or girls, according to which designation seems likely to offer the child the greatest future sense of comfort. Advocating gender assignment without resorting to normalizing surgery is a radical position given that it requires the willful disruption of the assumed concordance between body shape and gender category. However, this is the only position that prevents irreversible physical damage to the intersex person's body, that preserves the intersex person's agency regarding their own flesh, and that recognizes genital sensation and erotic functioning to be at least as important as reproductive capacity. If an intersex child or adult decides to change gender or to undergo surgical or hormonal alteration of his/her body, that decision should also be fully respected and facilitated. The key point is that intersex subjects should not be violated for the comfort and convenience of others.

One part of reaching ISNA's long-term goal has been to document the emotional and physical carnage resulting from medical interventions. As a rapidly growing literature (see the bibliography on our Web-site, <http://www.isna.org>) makes abundantly clear, the medical management of intersexuality has changed shockingly little in the more than forty years since my first surgery—doctors still cut up children's genitals and still perpetuate invisibility and silence around intersex lives. Kessler expresses surprise that "in spite of the thousands of genital operations performed every year, there are no meta-analyses from within the medical community on levels of success." Surgeons admit to not knowing whether their former patients are "silent and happy or silent and unhappy." There is no research effort to improve erotic functioning for adult intersex people whose genitals have been cut, nor are there psychotherapists who specialize in working with adult intersex clients trying to heal from the trauma of medical intervention. To provide a counterpoint to the mountains of professional medical literature that neglect intersex experience and to begin compiling an ethnographic account of that experience, ISNA has worked to make public the lives of intersex people through our own publications (including our video, Hermaphrodites Speak!) and by working with scholars and the popular media.

ISNA's presence has begun to be effective. It has helped politicize the growing number of intersex organizations as well as intersex identities themselves. When I first began organizing ISNA, I met leaders of the Turner's Syndrome Society, the oldest known support group focusing on atypical sexual differentiation founded in 1987. (Turner's Syndrome is defined by an XO genetic kary-

otype that results in a female body morphology with nonfunctioning ovaries, extremely short stature, and, variably, a variety of other visible physical differences still described in the medical literature with such stigmatizing labels as "web-necked" and "fish-mouthed.") Each of these women told me what a profound, life-changing experience it had been simply to meet another person like herself. I was inspired by their accomplishments (they are a national organization serving thousands of members) but wanted ISNA to have a different focus—less willing to think of intersexuality as a pathology or disability, more interested in challenging the medicalization of sexual difference entirely, and more interested in politicizing a pan-intersexual revolt across the divisions of particular etiologies in order to destabilize the heteronormative assumptions that underlie the violence directed at our bodies.

Public Discourse on Pediatric Genital Surgeries

Because the politicized intersex community is still quite young, and most intersex people remain too burdened by the crippling emotional consequences of what has been done to them to come out publicly, ISNA has deliberately cultivated a network of non-intersexed advocates who command a measure of social legitimacy and can speak in contexts where uninterpreted intersex voices will not be heard. Because there is a strong impulse to discount what intersex people have to say about themselves (as if we are too close to the issues to offer objective opinions), this sort of sympathetic representation has been welcome—especially in helping intersex people reframe intersexuality in nonmedical terms. Some gender theory scholars, feminist critics of science, medical historians, and anthropologists have been quick to understand and support intersex activism. Feminist biologist and science studies scholar Anne Fausto-Sterling—who wrote, years before ISNA came into existence, about intersexuality in relation to intellectually suspect scientific practices that perpetuate masculinist constructs of gender—became an early ISNA ally. Likewise, social psychologist Suzanne Kessler wrote a brilliant ethnography of surgeons who specialize in treating intersex. After speaking with a number of the normalized "products" of these medical programs, she, too, became a strong supporter of intersex activism. Historian of science Alice Dreger, whose work focuses not only on hermaphroditism but also on other forms of atypical embodiment that become subject to destructively normalizing medical interventions (as in her discussion of conjoined twins in "Limits of Individuality"), has been especially supportive. Fausto-Sterling, Kessler, and

Dreger have each written books that analyze the medical treatment of intersexuality as being culturally motivated and criticize it as often harmful to its ostensible patients.

Allies who help contest the medicalization of intersexuality have been especially important, because ISNA initially found direct, nonconfrontational interactions with medical specialists who determine policy on the treatment of intersex infants and actually carry out the surgeries to be both difficult and ineffective. Joycelyn Elders, the Clinton administration's first surgeon general, is a pediatric endocrinologist with many years of experience in managing intersex infants. In spite of a generally feminist approach to healthcare and frequent overtures from ISNA, she rejected the concerns of intersex people themselves.

Surgeon Richard Schlussel, at a pediatric plastic surgery symposium (which had rejected ISNA's offer to provide a patients' panel) at Mount Sinai Medical Center in New York City in 1996 proclaimed, "The parents of children with ambiguous genitals are more grateful to the surgeon than any—more grateful even than parents whose children's lives have been saved through open heart surgery."

Another pediatrician remarked in an Internet discussion on intersexuality, "I think this whole issue is preposterous. . . . To suggest that [medical decisions about the treatment of intersex] are somehow cruel or arbitrary is insulting, ignorant and misguided. . . . To spread the claims that [ISNA] is making is just plain wrong, and I hope that this [on-line group of doctors] will not blindly accept them." Yet another physician participating in that same chat, in a marvelous example of the degree to which practitioners of science can be blind to their complicity in constructing the objects they study, asked what was for him obviously a rhetorical question: "Who is the enemy? I really don't think it's the medical establishment. Since when did we establish the male/female hegemony?" Johns Hopkins surgeon Gearhart, quoted in a New York Times article on ISNA, summarily dismissed us as "zealots," but professional meetings in the fields of pediatrics, urology, genital plastic surgery, and endocrinology are abuzz with anxious and defensive discussion of intersex activism. In response to a 1996 protest by Hermaphrodites with Attitude at the American Academy of Pediatrics annual meeting, that organization felt compelled to hold a press conference and issue a statement: "The Academy is deeply concerned about the emotional, cognitive, and body image development of intersexuals, and believes that successful early genital surgery minimizes these issues." The academy refused, however, to speak with intersex people picketing its meeting.

The roots of resistance in the medical establishment to the truth-claims of intersex people run deep. Not only does ISNA's existence imply a critique of the normativistic biases couched within most scientific practice but it also advocates a treatment protocol for intersex infants that disrupts conventional understandings of the relationship between bodies and genders. On a level more personally threatening to medical practitioners, ISNA's position implies that they have—unwittingly at best and through willful denial at worst—spent their careers inflicting a profound harm from which their patients will never fully recover. ISNA's position threatens to destroy the foundational assumptions motivating an entire medical subspecialty, thus jeopardizing their continued ability to perform what surgeons find to be technically fascinating work. Science writer Melissa Hendricks notes that Gearhart is known to colleagues as an "artist" who can "carve a large phallus down into a clitoris" with consummate skill. Given these deep and mutually reinforcing reasons for opposing ISNA's position, it is hardly surprising that medical intersex specialists have, for the most part, turned a deaf ear toward us.

Thus, the most important aspect of our current activities is the struggle to change public perceptions. By using the mass media, the Internet, and our growing network of allies and sympathizers to make the general public aware of the frequency of intersexuality and of the intense suffering that medical treatment has caused, we seek to create an environment in which many parents will have already heard about the intersex movement when their intersex child is born. Such informed parents have proved better able to resist medical pressure for unnecessary genital surgery and secrecy and to find their way to a peer-support group and counseling rather than to a surgical theater.

The Double Standard: First-World Feminism, African Clitoridectomy and Intersex Genital Mutilation, and the Media

African practices that remove the clitoris and other parts of female genitals have lately been a target of intense media coverage and feminist activism in the United States and other industrialized Western societies, and the euphemism *female circumcision* has been largely supplanted by the politicized term *female genital mutilation* (FGM). Analogous medical (rather than folk) operations performed on intersex people in the United States have not been the focus of similar attention—indeed, attempts to link the two forms of genital cutting have met with multiform resistance. Examining the way that first-world feminists and mainstream media treat African practices and comparing that treatment with their response to intersex genital mutilation (IGM) in North America exposes some of the complex interactions between ideologies of race, gender, colonialism, and science that effectively silence and render invisible intersex experience in first-world contexts. Cutting intersex genitals becomes yet another hidden mechanism for imposing normalcy upon unruly flesh, a means of containing the potential anarchy of desires and identifications within oppressive heteronormative structures.

In 1994 the *New England Journal of Medicine* paired an article on the physical harm resulting from African genital cutting with an editorial denouncing clitoridectomy as a violation of human rights but declined to run a reply drafted by University of California at Berkeley medical anthropologist Lawrence Cohen and two ISNA members detailing the harm caused by medicalized American clitoridectomies. In response to growing media attention, Congress passed the Federal Prohibition of Female Genital Mutilation Act in October 1996. That act specifically exempted from prohibition medicalized clitoridectomies of the sort performed to "correct" intersex bodies. The bill's principal author, feminist Congresswoman Pat Schroeder, ignored multiple letters from ISNA members and Brown University professor of medical science Anne Fausto-Sterling asking her to recast the bill's language. "New Law Bans Genital Cutting," the *New York Times* proclaimed and refused to address documentation from ISNA and Michigan State University professor Alice Dreger pointing out that genital cutting continues to be standard medical practice in the United States.

The *Boston Globe's* syndicated columnist Ellen Goodman has been one of the few journalists covering African genital cutting to make any response to ISNA overtures. "I must admit I was not aware of this situation," she wrote to me in 1994. "I admire your courage." She continued, however, to discuss African genital cutting in her column without mentioning similar American practices. Ironically, Goodman is based in Boston, a Mecca of sorts after Johns Hopkins for the surgical management of intersex children, with prominent specialists operating at Harvard, Massachusetts General Hospital, and Boston Children's Hospital. An October 1995 Goodman column on genital cutting was promisingly entitled "We Don't Want to Believe It Happens Here" but discussed only practices imported to the United States by immigrants from third-world countries.

While anti-excision African immigrant women within the United States have been receptive to the claims made by intersex opponents to medicalized clitoridectomies, first-world feminists and organizations working on African genital cutting have totally ignored us. Only two of the many anti-genital-cutting activist groups contacted have bothered to respond to repeated overtures from intersex activists. Fran Hosken, who since 1982 has regularly published a catalog of statistics on female genital cutting worldwide, wrote me a terse note saying that "we are not concerned with biological exceptions."

Forward International, a London-based, anti-female-genital-cutting organization, replied to German intersex activist Heike Spreitzer that her letter of inquiry was "most interesting" but they could not help because their work focuses only on genital cutting "that is performed as harmful cultural or traditional practice on young girls."

As Forward International's reply to Spreitzer demonstrates, many first-world, anti-FGM activists seemingly consider Africans to have "harmful cultural or traditional practices," whereas we in the modern industrialized West presumably have something better. We have science, and science is linked to the meta-narratives of enlightenment, progress, and truth. Genital cutting is condoned to the extent that it supports these cultural self-conceptions.

Robin Morgan and Gloria Steinem set the tone for much of the first-world feminist analysis of African genital cutting with their pathbreaking article in the March 1980 issue of *Ms.* magazine, "The International Crime of Genital Mutilation." A disclaimer atop the first page warns, "These words are painful to read. They describe facts of life as far away as our most fearful imagination—and as close as any denial of women's sexual freedom." For *Ms.* readers, whom the editors apparently imagine are more likely to experience the pain of genital mutilation between the covers of their magazine than between their own thighs, clitoridectomy is presented as a fact of foreign life whose principal relevance to their readership is that it exemplifies a loss of "freedom," that most cherished possession of liberal Western subjects. One-half of the article's first page is filled with a photograph of an African girl seated on the ground, her legs held open by the arm of an unseen woman to her right. To her left is the disembodied hand of the midwife, holding the razor blade with which she has just performed a ritual clitoridectomy. The girl's face is a mask of pain, her mouth open, her eyes bulging.

In some twenty years of coverage, Western images of African practices have changed little although they have found their way into more mainstream publications. "Americans made a horrifying discovery this year," the January 1997 issue of *Life* soberly informed readers. The two-page photo spread shows a Kenyan girl held from behind, a hand clamped over her mouth, her face contorted in pain as unseen hands cut her genitals. Interestingly, the girl in this photo is adolescent, her breasts are shown, covered with rivulets of sweat, and there is a definite air of sensuality in the presentation. The 1996 Pulitzer prize for feature photography went to yet another portrayal of a Kenyan clitoridectomy. And, in the wake of Fauziya Kassindja's successful bid for asylum in the United States after fleeing clitoridectomy in Togo, the number of related images from her country skyrocketed. One wonders if Western photojournalists in search of sensational clitoridectomy photos do not represent a veritable tourism boom for a country the size of West Virginia.

These representations manifest a profound act of "othering" African clitoridectomy that contributes to the silence surrounding similar medicalized practices in the "modern," industrialized West. "Their" genital cutting is barbaric ritual; "ours" is scientific. Theirs disfigures; ours normalizes the deviant. The colonialist implications of these representations of genital cutting are even more glaringly obvious when contemporaneous images of intersex surgeries are juxtaposed with images of African practices. Medical books describing how to perform clitoral surgery on intersex children are almost always illustrated with extreme genital close-ups, disconnecting the genitals not only from the individual intersexed person but also from the body itself. Full body shots always have the subject's eyes blacked out. Why is it considered necessary—or at least polite—to black out the eyes of American girls but not the eyes of the African girls used to illustrate Steinem's "International Crime" or *Life*'s more recent "Ritual Agony"? I suspect one reason is that a Western reader is likely to identify with an American but not an African girl. Blacking out the American girl's eyes allows the reader to remain safely on this side of the camera.

First-world feminist discourse locates clitoridectomy not only elsewhere in African but also "elsewhen." An *Atlantic Monthly* article on African clitoridectomy, for example, asserted that the "American medical profession stopped performing clitoridectomies decades ago," and the magazine declined to publish a letter from ISNA contradicting that claim. Academic publications are as prone to this attitude as the popular press. Feminist Martha Nussbaum, in a discussion of judging other cultures, acknowledges, "If two abuses are morally the same and we have better local information about one and are better placed politically to do something about it, that one seems to be a sensible choice to focus on in our actions here and now." But then she counterfactually locates U.S. genital surgeries solely in the past: "As recently as the 1940s, [genital surgeries] were performed by U.S. and British doctors to treat female 'prob-

lems' such as masturbation and lesbianism." By collaborating in the silence about intersex genital surgeries, Nussbaum excuses first-world feminists from any obligation to challenge their own cultural practices as rigorously as they do that of others.

In the influential *Deviant Bodies* anthology, visual artist Susan Jahoda's "Theatres of Madness" juxtaposes nineteenth- and twentieth-century material depicting "the conceptual interdependence of sexuality, reproduction, family life, and 'female disorders.'" To represent twentieth-century medical clitoridectomy practices, Jahoda quotes a 1980 letter to the editor of *Ms.* magazine prompted by the Steinem and Morgan article. The writer, a nurse's aid in a geriatric home, says she had been puzzled by the strange scars she saw on the genitals of five of the forty women in her care: "Then I read your article. . . . My God! Why? Who decided to deny them orgasm? Who made them go through such a procedure? I want to know. Was it fashionable? Or was it to correct 'a condition?' I'd Like to know what this so-called civilized country used as its criteria for such a procedure. And how widespread is it here in the United States?"

While Jahoda's selection of this letter does raise the issue of medicalized American clitoridectomies, it again safely locates the cutting in the past, as something experienced a long time ago by women now in their later states of life. Significantly, Jahoda literally passes over an excellent opportunity to comment on the continuing practice of clitoridectomy in the contemporary United States. Two months earlier, in the April 1980 issue of *Ms.,* noted feminist biologists Patricia Farnes (a medical doctor) and Ruth Hubbard also replied to Morgan and Steinem:

> We want to draw the attention of your readers to the practice of clitoridectomy not only in the Third World . . . but right here in the Untied States, where it is used as part of a procedure to "repair" by "plastic surgery" so-called genital ambiguities. Few people realize that this procedure has routinely involved removal of the entire clitoris and its nerve supply—in other words, total clitoridectomy. . . . In a lengthy article, [Johns Hopkins intersex expert John] Money and two colleagues write, "There has been no evidence of a deleterious effect of clitoridectomy. None of the women experienced in genital practices reported a loss of orgasm after clitoridectomy." The article also advises that "a three-year old girl about to be clitoridectomized . . . should be well informed that the doctors *will make her look like all other girls and women*" (our emphasis), which is not unlike what North African girls are often told about their clitoridectomies. . . . But to date, neither Money nor

his critics have investigated the effect of clitoridectomies on the girls' development. Yet one would surely expect this to affect their psychosexual development and their feelings of identity as young women.

Although Farnes and Hubbard's prescient feminist exposé of medicalized clitoridectomies in the contemporary United States sank without a trace, there has been a veritable explosion of work like Nussbaum's and Jahoda's that keeps "domestic" clitoridectomy at a safe distance. Such conceptualizations of clitoridectomy's cultural remoteness—both geographically and temporally—allow feminist outrage to be diverted into potentially colonialist meddling in the social affairs of others while hampering work for social justice at home.

Conclusion

Feminism represents itself as being interested in unmasking the silence that surrounds violence against women and in providing tools to understand the personal as political. Most medical intersex management is a form of violence based on a sexist devaluing of female pain and female sexuality: Doctors consider the prospect of growing up male with a small penis to be a worse alternative than living as a female without a clitoris, ovaries, or sexual gratification. Medical intervention literally transforms transgressive bodies into ones that can safely be labeled female and subjected to the many forms of social control with which women must contend. Why then have most feminists failed to engage the issue of medical abuse of intersex people?

I suggest that intersex people have had such difficulty generating mainstream feminist support not only because of the racist and colonialist frameworks that situate clitoridectomy as a practice foreign to proper subjects within the first world but also because inter-

sexuality undermines the stability of the category "woman" that undergirds much first-world feminist discourse. We call into question the assumed relation between genders and bodies and demonstrate how some bodies do not fit easily into male/female dichotomies. We embody viscerally the truth of Judith Butler's dictum that "sex," the concept that accomplishes the materialization and naturalization of culturally constructed gender differences, has really been "gender all along." By refusing to remain silenced, we queer the foundations upon which depend not only the medical management of bodies but also widely shared feminist assumptions of properly embodied female subjectivity.

In 1990 Suzanne Kessler noted, "[T]he possibilities for real societal transformations would be unlimited [if physicians and scientists specializing in the management of gender could recognize that] finally, and always, people construct gender as well as the social systems that are grounded in gender-based concepts. . . . Accepting genital ambiguity as a natural option would require that physicians also acknowledge that genital ambiguity is 'corrected' not because it is threatening to the infant's life but because it is threatening to the infant's culture."

To the extent that we are not normatively female or normatively women, we are not the proper subjects of feminist concern. Western feminism has represented African genital cutting as primitive, irrational, harmful, and deserving of condemnation. The Western medical community has represented its genital cutting as modern scientific, healing, and above reproach. When will Western feminists realize that their failure to examine either of these claims "others" African women and allows the violent medical oppression of intersex people to continue unimpeded?

REFERENCES
A list of references is available in the original source.

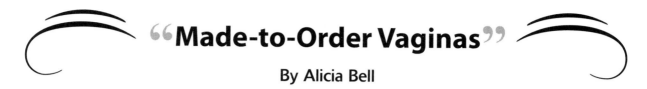

"Made-to-Order Vaginas"

By Alicia Bell

"A sexy surgery that can make you like a virgin . . . women all over the world are discovering a new fountain of youth."[1] This is how "vaginoplasty", a surgical procedure that involves cutting or burning the vaginal wall, is being described in the media. Gynecologists offering the procedure promote the idea that women can get a "designer vagina" by undergoing "vaginal rejuvenation."

These doctors are telling women that the surgery can make sex more pleasurable for them, though there's no science or data to back that up. In an Internet YouTube video, one gynecologist claims: "We can enhance sexual gratification because what we are doing is enhancing the muscles of the upper and lower parts of the vagina. We're decreasing the internal diameter [of the vaginal canal]." This doctor states that vaginoplasty is for women who have experienced "vaginal relaxation as a result of childbirth."[2] He continues, "Our whole mission is to empower women with knowledge, choice, and alternatives."[2] Another doctor says, describing women who undergo this surgery, "Even though nobody sees it, they wear it on their face and they walk down the street self-assured. They feel good about themselves."[1]

In a TV interview, one doctor asserted that vaginal rejuvenation will "stimulate your love life" by "restoring, recreating, rebuilding the entire vaginal wall, the vagina itself." He indicated that women who have the procedure will experience a rejuvenated sex life, commenting that "If at age 20, pre-childbirth, they've reached certain levels of sexual excitement, that will come back again."[1] Another doctor solemnly counsels in his YouTube video, "the reality of the matter is this—cosmetic surgery may make you look good. However, laser vaginal rejuvenation will make you feel good. One without the other is like the cake without the icing."[2]

Despite this language of sexual and emotional empowerment, the assertion that vaginoplasty leads to a better sex life is completely unproven. No studies on the procedure's use to enhance sexual pleasure appear in the medical literature and there is no evidence that the procedure is effective for enhancing female sexual pleasure. No *bona fide* medical journals or societies even discuss vaginoplasty as a way to enhance sexual plea-

sure. (Medical literature, in fact, uses the term "vaginoplasty" only to describe the creation of a vagina in women born without one and for male-to-female sex reassignment surgery.)[3,4]

The underlying logic for doing this surgery is the assumption that vaginal diameter is a determining factor in women's sexual pleasure. But there is no evidence either that vaginoplasty increases sensation or that vaginal tightness is proportional to sexual pleasure; this is a myth that stems from associating enhanced sexual pleasure with virginity and youthfulness. In fact, the surgery traumatizes the vaginal walls and any scarring that results can decrease sensitivity to sexual stimulation: not exactly a recipe for better sex. These doctors are playing on the cultural biases that already undermine women's confidence in sexuality as they age to encourage them to undergo an expensive, risky surgical procedure. (Cosmetic vaginoplasty costs about $6,500 and is not covered by health insurance.)[5,6]

Promoting surgery as a solution to bad sex or poor self-image is dangerous and perpetuates myths about women's psycho-social health and sexuality. Feminist sexologists have pointed out that: "there are no magic bullets for the socio-cultural, political, psychological, social or relational bases of women's sexual problems."[7] Even sex therapists who promote medical solutions to women's sexual concerns have been critical of this procedure, pointing out the serious risks that it will make an existing problem worse or create a problem where none existed.[8]

Why have professional medical associations not stepped up to tell women that there is no evidence to support vaginoplasty for enhanced sexual pleasure? Why are they not chastising doctors who promote and perform this pointless surgery? In response to these questions, Anthony Scialli, MD, Professor of Obstetrics and Gynecology at Georgetown University School of Medicine, said: "ACOG [the American College of Obstetricians and Gynecologists] represents gynecologists, not women."

Some doctors pushing vaginoplasty admit that it is not for every woman. But without evidence of sexual benefit this surgery should not be performed for any

---

"Made to Order Vaginas," by Alicia Bell, originally published in the *Women's Health Activist*, September/October 2007, pp. 4 & 7, the newsletter of the National Women's Health Network (NWHN). It is reprinted with the permission of the author and the NWHN.

woman. Women with concerns about sexual satisfaction need support and guidance from healthcare providers who will help them consider the full range of factors that may be affecting their sexual experiences and offer solutions that are responsive to their needs. Vaginoplasty should not be an option since it has potential harm and no evidence of benefit.

REFERENCES

1. ABC Action News WFTS TV, "Like a Virgin", November 6, 2006. Online: http://cosmeticsurgery2.com/cs2-stern.htm. Accessed 7/26/07.

2. Dr. Matlock Promo, added to YouTube on 6/7/07. Online: http://www.youtube.com/watch?v=HokEe7bE7ul&eurl. Accessed 7/25/07.

3. Selvaggi G, Ceulemans P, De Cuypere G, et. al. "Gender identity disorder: general overview and surgical treatment for vaginoplasty in male-to-female transsexuals," *Plastic & Reconstructive Surgery* 2005; 116(6):135e–145e.

4. Fedele L, Bianchi S, Berlanda N, et. al. "Neovaginal mucosa after Vecchietti's laparoscopic operation for Rokitansky syndrome: structural and ultrastructural study," *American Journal of Obstetrics & Gynecology* 2006; 195(1):56-61.

5. No author, "Pricing," Labiaplasty Surgery.com. Online: http://www.labiaplastysurgeon.com/dr-stern.html. Accessed 7/24/07.

6. Navarro M, "The Most Private of Makeovers," *New York Times*, November 28, 2004. Online: http://www.nytimes.com/2004/11/28/fashion 28PLAS.html?pagewanted=1&ei=5070&en=7321829bf4422c81&ex=1185595200. Accessed 7/25/07.

7. The Working Group on a New View of Women's Sexual Problems, *The New View Manifesto*, Online: http://www.fsd-alert.org/manifsto1.asp. Accessed 7/30/07.

8. Sandra G. Boodman, "Cosmetic Surgery's New Frontier: Procedures Popularized In L.A.'s 90210 Come to D.C.'s 20037", *The Washington Post*, March 6 2007, page HE01.

"How to Stop Female Genital Mutilation"

By Magggie Mortimer

Female genital mutilation (FGM) is a widely practised procedure that involves the removal of all or most of the clitoris (clitoridectomy), all or part of the labia minora (excision) or both (infibulation). While international efforts are underway to stop the practice, FGM still flourishes, killing many young girls and maiming millions more.

Waris Dirie, who fled Somalia at 13 and later became a model in London, is the UN special ambassador for the elimination of female genital mutilation. She is also head of the Waris Dirie Foundation, an international organization dedicated to eradicating FGM. She has written a book—her third—*Desert Children* (Virago Books) about the movement to end FGM.

Herizons: *In a 1988 Barbara Walters interview for* Marie Claire *magazine, you recounted your experience of female genital mutilation in public for the first time. Was it the initial public feedback after this personal disclosure that led to a larger social activism and your eventual appointment as UN special ambassador for the elimination of female genital mutilation in 1997?*

Waris Dirie: I didn't expect the reaction on that interview to be so overwhelming. It really frightened me, be-

cause I didn't know where it would lead me. After the interview, my mutilation had become a public matter and I didn't know if I should be proud of being the first woman talking about that, because I wasn't sure if this could save some girls from undergoing FGM or not—not because I was a successful model in those days—and from that day on I was often reduced to being a victim of barbaric traditions. But, after I thought about it for awhile, the idea of saving some girls from being mutilated had a major impact on me and I took that possibility as a great challenge in my life.

How has your strategy evolved/diverged in the years since?

Waris Dirie: When I started to fight against FGM, I was sure that the international solidarity would help me to erase that torture within a couple of years. I was young at that time, so I didn't expect that it would maybe take my whole life or even longer until it is eliminated. I was depressed sometimes when I realized that, but now I know that we already saved some girls and I'm satisfied about every single girl that is not affected by FGM due to our work.

The practice of FGM outside the social customs of African, Arab and Asian countries continues to migrate with the population. Often, daughters are sent back to their country of origin, and it is performed in the girl's new homeland.

Here in Canada, FGM is defined as aggravated assault under Section 268 of the Criminal Code. In other countries, legislation is similar, yet FGM still happens. With this in mind, what do you think are the most effective preventative measures?

Waris Dirie: Laws are important. But they can only be effective if the people know about the particular laws. And we also need more specific laws, which include the fact that girls are sent abroad to become mutilated. I'm deeply convinced that information and education are our strongest weapons to fight FGM. Therefore, my foundation works with opinion leaders, journalists and politicians, because they are the ones who inform others. During my research for *Desert Children*, I was really shocked about the lack of information among medical and social workers who are in direct contact with affected women. If they don't know how to deal with the topic, who should know? We also need more studies which deal with the psychological effects of FGM to help women to overcome their traumatic wounds.

Do you feel that there is one model that can be used in places where FGM is indigenous, as well as in countries in Europe or North America where the practice has migrated?

Waris Dirie: We need a worldwide campaign against FGM which includes legislative measures, information and education. The religious leaders could play an enormous role in that fight. With five words—"It is against our religion"—they could help to erase FGM for real! So, if we succeed in making FGM a matter of international interest, we could develop campaigns for specific groups affected by FGM.

There should be a medical examination in every school and kindergarten—where girls and boys are examined—which is not only focused on FGM, but also on sexual abuse and physical violence against children. If all parents are informed that we care about our children and are ready to do anything we can to save them from being abused in any form, I'm sure that the level of abuse would decrease.

We also need specific information for social workers and medical workers and we need a reporting requirement for professionals who notice a mutilation or who fear that a girl is at the risk of undergoing FGM. We also need a network for women who have undergone FGM. They should know that there is a reversal operation, which can decrease their pain—it can help to improve their permanent health complications.

What astounds me is the extent of FGM in one area and the almost unheard of numbers in another. In the horn of Africa—Somalia, Sudan, Ethiopia—it is estimated at 90 percent, while in Egypt, Liberia and Togo it is 50 percent, and takes a dramatic drop in other countries. I was also surprised that in Muslim countries outside Africa the practice has relatively low numbers, if none at all. Why such disparity?

Waris Dirie: The reason is that FGM is a pre-Islamic phenomenon. You will not find any word in the Koran which mentions FGM. In fact, there are some Hadiths where FGM is mentioned, but most of the Islamic scholars have proven them as being weak ones. Only one out of four Islamic schools preaches that FGM is *sunna*, which means it is the duty of every Muslim. This Islamic school is especially active in the horn of Africa.

All Muslims need to take this challenge to overcome FGM, but it is not only the religion which leads to the mutilations. We need information campaigns which work with the specific groups involved. For instance, I talked to a lot of men who didn't know anything about their women's mutilation, and especially not about the medical and physical health complications they suffer from.

What seemed a point of contention in articles I came across was the notion of FGM as a contributing vehicle to the transmission of HIV/AIDS? What is your take?

Waris Dirie: FGM is a contributing vehicle to the transmission of HIV/AIDS because of the dirty instruments used. But if we only focus on that part, it would lead to the argument that doctors should mutilate girls under hygienic and sterile circumstances. And this is not the right direction in our fight.

The Inter-African Committee has set a goal of 2010 for the eradication of FGM in Africa, and I will do everything I can to help them achieve their goal. I don't know whether it is realistic to erase FGM by 2010, but I'm convinced that we need this optimistic goal to fight against this torture!

Your book discusses many difficult topics. The statistics. The mutilations. The medical complications. The deaths. The emotional and mental turmoil. Little girls packed off on holiday to meet such a fate. There is also discussion on surgical options, including a technique to rebuild the clitoris. Stopping mutilation is obviously important, but what about surgical procedures for women who have been mutilated?

Waris Dirie: When I visited Dr. Pierre Foldes in France, who is the only doctor who does this reversal operation rebuilding the clitoris, I met my whole traumatic mutilation again. There was no way to think about it rationally, for me, while he showed me photos from this operation—it was just like being mutilated one more time. I'm still searching for women who have undergone this operation to talk to them about their experiences. I would appreciate it if there were a possibility to rebuild the clitoris—but only if it is accompanied with a psychological program for women who want to do this.

One thing we should do immediately is to send doctors to FGM practising communities who can offer a reversal operation without rebuilding the clitoris. A reversal operation for women like me who are affected by infibulation—the most severe form of FGM—could take a lot of pain and health complications away from women. It is just a little operation, where the woman is cut open again, and it takes only some minutes. It should be offered everywhere and without being charged for.

You have made a firm stance against FGM as "cultural identity." In many places, not being cut is identified with being unclean and unworthy of marriage. Has there been a movement to replace FGM with positive celebratory rituals accepted by the community as a girl's rite of passage?

Waris Dirie: I have a dream concerning this. I would appreciate it if we could turn the barbaric torture of girls to an educational program instead. We could try to take the girls away for a month, or even more, and start to teach them how to write and read. If the fact that a girl is able to write could make her a woman, we all could be satisfied with it.

FGM is often said to be necessary to turn a girl into a woman, so we need to change these attitudes to something positive. It would help to overcome these barbaric rites.

Name _____   Date_____

Sex, Gender, Roles, and Health

1. Demonstrate that you have an understanding of the differences between biologically determined sex differences and socially/culturally determined gender differences by filling in one or more examples on this table:

	Male/Masculine	**Female/Feminine**
Biologically determined sex differences		
Socially/culturally influenced gender differences		

2 For characteristics listed on this chart (and for others you think to add) identify whether that characteristic is more associated (accepted or expected) for one gender or the other and whether *in general* that characteristic is valued or devalued by society:

	Associated with women more than men	**Associated with men more than women**	**Valued**	**Devalued**	**Comments**
passive					
aggressive					
independent					
dependent					
stable					
easily excitable					
strong					
weak					
competitive					
non competitive					
always knows answer					
OK not to know answer					
cares about things more than people					

	Associated with women more than men	Associated with men more than women	Valued	Devalued	Comments
cares about people more than things					
earning $ Very important					
other things more important than $					
hides emotions					
shows emotions					
other					
other					
other					

3. Because gender roles are socially/culturally influenced, what is considered masculine or feminine may change from one historical moment to another or from one country to another. Can you think of an example of this?

4. A long time peace activist has said, "A prerequisite for being president of the USA should be that a person has to be a mother before they can be president." Describe your reaction to this statement and problems with such statements.

5. Check below which strategies you think are likely to help improve the role of women in society.

_____ Trying to eliminate differences between sexes/genders

_____ Trying to make men more like women

_____ Trying to make women more like men

_____ Making it possible for both men and women to explore both masculine and feminine sides of themselves

_____ Trying to make society value a much wider range of characteristics and behaviors

Briefly comment on why you made the choices you made:

6. Compare the messages girls and boys in your family received about "appropriate" and "inappropriate" behavior for their sex. When were girls praised for feminine behavior? for masculine behavior? Were boys ever praised for feminine behavior?

7. Many people observe that there is more social acceptance for girls to be "tomboys" than there is for boys demonstrating "sweet," "sensitive," "doesn't like to fight" behaviors. Explain why this might be.

8. The authors of the articles on intersex people would like doctors to say to parents of babies with genitals that are ambiguous—don't conform to male or female, "Your child is intersex, in other words, neither a boy nor a girl. There are resources available to help you raise your child in a healthy way. Go home and love your child as you would any other." Identify ways a community and parents could be educated to better prepare for intersex individuals and think of very practical suggestions (i.e. single-stall, gender-neutral bathrooms) to make life easier for intersex people. Also identify any other groups who might benefit from your suggestions.

9. In recent years, various states, cities, and universities have passed amendments to their anti-discrimination policies (prohibiting the discrimination on the basis of race, religion, marital status, etc.), adding the categories of gender (or gender identity and gender expression). Discuss how these changes would protect people who are not protected under the categories of sex or sexual orientation/sexuality. How might such anti-discrimination laws in healthcare protect transgender people (see Feinberg article in Chapter 2)?

10. The concept of informed consent in medical practice means that people: have a right to full information about all the risks and benefits of the treatment or procedure; are capable of understanding the risks and benefits and all the implications of those; are in a position to be able *not* to consent or to consent (think about different power differentials). Discuss how informed consent would apply to the different forms of genital surgery discussed in this chapter.

11. **Male and female physical fitness:** If average untrained college-age men and women are tested for physical fitness, the men are likely to appear to be more fit, particularly in the area of strength. These results fit with the assumption that many make that women naturally have less physical potential than men. However, exercise physiologists find very different results. For example, men tend to have greater strength in both upper (back, arms, shoulders) and lower body, but when the measurement is adjusted relative to body weight, the differences in lower body strength disappear. When untrained men and women begin to do weight-training, the women often progress much faster because they are farther below their potential. Androgens are needed for muscle proliferation, so the fact that the average woman has lower levels of androgens than the average man means there is some limit on her muscle bulk. However, this does not mean much in terms of strength limitation, since women can increase greatly in strength without "bulking" (muscles increasing in size). Right now we have no idea what the strength capability of women is, since women are so undertrained in terms of strength.

Women have a great capacity for developing endurance. Leading women marathoners can beat all but the best male runners and would, in fact, have won many past Olympic men's marathons with their current times. Women do even better in relation to men in ultra marathons (50 to 100 miles). Women hold many long-distance swimming records and compete directly with men.

When boys and girls are tested for physical performance, they are matched up to ages 10 to 12. In fact, girls are often faster than their male classmates in elementary school. After age 12, boys increase in strength and cardiovascular fitness more than girls. Exercise physiologists believe these differences may be social rather than biological in origin. It is not hormones that make women weaker but social and cultural processes.

a. Untrained males and females show little difference in lower-body strength but larger differences in upper-body strength. Show how this situation might arise by examining the activities from early childhood through adulthood that males and females might engage in that are likely to develop upper- or lower-body strength.

b. Differences in physical performance between males and females generally first appear around puberty. What are the changes in physical activity around puberty that might affect this? What are social and cultural messages that may limit girls' activities at puberty? Compare your own forms of exercise before and after puberty.

c. How does the definition of woman as "weaker" limit women's lives? Examine such issues as work, recreation, and safety. Who benefits from the definition of women as weaker?

MEDICALIZATION, MARKETING, *and the* POLITICS *of* INFORMATION

Consumer literacy, having access to good information and knowing how to use it, is essential to good women's health decision-making and activism. With more and more information available, much of it sophisticatedly designed to sell us perspectives, products, and procedures that may not be healthy for us, the skills to evaluate information and ask critical questions are more important than ever. This chapter specifically highlights key themes about medicalization, marketing, and the politics of information that are core throughout this book.

The **medicalization** of women's health refers to normal healthy physiological events in women's lives being defined as medical conditions to be "fixed" by a particular medical product or procedure. Such "medical answers" are often presented to women in a "one size fits all" protocol. We certainly feel grateful to modern medicine for the medical knowledge and products that save lives, lengthen lives, and improve the quality of lives. However, women's health activism requires us also to explore the "down sides" of medicalization.

Understanding and encouraging a range of normal, healthy physiological events may not get the attention or research it needs if no one is going to make much money from promoting natural events. For example, the significant health benefits for women and babies of breast-feeding are well recognized. But, relatively little attention is given to promoting breast-feeding or combating the obstacles to breast-feeding, because this area is so dominated by commercial infant formula makers who earn $5 to $6 billion each year on women *not* breast-feeding. (See "Formula for Profit: How Marketing Breastmilk Substitutes Undermines the Health of Babies" in Chapter 11.) In 1972, Doris Haire's "The Cultural Warping of Childbirth" (See Chapter 11) exposed how medical interventions often complicated childbirth. In the long run, we now also see that the U.S.'s overdependence on these medical interventions has left the U.S. far behind other countries in understanding and supporting healthy normal childbirth: The U.S. ranks 15th in the world for maternal mortality and ranks only 27th in terms of infant mortality rate. U.S. women experience the highest rate of postpartum depression in the world. (See "Overview of Maternity Care," Chapter 11.)

Too often the reliance on finding a new medical "solution" to an issue means that that issue is ignored or dismissed until clinicians have a "medical answer." We remember a time when women felt that infertility and miscarriage were not taken seriously by health practitioners because there were not medical answers. Now, as the infertility articles (See Chapter 10) identify, high-tech medical answers so dominate the field that practically no attention is paid either to the causes/prevention of infertility or less invasive, holistic answers. (See Elizabeth Ross, Chapter 10.) Many women still feel that miscarriage is too easily dismissed because there are seldom quick-fix medical answers.

In a capitalist economy, with a capitalist health system, there is another major down side to medicalization. Whenever there is a profit to be made, profit-making "solutions" will be pushed on people who do not really need them but have the money or health insurance to pay for them. On the other side of the economic divide, people who really need important medical interventions will not have access to them if they do not have insurance or resources to pay for them. Consumer literacy is essential for people to evaluate whether "solutions" being promoted to them are appropriate. Activism is essential to ensure that good medical solutions are equally available to all the people who would benefit from them.

Of course, the most obvious problem with medicalization is that most medicines and medical procedures have some side effects. If someone is making a decision about something that will or could save her/his life, mild or even serious side effects are a small price to pay for that. However, we should have very high standards for the safety issues and should expect long-term safety studies have been done on any product or procedure that will be used by healthy women. Because there are safe, non-medical ways to handle changes associated with menstrual cycles, to improve sexuality, to have babies, or to thrive during menopause, "it is a triumph of marketing over science and advertising over common sense" (National Women's Health Network) that this book is full of examples of the medicalization of PMS, sexuality, childbirth, and menopause. How is it that consumers and their health practitioners keep being swayed to use products or procedures with unnecessary or unknown hazards? (See "Lessons from the Past Should Be Informing Present Debates" in "HRT: Getting to the Heart of the Politics of Women's Health.") It is a history all women need to know about. For example, read Andrea Eagan's *1983* (see menstruation chapter) response to women taking progesterone for PMS:

> because of the work of the women's health movement and of health activists like Barbara Seaman, we have presumably learned something: we have become cautious about medical miracles and scientific breakthroughs. To suddenly discover, then, that thousands of women are rushing to get an untested drug to cure a suspected but entirely unproved hormone deficiency . . . is a little shocking.

This sounds way too much like Cindy Pearson's reaction (see "Hormone Therapy: Six Steps Toward a Better Future" in this chapter) to studies proving that the risks outweighed benefits of menopausal "hormonal therapy":

> Millions of healthy women were taking long-term hormone therapy for a preventative benefit not yet proven because medical practice was determined under the influence of industry rather than under the influence of (scientific) evidence . . . Drug companies, professional societies, women's groups, policy makers, and government agencies had all been complicit in creating a "climate of enthusiasm for hormone therapy" and allowing the needless suffering of tens of thousands of women.

The illustration below is a visual summary of the information I (NW) give readers in "HRT: Getting to the Heart of the Politics of Women's Health" (See Chapter 13) to show how many factors increasingly come together to promote the medicalization of many parts of women's lives.

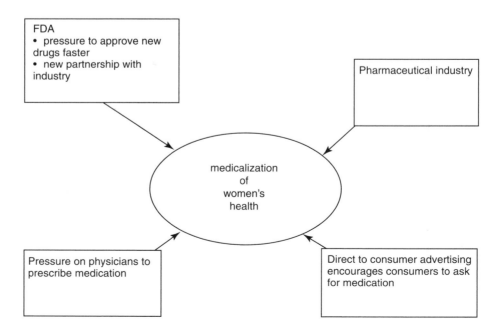

The unhealthy narrow definition of health itself is examined in the "Picture of Health" through the lens of how health is represented in photographs in health textbooks. In images very similar to those seen in advertising, those portrayed as "healthy" exclude large segments of the population, leaving a group that is young, white, thin, and physically abled to represent health. Health is presented in these images as a commodity that many will not be able to attain, in other words, a privilege, not a right.

"Manufacturing Need, Manufacturing Knowledge" (excerpted from *The Truth About Hormone Replacement Therapy*) introduces the reader to some of the techniques used to market products and the need for those products, to both consumers and clinicians. "Overdosed America," a book review of *How the Pharmaceutical Companies Distort Medical Knowledge, Mislead Doctors, and Compromise Your Health,* demonstrates the powerful influence drug companies have in "everything from the sponsoring of continuing medical education to the latest treatment guidelines that make an ever-expanding number of Americans candidates for life-long drug therapy." The point is also made that the pharmaceutical industry, even with its extremely high profit margin, spends considerably more money on marketing than on research. "Doctors Still Chummy with Drug Sales Reps" informed *AARP* (American Association for Retired People) *Bulletin* readers of how much of their medical advice and expenses are influenced by drug reps, by sharing how an ex-AstraZeneca manager described the incentives in promoting his company's products to doctors:

> Here's a big bucket of money sitting in every office . . . Every time you go in, you reach your hand in the bucket and grab a handful!

For the most insightful, thoroughly researched information on the role of the pharmaceutical industry in our lives and our medicine, the reader should check out http://www.pharmedout.org/

The next set of articles use the marketing of specific women's health issues to teach how marketing techniques work in almost incredible, too seldom recognized ways. "Advertising Disease," from the excellent *Selling Sickness: How the World's Biggest Pharmaceutical Companies Are Turning Us All into Patients*, uses Premenstrual Dysphoric Disorder (PMDD) to illustrate the power of the more than $3 billion per year spent on direct-to-consumer advertising. While the U.S. is only one of two developed countries in the world to allow drug companies to advertise their products directly to consumers, this article concentrates less on the pushing of particular drugs and instead describes the even bigger issue of how this form of marketing is used to define "everyday human experiences (as) symptoms of medical conditions requiring treatment with drugs." Researchers have found that nearly half of drug ads "tried to encourage consumers to consider medical causes for their common experiences . . . ads targeted aspects of ordinary life including sneezing, hair loss, or being overweight . . . and portrayed them as if they were a part of a medical condition." Following through the PMDD example, this article shows how the drug company, Lilly, needing a new way to market Prozac, managed to convince the public that a condition they essentially invented was real and "a problem" and that a different color and name of Prozac (Sarafem) was "the answer." Equally worrying is the fact that it only took a small group of industry-connected folks meeting and inspiring an article in a scientific journal for the FDA to approve renamed Prozac for this questionable "disease." (See "You, Too, Can Hold a Congressional Briefing" in Chapter 6, for activism on this issue.) This PMDD example also demonstrates how the medicalization (pushing a profit-making pill as "the answer") of a woman's health issue can dangerously distract from research and clinical attention to better understand what is happening in women's lives/women's bodies. Paula Caplan, the psychologist well known for her work opposing the PMDD diagnosis, "worries that a psychiatric label of PMDD can be used to cover up or mask the real sources of pain and anguish for some women at the time of their period. Such sources may include a history of violent relationships, stressful life circumstances, poverty, or harassment—problems that clearly cannot be fixed with a pill."

In an article written specifically for this book, women's health educator Ronna Popkin analyzes the "big picture" of how many factors come together to influence women's health or ill-health. Bringing together the history of both direct-to-consumer advertising and abstinence-only education, she paints the picture of how advertising for hormonal contraceptives, "far more than other direct-to-consumer advertising, raises concerns and has potentially serious implications for *young* women's health." She shows that the combination of teens, particularly teens with lower levels of education, being strongly influenced by the media, and the fact that many teens are not learning facts about contraception, how to protect themselves from sexually transmitted infections (STIs), or the skills to evaluate media information, makes young women especially vulnerable to drug company-inspired pressure to be on hormonal contraceptives without considering STI protection or potentially safer alternatives. (These themes are also emphasized in "Acquiescence in the Contraceptive Marketplace" in Chapter 10.)

"How Vaccine Policy is Made: The Story of Merck and Gardasil" presents yet another problem in how the pharmaceutical industry influences women's health. This time, "the company moved from the usual pharmaceutical industry huckerism (hype the disease, hype the new drug) to blatantly purchasing . . . public policy." Merck made donations to the Texas governor, who mandated that 6th grade girls be given Merck's anti-HPV Gardasil vaccination, and politicians in at least 20 other states. This article, similar to the previous one showing what Lilly did to get a new market for Prozac, shows the lengths companies will go to get their share of a highly profitable market. The Merck-goes-to-6th-grade story was all about that company trying to reach as many customers as possible in the short time before their competitors have a similar product on the market. (See Chapter 13 for more on Gardasil.)

The good news? The articles and websites in this chapter and book are examples of the information and activism now generated to empower consumers to critically examine how medicalization and marketing are influencing their lives, their decisions, their health practitioners, the FDA, and public policies. The politics of information—having access to scientifically accurate and personally empowering information and making certain that good information is available and accessible to all women—continues to be a key issue for women's health movements. The next articles in this chapter are examples of "good news" and skill building to promote increased consumer health literacy.

In a powerful example of resistance, the American Medical Student Association's Pharm Free Campaign demonstrates how medical students (our future doctors!) are organizing against the influence drug companies have on their medical education. The excellent Center for Medical Consumers' *HealthFacts* provides two different sets of guidelines for consumers on what to look for in drug ads, and how to read drug ads. Then, the National Women's Health Network's Clearinghouse Coordinator guides us on "Finding Good Health Information on the Web."

We conclude this chapter with "Hormone Therapy: Six Steps Toward a Better Future." Although Cindy Pearson delivered this "call to action" in response to the pharmaceutical industry-inspired hype for menopausal hormone therapy, we ask readers to think of this article more generally as, "Women's Health: Six Steps Toward a Better Future."

The Picture of Health
How Textbook Photographs Construct Health

by Mariamne H. Whatley

Photographs in textbooks may serve the roles of breaking up a long text, emphasizing or clarifying information in the text, attracting the buyer (the professor, teacher, or administrator who selects texts), and engaging the reader. But photographs cannot be dismissed merely as either decorative additions or straightforward illustrations of the text. Photographs are often far more memorable than the passages they illustrate and, because they are seen as objective representations of reality, rather than artists' constructions (Barthes, 1977), may have more impact than drawings or other forms of artwork. In textbooks, photographs can carry connotations, intentional or not, never stated in the text. The selection of photographs for a text is not a neutral process that simply involves being "realistic" or "objective"; selection must take into account issues such as audience expectations and dominant meanings in a given cultural/historical context (Whatley, 1988). In order to understand the ideological work of a textbook, a critique of the photographs is as crucial as a critique of the text itself.

Using ideological analysis to identify patterns of inclusion and exclusion, I examined photographs in the seven best-selling, college-level personal health textbooks. This chapter presents the results of that research. In the first part of the analysis, I examined the photographs that represent "health," describing who and what is "healthy," according to these representations. In the second part of the analysis, I determined where those excluded from the definition of health are represented in the approximately 1,100 remaining photographs in the texts.

Selling Health in Textbooks

Generally, textbook authors do not select specific photographs but may give publishers general descriptions of the type of photographs they wish to have included (for example, a scene showing urban crowding, a woman in a nontraditional job). Due to the great expense involved, new photographs are not usually taken specifically for texts. Instead publishers hire photo researchers to find appropriate photographs, drawing on already existing photographic collections. The result is that the choice of photographs depends on what is already available, and what is available depends to some extent on what has been requested in the past. In fact, because the same sources of photographs may be used by a number of different publishers, identical photographs may appear in competing books. Although authors may have visions of their books' "artwork," the reality may be limited by the selection already on the market. In addition, editors and publishers make decisions about what "artwork" will sell or is considered appropriate, sometimes overruling the authors' choices.

Photographs, especially cover-photos and special color sections, are considered features that sell textbooks, but they also can work as part of another selling process. Textbooks, in many cases, sell the reader a system of belief. An economics text, for example, may "sell" capitalism, and a science text may "sell" the scientific method, both of which help support dominant ideologies. Health textbooks may be even more invested in this selling process because, in addition to convincing readers to "believe" in health, their "success" depends on the readers' adoption of very specific personal behavioral programs to attain health. Health textbooks hold up the ideals of "total wellness" or "holistic fitness" as goals we can attain by exercising, eating right, reducing stress, and avoiding drugs. The readers' belief in health and their ability to attain it by specific behaviors is seen by many health educators as necessary to relevant educational goals; the belief in a clearly marked pathway to health is also part of a process of the commodification of health.

In North America and Western Europe, health is currently a very marketable commodity. This can be seen in its most exaggerated form in the United States in the proliferation of "health" clubs, in the trend among hospitals and clinics to attract a healthy clientele by advertising their abilities to make healthy people healthier (Worcester & Whatley, 1988), and in the advertisements that link a wide range of products, such as high fiber cereals and calcium rich antacids, to health. In a recent article in a medical journal, a physician examined this commercialization of health:

> Health is industrialized and commercialized in a fashion that enhances many people's dissatisfaction with their health. Advertisers, manufacturers, advocacy groups, and proprietary healthcare corporations promote the myth that good health can be purchased; they market products and services that purport to deliver the consumer into the promised land of wellness. (Barsky, 1988, p. 415)

Photographs in health textbooks can play a role in this selling of health similar to that played by visual images in advertising a product in the popular media. According to Berger (1972), the role of advertising or publicity is to

> make the spectator marginally dissatisfied with his present way of life. Not with the way of life of society, but with his own place within it. It suggests that if he buys what it is offering, his life will become better. It offers him an improved alternative to what he is. (p. 142)

The ideal of the healthy person and the healthy lifestyle can be seen as the "improved alternative" to what we are. It can be assumed that most of us will be dissatisfied with ourselves when measured against that ideal, just as most women are dissatisfied with their body shapes and sizes when compared with ideal media representations.

In effective advertising campaigns the visual image is designed to provoke powerful audience responses. In health textbooks the visual representation of "health" is calculated to sell, and it is likely to have a greater impact on the reader than discussions about lengthened life expectancy, reduction in chronic illness, or enhanced cardiovascular fitness. The image of health, not health itself, may be what most people strive for. In the attempt to look healthy, many sacrifice health. For example, people go through very unhealthy practices to lose "extra" weight that is in itself not unhealthy; being slim, however, is a basic component of the *appearance* of health. A recent survey found that people who eat healthy foods

do so for their appearance and *not* for their health. "Tanning parlors" have become common features of health and fitness centers, though tanning in itself is unhealthy. As with being slim, having a good tan contributes to the appearance of what is currently defined as health.

The use of color photographs is particularly effective in selling the healthy image, for, as Berger (1972) points out, both oil painting and color photography "use similar highly tactile means to play upon the spectator's sense of acquiring the *real* thing which the image shows" (p. 141). The recent improvement in quality and the increase in number of color photographs in textbooks provide an opportunity to sell the image of health even more effectively than black and white photographs could.

Selection of Textbooks

Rather than trying to examine all college-level personal health (as opposed to community health) textbooks, I selected the best-selling ones, since those would have the widest impact. Based on the sales figures provided by the publisher of one popular text, I selected seven texts published from 1985 to 1988. Sales of these textbooks ranged from approximately 15,000 to 50,000 for each edition. (Complete bibliographic information on these textbooks is provided in the Appendix. Author-date information for these textbooks refer to the Appendix, rather than the chapter references.) Obviously, the sales figures depend on the number of years a specific edition has been in print. For one text (Insel & Roth, 1988), I examined the newest edition (for which there could be no sales figures), based on the fact that its previous editions had high sales. A paper on the readability of personal health textbooks (Overman, Mimms, & Harris, 1987), using a similar selection process, examined the seven top-selling textbooks for the 1984–85 school year, plus three other random titles. Their list has an overlap with mine of only four texts, which may be due to a number of factors, including differences in editions and changing sales figures.

Analysis I: Healthy-Image Photographs

The first step in my analysis was a close examination of the photographs that I saw as representing "health," the images intended to show who is healthy and illustrate the healthy lifestyle. These included photographs used on covers, opposite title pages, and as openers to units or chapters on wellness or health (as opposed to specific topics such as nutrition, drugs, and mental health). While other pictures throughout the texts may represent healthy individuals, the ones selected, by their placement in conjunction with the book title or chapter title, can be seen as clearly connoting "health." I will refer to these as healthy-image photographs. I included in this analysis only photographs in which there were people. While an apple on a cover conveys a message about health, I was interested only in the question of who is healthy.

A total of 18 different photographs fit my criteria for representing health. I have eliminated three of these from discussion: the cover from Insel and Roth (1988) showing flowers and, from Dintiman and Greenberg (1986), both the cover photograph of apples and the health unit opener of a movie still from the *Wizard of Oz*. (This textbook uses movie stills as openers for all chapters; this moves the photograph away from its perceived "objective" status toward that of an obvious construction.)

There are a number of points of similarity in the 15 remaining photographs. In several photographs (windsurfing, hang gliding), it is hard to determine race, but all individuals whose faces can clearly be seen are white. Except for those who cannot be seen clearly and for several of the eight skydivers in a health unit opener, all are young. No one in these photographs is fat or has any identifiable physical disability. Sports dominate the activities, which, with the exception of rhythmic gymnastics and volleyball played in a gym, are outdoor activities in nonurban settings. Five of these involve beaches or open water. All the activities are leisure activities, with no evidence of work. While it is impossible to say anything definitive about class from these photographs, several of the activities are expensive (hang gliding, skydiving, windsurfing), and others may take money and/or sufficient time off from work to get to places where they can be done (beaches, biking in countryside); these suggest middle-class activities, whether the actual individuals are middle class or not. In several photographs (windsurfing, hang gliding, swimming) it is hard to determine gender. However, excluding these and the large group of male runners in a cross-country race, the overall balance is 23 males to 18 females, so it does seem that there is an attempt to show women both as healthy individuals and in active roles.

How Health Is Portrayed

A detailed analysis of three photographs can provide insight into how these text photographs construct health. The first is a color photograph of a volleyball game on a beach from the back cover of *Understanding Your Health* (Payne & Hahn, 1986). As with most of these images of health, the setting is outdoors, clearly at a distance from urban life. The steep rock walls that serve as a backdrop to the volleyball game additionally isolate the natural beach setting from the invasion of cars[1] and other symbols of "man-made" environmental destruction and ill health. The volleyball players appear to have escaped into a protected idyllic setting of sun, sand, and, we assume, water. They also have clearly escaped from work, since they are engaged in a common leisure activity associated with picnics and holidays. None of them appears to be contemplating the beauty of the natural setting, but merely using it as a location for a game that could go on anywhere in which there is room to set up a net.

The photograph is framed in such a way that the whole net and area of the "court" are not included, so that some players may also not be visible. On one side of the net are three women and a man, on the other two women and a man. While this is not necessarily a representation of heterosexual interactions, it can be read that way. Two players are the focus of the picture, with the other five essentially out of the action. The woman who has just hit the ball, with her back toward the camera, has her arms outstretched, her legs slightly spread, and one foot partly off the ground. The man who is waiting for the ball is crouched slightly, looking expectantly upward. Her body is partially superimposed on his, her leg crossed over his. This is essentially an interaction between one man and one woman. It would not work the same way if the key players were both female or both male, since part of the "healthiness" of this image appears to be the heterosexual interaction. For heterosexual men, this scene might be viewed as ideal—a great male-female ratio on an isolated beach; perhaps this is their reward for having arrived at the end of this book—this photograph is on the *back* cover—attaining their goal of health.

All the volleyball players are white, young, and slim. The woman farthest left in the frame appears slightly heavier than the others; she is the only woman wearing a shirt, rather than a bikini top, and is also wearing shorts. Besides being an outsider in terms of weight, dress, and location in the frame, she is the only woman who clearly has short hair (three have long hair tied back in ponytails, one cannot be seen completely). Perhaps she can move "inside" by losing weight and changing her image. As viewers, we are just a few steps beyond the end of the court and are also outsiders. As with pick-up games, there is room for observers to enter the game—if they are deemed acceptable by the other players. By achieving health, perhaps the observer can step into the game, among the young, white, slim, heterosexual, and physically active. But if the definition of health includes young, white, slim, heterosexual, and physically active, many observers are relegated permanently to the outside.

If this photograph serves as an invitation to join in the lifestyle of the young and healthy, the second photograph, facing the title page of another book, serves the same function, with the additional written message provided by the title of the book—*An Invitation to Health* (Hales & Williams, 1986). The photograph is of six bicycle riders, three women and three men, resting astride their bicycles. This photograph is in black and white, so it is perhaps not as seductive as the sunny color of the first cover. However, the people in this photograph are all smiling directly at the viewer (rather than just leaving a space in back where the viewer could join in). Two of the women, in the middle and the right, have poses and smiles that could be described as flirtatious. They are taking a break from their riding, so it is an opportune moment to join the fun of being healthy.

As with the volleyball players, all the bicycle riders are young, slim, white, and apparently fit. Another similarity is the amount of skin that is exposed. Playing volleyball on the beach and riding bikes in warm weather are activities for which shorts and short-sleeved shirts are preferable to sweatpants and sweatshirts. The choice of these types of activities to represent health results in photographs in which legs and arms are not covered. Appearing healthy apparently involves no need to cover up unsightly flab, "cellulite," or stretch marks. A healthy body is a body that can be revealed.

The bikers are in a fairly isolated, rural setting. While they are clearly on the road, it appears to be a rural, relatively untraveled road. Two cars can be seen far in the distance, and there may also be a house in the distance on the right side of the frame. Otherwise, the landscape is dominated by hills, trees, and grass, the setting and the activity clearly distance the bike riders both from urban life and from work.

In a third photograph, a health unit chapter opener (Levy, Dignan, & Shirreffs, 1987), we can see a possible beginning to alternative images of health. The players in this volleyball game are still slim, young, and apparently white. However, the setting is a gym, which could be urban, suburban, or rural. While four players are wearing shorts, one woman is wearing sweatpants; there are T-shirts rather than bikini tops, and gym socks rather than bare legs. The impression is that they are there to play a hard game of volleyball rather than to bask in the sun and each other's gaze. Two men are going for the ball from opposite sides, while a woman facing the net is clearly ready to move. Compared with the other volleyball scene, this photograph gives more of a sense of action, of actual physical exertion, as well as a sense of real people, rather than models.

It is interesting to imagine how healthy the volleyball players and bike riders actually are, underneath the appearance of health. The outdoor groups, especially the beach group, are susceptible to skin cancer from overexposure to the sun. Cycling is a healthy aerobic sport, though it can be hard on the knees and back. It is particularly surprising, however, to find that the bikers represented in a health text are not wearing helmets, thus modeling behavior that is considered very risky. Compared with biking, volleyball is the kind of weekend activity that sends the enthusiastic untrained player home with pulled muscles, jammed fingers, and not much of a useful workout. The question also arises as to how the particularly thin women on the beach achieved their weight—by unhealthy weight-loss diets, by anorexia, by purging? The glowing image of health may have little to do with the reality.

Similarities to Advertising

Shortly after I began the research for this chapter, I was startled, while waiting for a movie to begin, to see a soft drink advertisement from which almost any still could have been substituted for a healthy-image photograph I had examined. There were the same thin, young, white men and women frolicking on the beach, playing volleyball, and windsurfing. They were clearly occupying the same territory: a never-never land of eternal sunshine, eternal youth, and eternal leisure. Given my argument that these textbook photographs are selling health, the similarities between soft drink advertising images and textbook healthy images are not surprising. They are appealing to the same groups of people, and they are both attempting to create an association between a desirable lifestyle and their product. You can enjoy this fun in the sun if you are part of the "Pepsi generation" or think "Coke is it" or follow the textbook's path to health. These can be considered one variant of the lifestyle format in advertising, as described by Leiss, Kline, and Jhally (1986).

> Here the activity invoked in text or image becomes the central cue for relating the person, product, and setting codes. Lifestyle ads commonly depict a variety of leisure activities (entertaining, going out, holidaying, relaxing). Implicit in each of these activities, however, is the placing of the product within a consumption style by its link to an activity. (p. 210)

Even a naive critic of advertising could point out that drinking a carbonated beverage could not possibly help anyone attain this lifestyle; on the other hand, it might be easier to accept that the same lifestyle is a result of achieving health. However, the association between health and this leisure lifestyle is as much a construction as that created in the soft drink ads. Following all the advice in these textbooks as to diet, exercise, coping with stress, and attaining a healthy sexuality will not help anyone achieve this sun-and-fun fantasy lifestyle any more than drinking Coke or Pepsi would.

These healthy-image photographs borrow directly from popular images of ideal lifestyles already very familiar to viewers through advertising[2] and clearly reflect the current marketing of health. The result is that health is being sold with as much connection to real life and real people's needs as liquor ads that suggest major lifestyle changes associated with changing one's brand of scotch.

Analysis II: Where Are the Excluded?

For each textbook, the next step was to write brief descriptions of all other photographs in the books, totaling approximately 1,100. The results of the analysis of the healthy image photographs suggested a focus on specific aspects of the description of the individuals and activities in examining the remaining 1,100 photographs. The areas I selected for discussion are those in which "health" is linked to specific lifestyles or factors that determine social position/power in our society. I described the setting, the activity, and a number of observable points about the people, including gender, race, age, physical ability/disability, and weight. These photographs were all listed by chapter and when appropriate, by particular topic in that chapter. For example, a chapter on mental health might have images of positive mental health and also images representing problems such as severe depression or stress. These descriptions of photographs were used to establish whether there were images with characteristics not found in the healthy images and, if so, the context in which these characteristics were present. For example, finding no urban representations among the healthy images, I identified topic headings under which I did find photographs of urban settings.

White, young, thin, physically abled, middle-class people in the healthy images represent the mythical norm with whom the audience is supposed to identify. This not only creates difficulties in identification for whose who do not meet these criteria, but also creates a limiting and limited definition of health. I examined the photographs that did not fit the healthy-image definition to find the invisible—those absent from the healthy images: people of color, people with physical disabilities, fat people, and old people. I also attempted to identify two other absences—the urban setting and work environment. Because there were no obvious gender discrep-

ancies in the healthy images, I did not examine gender as a separate category.

People of Color

After going through the remaining photographs, it was clear that there had been an attempt to include photographs of people of color in a variety of settings, but no obvious patterns emerged. In a previous paper, I examined representations of African-Americans in sexuality texts, finding that positive attempts at being nonracist could be undermined by the patterns of photographs in textbooks that, for example, draw on stereotypes and myths of "dangerous" black sexuality (Whatley, 1988). Rather than reviewing all the representations of people of color in these health textbooks, I will simply repeat what I pointed out earlier—that there is a strong and clear *absence* of photographs of people of color in the healthy-images category. People of color may appear as healthy people elsewhere in the text, but not on covers, title pages, and chapter openers. If publishers wanted to correct this situation, they could simply substitute group photographs that show some diversity for the current all-white covers and title pages.

People with Disabilities

From the healthy-image photographs, it is apparent that people with visible physical disabilities are excluded from the definition of healthy. Therefore, I examined the contexts in which people with disabilities appear in the other photographs. Out of the approximately 1,100 photos, only 9 show people with physical disabilities, with 2 of these showing isolated body parts only (arthritic hands and knees). One shows an old woman being pushed in a wheelchair, while the six remaining photographs all are "positive" images: a number of men playing wheelchair basketball, a man in a wheelchair doing carpentry, a woman walking with her arm around a man in a wheelchair, a man with an amputated leg walking across Canada, children with cancer (which can be seen both as a disease and a disability) at a camp (these last two both in a cancer chapter), and a wheelchair racer. However, three of these six are from one textbook (Payne & Hahn, 1986), and two are from another (Levy, Dignan, & Shirreffs, 1987), so the inclusion of these few positive images is over-shadowed by the fact that three books show absolutely none. In addition, none of these positive images are of women, and the only disabilities represented are those in which an individual uses a wheelchair or has cancer.

This absence of representation of disabled people, particularly women, clearly reflects the invisibility of the physically disabled in our society.

It would be easy to blame the media for creating and maintaining many of the stereotypes with which the disabled still have to live. But the media only reflect attitudes that already exist in a body-beautiful society that tends to either ignore or ostracize people who don't measure up to the norm. This state of "invisibility" is particularly true for disabled women. (Israel & McPherson, 1983, pp. 4–15)

In a society that values the constructed image of health over health itself, a person with a disability does not fit the definition of healthy. In addition, since the person with a disability may be seen as representing a "failure" of modern medicine and healthcare (Matthews, 1983), there is no place for her or him in a book that promises people that they can attain health. The common attitude that disability and health are incompatible was expressed in its extreme by a faculty member who questioned the affirmative action statement in a position description for a health education faculty member; he wanted to know if encouraging "handicapped" people to apply was appropriate for a *health* education position.

Looking at the issue of health education and disabilities, it should be clear that it is easier for able-bodied people to be healthy, so more energy should be put into helping people with disabilities maximize their health. Able-bodied people often have more access to exercise, to rewarding work (economically[3] as well as emotionally), to leisure activities, and to healthcare facilities. Healthcare practitioners receive very little training about health issues relating to disability (self-care, sexual health), though they may receive information about specific pathologies, such as multiple sclerosis or muscular dystrophy. The inability to see, hear, or walk need not be the impairments to health they often are considered in our society. Health education is an obvious place to begin to change the societal attitudes toward disability that can help lead to poor physical and emotional health for disabled people. Health textbooks could present possibilities for change by showing ways that both disabled and able-bodied people can maximize health, and this could be done in both the text and the photographs. For example, one of those color chapter openers could include people with disabilities as healthy people. This might mean changing some of the representative "healthy" activities, such as windsurfing. While there are people with disabilities who participate in challenging and risky physical activities, there is no need for pressure to achieve *beyond* what would be expected of the able-bodied.[4] Showing a range of healthy activities that might be more accessible to both the physically dis-

abled and the less physically active able-bodied would be appropriate.

Fat People

There are no fat people in the healthy-image photographs. Some people who agree with the rest of my analysis may respond here, "Of course not!" because there is a common assumption in our society that being thin is healthy and that any weight gain reduces health. In fact, evidence shows that being overweight (but not obese) is *not unhealthy.* In many cases, being very fat is a lot healthier than the ways people are encouraged to attempt to reduce weight—from extreme low-calorie diets, some of which are fatal, to stomach stapling and other surgeries (Norsigian, 1986). In addition, dieting does not work for 99 percent of dieters, with 95 percent ending up heavier than before they started. Repeated dieting stresses the heart, as well as other organs (Norsigian, 1986). Our national obsession with thinness is certainly one factor leading to an unhealthy range of eating behaviors, including, but not limited to, bulimia and anorexia. While health textbooks warn against dangerous diets and "eating disorders," and encourage safe, sensible weight-loss diets, they do nothing to counter the image of thin as healthy.

Defining which people are "fat" in photographs is obviously problematic. In doing so, I am giving my subjective interpretation of what I see as society's definition of ideal weight. The photographs I have identified as "fat" are of people who by common societal definitions would be seen as "needing to lose weight." In the United States most women are dissatisfied with their own body weight, so are more likely to place themselves in the "need to lose weight" category than to give that label to someone else of the same size.

Not counting people who were part of a crowd scene, I found 14 photographs that clearly showed people who were fat. One appeared in a chapter on the healthcare system with a caption referring to "lack of preventive maintenance leading to medical problems" (Carroll & Miller, 1986, p. 471), one in a chapter on drinking, and one under cardiovascular problems. The remaining 11 appeared in chapters on weight control or diet and nutrition. Of the 11, one was the "before" of "before and after" weight-loss photographs. One showed a woman walking briskly as part of a "fat-management program" (Mullen, Gold, Belcastro, & McDermott, 1986, p. 125); that was the most positive of the images. Most of the photographs were of people doing nothing but being fat or adding to that fat (eating or cooking). Three of the photographs showed women with children, referring by caption or topic heading to causes of obesity, either genetic or environmental. Only 3 of the 11 photographs were of men. In these photographs, it seems we are not being shown a person or an activity, but a disease—a disease called obesity that we all might "catch" if we don't carefully follow the prescriptions for health. Fat people's excess weight is seen as their fault for not following these prescriptions. This failure results from a lack of either willpower or restraint, as implied by the photographs that show fat people eating and thus both draw on and lend support to the myth that fat people eat too much. The only health problem of fat people is seen as their weight; if that were changed, all other problems would presumably disappear. As pointed out earlier, the health problems of losing excess weight, particularly in the yo-yo pattern of weight loss/gain, may be greater than those created by the extra weight. In addition, the emotional and mental health problems caused by our society's fatphobia may be more serious than the physical problems (Worcester, 1988). These texts strongly reinforce fatphobia by validating it with health "science."

Health educators who consciously work against racism and sexism should carefully reevaluate how our attitudes help perpetuate discrimination against all groups. As Nancy Worcester (1988) points out,

> The animosity towards fat people is such a fundamental part of our society, that people who have consciously worked on their other prejudices have not questioned their attitude towards body weight. People who would not think of laughing at a sexist or racist joke ridicule and make comments about fat people without recognizing that they are simply perpetuating another set of attitudes which negatively affect a whole group of people. (p. 234)

An alternative approach would be to recognize that people would be healthier if less pressure were put on them to lose weight. Fat people can benefit from exercise, if it is accessible and appropriate (low impact aerobics, for example), without the goal needing to be weight loss (Sternhell, 1985). Photographs of "not thin" people, involved in a variety of activities, could be scattered throughout the text, and the pictures of those labeled obese could be eliminated completely. We all know what an obese person looks like; we do not need to have that person held up as a symbol of both unhealthiness and lack of moral character.

Old People

The healthy-image photographs show people who appeared to be predominantly in their teens and twenties, which is the age group toward which these college texts would be geared. Rather subjectively, as with the issue of weight, I will describe as old[5] those who appear to be about 65 or older. Obviously I probably judged incorrectly on some photographs, but since the representations seem to be skewed toward the young or the old, with the middle-aged not so prominent, my task was relatively easy. I identified 84 photographs that contained people I classified as old. Of these, 52 appeared in chapters specifically on aging or growing older, 10 appeared in chapters on death and dying, and the remaining 22 were distributed in a wide range of topics. Of these 22, several still focused on the issue of age. For example, a photograph of an old heterosexual couple in a chapter entitled "Courtship and Marriage" is captioned, "While some people change partners repeatedly, many others spend their lifetime with a single spouse" (Carroll & Miller, 1986, p. 271). One text showed a similar photo and caption of a heterosexual couple, but also included an old gay male couple on the next page (Levy, Dignan, & Shirreffs, 1987). This represents an important step in terms of deghettoization of gay and lesbian images, and a broadening of views about sexuality and aging. Two photos showed old people as "non-traditional students;" another depicted a man running after recovering from a stroke; and yet another featured George Burns as a representative of someone who has lived a long life. In others of the 22, the age is incidental, as in a man painting (mental health), people shopping in an open market (nutrition), people walking (fitness), a man smoking.

As the societally stereotyped *appearance* of health diminishes, as occurs with aging, it is assumed that health unavoidably diminishes. In fact, while there is some inevitable biological decline with age, many health problems can be averted by good nutrition, exercise, and preventive healthcare. Many of the health problems of aging have economic, rather than biological, causes, such as lack of appropriate health insurance coverage (Sidel, 1986). In a society that is afraid to face aging, people may not be able to accept that they will experience the effects of aging that they so carefully avoid (if they are lucky enough to live that long). In addition, as with disability, the people who may need to do more to maintain health are those being most ignored.

It is significant that these texts have sections on aging, which contain many positive images, but it is also crucial that health be seen as something that can be attained and maintained by people of all ages. The attempt to include representations of aging in these books must be expanded so that people of all ages are seen to be able to be healthy—a state now seemingly, in those images of health, to be enjoyed only by the young.

Urban Setting

The healthy-image photographs showing outdoor scenes are situated at the beach or in other nonurban settings; it is possible some were set in city parks, but there are no urban markers in the photographs. Bike riding, running, kicking a soccer ball, playing volleyball can all be done in urban settings, though the hang gliding and sky diving would obviously be difficult. Considering the high percentage of the U.S. population that lives in cities (and the numbers of those that cannot easily get out), it seems that urban settings should be represented in the texts. Of the 28 other photographs I identified as clearly having urban settings, I could see only 4 as positive. Two of these showed outdoor vegetable/fruit markets, one showed bike riding as a way of both reducing pollution and getting exercise in the city, and one showed a family playing ball together. Of the rest, 9 appeared in chapters on the environment, with negative images of urban decay, smog, and crowded streets; 10 were in chapters on mental health or stress, showing scenes representing loneliness, stress, or anger, such as a crowded subway or a potential fight on a street corner. Drinking and drug chapters had two urban scenes: "skid row" alcoholics and an apparently drunk man unconscious on the street. There were also three urban scenes in sexuality chapters—two of streets with marquees for sex shows and one showing a "man 'flashing' Central Park" (Payne & Hahn, 1986, p. 348).

There is a clear message that it is unhealthy to live in the city. While this is partly true—that is, the city may have increased pollution of various kinds, specific stresses, less access to certain forms of exercise, and other problems—there are healthy ways to live in a city. One of the roles of health education should be to help us recognize healthier options within the limits imposed on us by economic or other factors. Rather than conveying the message that urban dwelling inevitably condemns people to ill health (unless they can afford to get away periodically to the beach or the mountains), scenes showing health within the city could be presented.

Options for positive images include scenes of outdoor activities in what are clearly city parks, people enjoying cultural events found more easily in cities, gardening in a vacant lot, or a neighborhood block party. Urban settings are excellent for representing walking as a healthy activity. City dwellers are more likely to walk to work, to shopping, and to social activities than are suburbanites, many of whom habitually drive. Urban walking can be presented as free, accessible, and healthy in terms of exercise, stress reduction, and reducing pollution. More indoor activities could be shown so that the external environment is not seen as a determinant of "healthy" activity. These might give a sense of the possibilities for health within what otherwise might appear to be a very dirty, dangerous, stressful place to be.

Work and Leisure

The healthy-image photographs I analyzed were all associated with leisure activities, so I tried to establish how these texts represent work in relationship to health. For this analysis, all photographs of healthcare workers were excluded, since these are used predominantly to illustrate health or medical issues. Of the 16 other photographs showing people at work, 4 were related to discussions of sex roles and women doing nontraditional work (phone "lineman," lawyer). This seems part of a positive trend in textbooks to reduce sexism. An obvious next step would be to show women in nontraditional work roles without commenting on them, as is done with a number of photographs of women as doctors. Six of the photographs of work accompany discussions of stress. Besides stress, there are no illustrations of health hazards at work except for one photograph of a farm worker being sprayed with pesticides. Three positive references to work show someone working at a computer (illustrating self-development), a man in a wheelchair doing carpentry, and an old man continuing to work.

Overall, the number of photographs representing work seems low, considering the amount of time we put into work during our lifetime. Blue-collar work is represented by trash collectors in an environmental health section, police officers in a weight control chapter, firefighters under stress, a construction worker in the opener for a stress chapter, the farm worker mentioned above, and women in nontraditional work. Blue-collar work is seen in terms of neither potential health hazards beyond stress nor the positive health aspects of working. The strongest connection between health and work presented involves the stress of white-collar jobs (symbolized by a man at a desk talking on the phone). The message seems to be that health is not affected by work, unless it is emotionally stressful.

The photographs in this book seem to be aimed at middle-class students who assume they will become white-collar workers or professionals who can afford leisure activities, both in terms of time and money. Those who work in obviously physically dangerous jobs, such as construction work, or in jobs that have stress as only one of many health hazards, are rarely portrayed. These people are also likely not to be able to afford recreation such as hang gliding (and also might not need the stimulus of physical risk taking if their job is physically risky in itself). These photographs serve to compartmentalize work as if it were not part of life and not relevant to health.

Rather than selecting photographs that reinforce the work-leisure split and the alienation of the worker from work, editors could include photographs that show the health rewards of work and the real health risks of a wide variety of work. For example, a photograph of a group of workers talking on a lunch break could be captioned, "Many people find strong support networks among their co-workers." Another photograph could be of a union meeting, illustrating that work-related stress is reduced when we have more control over the conditions of our work. In addition the mental health benefits of a rewarding job might be emphasized, perhaps in contrast with the stress of unemployment. Health risks, and ways to minimize them, could be illustrated with photographs ranging from typists using video display terminals to mine workers. A very important addition would be inclusion in the healthy-image photographs of some representation of work.

Conclusion

The definition of health that emerges from an examination of the healthy-image photographs is very narrow. The healthy person is young, slim, white, physically abled, physically active, and, apparently, comfortable financially. Since these books are trying to "sell" their image of health to college students, the photographs presumably can be seen as representing people whom the students would wish to become. Some students, however, cannot or may not wish to become part of this vision of the healthy person. For example, students of color may feel alienated by this all-white vision. What may be most problematic is that in defining the healthy person, these photographs also define *who can become healthy.* By this definition many are excluded from the potential for health: people who are physically disabled, no longer young, not slim (unless they can lose weight, even if in unhealthy ways), urban dwellers, poor people, and people of color. For various social, economic, and political reasons, these may be among the least healthy groups in the United States, but the potential for health is there if the healthcare and health education systems do not disenfranchise them.

The healthy-image photographs represent the healthy lifestyle, not in the sense of the lifestyle that will help someone attain health, but the white, middle-class, heterosexual, leisure, active lifestyle that is the reward of attaining health. These glowing images imitate common advertising representations. An ice chest of beer would not be out of place next to the volleyball players on the beach, and a soft drink slogan would fit well with the windsurfers or sky divers. It must be remembered, however, that while college students may be the market for beer, soft drinks, and "health," they are not the market for textbooks. Obviously, the biggest single factor affecting a student's purchase of a text is whether it is required. The decision may also be based on how much reading in the book is assigned, whether exam questions will be drawn from the text, its potential future usefulness, or its resale value.

The market for textbooks is the faculty who make text selections for courses (Coser, Kadushin, & Powell, 1982). While the photographs may be designed to create in students a desire for health, they are also there to sell health educators the book. Therefore, health educators should take some time examining the representations in these texts, while questioning their own definitions of who is healthy and who can become healthy. Do they actually wish to imply that access to health is limited to young, white, slim, middle-class, physically abled, and physically active people? If health educators are committed to increasing the potential for health for *all* people, then the focus should not be directed primarily at those for whom health is most easily attained and maintained. Rethinking the images that represent health may help restructure health educators' goals.

It is an interesting exercise to try to envision alternative healthy-image photographs. Here is one of my choices for a cover photograph: An old woman of color, sitting on a chair with a book in her lap, is looking out at a small garden that has been reclaimed from an urban backlot.

Acknowledgments I would like to thank Nancy Worcester, Julie D'Acci, Sally Lesher, and Elizabeth Ellsworth for their critical readings of this chapter and their valuable suggestions.

NOTES

1. Cars appear in health textbook photographs primarily in the context of either environmental concerns or the stresses of modern life.

2. Occasionally, photographs used were actually taken for advertising purposes. For example, in a chapter on exercise there is a full-page color photograph of a runner with the credit "Photo by Jerry LaRocca for Nike" (Insel & Roth, 1988, p. 316).

3. Examining the wages of disabled women can give a sense of the potential economic problems: "The 1981 Census revealed that disabled women earn less than 24 cents for each dollar earned by nondisabled men; black disabled women earn 12 cents for each dollar. Disabled women earn approximately 52 percent of what nondisabled women earn" (Saxton & Howe, 1987, p xii).

4. "Supercrip" is a term sometimes used among people with disabilities to describe people with disabilities who go

beyond what would be expected of those with no disabilities. It should not be necessary to be a one-legged ski champion or a blind physician to prove that people with disabilities deserve the opportunities available to the able-bodied. By emphasizing the individual "heroes," the focus shifts away from societal barriers and obstacles to individual responsibility to excel.

5. I am using "old" rather than "older" for two reasons that have been identified by many writing about ageism. "Older" seems a euphemism that attempts to lessen the impact of discussing someone's age, along with such terms as senior citizen or golden ager. The second point is the simple question: "Older than whom?"

REFERENCES
A list of references is available in the original source.

Appendix: Textbooks Examined for This Chapter

Carroll, C., & Miller, D. (1986). *Health: The science of human adaptation* (4th ed.). Dubuque, IA: Wm. C. Brown.

Dintiman, G. B., & Greenberg, J. (1986). *Health through discovery* (3rd ed.). New York: Random House.

Hales, D. R., & Williams, B. K. (1986). *An invitation to health: Your personal responsibility* (3rd ed.). Menlo Park, CA: Benjamin/Cummings Publishing Company.

Insel, P. M., & Roth, W. T. (1988). *Core concepts in health* (5th ed.). Mountain View, CA: Mayfield Publishing.

Levy, M. R., Dignan, M., & Shirreffs, J. H. (1987). *Life and health.* (5th ed.). New York: Random House.

Mullen, K. D., Gold, R. S., Belcastro, P. A., & McDermott, R. J. (1986). *Connections for health.* Dubuque, IA: Wm. C. Brown.

Payne, W. A., & Hahn, D. B. (1986). *Understanding your health,* St. Louis: Times Mirror/Mosby.

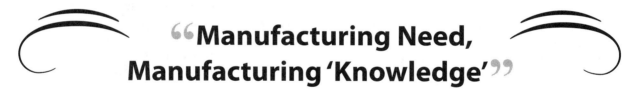

"Manufacturing Need, Manufacturing 'Knowledge'"

by the National Women's Health Network Writing Group (Adriane Fugh-Berman, Cynthia Pearson, Amy Allina, Jane Zones, Nancy Worcester, Mariamne Whatley, and Charlea Massion)

Several major medical journals recently announced a jointly created policy to refuse to publish research sponsored by pharmaceutical companies unless the researchers involved were guaranteed scientific independence.[1] While laudable, such a move addresses only a tiny part of a pervasive problem: pharmaceutical companies influence almost every piece of information available to doctors and consumers. Consumers may be totally unaware of the diverse ways that their healthcare providers have been influenced by pharmaceutical companies and medical device manufacturers; practitioners themselves may not be aware of how their ideas and "education" on drug treatments have been manipulated by the companies that sell these products.

Ersatz or Co-opted Consumer Groups

Ads are reinforced by educational campaigns that appear to be independent but are also paid for—and influenced by—the same companies. Companies seek out—or even invent—nonprofit groups and offer them money to do specific educational campaigns that they believe will help sell their products. These decoy organizations produce and distribute educational materials under their own name, and consumers can't tell who wrote the text or who paid for it. One example is a series of fact sheets on women's health produced by the Coalition of Labor Union Women and paid for by Eli Lilly. The fact sheets cover a range of health issues including menopause, cancer, osteoporosis and heart attack. It's surely no coincidence that Eli Lilly's drug Evista has been promoted (often misleadingly) as having potential uses for all of those health problems.

Sometimes these fact sheets are accurate and well balanced, and sometimes they are simply thinly disguised advertisements. What matters is that a health issue is raised as a concern that appears to be coming from an independent group concerned only with promoting women's health, rather than a corporation bent on making a profit. This is a particularly pernicious strategy because it undermines consumer trust in groups that were created to work for the public interest.

The NWHN surveyed women's health organizations, including disease-specific organizations (such as the Arthritis Foundation and the American Heart Association) that influence policy for substantial segments of the female population. Fifty-one of 80 groups that were approached responded. Ten of 17 professionalized women's health organizations (run by clinicians or researchers) acknowledged financial support from companies that provide services or products to their constituencies. The National Alliance of Breast Cancer Organizations (NABCO), for example, lists over 50 sponsors in its annual report; Bristol Myers Squibb, a major manufacturer of chemotherapy drugs, contributed over $100,000 to NABCO in 1996. Five professionalized organizations accepted no corporate donations, and two receive money from industries that do not have a direct financial interest in their issues.

Grassroots organizations (consumer-run) were less likely to accept industry donations; 19 of 31 (61.3%) grassroots organizations received no money from industry, and four (13%) accepted non-compromising corporate donations. Three provided no financial information, and five (16.3%) (four of them disease-specific) accepted donations from companies whose business interests intersect with the health issues of their constituencies.

News Stories

When you opened up your Sunday paper and read in a *Parade* magazine cover story that supermodel Lauren Hutton calls estrogen her favorite beauty secret, did you know that she is a paid spokesperson for Wyeth Ayerst, manufacturer of the biggest-selling estrogen (and in fact biggest-selling drug)? This is just one example of the ways that drug companies spend money to influence consumer opinions about their products.

Drug companies are working to influence every source of consumer health information, including the actual news. In addition to traditional press releases and

press conferences announcing the results of new studies or the launch of new products, companies now produce what look like actual news stories in the form of video news releases and sample articles, which television and radio stations, newspapers and magazines can broadcast or print directly. This tactic is very effective. In one survey, every one of more than 100 television news stations surveyed had used some part of a video news release. While responsible journalists will not use the company-sponsored materials without putting them in the context of a fuller story, they are still putting the company's materials, and importantly the product name, in the news and into the minds of their viewers and readers. When Pfizer launched Viagra, more than 210 million viewers saw some part of the company's video news release.

Even when reporters decide on their own that a new study is worth covering as news, they don't always do a good job of covering the story in a way that's useful for women. Reporters may take the company's promotional materials at face value, presenting beneficial findings in the most positive light and down-playing or ignoring entirely any potential risks. For example, a study that reviewed 70 news stories about positive new findings about Merck's osteoporosis drug Fosamax found that barely 50 percent mentioned adverse effects, and 70 percent quoted experts or studies with a financial tie to the company (only a third pointed this out to the viewer or reader).[2]

Websites

Websites have quickly become a critical source of health information for consumers. Like any other information source, information on the Web is subject to influence by corporate advertising efforts. For example, *womensorganizations.org*, a website that presents itself as a source of information on important women's health issues sponsored by a coalition of national women's groups, is paid for in part by a grant from Eli Lilly. Even though the Web is a new source of information, women need to be aware that it is just as subject to influence as any other and in some cases is more so since regulatory oversight procedures have not yet been established.

New Drug Campaigns

When a new drug is launched, pharmaceutical companies often mount an all-out assault on all these fronts. The goal of these efforts is to make sure that consumers hear about the new drug as often as possible, and always in the most positive terms possible. The more control the companies have over consumer information sources, the better they like it.

Before Merck launched a campaign for its osteoporosis drug Fosamax, it gave a large grant to a leading consumer group for older women with the explicit understanding that the grant would be used to "educate" older women with the message that they should worry about osteoporosis. Merck obviously hoped that this investment would raise the level of women's concern about the strength of their bones. To reinforce this concern, Merck began running direct-to-consumer ads featuring frail older women in pain contrasted with vivacious, active seniors in control of their lives, and used text to imply that medication was needed to prevent disability.

Next, Merck took this newly created fear and concern on the part of older women and translated it into action. They began marketing bone density testing, first by making it more available, then by making it more affordable.[3] Even before Fosamax was approved, Merck purchased a small company that manufactured bone density testing equipment and expanded its production, so that many more bone density machines were available.[4] Merck also gave the National Osteoporosis Foundation a large grant to promote a toll-free number through which consumers motivated by supposedly independent educational campaigns could find the location of nearby bone density screening.

And because bone density screening isn't cheap, Merck added a final piece to its campaign, a public policy initiative to persuade the federal government to pay for bone density screening tests through Medicare. This component of the campaign was replicated at the state level targeting private insurers.

Having successfully frightened women into worrying about bone strength and to get that strength measured, Merck had created the perfect environment to sell its product. Every component of its campaign contributed to sales of Fosamax, the only non-hormonal drug approved at the time for osteoporosis prevention. Yet, the vast majority of women affected by Merck's effort would never know the true motivation for that information, much less who paid for it.

This article is excerpted from *The Truth about Hormone Replacement Therapy: How to Break Free from the Medical Myths of Menopause* (National Women's Health Network, Prima Publishers, Rosedale, California, 2002).

REFERENCES

1. Okie S. *Washington Post,* August 5, 2001, A1.

2. Moynihan R, Bero L, Ross-Degnan D et al. "Coverage by the news media of the benefits and risk of medications." *New England Journal of Medicine* 1999; 342(22):1645-50.

3. Tanouye E. "Merck's osteoporosis warnings pave the way for its new drug." *Wall Street Journal,* July 28, 1995.

4. Sherwood L. Presentation to FDA Radiological Devices Panel meeting, May 17, 1999.

 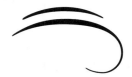

Overdosed America
"The Broken Promise of American Medicine"

from *HealthFacts*

No, this isn't another book about Americans popping too many pills and paying exorbitant prices for them. Its far more worrisome premise is summed up in the long subtitle: *How the Pharmaceutical Companies Distort Medical Knowledge, Mislead Doctors, and Compromise Your Health*. Author John Abramson, MD, is troubled by the commercial influences that pervade all aspects of American medical care. The pharmaceutical industry's influence can be seen in everything from the sponsoring of continuing medical

New Book Review of *Overdosed America—The Broken Promise of American Medicine* from *HealthFacts*, December 2004, pp. 2–3. Reprinted by permission of Maryann Napoli.

education to the latest treatment guidelines that make an ever-expanding number of Americans candidates for life-long drug therapy.

A Harvard Medical School faculty member, Dr. Abramson writes that he thoroughly enjoyed practicing family medicine for over 20 years. But he had become increasingly disturbed by the new brand of medical consumerism, typified by the middle-aged male patient who came in demanding an expensive, widely advertised prescription drug (Celebrex). No amount of explaining about cheaper, safer and equally effective alternatives could change his patient's mind.

It is not only his patients who get a skewed view of new drugs, observed Dr. Abramson, his fellow physicians were influenced by the same promotional campaigns, often masquerading as education. Whereas taxpayers once funded most medical research, the pharmaceutical industry now pays the lion's share. By now, many Americans know that the pharmaceutical industry has one of the highest profit margins of the Fortune 500 companies. How many know that the industry spends more money on marketing (from advertising to free drug samples for doctors) than on research?

Dr. Abramson left his practice to spend the next two and a half years doing what most practicing doctors have little time to do—"researching the research." What he found will not surprise HealthFacts readers. Drug companies: design clinical trials in such a way that ensures their products will come out on top; withhold the trials that show negative results; focus attention on the benefits while giving short shrift to the harms; and 'spin' equivocal results in a way that puts their drugs in a favorable light.

What's more, the people selected for clinical trials are often unrepresentative of the majority for whom the drug will ultimately be prescribed. Cancer drugs are offered as an example. "Nearly two-thirds of all cancer patients are 65 or older," observes Dr. Abramson, "but only one-quarter of the people in cancer studies have reached 65." Many of the articles published in medical journals, even the most prestigious ones, he found, are little more than infomercials for the drug.

In time, Dr. Abramson began to detect the frequent use of overblown statistics guaranteed to scare people into a life-long drug regimen. Two years ago, The New England Journal of Medicine published a study about a new, inexpensive blood test that measures blood levels of inflammation in the body called C-reactive protein, or CRP, which supposedly can predict a person's risk of heart disease. The study followed 28,000 women over eight years and found that those with the highest CRP levels were more than twice as likely to develop heart disease. The study's authors concluded that identifying people with elevated CRP would allow "optimal targeting of statin therapy." In other words, a way to identify future customers for cholesterol-lowering drugs.

What's wrong with this picture, asks Dr. Abramson after the largely uncritical media picked up the CRP story and ran with it as "ground-breaking" and "extremely important." A closer look at the statistics from this study showed that the 28,000 female participants were less than 55 years old and healthy. Their risk of heart attack, stroke, etc. was quite small. For "every 1000 women with the highest CRP levels, there was only slightly more than one (1.3) additional episode of cardiovascular disease each year than among the 1000 women with the lowest CRP levels." In other words, the twice-as-likely-to-develop-heart-disease statistic boiled down to a doubling of odds that were tiny to begin with.

With the relentless focus on drugs, Dr. Abramson suggests that doctors and the general public tend to overlook the considerable body of research showing that regular exercise, smoking cessation, and a healthy diet trump nearly every medical intervention as the best way to keep heart disease at bay.

Americans tend to have faith in the latest high-tech medical care, but a large Medicare study challenged some common assumptions. Areas of the country with higher concentrations of specialists have both higher healthcare costs and worse healthcare outcomes.

"The public needs access to independent expert opinion that can counterbalance the enormous influence that the medical industry wields over our beliefs about the best approach to health and medical care," writes Dr. Abramson. (Full disclosure: The Center for Medical Consumers is mentioned twice in this book as one of the rare sources of unbiased information.) A new national public body with the independence and expertise of the Institute of Medicine, he suggests, is the only way that will ever be accomplished.

"Doctors Still Chummy with Drug Sales Reps"

from *AARP Bulletin*

"There's a big bucket of money sitting in every office . . . Every time you go in, you reach your hand in the bucket and grab a handful." That's how a sales manager at AstraZeneca described to colleagues the rewards of pitching the company's products to doctors. His unguarded remarks showed up on the Internet—and got him fired, as the company confirmed—just as a new storm is brewing over tactics drugmakers use to influence doctors' prescribing habits.

A two-year Senate Finance Committee investigation, for example, has concluded that the companies, by funding continuing medical education programs for doctors, have been able to "increase their market for new products" and to illegally promote off-label uses for their drugs. The committee is concerned that persuading doctors to prescribe the newest, costliest drugs hikes government spending for Medicare and raises safety issues.

The drug industry in 2002 issued its own code of conduct declaring that interactions between sales reps and doctors should benefit patients and that meals—but not entertainment—are allowable if modest and connected to educational presentations. Today, 94 percent of doctors report a relationship with drug reps, according to a survey led by Harvard Medical School and published in the April 26 *New England Journal of Medicine*. The interactions range from receiving drug samples (78 percent) to getting free meals (83 percent) and expenses for attending industry-sponsored meetings (35 percent).

The authors of a second study wrote in the Public Library of Science's April medical journal that "reps scour a doctor's office for objects—a tennis racquet, Russian novels, '70s rock music"—to establish personal ties, and some give doctors food and gifts.

Advertising Disease "Premenstrual Dysphoric Disorder"

by Roy Moynihan and Alan Cassels

An anonymous woman tries to disentangle a shopping cart from an interlocked row of them, outside a suburban store. She is frustrated and angry. She becomes even more exasperated when another shopper enters the frame, calmly unhooks a cart, and glides smoothly on her way. Watching this TV advertisement unfold, it might look like the woman is experiencing little more than a normal bout of tension or stress. But the folks at the drug company Lilly know better. This woman may need a powerful antidepressant because she is suffering a severe form of mental illness called premenstrual dysphoric disorder—a new condition approved in the United States just months before the advertisement's broadcast.

Think it's PMS? It could be PMDD.

—Lilly TV commercial

Columbia University Professor Jean Endicott tells us PMDD is a psychiatric condition suffered by up to 7 percent of women. Brown University Professor Paula Caplan claims the condition has essentially been invented, and there is no strong scientific evidence to distinguish it from normal premenstrual difficulties. Even worse, argues Caplan, using a medical label to explain away the severe distress some women experience in the lead-up to their period runs the risk of masking the underlying causes of their suffering.

In the U.S., the FDA has accepted that the condition PMDD exists and has approved Lilly's Prozac and several similar antidepressants for its treatment, yet in other parts of the world it is not even a recognized disease. It is simply not listed as a separate disorder in the World Health Organization's International Classification of Diseases.[1] And even in the U.S., despite the hard work of Endicott, Lilly, and others, PMDD still only has a partial listing in the psychiatrists' manual of diseases, the *DSM*, and is therefore not strictly seen as a fully official category of illness.[2]

Yet this scientific controversy is invisible in the avalanche of television and magazine advertisements about PMDD in the U.S.—much of it targeting young women. The $500-billion pharmaceutical industry has identified another new mega-market—women of childbearing age—and the world of marketing demands simple, clear messages. The emotional ups and downs preceding your period are no longer a part of normal life—they are now a telltale sign you could have a psychiatric condition. As Caplan puts it, by watching these ads "women are learning to consider themselves mentally ill."[3]

A friendly and hardworking academic, Jean Endicott operates from a small office buried in the basement of a psychiatric hospital in New York City. In stark contrast to Caplan, she insists PMDD is a genuine disorder that can be "very disabling," and often not properly diagnosed or treated. She welcomes drug company efforts to have the condition taken more seriously. It was Endicott who led the key scientific meeting—funded by Lilly and attended by company representatives—that paved the way for two of the most important developments in the life of this young disorder: FDA acceptance of the condition, and approval of Lilly's antidepressant as the first drug to treat it. As to the appropriateness of drug companies advertising disorders like this on television, Endicott is a strong believer. "I think it educates people."[4]

The pharmaceutical industry in the U.S. now spends more than $3 billion a year on direct-to-consumer advertising, promoting its most lucrative brands. Promotional budgets that once exclusively targeted doctors with doughnuts and free samples, and cultivated thought-leaders, are now aimed very much at the general public as well. Prime-time television news bulletins are dominated by drug ads.[5]

Increasingly, however, these commercials are not just selling drugs, but also the diseases that go with them. The shopping cart ad for PMDD is part of a new form of TV advertising, designed to introduce millions of people to previously unheard-of conditions. While the advertising claims made about the benefits and risks of medicines are regulated by law—albeit very loosely—claims about diseases remain a virtual free-for-all.

The U.S. and New Zealand are the only developed countries in the world that allow full-blown advertising of drugs to consumers. However, many nations—including Australia, Canada, and Britain—allow companies to sponsor disease "awareness-raising" campaigns that involve advertising and other media attention. With prescription drug expenditures rising dramatically in many nations, and a growing view that these disease "awareness-raising" campaigns are really only a form of backdoor drug advertising, debates about tougher regulation of all these marketing activities have been taking place everywhere.

In Britain these issues have been treated so seriously a major parliamentary inquiry has investigated them, and in New Zealand there has been a strong push within the national government to tighten the rules on the advertising of both drugs and diseases. In Canada, Australia, and across Europe, national governments are juggling growing consumer concerns about this mass marketing with the pressure from the pharmaceutical industry and sometimes part of the media industry as well to open up the airwaves, just as they are in the U.S.

One of the world's best-known and most informed critics of the industry's advertising is Australian general practitioner Dr. Peter Mansfield, who helps run a globally recognized group called Healthy Skepticism, from his base in Adelaide. According to the indefatigable Mansfield, trying to find good consumer information about health is like searching for a needle in a haystack. Drug company advertising, says Mansfield with his trademark smile, "just makes the haystack bigger."[6]

Until very recently, much of the criticism of advertising has focused on the way ads can mislead people about the risks and benefits of new medicines—not surprisingly many commercials tend to exaggerate benefits and play down side effects.[7] In fact, the FDA, which regulates drug advertising in the U.S., frequently writes to drug companies warning them their advertisements are so misleading they may have broken the law. As it turned out, Lilly's shopping cart commercial was one that attracted such a letter. In this case the FDA alleged the ad was "lacking in fair balance" because it minimized information about the drug's side effects.[8] In the end, as is usually the case, Lilly was simply asked by the FDA, politely, to withdraw the offending ad. Despite repeated violations across the industry, and tens of millions of Americans being regularly exposed to misleading information about the risks and benefits of widely prescribed drugs, companies are not fined and executives are not held accountable.[9]

These days, though, another theme has emerged in the analysis of pharmaceutical industry advertising. Researchers are finding more and more ads are helping sell the idea that everyday human experiences are symptoms of medical conditions requiring treatment with drugs. Together with colleagues, the Dartmouth Medical School duo Drs. Steve Woloshin and Lisa Schwartz recently analyzed seventy drug company ads in ten popular U.S. magazines. They found that almost half tried to encourage consumers to consider medical causes for their common experiences, most often urging them to consult a physician.[10] The ads targeted aspects of ordinary life including sneezing, hair loss, or being overweight—things many people could clearly manage without seeing a doctor—and portrayed them as if they were part of a medical condition. The researchers speculated that advertising was increasingly medicalizing ordinary experience, and pushing the boundaries of medical influence far too wide.

Watching these trends closely is Canadian researcher Dr. Barbara Mintzes, who included in her Ph.D. at the University of British Columbia in Vancouver a rigorous examination of drug company advertising. She also discovered that many ads now promote medical conditions, rather than just drugs, and are helping to medicalize life, as she puts it. "To an unprecedented degree they portray the educational message of a pill for every ill—and increasingly an ill for every pill.[11] It's a shift from a drug that's approved to treat people who are actually suffering from an illness to the idea that you just take a pill to deal with normal life situations."[12]

Mintzes is particularly outraged by the promotion of PMDD, which has been aggressively advertised in magazines read by teenagers, as well as in TV commercials. In her view it seems designed to make younger women feel there is something wrong with the normal emotional fluctuations they experience in the lead-up to their monthly period. While accepting that for some people the problem can be severe, Mintzes worries that the ads paint a shallow picture of what it means to be a young women. "There is pressure on people to be someone other than who they are."[13]

With all treatments there is a balance between benefits and harms. For someone who is very sick, the chances of a great improvement may easily outweigh the risks of side effects from a drug. The antidepressants like Prozac that are being prescribed for PMDD carry many side effects, including serious sexual difficulties, and for teenagers an apparent increase in the risk of suicidal behavior.[14] Such risks might be worth taking for someone severely debilitated by chronic clinical depression, but for a woman arguing with a boyfriend, or frustrated by a shopping cart?

"When you're giving drugs to healthy people you're shifting the balance," says Mintzes. "If you're already healthy, the likelihood of benefit becomes much, much smaller and then there's a concern that what we are actually doing at a population level is causing much more harm than benefit through drug treatment."[15]

New York professor Jean Endicott bluntly rejects the concern that PMDD is an example of ordinary life being medicalized. "It's an insult to suggest that women with less severe symptoms would even be seeking treatment. Women are not running around saying, 'Give me a pill for everything.' "[16]

Looking for good hard scientific evidence to help settle this difference of opinion is difficult. Mintzes's view is based on a belief that the aggressive promotion of conditions like PMDD is causing too many otherwise healthy people to see themselves as ill and opt for drug therapies that may cause them more harm than good. Her research has added to a body of evidence showing that these ads do in fact drive many people into doctors' offices, and that some doctors will prescribe the advertised drugs even when they may doubt their appropriateness for the problem at hand.[17] But there have been few, if any, large studies that rigorously investigate whether direct-to-consumer advertising causes unnecessary medical labeling or leads to inappropriate or harmful prescription of drugs. What is crystal clear, however, is that these ads boost drug sales.

Industry executives argue that the most powerful case for direct-to-consumer advertising is evidence of underdiagnosis and undertreatment among those people with serious health problems, including high cholesterol, high blood pressure, depression and, presumably, PMDD.[18] In a special issue of the *British Medical Journal* devoted to the topic of medicalization, and titled "Too Much Medicine?," two senior officials from the drug company Merck wrote that the rules governing drug advertising should be loosened in Europe to help fix the urgent problem of undertreatment. They claimed there was little good evidence to support the view of Mintzes and others that advertising leads to inappropriate prescribing or harm: "unfounded fears" about advertising, they wrote, were restricting peoples' rights "to have all the information they need to make informed choices about their healthcare."

One of the weaknesses in this argument is the failure to acknowledge the controversy and uncertainty surrounding the definitions of the common conditions said to be massively underdiagnosed. If the estimates of the numbers of people suffering these conditions and requiring treatment are inflated to start with, as some observers consider to be the case with high cholesterol and depression for example, then claims of widespread undertreatment deserve to be taken with extra-large doses of scrutiny and skepticism. With PMDD, claims of underdiagnosis and undertreatment make little sense if the condition itself doesn't even exist.

A major report on medicines prepared for the European pharmaceutical industry, as part of the push to loosen the advertising rules there, claimed there is strong evidence of undertreatment in many conditions including heart disease, Alzheimer's, depression, and cancer.[19] Two Italian researchers analyzing that report, however, directly countered those claims, arguing that the industry's report selectively cited the scientific evidence—making reference to studies showing undertreatment, but overlooking studies that demonstrate examples of overtreatment. "Not a single study on overuse . . . is quoted, and only research looking at under-use is mentioned," wrote the Italian researchers.[20]

There is little doubt that many people in genuine need are not getting the medical attention or medication they require, particularly among the poor of wealthy nations and the wider developing world. Whether spending billions advertising disorders like PMDD on television and in women's magazines is the best way to correct that problem is highly questionable. Undertreatment may often have more to do with a lack of money or access than a lack of information. And as to the claim that advertising is the best way to inform, educate, and encourage more choice, the high-profile deputy editor at *JAMA*, Dr. Drummond Rennie, disagrees. "Direct-to-consumer advertising has got nothing to do with the public's education and it has got absolutely everything to do with . . . boosting product sales."[21]

The recent history of the controversial young disorder PMDD also has a lot to do with boosting product sales—in this case antidepressants. Taking a closer look at that history offers some fascinating insights into how a new condition is brought into the world, and the various players who nurture it in the years leading up to its debut on the world stage in highly produced TV advertisements. And just to underline how controversial this disorder really is, the European health authorities ultimately stopped Lilly promoting Prozac for PMDD, because it was "not a well established disease entity across Europe."[22]

Like the notion that menopause is a disease of estrogen deficiency, scholars trace the origins of the modern concept of PMDD back to the 1930s, when the term "premenstrual tension" was first being coined. By the 1960s the medical community was describing a "premenstrual syndrome" (PMS) that featured common symptoms like fluid retention, irritability, and moodiness. Writing about the history of PMS, feminist researchers Joan Chrisler and Paula Caplan find there are so many different definitions as to make any one overall definition almost impossible. What's more, they counted up almost 150 symptoms supposedly associated with the condition. "The concept of PMS is so vague and so elastic that almost every woman can see something of her own experience within it," they wrote.[23]

Examining references to PMS in popular culture and the medical literature Chrisler and Caplan found that it was very much a western notion, with most medical research having been done in Europe, North America, and Australia. While women everywhere experience tension, irritability, or water retention prior to monthly periods, many do not believe this is abnormal or feel any need for professional intervention. The two authors argue that long before PMDD was created, the widespread use of the term PMS had already medicalized women's menstrual cycles—the cycle itself had become the medical problem that needed to be solved.

While clearly critical of what they see as a strong example of unnecessary medicalization, the pair acknowledges that many women may feel their concerns will not be taken seriously if they aren't given a medical explanation. Similarly, they argue, many people may see the medical discussion of PMS as being friendly to women, and cast those who reject the idea of the medical label as being insensitive and uncaring.

Against this backdrop of uncertainty and debate about the very definition and meaning of PMS, in the mid 1980s a small group of psychiatrists and others working with the American Psychiatric Association came together to try to define a new condition. The idea was to separate out normal premenstrual complaints from a severe form of mood disturbance that came and went every month, but was serious enough in some women to be disabling and warrant treatment. The group was pulled together by the imposing figure of Dr. Robert Spitzer, the man then responsible for revising the psychiatrist's bible, the *Diagnostic and Statistical Manual of Mental Disorders (DSM)*.[24]

Each time the *DSM* is revised, new disorders are added and over the last few decades the numbers have expanded dramatically. Physically, the book started out as a slim volume, but has since morphed into a massive tome. Under the direction of Robert Spitzer—Jean Endicott's colleague at the New York State Psychiatric Institute—the numbers of new conditions listed in the *DSM* exploded. So keen was he on adding new diseases to the manual, the now elderly Spitzer confesses to having been teased by some of his younger colleagues as being someone who never saw a disorder he didn't like.[25] PMDD was one of the most controversial disorders ever added, and it was known at first by the very awkward name of late luteal phase dysphoric disorder (LLPDD) when Spitzer's committee sat down to discuss it back in the summer of 1985.

According to Spitzer's account of the heated debates of the time, even within his committee there were disputes about whether to include this supposed new mental disorder in the *DSM*. Part of the concern was that so little was known about its causes, or how to treat it— criticisms acknowledged by Spitzer and his colleagues. Yet ironically, this lack of knowledge became one of the powerful reasons to create the new condition, with enthusiasts arguing that a listing in the *DSM* would facilitate more research on its causes and treatment.[26]

Another key concern raised from the beginning by some of Spitzer's committee was that because all women experience some degree of premenstrual symptoms, there was a danger the psychiatrists were going to label aspects of ordinary life as a mental disorder. Again acknowledging the concern, Spitzer and his supporters responded that similar arguments could be made about many established mental disorders. For example, they argued, depression was simply an extreme form of sadness. Spitzer's point was that with these sorts of disorders, a lot of care must always be taken in defining the boundary between what is normal and what is sick. But Spitzer did not explain how those boundaries are supposed to survive the whirlwind of mass marketing deliberately designed to blur them. While the strict criteria for a disabling impairment might look like a reasonable boundary on paper in front of a group of psychiatrists, in the real world of drug promotion a woman having

trouble with a shopping cart becomes the definition of a new disorder seen by tens of millions across America.

Despite the objections of two of its members, Spitzer's original committee recommended including the condition then known as LLPDD in the *DSM*. The recommendation sparked a chorus of criticism from some women's groups and professional societies—underlining the premature nature of such an addition. The compromise solution was to include the new disease, but only in the appendix to the manual, as a disorder requiring further research. It was therefore not even an *official* category when the next version of the manual was published in 1987.[27]

Six years later, in preparation for the following revision of the *DSM*, another committee revisited the same debate. Despite reviewing hundreds of studies, committee members found there was still much uncertainty about how to define this condition. There was still no consensus about whether it existed as a separate mental disorder, and more research was needed to resolve the dispute. At that time the name late luteal phase dysphoric disorder was replaced with premenstrual dysphoric disorder, but the disorder would remain listed in the appendix of the *DSM* as a condition requiring further research.

There was, however, another highly significant development at this point. Despite the ongoing doubts and disputes within the committee, the publishers of the manual took the unusual step of classifying PMDD as a bonafide depressive disorder and listing it in the main body of the *DSM*, at the same time as it was still listed in the manual's appendix as a tentative unofficial condition needing more research. While appearing somewhat contradictory this move was important commercially because it gave PMDD a precious item number—allowing doctors to prescribe drugs to treat the condition, and health insurers to fund them.[28]

It was here that the rifts between the scientists debating this new condition became major disagreements. Psychiatry professor Sally Severino—a member of the committee trying to define the new condition—says it was at this point that she parted company with her colleagues Spitzer and Endicott. "The data did not prove PMDD existed as a valid diagnosis," she said. "The decision to make it a depressive disorder was driven more by politics than science."[29] Making the condition look more like a legitimate mental illness, Severino explained, opened it up for lucrative research funding from pharmaceutical companies. "As far as I was concerned the decision was not based on anything in the data we looked at." So does PMDD really exist? "That's a good question," she laughed.

What happened next would help push an unknown, unofficial and for some, an unreal condition from the back pages of the psychiatrist's manual into glossy magazines and television screens everywhere, thanks to Lilly, the company best known for its blockbuster antidepressant Prozac. By the late 1990s Prozac—whose chemical name is fluoxetine—was about to lose its patent, and Lilly stood to lose hundreds of millions of dollars because of the emergence of cheaper generic competitors. Winning approval for the drug for a new disease might re-energize sales of this blockbuster chemical.

In late 1998 Lilly helped fund a small meeting, impressively titled as a "Roundtable" of researchers, which came together and discussed PMDD. The meeting of just sixteen key experts took place in Washington, D.C., and it was attended by a group of FDA staff and at least four Lilly representatives. The chair was Columbia University's Jean Endicott, who had by then been pushing for the acceptance of this disorder for over a decade. This time, though, Endicott had a giant pharmaceutical company on her side.

Within twelve months the minutes of that "Roundtable" would appear in a medical journal article claiming there was now a scientific consensus that PMDD was a "distinct clinical entity."[30] Even though the article appeared in a very minor journal, its publication would lend credibility to the claims that this was a real disorder and help convince the FDA to approve Lilly's drug for the treatment of PMDD just a few months later. Despite requests, neither Lilly nor FDA officials would talk publicly about the Roundtable meeting. They have offered no explanation as to how a company-sponsored gathering can apparently play such a key role in regulatory acceptance of a new condition and simultaneous approval of that sponsor's drug. While the Roundtable was obviously designed to help win regulatory approval for Prozac's new use, it was also designed to try to end the scientific uncertainty about whether PMDD really exists. As it turned out the meeting only served to highlight the continuing uncertainty and controversy.

The meeting was held in the shadow cast by just one company, Lilly. It was supported by just one company, and representatives from just one company were in attendance. Turning down repeated requests for interviews, Lilly has refused to answer one of the most critical questions here: what role did it play in transforming those Roundtable meeting minutes into a medical journal article that helped provide the scientific rationale for the approval of the company's antidepressant for this controversial condition? Company-sponsored ghostwriting of scientific articles is widespread within the medical establishment, particularly within the world of psychiatry.[31] Asked about the fact that drug companies were now funding such vitally important scientific activities—where the very existence of new disorders was being debated—Endicott said simply, "It's a way of life."[32]

Critics like Paula Caplan argue no important new scientific evidence had emerged since the early 1990s to prove this was a separate condition, so at the time of the Roundtable in 1998 PMDD still didn't deserve the status of a separate mental disorder. Psychiatrist Sally Severino agrees. Jean Endicott disagrees and says there was significant new evidence, though not a lot of it. Yet even with the limited new evidence that Endicott points to, it is clear even from the published journal article that enormous uncertainties still existed about this so-called disorder—even among the tiny group of handpicked experts who attended the meeting.[33]

Endicott's summing up at the conclusion of the Roundtable had an important qualification, hinting at lingering doubts. "Most present are convinced (maybe in different ways) that PMDD is a distinct entity." But despite the doubts and disagreements the Lilly sponsored meeting had two important bottom-line conclusions, both highly favorable to the meeting's sponsor: there was now an alleged consensus that the disorder existed, and most people present thought there was sufficient evidence to support the use of antidepressants like Prozac to treat it.

By Christmas of 1999, a meeting of advisers to the FDA had voted unanimously to approve Lilly's fluoxetine for the treatment of PMDD. Soon after the FDA formally gave Lilly the green light to market its drug for PMDD and Lilly organized a launch to do just that. But in an extraordinary turn of events, the pill was not launched under the name Prozac. Lilly had done some sophisticated market research with doctors and potential patients, and as a result it had decided to repaint Prozac with attractive lavender and pink colors and rename it Sarafem.

For specialists in pharmaceutical marketing like Vince Parry, the story of PMDD and Sarafem is a great example of a company "fostering the creation of a condition and aligning it with a product."[34] He worked for Lilly on the campaign, which he describes as helping to "build awareness for both the condition and the drug." To kick it off, he says, the company sponsored a "pre-launch initiative" to raise awareness of the condition. "By changing the brand name from Prozac to Sarafem—packaged in a lavender-colored pill and promoted with images of sunflowers and smart women—Lilly created a brand that better aligned with the personality of the condition for a hand-in-glove fit."[35]

With Sarafem and PMDD, Parry explains, Lilly's market research investigated how best to brand both the drug and the condition, to come up with language women felt most comfortable with. PMDD, he says, "has a certain kind of personality that they can see themselves in . . . even the advertising that was done to support it, the women weren't sort of these spooky women who looked depressed. The advertising featured women who were confident, self-assured, were unafraid of asking for help and recognizing that this is a condition they shouldn't feel ashamed of or anything . . . all those things are developed in conjunction with the very patients themselves to make sure that there is a lock and key result."[36]

Somehow, though, despite Parry's and Lilly's best efforts, the *personality* of both Sarafem and PMDD became a little confused, partly because of some strong negative reactions to the shopping cart ad screened across America. Even the industry-friendly FDA reacted, arguing that the TV ad trivialized the seriousness of this alleged new mental disorder by associating it with normal premenstrual problems. In a letter to Lilly the FDA was particularly critical of the catchy tag line, "Think it's PMS? It could be PMDD."[37]

The letter stated that the ad never clearly defined the difference between PMS and PMDD, and it therefore "broadens" the condition unreasonably. While the FDA had clearly accepted the view that PMDD exists, ironically its criticisms of the ad reinforced the concerns of those who felt ordinary life was being made into a medical condition. Says drug researcher Barbara Mintzes, "These ads are really selling the magical solution that you won't have to deal with something that was a normal part of life any more."[38] Says psychologist Paula Caplan, "In a nutshell, you see them taking a very common kind of experience and making that very thing into a mental disorder."[39]

Caplan's concern that serious problems were being trivialized comes from a different perspective than that of the folks at the FDA. She worries that a psychiatric label of PMDD can be used to cover up or mask the real sources of pain and anguish for some women at the time of their period. Such sources may include a history of violent relationships, stressful life circumstances, poverty, or harassment—problems that clearly cannot be fixed with a pill.[40]

Despite the concerns, the marketing of both the new condition and the antidepressants to treat it has continued apace in the U.S. In Europe, however, Lilly's marketing of Sarafem/Prozac (fluoxetine) for PMDD came to a very abrupt stop. In mid-2003, following deliberations about standardizing product labels across Europe, the central drug regulator issued a devastating statement raising serious questions about the disorder's existence. It also fiercely criticized the quality of the company's

clinical trials that purported to show the benefits of the drug.

A panel from the European Agency for the Evaluation of Medicinal Products noted that "PMDD is not a well-established disease entity across Europe. It is not listed in the International Classification of Diseases and remains only a researcher diagnosis in *DSM IV*." But their next finding was the most powerful reason advanced for halting the promotion of Prozac for PMDD, and it echoed the now familiar arguments of feminist critics. "There was considerable concern that women with less severe premenstrual symptoms might erroneously receive a diagnosis of PMDD resulting in widespread inappropriate short and long-term use of fluoxetine."[41]

The regulators then vigorously criticized two of Lilly's key studies of Prozac/fluoxetine for PMDD, finding them to have major deficiencies. The trials were too short, the patients were not representative of those who would be prescribed the drug and, worst of all, it was not exactly clear what the trials were measuring so the results were of questionable value anyway. The damning findings of this panel were in stark contrast to the conclusions of the Lilly-sponsored Roundtable of experts in the U.S.: the European regulator was not at all convinced there was enough evidence to justify the use of Lilly's Prozac for PMDD.

Paula Caplan welcomed the move. "I think it's a wonderful decision," she said. "This kind of scrutiny of the science or lack of science behind trials of drugs is all too rare and it is to be praised." Jean Endicott was not at all impressed, saying the decision did a disservice to women. Lilly was forced to inform physicians in Europe of the regulator's decision banning Prozac for PMDD via letters, a decision that a spokesperson described as "unfortunate."[42]

While the FDA may have criticized Lilly's initial round of ads, the U.S. regulator has gone on to approve several other similar antidepressant medications for PMDD, including Pfizer's Zoloft and GSK's Paxil. And as with many new drug approvals these days, they are accompanied by much company-funded "awareness-raising" about the disorder the drugs have been approved to treat. Pfizer's marketing of PMDD even employs some of the words and concepts used by Lilly.

Are you giving up days to what you think is PMS? If you are, it could be PMDD.

—Zoloft ad

It's likely these more recent advertisements have not received the same level of scrutiny from the regulators as the initial Lilly ad received back in 2000. Soon after winning office that year, the Bush administration appointed an attorney to be the official counsel for the FDA who had in the past worked as a legal counsel on the side of the drug companies against the FDA. His arrival brought new procedures requiring that any warning letters to be sent to drug companies had to be first approved by his office, where inevitably a bottleneck formed. The steady stream of warning letters to companies slowed to a trickle, sometimes sent so belatedly they did not arrive at the company's offices until well after the offending ad campaign had finished.[43]

GSK's advertisements for Paxil and PMDD are even more blatant in their attempt to blur the boundaries between ordinary life and mental illness.

> I always thought it was just PMS. Now I know otherwise. Grouchy? Emotional? Irritable? It may be PMDD.[44]

As advertising campaigns like these are clearly targeting relatively normal and healthy women experiencing common problems, the issue of side effects becomes ever more important. For these three drugs, serious sexual problems are a major and common side effect. And as the world has learned, many years after its original approval, with Paxil side effects can be particularly worrying, including withdrawal problems that are in some cases severe.[45]

But the problem of withdrawal is just one of many challenges to the blockbuster Paxil—also known as Seroxat and Aropax. One of the world's top-selling antidepressants, the drug was also one of the biggest money-spinners ever for the giant Anglo-American pharmaceutical company GSK. A large part of Paxil's extraordinary success was because it has been approved to treat more conditions than almost all of its competitor antidepressants.

The most controversial of those conditions, though, was ultimately not PMDD, but another obscure psychiatric disorder ("Social Anxiety Disorder") the drug giant has pushed into the spotlight with claims it affects one in eight people. To help launch the new disorder, GSK turned to one of the world's giant communications corporations. That company would run what would become an award-winning public relations campaign, and produce a historic case study in selling sickness.

REFERENCES
A list of references is available in the original source.

A Dangerous Combination
"Direct-to-Consumer Advertising, Abstinence-Only Education, and Young Women's Health"

by Ronna Popkin

In recent years, advertisements for hormonal contraceptives have become an increasingly noticeable presence in popular women's magazines. These ads are colorful, multi-page spreads with catchy slogans and images of attractive women or couples, and they often include coupons, special offers, or information on obtaining free samples. The explosion in contraceptive advertising is part of a larger, overall increase in direct-to-consumer (DTC) prescription drug advertising that began in 1997, when the U.S. Food and Drug Administration (FDA) loosened drug ad regulations through the FDA Modernization Act. As many health advocates and media critics have argued, all DTC drug advertising has the potential to impact consumer health negatively (Laurence & Weinhouse, 2000; Pearson, 1995; Wilkes *et al.*, 2000). However, DTC hormonal contraceptive advertising, far more than other DTC drug advertising, raises specific concerns and has potentially serious implications for young women's health.

Since 1997, prescription drug advertising has become the fastest growing segment of the advertising industry (Headden & Melton, 1998). Spending on drug advertising has increased exponentially—drug manufacturers spent $791 million on DTC drug ads in 1996, but by 2001 spending had risen to nearly $2.7 billion (Kaiser Family Foundation, 2003a; Levitt, 2001). A study conducted by the National Institute for Healthcare Management (NIHCM) found that DTC advertising of prescription drugs is heavily concentrated on about 50 drugs, and that consumer spending on just these 50 drugs accounted for almost half—$9.9 billion—of the overall $20.8 billion increase in retail prescription drug spending in 2000. Furthermore, the sales growth of these 50 drugs in 2000 was over 32%, more than double the 14% sales growth for all other drugs, and doctors wrote nearly 25% more prescriptions for these 50 most heavily advertised drugs in 2000 than in 1999, while they wrote only 4% more prescriptions for all other drugs (National Institute for Healthcare Management, 2001). What these statistics demonstrate is that DTC advertising of prescription drugs works—it increases prescription rates, sales growth, and consumer spending on drugs.

While the FDA technically requires that DTC ads provide a fair balance of risk and benefit information in the main copy of the advertisement, the agency neither requires prior approval of DTC ads nor monitors the ads once they are released. As a result, drug companies often fail, or do the bare minimum required, to comply with this regulation. Several content analyses of DTC ads have demonstrated that they frequently contain vague, misleading, confusing, and unbalanced messages and present information in a manner that makes the benefits of using the drugs appear to outweigh the risks (Bell *et al.*, 2000; Roth, 1996; Welch Cline & Young, 2004; Woloshin *et al.*, 2001).

The misleading and manipulative messages in DTC drug ads could negatively impact any individual's health; however, they have a disproportionate potential to influence young women because teens often cite the media as important sources of sexual health information. In a recent survey conducted by the Kaiser Family Foundation on teen sexuality, 74% of teenage girls reported that they got "a lot" or "some" information on birth control and STD protection from magazines, and 68% reported getting "a lot" or "some" information on those topics from product advertising. Furthermore, those numbers were higher than the percentage of young women who reported learning "a lot" or "some" about birth control

and STD protection from their healthcare providers (64%), teachers (53%), and siblings (47%) (Kaiser Family Foundation, 2004). These statistics illustrate that young women view magazines and advertising as important sources of sexual health information, and since hormonal methods of birth control are some of the most widely promoted drugs in the U.S. (Wilkes et al., 2000), young women are likely to be heavily influenced by DTC ads for hormonal contraception.

Another reason DTC ads might be more likely to impact young women is that since 1997, the same year the FDA loosened prescription drug advertising restrictions, the federal government has poured over 1.5 billion dollars into abstinence-only sexuality education programs (Sexuality Information and Education Council of the United States, 2008). These programs, which several recent studies have found to be ineffective, provide young people with absolutely no information about contraception or protection against STDs except for potential—and often exaggerated—side effects and failure rates (Bennett & Assefi, 2005; Hauser, 2004; Kirby, 2002; Trenholm *et al.*, 2007; Waxman, 2004). The increases in abstinence-only sexuality education in schools means that many young women are being denied, at an institutional level, access to accurate and objective information on the health effects of taking hormonal contraception, which may make them more likely to believe and trust the potentially misleading messages in the ads.

As media critic Douglass Kellner explains, the promotional strategy of highlighting benefits and downplaying risks is used in all advertising: "Ads form textual systems with basic components which are interrelated in ways that positively position the product" (Kellner, 1995). However, manipulating and influencing consumers to buy a specific product is not that damaging when the choice is between buying Revlon or L'Oreal mascara. But when young women are being targeted and influenced to demand and use drugs that have widespread, systemic bodily effects, and they are simultaneously denied, in their schools, objective, unbiased information about the potential health consequences of taking those drugs, this manipulation has serious, dangerous implications.

An Unparalleled Presence

To more effectively assess the potential impact of DTC birth control advertising on young women's health, I tracked and examined the prevalence and content of ads for hormonal contraception printed in *Cosmopolitan, Essence,* and *Glamour* between 2001 and 2004. This detailed analysis revealed that hormonal contraceptives are, by far, the category of drugs most heavily promoted to young women. During this period, pharmaceutical companies printed a total of 148 advertisements for nine brands of hormonal contraception in the magazines, with the contraceptive ads occupying a total of 418 pages. Drugs that treat mood disorders were the second most heavily advertised category of drugs, with 44 advertisements occupying 106 total pages. Thus, hormonal contraception was advertised at more than three times the rate of the next most heavily advertised category of drugs.

The consistent and dominating presence of birth control ads in these magazines is one reason why these DTC ads have the potential to impact young women's health. Over the four year period, young women interested in treating their asthma would have come across only 13 DTC asthma drug ads: two in *Glamour*, six in *Cosmopolitan*, and five in *Essence*. Most of these ads had only one page of graphic content, and no issue of any magazine contained more than one DTC asthma drug ad. The DTC advertising for asthma drugs is therefore sporadic enough that women are not likely to be heavily influenced by the ads.

In contrast, over the same period of time, women would have been exposed to 148 hormonal contraceptive ads: 70 in *Glamour*, 53 in *Cosmopolitan*, and 25 in *Essence*. More than 2/3 of these ads had two or more pages of graphic content and many contained postcard or special offer inserts that encouraged the magazines fall open to those pages. Furthermore, approximately 1/3 of the issues of *Cosmopolitan* and *Glamour* printed DTC ads for two or more brands of hormonal contraceptives. Issues with several birth control ads and advertisements occupying multiple page spreads are far more likely to effectively capture readers' attention than shorter or less frequently printed ads. Clearly DTC hormonal birth control advertisements are a consistent presence in women's magazines that is significantly larger and more captivating than that of DTC ads for other drugs, and this presence enables the messages in DTC birth control ads to have a much greater impact on women and their health. But what messages are these ads sending to young women?

Ortho Tri-Cyclen: Skin Medication or Birth Control?

Ortho Tri-Cyclen was the first hormonal contraceptive to be heavily marketed to women through DTC ads, and advertisements for the brand heavily stressed and promoted the potential beauty benefits of using this form of hormonal contraception. "It's the #1 prescribed birth control pill. And it's clinically proven to help your skin look better," was the slogan plastered boldly across all 30 of the Ortho Tri-Cyclen advertisements. Thus, the first piece of information that readers were likely to absorb about Ortho Tri-Cyclen had nothing to do with contraception, its primary use and purpose; rather, women were likely to learn that that the drug has a positive effect on appearance. In fact, the emphasis on beauty in the Ortho Tri-Cyclen ads was so pervasive that none of the highlighted information on the main page of one of their most frequently used advertisements directly, clearly, or explicitly related to its use as a contraceptive. Instead, highlighted and bolded phrases emphasized that "nearly 9 out of 10 women saw significant improvements in their skin," conveyed that women taking the drug "showed no change in weight," and explained that the drug may work to make women's "periods shorter and more regular, and to reduce cramps."

Ortho McNeil, the manufacturer of Ortho Tri-Cyclen, also downplayed any health risks associated with taking the drug. None of the phrases in bold type were about major risks, side effects, or contraindications to the drug. Instead, the information about health risks that the FDA requires was printed in extremely small type at the very bottom of the page. In this brief section on risks and side effects, the first thing mentioned was that "most side effects of birth control pills are not serious. Those that are occur infrequently." Leading with this statement softens the impact of the subsequent information, which explained that the serious risks include blood clots, stroke, and heart attacks. While fewer than 5% of women do experience such serious side effects, these can be life threatening, so it is vital that women considering taking the drug be clearly alerted to these potential health issues (Boston Women's Health Book Collective, 1998). Yet the only risk information in the ad that was even remotely highlighted was a lightly underlined phrase printed at the bottom of the page that warned smokers over 35 not to take oral contraceptives. This phrase, however, was nowhere near as visible as the health and beauty benefit phrases printed in bold type. Because the information in the ad on beauty and health benefits outnumbered and was far more visible than the information on risks, the ad leaves women with the impression that taking hormonal contraceptives has many benefits and few health consequences.

Reading the Fine Print?

In contrast to the primary page of the ad, the back page, which contains the full product-labeling insert that comes with the drug, makes the actual potential dangers of using Ortho Tri-Cyclen eminently clear. This page lists 12 major warnings about using Ortho Tri-Cyclen, 13 serious precautions to consider, and over 50 adverse reactions that have been demonstrated in conjunction with the use of hormonal contraceptives. These risks and contraindications include milder problems like nausea and headaches, and more severe health issues like breast cancer, cervical cancer, and gallbladder disease. Only one short sentence amidst the sea of information on this page is the only place where the ad explains that the pill does not protect against the spread of HIV or STDs.

Alarmingly, research demonstrates that the majority of consumers do not read the important information printed on the back of DTC ads. When the FDA asked consumers in a 2002 survey how much of this small print information they usually read, only 16% said they read almost all or all of the information, while 73% said they read little to none of the small print information (Aikin, 2003). In addition, a recent study revealed that the literacy demands of the information on these summary pages is at a college or graduate level (Kaphingst *et al.*, 2004), so even if younger women were attempting to read this information they might not have the literacy skills to fully comprehend it.

These studies demonstrate that ads for birth control are not clearly and explicitly giving women all of the information they need to consider when deciding whether or not they want to use the pill. Technically the ads follow FDA regulations because the information on risks is printed somewhere in the advertisement; however, information on benefits is stressed and highlighted, while the risk information is presented in a manner that seriously discourages women from reading it. As a result, a majority of physicians surveyed by the FDA have noticed a dramatic difference in their patients' comprehension of drug benefits vs. risks after viewing DTC ads. While 78% of doctors felt that their patients were somewhat or very clear on the possible benefits and positive effects of advertised drugs, 60% felt that patients understood little or none of the risks and negative side effects (Aikin, 2003).

Seasonale: A False Sense of Freedom

Ads for Seasonale, another brand of hormonal contraceptives, also tended to highlight benefits while downplaying risks. Seasonale was approved by the FDA in 2004, and it is not a new formulation of birth control pills, but rather is a repackaging of traditional birth control pills that only includes placebo pills once every three months instead of once a month. Because it is the brief withdrawal of hormones during the placebo week that creates a pseudo-menstruation when women are on oral contraceptives, women taking Seasonale will have, as

the advertisements state, "just four periods a year." There is absolutely no increased contraceptive benefit to Seasonale—birth control pills are just as effective at protecting against pregnancy whether or not a placebo week is included on a monthly basis.

Since the only advantage to Seasonale is that women taking it will menstruate less frequently, this is what advertisements for the drug promoted. Yet Barr Laboratories, the manufacturer of Seasonale, didn't just promote the drug to women who would most benefit from using it, like those who were already heterosexually active and experienced severe menstrual pain or difficulties. Instead, they glorified the notion of fewer periods for *all* women, conveying through both the imagery and copy that women will be happier and freer if they have fewer periods. For example, every Seasonale ad contained a wildly dancing woman with a beaming smile and hair soaring in the wind. These women appeared absolutely ecstatic about the fact that they were menstruating less frequently. The copy in the ads reinforced the notion that Seasonale could liberate women, as the trademarked slogan for the product is "Fewer periods. More possibilities." This statement makes it perfectly clear that reducing the frequency of menstruation will provide women with more freedom and options, which adds to the widespread cultural notion that menstruation is a shackle and burden for women. These negative messages about menstruation could have a stronger impact on younger women who are still learning about, and becoming comfortable in, their changing bodies.

Many of the other messages in Seasonale ads, like those in Ortho Tri-Cyclen ads, were misleading and downplayed the negative side effects of the drug. First, the main copy in the ad touted the fact that Seasonale is "the only FDA-approved birth control pill that lets you have just 4 periods a year." Technically this is true, as Seasonale is the only contraceptive pill packaged with twelve weeks of active hormones and one week of placebo pills. However, women actually can use any birth control pill in the same manner as Seasonale and they will get the same main result: fewer periods. All they have to do is skip the placebo pills at the end of one package and then immediately begin taking the active pills from their next pack. So while the ads for Seasonale portrayed it as an innovative concept in contraceptives that "has changed the way you take the Pill," women can make this change whether or not they buy this specific product.

Another very misleading statement printed in every ad for Seasonale was that "leading women's healthcare experts agree you don't need a monthly period when you're on the Pill because you're not ovulating." First, this statement is scientifically inaccurate. Ovulation is a physiological process that occurs in the ovaries and has little bearing on the build up of women's uterine lining, which is the main tissue that is shed during menstruation. In fact, women not taking hormonal contraceptives sometimes have anovulatory cycles in which they still menstruate, so clearly a lack of ovulation does not make menstruation unnecessary. But even more misleading is the fact that women's health experts do *not* agree on this issue—there is actually widespread debate among healthcare providers about the safety of continuously suppressing menstruation, not only because they are unsure of what changes it might cause in women's endometrial tissue, but also because it requires significant additional hormone exposure (Rabin, 2004).

Having only four periods a year means that women will annually be exposed to nine additional weeks of hormones, a potentially risky aspect of Seasonale that was heavily downplayed in ads for the product. When using regular birth control pills, women take active hormones for 39 weeks a year, so the extra nine weeks of hormones in Seasonale amounts to a 23% annual increase in women's hormone exposure. Ads for Seasonale did, in the small copy at the bottom of the page, present this information by stating that "Seasonale users receive 9 more weeks of hormones every year than with a same-dose 28 day pill." Yet, immediately after that statement, Barr Laboratories also claimed that, "While this may increase the chance of serious health risks, current studies have not shown an increased risk." This statement is extremely misleading because it falsely implies that studies of the long-term health effects of the additional annual hormone exposure have been done and showed no increased risks. However, in reality, Seasonale was only studied for one year on a total of 261 women (Rabin, 2004), so the reason "current studies have not shown an increased risk" is that adequate studies have not been completed. Barr Laboratories leaves women with the impression that their product has been proven safe, when all that's really been proven about Seasonale is that it is an effective contraceptive.

The fact that the Seasonale ads played on and reinforced women's negative attitudes toward menstruation is also incredibly ironic, because, while women taking the drug may get only four official "periods" a year, they are much more likely to frequently spot or experience heavy breakthrough bleeding between periods. This information, like the most serious risk and side effect information in the Ortho Tri-Cyclen ads, was displayed non-prominently at the bottom of the page, and the alarming frequency of the intermenstrual bleeding wasn't at all clear. The main study done on Seasonale

found that, during their first 13-week cycle on the drug, 65% of women experienced at least 7 days of bleeding between periods and 35% bled for a total of 20 or more days. While, as the primary page of the ad claimed, this frequency did "decrease over time," at the end of the year 42% of women still experienced at least 7 days of bleeding between periods and 15% experienced 20 or more days. Yet these statistics were only presented on the back page of the ad that people are very unlikely to read. Given that Seasonale is being primarily promoted as a product that will free women from the burden of menstruation, it is highly misleading to conceal the fact that over half of the women taking the drug are actually bleeding more than just four times a year.

Ortho Evra: Feigning Cultural and Racial Sensitivity

Out of the seven pharmaceutical companies who printed contraceptive advertisements in *Cosmopolitan, Glamour*, and *Essence* between 2001 and 2004, only Barr Laboratories and Ortho McNeil used women of color in their ads. In fact, in stark contrast to the other manufacturers who made little or no attempt to reflect the racial and ethnic diversity of women in the United States, Ortho McNeil actually printed more ads with images of black women than with white women. Ortho McNeil also was one of only two contraceptive manufacturers to advertise in *Essence*, and ads for the company's three different contraceptive products accounted for 23 of the 25 birth control ads printed in *Essence* over the four year period.

Given their consistent use of women of color in their promotional materials and their choice to purchase advertisements in *Essence*, it appears that Ortho McNeil is more sensitive to women's diversity and is targeting black women more than other contraceptive manufacturers. Yet, while their marketing approaches and strategies indicate greater sensitivity to racial and ethnic diversity in the United States, one of their major products does not. Ortho Evra, the transdermal birth control patch developed by Ortho McNeil and released in the U.S. market in 2002, is available *only* in a beige color. Not surprisingly, a number of African-American women have cited the patch's visibility on their skin as the main reason they have chosen not to use Ortho Evra (Kaiser Family Foundation, 2003b).

Ortho McNeil's choice to manufacture Ortho Evra, a product that they market as concealable, in a shade that will match relatively few women's skin obviously greatly lacks cultural and racial sensitivity, but it is also radically incongruent with the company's marketing approach for the product. Over 60% of the ads printed for Ortho Evra in *Essence, Cosmopolitan*, and *Glamour* between 2001 and 2004 contained images of black women. Furthermore, with 13 advertisements in *Essence*, Ortho Evra was by far the most frequently advertised contraceptive product in the magazine and was the second most heavily advertised drug overall.

The possible motivation behind Ortho McNeil's contradictory approach of targeting young, African-American women with a product that illustrates insensitivity toward them was, initially, baffling. In order to justify the company's racially insensitive choice of patch colors, a vice president of Ortho McNeil claimed that the company had attempted to make the patch clear, but that it looked "grimy" in clinical trials. She also claimed that their manufacturing technology at the time they released the patch did not give them "color options" (Kaiser Family Foundation, 2003b). While their justification is suspect, even if one accepts the company's statements as true, they do not explain why or how executives felt that young, African-American women would still be a lucrative market for their product.

However, Ortho Evra is a longer-acting contraceptive than either Ortho Tri-Cyclen or Ortho Tri-Cyclen Lo, which may help explain why it is being marketed more heavily to black women than other contraceptive products. Unlike the various formulations of birth control pills, which women should take at the same time every day, Ortho Evra slowly releases hormones into a woman's body over the course of a week. Women using the patch need to change it only once a week for three consecutive weeks, and then wear no patch on the fourth week so that they will still get their periods. The convenience of a longer acting hormonal method like Ortho Evra is certainly something that is likely to please a number of women, as many women find it challenging to remember to take a pill at the same time every day.

Yet, for many women of color and poor women, Ortho Evra might raise some concerns, as there is a well-documented history of other longer acting hormonal contraceptive methods, such as Norplant and Depo-Provera, being inappropriately promoted or distributed within their communities. The disproportionate promotion of long acting contraceptives to poor women and women of color has mostly been due to grossly inaccurate racist and classist stereotypes that they cannot be relied upon to use contraceptives that require daily effort, yet need to limit their reproduction because they have too many children who become dependent on social services (Collins, 2004; Roberts, 1997). While none of these stereotypes are true—poor women and women of color do not have more children, on average, than wealthy or

white women, nor have they ever been proven to have higher failure rates with other contraceptive devices—these notions continue to circulate in public ideology. These stereotypes were also reflected in the rates at which longer acting methods were promoted within *Cosmopolitan, Glamour*, and *Essence*, and therefore might help explain Ortho McNeil's choice to target black women in their promotion of Ortho Evra. Ads for longer acting methods accounted for 60% of the contraceptive ads printed in *Essence*, but only 27% of those printed in *Glamour* and 36% of those in *Cosmopolitan*.

Because Ortho Evra contains similar hormones to daily birth control pills, its longer acting nature is its primary advantage over other hormonal products, and therefore the convenience of using weekly birth control is what Ortho McNeil chose to emphasize in their marketing campaign. The trademarked slogan for Ortho Evra, printed in every advertisement for the product, is "On your body. Off your mind." This message required marketing it directly as a contraceptive device, which might also help explain Ortho McNeil's choice to target black women more heavily with the patch. As the content in Ortho Tri-Cyclen and Seasonale ads shows, many hormonal methods of contraception are promoted mostly for their non-contraceptive advantages. But advertisements for Ortho Evra, unlike ads for nearly every other contraceptive product promoted in *Cosmopolitan, Essence*, and *Glamour*, did not highlight a single non-contraceptive benefit of the patch, despite the fact that it possesses the same advantages of most other hormonal products. Ortho McNeil's choice to market Ortho Evra only for its role as a contraceptive, combined with the fact that they promoted it in *Essence* far more heavily than any of their other contraceptive products, sends a subtle, disturbing message that both reflects and reinforces existing stereotypes: black women are more likely to need and use birth control to prevent pregnancy and limit their reproduction, while white women are more likely to use hormonal contraceptives for a whole host of other reasons.

Operating from stereotypes similar to those about women of color and poor women, some public health and health education professionals have suggested that Ortho Evra and other longer acting methods of contraception might be especially beneficial for younger women, whom they speculate might be more likely to have increased rates of user error with other contraceptives. If preventing pregnancy were our only public health goal with young women, this might be a valid assessment. However, little testing has been done regarding the long-term safety of the use of hormonal methods by young women. Furthermore, while teen pregnancy rates have been consistently dropping, rates of most sexually transmitted infections in young people have been slowly climbing (Centers for Disease Control and Prevention, 2004, 2004b). Thus, disassociating sexual activity from the risks it presents and responsibilities it requires might not be the soundest approach for young women. Encouraging them to use a contraceptive product that they can "take off their minds" might make them even more likely to also take disease protection measures "off their minds." In fact, research suggests that this is true, as longer-acting hormonal contraceptives have a stronger inverse relationship with condom use than daily oral contraceptive pills (Cushman et al., 1998).

The Dangers Revealed

The misleading and persuasive messages in these contraceptive advertisements are likely to have a disproportionately negative impact on the nearly 1/3 of young American women who are being taught about sexuality through abstinence-only programs. When students are openly taught about different contraceptive methods in schools, they learn accurate and valuable information about each method that they can use whenever they become sexually active: what it is; how it works; how to use it; and its benefits, drawbacks, efficacy, and safety. Abstinence-only approaches to sexuality education not only restrict such information on contraception in the classroom, but also convey to young people that they should not be sexually active at all, which could discourage them from actively seeking out other reliable sources of contraceptive information.

Without alternate sources of information on birth control, the advertisements that young women regularly see in magazines are likely to be one of their primary sources of sexual health information. In fact, in a recent survey of teens about birth control and sexual health, product advertising was the second most frequently cited source of information about birth control and STD protection, surpassing parents, siblings, teachers, healthcare providers, partners, television, the internet, and even magazine articles; only friends were cited more frequently (Kaiser Family Foundation, 2004). Other studies have shown that individuals with lower levels of education are more likely to seek information from media sources and have more positive attitudes toward advertising (Robinson *et al.*, 2004). Yet abstinence-only programs leave young women ill equipped to understand and critically evaluate the benefit and risk information in DTC birth control ads. These programs rarely teach media literacy skills, so young women educated through these programs might be even more likely to be influenced by the ads' misleading messages and choose to take hormonal products to clear up their skin or eliminate their periods without being fully informed of the potential risks the drugs pose to their health.

In addition, because abstinence-only programs often use scare tactics and exaggerate the risks of using contraceptives, these programs might actually lead young women to disregard the minute amount of risk information that is presented in the ads. Research has repeatedly indicated that, in any area of health education, scare tactics are ineffective, because once students discover that adults have exaggerated risk information, they become very skeptical of any other warnings they are issued (Hedgepeth & Helmich, 1996; Telljohann *et al.*, 2004). Young women educated through abstinence-only programs who are actively reading or seeking information about birth control are also likely to be, or soon become, sexually active. These young women, therefore, may already feel lied to or misled by the greatly exaggerated dangers of sexual activity and safer sex measures that are presented in these programs. As a result, even if these women read the finely printed risk information in birth control ads, they might also be more likely to disregard these warnings.

The failure of several manufacturers of hormonal contraceptives to clearly and explicitly present the lack of STD protection is also particularly dangerous for young women. Given that one out of four sexually active teenagers contracts an STD before the age of 20 (Centers for Disease Control and Prevention, 2004), STD protection is clearly a crucial component of young people's sexual health. Using a method of birth control that does not provide STD protection also disproportionately affects young women. Women are twice as likely as men to contract an STD in an unprotected act of heterosexual intercourse, and they are far more likely to go undiagnosed for longer because initial symptoms of STDs in women are often internal. When STDs go untreated in women, the consequences, such as pelvic inflammatory disease and infertility, are far more severe than those for men (Sloane, 2002). In addition, the cervixes of women in their teens and early twenties are still undergoing changes that make them more susceptible to infection than those of older women (Centers for Disease Control and Prevention, 2004).

Yet, despite these greater risks, many young women are unaware that hormones do not protect against STDs. In one recent survey, nearly half of teens who felt knowledgeable about hormonal methods of contraception also believed that these methods conferred some protection against disease transmission (Kaiser Family Foundation, 2004). Due to their lack of access to accurate education about contraception, young women educated through abstinence-only sexuality education programs may be especially likely to have misconceptions about hormones and STD protection. Thus, many teen girls could be unknowingly putting themselves at risk because they incorrectly believe that hormonal contraceptives also provide them with disease protection, and unfortunately the DTC ads they see often fail to clearly inform them otherwise.

The lack of STD information in hormonal birth control ads might not be so problematic if there were also a similar quantity of advertisements for condoms, which don't pose any serious health risks and do protect against STD transmission. However, not a single condom advertisement was ever printed in *Essence* during the four years of my analysis, and from 2001 through 2003, none were printed in either *Cosmopolitan* or *Glamour*. In fact, Trojan, the only condom manufacturer to advertise in the magazines, printed only three ads in total: one in the May and July 2004 editions of *Glamour*, and one in the August 2004 edition of *Cosmopolitan*. Compared to the 148 ads for hormonal contraception printed in the magazines over the same four-year period, the Trojan ads were an insignificant presence.

The Trojan advertisements also failed to provide factual information about condoms' effectiveness at protecting against both pregnancy and STDs. Abstinence-only programs that make references to condoms often present inaccurate and greatly exaggerated information about condom failure rates (Waxman, 2004). Since nothing printed in the Trojan ads countered those erroneous teachings, even young women who saw these three condom advertisements would not have learned about the benefits of using condoms over the hormonal methods that are so pervasively being marketed to them. Teens taught inaccurate information about condom failure rates might, in fact, be more heavily persuaded by ads for hormonal birth control since these ads consistently stress hormones' high rates of effectiveness. Incorrectly believing that condoms will not effectively protect them against pregnancy could lead them to choose products that they have been assured will.

Conclusion

DTC ads for hormonal contraception occupy many more pages and are far more prevalent than ads for other drugs in women's magazines. Hormonal birth control ads, like all advertisements, are primarily designed to increase sales of products and to generate profits, not to educate consumers, and they therefore contain misleading and manipulative messages designed to favorably position the products in consumers' eyes. The pharmaceutical manufacturers of these drugs do abide by FDA regulations and print serious risks, contraindications, and side effects associated with the drugs, but they do so in a manner that downplays these risks and strongly highlights other potential benefits. Therefore, the dominating presence of DTC hormonal birth control ads, coupled with the dramatic increase in abstinence-only sexuality education, poses serious risks to young women's health.

Young women adequately educated about the risks and benefits of hormonal contraception through school or community programs are better equipped to critically evaluate these misleading messages because they can negotiate the information that the ads provide with information they already have about sexual health. However, nearly one-third of young American women are taught sexuality in schools through an abstinence-only model, and therefore the birth control ads that are consistently and widely printed in women's magazines are likely to become primary sources of sexual health information for these women. Women who don't readily have access to non-promotional sources of information about contraception can't adequately evaluate the accuracy of the information provided in these ads and are therefore more susceptible to the misleading and persuasive messages in them.

DTC advertisements for hormonal birth control are relatively new, yet increasingly prevalent, voices in the sea of mixed messages and blurry information that young women receive about their sexuality and bodies. If, as a society, we want young people to safely navigate through those mixed messages and grow into sexually healthy adults, we have to model and teach them the principles of healthy relationships; help them build communication, critical thinking, decision-making, and media literacy skills; and provide them with accurate and current information about safer sex practices and sexual health. Both abstinence-only sexuality education programs and DTC birth control advertising fail on most of the above accounts, so the combination of distorted information from both of these sources poses a serious potential threat to young women's health. Yet, despite research illustrating their negative effects, funding for abstinence-only programs and spending on DTC advertising have both continued to increase annually at dramatic rates, and this is unlikely to change in the near future. Thus, it is vital that media critics, health researchers, sexuality educators, and youth advocates further investigate and address the joint impact of DTC birth control advertising and abstinence-only education on young women's sexual knowledge, behavior, and health.

REFERENCES

Aikin, K. J. (2003). The impact of direct-to-consumer prescription drug advertising on the physician-patient relationship. *Presentation at Direct-to-Consumer Promotion Public Meeting* Retrieved April 5, 2005, from http://www.fda.gov/cder/ddmac/aikin/sld001.htm

Bell, R. A., Wilkes, M. S., & Kravitz, R. L. (2000). The educational value of consumer-targeted prescription drug print advertising. *The Journal of Family Practice, 49*(12), 1092–1098.

Bennett, S. E., & Assefi, N. P. (2005). School-based teenage pregnancy prevention programs: A systematic review of randomized controlled trials. *Journal of Adolescent Health, 36*(1), 72–81.

Boston Women's Health Book Collective. (1998). *Our bodies, ourselves for the new century.* New York: Simon & Schuster.

Centers for Disease Control and Prevention. (2004). *Sexually transmitted disease surveillance, 2003.* Atlanta: U.S. Department of Health and Human Services.

Centers for Disease Control and Prevention. (2006). Youth risk behavior surveillance: United States, 2005. *Morbidity and Mortality Weekly Report, 55*(SS–5).

Collins, P. H. (2004). *Black sexual politics: African Americans, gender, and the new racism.* New York: Routledge.

Cushman, L. F., Romero, D., Kalmuss, D., Davidson, A. R., et al. (1998). Condom use among women choosing long-term hormonal contraception. *Family Planning Perspectives, 30*(5), 240–243.

Hauser, D. (2004). *Five years of abstinence-only-until-marriage education: Assessing the impact.* Advocates for Youth.

Headden, S., & Melton, M. (1998, July 20). Madison Ave. loves drug ads. *U.S. News and World Report*, 56.

Hedgepeth, E., & Helmich, J. (1996). *Teaching about sexuality and HIV: Principles and methods for effective education.* New York: New York University Press.

Kaiser Family Foundation. (2003a). *Impact of direct-to-consumer advertising on prescription drug spending.* Menlo Park, CA.

Kaiser Family Foundation. (2003b). Some African-American women avoid Ortho Evra birth control patch citing patch's visibility on skin. *Kaiser Daily Reproductive Health Report* Retrieved January 23, 2005, from http://www.kaisernetwork.org/daily_reports/rep_index.cfm?hint=2&DR_ID=19141

Kaiser Family Foundation. (2004). Birth control and protection. *SexSmarts* Retrieved April 13, 2005, from http://www.kff.org/entpartnerships/7106.cfm

Kaphingst, K. A., Rudd, R. E., DeJong, W., & Daltroy, L. H. (2004). Literacy demands of product information intended to supplement television direct-to-consumer prescription drug advertisements. *Patient Education and Counseling, 55*(2), 293–300.

Kellner, D. (1995). Reading images critically: Toward a postmodern pedagogy. In G. Dines & J. M. Humez (Eds.), *Gender, race, and class in the media: A text-reader* (pp. 126–132). London: Sage Publications.

Kirby, D. (2002). *Do abstinence-only programs delay the initiation of sex among young people and reduce teen pregnancy?* Washington D.C.: National Campaign to Prevent Teen Pregnancy.

Laurence, L., & Weinhouse, B. (2000). Drug marketing: Selling women out. In N. Worcester & M. H. Whatley (Eds.), *Women's health: Readings on social, economic, and political issues* (3rd ed., pp. 166–174). Dubuque, IA: Kendall/Hunt Publishing Company.

Levitt, L. (2001). *Prescription drug trends.* Menlo Park, CA: Henry J. Kaiser Family Foundation.

National Institute for Health Care Management. (2001). *Prescription drugs and mass media advertising, 2000.* Washington, D.C.: National Institute for Health Care Management.

Pearson, C. (1995). Direct-to-consumer promotion of prescription drugs. Retrieved November 18, 2002, from http://www.womenshealthnetwork.org/advocacy/fulltext/tdtc.htm

Rabin, R. (2004, February 9). A hard pill to swallow: Menstrual suppression worries many. *Milwaukee Journal Sentinel*, pp. 1G, 16G.

Roberts, D. (1997). *Killing the black body: Race, reproduction, and the meaning of liberty.* New York: Random House, Inc.

Robinson, A. R., Hohmann, K. B., Rifkin, J. I., Topp, D., Gilroy, C. M., Pickard, J. A., et al. (2004). Direct-to-consumer pharmaceutical advertising: Physician and public opinion and potential effects on the physician-patient relationship. *Archives of Internal Medicine, 164*(4), 427–432.

Roth, M. S. (1996). Patterns in direct-to-consumer prescription drug print advertising and their public policy implications. *Journal of Public Policy & Marketing, 15*(1), 63–75.

Sexuality Information and Education Council of the United States. (2008). Spending for abstinence-only until marriage programs. Retrieved April 9, 2008, from http://www.siecus.org/policy/states/2006/federalGraph.html

Sloane, E. (2002). *Biology of women* (4th ed.). Albany: Delmar Publishing.

Telljohann, S. K., Symons, C. W., & Pateman, B. (2004). *Health education: Elementary and middle school applications* (4th ed.). Boston: McGraw Hill.

Trenholm, C., Devaney, B., Fortson, K., Quay, L., Wheeler, J., & Clark, M. (2007). *Impacts of Four Title V, Section 510 Abstinence Education Programs: Final Report.* Princeton, NJ: Mathematica Policy Research, Inc.

Waxman, H. A. (2004). The content of federally funded abstinence-only education programs (pp. 1–22): Committee on Government Reform—Minority Staff, United States House of Representatives.

Welch Cline, R. J., & Young, H. N. (2004). Marketing drugs, marketing healthcare relationships: A content analysis of visual cues in direct-to-consumer prescription drug advertising. *Health Communication, 16*(2), 131–157.

Wilkes, M. S., Bell, R. A., & Kravitz, R. L. (2000). Direct-to-consumer prescription drug advertising: Trends, impact, and implications. *Health Affairs, 19*(2), 110–128.

Woloshin, S., Schwartz, J. T., & Welch, H. G. (2001). Direct-to-consumer advertisements for prescription drugs: What are Americans being sold? *Lancet, 358*(9288), 1141–1146.

How Vaccine Policy Is Made
# "The Story of Merck and Gardasil"

from *HealthFacts*

Much has happened since the November Health-Facts took the position that the new cervical cancer vaccine should not be mandated. By now, most of the U.S. is probably aware that donations from Merck, maker of the Gardasil vaccine, influenced Governor Rick Perry's decision to make Texas the first state to mandate Gardasil vaccinations for all girls entering the sixth grade.

Merck had been bankrolling similar mandates under consideration in at least 20 other states. In doing so, the company moved from the usual pharmaceutical industry hucksterism (hype the disease, hype the new drug) to blatantly purchasing a public policy that is clearly a windfall for the one and only company that sells a cervical cancer vaccine.

The prolonged nationwide publicity given Merck's actions frequently overlooked a key element to the question of whether mass cervical cancer vaccinations make sense whether they are mandated or voluntary. Cervical cancer is, by any measure, a rare disease in the U.S., afflicting fewer than 10,000 women and causing about 3,700 deaths each year.

And then there's the proverbial elephant in the room that no one seems to want to address. It has been known for over three decades *who* is most likely to get cervical cancer. In fact, it is known by geographical region. So why not save taxpayers' money, especially at a time when the states are running out of health dollars for children, and provide the vaccine for the girls most in need?

All medical decisions made by and for healthy people boil down to probabilities. What are the odds of dying of the disease that the vaccine protects against? (There are three cervical cancer deaths for every 100,000 women in the U.S.) How protective is the vaccine? (70%, according to Merck) What are the odds of serious harm from the vaccine itself?

The last question is not answerable because the vaccine has only been available for eight months, and several hundred thousand girls must be vaccinated and followed for many years before any rare or even uncommon serious adverse reactions can be documented. The longest follow-up is 4½ years, so how long the protection lasts is another unknown.

What makes this vaccine different from virtually all others currently given to babies and young children is the fact that cervical cancer is a sexually transmitted disease. (The hepatitis B vaccine given to newborns since 1991 is the other exception.) There are more than 100 different types of human papilloma virus (HPV), but only four to six are cancer-causing—that is, high risk. "Rarely can an infection with high-risk HPV develop into precancer or cancer. The majority of HPV infections go away on their own and do not cause any abnormal cell growth," according to the National Cancer

"How Vaccine Policy is Made: The Story of Merck and Gardasil," from *HealthFacts*, March 2007, pp. 1–3. Reprinted by permission of Maryann Napoli.

Institute's Edward L. Trimble, MD. Gardasil protects against two of the cancer-causing strains that account for about 70% of all cases of cervical cancer

Typically, a new vaccine goes into use gradually, and a mandate comes only after several years. The haste with which Gardasil became mandatory in Texas is challenged. "This [cervical cancer] is not a public health emergency, so the government has no right tell parents or kids to have the vaccine or even to opt out," said Michael Policar, MD, associate clinical professor of Obstetrics, Gynecology and Reproductive Science at the University of California, San Francisco. "You can't get this disease from someone sitting next to you on a bus. If you have TB, a judge can tell you to take your drugs because you can give the disease to other people and if you don't take the drugs, the judge can have you confined," Dr. Policar said in a telephone interview.

Physicians and public health experts quoted in the media were unanimous in their recommendation of the vaccine, though some, like Dr. Policar, do not like the mandate. And all insist that strong evidence supports its safety and efficacy. Physicians seem untroubled by the fact that no *published* HPV vaccine trial had participants under the age of 15. The CDC recommends the HPV vaccine for 11- and 12-year-old girls, and the American Cancer Society sees the vaccine as appropriate for girls as young as nine years of age. The girls must receive the vaccination before they become sexually active or else it will not be effective.

Why is there so little public discussion among doctors about the wisdom of vaccinating *all* young girls for a rare disease? "Great question," responded Dr. Policar. "Certain people are very tied into vaccines—pediatricians, infectious disease doctors, public health doctors—these people have never seen a vaccine they didn't like. The pressure to vaccinate comes not only from them, but also from industry."

The rush to make a new vaccine compulsory appears to be all about Merck making as much money as possible before Cervarix, GlaxoSmithKline's version of the HPV vaccine, comes on the market. "Merck started three to four years ago convincing us that HPV is a dangerous infection," said Dr. Policar, noting that the company has been overdoing it. "HPV is a marker for sexual activity. The majority of us are infected with it and that doesn't mean we'll all get cancer. This is another industry-created disease," he explained, stressing that all HPV-vaccinated women should have regular Pap tests. Dr. Policar is favorably inclined toward the vaccine, but has reservations about the excessive cost and possible need for booster shots ("it took 30 years to learn that the pertussis vaccine needs a booster"). Dr. Policar said he has

been "a paid lecturer on occasion for Merck regarding Gardasil."

More and more parents worry about the growing number of vaccines now given to babies and young children, according to Barbara Loe Fisher of the National Vaccine Information Center, who notes that 40 vaccine doses are already mandated for babies and young children. Fisher, an advocate for vaccine safety, is concerned that doctors are not giving enough attention to possible harmful effects of Gardasil when combined with other vaccines.

She advises parents to inform themselves. But this is difficult when the trials are funded by the vaccine companies and the last place parents will get an unbiased evaluation of any vaccine are the U.S. Centers for Disease Control and Prevention (federal promoters of vaccines in general) or the American Academy of Pediatrics (specialty that sees all vaccines as a medical triumph). In fact, Fisher's Web site www.909shot.com is the only evidence-based independent Web site on this topic.

Science seemed to take a back seat in the prolonged media coverage last month. The one trial that proved "sustained efficacy up to 4.5 years" was funded by GlaxoSmithKline, and published last year in The Lancet. The majority of the participants were over 18. About half of these 776 study participants were randomly assigned to receive the HPV vaccine, thus the longest follow-up involves less than 400 women.

And now for the elephant in the room. Cervical cancer is largely a disease associated with extreme poverty, smoking, lack of education, and less than sanitary living conditions. According to a 2005 National Cancer Institute report, most cervical cancer deaths occur in black women in the rural South, Hispanic women living along the Texas-Mexico border, white women in Appalachia, American Indians in the Northern Plains, Vietnamese-American women and Alaskan Natives. These groups are also more likely than other U.S. women to be diagnosed with other diseases like breast cancer, colorectal cancer and heart disease.

Wouldn't it make sense to aim the Gardasil vaccine recommendation at these women? Or better yet, given the limited federal health dollars, why not spend some money to improve their health in general? The answer, of course, is that this would not suit Merck, who appears to be setting the national agenda on cervical cancer. Nor does it suit the federal government and the special interests—so aptly represented in Congress—who want to do everything to keep companies from shunning the vaccine business as risky and unprofitable. Merck needs to make as much money as quickly as possible from Gardasil before Cervarix goes on the market. Each year in the U.S., about a million girls turn 11. Mandating a $360* series of three injections means an estimated $360 million-a-year market.

It didn't take long for Merck to experience a well-deserved backlash. Within three weeks of Governor Perry's announced mandate at the end of January, Merck revealed that it would stop lobbying state legislatures to mandate Gardasil. (Texas legislators are reportedly at work undoing the mandate.) But Merck is not the only company to provide "unrestricted educational grants" to Women in Government, a Washington, DC based advocacy organization of female state legislators. This group, the conduit for the Merck-purchased mandates, has also received funding from

Glaxo, as well as Digene, a company that makes a test that detects HPV.

The funding paid off as female state legislators were highly visible in the media coverage given Gardasil last month. The legislators were presenting themselves as champions of women's health and spreading the word about the dangers of HPV, often quoting worldwide cervical cancer statistics (500,000 deaths annually!! Second leading cause of cancer deaths!!) as if these numbers pertained to U.S. women.

The Merck people probably knew that a vaccine company presenting itself as champions of women's health wouldn't fly with the public. Much better to send in the female legislators to shill for them.

---

*This is the most widely quoted price, but a random survey by the National Vaccine Information Center found the price varies considerably and can be as high as $825 plus office charges.

"AMSA's PharmFree Campaign"

from American Medical Student Association

The pharmaceutical industry has ramped up its spending on marketing dramatically over the past few years. In 2000, according to IMS Health, the pharmaceutical industry spent $13 billion, more than 10 cents of every prescription dollar, on marketing and promotion to health providers contributing to the astronomical prescription costs our patients must bear.

On the wards, we are often expected to attend pharmaceutical company sponsored "educational" conferences. Research has shown that these conferences are associated with learning and disseminating inaccurate information, and with inappropriate prescribing.

AMSA PharmFree Timeline

Jan 2002: *Excerpt from President's Column*

March 2002: *AMSA House of Delegates passes groundbreaking no free lunch association policy*

April 2002: *AMSA President and Executive Board draft Model Oath and launch Revitalizing Professionalism Campaign*

There Is No Such Thing as a Free Lunch

As medical students, we must advocate for better professionalism training and in particular resist the penetration of medical education by the pharmaceutical industry. To this end, we would like to announce the AMSA PharmFree Campaign to educate and train our members to professionally and ethically interact with the pharmaceutical industry.

The Rx Industry and Persephone

Persephone was the beautiful daughter of the ancient Greek goddess Demeter. As the story goes, Hades, Lord of the Underworld, kidnapped her and brought her to his lair in Hell, guarded by Cerberus, the three-headed dog. While she was in captivity, she wisely refused the gifts and jewelry Hades lavished upon her to win her favor; but out of hunger, she said yes to six pomegranate seeds. When she was liberated and returned to her mother, Hades protested and pointed out that she had accepted the seeds.

Though she was a cheap date, she had let him pay for dinner and thus she "owed him something." To repay her debt, she was required to live with Hades as his wife in the realm of the dead for six months out of the year, and she was forever dubbed "Queen of the Underworld."

It's hard to blame Persephone, the poor thing. And you may even identify with her on days when you feel like a prisoner in the hospital, wandering through the halls of an Underworld you still can't believe you willingly entered. You are starving, but there is no one to liberate you. You must go to the noon conference; your attending and your team are waiting for you and would notice your absence. You arrive at the noon conference and there at the gate is Celebrex, a three-headed dog, and his master, Steven, a smiling drug representative from Pennsylvania. You peek through the gate and see the greatest wonders that Hades has to offer—a delicious meal complete with brownies. Steven holds something out to you; it's the key to the Underworld, in the shape of a pen bearing the name of his dog. "Why not?" you ask yourself.

There are those who say there has been no new information in the world since 800 B.C. There have been numerous studies done to prove what the ancient Greeks knew all along—"There is no such thing as a free pomegranate seed." Since we can't defend our positions with ancient wisdom alone, I encourage you to visit www.nofreelunch.org. After clicking on "Required Reading," you will find studies that demonstrate that accepting gifts and hospitality from pharmaceutical companies affects prescribing patterns to the benefit of the drug company (because you prescribe more expensive drugs than you would otherwise) and often to the detriment of the patient.

The drug industry tells us that the cost of their drugs is high and rising because they spend so much on research and development (R&D). The truth is that the actual amount spent on promotion is much higher than the amount spent on R&D. Rising drug costs are responsible for a good portion of the increase in health-care spending in the United States. There is a correlation between the rising costs and the money spent on promotion: Just four categories of drugs accounted for 31 percent of the $42.7 billion increase in drug costs form 1993 to 1998. These include seven of the 10 drugs most heavily advertised to consumers in 1998.

I encourage you to take the pledge on the "No Free Lunch" Web site. I know it's not easy, but it will liberate you and your patients from the Underworld. If you have already taken from Hades, no worries—you can still participate in the Pen Amnesty Program, as directed by the site.

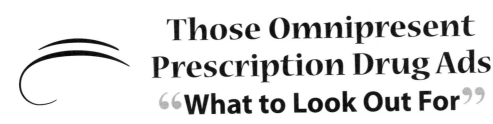

Those Omnipresent Prescription Drug Ads
"What to Look Out For"

from *HealthFacts*

Turn on the TV, pick up a magazine, pass a bus shelter. You're bombarded with prescription drug advertising. Keep the following in mind the next time you think a prescription drug ad appears convincing:

- Ads are not about educating the public; they're about marketing a product. Anyone trying to sell

you something isn't going to give you the most balanced picture of the product's effectiveness and risks.

- You are being sold the newest—and therefore, the most expensive—drug of its kind. New is not necessarily better. Pharmaceutical companies need only prove that their drug is better than a placebo; they are not required to prove that it is any better than older, less expensive drugs for the same condition.

Taking a new medication on a long-term basis is like going into uncharted territory. Most drug trials last only a few months, at best. It takes years and a broader level of usage than usually found in clinical trials before adverse interactions and rare side effects can be identified.

- Notice how unusual it is for an ad to tell you what percentage of people showed improvement taking the drug during clinical trials. This is because many of the most heavily promoted drugs are only moderately effective.

- Much of the advertising dollar goes to "me too" drugs, designed to cut into the market share of a competing blockbuster medication. Think Zoloft and Prozac, Vioxx and Celebrex, Pepsi and Coke.

- If an ad tells you that a drug cuts your risk by 50%, always ask "50% of what?" Daily aspirin cuts the risk of heart attack by 50%. Look carefully at the study results, you might find that halving the risk is less than meets the eye. For example, a five-year study showed that heart attacks occurred in 1% of the participants taking aspirin, as compared with 2% of those taking the placebo.

- Be aware that an ad's graphics alone can be misleading. No one looks sick in these ads. You'll see men with AIDS hiking up mountains and elderly people with osteoarthritis running around with their grandchildren. One might get the impression that a cure has been found for AIDS, osteoarthritis, and chronic pain in general.

- The next time you see an ad featuring a happy woman walking along the beach, be on the alert for a weight loss drug. Notice that the drug's effi-

cacy is contingent upon cutting calories and regular exercise.

- Ads need not be pre-screened for accuracy by the Food and Drug Administration (FDA), though drug manufacturers may voluntarily submit ad copy to the agency beforehand.

- The FDA has issued over 90 warning letters to drug companies about misleading ads in the last year alone. You can learn the names of the offending companies and why the FDA acted by visiting the agency's web site (www.fda.gov), click on drugs, and continue to "Warning Letters and Notice of Violation Letters."

- Once the FDA has been alerted that a pharmaceutical company is running a misleading ad, it takes the agency about six months to verify the charge. Then, the offending company is allowed another six months grace period before retracting the ad. Drug companies usually change their ads yearly anyway.

- A drug company incurs no penalty for having run a misleading ad. In rare circumstances, the company may be required to run a corrective ad.

- The few studies exploring the effect of pharmaceutical promotional activities aimed at physicians show that they can be seriously misled. If they can be fooled, why not us?

- Don't take a drug without reading about it first. Ask for the labeling information from the pharmacist. Go to the local library and consult *The Physicians' Desk Reference*. And for your home library, buy *The Essential Guide to Prescription Drugs 2001* by James J. Rybacki, Pharm.D, and James W. Long, MD, and *Worst Pills, Best Pills* by Sidney M. Wolfe, MD, Larry D. Sasich, Pharm.D, Rose-Ellen Hope, R.Ph, and Public Citizen's Health Research Group.

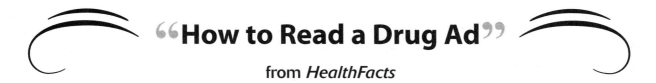

"How to Read a Drug Ad"

from *HealthFacts*

Fear mongering is the subtext of many of the prescription drugs ads you see on TV and in print. These ads might just as well come out and say: OK, you're healthy now, but any time in the near future you can die from a heart attack, cancer, or hip fracture. The surest route to high profits is the expensive drug that must be taken daily for years, preferably for life, out of fear of a disease that might create symptoms 10, 20, 30 years down the road.

Many of the ads play on fears of aging. Middle-aged people (with the necessary drug-coverage) are the natural targets. It helps to read these ads skeptically because many are riddled with half-truths. Here are some representative examples of the different approaches to advertising prescription drugs to the public. All are bound by the rules of the Food and Drug Administration (FDA).

Sell Fear of the Disease

"Osteoporosis—Could you be at Risk" This is the headline of the current ad campaign sponsored by Eli Lilly, which does not mention its osteoporosis drug, Evista (generic name: raloxifene). Anytime the drug *and* its purpose appears in an ad, then the side effects and adverse reactions must also be included. But Eli Lilly's ad illustrates another option in drug advertising. Instead of identifying its drug, a company can choose to sell the dangers of a given disease, in this case, osteoporosis. Ads like this one must list an 800 number that will generate a free packet of information and your name on the company's mailing list for life.

"Up to half of women over age 50 will break a bone due to osteoporosis in their lifetime. And the risk increases when menopause ends," warns the Eli Lilly ad, which features a fiftyish woman. The statement is true, but choosing the age of 50 as the cut-off is guaranteed to instill fear. The following statements are not found in the ad, but they are also true: A woman's odds of having an osteoporosis-related hip fracture between the ages of 50 and 70 are low. Half of all hip fractures in women occur after the age of 80.

Years ago, the diagnosis of osteoporosis was made only after the person experienced a fracture due to thin-ning bones. Now, the definition of osteoporosis has changed to simply mean low bone mass. In other words, what was once a risk factor for fracture is now a disease. Susan M. Love, MD, author of *Dr. Susan Love's Hormone Book,* writes that the panel of experts that changed the definition of osteoporosis was funded in part by pharmaceutical companies.

Sell a Test

"See how beautiful 60 can look? See how invisible osteoporosis can be?" This is the headline for Merck's ad, featuring an older woman. It's a good example of the indirect approach to selling drugs: Encourage people to go for testing and invariably you will create many new customers for your drug. Several years ago, Merck announced that it had entered a financial agreement with a major bone density measurement equipment company, in order to get these expensive machines into as many doctor offices as possible.

Merck does not mention its osteoporosis drug, Fosamax, in this ad which simply advises, *"Ask your doctor if a bone density test is right for you."* It almost comes across as a public service announcement. To prompt the hesitant women into action, Merck adds, ominously, *"The fact is, if you're 60 or older, there's a nearly 1 in 2 chance you have osteoporosis."* Yes, this statement is probably true given the above, expanded redefinition of the "disease." However, there is a debate among osteoporosis researchers about the value of measuring bone density because the test can't predict who will eventually have a fracture. Some evidence indicates that bone turnover may be more relevant, but there is no available test for it.

Name the Drug . . . and Its Side Effects

HIGH CHOLESTEROL ISN'T JUST A NUMBER IT'S A WARNING. The message screams out from Bristol-Myers Squibb's ad for its cholesterol-lowering drug, Pravachol (generic name: pravastatin sodium). This represents the type of ad that identifies the drug and its purpose ("protect your heart"), so it must also list side effects and adverse reactions. In the case of a print ad, the side effects appear in tiny type on the next page. Surveys show that few people read the fine print, and this includes doctors.

The ad emphasizes the Pravachol's safety because a competing cholesterol-lowering drug, Baycol, was withdrawn last summer after it caused 31 deaths. The ad attempts to get the people who just went off Baycol to: *"Ask your doctor to tell you more about high cholesterol, the risk of heart attack, and if Pravachol is right for you."*

The safety claims in this ad are: *"Pravachol is no more likely to cause side effects than a placebo (sugar pill) in landmark clinical studies."* Well, yes, that's true, but only the people who turn the page and read the fine print will learn that this refers solely to the FDA-required trials that lasted only four months. Most people who take cholesterol drugs do so indefinitely, and the fine print has 16 lines of side effects experienced by drug-treated people in the longer trials that lasted five to six years.

The long list of side effects was attributed to the entire class of "statin" drugs, which includes Pravachol (pravastatin) and Baycol (cervistatin), Mevacor (lovastatin), and Zocor (simvastatin). The 31 deaths attributed to Baycol were due to a rare condition called rhabdomyolysis, which causes a breakdown of muscle tissue. All statin drugs have this rare risk, according to *The Medical Letter* (9/10/01), a physician publication with no drug advertising.

Name the Drug, but Not the Condition

This is the strangest approach to drug advertising because it mentions the name of a drug but not what it's for. This type of ad circumvents the FDA-requirement of listing side effects once the drug's purpose is identified. It is best exemplified by Schering-Plough Corporation's ads for Claritin, a drug for seasonal allergies. They usually feature a close-up of a young woman's face against a bright blue sky and often some flowers in the background. The message is simply: "Ask your doctor about Claritin."

Claritin stands as a testament to the power of advertising and as a classic example why a drug doesn't have to be any good to become a big seller. Schering-Plough spent a record $136.8 million advertising Claritin directly to consumers in 1999 alone. It paid off. Claritin is the most profitable antihistamine of all time, with annual sales of more than $2 billion, according to *The New York Times*. A month's supply costs about $85.

Claritin is no more effective than older, cheaper antihistamines. Its much-touted advantage is the lack of drowsiness that comes with other antihistamines. Two FDA-required trials showed that Claritin is better than a placebo, but not much better. At 10-milligram doses, Claritin was only 11% more effective than a placebo. Taken at higher, more effective doses, the drug causes drowsiness.

End-Run Around the FDA

TV ads are generally bound by rules similar to those of print ads. In 1997, however, the FDA relaxed the rules for broadcast advertising where it concerns side effects. From that year on, only the major side effects had to be mentioned in radio and TV ads that name the drug and its purpose. This accounts for the massive increase in TV ads for prescription drugs.

But some major side effects can be a major turn-off, and that has led to some creative bending of the FDA rules. And this is best illustrated by Roche's ads for Xenical, a weight-loss drug. How many people would run out and ask their doctors for Xenical after hearing that anal leakage is a common side effect?

Roche has found a way to avoid this information with its two-part TV commercials for Xenical. The first ad does not mention Xenical; it simply shows quick images of a baby growing up to be a heavy-set woman while describing excess weight as unhealthy. The second ad names the drug but not the condition, using the same background music and images. By separating the two ads with brief unrelated commercials, Roche has circumvented FDA rules about describing side effects. The ads appeared early this year, and thus far, no warning letter to Roche from the FDA has appeared on the agency's Web site.

What to Consider When Reading a Drug Ad

- Many ads leave the impression that everyone who takes the drug will benefit from it. You will want to know how effective the drug has been proven to be in terms of, say, reducing heart attacks, fractures, or cancer recurrences, etc. Rarely, will a drug ad ever provide this crucial information. Consult the *Physicians' Desk Reference,* which is available at most community libraries. It can also be purchased at most chain bookstores. The book is difficult to read, but it is the only readily available source of data concerning what has been proven in drug trials and how long the trials lasted.

- Avoid taking any newly approved drug when there is an alternative. The pre-approval studies required by the FDA usually last only a few months and do not include enough participants to uncover rare side effects. In the last decade, a number of prescription drugs have been withdrawn within five years of becoming available due to life-threatening side effects. This has led many consumer advocates to advise people to wait at least five years from the date of release before taking any new drug. This also allows time for follow-up studies to determine whether the new drug is truly an improvement over the older versions of the same medication.

- These ads are increasing the cost of healthcare for everyone. The 50 most-advertised prescription medicines contributed significantly last year to the increase in the country's spending on drugs, according a new report. It also found that these 50 drugs accounted for almost half of the $20.8 billion increase in drug spending last year. The report was prepared by the National Institute for Healthcare Management, a nonprofit research foundation. Only the drugs still under patent, and therefore expensive, are advertised directly to the public.

- Drug ads are not checked by the FDA for accuracy beforehand, though drug companies are free to do so voluntarily. This occurs infrequently. Instead, the ads are pulled only after complaints are made and verified. This usually takes about six months, and the drug company is given several additional months grace period. Companies whose ads are judged to be misleading will receive a warning letter that is published on the FDA Web site. Offending drug companies incur no penalty for misleading the public. They are merely told to withdraw the ad. Many drug companies change their ads every six to 12 months anyway. On rare occasions, a company may be required to run a corrective ad.

- Go to the FDA's Web site (www.fda.gov). You will find a wealth of information about drugs, as well as dietary supplements (herbs and vitamins). On the home page alone, you can go to "Safety Alerts" and see the latest recalls; "Product approvals" for information about the new drug approvals; "How to Report a Problem to the FDA;" and "Drug Information" for standard labeling facts, such as side effects, purpose, warnings for specific drugs.

"Finding Good Health Information on the Web"

by Electra Kaczorowski

When looking for health formation on the Internet, most of us type the name of a condition or procedure into Google or another search engine, then wait for the results to pop up onto the screen.[1] While this method immediately yields many results, it also can generate inaccurate, unreliable, or biased health information. This is of particular concern to women, who are more likely than men to seek health information on-line.[1] There are several women's health topics that are currently controversial, but are hard to find evidence-based, feminist information about. This makes it even harder for women to rely on web resources when making healthcare decisions. Nevertheless, the Internet can be a great tool for becoming more informed about your health. But, to get the best information, you have to take a critical look at your search results and use the best information available. Here are our guidelines for becoming a web-savvy health researcher:

Beware of Drug Ads

When a health site includes drug advertisements it's an obvious red flag that the health information is, at best,

"Finding Good Health Information on the Web," by Electra Kaczorowski, originally published in the *Women's Health Activist*, March/April 2006, pp. 4–5, the newsletter of the National Women's Health Network (NWHN). It is reprinted with the permission of the author and the NWHN.

biased, and at worst, factually incorrect. This is because the drug companies who run ads on the site are also likely to sponsor site's health information. The information presented will have been reviewed and selected to ensure it meets the standards of the drug companies rather than the consumer. It's not always easy to spot the advertisement on health sites, though. Drug ads are often ingeniously placed to be as unobtrusive as possible; sometimes they even merge seamlessly with the site itself. This is especially true on mainstream, general health websites heavily promoted on TV and in other media. While it is usually easy to access basic information on these large, popular sites, it is difficult to avoid the barrage of ads that come with it. Be on the lookout for product promotions that are disguised as health information, an essential skill in conducting good web research. Being aware of the presence of drug ads will help you review the site's information carefully and with a critical eye.

Look Behind the Scenes

Even if a website has no overt advertisements, the agency that runs it may be sponsored or supported by the pharmaceutical industry. Creating and maintaining a website costs money, so many companies seek support from drug and device manufacturers. Just like in politics, these financial contributors have a say in the information and research their money supports. It can be hard to tell if an agency or organization (and, thus, its website) has corporate ties, as the information may be hidden well within the site. Try looking for links to "sponsors," "partners," or "advisory boards" to get more information. A long list of pharmaceutical companies or medical device manufacturers indicates that the site's content is subject to corporate influence. Even if the information you're looking for is factually correct, there's an excellent chance that other information (e.g., alternate, non-pharmacological treatments or risk factors and complications) has been downplayed or omitted.

Read Between the Lines

When looking at web-based information, it is important to identify the intended purpose of the information provided. Is the site trying to sell a specific treatment, or convince the viewer that one particular procedure is the best way to go? Is the information provided in a way that informs and educates the reader? Reliable health information should help individuals make informed decisions, not to promote specific health procedures. If a website includes numerous mentions of one specific approach without also discussing risks, side-effects, or alternatives, it may not be the best tool to use in making a health decision.

For example, one popular menopause site features Q&A sessions with a physician who essentially prescribes specific regimens of bioidentical hormones to women who write in, complete with dosage information and referrals to specific businesses. This is clearly intended to be a substitute for a doctor's visit, and leaves no room for questions that do not end with a specific recommendation. The women who write in are encouraged to follow this particular doctor's orders in lieu of gathering information to make their own informed decision. Look for information that is balanced, well-organized, and comprehensively addresses all aspects of the topic.

Check the Address

Before going to a link, it's a good idea to assess if the website is a commercial site (ending in *.com* or *.net*), a non-profit site (ending in *.org*), an educational institution site (ending in *.edu*), or a governmental site (ending in *.gov*). (Internet addresses are expanding, but these are the most common suffixes.) Commercial sites aim to sell products and may contain many ads. Or, they may be simply trying to promote one type of treatment over another, as do many commercial sites on fibroids. Organizational sites are run by an agency and reflect the group's perspective and that of any sponsors. Finding out more about the agency's philosophy and approach to women's health can help visitors take a critical look at the site's health information. Governmental sites on women's health generally contain accurate information, but may not always be comprehensive, and often lack analysis. Knowing the kind of website from which the information is coming is helpful in making informed decisions and learning more about a health topic.

Watch for Hype

Health information on the web is just like any other kind of information: subject to bias and inaccuracies. Some hot-button women's health topics have been getting a lot of attention recently, the most prominent being menopause hormone therapy, bioidentical or 'natural' hormones, hysterectomy, osteoporosis, and infertility. Websites that cover any of these topics should be looked at very carefully to ensure that their information is based on scientific evidence (with clear references), not just testimonials or theories. Information on these hot-button issues abounds; even TV stations may have auxiliary websites featuring 'experts' on these topics. While consumer education is important, the views represented on these sites usually reflect those of corporate sponsors and the information is rarely presented in a balanced way. The more controversial a health topic is, the more essential it is for the reader to be vigilant and discerning.

Keep an Eye on the Evidence

There are places out there that are committed to providing individuals with the information they need to make decisions about their healthcare. Supporting individual decision, making is very important to the NWHN, and we plan to expand our website to make even more information available on-line. Other sites with feminist, evidence-based health information are www.bcaction.org (Breast Cancer Action), www.ourbodiesourselves.org (Our Bodies, Ourselves), www.stopbreastcancer.org (National Breast Cancer Coalition), www.desaction.org (DES Action), www.susanlovemd.org (Susan Love's website, and www.center4research.org (National Research Center for Women and Families), to name just a few. The Network also appreciates the good work of the Cochrane Collaboration (www.cochrane.org), which produces and disseminates reviews on evidence-based healthcare interventions. For a more comprehensive list of sites NWHN likes, please visit the *links* section of our website.

Women can also access journal articles and studies on their own through www.pubmed.gov or www .medlineplus.gov (both services of the National Institutes of Health), although it is essential to be aware that even these sources are subject to bias and industry influence.

A Final Word

Being aware of all of these factors is the key to solid web research. Sometimes it's impossible to find information on a certain topic that is free of product promotions or pharmaceutical-sponsored studies. Just knowing about these potential influences can make a big difference when sifting through information, however. The Internet is a wonderful way for individuals to quickly and privately become more informed and educated about their health. As with any tool, it is important to know how to use it well and to the best advantage.

NOTES

1. Fox, S., Rainie L. 'Vital Decisions: How Internet Users Decide What Information to Trust When They or Their Loved Ones Are Sick.' Pew Internet and American Life Project, May 2002. On-line at http://www.pewinternet .org/pdfs/ PIP_Vital_Decisions_May2002.pdf.

 # Hormone Therapy "Six Steps Toward a Better Future"

by Cindy Pearson

On October 24, 2002, Network Executive Director Cindy Pearson discussed the implications of the Women's Health Initiative at a Scientific Workshop on Menopausal Hormone Therapy at the National Institutes of Health. More than 500 physicians, researchers and activists were in the audience. Before concluding with the recommendations excerpted below, Pearson warned that drug companies, professional societies, women's groups, policy makers and government agencies had all been complicit in creating a "climate of enthusiasm for hormone therapy" and allowing the needless suffering of tens of thousands of women.

To consider the implications for future research, we need to consider current research. The Women's Health Initiative's controlled trials of hormone therapy took place in the context of massive off-label use of hormone therapy. Millions of healthy women were taking long-term hormone therapy for a preventive benefit not yet proven because medical practice was determined under the influence of industry rather than the influence of evidence. . . .

To prevent more tragedies like this, and to make sure that future research is able to make as big an impact as possible, significant changes are needed in policy and practice within the regulatory agencies, media, professional societies, consumer groups with financial ties to industry, and the behavior of industry itself.

Future research will be undercut before it is underway unless we as a society muster the necessary will to take the following steps:

- Get drug company money out of medical education.
- Give the FDA the authority to pre-approve direct-to-consumer advertisements for prescription medications.
- End industry payments to physicians for writing papers that appear in medical journals.
- Stop quoting medical experts in media reports on health without reporting on their financial relationship with industry.

- Clean up consumer groups' health education efforts so that the all-too-common and dangerous influence of drug company money is replaced with a healthy skepticism.
- Bar anyone with significant financial ties to industry from involvement in the development of professional guidelines.

The National Women's Health Network calls on the policy makers, researchers, clinicians and leaders assembled here to take steps to make these changes a reality.

WORKSHEET—CHAPTER 4

Medicalization, Marketing, and the Politics of Information

1. After reading "The Picture of Health," go through a number of health textbooks, health ads, or other health information. Describe who is and who is not included in the images, and how the images create the definition of health. Describe alternative healthy image photographs that you would like to include if you were designing a health textbook.

2. Identify a time when you or a family member made a decision about whether to use a drug or have a medical procedure. What information did you/they use to make the decision? What information do you wish you had had available?

3. Collect several drug ads or ads related to health issues aimed at women as consumers from popular women's magazines. Compare what you find with the issues raised in articles in this chapter.

4. Collect several ads about women's health issues/products from medical journals aimed at health practitioners. What messages/stereotypes do the ads give to practitioners about women as consumers?

5. "Advertising Disease" describes how drug ads turn ordinary human experiences into "diseases" that need a medical fix. Describe examples you find of this.

6. Choose to track ads on any one specific product. Make notes on ads for that product as they appear in different sources (print ads, television ads, ads in medical journals, ads in magazines for mainstream vs specialized audiences). How are ads the same or different when aimed at different audiences?

7. Collect a number of ads for contraceptive products. (Be sure to note which source each ad is from.) Compare what you observed in collecting the ads with what Ronna Popkin found in her analysis of contraceptive ads in "Dangerous Combination: Direct-to-Consumer Advertising, Abstinence Only Education, and Young Women's Health."

MENSTRUATION

We begin this chapter with the classic "If Men Could Menstruate" by Gloria Steinem. Besides demonstrating that feminists *do* have a sense of humor, this enjoyable, popular article really sets the framework for this chapter. Indeed, it is often the first article discussed in our women's health courses because it so perfectly sets a theme to be addressed throughout the semester: when there are inequalities in a society, everything associated with the valued group will be valued and anything connected with the less valued group will be less valued.

The normal physiological process of menstruation has been defined and redefined by male "experts" throughout history. It has been labeled a disability or illness, as a barrier to higher education for women, as a weakness that justified keeping middle-class women from working outside the home (working class women were expected to continue their work.) Later, menstrual cramps were identified as psychogenic in origin, brought on by the fear of femininity or sexuality. Now hormonal flucuations are blamed for a wide range of symptoms premenstrually, from acne and water retention to depression, homicidal behavior, and self-mutilation. Readers interested in more background on the changing meanings of menstruation are referred to two articles which appeared in earlier editions of this book: "Women, Menstruation, and Nineteenth Century Medicine" by Vern Bullough and Martha Voght, in the excellent *Women's Health in America* edited by Judith Walzer Leavitt, puts the changing definitions and meanings of menstruation within their historical contexts, while at the same time addressing a recurring theme in medical history—"the reluctance of physicians to accept new scientific findings" and Louise Lander's thought-provoking *Images of Bleeding: Menstruation as Ideology* examines what the social sciences say about the meaning of menstruation, concluding that the meanings will always change because menstruation will always be one aspect of what it means to be a woman in a given cultural and historical context.

An entire volume (Volume 46, numbers 1 and 2, January 2002) of the *Sex Roles* journal is devoted to new research on menstruation, which was presented at a 2001 conference of the Society for Menstrual Cycle Research. Yes! There is an entire organization devoted to the study of menstruation and menstruation-related issues. The Society for Menstrual Cycle Research (SMCR) is an excellent example of the changing face of science as more women have opportunities to become scientists, and as women, as both scientists and activists, push for different types of questions to be asked in scientific research. Bi-annual conferences of SMCR are interesting, stimulating opportunities to see feminist science at work and to learn more about menstruation than we ever knew there was to know. (Society for Menstrual Cycle Research website = http://menstruationresearch.org/)

"Female Adolescence: Puberty and Growing Up" describes the history of the discovery that the average weight of girls (whether they mature early or late) at menarche is approximately 103 pounds because a critical, minimum amount of body fat is required before the body is capable of reproduction. This chapter traces some of the science of understanding this phenomena from the days (pre 1970) when the author, Rose E. Frisch, observed the critical menarche weight based on data from 181 girls and Gordon C. Kennedy was postulating that there must be a "lipostat" (a sort of internal measurement of body fat which signals that a young woman is "ready" for reproduction), to the 1995 discovery that indeed leptin, a protein hormone produced by fat cells, seems to play this role in controlling reproduction. This article could stimulate discussions on important issues related to what it means that young women's age of menarche and potential pregnancy is so related to body fat composition. The average age of menarche today is 12.6-12.8 years compared to 14.7 years in 1880. Similarly, other chapters in the book (*Female Fertility and the Body Fat Connection* by Rose E. Frisch), which this article is taken from, provide fascinating, thought-provoking information on how body fat is a crucial factor in determining a woman's fertility (gaining a few pounds can make the difference between fertility and infertility for a thin woman) and asks whether the incidence of breast cancer in women can be reduced by encouraging delayed menarche in adolescents through promoting a healthier amount of exercise in girls before menarche. In addition to learning the science of the body fat-fertility connection from Rose E. Frisch's book, the reader is treated to one woman's personal story of the rewards of being a scientist. Few scientific books are so personal and honest as Frisch's in describing the pure pleasure of scientific discovery.

The economics of menstruation is a useful reminder of an overall theme in women's health: there is a huge market, and much money to be made any time a company can sell something to groups of healthy women. The worksheet on menstrual products requires the calculation of the financial costs of menstruation related products for one woman in her lifetime. Any reader who multiplies that figure by the number of menstruating women will see the dollar signs that tempt companies to get a piece of the menstruation product market.

Since women went "off the rag" and began using disposable menstruation products, there has been a large profitable business in tampons, napkins, and pads. While these are products most women want to keep on the market, the competition and profit motives sometimes mean that consumer health and safety receive minimal attention. The most obvious example was the Rely super absorbent tampon, marketed by Proctor and Gamble, which was associated with toxic shock syndrome deaths in the late 1970s and 1980s. In *The Price of a Life*, Tom Riley, the lawyer for the family of Pat Kelm, a young woman from Cedar Rapids, Iowa, who died from toxic shock syndrome four days after using her first Rely tampon, describes how Proctor and Gamble intentionally ignored reports of problems and instead chose to spend more than all other tampon manufacturers combined marketing their product as the tampon that "even absorbs the worry." Now that toxic shock syndrome (TSS) is no longer the women's health issue in the headlines and in women's magazine, we are concerned that young women (TSS mainly strikes menstruating women under age 30 using tampons) are not learning what they need to know to protect themselves from products (high absorbency products) or circumstances (leaving a tampon in for many hours) which increase risks of TSS.

"Don't Just Go with the Flow," from *Teen Voices*, is an excellent example of the type of women's health information which should be available to all women, not just the young women lucky enough to subscribe to this magazine, which deliberately works to be an alternative ("Because you're more than just a pretty face." Web-site = http://teenvoices.com/) to mainstream teen magazines. This little article, jam-packed with information, manages to critique the menstrual products available in most grocery stores and pharmacies, introduce a range of menstrual products that are safer for women's bodies and the environment, encourage a campaign to get natural feminine hygiene products more widely distributed, give a "herstory" of menstrual products, provide information on toxic shock syndrome, and introduce readers to websites on natural menstruation products.

When any product will be marketed to large numbers of healthy women, safety standards for that product must be extremely high. As the Rely tampon example above demonstrates, there is a growing history of profits put before safety, and women used as guinea pigs for products (high dose oral contraceptives, DES, the Dalkon Shield, hormone replacement therapy) for which promises were too good to be true. The next article is a favorite classic, "The Selling of Premenstrual Syndrome" by Andrea Eagan, which both introduces the topic of premenstrual syndrome and provides an analysis for critiquing the increasing number of products that are getting to the market and hyped to women and their practitioners (see articles on advertising in Chapter 4 and articles on hormone replacement therapy in Chapter 12) before their long-term safety has been studied/proven. This article uses PMS to symbolize the "double-edged sword" women and women's health activists face more generally when we ask that women's health issues be taken seriously: we want good scientific research and health system response to the health issues that affect us, but we do not want these issues to be medicalized or used against women. The words of Andrea Eagan seem as urgent today as they were when they were written in 1983:

> To suddenly discover that thousands of women are rushing to get an untested drug to cure a suspected but entirely unproven hormone deficiency . . . is a little shocking . . . I'm ashamed to see women flocking to use an untested substance about which there is substantial suspicion, whose mode of action is not known, to treat a condition whose very cause is a mystery.

These 1983 words bring us full circle to new examples of the concept that meanings of menstruation will always change because menstruation is always one aspect of what it means to be a woman in changing cultural and historical contexts. In articles alarmingly similar to Eagan's classic PMS article, the previous (Chapter 4, "Advertising Disease") and following (Chapter 6, "You, Too, Can Hold a Congressional Hearing") chapters explore the marketing of mood altering drugs for the treatment of Premenstrual Dysphoric Disorder, which has not even been proven to exist.

Seasonale, a new packaging of birth control pills so that women have "menstruation" just 4 times a year, was brought onto the market just as the previous (4th) edition of this book went to press. At that time, we encouraged readers to watch how the marketing of Seasonale represents society's views of menstruation—and women. We end the chapter with an update on this topic, with an article examining "menstrual suppression" products, which have grown in numbers and marketing since Seasonale first hit the market. The author, Kiesha McCurtis, places the concepts of drugs used for suppressing menstruation in the context of the increasing "medicalization of women's bodies and lives," a key theme of this book, stating:

> We are concerned about this process, in which natural experiences and socially created problems are treated as biological diseases that require medical (preferably pharmaceutical) intervention to "protect" women's health.

The manufacturers of Lybrel, which is designed to eliminate menstruation completely, is another step in "protecting" women from the natural process of menstruation.

IF MEN COULD MENSTRUATE
A Political Fantasy

by Gloria Steinem

A white minority of the world has spent centuries conning us into thinking that a white skin makes people superior—even though the only thing it really does is make them more subject to ultraviolet rays and to wrinkles. Male human beings have built whole cultures around the idea that penis-envy is "natural" to women—though having such an unprotected organ might be said to make men vulnerable, and the power to give birth makes womb-envy at least as logical.

In short, the characteristics of the powerful, whatever they may be, are thought to be better than the characteristics of the powerless—and logic has nothing to do with it.

What would happen, for instance, if suddenly, magically, men could menstruate and women could not?

The answer is clear—menstruation would become an enviable, boast-worthy, masculine event:

Men would brag about how long and how much.

Boys would mark the onset of menses, that longed for proof of manhood, with religious ritual and stag parties.

Congress would fund a National Institute of Dysmenorrhea to help stamp out monthly discomforts.

Sanitary supplies would be federally funded and free. (Of course, some men would still pay for the prestige of commercial brands such as John Wayne Tampons, Muhammad Ali's Rope-a-dope Pads, Joe Namath Jock Shields—"For Those Light Bachelor Days," and Robert "Baretta" Blake Maxi-Pads.)

Military men, right-wing politicians, and religious fundamentalists would cite menstruation ("*men*struation") as proof that only men could serve in the Army ("you have to give blood to take blood"), occupy political office ("can women be aggressive without that steadfast cycle governed by the planet Mars?"), be priests and ministers ("how could a woman give her blood for our sins?"), or rabbis ("without the monthly loss of impurities, women remain unclean").

Male radicals, left wing politicians, mystics, however, would insist that women are equal, just different, and that any woman could enter their ranks if only she were willing to self-inflict a major wound every month ("you *must* give blood for the revolution"), recognize the pre-eminence of menstrual issues, or subordinate her selfness to all men in their Cycle of Enlightenment.

Street guys would brag ("I'm a three-pad man") or answer praise from a buddy ("Man, you lookin good!") by giving fives and saying, "Yeah, man, I'm on the rag!"

TV shows would treat the subject at length. ("Happy Days": Richie and Potsie try to convince Fonzie that he is still "The Fonz," though he has missed two periods in a row.) So would newspapers. (SHARK SCARE THREATENS MENSTRUATING MEN. JUDGE CITES MONTHLY STRESS IN PARDONING RAPIST.) And movies. (Newman and Redford in "Blood Brothers"!)

Men would convince women that intercourse was *more* pleasurable at "that time of the month." Lesbians would be said to fear blood and therefore life itself—though probably only because they needed a good menstruating man.

Of course, male intellectuals would offer the most moral and logical arguments. How could a woman master any discipline that demanded a sense of time, space, mathematics, or measurement, for instance, without that in-built gift for measuring the cycles of the moon and planets—and thus for measuring anything at all? In the rarefied fields of philosophy and religion, could women compensate for missing the rhythm of the universe? Or for their lack of symbolic death-and-resurrection every month?

Liberal males in every field would try to be kind: the fact that "these people" have no gift for measuring life or connecting to the universe, the liberals would explain, should be punishment enough.

And how would women be trained to react? One can imagine traditional women agreeing to all these arguments with a staunch and smiling masochism. ("The ERA would force housewives to wound themselves every month": Phyllis Schlafly. "Your husband's blood is as sacred as that of Jesus—and so sexy, too!": Marabel Morgan.) Reformers and Queen Bees would try to imitate men, and *pretend* to have a monthly cycle. All feminists would explain endlessly that men, too, needed to be liberated from the false idea of Martian aggressiveness, just as women needed to escape the bonds of menses-envy. Radical feminists would add that the oppression of the nonmenstrual was the pattern for all other

oppressions ("Vampires were our first freedom fighters!") Cultural feminists would develop a bloodless imagery in art and literature. Socialist feminists would insist that only under capitalism would men be able to monopolize menstrual blood. . . .

In fact, if men could menstruate, the power justifications could probably go on forever.

If we let them.

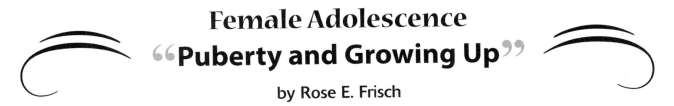

Female Adolescence
"Puberty and Growing Up"
by Rose E. Frisch

You may never have heard of the adolescent "growth spurt"—a sudden, rapid growth first in height, then in weight—but if you are grown up, you have had it. A girl's growth spurt always occurs before menarche. In well-nourished populations like that of the United States, girls experience the spurt beginning at about age 9; boys experience it at about age 11.

Some researchers and the media use the word *puberty* to include all the physical changes that happen around and during the time of the growth spurt. Puberty is a rather fuzzy term that can denote the years of rapid adolescent growth, the appearance of secondary sex characteristics such as breast development and pubic hair, and menarche. Instead of using the category "puberty," I will refer separately to the adolescent growth spurt, the first "growing up" event that lasts for about three years; the development of secondary sex characteristics; and menarche, which follows the spurt.

Together with Roger Revelle (former director of the Harvard Center for Population Studies, where I conduct my research), I spent several years in the late 1960s and early 1970s learning about the weight changes that occur in girls during the adolescent growth spurt. (I'll tell you why shortly.) In that phase of the research, we made a new and important finding: menarche was closely related to a "critical" body weight. We were totally surprised at the connection to body weight. I soon found

by reading about other species, however, that girls are just like other mammals, including monkeys and apes, in that sexual maturity is more closely related to body weight than to chronological age.

How did we ever come to research something so crude as kilograms of body weight? (A kilogram is equivalent to 2.2 pounds.) I was trained as a geneticist, and Roger was a well-known oceanographer; neither of us had been interested in body weights. We were inspired to look into adolescence and sexual maturation by our studies of body weight that had nothing to do with either topic—a good way to discover something new in science. At the time we were working on a Harvard project to calculate future world food needs. To estimate calorie requirements, you first have to know the body weights of the population you are planning to feed, so I collected body weight data for females and males of all ages, from birth to age 65 and older, from many developing countries.

An Unexpected Finding

Collecting all those body weights was somewhat boring, so I looked for the age of the largest yearly gain in weight of girls in various populations of developing countries. I knew that this "peak weight gain" always took place before menarche, and I was curious to know at just what age it took place. (Age of menarche was not reported.) For example, I found that Pakistani girls had their largest weight gain at age 13. I could infer, then, that menarche would occur for these girls sometime after that age, probably at 14 or 15.

But then something quite intriguing turned up. Within a generally undernourished population like Pakistan, poor rural girls experienced this peak weight gain at a later age (14) than did better-nourished urban girls (12). This finding agreed with previously published reports showing that poorly nourished girls had their growth spurt and menarche later than did well-nourished girls. What was unexpected was that the rural and urban girls had the *same average weight* at the time of the peak weight gain, although they peaked at different ages. Did the weight itself mean something? If so, what did it represent?

I decided to pursue this interesting discovery. I repaired to the library and began reading the literature on body size at all stages of a girl's sexual maturation. I found many research papers, but most of them focused on height rather than weight. When I inquired among anthropologists and pediatricians about the reason for the lack of detailed research on body weight, I was told that body weight was so variable that it was not worth studying in relation to sexual maturation. But as newcomers to the subject, neither Roger nor I had any such prejudice, so we did look at body weight.

Analyzing Growth Data: The Girls' Spurt

To use the most accurate growth data, we relied on longitudinal growth studies in which the same girls were measured regularly as they grew up. In the studies we analyzed, the height and weight of each girl was measured every six months from birth to age 18, and her age of menarche was recorded. There were three such studies of girls and boys in the United States, one in Berkeley (California), one in Boston, and one in Denver. In all three, the subjects were well nourished and middle class.[1] The studies were completed in 1940–1950. We needed all three studies to get a large enough sample because there is always a great deal of variability in human growth.

Figure 1 shows the annual weight gain of one of the girls from birth to age 18. (I plotted similar curves of height and weight gain for each of the 181 girls in the studies.) This girl was a rapid grower and an early maturer. The arrow in the diagram indicates when her growth spurt in weight began at age 10; that sudden, rapid rise in weight gain is "the spurt." The girl's fastest growth in weight occurred at age 12. As you can see in the diagram, menarche occurs after weight gain starts to slow down; in this girl, menarche occurred at 12 years

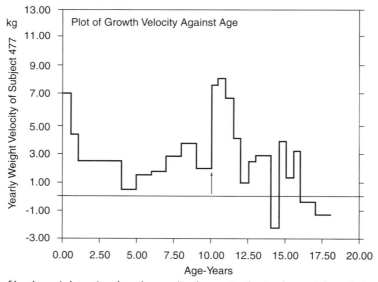

FIGURE 1 The amount of body weight gained each year (in the vertical axis, the weight gain is measured in kilograms; one kilogram equals 2.2 pounds), from birth to age 18, of one girl in the Denver study. The arrow shows the initiation of the adolescent growth spurt in weight at age 10. The rapid rise in weight gain is the spurt, which occurs before menarche, the first menstrual cycle. This girl, a rapid grower, had menarche at age 12.3. As the diagram shows, weight gain slows before menarche.

From R. E. Frisch, "The Critical Weight at Menarche and the Initiation of the Adolescent Growth Spurt, and the Control of Puberty," in *Control of the Onset of Puberty*, ed. M. M. Grumbach, G. D. Grave, and F. E. Mayer (New York: John Wiley & Sons, 1974), 404.

and 4 months (12.3 years). The average age of menarche of the 181 girls was 12 years and 10 months (12.8 years).

What starts that rapid acceleration in growth before menarche? Researchers are still not sure of the control mechanisms, but two things are certain: every normal adolescent girl and boy has the growth spurt before maturing sexually, and adolescents starting the growth spurt eat, eat, and eat; it's hard to keep enough food in stock. Then, after the peak gain in weight, both weight gain and food intake decrease. Little is known about what controls the reduction in food intake. In fact, we still don't know why human beings have an adolescent growth spurt at all. Why not idle along at the same growth rate until menarche?

All mammals seem to have a growth spurt before sexual maturation, but we don't know why this happens, either. One possible reason for the growth spurt in humans is that the rapid growth for girls is accompanied by a large increase in stored, easily mobilized energy—body fat—useful for successful reproduction.

Timing of the "Spurt" and Menarche

In the studies we analyzed, girls began the adolescent growth spurt at 9.5 years of age on average. Menarche occurred about three years after the start of the spurt, at 12.8 years. Many teachers and parents are still surprised at these early ages. Girls experienced the fastest growth in height at 11.5 years of age on average, and their peak weight gain occurred about six months later, at age 12. However, there is a lot of variability around these average ages; this variability is measured statistically by the *standard deviation* (often abbreviated as SD).

In our study, the standard deviation of the ages for each of these adolescent events was about one year. For example, the average age of menarche was 12.8 years with a standard deviation of one year. This means that two-thirds of the girls had menarche between the ages of 11.8 (the average age, 12.8, minus one year) and 13.8 (the average age, plus one year).

Growth rates are so variable because how quickly or slowly you grow at all ages is controlled genetically; you inherit your growth rate. But growth rate can also be affected by environmental factors such as the quality and quantity of food you eat and the amount of energy you expend. Two girls in the same family who eat the same food and have the same environment can grow at very different rates, one fast and one slow. The genetically fast grower will mature sexually before the slow grower does. However, the fast grower will mature later if she diets to become super slim or if she runs twenty miles a week. And the slow grower will mature even later if she changes her life style similarly. Nu-

trition and energy outputs interact with the genetic control.

Weight at Menarche

Pediatricians conduct growth studies of healthy, normal children, like the studies I analyzed, to establish standards of height and weight for girls and boys at each age. Then they are able to assess whether a girl or boy is growing normally.

Oddly, even though the age of menarche was noted precisely for each of the girls in the growth studies we analyzed, apparently no one had ever asked the simple question, what is the height and weight of girls at menarche? After we determined the average height and weight, we especially wanted to know whether early and late menarcheal girls had the same weight at menarche. This was easy to find out because we had each girl's exact age of menarche and her height and weight at every age up to 18. It just took time to gather the data for 181 girls.

We were excited by the answers. For all the girls, the average weight at menarche was 103 pounds (47 kg), and the average age of menarche was 12 years and 10 months (12.8 years). And eureka! Similar to our earlier results on peak weight gain, the early- and the late-maturing girls had the *same* average weight, 103 pounds (47 kg), whether they were younger than 12.8 years or older than 12.8 years at menarche. In 1970 Roger and I published this unexpected result in *Science* magazine, with some speculations as to what it could mean. The reaction to our article was usually incredulity: how could body weight matter? A good question that I set out to answer.

It was already known that height at menarche differed for early and late maturers. The average height for all girls at menarche was 62 inches (158 cm), but late-maturing girls were on average taller at menarche than the earlier maturers. I could now explain why many researchers reported that early maturers had more weight for height than did late maturers: average weights at menarche of early and late maturers are the same, but early maturers are shorter at menarche than late maturers.

When I reported these menarcheal height and weight results and their possible significance at a conference of pediatricians, I was greeted at first with dead silence. Then I was asked, "What is your background, Dr. Frisch?" (the tone of voice implying, how come are you here?). "I have my doctoral degree in genetics," I replied. "And who is Roger Revelle?" someone asked, mispronouncing "Revelle" to rhyme with "jelly." "Oh, Roger is an oceanographer," I answered, "and the director of the Population Center, where I work." More silence. No one apparently thought our new findings on weight at menarche mattered, and my presence was considered one of those aberrations that can happen at a conference. The response didn't trouble me. I had presented my message, and the doctors were polite.

I had been invited to speak at the conference by Dr. Thomas E. Cone Jr., then of Children's Hospital in Boston. Dr. Cone had read our published papers on the weight of girls and the adolescent spurt, including menarche. He was an expert on children's growth, and he found our results provocative and interesting. There were other doctors who also thought, as we did, that we were on to something, and they encouraged us to continue. But soon I learned that clinical doctors and researchers in any field, be it pediatrics, gynecology, or anthropology, are often uninterested in new ides. Some scientists are even hostile to them, especially if the ideas come from a researcher they've never heard of who works in an unrelated discipline (like me). A famous biochemist at Harvard Medical School once asked me, perhaps overly pessimistically, "How do you think new ideas advance, Dr. Frisch?" "I'm not too sure," I replied, thinking of some of my recent experiences. "Funeral by funeral is the answer," he said.

Overall, I had an exciting time pursuing this research. I found that when I had good questions to ask, I could call or write experts in a field, and most would respond generously with answers and advice. In fact, that is how I met some of my co-investigators and mentors. I also followed the sage advice I read in a scientist's memoir (I can't remember whose): choose the experts in a field whom you respect most for knowledge and advice, and ignore the reactions of everybody else.

Earlier Menarche: Girls "Grow Up" Faster

Even before being able to predict menarche for an individual girl, I could explain the well-known but unexplained fact that menarche had occurred progressively earlier during the past one hundred years. As I found, historical studies showed that the average weight at menarche of girls in the United States was the same in the past as it is now, 103 pounds (47 kg). What happened about a century ago was that girls began to grow more quickly in both height and weight because of improved nutrition and a decrease in childhood disease. They became larger sooner and therefore reached the average weight at menarche at an earlier age.

As shown in Figure 2 below, the average age of menarche in Europe has become earlier by two to three months per decade over the past century and a half. In the mid-1800s, for example, menarche occurred as late as age 17 in Scandinavia; one hundred years later, the average age had declined to about 14.5. In the United States, the average age of menarche was 14.7 in 1880 and declined to age 14 by 1900. Thereafter menarche occurred earlier by about three months per decade until 1945, when it leveled off at age 12.6 to 12.8.

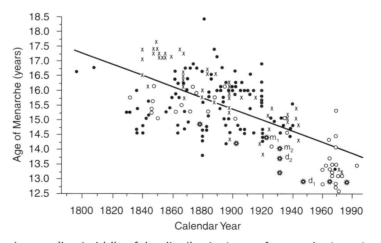

FIGURE 2 Mean (average) or median (middle of the distribution) age of menarche (years) as a function of calendar year from 1790 to 1980. The symbols refer to England (◎); France (●); Germany (⊗); Holland (□); Scandinavia (Denmark, Finland, Norway, and Sweden) (x); Belgium, Czechoslovakia, Hungary, Italy, Poland (rural), Romania (urban and rural), Russia, Spain, and Switzerland (all labeled ○); and the United States (✳) (U.S. data not included in the regression line). The age of menarche has already leveled off in some European countries as it has in the United States (see U.S. data and text).

Reprinted from G. Wyshak and R. E. Frisch, "Evidence for a Secular Trend in Age of Menarche," *New England Journal of Medicine* 306 (1982): 1033.

Since the average age of menarche was 15.5 or 16 a century and a half ago, doctors then defined precocious puberty (abnormally early menarche) as menarche at age 11 or 12. Those ages are now close to the present average age of menarche, 12.6 to 12.8. Doctors now define precocious puberty as menarche at age 8 or 9.

I once heard an eminent anthropologist predict that menarche would become earlier and earlier, so eventually menarche might occur at age 6. First graders! What a thought! It cannot be so.

Age of Menarche Now Leveled Off

Because menarche is a measure of how quickly girls grow, when girls' growth rates level off, the average age of menarche also levels off. As shown in the figure above, this is what has happened in the United States. Twelve-year-old girls have been the same average height and weight for more than fifty years. They have had good nutrition, and they no longer contract many of the childhood diseases that might slow their growth. Therefore, the average age of menarche has remained the same for the past fifty years as well.

Parents are apparently just becoming aware that the age of menarche is earlier now than it was a century ago. Puberty has become a popular subject in the media, and journalists often consult me to find out the facts. Confusion reigns about the timing of the "first menses," as one interviewer hesitantly described it. In summary, menarche is earlier today than in 1890 and 1900 for girls in the United States, but the trend to an earlier age of menarche has stabilized at 12.6 to 12.8 years.

Factors Delaying the Age of Menarche

Confirming the connection between the age of menarche and how rapidly or slowly girls grow in a particular population, any factor that slows weight growth before or after birth delays the age of menarche. Menarche occurs later in twins than in single-born children, for example, because twins grow more slowly. Malnutrition and undernutrition, both widespread among children in developing countries, delay menarche. Chronic childhood diseases in the United States, such as juvenile diabetes, sickle cell anemia, and cystic fibrosis, also slow growth and delay menarche. High altitude delays menarche by slowing the rate of weight growth both before and after birth; some of the latest average ages of menarche in the world, 17 and 18, occur in poorly nourished girls living at high altitudes in Peru and New Guinea. Then there are the athletes and dancers, who, as we found, fit the same model by undereating and overexercising, thus delaying menarche to the age of 15, 16, 17 or even 20.

A Mile High: Later Menarche of Denver Girls

Girls from Denver provide a particularly good example of how the natural environment can affect growth rate and thus the age of menarche. In the studies we analyzed, Denver girls were well nourished and middle class, as were the Berkeley and Boston girls. But Denver girls had menarche later, at an average age of 13, compared to 12.8 years for the two other groups. Although small, this difference was statistically significant. I couldn't figure out the reason for it until I read that at high altitudes growth in the uterus is slowed, resulting in lighter birth weights for both girls and boys.

But Denver is only a mile above sea level; would that be enough to affect birth weight? Indeed it is. When I added up the birth weights of the girls from Denver, they were 200 grams (7 oz) lighter on average than the birth weights of the girls in the sea-level cities of Berkley and Boston. Birth weights of the boys from Denver averaged 400 grams (14 oz) lighter than the birth weights of the sea-level boys. (Note that boys showed a bigger difference in birth weight than girls. Boys are more sensitive to "environmental insults"—under-nutrition, toxic substances, radiation, and high altitude. No one yet knows why this is so, but the effect of altitude on birth weight is a clear example of the phenomenon.)

How does altitude affect birth weight? The air has less oxygen at high altitudes, and therefore the fetus grows more slowly in the uterus. Consequently, high-altitude newborns weigh less than sea-level babies. But do the high-altitude babies eventually catch up? To find out, I compared the height and weight at every age of the Denver girls and the Berkeley girls, and I discovered that the Denver girls did not catch up in weight. Denver girls weighed less at every age than Berkeley girls, even though both groups of girls were similar in height at every age. Interestingly, during the adolescent spurt, the Denver girls gained the same amount of height (8.7 in; 22.1 cm) and the same amount of weight (37 lb; 17 kg) as did the Berkeley girls. It was the growth in weight up to the beginning of the spurt that was slowed. This suggests that the rapid growth during the spurt is controlled independently from the growth before the spurt.

Faster Growth, Earlier Menarche

It is clear that, in general, any environmental—or genetic—factor that slows weight growth also delays menarche. Conversely, any factor that speeds up weight growth, such as ample food and fatty food, is associated with earlier menarche. For example, obese girls have menarche earlier than the average age unless their obesity is associated with pathology.

Individual girls have menarche at all different weights, though. What connects the slow or fast growth rates with the age of menarche? I had no explanation. But I did have an idea as to why body weight at the time of the first menstrual cycle could matter.

Body weight at menarche is close to adult body weight. Remember, for maintenance of the species it is a smart strategy to connect body weight and menarche. The survival of a newborn depends on the infant's birth weight, and the infant's birth weight is correlated with the mother's prepregnancy weight and her weight gain during pregnancy.

What Is the Clue in Body Weight?

What did body weight represent? What was the connection between body weight and sexual maturation? When I discussed these questions with Dr. J. M. Tanner, an expert on adolescent growth at the Institute of Child Health in London, he suggested that I consult the work of Gordon C. Kennedy of Cambridge University. I still recall the excitement of reading Kennedy's papers. He was one of the few researchers who combined the two fields of nutrition and reproduction. Kennedy had found that he could delay sexual maturation (called *estrus* in nonprimate mammals) in rats indefinitely by underfeeding them.

Kennedy stated, "Everybody knows you 'grow up' before you mature sexually." But then he asked the important question, "How do you define being 'grown up'?" (Roger used to say, "In the navy, they said if you are big enough, you are old enough." Kennedy was more precise.)

Based on his research connecting body weight, food intake, and puberty in rats, Kennedy proposed that the signal the brain receives indicating that a female is grown up enough to reproduce successfully is related to the amount of fat stored in the body. Kennedy also proposed that there is a "lipostat," some sort of internal measurement of body fat that is perceived by the hypothalamus, the part of the brain that controls food intake and reproduction. I was so inspired by Kennedy's work that I wrote him to ask if I might visit him; I had the good fortune to visit him twice. I came away from our discussions convinced that a lipostat was somehow involved in female sexual maturation. I decided to follow this "fatness" clue based on the idea that a critical, minimum amount of body fat is necessary for reproduction.

After reading the human and animal body composition literature for about two years (the data for humans were very difficult to follow because at that time there were no direct measures of human body fat), I found that I could indeed predict a minimum weight for height necessary for menarche or regular menstrual cycles from a fatness indicator. I was cheered by this result; when you can predict, nature is telling you something.

I am writing this about three decades after Kennedy published his lipostat idea and more than twenty-five years after my controversial 1974 *Science* article. In 1995, I opened the July issue of *Science* and read of Jeffrey Friedman's cloning of the "obese" gene at Rockefeller University and of the strong evidence for a lipostat. Freidman and other researchers reported that body fat cells produced a protein hormone called leptin (from *leptos*, the Greek word for "thin"). Leptin is perceived by special cells, called receptors, in the hypothalamus. Kennedy's paper of three decades earlier was the first publication cited in the references section of Friedman's article.

After reading Friedman's *Science* article, I sent him some of my articles on body fat, menarche, and ovulation. I also mentioned that I had visited Gordon Kennedy twice. Not long after that I was amazed to receive a call from Friedman. First he asked me about Gordon Kennedy. Then he said, "I thought you would be interested to know that you can make an infertile mouse fertile by injecting leptin," indicating that indeed leptin, and thus body fat, has a role in reproduction. (Dr. Farid Chehab of the University of California Medical Center in San Francisco published this result in *Science* in 1997: prepubertal mice—mice without fat—became pubertal after the injection of leptin.)

I was present when Friedman delivered three lectures on leptin at Harvard Medical School in 1996, and he mentioned my research on the critical-fatness connection to menarche and ovulation. During the question period following one of the lectures, a man asked, "What about weight loss in men? Does it affect their reproductive ability?" "I don't know," replied Friedman. "Does anyone in the audience know?" Silence reigned in the well-filled, sizable amphitheater. I raised my hand. "I do," I said.

"As men lose weight, the first thing to go is libido—as in bulls. Then, as testosterone levels fall further, there is a loss of prostate fluid; then sperm motility and mobility are affected. Then, with an extreme, 25 percent weight loss (the men look like skeletons), sperm production is also affected. Weight gain reverses all of these effects." I was quite surprised that facts known three decades ago were new to this large medical audience, but then, this is a molecular, DNA age.

A Paradox of Population Growth

A question may have occurred to you as you read about a direct link between nutrition and fertility. If undernourishment decreases fertility, how do we explain the rapid population growth of undernourished populations in developing countries? Fertility rates in many developing countries (6 to 7 children per couple) are actually far *below* the maximum human fertility (11 to 12 children per couple) found in well-nourished, noncontracepting populations. Populations of many developing countries are growing rapidly because death rates have decreased (thanks to modern public health measures) while fertility rates have remained the same.

Not to Neglect the Boys

My research focused on girls, but I did compare some of the adolescent events for boys who were in the same longitudinal growth studies.

Boys in the United States begin their rapid growth in height and weight simultaneously, at about age 11 on average, two years later than girls. In developing countries and historically, boys experience the spurt three years later than girls. The rapid growth continues for about three years in boys, as it does in girls, and it decelerates before *genarche*, the boys' equivalent of menarche, at about age 14.6 to 14.8. Genarche is not precisely timed because there is not a clear endpoint for boys such as the first menstrual cycle for girls. Nocturnal emissions usually begin at this time, but this event is not easy to document.

John Crawford, a pediatric endocrinologist then at Massachusetts General Hospital, suggested a possibly more precise endpoint when he urged me to study boys in detail in addition to girls. Crawford noted that apocrine sweat, which has an odor, appears at the time of genarche, so one could determine the timing of genarche by smelling the underarm sweat of boys. I declined the opportunity, and as far as I know, no one else has leaped to do it.

Why do boys start their rapid growth later, and therefore reach sexual maturation later, than girls? One possible reason may be that when girls have menarche, regular ovulatory cycles do not begin immediately. There are often irregular, anovulatory periods. Boys do not have this period of relative infertility; once they are sexually mature, sperm production is at the adult level. Later maturation for boys would therefore be an advantage for successful reproductive outcome—useful in the past, but not now! Whatever the reason, the later growth spurt for boys means that during elementary school there is a period when girls are bigger than boys at the same age. I have been amazed at the large number of men (including my husband) who remembered this time, even thirty or forty years later.

NOTES

1. It is important to compare persons of similar socioeconomic backgrounds, as studies have shown that age of growth and maturation differ by social class. See H. P. Bowditch, *Eighth Annual Report* (Boston: Massachusetts State Board of Health, 1877); V. Kiil, *Skrifter utgitt av det Norske Videnskaps-Akademi i Oslo 2*, no. 1 (1939). Kiil's data, collected from different social classes and geographic regions in Norway over 100 years, show "an undoubted connection between the age of the individual at the time sexual maturity commenced and the social conditions under which that person lives" (p. 145).

"Don't Just Go with the Flow"

from *Teen Voices*

Did you ever stop to think about the feminine product(s) you use during your special time of the month? Is it the same product your mom or friends introduced to you when you first got your period? Disposable, bleached pads and tampons you find in the grocery store or local pharmacy . . . that's about all that's out there in period world, right? Wrong! There's a whole other world of menstrual products to choose from. And it doesn't stop there! There are menstrual products out there that are not only safer for our bodies, but will make the environment happy too!

Read on to find out more about these fabulous alternatives, why they're not in stores near you (and how you can get them there).

> ### Words to Know
>
> **Shelving or "Slotting" fees.** Payments product manufacturers must make to retailers to be able to sell their items on store shelves. They range from hundreds to thousands of dollars per item based on the items' placement on shelves. [Eye level costs more.]
>
> **Food cooperatives.** Locally owned stores run by community members that usually offer a wide variety of products and environmentally safe options like recyclable bags and food in bulk.
>
> **Natural health food stores.** Markets or specialty shops offering a variety of natural and organic foods and healthcare products.

Have You Heard of Any of These?

That's right, there are menstrual products you can buy that are safer for you and the environment. There are products actually out there that are chlorine-bleached-rayon-free. Chlorine-bleached rayon is currently found in menstrual products sold in big stores across the country. These two ingredients together are said to make dioxin, which according to a 1994 U.S. Environmental Protection Agency EPA study is found to be cancerous [an estimated 100 of the roughly 1,400 daily cancer deaths in the U.S. are said to be caused by dioxin]. Differences in opinion still surround whether the levels of dioxin found in pads and tampons are high enough to be of any risk to you. But why add any risk, and why contribute to environmental harm?

Start Your Own Campaign!

The sooner we speak out, the sooner change will happen! Tear out this letter, sign your name, get your friends to sign it, and walk it over to your nearby grocery store or pharmacy. Demand that all your menstrual product choices be on the shelves of your grocery store!

Why Aren't They Sold in Most Stores?

Teen Voices asked GladRags, Natracare, and Organic Essentials (three companies that sell a variety of natural menstrual products) why their menstrual products aren't sold in most major grocery stores or pharmacies. Here's what they had to say. Do you want to do something about it?

> To Whom It May Concern,
>
> I shop at your store regularly and I am bothered that you fail to carry any natural feminine hygiene products. I can't believe you're leaving so many of us to have to travel miles out of our way to natural food stores to buy products we should be able to buy on your shelves.
>
> I am well aware that most of these natural feminine hygiene products are produced by small companies that cannot afford high shelving costs like the major brands—but what about the health of your customers? Perhaps your store might consider reducing fees for shelf space for these companies until their sales go up, or help them to advertise their products in your store.
>
> I think you should be more than willing to provide all of us with all our menstrual choices. After all, I'm sure you have women in your lives and care about their health and choices.
>
> Sincerely,

Not in the Majors

Menstrual Product	How does it work?	Pro-you	Not good for you	Environment friendly?
Bleached with Chlorine-free methods, Cotton Pad	• Disposable. • Can attach to your under wear with its sticky back.	• No harmful dyes. • Dioxin-free	• Harmful pesticides may have been used to grow cotton. • Usually found only in natural health food stores or on the web. • More expensive.	• Better for the environment than commercial pads, but still not too great. • Environment is OK, but could be happier.
Cloth Pad	• Reusable. • Can wrap around your underwear with the help of its buttons or clips.	• It's cheaper. You can just buy one or two and you're set for months.	• Need to wash. • Usually found only in natural health food stores and co-ops.	• Environment is very happy.
Organic Tampon	• Disposable, 100% compressed cotton grown without the use of pesticides or chemical fertilizers. Unbleached and undyed.	• Dioxin-free	• Usually found only in natural health food stores, in co-ops, or on the Web. • More expensive.	• Environment is OK, but could be a bit happier.
Menstrual Cup	• Reusable, flexible rubber cup [usually made out of natural gum rubber] that you insert inside your vagina.	• Dioxin-free • Very cheap. One is enough to have.	• A sink is needed to rinse it out. • Usually have to order through a mail catalog, may be available in certain natural health food stores, in co-ops, or on the Web.	• Environment couldn't be happier!
Sponge	• Reusable, natural sponge found in the ocean!, with a string attached to it.	• Dioxin-free • Cheaper. Can just buy one or two and you're set for months.	• Need to boil it to clean. • Usually have to order through a mail catalog, may be available in certain natural health food stores or on the Web.	• Environment very happy!

Source: "EPA Links Dioxin to Cancer," *The Washington Post,* 17 May 2000: "The Trouble With Tampons," *Vegetarian Times,* July 1996.

In the Majors

Menstrual Product	How does it work?	Pro-you	Not good for you	Environment friendly?
"Common Pad" (**Bleached, Dry-weave Pad**)	• Disposable. • Can attach to your underwear with its sticky backing.	• Can be thrown right away after use. • Can be found in almost all convenience stores, grocery stores, and some public bathrooms.	• Has pesticides and dyes. • Dry-weave portion of pad is often made out of plastic. • Some contain dioxins.	• No Way!
"Common Tampon" (**Bleached Tampon**)	• Disposable compressed cotton mixtures that you insert into your vagina.	• Can be thrown away after use. • Can be found in almost all convenience stores, grocery stores, and some public bathrooms.	• Could have pesticides and dyes or could be bleached. • Dioxin risk.	• Very bad for the environment.
Lubricated Tampon	• Disposable tampons with a wet film on them to make inserting them more comfortable.	• The film is sterile and kills the bacteria that cause T.S.S.	• Lubrication could disrupt the body's natural lubrication.	• No Way!

GladRags

"Alternative feminine hygiene products are not yet sold in most stores because the customers aren't interested in or ready for them. [In particular], I don't think department store shoppers are ready for reusable menstrual alternatives; they are used to disposable products because that's what they see on TV and in magazines.

Women are also seldom actually comfortable with menstruating. Unfortunately few women view their bleeding as a positive empowering experience and don't want to touch or see it happen. When women learn to like menstruating, they will most likely switch to washable pads or healthy options."—Carmen de la Cruz, General Manager

Brenda Mallory founded GladRags in 1992 in Portland, Oregon. She got the idea from the cloth diapers she used for her baby daughter Emma. She first thought she would be making cloth pads from home on her own sewing machine, but orders got too big and now GladRags is sold nationally in natural food stores, food co-operatives, and by its catalog and Web site.

Natracare

"In Canada, the Northwest, and other parts of the U.S., Natracare is sold in some grocery stores. Grocery stores usually ask for a lot of money for products to be placed [on their shelves], and because we're a small company, we don't have the resources to pay these high fees. It's not until the demand [from] women and young women actually going into stores and asking for it that they would actually get it [there]."—Susan Carskadon, Manager in North America.

In Great Britain in 1989, a British national network aired a program on the effects of dioxin pollution and its influences on women's menstrual products. After its airing, many women began boycotting the disposable, bleached pads and tampons they had been using to demand change. Susie Hewson then developed Natracare for the women of Great Britain. It then spread throughout Europe, New Zealand, Canada, and the Sultanate of Oman in the Middle East. Natracare made its way to the U.S. in 1993.

Organic Essentials

The reason you cannot find Organic Essentials in other major retail stores and discount stores is simply because of lack of education and demand. We believe that every family had their cotton farm certified organic by the Texas Department of Agriculture in 1991.

The Herstory of Our Monthly Visitor

Julia Steinberg, 19
Newton, Massachusetts

So what did women do back in the day about their periods?

- 15th century Egyptian women used tampons too! But their tampons were made of soft papyrus [a tall, grassy plant found on the shores of the Nile River that ancient civilizations used to make paper].
- For centuries, women all over the globe who lived by the sea used natural sponges to absorb their periods.
- Native American women made pads from buffalo and deer skins, cattail down, moss, and even tree bark!
- 19th century American women were really "on the rag" when they got their periods. They did use old rags!

Check Out These Sites
For more info on how and where to get natural menstrual products for yourself, visit these sites for listings and links:
www.critpath.org/tracy/healthy.html
www.borntolove.com/d-list.shtml
www.bloodsisters.org

Check These Books Out!
A Girl's Story by Toni Cade Bambara
The Vagina Monologues by Eve Ensler
Quilting: Poems 1987–1990
See "poem in praise of menstruation," "poem to my uterus," and "to my last period."
by Lucille Clifton

- By 1886, disposable towels were invented in the U.S. but couldn't be marketed because menstruation was considered immoral [evil]! Instead, women wore menstrual pad belts that sometimes even had suspenders.
- In 1922, hundreds of American women bought "sanitary bloomers" [diaper-like undies] from Sears Robuck & Co. catalogue.

The Lowdown on T.S.S.

While on the topic of menstrual products, if you're a tampon user, stories of Toxic Shock Syndrome may have come up once or twice in conversation. Here's the quick lowdown: T.S.S. is caused from the bacteria Staphylococcus aureus. It has been reported that most cases of this bacteria entering the body and spreading its toxins have been through tampon use. Some health experts believe that tampons may produce small cuts along our vaginal walls that can allow this bacteria to enter our bodies. Others believe that the menstrual blood left within or behind tampons may permit the bacteria to grow.

Symptoms of T.S.S.

These symptoms can occur suddenly and may be confused with illnesses like the flu or measles. If you suffer from any of these during your time of the month while wearing a tampon, remove it right away. This can stop the bacteria from growing in 80% of cases. Also see your doctor right away.

- Fever greater than 101 degrees F
- Low blood pressure that may cause you to faint
- Vomiting
- Diarrhea
- Aching muscles
- Sunburn-like rash that results in severe peeling in 1-2 weeks

Easy Ways to Prevent T.S.S.

- Change your tampons every 4 to 5 hours
- Wash your hands before inserting tampons
- Try alternating between tampons and pads, or other alternatives
- Try not to wear tampons while you sleep

Source: Women's Health Interactive; Calgary Regional Health Authority

- While bandaging up patients during World War I, French nurses discovered gauze materials were much better for absorbing periods than cloth diapers.

- With the increased number of working women during the 1920s and 1930s in the U.S., companies began manufacturing the first "tampons" to meet the demand for comfortable period protection.

- During the 1970s, the self-adhesive pads we know today were invented and put on the market, "Beltless freedom."

- By the 1980's women were buying snap-on flannel pads with removable fillers.

- Today, over 50 brands of menstrual products are on the market in the U.S., and are a half billion dollar industry! Products like thong panty pads are even on the market–talk about women refusing to let menstruation into their everyday lives!

Source: Red Flower: Rethinking Menstruation *by Dena Taylor*

The Selling of Premenstrual Syndrome
Who Profits from Marketing PMS "The Disease of the 80s"?

by Andrea Eagan

In the summer of 1961, I was working as a laboratory assistant at a major pharmaceutical firm. Seminars were regularly given on recent scientific developments, and that summer, one of them, on the oral contraceptive, was given by an associate of Dr. Gregory Pincus, who was instrumental in the development of the Pill. As a rule, only the scientists went to the seminars. But for this one, every woman in the place—receptionists and bottle washers, technicians and cleaners—showed up. Oral contraception sounded like a miracle, a dream come true.

During the discussion, someone asked whether the drug was safe. Yes, we were assured, it was perfectly safe. It had been thoroughly tested in Puerto Rico, and besides, you were only adjusting the proportions of naturally occurring substances in the body, putting in a little estrogen and progesterone to fool the body into thinking that it was "just a little bit pregnant." The Food and Drug

Administration had approved the sale of the birth-control pill in the United States the year before. News of it was everywhere. Women flocked to their doctors to get it. The dream, we now know, was much too good to be true. But we learned that only after years of using the Pill, after we had already become a generation of guinea pigs.

Since then, and because of similar experiences with DES and with estrogen replacement therapy (ERT), because of the work of the women's health movement and of health activists like Barbara Seaman, we have presumably learned something: we have become cautious about medical miracles and scientific breakthroughs. To suddenly discover, then, that thousands of women are rushing to get an untested drug to cure a suspected but entirely unproved hormone deficiency which manifests itself as a condition with a startling variety of symptoms—known by the catchall name premenstrual syndrome (PMS)—is a little shocking.

Often when a drug suddenly makes the news, or when a new "disease" for which there is a patented cure is discovered, it is fairly easy to find the public relations work of the drug manufacturers behind the story. As just one example, estrogen replacement therapy for the symptoms of menopause had been around since the 1940s. But in 1966, a Brooklyn physician by the name of Robert Wilson wrote a book called *Feminine Forever*, which extolled the benefits of ERT in preventing what the author called "living decay." Wilson went on TV and radio, was interviewed for scores of articles. He claimed that *lifelong* ERT, starting well before menopause, would prevent or cure more than 20 different conditions, ranging from backaches to insomnia and irritability. Wilson ran an operation called the Wilson Research Foundation that put out information to the media and received grants from drug companies. Among those contributing to the Wilson Foundation was Ayerst Laboratories, the largest manufacturer of the estrogen used in the treatment of menopause symptoms. Ayerst also funded a group called the Information Center on the Mature Woman, from which regular information bulletins were sent to the media.

Many doctors had misgivings about ERT (the link between estrogen and cancer had been reported since the 1930s), but the information that the public received about ERT was almost entirely positive. One of the few warnings against ERT appeared in *Ms.* in December, 1972. Three years later, in 1975, a study was published in the *New England Journal of Medicine* reporting that estrogen users had a five to 14 times greater incidence of uterine cancer than did nonusers. This was news, and it made the papers. (*The New England Journal*, like several other prestigious medical journals, sends out advance issues to some news services, which is why the networks all have the same story on the same day.)

Women, needless to say, were concerned about ERT. Many simply stopped taking the drug, and sales of Premarin (the brand name of Ayerst's ERT preparation, which accounted for 80 percent of the market) dropped.

Soon after this, Ayerst received a memo on media strategy from Hill & Knowlton, its public relations firm. This memo, the sort that is supposed to be absolutely confidential, became public when someone sent a copy to the New York women's newspaper, *Majority Report*. *MR* published the entire memo under the headline, "New Discovery: Public Relations Cures Cancer." The first part of the plan was to take the spotlight off estrogen and refocus it on menopause. The "estrogen message," said the memo, "can be effectively conveyed by discreet references to 'products that your doctor may prescribe.'" Articles on menopause were to be placed in major women's magazines. Information was also to be fed to syndicated women's page columnists, general magazines and prominent science writers and editors.

The second part of Hill & Knowlton's plan was to counter anticipated negative publicity. A list of potentially damaging events—research reports (one was expected from the Mayo Clinic), FDA announcements, lawsuits—was given. News releases were to be prepared in *advance* of the "damaging commentary . . . in as much detail as possible." When this memo became public (Jack Anderson picked it up after *MR*'s publication), Ayerst denied any intention of following its recommendations, but the memo actually outlines the kinds of steps some drug manufacturers take to bring their products to the attention of the public and to counteract criticism.

The same story, with only minor changes, can be told for a number of other drugs, so when I began seeing articles about PMS and progesterone treatment, I immediately had some questions. Why was PMS suddenly "news"? What do we really know about progesterone? And who are the advocates of this treatment?

PMS stories began appearing rather suddenly about two years ago, after two Englishwomen claimed PMS as a mitigating factor in their defense against murder charges. When the stories about these cases appeared, many American women who suffer from cyclical problems naturally became interested in finding out all they could about the condition.

PMS itself is not news. It was first mentioned in the medical literature in the 1930s, and women presumably had it before then. Estimates on the numbers of women affected by PMS vary wildly. Some claim that as many as 80 percent are affected while others place estimates at only 20 percent. Similarly, doctors' opinions vary on the number and type of symptoms that may indicate PMS. They cite from 20 up to 150 physical and psychological symptoms, ranging from bloating to rage. The key to recognizing PMS and differentiating it from anything else that might cause some or all of a woman's symptoms is timing. The symptoms appear at some point after ovulation (around mid-cycle) and disappear at the beginning of the menstrual period. (It should not be confused with dysmenorrhea or menstrual discomfort, about which much is known, and for which several effective, safe treatments have been developed.)

While PMS is now generally acknowledged to be a physical, as well as a psychological disorder, there is little agreement on what causes it or how it should be treated. There are at least half a dozen theories as to its cause—ranging from an alteration in the way that the body uses glucose to excessive estrogen levels—none of which have been convincingly demonstrated.

One of the most vocal proponents of PMS treatment is Katharina Dalton, a British physician who has been treating the condition for more than 30 years. Dalton believes that PMS results from a deficiency of progesterone, a hormone that is normally present at high levels during the second half of the menstrual cycle and during pregnancy. Her treatment, and that of her followers, relies on the administration of progesterone during the premenstrual phase of the cycle.

Progesterone is not absorbed effectively when taken by mouth. Powdered progesterone, derived from yams or soybeans, can be dissolved in oil and given in a deep, painful muscular injection. Or the powder can be absorbed from vaginal or rectal suppositories, a more popular form. (In this country the Upjohn Company is the major manufacturer of progesterone, which they sell only in bulk to pharmacies where pharmacists then package it for sale. Upjohn makes no recommendation for the use of progesterone and is conducting no tests on the product.)

Although she promotes the progesterone treatment, Dalton has no direct evidence of a hormone deficiency in PMS sufferers. Because progesterone is secreted cyclically in irregular bursts, and testing of blood levels of progesterone is complicated and expensive, studies have been unable to show conclusively that women with PMS symptoms have lower levels of progesterone than other women. Dalton's evidence is indirect: the symptoms of PMS are relieved by the administration of progesterone.

Upon learning about Dalton's diagnosis-and-cure, many women concluded that they had the symptoms she was talking about. But when they asked their doctors for progesterone treatment, they generally got nowhere. Progesterone is not approved by the FDA for treatment of PMS (the only approved uses are for treating cessation of menstrual flow and abnormal uterine bleeding due to hormone imbalance); there is *nothing* in the medical literature showing clearly what causes PMS; and there has never been a well-designed, controlled study here or in England of the effect of progesterone on PMS.

Despite some doctors' reluctance to prescribe progesterone, self-help groups began springing up, and special clinics were established to treat PMS. Women who had any of the reported symptoms (cyclical or not) headed en masse for the clinics or flew thousands of miles to doctors whose willingness to prescribe progesterone had become known through the PMS network. And a few pharmacists began putting up progesterone powder in suppository form and doing a thriving business.

How did PMS suddenly become the rage, or what one New York gynecologist called "the hypoglycemia of the 1980s"? At least part of the publicity can be traced to an enterprising young man named James Hovey. He is reported to have claimed he had a B.A. in public health from UCLA despite the fact that, aside from extension courses, he had been there less than a year. (UCLA does not even have a B.A. program in public health.) He met Katharina Dalton in Holland several years ago at a conference on the biological basis of violent behavior. Returning to the United States, he worked with a Boston physician who opened the first PMS clinic in Lynnfield. A few months later, Hovey left the clinic. He then started The National Center for Premenstrual Syndrome and Menstrual Distress in New York City, Boston, Memphis, and Los Angeles—each with a local doctor as medical director.

For $265 (paid in advance), you got three visits. The initial visit consisted of a physical exam and interview, and a lengthy questionnaire on symptoms. During the second visit, the clinic dispensed advice on diet and vitamins, and reviewed a monthly record the patient was asked to keep. On the third visit, if symptoms still persisted, most patients received a prescription for progesterone.

Last year, James Hovey's wife Donna, a nurse who was working in his New York clinic, told me that they were participating in an FDA-approved study of progesterone, in conjunction with a doctor from the University of Tennessee. In fact, to date the FDA has approved only one study on progesterone treatment of PMS, which is conducted at the National Institute of Child Health and Human Development, an organization unrelated to James Hovey.

Similar contradictions and misrepresentations, as well as Hovey's lack of qualifications to be conducting research or running a medical facility, were exposed by two journalists last year. Marilyn Webb in the *Village Voice* and Jennifer Allen in *New York* magazine both dug into the operation of the clinic and Hovey's past to reveal him as a former Army medical corpsman turned entrepreneur. Hovey left New York and gave up his interest in the New York and Boston clinics. He is currently running a nationwide PMS referral service out of New Hampshire.

In a recent interview, Hovey said that the clinic business is too time-consuming, and that he is getting out. His "only interest is research" he says. He was associated with two scientists who applied to the FDA for permission to do progesterone studies but who were rejected because the FDA considered the doses of progesterone to be too high. At last report, Hovey still headed H and K Pharmaceuticals, a company founded in 1981 for the manufacture of progesterone suppositories, and it is as a supplier that his name has appeared on FDA applications.

Hovey's involvement in PMS treatment seems to have centered on the commercial opportunities. Others, such as Virginia Cassara, became interested in PMS for more personal reasons.

Cassara, a social worker from Wisconsin, went to England in 1979 to be treated by Dalton for severe PMS. The treatment was successful and Cassara returned to spread the good news. She invited Katharina Dalton to Wisconsin to speak and notified the press. Though only one article appeared, it brought women "out of the closet," Cassara says. Cassara began counseling and speaking, selling Dalton's books and other literature. Her national group, PMS Action, now has an annual budget of $650,000, 17 paid staff members, and 40 volunteers. Cassara spends most of her time traveling and speaking.

Cassara's argument is compelling, at least initially. She describes the misery of PMS sufferers, and the variety of ineffective medical treatments they have been subjected to in their search for relief. For anyone who is sensitive to women's health issues, it is a familiar tale: a condition that afflicts perhaps millions of women has never been studied; a treatment that gives relief is ignored. Women, says Cassara, are pushed into diet and exercise regimens that are difficult to maintain and don't always work. One valid solution, she feels, lies in progesterone.

According to FDA spokesperson Roger Eastep, Phase I studies—those that determine how much a particular substance is absorbed by the body and how it works—have yet to be done for progesterone. But in the meantime, more and more doctors are prescribing the hormone for PMS.

Dr. Michelle Harrison, a gynecologist practicing in Cambridge, Massachusetts, and a spokesperson for the National Women's Health Network, is one physician who does prescribe progesterone to some women, with mixed feelings. "I've seen it dramatically temper women's reactions," she says. "For those women whose lives are shattered by PMS, who've made repeated suicide attempts or who are unable to keep a job, you have to do something. But I have a very frightening consent form that they have to sign before I'll give progesterone to them." Harrison also stresses that a lot of PMS is iatrogenic; that is, it is caused by medical treatment. It often appears for the first time after a woman has stopped taking birth-control pills, after tubal ligation or even after a hysterectomy, in which the ovaries have been removed.

When doctors do prescribe progesterone, their ideas of the appropriate dosage can vary from 50 to 2,400 mg. per day. For some women, dosages at the lower end of the scale do not bring relief from their symptoms. It has also been reported by women taking progesterone and in medical literature that the effect of a particular dose diminishes after a few months. Some women are symptom-free as long as they are taking the drug, but the symptoms reappear as soon as they stop, regardless of where they are in the menstrual cycle.

For all these reasons, some women are taking much higher doses than their doctors prescribe. Michelle Harrison had heard of women taking 2,400 mg. per day; Dalton had heard about 3,000; Cassara knows women who take 4,000. Because PMS symptoms tend to occur when progesterone is not being taken, some women take it every day, instead of only during the premenstrual phase. Some bleed all the time; others don't menstruate at all. Vaginal and rectal swelling are common. Animal studies have shown increased rates of breast tumors and cervical cancer. Marilyn Webb, a reporter who began taking progesterone while working on a story about PMS, developed chest pains after several months. She asked all the doctors she interviewed whether any of their patients had experienced chest pains. Every one said that she or he had at least one patient who had.

Reminding her of the history of the Pill, of DES, and of ERT, I asked Virginia Cassara whether she was concerned about the long-term effects of progesterone on women. "I guess I don't think there could be anything worse than serious PMS," she responded. "Even cancer?" I asked. "Absolutely. Even cancer." Later, she said, "I think it's paternalistic of the FDA to make those choices for us, to tell us what we can and cannot put in our bodies. Women with PMS are competent beings, capable of making their own choices."

I don't have severe PMS, and I don't think I fully understand the desperation of women who do and who see help at last within reach. But given our limited understanding of how progesterone works, I do not understand why women like Cassara are echoing drug company complaints of overregulation by the FDA. I'm alarmed to see women flocking to use an untested substance about which there is substantial suspicion, whose mode of action is not known, to treat a condition whose very cause is a mystery. And I fear that, somewhere down the line, we will finally learn all about progesterone treatment and it won't be what we wanted to know.

One doctor, who refused to be quoted by name, cheerfully assured me that progesterone was safe. "Even if a woman is taking 1,600 milligrams per day, the amount of circulating progesterone is still only a quarter of what is normally circulating during pregnancy." And I couldn't help but think of the doctor at the seminar more than 20 years ago: "Of course it's safe. It's just like being a little bit pregnant."

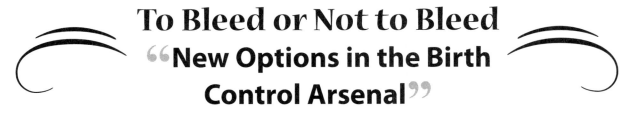

To Bleed or Not to Bleed
"New Options in the Birth Control Arsenal"

By Kiesha McCurtis

"Menstruation is not a normal, healthy thing to happen."[1]

Since the recent introduction of "menstrual suppression" products to help women avoid or limit their periods, some physicians and scientists have made grossly unsupported claims—like the one above—with respect to menstruation. While the NWHN supports the availability of menstrual suppression products as an option for women, we have strong concerns about the unsavory manner in which these products are being marketed by manufacturers and healthcare providers alike.

As part of the menstrual suppression trend, in late May, the Food and Drug Administration (FDA) approved a "new" form of hormonal contraception—Lybrel—that is not quite as new as women might be lead to believe. Lybrel is the first birth control designed to completely eliminate a woman's monthly period, the concept known as "menstrual suppression". The idea isn't new; for years, women have taken their traditional birth control pills on a non-traditional schedule in order to manipulate the timing of their periods. In fact, Lybrel is not the only product on the market that has been designed to attract women who wish to avoid menstruation. Two other products—Seaonale and Seasonique—are intended to alter a women's bleeding pattern so that she has just four periods in a year's time, instead of the typical dozen.

The common thread for all of these menstrual suppression products is that they are chemically identical to traditional oral contraceptive (OC) pills. The active tablets in all of these pills contain a combination of levonorgestrel and ethinyl estradiol. The difference lies in the way a woman takes her pills: traditional OC is taken for 21 days, followed by 7 days of placebo pills, during which time the woman has her period. Lybrel uses the same hormones in a slightly lower dose, but has no change in hormone dose throughout the year and no placebo pills—thus, the woman has no periods at all. With Seasonale and Seasonique, a woman takes one pill every day for three months then, during the final week of the pack, she takes placebo pills and has her period.

From a safety perspective, menstrual suppression products are probably an acceptable option for most women. The effectiveness of menstrual suppression products in terms of preventing pregnancy is very similar to regular OC pills. Women who can safely take traditional OC are unlikely to experience problems or difficulties with these new products. Although women who use menstrual suppression pills will take a few dozen more active hormone pills over the course of a year than do women who use 21-day OC, no evidence has been found that shows a meaningful or increased health risk from doing so. The small risks of stroke and blood clots that are associated with traditional OC (which are increased in women who smoke) are also associated with extended-use pills like Lybrel, Seasonale, and Seasonique.

The pill is arguably one of the most researched drugs that is available on the market today. Nonetheless, OC products designed for menstrual suppression are still new products that could, potentially, develop unanticipated side effects over the long-term. There were high drop-out rates in the product safety and effectiveness trials for all of these menstrual suppression products, so the number of women who were observed and monitored was smaller than might be desired. One of the more important downsides is likely to be the high rate of break-through bleeding—which can last as long as a regular period but occurs without the predictability of a monthly cycle. Another concern is that women taking menstrual suppression pills will not be able to use a missed period as a sign of possible pregnancy; for this reason, the FDA recommends that women taking Lybrel

"To Bleed or Not to Bleed: New Options in the Birth Control Arsenal," by Kiesha McCurtis, MPH, originally published in the *Women's Health Activist*, November/December 2007, pp. 1, 3, 6, the newsletter of the National Women's Health Network (NWHN). It is reprinted with the permission of the author and the NWHN.

or other menstrual suppression products use pregnancy tests if they suspect they might have gotten pregnant.

As women's health activists, the Network regularly analyzes and criticizes the increasingly common process of medicalization of women's bodies and lives. We are concerned about this process, in which natural experiences and socially created problems are treated as biological diseases that require medical (preferably pharmaceutical) intervention to "protect" women's health. Disease creation has morphed; pharmaceutical companies are now considered to be the creative geniuses responsible for mending the "broken" female form. Examples of this process include premenstrual dysphoric disorder (e.g., PMS as a mental health condition); thin bones; and female sexual dysfunction (to be treated by drugs).

Menstrual suppression products are another option in the arsenal of fertility control, yes, but the manner in which they are being marketed is disconcerting. Pharmaceutical companies have begun to promote menstrual suppression products using the bogus assertion that monthly periods are somehow dangerous or unhealthy. Some scientists have even speculated that reducing the frequency of menstruation (and ovulation) reduces the risk of breast, endometrial, and ovarian cancers—but none of these claims have been substantiated by scientific evidence.[2,3] The fact is, there is no scientific evidence to support the hypothesis that the frequency of menstruation and ovulation directly causes reproductive cancers. It is precisely this type of false and misleading advertising that generates profit for pharmaceutical companies to the detriment of women's health.

Greater variety in the available options on the birth control spectrum is a positive move forward, but it should not come at the risk of further medicalizing women's bodies. Misleading information about the inherent "danger" of menstruation is not helpful, and actually harms young girls' and women's understanding of their bodies and natural bodily functions. Introducing menstruation to pre-adolescents and newly menstruating girls as a negative (and potentially dangerous) experience that is best avoided could strongly affect their body image and self-perception in negative and lasting ways. Young girls have their work cut out for them as it is in our culture; they shouldn't have to battle a barrage of negative and misleading messages about a natural bodily process on top of the other challenges they face.

Women's individual experiences of, and attitudes about, menstruation play an important role in determining their interest in menstrual suppression and may also affect the level of satisfaction with the method among women who use these products. Some women find the thought of not having a period (or as many periods) appealing for convenience, while others rely on monthly menstruation as a sign of a healthy body or a signal that they are not pregnant. For women who have monthly menses accompanied by pain, discomfort, or extremely heavy bleeding, menstrual suppression offers an accessible health benefit.

These products are yet another contraception option among many, and have the potential to expand options and increase convenience for some women. This advance should not be undermined, however, by stigmatizing menstruation or by passing products off as new and innovative, when they are really just newly packaged and promoted.

REFERENCES

1. Rabin R, "The New Pill in Town: Controversial Form of Birth Control Delays Monthly Cycle," *Newsday*, January 25, 2004, p. 4.

2. Eaton SB, Pike MC, Short RV, et al., "Women's Reproductive Cancers in Evolutionary Context," *Q Rev Biol.* 1994; 69: 353–367.

3. Arthur C, "New Pill Will Allow Women to Have Just Three Periods a Year," *The Independent*, March 14, 2002, p. 6.

WORKSHEET—CHAPTER 5

Menstruation

This worksheet must be optional. Some parts of this worksheet are designed for women who go through reproductive cycles. Women who do not have reproductive cycles and men may or may not want to interview women with reproductive cycles about the personal questions asked in 1 and 3.

1. **Your menstrual cycle.** Observe changes your body goes through during a menstrual cycle. Here are a few things you may want to note. You may think of others you would find interesting to record (cravings, water retention, etc.) See if you can identify when you are ovulating/have ovulated. If you are on oral contraceptives, how will your observations differ from those of women not on synthetic hormones?

   Temperature: Record body temperature (by mouth is fine) first thing in the morning before you get up, before you have anything to drink or smoke. You are more likely to note changes if you have a fairly regular schedule and use a very accurate thermometer.

   Mucus (secreted by the cervical glands): Observe changes in mucus. Choose your own words to describe what you feel. Words like much, some, scant, clear, watery, like egg-whites, and sticky are sometimes useful. Remember that contraceptive gels, foams, and semen in the vagina will mask much of what you might notice about mucus.

   Breasts: Fuller, less full, lumpier, tender, "What I think of as 'normal'," and sore may be words useful to describe breast changes.

	Date	Temperature	Mucus	Breasts	Other observations
1					
2					
3					
4					
5					
6					
7					
8					
9					
10					
11					
12					
13					
14					
15					
16					
17					
18					
19					
20					
21					
22					
23					
24					
25					
26					
27					
28					
29					
30					
31					
32					
33					
34					
35					

2. **Menstruation Products.** Calculate how much you or an "average" woman spends on menstruation products in a lifetime. (These calculations can be based on today's prices.) Check current prices for one or two brands of tampons, napkins, or other "menstruation hygiene products." Estimate how much of this product is used for each menstrual cycle. (A woman with a heavy flow will use many more than a woman with a light flow.) For your calculations you will need to figure how many years a woman will menstruate (age of menopause— age of menarche), and how many times a year a woman menstruates. Show your work. (For a very accurate estimation, you would want to think about how pregnancies, lactation, choice of contraception and menstrual changes at different ages would influence your calculations, but you do not need to do this for this question.)

3. **Premenstrual syndrome.** The publicity about premenstrual syndrome (PMS) and premenstrual dysphoric disorder (PMDD) and advertising for drugs promising medical-fixes for these have helped make women and men regard the premenstrual days as "the bad time of the month" for women.

   a. If a few days are regarded as the relatively "bad" days, then other parts of the cycle must be viewed as relatively "good." Identify "good" things you associate with different parts of your cycle. (These might include such things as times of high energy, times when you require less sleep, times when you most enjoy how your body feels, times when you especially enjoy exercising, times when you find it easy to resist sweet or salty foods, times when you especially enjoy your sexuality.)

   b. Some women identify very positive things about premenstrual days. For many women this is a time when they are most creative, their dreaming is most vivid, they are the most sexually aroused, they find it easiest to "justify" taking time for themselves, they feel most in touch with things in their life that need changing. Identify positive things you, your friends, or your mother notice about premenstrual days.

4. Describe how you learned about menarche/menstruation and compare this to how you wish you had learned about it.

5. Think about ways in which menarche/menstruation could be introduced to young people as a positive part of women's and men's lives.

   a. Suggest one or more ways to introduce menarche/menstruation as positive to young women.

   b. Suggest one or more ways to introduce menarche/menstruation as positive to young men.

6. **Menstrual suppression products.** Collect ads, articles, or friends' comments about Seasonale, Seasonique, Lybrel, and any other similar products, which are basically contraceptive pills packaged so that women have periods just once a season or not at all. What patterns do you see in these messages about attitudes toward menstruation and concerns about the safety of new products on the market that have not been extensively studied?

MENTAL HEALTH

Many formerly battered women who have been close to death with life-threatening physical injuries have said the physical violence had less impact on them than day-to-day psychological/emotional abuse they survived. Many women with chronic fatigue syndrome so severe that taking a shower became a major goal have said that the worst part of their condition was that people (including doctors) would not believe they were ill and had said that their condition was "all in their heads." Mental and physical health issues have so much impact on each other that in many cases it may be misleading to try to make a distinction and in other cases it can be very dangerous to confuse mental and physical ramifications of a situation. Readers will notice that mental health components are central to every women's health topic.

"Women and Mental Health" by Marian Murphy, provides an overview of definitions of mental health, gender differences in patterns of mental ill health, women and depression, women and mental health services, and positive suggestions for change. This classic article argues that women's ill health (particularly depression) is very clearly related to the fact that women find themselves in depressing situations. Being active agents to change those situations goes against how women/girls are socialized and the types of activities which are accepted as "suitably feminine" in a world where healthy females are defined as being submissive, dependent, easily influenced, and not competitive.

Going into more depth on the same themes, Fiona Rummery provides specific examples of how femininity is socially constructed. She explains that what "is generally regarded as the women's role happens to coincide with what is regarded as mentally unhealthy" so that "whether women comply with or rebel against traditional precepts of femininity, we risk being labeled as 'dysfunctional'." Of course, the dilemma then, as described by both Murphy and Rummery, is that mental health services also reflect the values of society. Consequently, a woman's mental health issues get her labeled and treated (often medicalized) as having an individual problem unrelated to the social context of the oppression of trying to "adjust/accept" an inferior role in life.

Focusing on the important issue of depression, the next two articles, excerpted from the *Report of the Task Force on Women and Depression in Wisconsin,* bring depression, one of the topics in the previous two articles, up to date, with recent research on risk factors, possible causes, and policy recommendations. While the report examines biological factors, it also explores the role of social factors, pointing out that, "Higher rates of depression in women have also been linked to other forms of chronic stress, including poverty, little education, inequality, immigration, and discrimination." The report also emphasizes that "women are more likely than men to experience depression in response to stressful life events. Traumatic stressors such as childhood sexual abuse, adult sexual assault, and male partner violence are consistently linked to higher rates of depression, other psychiatric disorders, and physical illness in women." Postpartum depression, an issue that is often ignored, individualized, or sensationalized, is highlighted in this report as needing attention from policy makers and is also discussed in depth in the "What Is Postpartum Depression?" article in Chapter 11.

Moving into a very different cultural context, the next article, "Healing and Public Policy," focuses on similar complex interactions and impacts of social, economic, and individual factors on mental health, and what healing means for Aboriginal communities in Australia, often relating these issues to those of North American indigenous peoples. The article was written specifically in response to some harsh and punitive government policies that were developed to deal with alleged dysfunction in some Aboriginal communities. Those developing these policies would have done a much more appropriate job if they had taken the advice in the article "Cultural Humility versus Cultural Competence" in Chapter 2. The author of "Healing and Public Policy," Gregory Phillips, points out that some of this "dysfunction" is due to trauma:

> This does not mean that trauma is an excuse for socially unacceptable behavior. It is a critical part of the explanation though, and cannot be ignored. If a people have been told for generations that they are worthless, and if they have seen people constantly abused or dying, they often believe these messages, internalise them, and become traumatised or psychically numbed.

The article emphasizes the need for healing in many ways, recognizing historical and cultural factors, and on many levels from the personal to national.

Continuing to focus on healing, the good news is the availability of feminist therapy, women's self-help groups, and other resources very specifically supporting women to explore and confront the social and cultural contexts of what is making them unhealthy. Now that women who choose to be in therapy have identified that they want counseling that relates to their socialization in a sexist society, consumers need to be alerted to the trend for some therapists to market themselves as "feminist therapists" even if their therapy techniques are fairly traditional. Both the Murphy and Rummery articles describe guiding philosophies a woman seeking feminist therapy should be able to expect. Although the Rummery article is titled "Mad Woman or Mad Society: Towards a Feminist Practice with Women Survivors of Child Sexual Assault," it is included in this chapter because it so well describes wider mental health issues and feminist theory and practice addressing the core social context of women's mental ill health.

"Co-dependency: A Feminist Critique" looks at how the co-dependency label is put on many of the same behaviors which our society encourages as positive for women and then, "because co-dependency so accurately describes what many of us experience in our lives, we blame ourselves for the behaviors." Bette Tallen's classic thought-provoking article looks at how the concept of co-dependency depoliticizes feminism (or any other movement by people who fight against sexism and racism) but also appeals to many women. She also argues that "with the concept of co-dependency the therapeutic community attempts to co-opt both the feminist movement and the Twelve Step movement represented by Alcoholics Anonymous," the latter of which was designed to be "a grassroots, member-focused organization," and not one run by the "experts."

Charlotte Davis Kasl, a psychologist and former member of 12-step programs, contributes to this discussion by examining different aspects of the programs modeled after Alcoholics Anonymous, which was originally designed for and by men. In her 1990 classic article, "The Twelve Step Controversy," Kasl proposed a 12-step model built on the reality of women's lives, which would be more useful to women trying to heal and move from "*re*covery to *dis*covery." The good news is that this article and others like it have influenced 12-step programs in many communities to be much more appropriate to women's needs.

Mood-altering drugs are prescribed for women twice as often as for men. There are certainly many times when mood-altering drugs are beneficial to women, particularly for short periods of time in conjunction with therapy. However, the overall pattern of high prescription rates for women is of concern and is symbolic of how often women are told directly or indirectly that their problems are "all in their heads." Just as Greaves identifies (in Chapter 3) that many women use cigarettes as a way to cope with their lives, mood-altering drugs have often been a physician's way of calming a woman down without addressing the real-life issues that are upsetting her. The problems of such a pattern are particularly well documented for battered women when mood altering drugs do nothing to stop her abuser's violence but may actually increase her danger by making her miss warning signs of escalating violence, reinforce what her batterer told her about "it's all in your head/you are crazy," and also become the tools with which to commit suicide.

The next article follows up on a specific drug, Sarafem or, as some call it, "born-again Prozac," which was discussed in chapter 4 in the article "Advertising Disease: Premenstrual Dysphoric Disorder." The critique should not be viewed as of Prozac/Sarafem per se, but instead of the dangerous patterns of the over-use of a wide range of mood-altering drugs. In an excellent *New York Times Magazine* article (October 1, 2000, pp. 17–18, not reprinted here), "Female Troubles" which first exposed how Eli Lilly was repackaging Prozac as a pink-and-lavender capsule to market for pre-menstrual syndrome, Peter D. Kramer, author of *Listening to Prozac*, observed and asked:

> If drugs are carriers of cultural values, Sarafem looks like a harbinger of change. Women are the primary users of drugs that alter mood. At mid-century, Miltown and Valium were infamous for helping housewives cope, if sluggishly, in settings where discomfort may have been in order. By contrast, at Century's end, when women's place had moved from home to office, the drugs of the moment were the ones that seemed to confer energy and resilience—Prozac and its peers. . . . What does it mean that, as the start of a new century, a drug so many women say has caused them to be less retiring, more confident is being repackaged as a "mother's little helper?"

Paula Caplan, whose critique of PMDD and related marketing is discussed in "Advertising Disease," describes in her article, "You, Too, Can Hold a Congressional Hearing," how anyone can learn to use political processes to become an activist for women's health. This article traces the steps a group of women, representing many women's health organizations, took to alert congressional members to the problems of approving Sarafem for the treatment of Premenstrual Dysphoric Disorder (PMDD). The problems were both that it was simply a way for the drug company to get around the fact that the patent was running out on Prozac, so it reappeared as Sarafem—renamed and repackaged in different colors—and, more importantly, that there is no evidence that PMDD exists. Using this specific example, this hearing was able to address the broader issues of the dangers of direct-to-consumer advertising and "the entirely unregulated nature of psychiatric diagnosis." Caplan notes that Europe is ahead of the U.S. in not allowing Sarafem to be marketed for PMDD because it was determined that PMDD is not a proven condition.

Women and Mental Health

by Marian Murphy

What We Mean by Mental Health

Mental health, as opposed to mere absence of mental illness, is a complex and often controversial subject. What defines mental health? Who defines it? In terms of women, notions of mental health carry an added burden of value judgments and traditional beliefs. It is my view that mental health is a concept that needs constant redefinition in the light of new knowledge and, within the framework of this discussion, mental health refers not simply to the absence of symptoms or problems but to the presence in a woman of *well-being* and *growth* and the ability of a woman to solve problems in a reality-based way.

A healthy and growing person can be described as moving towards increased acceptance of and openness to herself and others; increased self-support and self-esteem; growing capacity to give and receive love; increased intellectual competence and creativity; greater freshness of perception and richness of feelings (both joy and pain); a more aware, autonomous, and caring value system; a growing sense of closeness to the natural world; a greater frequency of moments of transcendence; a growing enjoyment of living in her present experience. Using this kind of standard, most people live in a state of permanent mental ill health. At the very least, it is estimated that on average we each fulfil less than 10 per cent of our potential for this kind of growth. The extreme forms of this general ill health are reflected in the increasing numbers of people using psychiatric and counselling services and increasing rates of suicide, alcohol/drug abuse and crime.

In the case of women, this situation is compounded by the very standards used to define mental health/illness. There are differing standards of mental health for women than for men among mental health professionals. An often-cited study carried out by Broverman and colleagues (1970) showed that a double standard is employed when assessing the mental health of women and men. Behaviour that was regarded as healthy for an adult, sex unspecified, and thus viewed from an ideal absolute standpoint, was identical to behaviour considered healthy for men, but not for women. This finding that psychiatrists, psychologists and social workers ascribe male-valued stereotypic traits more often to healthy men than to healthy women conceals a powerful, negative assessment of women in general. For instance, these professionals were more likely to suggest that healthy women differ from healthy men by being more submissive; less independent; more easily influenced; more excitable in minor crises; less competitive. Such a combination of traits is a most unusual way of describing any mature, healthy individual.

Another important factor here is the notion of health itself that is used by many professionals working in health services, i.e., an adjustment notion of health. This would suggest that one of the most important factors involved in mental health is adjustment to one's environment. This, together with the existence of different norms of female and male behaviour, also leads to different standards of mental health for women and men. Thus for women to be healthy from an adjustment viewpoint, we must adjust to and accept the behavioural norms for our sex, even though these behaviours are generally less valued socially and are considered less healthy for the generalised competent, mature adult. Acceptance of this adjustment notion of health places women in the difficult position of having to decide whether to exhibit those positive characteristics considered desirable for men and adults such as assertiveness and ambition, thus calling our 'femininity' into question; or to behave in the prescribed 'feminine' manner, accept second-class adult status and possibly live a lie to boot. This strongly suggests that mental health professionals should be concerned that the influence of sex-role stereotypes on their professional activities actually reinforces social and psychological conflict.

Thus, before we even get to the point of looking at the different mental health statistics of women and men, we can begin to consider the possible effects of this double standard of health. A possible implication is that (a) behaviours and feelings exhibited by women and considered 'normal' for us, (e.g., low self-esteem, feelings of depression) and thus not requiring treatment, would

Reprinted with permission from *Personally Speaking* ed. Liz Steiner Scott, Attic Press: Dublin, Ireland 1985.

be seen as 'symptoms' in men and would be treated; (b) women exhibiting behaviour which did not conform to these female stereotypes (non-nurturing, lack of interest in childbearing) would be considered 'abnormal' and in need of psychiatric treatment. There is much evidence that this is in fact the case. There are, therefore, numerous implications for both sexes, in the way in which they view themselves and how they should deal with life problems and also in the kinds of treatment they receive from the mental health and medical professions.

Differences in Patterns of Mental Ill Health

The worldwide picture is that the majority of clients for mental health services are women. In North America, for example, women comprise 60–75 percent of clients. In Canada, it has consistently been demonstrated that women receive more prescriptions for all drugs than men and this difference is even more noticeable in the case of psychotropic (mood-changing) drugs, with between 67–72 per cent of these drugs going to women. In Britain, 12 per cent of women take tranquillisers daily for a month or more each year. Although there are no statistics for Ireland, doctors' reports would suggest an equally high level of usage of tranquillisers by women. Women have consistently higher levels of medical consultations than men, both with general practitioners and specialist consultants. What is even more striking than these overall rates of usage of mental health services, which, after all can sometimes be dismissed as differences in help-seeking patterns and willingness to talk about distress etc., is the different patterns of illness displayed by women and men.

In community studies in Britain and the USA where people who have not sought help at all are studied, women consistently report more distress, anxiety and depression. In diagnostic terms, doctors are treating large numbers of women with such clinical conditions as hysteria, eating disorders such as anorexia nervosa (under eating) and bulimia (binge eating) and, most particularly, depression. The incidence of depression in women (matched only by rates of alcoholism in men in Ireland) illustrates the internalised way in which women deal with problems, whereas it appears that men cope by externalising their frustrations. As depression is the most prevalent mental illness among women and has been extensively studied, it may be useful to spend some time on it here.

Women and Depression

Is there something inherent in being a woman that predisposes us to developing an emotional illness? There are a number of possible answers to this question. Firstly, it is suggested that the incidence of depression is actually more equally divided between women and men but that each sex expresses it differently. It is suggested that men often develop mechanisms such as excessive drinking, or have outbursts of violence. Many treated alcoholics do have symptoms of depression so it would not be unreasonable to infer that men may use alcohol to hide their symptoms of depression. For others, chronic alcohol abuse and the cause and effect factors have not yet been sorted out and, although it is possible to speculate that there are large numbers of depressed men in the community who are simply not visible because of the masking effects of alcoholism, there is no evidence that this is the case.

The differing ratios of depressive ill health in women and men is often accounted for by the fact that women perceive, acknowledge, report and seek help for stress and its related symptoms more readily than men. However, recent studies have shown that women do not experience or report more stressful events than do men nor do we evaluate the standard lists of life events (death of a spouse, separation, change in jobs, etc.) as having greater impact than do men. We must, therefore, conclude that women do actually experience more frequent and more severe symptoms of depression than men.

Could women's depression be accounted for by biological factors? While there is now some evidence to suggest that there is a genetic factor operating in depression, the samples that have been studied are few and there is insufficient evidence to draw conclusions about the way depression is transmitted or to explain the sex differences. Similarly, while there is good evidence that premenstrual tension (PMT) increases rates of depression, it is not a major cause. Also, the amount of female depression that is attributable to the possible effects of oral contraceptives is extremely small indeed. There is excellent evidence that the period following childbirth does induce an increase in depression. However, contrary to widely held views, there is now evidence to show that the menopause has virtually no effect in increasing depression rates. While, therefore, some portion of the sex differences in depression, probably during the child-bearing years, may be explained by reference to biological and hormonal factors, it is not sufficient to account for the consistently large differences.

Sociologists, psychologists, feminists and others concerned with women have become increasingly occupied with explaining why more of us become depressed. The conventional belief is that our long-standing disadvantaged social status causes women to become depressed. The persistence of social status discrimination for women therefore is proposed to explain the greater numbers of us suffering from depression. One extensive study on depression in women suggests that there are two main reasons why we become depressed. This study holds that many women find their situations depressing because of the real social discrimination we experience in our everyday lives; this makes it difficult for us to achieve control by direct action and self-assertion, further contributing to our psychological distress. Such discrimination leads to legal and economic helplessness, dependency on others, chronically low self-esteem, low aspirations and ultimately clinical depression. The second reason why women become depressed is that our socialisation discourages assertiveness. Young women learn to be helpless while we are growing up and thus develop a limited ability to respond when under stress. Instead of learning to act out in frustration or anger as young men do, young women internalise these feelings and become depressed.

Attempts to test these hypotheses have focused on the different rates of mental illness among married and unmarried women.

If these hypotheses are correct, marriage should be of greater disadvantage to women than to men, and since married women are more likely to embody or find themselves in the traditional stereotyped role, they should, therefore, have higher rates of depression. In one study it was found that the higher overall rates of many mental illnesses for women are largely accounted for by higher rates for married women. In every other marital status category, single, divorced and widowed women have lower rates of mental illness. It concludes that being married has a protective effect for males but a detrimental effect for women. Similar conclusions have been reached by researchers in several different countries.

This study and others attribute the disadvantage of the married women to several factors: role restrictions (most men occupy two roles and therefore have two sources of gratification whereas many women have only one); the low prestige of housekeeping and its frustrating effect for many women; the unstructured role of 'housewife', allowing time for brooding and the fact that even if a married woman works, her position is usually less favourable than a working man's.

There are, of course, other important intervening factors such as family size and financial resources. Other researchers have examined the relationship between psychological stress and subsequent affective disorders. They found that working-class married women with young children living at home had the highest rates of depression. Subject to equivalent levels of stress, working-class women were five times more likely than

middle-class women to become depressed. Four factors were found to contribute to this class difference: loss of a mother in childhood; three or more children under the age of fourteen living at home; absence of an intimate and confiding relationship with partner; lack of full- or part-time employment outside the home. The first three factors were more frequent among working-class women. Employment outside the home, it was suggested, provided some protection by alleviating boredom, increasing self-esteem, improving economic circumstances and increasing social contact.

From these studies, it can be concluded that the excess of depressive symptoms in women is not entirely due to biological factors inherent in being female, but is contributed to by the conflicts generated by the traditional female role, and the isolation that this role may bring.

The Mental Health Services: How Women Use Them and How Women Are Treated by Them

Given that more women than men experience symptoms of depression and other mental ill health, how is this manifested when we look at the mental health services? To begin with, as already noted, rates of consultation are higher. The usual avenue to the health services is through contact with general practitioners. In this country general practitioners say that at least 25 percent of the consultations are due to psychological factors and that they have neither the training, the time nor the resources to provide appropriate treatment. Moreover, many problems which result from a way of life or a particular difficulty or habit have come to be regarded as diseases rather than problems. Some women's problems which may actually be social, economic, ethical or legal, may be misidentified or wrongly regarded as psychiatric disturbances.

However, there have been few attempts by any western governments to introduce professionals with other than medical training into the first line of contact with people suffering from these kinds of problems and similarly, no attempts have been made to implement programmes of primary prevention and mental health education. The most likely form of treatment, therefore, that a woman will receive for a variety of these problems, is medical, in the form of mood-changing drugs. In fact doctors are more likely to offer tranquillisers to us than to men who present the same complaints, specifically complaints which involve the client being: unhappy, crying, depressed, nervous, worried, restless and tense. For these kinds of complaints men are more likely to receive more physical therapies, laboratory tests and referrals to specialists. Here again the double standard is apparent.

A major contributing factor to this scenario is women ourselves who, in fact, frequently request our doctors to prescribe drug treatment for such symptoms. It has been suggested that this comes about as a result of women's view of our situation, a view which society teaches us. Women have learned to see our resentment and despair about our place in the social structure, as an individual problem, an emotional disorder. Women are trained to invalidate our own experiences, understanding and feelings and to look to men to tell us how to view ourselves. Ideas, concepts, images and vocabularies available to women to think about our experiences have been formulated from the male viewpoint by universities, professionals, industries and other organisations. These are reinforced by images of women in the media: women's magazines, women's novels, women as depicted in advertisements, children's stories and much more. These views are supported by the findings of a Vancouver study that questioned groups of women about their understanding of the uses of minor tranquillisers. Women felt that tranquillisers were sometimes needed to help them cope; coping, for them, meant the management of their roles as housewife and mother. In retrospect, some women expressed doubts about the role of illness that they had accepted and wondered about other options. One woman said: 'I feel that, essentially, when a doctor prescribes a pill for me, it's to put him out of my misery'. Another commented that a prescription for babysitters would have been more useful than a prescription for tranquillisers.

When we look at the training attitudes and practices of doctors and psychiatrists, we see even more blatant examples of sex-bias in treatment. In 1974 a study highlighted the process by which medical schools teach demeaning and derogatory attitudes to women, both as patients and as students. Physicians are taught that women's illnesses are not worth understanding, are unimportant and are of emotional origin. The woman 'patient' is objectified and made fun of. These assumptions about women are part of the very fabric of our society—this appears to be borne out by several studies in the USA on the amount of sex-bias and sex-role stereotyping involved in psychotherapeutic practice. In July 1974, responding to requests by the American Psychological Association Committee on Women in Psychology, a task force was established to look at this whole area. The task force identified four general areas affecting women as clients. The first of these was in the area of support for traditional sex roles. Here the therapists assumed that resolving of problems and self-

fulfillment for women come from marriage or perfecting the role of wife without any recognition of women's other potential roles in society. The second general area was the above-mentioned bias in the medical profession's expectations and devaluation of women. This was exemplified in practice by the use of theoretical terms and concepts (e.g., masochism), to ignore or condone violence towards and victimisation of women; and by the use of demeaning labels such as manipulative, hysterical, etc. when describing female patients. The third general area was the sexist use of psychoanalytic concepts, e.g. labelling assertiveness and ambition with the Freudian concept of penis envy. The fourth area of discrimination identified was the therapist's response to women as sex objects, e.g., heavily weighing physical appearance in the selection of patients or having a double standard for male and female sexual activities and even going as far as seducing female clients.

In view of these findings the American Psychological Association subsequently advocated a whole range of educational efforts to overcome these appalling practices and injustices. There is little evidence to show that these findings have had any effect on the practice of many psychiatrists. In fact, the realisation that 'feminine' characteristics can, in fact, be seen as those of any oppressed group of people tends to be astounding to the psychiatrist.

It is obvious then that the three interacting sets of factors briefly discussed here (a) the medical and mental health systems and the process of medicalisation; (b) the mental health professionals and their attitudes and theoretical backgrounds and (c) the woman and her socialisation; perpetuate a situation which predisposes women to mental, and particularly depressive, illness. Women's problems are treated only as psychological problems, without any prospect of addressing and dealing with the root causes.

Where Do Women Go from Here?

Internationally, the future for our mental health is bleak. In Ireland, as everywhere, additional stress factors such as high unemployment rates and the consequent lack of access to work outside the home for many women, interact with a traditionally male medical and psychiatric culture emanating from a society that clings stubbornly to a view of woman as homemaker and mother. Realisation of the need for a new medical model is appearing, however, and the supposed scientific basis of psychiatry has been greatly criticised. Psychiatrists are beginning to see sexism as a barrier to our understanding of the family and to acknowledge that 'much patriarchal rhetoric has masqueraded as theory.'

Theoretical and practical alternatives are emerging that approach women's problems in ways that are more closely connected with our life experiences. Worldwide, feminist therapy is developing to such a degree that it has been suggested that it has some of the characteristics of a school of psychotherapy. The increased equality of client and therapist, the main focus on environmental interpretations, the movement away from sex-role prescriptions are the features of this new therapy. In Ireland some alternatives to traditional psychotherapy are available but only in urban centres. Women's self-help groups and consciousness-raising groups can be particularly useful here. Women in groups can come to realise that cultural values we have accepted unquestioningly such as maternal success, complete devotion of self to motherhood, and consumerism, as a major source of our tensions and dissatisfactions. Researchers have found that consciousness-raising groups provide a forum in which mildly depressed women with low self-esteem can explore our feelings about ourselves and our life situations. Obviously, participation in such groups is not a substitute for psychotherapy for those women whose problems are long-standing and severe. However, they can provide a useful starting point for women who are beginning to take more personal responsibility for the quality of our lives.

A range of other resources has also begun to emerge which provide support and reduce the isolation of women in extended families. These include family and community resource centres which often provide mother and child clubs, pre-school and day-care facilities, discussion and personal development groups, employment counselling, assertiveness training and legal clinics. 'Return to work' courses, creches in a variety of educational facilities and opportunities for women to come together to work at co-operative ventures are playing a vital role in preventing the development of further mental illness among women. In Ireland, there are few counselling centres which provide education and treatment that is not sex biased, but beginnings are being made.

For women undergoing particular crises, facilities such as rape crisis centres supply practical help, enabling us to confront our anger and avoid chronic and disabling shame and embarrassment. Advice is also available on possible legal action and its implications. Transition houses provide shelter for battered women and their children and have served to alert the community to the enormity of this problem.

Notwithstanding these developments, a great deal still needs to be done. Generally, we need to be more aware of the factors leading to stress and mental ill health. Preventive programmes should be established to help peo-ple discover and use their own coping mechanisms and recognise the value of yoga, relaxation techniques, akido, a balanced lifestyle, and other alternatives to the traditional medical response to mental illness.

Caution must be exercised by women anxious to develop alternatives outside the traditional framework of 'the home'. They should not swing to the opposite extreme and create new kinds of 'career' and other pressures that can equally cause an imbalance—to behave like men under stress is not a solution. The ideal would be to redistribute nurturing and work roles between women and men allowing for more balanced lifestyles for all. It is also vital that the new kinds of services already discussed at some length be encouraged and recognised as viable sources of help for women who have hitherto all too often been seen as in need of psychiatric treatment.

Finally, it is imperative that those working in the mental health professions be encouraged, both at pre- and post-qualifying levels, to employ the following guidelines in their dealings with women and that we in turn begin to seek and insist upon a service that embodies the following principles: (1) an equal relationship with shared responsibility between counsellor and client; (2) provision of help in differentiating between the politics of the sexist social structure and those problems over which, realistically, we have personal control; (3) provision of help in exploring our personal strength and how we can use it constructively in personal, work and political relationships; (4) provision of help in confronting unexpressed anger in order to combat depression and to make choices about how to use our anger constructively; (5) provision for helping women to redefine ourselves apart from our relationships to men, children and home including exploration of fears about parental role changes; (6) encouragement to women to nurture ourselves as well as caring for others, thereby raising self-confidence and self-esteem; (7) encouragement of the development of a range of skills to increase women's competence and productivity. This may include assertiveness training, economic and career skills and advice on how to reeducate family and friends who resist change. Although not every counselling situation with women will necessarily incorporate all of these principles they provide a basis for mental health professionals as well as a standard which can be used by women to evaluate the treatment we receive. Women clients, no less than men, have a right to mental health services that are sex-fair, competent and ethical.

Conclusion

Moving from an 'ideal-type' definition of mental health, through some of the examples of ill health in women,

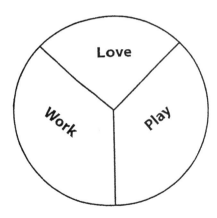

and how these are currently treated, I have arrived at suggestions which I believe would help to promote better levels of mental health in women. These suggestions are underlined by a view of people and their psychological needs which I, together with others, working in the mental health services, hold. This view presupposes that mental health involves a balance between three basic areas of life (see diagram): love, based on self-acceptance and self-esteem; work, providing opportunities for a sense of achievement, recognition and status; play, allowing for relaxation and forgetting of self and other preoccupations.

Traditionally, women have loved and worked, men have worked and played. This imbalance has impoverished the lives of both sexes. Ironically, now that some men are beginning to learn to feel and show emotions, affection in relationships is being awarded a status it did not enjoy when found predominantly among women. Women, however, must not only achieve recognition status for the work we do, we must also learn to look after our own needs for relaxation, play and satisfying work and above all for a sense of self that is not defined for us either by society or by our relationships with others. For each individual woman this means maximising existing opportunities for looking at and, if necessary, reordering her lifestyle. For members of the health profession, it means reorganising and eliminating sex-biased practices.

For the community as a whole, it not only means making a commitment to programmes of prevention in the mental health field, but also rejecting the rigid adherence to the stereotypical division of roles, responsibilities and acceptable behaviours between women and men.

It has been because of the growth of feminist thinking and 'psychotherapy' that changes and reanalysis of women and mental health have begun to take place. This development must be guided and supported. It is important for women to recognise our own strengths and contributions in this field and to look to each other for the shared experience and discussion which will allow greater control and responsibilities in our lives.

Questions for Discussion

1. Do you think that the family as we know it is to blame for a considerable amount of mental ill health in women? Discuss.

2. Some women become depressed after childbirth. Why? What other events in women's lives might be the cause of their depression?

3. From your own experience, how does the medical profession treat women as clients? How might you change that attitude?

4. Is it in women's 'nature' to be more prone to mental ill health, especially depression, than men? Discuss.

5. If you have ever taken tranquillisers for any length of time, can you assess how they affected you? Did they help? How? Was it difficult to stop taking them?

6. In what ways can women's groups be a positive force for mental health?

7. If you were in need of professional help, where would you go? Can you think of any alternatives to professional help that might be of use?

REFERENCES
A list of references is available in the original source.

Mad Women or Mad Society
"Towards a Feminist Practice with Women Survivors of Child Sexual Assault"

by Fiona Rummery

This chapter examines an aspect of structural violence as embodied in traditional psychiatric labels of mental ill health. Although this discussion revolves around the issues of child sexual assault (which is constituted by physical violation) it does not focus on the interpersonal aspects of such abuse. Rather, it explores the subtler abuse which often informs the framework of societal institutions, such as medicine. When considering violence against women, it is usually overt and direct experiences of violence which are highlighted. It is arguable that women's experiences of systemic violence when seeking assistance are as worthy of detailed assessment. As Irwin and Thorpe argue in the opening chapter in this collection, systemic violence plays a crucial role in allowing interpersonal violence to continue, partly through the processes of silencing and discrediting, as this chapter details.

This chapter considers the question of what it is about a feminist counselling practice that differentiates it from other, more traditional modes of working. It will thus utilise an illustrative discussion of an issue which arose for me whilst working as a sexual assault counsellor. This involved working with an incest survivor who had an extensive history with the psychiatric profession, and my subsequent investigation into this area. As such, this chapter encompasses discussions of the issues involved in child sexual assault generally; women and notions of madness and the way these intersect with constructions of femininity; as well as ideas about working as a feminist practitioner. This is not an exhaustive discussion but rather exists as an exploration of some of the more subtle ways in which we, as workers, must always consider and reconsider the theoretical underpinnings of any practice, as well as constantly analyzing the practical implications of any theoretical formulation.

Child Sexual Assault

Misconceptions, fear and denial surround the issue of child sexual assault, as its existence problematises popular ideas about the fundamental institution of the family. In most cases of child sexual assault the perpetrator is known to the child, and the abuse continues over some time (Waldby 1985). The dominant cultural discourses which attempt to deal with child sexual assault form a powerful and ubiquitous part of the social fabric. More importantly (and confusingly) they are bizarrely contradictory in their nature:

> It doesn't happen; it only happens to poor families; it doesn't happen to THIS family; men do it when their wives are frigid or otherwise unavailable; children are naturally seductive; it doesn't do any harm; it damages for life. (Linnell & Cora 1993, 24)

The sexual assault of children usually involves progressive intrusion over a long period of time, with gradual coercion or co-option of the child, and with disclosure not occurring until some time after the abuse has ended (Cashmore & Bussey 1988). Child sexual assault is a particularly silenced experience; still commonly eliciting responses of disbelief and stigmatisation. It is also a particularly silencing experience in that the intensity and intimacy of violation often leads women to such a state of depression, self-hatred and/or distrust that they are unable or reluctant to talk about it (Stanko 1985; Ward 1984). Much of the early literature on child sexual assault documented the ravages of abuse, focussing on the tragedy of supposedly ruined lives. More recently the focus has shifted towards the process of recovery, with the aid of appropriate intervention. Incest survivors need to be provided with appropriate supportive services that allow them to actively and consciously confront the legacy of their abusive history.

One of the issues that I experienced when I began working with incest survivors, was that a high number had some psychiatric history or diagnosis. Approximately seventy percent of the clients I had seen had been categorised with Borderline Personality Disorder, or as Manic Depressive or as having psychotic episodes and as a result had been hospitalised or prescribed medication. When I questioned these women as to the details of the exact nature of the causes of their depression—or psychotic episodes—I was again surprised by the manner in which the symptoms manifested by these women seemed to me to be normal reactions to abusive situations. This led me to do some reading into women and psychiatry so that I could better understand theoretically the unease I felt intuitively to such psychiatric labelling of women's distress. Moreover, I wanted to incorporate this unease more effectively into my practice.

Women and Madness

The history of the connections between women and madness has been examined by a number of feminist writers in the last twenty years. These have ranged from historians (such as Matthews 1984) through to psychiatrists and social workers (such as Penfold & Walker 1983) and to philosophers (Russell, 1986, 1995). They have examined the manner in which what is defined as "madness" has changed over time according to context. In addition, they have exposed the manner in which the mental health profession has been used as a mechanism of social control, inextricably intertwined with notions of what constitutes "femininity".

The "science" of mental health will be treated in this discussion as an elastic and value-driven social science. Whilst I acknowledge that some women may be genuinely suffering from psychiatric illnesses, there are also many whose emotions, responses and "symptoms" are unnecessarily deemed "sick" within a psychiatric framework. It is this process of pathologising women's behaviour with which this paper is most concerned.

Phyllis Chesler says of her interviews with sixty women aged 17–70 with regard to their experiences in both private therapy and mental asylums: "Most were simply unhappy and self-destructive in typically (and approved) female ways. Their experiences made it very clear to me that help-seeking or help-needing behaviour is not particularly valued or understood in our culture" (Chesler 1973, XXII).

Central to the definition of what constitutes madness then, is the manner in which femininity is socially constructed. Caplan like Chesler, asserts that: "A misogynist society has created a myriad of situations that make women unhappy. And then that same society uses the myth of women's masochism to blame the women themselves for their misery" (Caplan 1985, 9).

The traditional "psychology of women" correlates closely with the "characteristics of oppression" (Penfold & Walker 1983). Women's sane, average, even self-preserving responses to situations of abuse or oppression are often used as evidence of their own lack of mental health.

Debra

I want at this point to introduce a case example in order to highlight some of the issues referred to throughout. Whilst I am loathe to do this in some senses—as it easily becomes voyeuristic and simplistically condenses a woman's struggle and life—it elucidates my point at different stages of this discussion more effectively than any abstract discussion of "women" can.

Debra was a woman whom I saw for counselling after she referred herself to the sexual assault service. It was largely through my contact with her that I undertook this research into women and psychiatry. She was thirty-four at the time and had a nine-year-old daughter. She was chronically and sadistically sexually abused by a male family member from the age of approximately eight until sixteen. She has had extensive contact with the psychiatric profession, has had a variety of diagnoses and been prescribed nearly every type of medication. Her first contact with psychiatrists was at age eight when she attempted suicide. After hospitalisation she was labelled "depressed" and given Valium and sleeping tablets for a number of years.

Her first psychotic episode occurred after the birth of her daughter, at which time she was placed in a psychiatric institution for some months. Since then, intrusive flashbacks of the sexual abuse she had experienced as a child have increased and intensified. She regularly had bouts of depression, suicidal feelings and tendencies as well as repeated psychotic episodes during which time she was hospitalised. She had been prescribed a plethora of drugs, none of which alleviate either the psychotic episodes or her flashbacks. Debra sought counselling at the sexual assault service as her flashbacks had further intensified since the time her daughter turned eight, and she felt strongly that there were things about the sexual assault which she needed to resolve.

Although Debra had a history of extensive contact with health professionals, at no time was she asked about her childhood. Even at age eight, and during her adolescence when Debra was medicated and hospitalised a number of times, the safety and stability of her family life was not questioned. The psychiatrists she saw did not ask her whether she had any ideas about what might be causing her distress. Rather, the manifestations of her emotional distress in response to abuse were treated as symptoms of an illness which could be cured by psychiatric intervention, such as medication.

It became clear to me quite early on that the messages which I was giving Debra directly contradicted those of her psychiatrist, whom she was still seeing. The things that he said to her are best encapsulated in the following examples:

> You have no control over this.
>
> You don't know what you need, I know what's *best for you.*
>
> Just do as I say and take the medication.
>
> The sexual assault is not *particularly relevant.* You must not indulge in self-pity and dwell on it. Put it out of your mind, it is in the past now.
>
> You are psychotic and manic depressive. There is nothing you can do about it. You must learn to live with your mental illness.

The work that I undertook with Debra, some of which will be described here, focussed upon validating both her feelings and memories, believing her, and giving her control over the counselling relationship. This approach stems from the belief that the core experiences of child sexual assault are disempowerment and disconnection from self and others. Recovery, therefore, is based primarily upon the empowerment of the incest survivor and the creation of new relationships which are non-abusive. "No intervention that takes power away from the Survivor can possibly foster her recovery, regardless of how much it appears to be in her best interest" (Herman 1992, 133).

The way in which Debra's psychotic episodes were dealt with by psychiatrists provides an illuminating illustration of the manner in which women's distress is pathologised rather than validated. When I questioned Debra as to the exact nature of her psychotic episodes, these were revealed (over some time) to be a series of extremely distressing memory flashbacks. To label these "psychotic" effectively removes them from her reality, thereby denying her the opportunity of integration. Whilst these memories were extremely distressing and often bizarre in nature, it was only through exploring them fully that Debra was able to become less afraid of them. As one survivor of childhood sexual abuse wrote: "I've looked memories in the face and smelled their breath. They can't hurt me any more" (Bass & Davis 1988, 70).

The validation that her terror of flashbacks was an expression of the terror she had felt at the time of the abuse

enabled Debra to remove these from the realm of paranoia. By extension, she was then able to turn fear into (justifiable) rage toward a perpetrator who could do such cruel things to a child. This change was in direct contrast to her previous self-blame and confusion about feeling crazy due to her mood hallucinations. The process of remembering and mourning has been well-documented by feminist practitioners as a crucial stage in recovery from childhood trauma of any kind, as it is only through knowing what happened that women can begin to heal and recover from the damage done to them (Herman 1992, 155).

The Problems with Categorisation

A major part of the construction of femininity is the emphasis which is placed upon serving others. This is exemplified in the importance which is accorded to motherhood and women's roles in providing for children. This role, however, has gradually become devalued in western society, so women are ensnared within the paradox of being both glorified and trapped within an oppressive definition of what they should be. At its extreme, some feminist commentators have argued that concepts of femininity and madness are actually interchangeable.

Numerous psychological studies have pointed out that what in the west is generally regarded as the woman's role happens to coincide with what is regarded as mentally unhealthy (Russell 1986, 86; Russell 1995). *The Diagnostic and Statistical Manual of Mental Disorders* (DSM-IIIR), created by the American Psychiatric Association, lists symptoms of all psychiatric disorders and is considered to be the essential reference for those working in Mental Health in the western world. Whilst the length of this chapter prevents greater exposition, it is useful to compare the set of criteria for certain diagnoses, particularly those which are most often assigned to women.

Kaplan (cited in Russell 1986, 82–90) undertook a comparison of the DSM-III description of Histrionic Personality Disorder (which is far more frequently diagnosed in women than in men) with the findings of Broverman's (1972, in Russell) research into what constitutes a mentally healthy woman. The criteria for a diagnosis of Histrionic Personality Disorder are "self-dramatization, for example exaggerated expression of emotions, overreaction to minor events" (Spitzer & Williams 1987). Remarkably similar is the woman deemed mentally healthy in Broverman's research "being more emotional and more excitable in minor crises" (as cited in Russell 1986, 82–90).

This comparison illustrates the paradox in which women are placed, in that what are described as healthy feminine attributes can equally be seen as symptoms of psychiatric disorders. Thus, through assumptions about appropriate sex roles on the part of practitioners, a woman who is "successfully" fulfilling the feminine role by "revealing emotional responsibility, naivete, dependency and childishness" (Lerner & Wolowitz as cited in Russell 1986, 88) can be very easily diagnosed and labelled. The example used here is by no means the only one. A woman conforming to the female role can also be deemed to have a "dependent personality disorder", or "avoidant personality disorder". These definitions also include a high level of ambiguity, allowing for much interpretation on the part of the practitioner.

Whether women comply with or rebel against traditional precepts of femininity, we risk being labelled "dysfunctional". As the above examples reveal, compliance with femininity is not necessarily the safer option, as it can imply any variety of mental disorders; but rebellion against it can be seen as signifying aggressiveness, lack of gender identity, and social maladjustment. The "catch-22" inherent in this paradox is treacherous for women.

Constructing Reality

The dominant group in any society controls the meaning of what is valid information. For women and other subordinate groups, the version of the world which has been sanctioned as reality does not address their lived experience . . . (Penfold & Walker 1983, 56)

When there is a disjunction between the world as women experience it and the terms given them to understand the experience, women often have little alternative but to feel "crazy". Labels of mental ill-health thus create and authorise ways in which women can conceptualise their unhappiness and despair, in a societally acceptable manner. In struggling against this, rather than treating Debra's symptoms as hers alone, a feminist approach seeks to normalise these by placing them within a context. Whilst this does not necessarily alter the feelings she experiences, it does alleviate accompanying feelings of isolation and fault. For example, when I pointed out to Debra that many women experience an increase in intensity and number of memory flashbacks after the birth of a child, or when a daughter reaches the age that they were when the abuse began, she was relieved, and we were able to explore what a daughter's vulnerability might mean to her. I would stress again that this does not necessarily relieve the distress experienced during these flashback episodes, but rather that the panic of feeling "crazy" and out of control during and afterwards is alleviated. Thus, Debra was able to

view her symptoms as having a cause, rather than being something intrinsic to her as an individual which she needed to "learn to live with". It is important to remember that women's symptoms are real. Although this chapter criticises the fact that these symptoms are seen to constitute an identifiable (or classifiable) mental illness, this does not negate the fact that the symptoms as experienced by individual women can be intense and overpowering. Thus, the theoretical underpinnings of one's practice are revealed in the manner in which one defines women's distress. The psychiatrists who saw Debra acknowledged her distress, as did I. It is the framework in which we interpreted this that differed dramatically.

Mental Illness as Social Control

The institution of psychiatry presents itself as healing, benign and compassionate while obscuring its function as part of the apparatus through which society is ordered. (Penfold & Walker 1983, 244)

Depressed or subservient women serve a social function in that they are unlikely to question their subordinate gender roles nor challenge broader social structures. This is exemplified by Miles (1988) in her discussion of the role of housewife:

The stresses inherent in domestic work and the role of the housewife can lead to neurosis which in its turn is likely to make her even more home-centered and thus vulnerable to further stress . . . [T]he home can become . . . a setting which, by its peculiar strains, "drives her mad" yet which provides asylum from the impossible demands of the world outside with which she feels that she can no longer cope. (Miles 1988, 7)

If one accepts the premise that the construction of mental health reflects a social ordering of gender, one must then ask what purpose the pathologising of women's behaviour serves. To medicate Debra meant that she remained socially compliant. To label her as crazy enabled both professionals and her family to dismiss those disclosures she did make about the child sexual assault as imagined or exaggerated. This silenced her more effectively than any terror she may have felt.

Jordanova (1981, 106) expands upon this idea, by examining depression within the paradigm of an "illness". She compares those illnesses from which men most commonly suffer, with those of women, highlighting how rarely women are allowed to take on the "sick role": a role which provides relief from day-to-day burdens of work. This is not to negate the underlying framework which operates to posit the female condition as continuously or innately "sick". Rather, my point is that men are given societal access to a "legitimate" sick role. Jordanova effectively contrasts a woman who is depressed and on medication but still expected to perform familial duties, with the more "serious" illnesses which lead to time spent in bed, relaxation, holidays, and time off work for men. Again, Debra had been medicated and encouraged to "cope". For ten years her ability to care for her child and elderly relatives (including her and her partner's grandparents) domestically was actively rewarded, and the time that she spent in hospital frowned upon as indulgent. At no point was she offered the space, time or care to understand and deal with the cause of her distress.

Strategies for a Feminist Practice

Practicing from a feminist perspective will involve a variety of methodological approaches depending upon the context in which one is working. Thus, I do not intend to discuss method, but rather the underlying ideals informing a feminist approach. The ideal is to empower clients to challenge both external power structures and their own internalised oppression. This is necessary because both external and internal oppression can be equally debilitating and disempowering in the manner in which they are personally experienced (Fook 1990, 30).

A feminist approach cannot be a set of "how-to's" which can be easily adopted. A feminist framework is flexible and evolving, and involves as much an analysis of one's self, as that of the women with whom one is working. This is not to simplify feminism, nor to unify all feminist counsellors into the one category. I acknowledge the diversities within the existing definitions of feminism (and women) and the way in which these manifest in work practices. In order to establish and maintain a feminist practice, the worker must firstly be a feminist. This is in some senses stating the obvious, but I would reiterate that undertaking counselling in a feminist manner is not simply a job or framework which can be utilised and then discarded. Feminist practice is also not merely client-focused. Rather, it extends into all areas of work, examining and analysing the structures in which one is working and in the dynamics between staff members. An example which is pertinent is that of working within a psychiatric institution. In such an environment, one's feminist perspective would be of crucial motivation when interacting with other staff members in the organisation, particularly doctors, and others in positions of power in the hierarchy—in challenging the established frameworks in which they think and label people and which influence their practice.

A feminist approach values collective rather than hierarchical structures and seeks to deconstruct the "expert worker"—"client in need of help" dynamic, favoring instead empowerment of clients. This is particularly pertinent to a discussion on working with incest survivors. Working from a feminist perspective in essence allows women to be the expert of their own lives. This structuring of one's practices, so that the client is more than merely a recipient, allows the space for them to control the relationship. This is crucial as Herman points out, "The first principle of recovery is the empowerment of the Survivor. Others may offer advice, support, assistance, affection and care, but not cure" (Herman 1992, 133).

A feminist focus upon validating women's experiences is paramount—indicating to them that they have been listened to, heard, and believed, as this so rarely occurs elsewhere. This again is particularly pertinent to working with victims of sexual assault whose experiences of abuse may have been denied, trivialised or ignored—as in Debra's situation. The silence surrounding sexual assault makes it incredibly difficult for women to speak of their experiences; thus it is not possible to underestimate the impact on a personal level of a worker hearing and believing a woman's disclosure. Working with Debra involved providing constant reassurance that I did believe her memories and that I did not think that she was lying. At times, her fear of having spoken the abuse was palpable. This again reinforces the transformative power of merely disclosing the abusive experiences. It has been stressed that as workers we should never lose sight of the terror of disclosure, adding that on many occasions it is actually as if the perpetrator were in the room: "The terror is as though the patient and therapist convene in the presence of yet another person. The third image is of the victimiser, who . . . demanded silence and whose command is now being broken" (Herman 1992, 137).

This also highlights the importance of the manner in which the counsellor perceives of change. The worker should not view change simply as a change in behaviour, but rather expand this to create an environment in which it is recognised that change does not have to be structural or large to be of importance. The emphasis is therefore shifted so that an apparently slight change in awareness is valued and its ability to facilitate considerable difference in a woman's life is acknowledged. For Debra this type of change in awareness allowed her to begin to redefine her self and formulate a differing self-image from that previously provided to her. The creation of a new manner in which to perceive her self and her life allowed her to reinterpret her own life experience (Linnell & Cora 1993, 36).

This new-found ability to resist the dominant discourse of her experience facilitates the potential for both social and personal empowerment. Goldstein comments that the personal narrative has been the way in which women have attempted (often privately and without recognition) to link up their lived experiences and feelings in the face of social definitions: "The use of this method is most instructive for social work because it reveals how personal and social change may be spurred by the kind of consciousness raising that occurs when people explore their own stories" (Goldstein 1990, 40).

Another essential feature of a feminist practice is that the worker's values are stated, and there is no pretence at objectivity or impartiality: "The consciousness of oppression has implications for alternative approaches such as those developed in self-help groups, women's studies, political action and consciousness raising" (Penfold & Walker 1983, Xl).

In my practice, in order to challenge dominant constructions of power and knowledge, I take an overtly non-neutral position. This is achieved through providing the woman with the space, opportunity and information which is necessary for her to begin to consider her own experiences in the light of the broader cultural and social context. An example of this involves providing women with knowledge of the incidence of child sexual assault (as well as common reactions and experiences as detailed previously). This broader context allows the woman's perspective to encompass her own experience as well as the knowledge of a complex social dynamic. It is then possible to provide questions and possibilities which facilitate the reframing of personal experience within the context of this new knowledge (Linnell & Cora 1993, 34). Whilst this mode of working could be accused of not being "impartial" enough by traditional practitioners, it is important to differentiate here between making one's political and social ideologies clear without rupturing the boundaries of the counselling relationship, and importing the worker's own emotional personal agenda into the working relationship. Herman provides a poignant explanation of the difference between the technical neutrality of the practitioner as opposed to what she calls moral neutrality: "Working with victimised people requires a committed moral stand. The therapist is called upon to bear witness to a crime. She must affirm a position of solidarity with the victim" (Herman 1992, 135).

She further extends this notion to explain that it does not necessitate a simplicity which assumes that the victim can do no wrong and asserts that rather it involves an understanding of the fundamental injustice of the child sexual assault and the victim's subsequent need for "a resolution that restores some sense of social justice" (Herman 1992, 135).

If we see that the depression of women speaks their lived experiences and represents a feminised manner of calling for some kind of understanding, then "a detailed examination is called for which concerns itself not just with which women in the population get depressed, but how and why" (Jordanova 1981, 106–07).

Social analysis does not necessarily help those women who feel unable to cope with their day-to-day existence. Knowledge that their "illness" is part of broader structural problems, and attributable to their social situation does not automatically endow them with feelings of joy and liberation. Whilst this is an important long-term aim, it does little to alleviate the suffering women individually experience. It "highlights the immediacy of the problem for women, and the need to think in terms of immediate action, not just the distant solutions implied in abstract analysis" (Jordanova 1981, 105).

If counselling is about negotiating an adjustment between client and environment (Fook 1990), then the treatment undertaken for women deemed "mentally unhealthy" has largely sought to adapt them to their environment. A feminist approach, however, would necessitate an examination of the societal factors which have led to the level of emotional distress present. Essentially then, public and private struggles are as inextricably linked as are theory and practice. Most importantly, neither partner in either equation should be treated as superior as each is crucial to the other.

Conclusion

It is necessary for a feminist practice to examine the oppression of women in both private and public, individual and institutional, structural contexts. Although this chapter has utilised the example of parts of one woman's story, as stated earlier this is representative of the experiences of many of the women with whom I have worked. The process of labelling these women when they exhibit intense emotional distress as "disordered" or "sick", effectively silences their disclosures of abuse. To accept that there are extremely cruel and sadistic acts perpetrated against children within our society is confronting and difficult. The manner in which social institutions and scientific discourse interact with the ideologies of patriarchy, needs to be exposed, and such interactions condemned for the manner in which they subjugate women.

Labels of mental illness do not exist in a social vacuum. To deny the importance of an individual's abusive childhood is to abdicate the responsibility that we all have for the impact of our actions on others. Such denial contributes to the continuation of such abuse. Links between madness as a social construction, and madness as a subjective experience (or as a "sane" response to abusive or oppressive experiences) need to be explored. Further, the label of "madness" when applied to women

needs to be viewed with utter skepticism before being accepted as an appropriate diagnosis.

REFERENCES
A list of references is available in original source.

 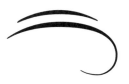

"Frequency, Causes, and Risk Factors for Depression"

from *Report of the Task Force on Women and Depression in Wisconsin*

Prevalence and Consequences of Depression

Depression is a common, under-diagnosed, yet highly treatable disorder. This section examines national data, and the next section reviews available data specific to Wisconsin. In any given 1-year period, 9.5% of the adult population in the United States, or almost 20 million adults, suffers from a depressive illness. There are similarly high rates of subclinical symptoms, which, although less debilitating, also interfere with psychological and interpersonal well being and can lead to the development of a depressive disorder. While the economic costs to society are enormous, the cost in human suffering is incalculable. Depressive illnesses and symptoms interfere with normal functioning. They cause pain and suffering not only to those with the problems, but also to partners, children, other family members, friends, and co-workers. Serious depression left untreated can irreparably damage family life as well as the life of the ill person.

Depression leads to workplace absenteeism twice as often as in non-depressed persons and interferes with work productivity. Compared with community samples, depressed persons are 7 times more likely to be unemployed, employed part-time, or in jobs below their education levels (Druss, et al., 2001). In addition to these occupational costs, the medical costs of depressed persons average twice those of non-depressed persons. Depression is one of the most common conditions found in the primary care setting. It can increase the risk of cardiac problems, cerebrovascular events, overall mortality, and other physical health-related problems (Van Rhoads & Gelenberg, 2005). Depressive disorders also raise the risk for suicide attempts and suicide completions.

> ### The Experience of Depression
>
> I felt like I would never stop crying. Everything around me felt like a blur. Everyday decisions were so difficult and when I finally did make a choice I would get so upset because it was always the wrong one. Once in a blue moon, though, I would have good days; I would be laughing and having fun and the next thing I knew things would seem even worse than before. Then I started having anxiety attacks. Sometimes it would be twice a week or none for two weeks. There was never a pattern.

Gender Differences in Depression

Women are at least twice as likely as men to experience depressive disorders and symptoms, and some studies report even higher ratios (Kessler, et al., 1993; Piccinelli & Wilkinson, 2000; Weissman, et al., 1988). Thus women and those close to them are much more likely than men to suffer the economic, psychological, and social consequences. Women consistently have higher rates of depression than men across all cultures (Kleinman & Cohen, 1997), though the ratios vary. For example, women in China have rates of depression nine times that of men and also higher rates of completed suicides.

Because depression is so much more common in women than men, the search for causes has begun to focus on reasons for their greater susceptibility. Before adolescence, rates of depression are low and similar for boys and girls. Depression becomes more prevalent in females than males beginning around ages 13–15, according to studies based both on diagnostic interviews and standardized self- reports (Hankin, et al., 1998; Zahn-Waxler, et al., 2004). By 15–18 years the gender disparity reaches the 2:1 ratio that persists throughout most of adulthood. Adolescence is a developmental period of high risk for many girls. Anxiety becomes more prevalent as do eating disorders. Depression is also linked with drug use, heavy alcohol use, and cigarette smoking, which may serve as ways to self-medicate for depression. Since girls are likely to become physiologically dependent on substances more quickly than boys (Andrews, 2005) and have greater difficulty stopping, there may be greater adverse consequences for their physical health as well as their mental health. Because depression co-exists with these and other problems in females more than males starting in adolescence (Loeber & Keenan, 1994), females are likely to become more functionally impaired with these symptoms earlier in their lives (Zahn-Waxler, et al., 2006).

Depression that begins in childhood and adolescence often continues into adulthood and is especially likely to be associated with risk for suicide. A large proportion of apparent new cases of depression in adulthood, in fact have origins in childhood or adolescence (Kessler, et al., 2005). At the same time, many new cases are diagnosed in women at different points in adult development. Depression has been called the most significant mental health risk for women, especially younger women of childbearing and child-rearing age, and the rate appears to be increasing in recent decades (Cross National Collaborative Group, 1992). Postpartum depression is particularly serious, both for the mother and for the offspring. Due to the dramatic increase in rates of depression in girls in adolescence, most explanations for the causes have focused on this period of development and beyond (as new cases of depression emerge in adulthood). Even in childhood, though, some risk factors are more common among girls than boys and may contribute to their later, greater vulnerability (Zahn-Waxler, et al., 2004).

There are gender differences in how adolescents and adults show their depression (Zahn-Waxler, et al., 2004). In addition to their greater anxiety, depressed females also show more physical symptoms, including excessive sleep, weight gain, increased appetite, fatigue, slowed motor activity, and body image disturbance. Higher rates of crying, sadness, self-control, and negative self-concept are also seen in depressed girls than boys, as well as less irritability and self-aggrandizement. Although many of the symptom differences are physiological in nature and could suggest biological differences, others are likely to reflect environmental processes.

Although some causes and risk factors for depression are similar for males and females, others are likely to differ. The explanations for higher rates of depression in females than males include a number of biological, psychological, and social factors.

Genetic and Other Biological Causes and Risk Factors

Genetic Factors   Major depression clusters in families and depression in a first-degree relative is a risk factor for depression. Although some investigators find similar levels of heritability of depression in women than men, several others have found higher genetic loadings for females. Moreover, some genetic linkage studies suggest that the impact of some genes on risk for major depression differ in women and men (Kendler, et al., 2001). Genes are also involved in the causes of depression through their effect on sensitivity to environmental events. Persons who are at greater genetic risk for depression are twice as likely to develop depression in response to severe stress as those at lower genetic risk.

Puberty and Sex Hormones   Because the unique biology of women may explain, in part, their greater prevalence of depression beginning in adolescence, early puberty and sex hormones are likely to play a role (Ge, et al., 1996, 2003; Zahn-Waxler, et al., 2004). Early puberty is a risk factor for depression for girls, but not boys. Genes, as well as environmental factors like nutrition, exercise, and weight, play a role in the onset of puberty. Depression in mothers may induce early puberty in daughters; the presence of unrelated male father figures in the home may also induce early puberty for girls. Animal studies suggest that chemicals known as pheromones produced by unrelated adult males accelerate female pubertal development. In addition to the hormonal and other biological changes that come with early menarche, young adolescent girls also may not have acquired sufficient skills for coping with the social pressures and stresses of early physical maturation. There is no biological counterpart for boys that creates a similar level of risk for depression.

The sex hormones testosterone and estrogen, which are associated with pubertal development and reproduction, are related to depression in adolescent girls (Angold, et al., 1999). Estrogen has been shown to predict depression in adolescent girls, even as long as a year later (Paikoff, et al., 1991). There is some support for the hypothesis that women may be vulnerable to disturbances in the interaction between the sex hormone system and brain chemistry (neurotransmitters such as serotonin). This dysregulation may also make women more sensitive to psychosocial, environmental, and other physiological factors (Mazure, et al., 2002).

Premenstrual Depressive Symptoms

As many as 75% of women experience some premenstrual behavioral and emotional symptoms (Mazure, et al., 2002). These depressive menstrual symptoms are disabling in small but sufficient numbers of women to warrant a diagnosis of premenstrual dysphoric disorder (PMDD). The positive response of these women to treatment with antidepressants (specifically, selective serotonin reuptake inhibitors or SSRIs) suggests that their serotonin may be altered via hormone-neurotransmitter interactions. Other treatment studies have shown that the female hormone progesterone may promote the cyclic symptoms of PMDD, while a metabolite of this hormone (allopregnanalone) may have a calming effect.

Postpartum and Menopausal Phases

Depression associated with the postpartum and menopausal times of life is now being studied in relation to hormonal factors and interactions between hormones, neurotransmitters, and other biological systems (Mazure, et al., 2002). The shifts in sex hormones and major changes in the stress-response physiological system (the hypothalamic-pituitary-adrenal [HPA] axis) during these periods are well known. Pregnancy and delivery produce marked changes in estrogen and progesterone levels as well as major shifts along the HPA axis. Depression in pregnancy is associated with biological disturbances that may affect the developing fetus. Postpartum depression may interfere with the development of a secure mother-child attachment and hence with the quality of the relationship that is established. Failures to reproduce, such as infertility, miscarriage, and surgical menopause, are also associated with depression. Natural menopause results in substantial fluctuations in estrogen and changes in other hormones as well. The effects of these changes have not yet been clearly linked to the onset of depression but the questions merit further inquiry.

While maternal depression is a consistent risk factor for childhood anxiety, depression and disruptive disorders, the positive news is that recent research shows that vigorous treatment of a mother's depression can reduce symptoms of anxiety and depression in her child. A 2006 study of 151 mother-child pairs, with children ranging from 7 to 17 years old, found 33% remission among children with a base-line diagnosis for depression whose mothers' depression remitted, compared to 12% remission among children whose mothers' depression did not remit (Weissman, et al., 2006).

Psychological and Social Factors

Socialization Experiences Parental depression (most often studied in mothers) creates substantial risk for depression in offspring and more so if both parents are depressed (Rohde, et al., 2005; Williamson, et al., 2004; Zahn-Waxler, et al., 2004). The lifetime risk for depression in children with a depressed parent has been estimated at 45%. It is often assumed that these children are at risk due to genetic risk factors; however, these children's experiences often differ markedly as well. Depressed mothers are less reciprocal, attuned, and engaged in interactions with their children beginning in infancy. Depressed mothers often model helpless, passive styles of coping and negative emotions that their children also then experience and may imitate. A number of problematic child-rearing and discipline practices have also been identified. In childhood and adolescence, girls of depressed mothers are more susceptible to the influences of maternal depression than boys, showing greater depression and anxiety.

The effects of maternal depression on adolescent girls' depression become stronger as girls mature (Zahn-Waxler, et al., 2004). Adolescent daughters provide more support to their depressed mothers than do the sons. They also express more sadness, worry and responsibility for the mother's depression. Parental conflict and divorce (which often accompany parental depression) are more likely to lead to depression and related problems in girls than boys. In adulthood, too, women's higher levels of caring for others more often become burdensome and create risk for depression. Maternal depression often occurs in the context of other environmental factors that create additional risk.

Socialization practices directed more often to girls than boys can reflect the beginnings of the adverse environments that create risk for depression (Zahn-Waxler, et al., 2006). Parents are less likely to encourage independence and more likely to foster interpersonal closeness in their daughters than their sons. Girls are more often socialized in ways that interfere with self-actualization, that is, to be dependent, compliant, and unassertive. Parents are more restrictive and demanding of mature interpersonal behavior in girls than boys and are less tolerant of girls' anger, aggression, and mistakes. Such practices may contribute to the development of maladaptive cognitive styles and coping patterns that can contribute to depression. In early adolescence, pubertal changes combine with intensified pressure for gender-role conformity increase the likelihood of depression in girls.

Life Stress, Trauma, and Violence Life stress and trauma throughout the life cycle play a major role in the onset and continuation of depression (Mazure, et al., 2002). More than 80% of cases of depression are preceded by a serious adverse life event. Women are more likely than men to experience depression in response to stressful life events. Traumatic stressors such as childhood sexual abuse, adult sexual assault, and male partner violence are consistently linked to higher rates of depression, other psychiatric disorders, and physical illness in women. National statistics indicate that the lifetime chance of a woman being raped is between 15 and 25 percent (Koss, 1993). The psychological impact of rape can be severe. It includes not only major depression and long-term depressive symptoms, but also smoking, alcohol use, reduced activity, and physical injury. Each year an estimated 588,000 women in the United States are beaten by their intimate partners (U. S. Department of Justice, 2003). Thus depression among women who experience male partner violence is very high and male partner violence is the greatest single cause of injury to women who require emergency medical treatment. Women more often experience other stressors associated with depression, including caring for elderly parents (often with severe physical and cognitive impairments), while simultaneously caring for their own children.

Higher rates of depression in women have also been linked to other forms of chronic stress, including poverty, little education, inequality, immigration, and discrimination. Depression is more common among low-income persons, particularly mothers with young children (Belle, 1982; Brown & Moran, 1997). The more children a woman has, the more likely she is to experience depression. Depression is more common in single mothers and women of color; women are also more likely than men to have incomes below the poverty line. Seventy-five percent of people living in poverty in the U.S. are women and children, reflecting a trend termed the feminization of poverty. Because adults in poverty are over twice as likely to experience major depression as adults who are not poor (Bruce, et al., 1991), poor women are disproportionately at risk. Poor women have more frequent and uncontrollable adverse life events than the general population, which are known to contribute to depression. In addition to dire poverty, economic inequality contributes to negative health outcomes and is linked to depression in women. Similarly, sex discrimination in the work place and elsewhere is associated with depression, anxiety, and an overall diminished sense of well being (Klonoff, et al., 2000). Refugee women, particularly those who escaped from traumatic situations such as war, are at heightened risk for depression or post-traumatic stress disorder (Fazel, et al., 2005).

The stress associated with discrimination can be particularly severe for women of color since they experience both racial/ethnic and sex discrimination (Reskin, 2000). The higher rates of depression for these women primarily reflect their poorer life circumstances rather than their ethnicity. That is, women from ethnic and racial minorities in the U.S. are more likely than White women to experience social and economic inequities that include greater exposure to racism, discrimination, violence, and poverty (U.S. Department of Health and Human Services, 2001). They also are more likely to experience lower educational and income levels, segregation into low-status and high-stress jobs, unemployment, poor health, larger family sizes, marital dissolution, and single parenthood.

Personality Characteristics Some psychological characteristics make people more likely to become depressed in the face of life stress (Abramson, et al., 1989; Mazure, et al., 2002; Nolen-Hoeksema, 2001). These include maladaptive beliefs (for example, that they are at fault for most of their own and others' problems), accompanied by feeling helpless and hopeless. One predisposing style seen more often in women than men is ruminative thinking. Rumination involves a repetitive and passive mental focus on one's symptoms of distress and their causes and consequences. It leads to impaired problem solving and difficulty engaging in actions that would allow one to take greater control over one's life. Excessive rumination predicts longer and more severe episodes of depression and an increased likelihood of being diagnosed with major depressive disorder (Nolen-Hoeksema, 2000).

In childhood girls are more likely than boys to experience anxiety that includes dwelling on problems even before depressive symptoms are identified. This may help to set the stage of later depression. Early socialization practices that emphasize gender-stereotyped roles for girls and discourage independence and active problem solving may contribute to dysfunctional beliefs and rumination, which help to create risk for later depression (Zahn-Waxler, et al., 2004).

By adulthood, women who build their identity narrowly, e.g. mainly around family (a possible consequence of assuming gender-stereotyped roles as children) are more prone to rumination and depression in part due to their narrow base for self-esteem and social support (Law, 2005). More generally, depression is associated with perfectionism and an excessive relational focus (Law, 2005). Excessive relational focus, more common to women than men, is the valuing of relationships to the point of maintaining them regardless of personal costs. Women are more sensitive than men to relationship-based stressors, which can lead to depression.

Other Factors   Family history and context also influence the expression of depression in women. Many depressed women were raised in dysfunctional families with parents who had mental health problems (Hammen, 1991). These conditions contribute to antisocial behavior in girls and antisocial girls are prone to depression (Gunter, 2004). Compared with nondepressed women, depressed women are more likely to experience conflict in their marriage and divorce, in part because depressed women are more likely to marry men with psychiatric disorders, which include antisocial behaviors that can be directed toward the woman (Hammen, et al., 1999). Depressed women also have fewer social networks and supports (Belle, 1982) and their friendships tend to be with other depressed women. Thus when their young children do get to play with other children, the mothers of their playmates are more often depressed. Although some of these factors are reflections rather than causes of depression, they tend to perpetuate problems by creating adverse experiences for children that contribute to intergenerational transmission of depression.

Section Highlights

- Depression is a very common, but under-diagnosed, disorder. Both nationally and in Wisconsin, twice as many women as men are depressed.

- One of the key factors contributing to depression is poverty. Policies that reduce poverty and that give greater access to treatment for those in poverty will reduce the number of cases of depression.

- The gender difference in depression is not present in childhood, but emerges by 15 years of age. Policies should address the risk factors for depression among adolescent girls.

- Women are especially at risk for depression during the postpartum period. Postpartum depression can be debilitating for the woman and can have negative effects on her child and other family members. Policies must focus on postpartum depression.

- Both biological factors (genetics, hormones) and stressors contribute to depression. Rape and battering are two extreme stressors that disproportionately affect women and increase their risk for depression. Policies that reduce the incidence of rape and battering will help to reduce women's depression.

- Chronic stressors, such as poverty and discrimination, also contribute to depression, putting poor women and women of color at greater risk.

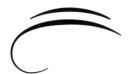 

"Depression in Wisconsin Women"

from *Report of the Task Force on Women and Depression in Wisconsin*

The research reviewed in the previous section is based on national data. What is known specifically about women and depression in Wisconsin? According to a 2001 national study, the gender difference found nationally is evident specifically in Wisconsin (National Center for Chronic Disease Prevention, 2005). Thirteen percent of Wisconsin women, compared with six percent of men, reported that they had been diagnosed with depression at least once in their lifetime. In raw numbers, this equates to 259,000 women and 124,000 men who have been diagnosed. This is an underestimate, of course, because many people with depression never seek treatment and therefore are never diagnosed. A longitudinal study conducted with all graduates of Wisconsin high schools from the class of 1957 also found a 2:1 ratio of depressed women to men when assessed at 54 years of age (Wisconsin Longitudinal Study, 2005).

In 2002, Wisconsin Lieutenant Governor Barbara Lawton launched the *Wisconsin Women=Prosperity Initiative* to improve the well-being of women in the state. The Initiative has its roots in a national report, *Status of Women in the States*, a biennial state-by-state comparison compiled by the Institute for Women's Policy Research (IWPR). Among other troubling findings, the IWPR gave Wisconsin a poor evaluation on women's mental health (Institute for Women's Policy Research, 2002).

As part of their overall health index, the Institute for Women's Policy Research used two measures to assess states on women's mental health: poor mental health days and mortality from suicide. On poor mental health days, Wisconsin ranked a low 48 of 51 states. Wisconsin women self-reported an average of 4.4 poor mental health days (depressed and anxious) per month compared with 3.8 for women nationally. On death from suicide, Wisconsin ranked more favorably at 16 of 51 states.

Caution should be used when interpreting the meaning of the IWPR rankings because they are based on few measures and a broad definition of mental health. These data cannot be viewed as a substitute for a more comprehensive, uniform assessment of depression in Wisconsin women, which is needed to assess the true extent of the problem. The findings, however, suggest that women in Wisconsin experience high levels of subclinical depression, which when ignored, often escalates to more severe clinical depression. At the end of this section we highlight a number of factors that may put Wisconsin women at greater risk for depression.

The other measure of mental health status in the IWPR report was suicide, which is most likely a result of depression. While the rates of suicide are relatively low in Wisconsin women, there is still cause for concern. Although men more often complete suicide attempts, women are much more likely to make them. In the past these attempts have been viewed as cries for help and not taken seriously; however, the reason women often do not "succeed" may have more to do with their inability to access methods that more likely guarantee completion of the attempt. As more women gain access to firearms and other more certain methods, these ratios may change. The most promising way to prevent suicide is through early recognition and treatment of depression (Wisconsin Department of Health and Family Services, 2002).

Suicide is the second leading cause of death for individuals between the ages of 15 and 34 years. Young people in Wisconsin may be particularly vulnerable. Suicidal thoughts among Wisconsin teenagers are high, with 1 in 5 high school students having considered suicide. While the rate of youth suicide has declined by 24% nationally over a 9 year period, the rate in Wisconsin declined by only 8% (Eisenberg, et al., 2005). As with older adults, young females are less likely than males to commit suicide; however, they are over twice as likely to be hospitalized for self-inflicted injuries and the medical costs are high. American Indian youth have the highest rates of suicide and hospitalization of all ethnic groups (Eisenberg, et al., 2005).

Other causal factors that increase risk for depression have special relevance to Wisconsin women, e.g. economics, location, education, employment status, reproductive control, and health risk behaviors. Although Wisconsin has a high proportion of high school graduates (ranking 21st in the nation), it ranks low (40th in the nation) relative to other states in terms of levels of higher education (graduate and post-graduate) (U.S. Census Bureau, 2004). Although this education deficit will affect incomes for both women and men, it may have a greater negative impact on women. Women in Wisconsin also rank low on self-owned businesses (33rd in the nation), and, compared with women in the nation as a whole, they work less frequently at higher level jobs such as managers or professionals.

Low income and poverty are associated with higher rates of depression and Wisconsin women have a lower income than women in most other states. Moreover, the wage gap—the *differential* between the income of men and women—is also greater in Wisconsin than the national average. Women's earnings as a percent of men's in 2004 was 80.3% in the United States as a whole and 75.2% in Wisconsin, with Wisconsin ranking 40th in the country on this measure (U.S. Department of Labor and U.S. Bureau of Labor, 2005). The wage gap would be expected to increase women's rates of depression and cause greater economic disadvantage and deprivation, as well as contributing to their lower status as members of society.

Because a relatively large proportion of Wisconsin women live in rural areas they may experience greater isolation, which also contributes to depression. Northern climates, with their shorter days and longer nights during part of the year, are associated with a seasonal form of depression. Another major risk factor for Wisconsin women involves substance abuse, particularly their rates of binge drinking that are almost twice as high as the national average. Alcohol use is commonly linked to depression. It may be a form of self-medication for existing depression, but it may also lead to the development of depression. There are physical health consequences as well, both for the woman and for her children, if she drinks during pregnancy. A risk factor particularly germane to Wisconsin women concerns their lack of control (a factor that contributes to depression) of their own bodies (Institute for Women's Policy Research, 2002). Wisconsin ranked near the bottom of all states (48th) on reproductive rights.

The vast majority of women in Wisconsin (90%) are White. In absolute numbers they represent most of the depressed women in need of treatment; however, as noted, women of color are disproportionately more likely to experience depression and are less likely to be in a

position to access treatment. Therefore, it is important to be sensitive to their special needs as can be seen in several examples. Although African American women make up only 6% of the Wisconsin population, they account for 20% of all sexual assault victims (Wisconsin Women's Health Foundation, 2001). They are also incarcerated at disproportionate rates (Gunter, 2004). Both violence against women and women's antisocial behavior are linked to higher rates of depression. These conditions occur most commonly in circumstances of poverty. The city of Milwaukee, with a large African American population, has the seventh highest poverty rate of all cities in the nation, with 26% of all individuals and 41% of children living below the poverty line (U.S. Census Bureau, 2004).

Poverty is also characteristic of large numbers of other ethnic minority women in Wisconsin. Hmong have an unemployment rate of 27% (Hmong Population Research Project, 2000). In a study conducted in western Wisconsin, among Hmong postpartum women, 43% met the criteria for depression (Schaper, 2000). Depression is also common among American Indians in Wisconsin. American Indian women have the highest rates of hospitalization for depression in Wisconsin—1.8 times greater than the rate for White women (Wisconsin Department of Health and Family Services, 2005b).

As ethnic minority populations in Wisconsin increase, more attention will need to be paid to depression in these groups. To the extent that women in Wisconsin, regardless of race/ethnicity, disproportionately experience risk factors for depression, their mental health will remain a significant problem unless these needs are further addressed. There is little reason to think that Wisconsin women differ from women in other states in terms of biologically based vulnerability factors; however, the environmental factors discussed here may contribute to even higher levels of depressive symptoms in Wisconsin women than women in most other states. Cumulatively these risk factors function to interfere with the self-actualization, independence, and positive contributions to society that help to prevent depressive experiences.

Reading Highlight

Several factors in Wisconsin specifically may increase women's risk for depression. These include a larger gender gap in wages compared with the nation, leaving women more economically distressed, and high rates of poverty in Milwaukee.

"Healing and Public Policy"

by Gregory Phillips

Aboriginal and Torres Strait Islander communities want to move from dysfunction and violence to growth and vitality. We have always wanted this positive change. This is the subtext of all our community development attempts, programs and policy responses in the last one hundred years—we want a fair go, and we want our kids to have the same opportunity and same life expectancy as other Australian children. Achieving this positive change has not been easy, and there have been volumes written about why.

Here I propose some solutions to move from dysfunction to vitality. I do this from the position of an Aboriginal community member, a health researcher, a policy strategist, and most importantly, as an uncle, a brother, a son and a friend. Positive change in Aboriginal and Torres Strait Islander communities will require many challenges to be met but among them the following three are critical: defining healing, measuring its effectivness, and developing appropriate public policy responses.

Defining "Healing"

In order to know whether healing is going to help make positive change, we must first define what we mean by the term. Healing has been used by different people to mean slightly different things, and the many usages of the word have contributed to confusion over its appropriateness as a public policy response.

Essentially, the term healing has been borrowed from our North American Native and First Nations brothers and sisters. They first started using the term to describe spiritual and cultural renewal as a part of the addictions recovery process. They discovered that when they started to get sober and deal with their alcohol addictions, they uncovered a lot of pain, trauma and self-hate. Once they dealt with those underlying issues, they were freed up to move from victimhood to empowerment. Most critically, they discovered that when sober they had more time to devote to cultural and spiritual pursuits—they actually felt like learning about the sacred drum, the medicine wheel and the sweat lodge ceremony. They rediscovered their sense of Native cultural identity. Furthermore, they actually felt like taking part in, but not being controlled

by, mainstream Canadian or U.S. lifestyles and values—they were engaged in broader society as productive citizens. In short, healing to them is a spiritual process that includes therapeutic change and cultural renewal.[1]

In Australia, Aboriginal people use the term healing loosely, but increasingly. Some use it to mean the process of healing from the trauma of being a member, or relation of a member, of the stolen generations. Some use it in the sense of recovering from alcohol and drug addictions, similar to the way it is used in North America. Some use it to mean healing in a national political sense—reconciliation between the Aboriginal and Torres Strait Islander peoples and others.

Confounding the confusion over definition is the so-called "new age" approach to healing. There are lots of charlatans, Aboriginal and non-Aboriginal, who assume the mantle of "healer" and seek to sell their dodgy charms and wares for money, ego or prestige. Some of them appropriate or steal sacred Indigenous cultural ceremonies and artefacts, such as the sweat lodge or didgeridoos, and pretend they can then teach or sell this knowledge to other unsuspecting buyers. This is not the type of spiritual renewal or cultural practice I regard as authentic Indigenous healing. As a wise elder said, "if people have to call themselves healers, they probably are not."

Having said that, some practices such as massage, acupuncture or reiki come from rich and deep spiritual traditions and, if practised appropriately, ethically and authentically, can complement successful contemporary Indigenous healing programs. Authenticity can be validated by respected elders and community people, and it is an axiom of Aboriginal worldviews that spiritual medicine must be respected and only taught to those ready to handle it with care—if you mistreat spiritual medicine, it will mistreat you. Aboriginal bush medicine, or bush healing, is another type of healing that must only be used with respect and care.

For the purposes of this chapter, I use the terms healing and holistic healing to refer to the four parts of our being and to the many tools that are available for work in these areas. We must work on all four areas of the person's being to achieve balance and healing. Some examples of these areas and the tools that might be used are:

- Physical being: bush medicine, traditional dance, physical detoxification from grog, withdrawal from gambling,[2] massage, yoga and reiki.
- Emotional being: therapy, talking circles, psychodrama, rituals and ceremonies that help us grieve and memorialise our losses, anger release.
- Mental being: anger management, education and awareness about the effects of harmful behaviour (health promotion), addictions training, yoga, positive affirmation, some *nangkari* (traditional healer) healing, and yarning with a trusted wise elder.
- Spiritual being: ceremonies, looking after the land, *nangkari* healing, Alcoholics Anonymous and other twelve-step programs, connection with a higher power, religion (if it is devoid of power and control).

Thus, for the individual and family, healing is a spiritual process that includes therapeutic change and cultural renewal. Later I will discuss what healing is for the community and nation.

Given that healing is a spiritual process, it cannot simply be understood or measured by Western linear thought processes, which are inherently culturally bound. As Mason Durie points out, Indigenous and Western scientific worldviews are different and equally valid. To judge one with the thought processes and measuring tools of the other would produce skewed analysis and conclusions.[3]

Yet healing in a modern Indigenous Australian context does not need to mean it is mysterious hippie hogwash that is hard to respond to in public policy. We can understand and measure it, albeit in slightly more innovative ways. Healing as it is used here really is quite simple.

Measuring the Effectiveness of Healing Programs

A range of healing programs will be needed to counter the mass dysfunction we are seeing in Indigenous and non-Indigenous communities. In Indigenous communities, issues like family violence, suicide, alcohol and drug addiction, and sexual abuse are often dealt with as if they are separate phenomena.

I assert that they are all symptomatic of a deeper underlying set of issues. These issues include loss of spirit and identity and post-traumatic stress syndromes, including collective intergenerational trauma.[4] This does not mean that trauma is an excuse for socially unacceptable behaviour. It is a critical part of the explanation though, and cannot be ignored. If a people have been told for generations that they are worthless, and if they have seen people being constantly abused or dying, they often believe these messages, internalise them, and become traumatised or psychically numbed.[5]

Pretending that making people start a small business or buy their own home will be an effective intervention, without also providing the means to deal with a person's underlying therapeutic issues, is ludicrous. Where is the support for that person to heal themselves internally so they feel like willingly participating in society? This does not mean we should prop them up or enable them to continue to abuse themselves and others. Reframing community social norms is critical work, but it only happens by example and also by having treatment and reintegration services available.[6] Successful addiction and trauma recovery models understand that treating the trauma will enable a person to move on to a more productive life. Without healing the trauma, the subliminal message often becomes that the person should just forget it, or even that it is the person's fault that they were abused. Even for those who have not been abused, the subliminal message often reinforces the person's internal self-hate and further makes them believe they will never be a 'good' person and can never change.[7]

Of course, each individual will have a different set of presenting issues, and clinicians and health workers will be required to gain skills in understanding which interventions are appropriate for which clients.[8] The point is, a full range of treatment interventions are required—harm reduction and health promotion to reduce physical and mental harm, along with therapeutic and culture-based programs to help heal people's shame and trauma and strengthen their sense of cultural identity.

There are some notable examples of healing programs producing marked success. The First Nations community of Hollow Water in Ontario, Canada, recovered from an epidemic of sexual abuse by community-led action in healing, child protection, corrections and education.[9] Yarrabah, an Aboriginal community just outside Cairns, turned around a suicide epidemic by community-led capacity building, awareness training and redefinition of community norms and services.[10] Alkali Lake in British Columbia, Canada, turned their community around from 100 per cent alcoholism (eight years and above) to 95 per cent alcohol-free in ten years.[11]

All of these programs had at their heart a community-led response. They redefined community norms and made sure their people got sober through appropriate treatment services. The government did not force change on the people; they simply supported healing as a spiritual process, and were flexible in their public policy responses.[12] Dr. Maggie Hodgson, a wise First Nations leader, said "if the government did not support us to make mistakes and learn from them, and if we were not genuine about learning and moving on, then we would never have got as far as we did".[13]

Appropriate Public Policy Responses

Public policy responses in Australia should support grassroots efforts, rather than seek to control or enforce change from afar. Public health experts, police, missionaries, politicians and some well-intentioned Aboriginal leaders have suggested prohibition. Reducing supply, employment, economic development and health promotion are the best and most cost-effective ways to bring about positive change and restore balance in Indigenous communities. While some of these interventions have their merits, some have produced more harm than good.[14] A full range of interventions are needed for the individual, family, community and nation.

I have already suggested some appropriate individual and familial types of healing. The following public policy responses will be required to support such work.

Treatment

- Indigenous healing services must be developed to deliver culturally appropriate therapeutic change programs. These services must be aimed at addressing 'the guts of the matter'—why, in the first place, the person took to drinking or being violent. These services can be delivered at a fixed location or via mobile treatment, where week-long treatment and training modules are delivered in a range of locations.

- Solid pre-treatment counselling and quality aftercare initiatives are required to help the person prepare for treatment and then to re-integrate successfully after they have finished. Without this, the likelihood of successful and positive change in the person's life is lessened. Round Lake Treatment Centre in Canada is an excellent example.[15]

- Indigenous-run correctional facilities need to be developed, where healing and change are part of the justice agenda. Stan Daniels Healing Centre in Edmonton, Canada, is an excellent example of maintaining standards while delivering effective inmate healing programs and reducing recidivism.[16]

- Cultural renewal programs are an important part of healing. Once a person has had treatment and started to deal with their demons, they will re-

quire support to find their true identity again. Programs that strengthen cultural identity are critical to the healing process and to maintaining a healthy lifestyle—a reason for living. Culture by itself will not be able to deal with addiction and dysfunction unless the cause of it has been identified and healing begun.

Workforce and Training

- Aboriginal community people and health professionals have to develop training modules that explain what healing is and how to treat trauma in a culturally appropriate way. Many biomedical mental health programs lack understanding of spirituality and how to deal with feelings in their training programs. Even some "indigenous" social and emotional well-being centres often are simply delivering a Western diagnostic and treatment regime in an Aboriginal setting.

- We will need to train the natural helpers[17] (grandmothers, brothers, aunts and parents) in basic suicide prevention, addictions interventions and the meaning of healing. "Mental health first aid" may merely be Western mental health understandings dressed up for a different client group.

- Alcohol and healing workers will need to be sober. Similar to the way anti-tobacco workers are supported to quit, addictions and healing workers must make a commitment to personal sobriety and modelling of healthy behaviours. They do not have to be perfect, but they do have to model the change they wish to see.

- Debriefing and support for workers who are on the front line of traumatised communities is critical. Workers are often vulnerable to traumatisation from dealing with traumatised clients, and ignoring this dynamic is dangerous. Simply paying them more or replacing them is not sustainable or effective.

Theory and Diagnostic Regimes

- Aboriginal community-led research will be required to work with Western-trained Indigenous clinicians to establish new psychological theories and bases for blended interventions in areas like dual diagnosis. Indigenous understandings of healing and spirituality must be equally respected in this redefinition of aetiological and intervention bases.

- Aboriginal community-led research will be required to develop more appropriate tools for measuring change in the psychosocial well-being of the individual, family and community.

- Healing programs need to be redefined as tertiary prevention. That is, when someone stops drinking and starts healing, it stops them hurting others and encourages their brothers and sisters to change too, thereby preventing further harm. It is usually the case that there is only limited funding—for prevention or treatment—and mantras such as 'prevention is better than cure' win out because treatment is often seen as cost-ineffective. Yet, prevention assumes the person is well and that we need to stop them getting unwell. But that does not work if a whole community is unwell from intergenerational trauma or violence already. We have to help people heal before we can prevent them doing more harm.

Redefining Social Norms

- Communities need to be supported in making hard discussions about socially acceptable standards. This needs to be done in a way that empowers the community on the basis of a strengths-based approach, rather than by using a deficit model of shame and blame.
- Communities of care need to be encouraged, where individual responsible and / or sober role models work with their brothers and sisters for change, and where newly healing or sober people can find support away from the "humbug" and old drinking / gambling circles and habits.
- Cultural renewal programs will help people who have begun dealing with their demons to build their self-esteem and sense of identity. These programs add to a collective sense of change, wellness and empowerment, similar to the way the arts in Western communities help people to understand their own stories.

Healing a Nation

For the community and nation, healing is a spiritual process that includes therapeutic change and cultural renewal—but it looks different from individual healing, and we might not use the same terms to describe it. Healing for the community and nation is about changing the terms on which society is based, such as foundation documents and agreements; acknowledgment of historical truths and their impacts on contemporary life; levelling the playing field of socio-economic development; rebalancing social norms and responsibilities; and implementing public policy programs based on genuine

mutual respect, shared decision making and the principles of freedom.

In Australia, our public policies have fallen short by focusing on these broader public debates and initiatives while failing to address individual and familial requirements for healing.[18] Most of the nation's public policy responses to dysfunction in Indigenous communities (as if non-Aboriginal people do not have a problem with alcohol) are in punitive legislative and administrative terms. We have not developed the means to support the spiritual process of therapeutic change and cultural renewal in individuals and families because we think it is too hard. Public policy makers and healthcare workers often cannot understand healing; sometimes they may avoid it because it triggers a response in them to do with their own personal issues. Without the appropriate training and debriefing supports in place, workers will continue to be at a loss to appropriately understand and deal with traumatised communities and individuals. Furthermore, many Australians do not want to deal with their guilt about the history of Indigenous—non-Indigenous relations and prefer to stay in denial, or blame Aborigines themselves for current predicaments. "Reconciliation" is unfortunately often a euphemism for denial because most Australians want the reconciliation part without the truth of history upon which it must be based.

Yet healing is possible. With the right services and public policy responses, individuals, families, communities and nations can change.

Making Things Right

The word healing is at risk of becoming another one of those important concepts that gets so abused and twisted in public policy debate that it ends up being almost meaningless—lacking strength and weight. Healing can mean many things to many people, yet at its heart healing is about restoring balance where wrong has been done—a spiritual process that includes therapeutic change and cultural renewal. It is about protection and care for the victims of violence and abuse, as well as the development of correctional services for perpetrators that are based on healing and change, not stigmatisation and shame. Healing is about a family finding its way home, and about communities finding their sense of pride and cultural vitality again. It is about making things right in a nation deeply divided about the principles of justice, equity and a fair go for Indigenous Australians.

Healing requires us to go beyond our personal limitations and "to reach through into the soul of the world"[19] for the answers we need in order to love each other and to live in peace. I strongly believe we will see this great change in Australia yet, and I hope you will join the efforts to meet this challenge.

NOTES

1. M. Hodgson, *Spirituality vs Religion and First Nations' Response to Healing of a Government's Decision to Set Social Policy to Dictate Christianity as the Solution to Assimilate Our People*, Edmonton, Nechi Institute on Alcohol and Drug Education, 1991; and C. Morrisseau, *Into the Daylight: A Holistic Approach to Healing*, Toronto, University of Toronto Press, 1998.

2. Withdrawal from gambling and/or other addictions may create anxiousness and shame until withdrawal is complete and healing has begun.

3. M. Durie, 'Understanding Health and Illness: Research at the Interface Between Science and Indigenous Knowledge', *International Journal of Epidemiology*, vol. 33, no. 5, 2004, pp. 1138–43.

4. G. Phillips, *Addictions and Healing in Aboriginal Country*, Canberra, Aboriginal Studies Press, 2003.

5. B. Raphael, P. Swan and D. Martinek, 'Inter-generational Aspects of Trauma for Australian Aboriginal People', in Y. Danieli (ed.), *International Handbook of Multigenerational Legacies of Trauma*, New York, Plenum Press, pp. 327–39.

6. E. Willie, 'The Story of Alkali Lake: Anomaly of Community Recovery or National Trend in Indian Country?', *Alcoholism Treatment Quarterly*, vol. 6, no. 3/4, 1989, pp. 167–74.

7. C. Black, *Double Duty: Dual Dynamics Within the Chemically Dependent Home*, New York, Ballantine Books, 1989; and J. Middelton-Moz and L. Dwinell, *After the Tears: Reclaiming the Personal Losses of Childhood*, Deerfield Beach, Health Communications Inc., 1986.

8. J. Timpson, S. McKay, S. Kakegamic, D. Roundhead, C. Cohen and G. Matewapit, 'Depression in a Native Canadian in Northwestern Ontario: Sadness, Grief or Spiritual Illness?', *Canada's Mental Health*, June/September, 1988, pp. 5–8.

9. Aboriginal Corrections Policy Unit, *The Four Circles of Hollow Water*, Ottawa, Public Works and Government Services Canada, 1999.

10. K. Tsey and A. Every, 'Evaluating Aboriginal Empowerment Programs: the Case of Family Well-Being', *Australian and New Zealand Journal of Public Health*, vol. 24, no. 5, 2000, pp. 509–14.

11. A. Chelsea and P. Chelsea, *The Honor of All—Parts I and II* (Video), Alkali Lake, Alkali Lake Band Council and Four Winds Development Corporation, 1985. Also E. Willie, 'The Story of Alkali Lake'.

12. Aboriginal Healing Foundation, *Final Report of the Aboriginal Healing Foundation*, Ottawa, Aboriginal Healing Foundation, 2006.

13. M. Hodgson, personal communications, 6th Healing Our Spirit Worldwide Conference, Edmonton, Canada, 2006.

14. J. O'Neil, J. Reading and A. Leader, 'Changing the Relations of Surveillance: The Development of a Discourse of Resistance in Aboriginal Epidemiology', *Human Organization*, vol. 57, no. 2, 1998, pp. 230–7.

15. Round Lake Treatment Centre, *Client Outcome Study*, Grandview Flats, Round Lake Treatment Centre, 1996.

16. Aboriginal Healing Foundation, *Final Report*; and *Stan Daniels Healing Centre, Stan Daniels Healing Centre Programs and Mission Statement*, Edmonton, Stan Daniels Healing Centre, 1999.

17. M. Kahn and C. Fua, 'Counselor Training as a Treatment for Alcoholism: the Helper Therapy Principle in Action', *The International Journal of Social Psychiatry*, vol. 38, no. 3, 1992, pp. 208–14.

18. G. Phillips, *Addictions and Healing*.

19. P. Coelho, *The Alchemist*, London, HarperCollins, 1988.

Co-dependency
A Feminist Critique

by Bette S. Tallen

I live in a community where co-dependency is big business, where women have had in-hospital treatment for it, where many belong to Co-dependents Anonymous, where therapists advertise in the women's community as specialists in co-dependent treatment. Many women have described themselves to me as co-dependent. This behavior is neither new nor unique. In 1989 when I worked in a Women's Studies Department in a state university in southern Minnesota, we offered a one-credit workshop on co-dependency, we were so flooded by student demand for the course that we had to schedule a second section. This was in a community of less than 40,000 people. Moreover, the more I talk to other women around the country the more I realize none of this behavior is all that unusual. Books on co-dependency are best sellers, not only in feminist bookstores but on national best-seller lists. Women-only and lesbian-only co-dependent groups abound. Treatment centers for women advertise in newspapers as well as on TV.

In short, co-dependency is an idea whose time has come. Sharon Wegscheider-Cruise defines co-dependents as "all persons who (1) are in a love or marriage relationship with an alcoholic, (2) have one or more alcoholic parents or grandparents, or (3) grew up in an emotionally repressive family." (Wegscheider-Cruise, as quoted in Anne Wilson Schaef, *Co-Dependence: Misunderstood—Mistreated,* p.14.) Feminists and non-feminists alike embrace the concept of co-dependency to describe a phenomena that, according to Wegscheider-Cruise affects 96% of the population. *(Ibid.)*

Startlingly few critiques of the concept of co-dependency have emerged from our lesbian and feminist communities. We have no sustained analysis of the history of the term and have had little or no discussion of the political implications of using it as a method of understanding women's lives. Recently, I heard a woman describe another woman who is dying of cancer as only sick because she was co-dependent (cancer being one of several fatal diseases that co-dependency "causes," at least according to Anne Wilson Schaef [*Co-Dependence,* p.8.]). I was enraged, both as a cancer survivor and as a teacher of courses on women and health, I know only too well about the environmental and political issues that are critical to any discussion of cancer. African-American women and men suffer from and die from cancer in far greater numbers than do white people. Women continue to die from such drugs as DES. Are we all co-dependent? Or are we all suffering from a system that systematically targets certain groups as expendable? In short, what do we as women gain from explaining aspects of our lives as stemming from co-dependency?

Who is a co-dependent person? Who gets to say? Who has the appropriate credentials and skill to label someone as co-dependent? The list of symptoms of co-dependency sounds like a catalogue of our lives. Anne Wilson Schaef, for example, lists the following as characteristics of co-dependency: dishonesty, not dealing with feelings in a healthy way, control, confusion, thinking disorders, perfectionism, external referencing, de-

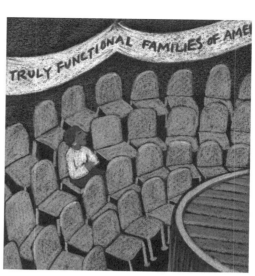

From *Sojourner: The Women's Forum,* (January, 1990). Illustration © 1990 by Linda Bourke.

pendency issues, fear, rigidity, judgmentalism, depression, inferiority/grandiosity, self-centeredness, loss of personal morality, stasis and negativism. (*Co-Dependence,* pp. 42–43.) Who hasn't experienced these feelings? John and Linda Friel argue,

> Is it not true that almost everyone had some form of dysfunction in their childhood that could lead to co-dependent symptoms? And if everyone has "it," does it not lose its conceptual and diagnostic meaning. . . . The [DSM-III-R] always describes symptoms, but asks us to look at length and severity of symptoms . . . before we make a definite diagnosis. (*Adult Children: The Secrets of Dysfunctional Families,* p.161)

Since apparently only the "experts" can label co-dependents and since all of us potentially suffer from "it," we are all forced to seek their "expert" advice, treatment, and workshops in order to "get well," or opinion to determine if we are sick in the first place.

Co-dependency as a concept emerged during the late 70's from the therapy community. Melody Beattie suggests that the term emerged simultaneously from several treatment centers in Minnesota. (*Co-dependent No More,* p. 29.) With the concept of co-dependency the therapeutic community attempts to co-opt both the feminist movement and the Twelve Step movement represented by Alcoholics Anonymous.

Alcoholics Anonymous, one of the most successful grassroots movements of our time, was founded in 1935 by two upper-middle-class white males, Bill Wilson and Dr. Robert Smith. It has literally saved the lives of thousands of men and women who would have otherwise died because of their drinking. Much is quite admirable about Alcoholics Anonymous, its offshoot organizations, and the Twelve Steps themselves. However, feminists and lesbians need to examine the roots of AA, et. al. We must also make distinctions between those groups that are under the AA umbrella (such as Al-Anon and Alateen) and are therefore governed by AA's Traditions and those that are not (such as Co-dependents Anonymous). Alcoholics Anonymous attempts to combine the medical knowledge of alcoholism with the pragmatism of William James ("Keep on coming back! It works!") and a form of Christian fundamentalism which is peculiarly American ("Let Go. Let God.")* The founders of AA believed in scaring the alcoholic by hitting "him" (in its early days AA did not admit women) with the medical facts about *his* "disease." Only when the alcoholic had sunk as low as possible, would *he* be amenable to treatment. Underlying the Twelve Step approach to the treatment of alcoholism is a conversion experience, being "born again," after one hits rock bottom. This can involve either a religious experience, as traditionally understood (belief in a patriarchal God) or can also mean an immersion in a community (the community of those recovering) or any number of possibilities in-between. AA historian, Ernest Kurtz, describes it as a, *"salvation attained through a conversion, the precondition of which was the act of surrender."* (Ernest Kurtz, *Not-God: A History of Alcoholics Anonymous,* p.182.) Critical to this conversion is not only an understanding of the Twelve Steps but also its grounding in the Twelve Traditions of Alcoholics Anonymous.

The Twelve Traditions are the governing principles of AA, they express many of the principles of first century Christian anarchism on which AA was based. They were designed to keep AA a grassroots, member-focused organization. Not only do the Traditions distance the organization from experts and from treatment approaches, but they also address the forms of self-aggrandizement and endorsement that are seen at the core of alcoholic behavior. They fully explain the Anonymous part of the AA name. Twelve Step groups not under the AA umbrella are not bound by the Traditions. And it is precisely these traditions, to my mind the most positive features of AA, that are getting lost in the Recovery Industry.

It does not take a particularly astute observer of American life to realize how big the Recovery Industry is, judging from its numerous publications, workshops, treatment centers, best-selling books, etc. Its big names are major media stars: their words and ideas come at us from all directions. We are literally bombarded with their messages. And what they have done to the Twelve Step movement is most interesting indeed.

Recently a friend and I visited one of the largest treatment centers for women in southern Minnesota, we were both suitably impressed by the presentation. It was slick, the brochures impeccable, the grounds immaculate, and of course, the facility spacious and inviting (providing the patient was not on medicaid or public assistance, they treat only those with adequate insurance or cash). Critical to the center's treatment program is its in-patient Twelve Step groups. In fact, one of the therapists mentioned that because the center was not given enough time and money from insurance companies to provide truly adequate de-tox (e.g., for some addicted to prescription medications it could take months to bring them safely off the drug but most insurance plans pay only for no more than thirty days in-hospital treatment), groups (along with individual counseling) were the primary treatment. When I questioned the head psychiatrist about requiring patients to attend Twelve Step meetings, since required attendance is antithetical to AA practice, she replied, "Yes, that is a problem," and changed the subject. Questions about how the therapists (many of whom were neither recovering substance abusers nor self-identified co-dependents) could participate in recovery groups were met with the same gracious stonewall of polite avoidance. The presence of therapists as experts, qualified only by training and not by experience, in such meetings, and the compulsory attendance contradict the Traditions and practices of AA (e.g., therapists cannot remain anonymous in group meetings when they see the same clients in individual counseling). Further, this takes place, not in a grassroots setting accessible to all who need help, but in an expensive facility which is enormously profitable. One of the therapists frankly admitted that she had never even heard of the Twelve Traditions. She stated that the only reason the hospital had started the women's unit was because they knew it would make money. And lots of money it makes.

Co-dependency and its treatment lie at the heart of how the Recovery Industry seeks to manipulate and control women. Ostensibly the concept arises out of the Al-Anon movement, the group started by Lois Wilson and Anne Smith that was initially composed of wives of men in AA. Al-Anon was founded on the concept that those who lived with alcoholics were affected by alcohol in some of the same ways as the alcoholic. However, at no time during its founding or since, was it held that alcohol affected the spouse physically, as it affected the alcoholic. The behaviors of the alcoholic were the primary issues. Enabling behaviors of the significant other were not seen as a disease or an addiction, but as a stumbling block to the alcoholic's recovery. The current concept of co-dependency varies from this quite significantly.

First, and perhaps most important, co-dependency is seen as a disease, a progressive, definable disease, with an inevitable outcome, and which, if not treated will result in death. Schaef even argues that, left untreated, the co-dependent will likely die before the addict. (*Co-Dependence,* p. 6.) There is the implication that co-dependency may actually be a more serious condition than addiction to a substance. Co-dependency is characterized as an addiction that produces significant physical symptoms, which some experts believe occur before the co-dependent becomes involved with the substance abuser. As the Friels argue, "[W]e are stating clearly that we do not believe that people become co-dependent because they have been living with an addict. Rather we are stating that they are in a relationship with an addict *because* they are co-dependent." (*Adult Children,* p.157.) The difference between the stance taken by the Recovery Industry and that of Al-Anon is huge. People in Al-Anon, are encouraged to create a healthy distance between themselves and the behaviors of the alcoholic, but they are not viewed as being ill prior to the relationship. Feminists and others who have critiqued Al-Anon say it too often focuses only on the alcoholic and not enough on the significant other.

Second, almost all the behaviors ascribed to co-dependents are traditionally seen as feminine behaviors in this society. How the experts on co-dependency handle this, I believe, underlies much of how the co-dependent movement itself seeks to de-politicize feminism. Melody Beattie, for example, describes the characteristics of co-dependent behavior as low self-worth, repression, obsession, controlling, denial, dependency, poor communication, weak boundaries, lack of trust, anger, and sex problems. (*Co-dependent No More,* pp. 35–47.) These behaviors form feminine identity in American culture. Growing up female means identifying ourselves as weaker, less-worthy, dependent on men, etc., in order to survive. If we resist these messages, we are penalized for our anger and lack of trust.

Because co-dependency so accurately describes what many of us experience in our lives, we blame ourselves for the behavior. In an introductory women's studies class I taught, a student talked about how much she learned from the book *Women Who Love Too Much* and how it helped her understand her feelings about her ex-husband, who battered her. I made an off-handed comment that perhaps the best book would not be on women who love too much but one on men who hit too much. In her journal, she wrote about how my comment "blew her away;" she never thought she could hold him responsible for his own behavior. Co-dependency, thus teaches

us that femininity is a pathology, and we blame ourselves for self-destructive feminine behavior, letting men evade any real responsibility for their violent and abusive behavior. The Friels state, "If someone tried to make love to me when I said I didn't want to, this would be an individual boundary invasion." (*Adult Children,* p. 58.) I would call that rape. (They consider incest the result of "weak intergenerational boundaries," p. 60.) Redefining rape as weak boundaries on the part of both victim and perpetrator blames the victim.

Critical to co-dependency analysis is the view that you cannot control the behavior of the addicted person. Although obviously it is true that no one can control anyone else's behavior, the extension of the argument is that a co-dependent cannot even criticize the behavior of the addicted person; rather they are taught to focus exclusively on their own health. Anne Wilson Schaef states that responsibility should no longer imply any kind of obligation, but rather should only be seen as the ability to respond, to explain one's own behavior. She writes, "responsibility is the *ability to respond.* In the Addictive System responsibility involves *accountability and blame.*" (*When Society Becomes an Addict,* p. 42.) In this view, women's responsibility is to look at their own behavior: they can neither blame nor hold men accountable for violent and abusive behavior. Sexism, and by extension, any system of oppression, becomes only the problem of the victim; the perpetrator can no longer be held responsible.

Third, the therapy community de-politicizes feminism by insisting that the root cause of co-dependent behavior is being raised in a dysfunctional family. The concept of dysfunctional family is based on the idea that it is possible to have a warm, loving, close nuclear family within the context of racist, capitalist, heteropatriarchy. It betrays the fundamental feminist insight that the patriarchal family itself is the primary institution in the oppression of women. As Simone de Beauvoir states, "Since the oppression of women has its cause in the will to perpetuate the family and to keep the patrimony intact, woman escapes complete dependency to the degree in which she escapes from the family." (*The Second Sex,* p. 82.) Not only does the concept of dysfunctional family ignore the sexism and heterosexism involved in the reality of family life, but it also renders invisible the racism and classism inevitably underlying the "warm, loving, family" conceived of by family therapists and psychologists. It creates, in Audre Lorde's term, a "mythical norm:" a standard by which we all judge ourselves to be wanting. ("Age, Race, Class and Sex: Women Redefining Difference," in *Sister Outsider,* p. 116.) The fantasy of the "functional" family imagines a well-employed father, and perhaps now, an equally well-employed mother, and children, able-bodied and well-adapted to society's definition of their race, class and gender. Families, such as the single-parent African-American family or gay and lesbian families, are seen as dysfunctional by definition and are therefore dismissed without any understanding of how those families may function far better for their members than the white, middle-class, "ideal" family. As Donna Langston has pointed out to me, many of the characteristics of co-dependent behavior, when seen in a working-class context, are actually critical aspects of survival skills. To learn to depend on others is what enables poor and working-class people to survive. To work only on healing the pain from having been raised in a "dysfunctional" family, holds out the hope that it is possible to achieve a fundamentally healthy family in this society without challenging the basic institutions of capitalism, heterosexism, sexism, racism, and classism that produced the patriarchal family in the first place. When we, as feminists, work on our issues of childhood abuse and neglect, part of the purpose is healing our own pain, but we also must seek to understand the political context that makes such abuse widespread, accepted, and an everyday occurrence, and fight collectively to stop it. The lack of any racial or class analysis in any of the literature on co-dependency underlines the white, middle-class nature of its roots in the therapy community and reinforces my belief that it represents an attempt to de-politicize feminism. Co-dependency adherents argue that we can get "well" without fundamentally altering the very institutions that created the situation in the first place. Beattie goes so far as to argue, that a preoccupation with injustice is a further proof of addiction. (*Co-dependent No More*, p.33.)

Why then is the concept of co-dependency so attractive to so many feminists and lesbians? A primary reason, in my view, is that co-dependency theory so accurately describes the reality of many of our lives. We feel powerless and unhappy. We live in a woman-hating culture where we pay a high price for resisting internalizing messages of feminine weakness and unworthiness. We are taught to depend on men for our survival. Co-dependency treatment offers hope that we can achieve our own private health. It allows those privileged by race, class, or sexual identity, among others to avoid looking at our privileged statuses. Co-dependency theory feeds on our complacency: we are no more responsible for behavior oppressive to others than any man is for his behavior to women. It teaches us that only we are responsible for our fate, that social activism and dis-

content are merely further symptoms of our "disease." When white women are confronted by women of color about their racism, they can now claim that racism is another symptom of their addiction, and their major task is to "get well." White people are not racist because they are sick, they are racist because they benefit from a system of racial superiority, they are privileged.

Co-dependency offers a relatively safe haven for those who can afford treatment. Its theory addresses many of the same concerns that we as feminists address, but without asking us to pay the high personal price of challenge and criticism. How many times have we felt judged wrongly or trashed in feminist groups without being given adequate space to explain? Co-dependency treatment offers a context of personal support that is all too often missing in our communities.

Co-dependency provides another way to resist the messages of femininity without fundamentally questioning the values of the racist, capitalist, heteropatriarchy we live with. We can get well, are encouraged to resist on a personal level, without ever really having to examine what made us "ill" in the first place. Therefore as we get "better," millions of other women will continue to be born into a culture that is misogynist to the core. Co-dependency theory offers a way to achieve a personal peace without examining the cost of that peace to others.

NOTE

*For a more detailed discussion of the history and roots of AA see my paper, "Twelve-Step Programs: A Lesbian-Feminist Analysis," in *NWSA Journal,* Summer 1990.

REFERENCES

Melody Beattie, *Co-dependent No More*. New York: Harper/Hazelden, 1987.

Simone de Beauvoir, *The Second Sex*. New York: Bantam, 1961.

John Friel and Linda Friel, *Adult Children: The Secrets of Dysfunctional Families*. Pompano Beach, Florida: Heath Communications, 1988.

Ernest Kurtz, *Not-God: A History of Alcoholics Anonymous*. Center City, Minn.: Hazelden, 1979.

Audre Lorde, *Sister Outsider*. Trumansburg, N.Y.: Crossing, 1984.

Anne Wilson Schaef, *Co-Dependence: Misunderstood—Mistreated*. Minneapolis: Winston,1986.

Anne Wilson Schaef, *When Society Becomes an Addict*. San Francisco: Harper & Row, 1987.

The Twelve-Step Controversy

by Charlotte Davis Kasl

Drug addiction, codependency, incest, compulsive eating, sex, gambling, and shopping—multitudes of people are using 12-step programs modeled after Alcoholics Anonymous (AA) to recover from these problems. But beneath the surface of this massive movement, women are asking, is this really good for women? While female dissatisfaction with AA is not new (Jean Kirkpatrick founded Women for Sobriety in 1976), widespread questioning of these programs has only begun recently.

In workshops and group interviews, women repeatedly expressed fear about opening up the sacrosanct 12-step institution to scrutiny: "I'm afraid if we talk about this I'll lose something that helped me," or "I questioned the steps in my training program and they said I'd have to leave if I kept that up."

Women who question "the program," as it's often called, have been shamed, called resistant, and threatened with abandonment. They have been trained to believe that male models of nearly anything are better than whatever they might create for themselves.

Some women are grateful for what 12-step programs have given them: a generally available peer model providing support and understanding at no cost. Yet no one way works for everyone. The steps were formulated by a white, middle-class male in the 1930s; not surprisingly, they work to break down an overinflated ego, and put reliance on an all-powerful male God. But most women suffer from the *lack* of a healthy, aware ego, and need to strengthen their sense of self by affirming their own inner wisdom.

Research strongly indicates that alcohol addiction has links to genetic predisposition. A vital point that seems overlooked in AA is that in the case of nearly all substance abuse, the brain chemistry and the body ecology need e xtensive healing in order to prevent the protracted withdrawal syndrome of depression, anxiety, volatile emotions, and obsessive thinking that can last for years. Too often women endlessly attend groups, have psychotherapy, or take antidepressants when their emotions are actually being influenced by a chemical imbalance that could be helped by proper nutrition and exercise.

Other addictions, and codependency (as well as the will to recover), are influenced by cultural *oppression,* which includes poverty, battering, racism, sexism, and homophobia. Treatment programs need to incorporate understanding—and advocacy—regarding these concerns.

As a psychologist and a former member of 12-step programs, I have encouraged women to write steps that resonate with their own inner selves, putting the focus on self-empowerment.

Here are the 12 steps (as published by AA World Services) followed by a critique and by some possible empowerment steps:

1. "We admitted we were powerless over [our addiction]—that our lives had become unmanageable." The purpose of this step is to crack through denial or an inflated ego and acknowledge a destructive problem. It can be helpful to say "I am powerless to change my partner," but many women abuse chemicals or stay in harmful relationships *because* they feel powerless in their lives. Thus, many women prefer to affirm that they have the power to *choose* not to use chemicals or have dependent relationships. So, alternatively: *We acknowledge we were out of control with _____ but have the power to take charge of our lives and stop being dependent on others for our self esteem and security.*

2. "Came to believe that a Power greater than ourselves could restore us to sanity." I believe that spiritual power is neither higher nor lower but all pervasive. I would replace the passivity implied in this step—that something external will magically restore us to sanity—with "affirmative action": *I came to believe that the Universe/Goddess/Great Spirit would awaken the healing wisdom within me if I opened myself to that power.*

3. "Made a decision to turn our will and our lives over to the care of God *as we understood Him.*" This conjures up images of women passively submitting their lives to male doctors, teachers, ministers, often with devastating consequences. Instead: *I declared myself willing to tune into my inner wisdom, to listen and act based upon these truths.*

The following steps are grouped together here because they all ask women to focus on negative aspects themselves:

4. "Made a searching and fearless *moral inventory* of ourselves."

5. "Admitted to God, to ourselves, and to another human being the exact nature of our *wrongs.*"

6. "Were entirely ready to have God remove all these *defects of character.*"

7. "*Humbly* asked Him to remove our *shortcomings.*"

8. "Made a list of all *persons we had harmed,* and became willing to *make amends to them all.*"

9. "*Made direct amends* to such people wherever possible, except when to do so would injure them or others." (All emphases mine.)

We women need to make a searching and fearless inventory of how the culture has mired *us* down with guilt and shame, recognizing how hierarchy has harmed *us* and how *we* have been complicit in harming ourselves and only then look at how we have harmed others. So, instead:

> *We examined our behavior and beliefs in the context of living in a hierarchal, male-dominated culture.*
> *We shared with others the ways we have been harmed, harmed ourselves and others, striving to forgive ourselves and to change our behavior.*
> *We admitted to our talents, strengths, and accomplishments, agreeing not to hide these qualities to protect others' egos.*
> *We became willing to let go of our shame, guilt, and other behavior that prevents us from taking control of our lives and loving ourselves.*

> *We took steps to clear out all negative feelings between us and other people by sharing grievances in a respectful way and making amends when appropriate.*

10. "Continued to take personal inventory and when we were wrong promptly admitted it." As one woman said in a group, "Admit that I'm wrong? I say I'm wrong for breathing air. I need to say I'm *right* for a change." *Continued to trust my reality, and when I was right promptly admitted it and refused to back down. We do not take responsibility for, analyze, or cover up the shortcomings of others.*

11. "Sought through prayer and meditation to improve our conscious contact with God *as we understood Him,* praying only for knowledge of His will for us and the power to carry that out." Instead of looking to an external power, women need to reach inside and ask, What do I believe, what feels right to me? For example:

> *Sought through meditation and inner awareness the ability to listen to our inward calling and gain the will and wisdom to follow it.*

12. "Having had a spiritual awakening as the result of these steps, we tried to carry this message to [others], and to practice these principles in all our affairs." The desire to reach out to others is a natural step that comes with healing, but women need to remember to first care for and love themselves and then to give from choice, not from guilt, emptiness, or to prevent abandonment.

Most important is that we not identify ourselves with such labels as codependent or addict, or get stuck in chronic recovery as if we were constantly in need of fixing.

The goal is to heal and move on, embrace life's ups and downs, and move from *recovery* to *discovery.* Then we can break through the limitations imposed by hierarchy, work together for a just society, and free our capacity for courage, joy, power, and love.

You, Too, Can Hold a Congressional Briefing

"The SMCR Goes to Washington about 'Premenstrual Dysphoric Disorder' and Sarafem"

by Paula J. Caplan

On February 22, 2002, a Congressional briefing was held on the topic, "Women, Drugs, and 'Premenstrual Dysphoric Disorder': What is Behind the Pathologizing of Mood Changes?" This is the story of how it came to happen and where we go from here.

I was ecstatic when Dr. Joan Chrisler invited me to the Society for Menstrual Cycle Research conference in June, 2001, to coordinate a session to "strategize about what to do about 'Premenstrual Dysphoric Disorder' and Sarafem." That session was the first step on the way to a Congressional briefing, though the latter had not yet entered our minds.

In Avon, Connecticut, the workshop drew many women who were passionately concerned about the topic. I know sometimes I come on like a Mack truck, and I'm not what you'd call a great facilitator, not much good at helping to find solutions the group will like. I had the feeling that my own suggestions, such as demonstrating in front of Eli Lilly's headquarters or the FDA, were not capturing people's imagination, but I hadn't a clue how to get people to say what they wanted.

In walked Joan Chrisler, who listened for a bit and then proposed that we draft a resolution for the SMCR business meeting, and we did that and then headed for the business meeting. Given the absence of evidence that PMDD exists, as well as the common negative effects of Prozac/Sarafem, we proposed that the FDA reconsider its approval of that drug to treat "PMDD", and until that is done, to enjoin Lilly from doing direct-to-consumer advertising (DTCA) about it.

The vote was strongly in favor of the resolution, perhaps helped by the knowledge that the National Women's Health Network (NWHN) was mounting a major campaign about DTCA, and Dr. Diana Taylor, Joan Chrisler, and I were chosen to do follow-through.

I still loved the idea of a demonstration, which would include presenting to the FDA head a large scroll with the resolution calligraphied on it. Diana lives on the West Coast, but Joan and I are both New Englanders and met in the summer of 2001 to brainstorm about the next steps to take. Joan noted that the FDA had no head, and as I write this George W. Bush still has not appointed its new Commissioner. We wanted to do something at the time of the Women's Health Conference, then scheduled for October, so people attending the conference could join us.

For more than two decades I had wanted to have a Congressional hearing about the whole enterprise of psychiatric diagnosis, because it is totally unregulated. We had no idea how or if we could arrange for a congressional hearing by October, but we came up with a couple of other ideas. One was to address the Congressional Women's Caucus, even briefly, to inform them about the existence of "PMDD" and Sarafem and alert them to our concerns. Another was to try to hold a Congressional briefing on the subject—not that we knew the first thing about how one makes a Congressional briefing happen. Joan wisely pointed out that, if we aimed to do either or both of those, it might be prudent to defer the FDA action for a while. We also planned to ask other organizations besides the SMCR and NWHN to support our efforts.

After September 11, the national Women's Health conference was postponed to late February. In late September, visiting my daughter's alma mater, Washington College of Law at American University, I ran into Professor Jamin Raskin and told him about our work. He urged me to race up to a lecture hall, where Congresswoman Jan Schakowsky had just given a talk, and tell her he had sent me. Raskin's immediate and serious re-

From *The Society for Menstrual Cycle Research—NEWSLETTER,* Summer 2002 by Paula J. Caplan, Ph.D. Copyright © 2002 by Paula J. Caplan, Ph.D. Reprinted by permission.

sponse to the mention of our aim to have a Congressional briefing was another crucial event. Had he laughed at that aim, it would have been harder to keep trying. I spoke briefly with Schakowsky, a progressive Democrat. She expressed interest in the subject and asked me to follow up with a letter providing her more detail. I did that but received no reply. I learned that it is important to keep phoning, faxing, or emailing because aides are overworked. They may not respond to an initial contact because your issue is not on their Representative's or Senator's legislative agenda, which will not change until after the next election.

Knowing I was going to D.C. right after Thanksgiving, I started making phone calls and requesting meetings with the health and/or women's issues legislative aides in a number of offices. The first was with Schakowsky's Chief of Staff, and with the help of Professor Raskin, I scheduled a talk with two aides for Congresswoman Connie Morella. The first time I entered a Congressional Office Building, I was surprised to find tears in my eyes. As an antiwar protester from 30 years ago, and again now, I would not have expected to be so moved; but it took my breath away to be in a place where an ordinary citizen, could just walk in (through the security machines), feel as though I had a right to be there, and feel that this was where the powerful ideals of democracy live . . . even if only in some of its occupants. Whether sitting in a beautiful inner office with Schakowsky's Chief or leaning on a hallway window ledge with Morella's aides because their office was crowded, I was spurred on to contact aides in other offices because those first ones listened carefully, made good comments, and suggested other leads. I learned quickly that the aides are the ones to ask to see, not the Senators and Congresspeople, who primarily meet with their constituents and colleagues. It struck me that what I was doing was lobbying, and I had no idea how to do it right. Over time, my shyness and sense of being an impostor lessened, but only a little.

In early December, I returned to D.C. to meet with aides in six more legislators' offices. The aides do the research and propose positions to their legislators. On the visit, I saw my Rhode Island Representative, Patrick Kennedy, on the sidewalk and told him I wanted to speak with someone in his office. He gave me the name of the appropriate aide, and saying that the Congressman had told me to call made it easy to get an appointment. Having spread the word about our campaign to friends of friends, I obtained appointments to meet with aides in still more offices but also made cold calls, asking for brief appointments.

As a lifelong Democrat, I had tended to assume that it would be a waste of time to talk to Republicans, but Morella is an outspoken advocate of progressive causes, and aides from both parties were positive about our concerns about the PMDD and Sarafem story.

I had assumed I'd have about 10 minutes to make our case and ask for support, but many aides gave me half an hour or more from their packed schedules. I explained that there was no evidence that "PMDD" exists and that Eli Lilly, Inc., had worked with the authors of the American Psychiatric Association's *Diagnostic and Statistical Manual of Mental Disorders* to convey the impression that "PMDD" is a real entity and is ameliorated by Prozac, an Eli Lilly product. I explained that Lilly's patent on Prozac was about to expire, but getting the FDA to approve it to treat "PMDD" enabled them to apply for a patent extension, ensuring them additional millions, if not billions, of dollars in future sales. I also said that Lilly had created a pink-and-purple version of Prozac, specially named Sarafem to appeal to women and had mounted a DTCA campaign. Further, I told them that the "PMDD" and Sarafem matter was of concern in and of itself and also was an example of three other major concerns:

1. DTCA advertising of drugs in general;

2. The entirely unregulated nature of psychiatric diagnosis:

3. The fact that, because so many *DSM* categories have not been scientifically shown even to be real entities, anyone assigning a patient an unvalidated diagnosis and then selecting treatment on the basis of that diagnosis is actually subjecting the patient to experimental treatment without their knowledge or consent. I said that many professionals using these labels have no idea that the *DSM* is based on little science.

I found out that Congresswoman Juanita Millender-McDonald was a co-chair of the Congressional Women's Caucus and met with Rae Nicholl, a New Zealander doing a fellowship in her office. Nicholl is an ardent feminist who immediately understood our concerns. My mother and grandmother had always told me that the way to make things happen is to go straight to the top, so—pretending I knew this was an appropriate request but really fearing that things were never done this way—I tried to sound matter-of-fact and asked if we could have ten minutes to address a meeting of the Congressional Women's Caucus. That request was never granted. Back in Rhode Island, well into January, I continued to phone legislative offices and ask to speak to their aides for women's and/or health issues. Often, I got to speak with them. I also contacted members of various women's groups, including the National Organization of Women, to request support. One such aide was Cindy Pelligrini, Chief of Staff and Legislative Director for New York Congresswoman Louise Slaughter, with whom I spoke briefly and to whom I then immediately sent a two-page fax presenting our concerns.

We never found out when the Women's Caucus would meet, but Rae Nicholl told me about a luncheon conference on women's health that was scheduled for January 30, sponsored by Women's Policy, Inc. Going to the latter's website, I learned that Women's Policy, Inc., "is a nonprofit, nonpartisan organization whose mission is to provide nonpartisan public policy research, legislative analysis, and information services to policymakers, the press, and the public on issues important to women and families. It was established in 1995 after the [Republican] House of Representatives voted to abolish . . . the congressional Caucus for Women's Issues. Following the January 1995 vote, the Congresswomen reorganized themselves into a Members' organization by the same name, to continue their bipartisan advocacy on behalf of women. With the encouragement of the Congresswomen, two former staff members of the Caucus started WPI." A phone call to Women's Policy, Inc., saying that Rae Nicholl had suggested I attend the luncheon garnered me an invitation. At the luncheon, I distributed a one-page description of our concerns. The same day, I also met with aides in two more offices, and I received a message from Cindy Pelligrini, saying that Congresswomen Slaughter would be glad to sponsor a briefing and would reserve a room in a House Office Building for us. Thus, we learned we had been wrong to assume we would first have to address the Congressional Women's Caucus in order to begin to garner enough support to find a sponsor for a briefing. (I don't know whether there is any way to have a Congressional briefing other than having a Representative or Senator sponsor it and book the room.) The national conference on Women's Health had been rescheduled for February 21–23, so we chose February 22 for the briefing.

It turns out that the people on the Hill who seem the most supportive and communicate with you the most are not necessarily the ones who will help you make things happen. It had taken only one telephone call and a fax to Cindy Pelligrini to get us a sponsor and a room. I had wrongly assumed that we needed to drum up support from several legislators in order to hold a briefing, but Pelligrini said that Congresswoman Slaughter never minds doing things on her own, a statement that I found both moving and inspiring.

In a three-way call among Joan Chrisler, NWHN Program and Policy Director Amy Allina, and me, and consulting with Judy Norsigian from the Boston Women's Health Book Collective (BWHBC), we chose the title of the briefing, and Allina designed an invitation. Between Amy and Judy, a list was compiled of the fax numbers for many Representatives and Senators, as well as U.S. legislators who serve on committees or subcommittees relevant to our topic, and NWHN interns Meg Rose and Christine Plummer helped fax them the invitations. At Pelligrini's suggestion, we sent out our invitation, and then the Congresswoman sent her colleagues a letter of her own.

Diana Taylor worked diligently to garner support from other groups, and ultimately the following groups were listed as members of the coalition temporarily created to work on this set of issues: The National Women's Health Network, The Boston Women's Health Book Collective, The Society for Menstrual Cycle Research, The Association for Women in Psychology, the National Association of Hispanic Nurses, The Women's Health Initiative, The Center for Medical Consumers, DES Action, The Working Group on Women and Health Protection, Breast Cancer Action, Prevention First, and The Massachusetts Breast Cancer Coalition. As of this writing, other groups are deciding whether to add their support for the next phase of the work.

The 90-minute briefing was held in beautiful, red-walled Room 1539 in the Longworth House Office Building and was attended by about 25 people—far more than we had dreamed would come—mostly legislative aides or people from government agencies or nongovernmental organizations. The view out the large windows behind the speakers' table was of the Capitol building. Cindy Pelligrini gave a brief welcoming speech and a strong statement of Congresswoman Slaughter's concerns about women's health. Joan Chrisler then spoke on behalf of the SMCR about "Prozac, Patents and Profits—What is PMDD?" Amy Allina spoke for the NWHN about. "Selling Sarafem: Direct to Consumer Advertising," and I spoke on behalf of the Association for Women in Psychology about "Psychiatric Diagnosis: Little Science and No Regulation." We made recommendations for action, including the following:

1. To begin to educate the people of this country about these concerns by appropriating funding for public service announcements, educational pamphlets, and materials about these matters for use in schools, colleges, universities, programs where mental health professionals are trained, and law schools.

2. To propose legislation holding publishers of diagnostic manuals in the mental health field to a standard of full disclosure of the quantity and quality of research behind the diagnostic labels in their books.

3. To propose healthcare legislation requiring professionals who assign diagnostic labels in the mental health field to be well-informed about the quantity and quality of research behind those labels.

4. To propose legislation that will improve the guidelines used by the Food and Drug Administration in assessing research before new drugs and new uses for existing drugs are approved. The guidelines would need to include powerful safeguards to ensure that FDA committees hear from people other than those who have the most to gain from drug approvals.

5. Because there is so much misinformation and disinformation and so little critical thinking about psychiatric diagnosis, to create a forum in which the variety and extent of problems can be presented and as many solutions as possible put forward. For that reason, it is important to schedule Congressional Hearings about the whole enterprise of psychiatric diagnosis.

Following the briefing, many attendees came up to ask questions, and a young woman on a Congressional fellowship to work on women's health until the late summer offered to assist in trying to implement some of the recommendations. A short summary of the briefing was sent to Congresswoman Slaughter. We are now gathering information about other important legislators and aides to whom we should speak about proposing legislation or, as a beginning, proposing House or Senate resolutions, which are much easier to pass than legislation. After the briefing, and exploring legislative routes to change, we have come to understand, even more deeply than before, how much the Congress is hamstrung by their fear of alienating the pharmaceutical companies, who donate huge sums to the campaigns of both Republicans and Democrats. We are also investigating which offices of the Executive Branch of the federal government, particularly Health and Human Services and the Justice Department, are charged with relevant tasks, although the Bush government has shown little interest in increasing regulation. Another possibility we have discussed is trying to persuade one or more state governments to do pilot projects, such as for recommendation #1 or #3.

We know that change takes a long time, but at the June, 2001, SMCR conference, who would have thought that less than nine months later, a large number of women's groups would have come together and had a Congressional briefing? The process of educating and galvanizing support from legislators is well under way, and we are committed to taking the next steps.

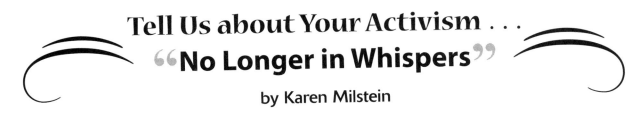

Tell Us about Your Activism . . . "No Longer in Whispers"

by Karen Milstein

A consumer is not just someone who buys products in our society. I am called a "consumer" because I receive mental health services. For quite some time I have worked as an activist in the mental health field in Madison, Wisconsin. I work to help consumers fight stigma and empower ourselves. This is an uphill fight against strong "phobic" forces around mental illness: societal stigma and self-stigma.

I wear many hats in this city. All of the places I work—for pay or as a volunteer—offer services to persons struggling with mental illness. The struggle is personal. It's where I've been, it's what I know, and helping others helps me. I work for pay at a consumer-run arts-and-computer-organization that provides classes for other consumers, ranging from oils to clay to writing. I am also both a part-time weekend staff worker as well as member of a "clubhouse," a place where people with mental illness rejoin the workforce. Finally, this fall I will be working also part-time as a "crisis aide," helping other consumers with various tasks in their lives through our local mental health agency. Wearing these many hats, my life is devoted to encouraging people with mental illness to further their dreams and ambitions.

The vision I work towards is helping people with mental illness to live lives of quality and be granted respect and dignity in our society. So many of the people I know and work with are gentle and highly creative. I also envision giving them a chance to have a life with more promise than hours of loneliness and boredom resulting from living on disability. Granted, I would probably be on the streets without the government support I have had. But it took great creativity to keep my mind alive before I found the local clubhouse, and my present jobs that now fill my time. Life without a respectable full-time job can be an empty, barren life, especially if you have few friends and are revolving through the hospital doors. The agencies I work for rebuild the dignity and pride lost after years of mental distress and hopelessness. So often when one "outs" one's self as a "person with mental illness" one is immediately given less respect and accord. This is certainly an injustice.

For me, activism is making a voice and acting up in the name of injustices done to one because of an aspect of one's identity. I can never forget where I've been and must always strive to go further. "Recovery" is a key word in the mental health field. Helping others find recovery is part of activism. "Thriving" is a word I heard at a workshop last fall in Chicago. "Thriving" is going beyond simply recovery. I hope to help others—and myself—thrive after our oftentimes desperate struggles with mental illness. Mental health problems can be among the most devastating to hit an individual, ripping away one's identity. I hope my efforts in the jobs I occupy make a difference in people's lives, helping them to find new avenues to venture down and finding pride in experiences that are looked down upon in this society, i.e. having been psychotic or hospitalized. At the agencies where I work we are able to talk openly about our experiences with mental distress. This a moving force for consumers. I envision a society in which this can happen. I try to encourage dialogue so the public can learn what mental illness is really about.

These are the things I do: for others, for my own sanity.

WORKSHEET—CHAPTER 6

Mental Health

1. Stress is defined as the non-specific response of the body to demands made on it. These demands can be physical or emotional. The response is non-specific in the sense that, no matter whether the stressor (cause of stress) is seemingly negative or positive, the body responds the same way physiologically. On scales that measure stress of life events, marriage, graduation, and promotion get high stress ratings, along with break-up of a relationship, death in the family, and a jail sentence. If we cannot find ways to manage stress, there can be many possible long-term health consequences, such as high blood pressure and high cholesterol (both of which increase the risk of heart disease), at least in men lowered resistance to infectious diseases, more migraines if prone to them, various disturbances of the digestive system (including ulcers and colitis), and sleep problems.

   a. List ways you know your body responds to stress.

   b. List several stressors in your life.

   c. List several ways you cope with or manage stress.

   d. If any of your answers to question C have potentially negative consequences, identify an alternative positive approach. For example, some people deal with stress by shopping, but a shopping spree can create more stress when the bills have to be paid. Others turn to alcohol or binge eating. What are "healthy" alternatives to these strategies?

   e. Do women and men experience different stressors? Are there differences in the way women and men may choose to or be able to deal with stress? Compare your answer to Marian Murphy's statement, "It appears that men cope by externalizing their frustrations."

2. Mental health is said to be related to a balance of work, play, and love in our lives.

    a. How do these elements balance out in your life?

    b. Thinking through the roles that women and men play in this society, and by rereading the article "Hazards of Hearth and Home" in Chapter 3, think of whether there are differences for women and men in trying to maintain a balance in their lives. If so, describe some specific differences.

3. What does it mean that mental health professionals give similar definitions for healthy adults and healthy men but describe healthy women as more submissive, less independent, more easily influenced, less competitive?

    a. Does this mean "the only mentally healthy women are the ones who adjust to a world where women are considered inferior?"

    b. Does questioning sexism mean that someone is mentally unhealthy?

4. If you are lucky enough to have health insurance, look at your health insurance policy to see what mental health coverage you have. If you wanted or needed counseling, how much counseling would your insurance cover? Can you imagine a situation in which you or a loved one would end up using mood-altering medication without appropriate or sufficient accompanying therapy?

5. Take one issue raised in the excerpts from "The Report of the Task Force on Women and Depression in Wisconsin" and suggest some government policies that might help improve that specific concern. How might the issues discussed in the article "Healing and Public Policy" be relevant for these policies in a U.S. context?

VIOLENCE *against* WOMEN

Many women define violence—both their actual experiences with violence and their fear of violence—as their number one health issue. "More women are injured each year in their homes by their spouses or male partners than by accidents or illness" (see Ritchie and Kanuha's article). Violence is certainly an issue that affects women's health, both mental and physical. In fact, the level of violence a woman has experienced has been found to be a very powerful predictor of her use of medical services, more predictive than demographic variables, other life stressors, self-perceived health, or injurious health habits (I. Schwartz, *American Journal of Preventive Medicine*, 1991, 7(6), pp. 363–373). Many women who have suffered severe physical pain and life-threatening injuries from violence have said that the emotional and psychological bruises from abuse take years or decades longer to heal than the physical injuries.

Violence manifests itself in girls' (and boys') and women's lives in many different forms including child abuse, incest, dating violence, sexual harassment, stalking, pornography, sexual assault, date rape, domestic violence, and elder abuse. Although each specific form of violence may be unique in its consequences and the knowledge needed to recognize it, respond to it, and prevent it, all forms of violence (against women) can be defined as issues of power and control where one person or a group takes power and control over another individual or group. This chapter concentrates primarily on a range of approaches to understanding and addressing the complexities of intimate partner violence. It is hoped that readers will draw on these approaches to develop a similar analysis of other forms of violence against women. (Men also get terribly hurt by violence, but men are predominately hurt by strangers, in contrast to women being hurt primarily by people they know and love/have loved. As this chapter concentrates on the health ramifications of violence against women, it does not address the important ways that men get hurt by living in a violent society, or the messages that support violence and unhealthy aggression as signs of masculinity.)

Organizing against violence against women has been among the most visible and successful work of modern women's movements. For the last three decades, women in all parts of the U.S. and the world have been putting much time, energy, and resources into rape crisis centers, domestic violence programs, incest survivors' groups, and "coordinated community responses" to violence against women. A sophisticated analysis has been developed to show how the abuse of individual women by individual men reflects and is perpetrated by the patriarchal dominance of men over women in a sexist society. Although social change work is always slower than we imagine, in some ways, the violence against women movements have had an almost "revolutionary" impact on the legal system, the criminal justice system, and the general public's awareness that this is a serious issue. This chapter includes examples of the excellent information that is now produced and distributed by activist groups working to end violence in women's lives.

The continuum of family violence chart demonstrates the relationship of subtle forms of physical, verbal/emotional, and sexual abuse, which society all too often tolerates or condones, to the forms more obviously recognized as serious and deadly. The more subtle forms can themselves have serious consequences and invariably lead to other means of control. It is important to understand that this continuum, an important teaching tool, would look different for different women. While being screamed at would be terribly hurtful for many women, others would be more hurt by "the silent treatment." Abusers usually pay enormous attention to details so that they *choose* to use the tactics most effective in controlling their partner specifically.

The power and control wheel (developed by battered women and formerly battered women to describe abuse in their lives) is a key tool for educating people that domestic violence is not "just about hitting" but is about an ongoing pattern where one person controls many or all aspects of another person's life. The power and control wheel reminds us that domestic violence is not about an "anger management problem" or "losing control;" it is about *choosing* to *use control*. The cleverest abusers may never get "caught" leaving physical injuries or breaking the law because they so effectively control their partners through the children, by controlling finances, playing mind games, and/or isolating them from their support systems. In contrast to the power and control wheel, the equality wheel (also developed by battered and formerly battered women) serves as an inspiring model of what we want to work for in creating healthy relationships, striving to equalize, rather than use or abuse, power.

Many college women learn about battered women as if domestic violence is something that might happen to them in the future, with too little acknowledgment that at least 1 in 4 young women experience power and control dynamics in dating relationships. An important study (*American Journal of Public Health*, Volume 93, 2003, pp. 1104–1109) stated that "88% of women reporting at least one incident of physical or sexual victimization between adolescence and their fourth year of college when victimization was defined broadly." It seems high school girls and college women are better at identifying one-time sexual assault by a stranger than identifying ongoing power and control (including sexual control) in dating relationships. "A More Hidden Crime: Adolescent Battered Women" identifies that the ramifications of intimate partner abuse may be even more serious for adolescent than adult women, but that there are far fewer resources or options available to young women.

In "Breaking the Silence," in sharing the experience of her own rape, which involved "date rape drugs," Megan Steffer, a college student, emphasizes that "the vast majority of rapes (80%) occur between people who know each other, and take place in environments that are generally considered to be safe." In recognizing the value of speaking out against sexual violence, Steffer urges other survivors to tell their stories and for everyone to "be ready to listen and support these women as their stories unfold."

Health practitioners can be key "listeners" in picking up signs that a patient is living with violence or that her health issues are related to previous abuse. The next articles and resources in this chapter specifically address the issue of the health system's response to violence against women. Although women who were victims/survivors of violence have long identified violence as a major health issue and have been aware of how violence impacted on their mental and physical health, the health system has been notoriously poor at addressing violence issues, and has often played a dangerous role in revictimizing survivors of violence. As articles in this chapter demonstrate, as a result of much activism, professional training, and national attention to medical standards and protocols, healthcare practitioners are increasingly aware of the health ramifications of violence, and of their responsibilities. In "The Unique Role Health Workers Can Play in Recognizing and Responding to Battered Women," I (Nancy Worcester) outline the key issues I teach health practitioners about the crucial roles they should play in routinely screening and appropriately responding to domestic violence.

Building on the analysis of the battered women's movement as demonstrated in the power and control and equality wheels, Amanda Cosgrove and Dr. Kevin Fullin (founders of Wisconsin's first hospital-based domestic violence program, in Kenosha) developed similar "Medical Power and Control" and "Medical Advocacy/Empowerment" wheels, which health workers can use to determine whether their response to victims/survivors is abusing their power (medical power and control) or whether they are using their positions to advocate for women and help them end the violence in their lives.

Violence against women affects women in *all* communities. Although activists have long been careful to emphasize this fact, more attention has been paid recently to going beyond the rhetoric to explore the unique issues faced by different groups of women. There is enormous pressure on women in some communities to hide the violence in their lives. In such communities, a woman may feel even more isolated and hopeless than in a community where violence is acknowledged. Battered women's programs see only a tiny percentage of all the women affected by violence, and domestic violence service providers are increasingly aware that they do a better job of serving some groups of women than others. For example, even though many women with disabilities, older women, and lesbians are hurt by domestic violence, disproportionately few victims/survivors in these groups make contact with domestic violence programs. Urgent attention needs to be paid to the unique barriers different women face in trying to end the violence in their lives. The next four articles in this chapter address this issue from different perspectives, in relation to specific groups of people. It is hoped that these articles will stimulate the reader to think about particular barriers to ending violence that other women (not included in these articles) face.

Beth E. Richie and Valli Kanuha's crucial article, "Battered Women of Color in Public Health Care Systems: Racism, Sexism, and Violence," synthesizes many of the key issues in this book specifically as they relate to violence in women's lives and what is needed for an appropriate public health system response. This article clearly articulates the urgency "to integrate an understanding of violence against women with other forms of oppression (such as racism, classism, ageism) in addition to sexism" and highlights how "women of color have actively and creatively challenged the discriminatory, institutional practices of healthcare and crisis intervention services."

"Anishinabe Values/Social Law Regarding Wife Battering" helps us see that "wife battering among the Ojibwe people emerged as a result of dissolution of traditional lifeways, including spirituality, the structure of government, laws, economics, relationships, values, beliefs, morals, and philosophy, that were in place in the pre-reservation era."

The article by Diana Courvant and Loree Cook-Daniels, "Trans and Intersex Survivors of Domestic Violence: Defining Terms, Barriers, and Responsibilities" (which includes a very useful definition of terms), helps us think through the barriers to living safely which are at work for many trans and intersex people. A fundamental issue for domestic violence programs which is important to many survivors, that of gender-segregated services, is a major obstacle for this group of survivors. The authors outline many suggestions for how to improve services for trans and intersex survivors.

The excellent article, "Ruling the Exceptions: Same Sex Battering and Domestic Violence Theory," obviously addresses the important issue of violence in lesbian and gay relationships, but also goes deeper to stimulate our broader analysis of intimate partner violence. Similar to the Richie and Kanuha article emphasizing that other forms of oppressions must be integrated with sexism for an understanding of violence against women, Gregory Merrill's article challenges gender-based domestic violence theory to explore "the many dimensions of power and explain(s) the phenomenon of domestic violence as it occurs in all relationship configurations." Three conditions for battering are identified as "learning to abuse; having the opportunity to abuse; and choosing to abuse." It becomes evident how violence is connected to privilege and oppression when one thinks about how society gives very clear messages about who has "the opportunity to abuse without suffering negative consequences":

> . . . would-be abusive individuals must perceive that they can "get away with it." Because of the pervasiveness of cultural sexism, homophobia, racism, classism, anti-Semitism, ageism, and ableism, some groups are empowered with privileges at the expense of others. For the battered heterosexual woman, the cultural context of sexism and other forms of oppressions which may affect her (such as racism in the instance of a woman of color), as enforced by friends, family members, hospital workers, mental health providers, and the criminal justice system, contribute to an environment in which her abusive partner can batter her without intervention or consequence. Likewise, homophobia, heterosexism, and other forms of oppressions operate in the same way to isolate the battered person in a same-sex relationship, permitting the violence to continue. While the social phenomenon

of prejudice does not cause battering, it does create an opportune environment that supports abusive behavior by its refusal to challenge it.

In a post 9/11 world where talk of "terrorism" dominates so many national policy decisions, the article "Sexual Terrorism" powerfully captures the reality of how violence and the fear of violence dominate many women's lives and women's decisions (even about staying at a laundromat.) The article is unique in observing the enormous impact of "the fear of violence" even for women who would never identify themselves as victims of violence, and how few men (or at least straight, white men) experience or recognize this. In a statement related to every topic in a women's health course, Sheffield provocatively concludes that "violence against the female body and the perpetuation of fear of violence form the basis of patriarchal power."

The final article in this chapter is a work-in-progress addressing the controversial topic of women's use of force. Much media attention has recently focused on "violent women" and "mean girls" but nearly all information on this topic has been from an anti-woman, backlash perspective or by people inappropriately misusing a gender-neutral approach. "Women's Use of Force," reflecting work of the Wisconsin Coalition Against Domestic Violence's Educating and Emerging Issues Committee, summarizes much of the present-day thinking of the battered women's movement as captured through a series of recent statewide and national think-tanks and workshops on this topic:

The challenge is to take violence by women seriously without losing sight of the fact that the pattern of male and female violence within adult intimate relationships are usually very different, often happen within different contexts, and generally have different consequences and that both violence itself and the barriers to ending violence are related to societal inequalities.

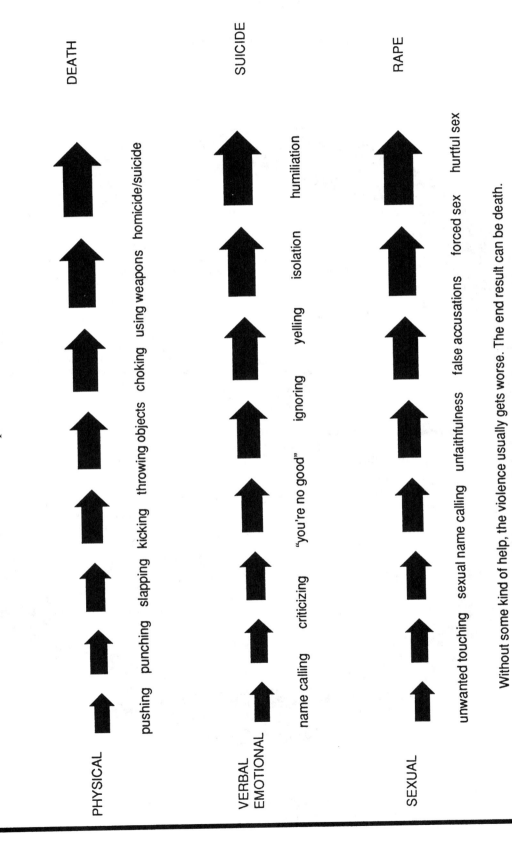

Continuum of Family Violence
from Alaska Department of Public Safety

PHYSICAL pushing punching slapping kicking throwing objects choking using weapons homicide/suicide DEATH

VERBAL EMOTIONAL name calling criticizing "you're no good" ignoring yelling isolation humiliation SUICIDE

SEXUAL unwanted touching sexual name calling unfaithfulness false accusations forced sex hurtful sex RAPE

Without some kind of help, the violence usually gets worse. The end result can be death.

"Power and Control Wheel"

by the Domestic Abuse Intervention Project, Duluth MN

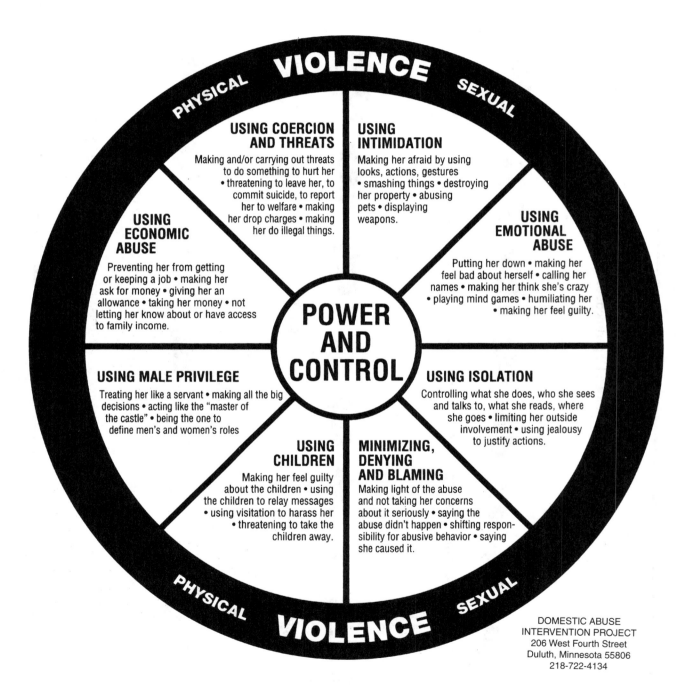

Based on the "Power and Control Wheel" and the "Equality Wheel" by the Domestic Abuse Intervention Project. Reprinted by permission of the Domestic Abuse Intervention Project and the Domestic Violence Project, Inc.

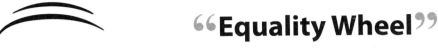

"Equality Wheel"

by the Domestic Abuse Intervention Project, Duluth MN

NONVIOLENCE

NEGOTIATION AND FAIRNESS
Seeking mutually satisfying resolutions to conflict • accepting change • being willing to compromise.

NON-THREATENING BEHAVIOR
Talking and acting so that she feels safe and comfortable expressing herself and doing things.

ECONOMIC PARTNERSHIP
Making money decisions together • making sure both partners benefit from financial arrangements.

RESPECT
Listening to her non-judgmentally • being emotionally affirming and understanding • valuing opinions.

EQUALITY

SHARED RESPONSIBILITY
Mutually agreeing on a fair distribution of work • making family decisions together.

TRUST AND SUPPORT
Supporting her goals in life • respecting her right to her own feelings, friends, activities and opinions.

RESPONSIBLE PARENTING
Sharing parental responsibilities • being a positive non-violent role model for the children.

HONESTY AND ACCOUNTABILITY
Accepting responsibility for self • acknowledging past use of violence • admitting being wrong • communicating openly and truthfully.

NONVIOLENCE

DOMESTIC ABUSE INTERVENTION PROJECT
206 West Fourth Street
Duluth, Minnesota 55806
218-722-4134

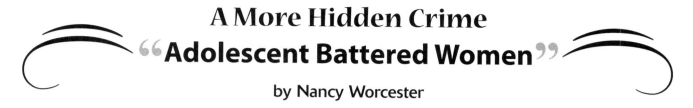

A More Hidden Crime
"Adolescent Battered Women"

by Nancy Worcester

Domestic violence has often been referred to as our nation's most hidden crime. However, after 15 years of activism and the establishment of more than 1000 battered women's shelter programs around the country, the battered women's movement has made many people and community services aware of the fact that huge numbers of women are entrapped in relationships of ongoing abuse of power, control, and physical coercion. The FBI estimates that a woman is battered every 15–18 seconds in this country and that approximately one of every three women experiences some physical violence in her long-term relationship(s). The pervasiveness of the violence may be best represented by the statement that one of every five women probably experiences five or more serious battering incidents each year.

Just as there is finally a public consciousness of the magnitude of the problem of women being battered, we are discovering an even more hidden, perhaps even more prevalent crime—violence against adolescent women. It turns out that most of the understanding of the dynamics of power and control in intimate relationships gained from the battered women's movement applies as much to adolescent women in dating relationships as it does to adult women. Tragically, the ramifications of violence for younger women are often exaggerated by a number of factors, but there are far fewer resources and options available to adolescent than adult women who are trying to end the violence in their lives.

Working to prevent violence in young people's lives must be a highest priority for any of us committed to creating a better world for the next generation and to helping young women maximize on their full potential. The isolation and lowered self-esteem which are so often a *consequence* of violence will have exaggerated ramifications for a young woman if they cause her to limit or eliminate skill-building, career opportunities or educational opportunities which could affect the rest of her life. (It is important to emphasize that the isolation, lowered self-esteem, and unhealthy coping mechanisms which are often observed in abused women are predictable *consequences* of violence and are not the *cause* of the violence. Confusing a consequence of violence with a cause can lead to dangerous, victim-blaming misunderstandings of the violence.)

If a woman is experiencing violence in her dating relationship(s), it will almost certainly be related to many other issues in her life. Anyone working with adolescents will benefit from seeing the connections between violence and the issues they already address. Why she is not always able to show up for study group, why she "had to go" to a concert instead of studying the night before an important exam, why she is no longer best friends with "the nice girl who seemed to have such a positive influence on her" or why she "suddenly" started dressing in a way which always or never shows off her figure may be explained by knowing that a young woman is in a relationship where someone else is taking control over almost all aspects of her life. Health educators need to recognize that many women are beaten up if they try to insist that male partners wear a condom or abstain from sexual activity. Because battering so often starts or accelerates during pregnancy and because sexual assault and other forms of violence are so intimately connected, anyone who works with adolescent pregnancy or sexual assault issues needs to be aware of the connections.

Ironically, many women learn about motherhood and battering at exactly the same time. Retrospective studies show that 25% of battered women experienced their first physical abuse during a pregnancy and that 40–60% of battered women were abused during a pregnancy or during pregnancies. The consequences are a much higher rate of miscarriage, stillbirth, premature delivery, and low birth weight infants in battered than non-battered women. The problem may be even more exaggerated in pregnant teens. A study looking specifically at physical abuse during teen pregnancy found that 26% of pregnant teens reported they were involved with a man who physically hurt them and 40–60% said that the battering had begun or escalated since their boyfriends knew they were pregnant. This study also provides an urgent reminder that services are not addressing the issue of violence for adolescent women: 65% of pregnant teens had not talked to anyone about the abuse.

Looking at the continuum of violence issues (The Power and Control and Equality Wheels by the Duluth Domestic Abuse Intervention Project (see pp. 259 & 260) and the Continuum of Family Violence Chart (see p. 258), by the Alaska Dept. of Public Safety are particularly useful), it becomes apparent how a range of forms of violence—physical, verbal, emotional, and sexual—are used by abusers to dominate their partners. The more subtle forms of sexual violence (unwanted touching, sexual name calling, unfaithfulness or threat of unfaithfulness, saying "no one else will ever love you", false accusations) are clearly emotionally as well as sexually controlling. These need to be identified as "violence issues" which are related to, and can escalate into, unwanted sex, unprotected sex, hurtful sex and other forms of sexual assault. Sexual violence is often the expression of violence which is the most painful for a woman to discuss. Emotional abuse is almost always present if there are other forms of abuse in a relationship but a clever abuser may achieve sufficient control by emotional abuse without ever resorting to other forms. Women consistently say that emotional abuse is the hardest form to identify (Is this really happening? Is this abuse? Am I making too much of this?) but recognize it as the form of abuse which has the most impact on their lives and their view of themselves. Many women who have been in life-threatening situations say, "The physical battering was nothing compared to the daily emotional abuse." Helping young women see the interconnectedness of verbal, emotional, physical, and sexual power and control issues may be the most useful information in empowering them to end *all* forms of violence in their lives.

By the time adolescents start experimenting with their own dating relationships, they have been bombarded with messages that violence against women is tolerated and even encouraged and that dominance, aggression, and abuse of power and control are appropriate masculine behaviors which are rewarded by society. Today's young people have been exposed to a tolerance and perpetuation of male violence which is unique to this generation. They grew up in the era when the average child was watching 24 hours of television a week with children's programming averaging 15.5 violent acts per hour. By the time they reach 18, the average US adolescent has witnessed approximately 26,000 murders, in their own homes, via the tv screen.

The role of television in sex-role socialization and the perpetuation of male violence has been grossly exaggerated for today's young people because changes in federal regulations, in the early 1980s, allowed the sale of toys directly connected to tv shows, removed regulations limiting the amount of advertising allowed on children's programming, and ruled that product-based shows

were legal. The result was a totally new integration of the tv and toy industries. By 1986 all of the ten best selling toys had shows connected with them and by 1988, 80% of children's tv programming was produced by toy companies. Parallel marketing promoted definitions of masculinity and femininity as clearly defined as the distinct lines of boys' toys vs. girls' toys. Because of the new integration of tv and toys, today's young people did not learn to explore their own creativity or imagination in healthy ways but instead learned to "act out their scripts" as dominant and competitive *or* caring, helpless, and concentrating on appearance, either as GI Joe or Ghostbusters vs. Barbie or My Little Pony.

With electronic video games, an even newer and unstudied phenomena, young people get to act out and be rewarded for playing their violent roles. The direct participation in "performing" the violence of video games is predicted to magnify whatever effect more passive tv viewing has on one's acceptance or perpetuation of violence. In a violence promoting and accepting culture, it is not surprising to find that *most* video games are very violent (a sampling of 120 machines in three arcades in Madison, Wisconsin, found that more than 70 involved either hand-to-hand combat or shooting to kill enemies) and that the most popular games in an arcade are the most violent.

Consequently, *unlearning* the tolerance of violence and *learning* how to achieve violence-free, equal relationships are skills which are now as crucial to *teach* young people as reading, writing, math and the use of computers. The way people learn, in their earliest experimentation, to be in intimate relationships can set the pattern for what they expect in future relationships. It is a time when the highest standards should be set! Adolescents need to see models of healthy, equal, violence-free relationships, in order to aim for that in their own lives and *to be able to model that for their peers.*

At this stage, many teens do not have the knowledge or skills to prevent or react against violence in their own lives or in their friends' lives. In fact, exactly the opposite is much more likely. Many young women have said that even when they have told friends they were being hurt by their boyfriends, the response was that they were lucky to have boyfriends. There is enormous peer pressure not to break up. Many teens regard violence as a normal part of dating and have no idea they deserve better. Extreme possessiveness, jealousy, dominance, and not being "allowed" to break up get wrongly identified as desirable, positive signs of caring, love and commitment, rather than strong warning signs that they are in an unhealthy, potentially dangerous relationship.

Figuring out what to expect in relationships may be particularly confusing for anyone who grew up in a home where there was violence. Many young men only see abusing males (in reality and in the media) as role models. Many young women who told their mother about being hurt by their boyfriend, have heard, "you have to learn to take the bad and the good in a relationship to make it work."

Many teens who have grown up in violent homes face the difficulty of trying to figure out how they want to be in their own young adult relationships while they are still learning (or not learning) to cope with being affected by the violence with which they grew up. The battered women's movement has very effectively identified that when a woman is battered, the children are almost always affected by the violence. Seventy-five percent of women who are battered in this country have children living at home. Children in homes where domestic violence occurs are physically abused or seriously neglected at a rate 1500% higher than the national average in the general population. Even witnessing domestic violence can have a tremendous impact on young people and may result in symptoms very similar to those seen in people who have been abused. Helping these young people learn healthy relationship skills can be particularly challenging as many teens do not recognize the impact the violence in their homes has had on them and many teens do not want to talk about witnessing or experiencing abuse.

Particularly crucial to how we help young people learn relationship skills *and* acknowledge that violence in their lives may have already influenced their attitudes and behaviors is how we address the impact of the "intergenerational transmission of violence." There is a confusing body of work which examines how the cycle of violence can be passed on through the generations. We now know the old "dad beats mom, mom beats the children, and the children beat the pets" picture was much too simplistic and inaccurate. Increasingly, it is being shown that the person beating mom may also be the one beating the children and protecting the mother is often the best way to protect the children. Although research is inconsistent in documenting the rates of intergenerational transmission of violence, there is a consistent trend which shows that boys who witness domestic violence as children are more likely to batter their female partners as adults than are men from non-violent homes.

How we use this information can be a key factor in determining whether we help break the intergenerational transmission of violence or actually contribute to its perpetuation. Too much of the literature deals with this data as if were inevitable. Central to breaking the pattern is addressing and researching a different set of questions. *If* 30% of boys who witness violence become abusers,

the question must be asked, "What can we learn from the 70% who witness violence but do not become abusers?" What factors help young people who have witnessed violence learn to resist violent behavior? Young people from violent homes who have experienced the ugliness of violence and have learned to value non-violent relationships can be exactly the people most committed to breaking the cycle of violence and can be incredibly effective peer leaders.

Most important, young people must *never* learn that violence is inevitable. Many dating violence resources (including some of the materials I highly recommend on other aspects) include information on the intergenerational transmission of violence without making it clear that the cycle can be broken. Information on warning signs of potential abusers almost always include "boys who grew up in violent homes." What does it feel like to see that information if you are a young man who witnessed violence at home? We must make certain that none of our materials or our messages ever contribute towards a young man feeling that he is destined to be violent.

Studies on dating violence consistently show that many teens in violent relationships have not talked to *any* adults about the violence in their lives. We need to start identifying the barriers which have made us so ineffective on this issue and acknowledge that we are only starting to have the language and tools for opening a dialogue on dating violence.

The good news is that a wide range of excellent resources, curricula, and videos have been produced on dating violence issues and violence-free relationships in recent years. It's a very exciting stage to be working on this issue because no one needs to "start from scratch." However, work needs to be done to make the excellent resources and services available to, and appropriate for, many more teens. Few of the resources address the issue in a way that has any meaning for lesbian, gay or bisexual teens or for young people of color. Many of the materials seem to have the underlying assumption that children grow up in homes where there is one male and one female adult. Special issues for teens with disabilities need to be addressed because of both the high rate of sexual assault of people with disabilities and the complexities of dating which arise from the myth that people with disabilities are "asexual." The obsession with body image and a very narrow definition of attractiveness can also be particularly cruel and abusive in adolescence.

"You deserve to be treated with respect."

"You are not alone if someone is hurting you. There are excellent resources to help you end the violence in your life."

These messages which we have been giving adult battered women for the last 15 years are now the same messages we have to give to much younger women.

REFERENCES
A list of references is available in the original source.

"Breaking the Silence"

by Megan Steffer

Rape and sexual assault are public health issues that most of us would prefer to ignore. In 1987, it was first reported that approximately 27 percent of college-aged women had been rape victims since age 14.[1] Further studies have gone on to specify that anywhere from 15–20 percent of women are raped during their time as an undergraduate student.[2] These numbers rise significantly when statistics also include attempted rape and sexual assault: studies report that as many as 57 percent of college women have been victims of some kind of sexual assault during their college careers.[2] Despite having rape prevention programs in place at almost every major university in the country, current figures still estimate that one in four college women are survivors of rape or attempted rape.[3]

When many people think of rape, they imagine a sinister-looking man sexually assaulting a woman in a dark alley. While these situations do occur, the vast majority of rapes (80%) occur between people who know each other, and take place in environments that are generally considered to be safe.[4] Rapists also do not match most stereotypes: men who commit rape are our friends, co-workers, neighbors, and relatives. In some groups (such as sports teams and fraternities) sexual aggressiveness is seen as a positive trait for men to have. From conversations I've had, it seems that many rapists don't even know what they have committed is rape, assuming that it was okay because a girl was drunk, provocatively dressed, or displaying "suggestive" behavior.

Something clearly needs to be changed in our society when this kind of violence towards women is accepted or ignored by the majority of the population. Even women at the highest risk of becoming victims of rape seem ultimately unconvinced that it could happen to them. Even me.

My story is all too typical. I am the one college woman in four. My experience began on an average Saturday night, partying with my roommates at a co-worker's house outside campus. Not in the mood to drink, I shared a beer with a roommate so people would stop pestering us about the fact that we weren't holding red cups of beer.

As the night wore on, my roommates grew bored and wanted to go home, but I was having fun with my co-worker and his friends. He assured me that he would get me home safely. I bid my roommates adieu, refilled my red cup with water, and returned to the party. Less than 15 minutes later, I had my last memory of the evening.

I opened my eyes the next morning, naked, in a room I had never seen before. Next to me was my co-worker, naked and sound asleep. Large purple bruises covered both of my arms and legs, two parallel lines were burned into my right forearm, and dried blood covered my thighs and the sheets all around me. I saw my clothes nearby. My only thought: "Get out now." As I climbed out of the bed, he opened his eyes and gazed at my bloody, bruised, and burned body. "Good morning, beautiful."

When I asked him what had happened he just laughed. "You had a good time," he told me, after grumbling about how he'd have to wash my blood out of his formerly

"Young Feminists: Breaking the Silence," by Megan Steffer, originally published in the *Women's Health Activist*, July/August 2006, pp. 8–9, the newsletter of the National Women's Health Network (NWHN). It is reprinted with the permission of the author and the NWHN.

clean sheets. "Take me home now," I demanded. After assuring him that I did not, in fact, want to stay for breakfast, he got his keys.

The following days were extremely difficult, as I tried to determine what actually happened. To me, it is pretty clear that "date-rape drugs" were involved. These sedatives, which include GHB, Rophynol, and Ketamine, usually are colorless and odorless when added to a drink. The sedatives often make the person who drinks them appear to drunk and makes them lose their memory; for this reason, they have become widely known for their use in conjunction with rape and sexual assault. Although I will never be completely sure that someone gave me such a sedative, the blood and pain clearly tell me I was raped.

Thankfully, although I knew him from work, our interactions there were few and far between. I saw him in the building two or three times after that night, and did my best to avoid him. When I saw him at work, he acted as if nothing had happened, asking: "Why haven't you called?" Some days he would show up in the parking lot or outside my apartment complex, but I refused to talk to him. The last time I saw him was when he showed up at a restaurant where I worked, told me he missed me, and kissed me on the cheek. I almost slapped him. He sat in another server's section, and I avoided that part of the restaurant until he was gone.

It has been a year and a half since that night. At first, I couldn't even think about what had happened, not wanting to face the reality of what I had been through. I did not report the crime. I knew that my lack of memory about the evening would weaken my case. I was also confused because I had once seen this man as a friend and wanted to believe that he had not betrayed my trust.

Eventually, I began talking about my experience. Some friends seemed hesitant to believe my story, suggesting that I could have been drunk and blacked out, or that I had led him on. Others did believe me, but continued to interact with him like nothing had happened.

Similar reactions have been documented across the country. We simply don't want to believe that rape happens. We especially don't want to accept that our friends or family members could be perpetrators or victims of rape. Before this experience, I didn't either.

As difficult as it was, I found that talking about what had happened was the most helpful thing in allowing me to move on with my life. Even after I had shared my story, it seemed as though I was talking about something I had seen in a movie or heard from a friend, not an experience that I had lived through. It wasn't until about

three months later, when I was beginning a romantic relationship with another man, that the reality of it all finally hit me.

When he touched me in certain ways, or even cast certain looks at me, it could cause bouts of uncontrolled panic and grief. Fortunately, he was very understanding, talked with me about my experience, and helped me to work through the pain. I was very lucky to have someone who was so patient and supportive of me as I tried to make sense of my feelings and reactions. After accepting the fact that this experience was not something that I could simply block out of my life, I decided to seek counseling at the campus health center. Through the support of some close friends and the counseling sessions, I am finally able to speak openly about my experience, and recognize the value of being able to share it with others.

If one benefit can come from this, it is that I can tell you that rape does happen, it is a problem, and we can make a difference. Please, if you are a victim of sexual violence, start talking about it. Ask your daughters and friends about their experiences. Most importantly, be ready to listen and support these women as their stories unfold.

REFERENCES

1. Koss MP, Gidycz CA, Wisniewski N. "The scope of rape: incidence and prevalence of sexual aggression and victimization in a national sample of higher education students." *Journal of Consulting and Clinical Psychology* 1987; 55(2): 162–170.

2. Koss MP, Dinero TE, Siebel CA et al. "Stranger and acquaintance rape: are there differences in women's experiences." *Psycholgy of Women Quarterly* 1988; 12: 1-24. Gary JM. "An overview of sexual assault on campus." In: Gary JM (ed). *The Campus Community Confronts Sexual Assault: Institutional Issues and Campus Awareness*, Holmes Beach, FL: Learning Publications, 1994, 1–9, Brener ND, McMahon PM, Warren CW et al. "Forced sexual intercourse and associated health-risk behaviors among female college students in the United States. *Journal of Consulting and Clinical Psychology* 1999; 67(2): 252–9; Fisher B, Cullen F, Turner M. *The Sexual Victimization of College Women.* Washington, DC: U.S. Dept. of Justice, 2000.

3. Fisher, Cullen, and Turner, see above.

4. Tjaden P, Thoennes N. *Full Report of the Prevalence, Incidence, and Consequences of Violence Against Women: Findings from the National Violence Against Women Survey* (Report NCJ 183781). Washington, DC: National Institute of Justice, 2000.

"The Unique Role Health Workers Can Play in Recognizing and Responding to Battered Women"

by Nancy Worcester

"Battering appears to be the single most common cause of injury to women—more common than automobile accidents, muggings and rapes combined."

Many women identify violence in their lives, and their fear of violence, as the number one health issue they face. For health workers responding to battering, it is important to remember that battering is *much* more than the physical injuries. Violence serves as an excellent reminder that mental and physical health issues cannot be separated. For a woman being abused, physical violence is but one of the tools that her abuser uses to have power and control over many, or all, aspects of her life. Many formerly battered women who have even suffered life-threatening injuries say that the physical violence was nothing compared to the psychological and emotional abuse they endured.

Now that many states have mandatory arrest laws, battered women have been quick to remind us that stopping abuse in a home is much more complex than simply stopping the hitting. Women have noted that a result of abuser counselling can be that abusers learn they can no longer get away with hitting their partners. However, unless larger issues of power and control are also addressed, the abuser may learn to shift to psychological/emotional forms of abuse and the woman continues to be battered even if she is no longer physically injured.

A wide range of chronic health issues including headaches, backaches, sleep disorders, anxiety, abdominal complaints, eating disorders, depression and chronic pain are particularly common in battered women and are clearly related to the stress of living in a violent relationship.

You See Battered Women Everyday

The FBI estimates that a woman is beaten every 15–18 seconds in this country. Violence affects women of all social groups, ages, races, rural and urban environments, and affects both rich and poor and both heterosexual and lesbian women. Many health workers and health workers' partners live with violence as a part of their lives.

Battered women regularly call upon the health system even though health workers have a poor record of identifying them. Studies have shown that abused women have more health problems than non-abused women, so those who trust the health system and have insurance probably seek healthcare at disproportionately high rates. Studies have shown that 22–35 percent of all women who use emergency room services are battered women and because the same women may need to return time and time again, almost half of all injuries presented by women in emergency rooms may be a result of abuse.

Although health workers do not regularly ask about battering during pregnancy, it is more common than and has as serious consequences (increased rates of miscarriage, stillbirth, low birth weight babies, and risk of homicide) as the conditions routinely tested for in prenatal care. Retrospective studies of battered women have found that 40–60 percent were abused during pregnancy; 25 percent of battered women say they were beaten for the first time during a pregnancy. The problems may be even more exaggerated in pregnant teenagers. One study found that 26 percent of pregnant teens were currently in a relationship with a man who was abusive; many stated that the abuse had started when they discovered they were pregnant. Most alarming, 65 percent of the battered teens had not talked to *anyone* about the violence in their lives.

Health Workers Can Play a Key Role

Many battered women would like to tell someone about the violence in their lives and would greatly benefit from knowing that their situation is not unusual and that there are a range of excellent resources available to them. Understanding common patterns of domestic violence makes it obvious that health workers who do recognize battered women and empower them to explore their options can play a key role in helping women end the violence in their lives.

Isolation

Isolation is a primary weapon that one person can use to gain control over another person's life. Battered women describe how abusers gradually isolate them from their other social/emotional support networks so that eventually the abuser is the main person in the abused woman's life giving her information about her own value. Messages like "No one else will ever love you" and "You deserve to be beaten" become very powerful when a woman is not hearing any other messages. Understanding that isolation is a *consequence* (*not* a cause) of battering can help health workers recognize that what they say to battered women can be extremely important. Health workers aware of power imbalances in health worker-patient relationships can see why this can be exaggerated when the patient is an abused woman. A health worker who implies that the woman is "the problem" will reinforce the messages she gets at home; the health worker who says "You don't deserve to be hit" will be giving a crucial, different message.

The Cycle of Violence

The cycle of violence is a pattern that many battered women start to recognize in their lives. The battering incident seldom comes from "nowhere," but is the expected "explosion" from a period of increasing tension. Women describe the stress of living in the tension-building stage, the waiting for the straw that will finally provoke the battering, as so awful that some women remember when even a severe battering was almost a welcome "release" from the unbearable tension.

Particularly in the early years of abusive relationships, the battering incident is often immediately followed by a good stage which some women call the "honeymoon stage." The honeymoon stage is the wonderful stage we *all* want in relationships. Understanding the importance of the honeymoon stage in battering relationships can help us understand the complexities of these (and all!) relationships. This is the stage at which abusers say (and think they mean) that they are very sorry and it will never happen again. This is the stage when loving sex, extravagant presents, and a renewing of dreams and life long plans/goals can be very enticing.

If the battering is severe enough to cause injuries, the health worker, particularly emergency service providers, may see the woman immediately after the battering and before the "honeymoon stage." This is a key time to make sure the woman knows her options and resources, because she may be the most open to exploring alternatives to staying in a violent relationship. Once the "honeymoon stage" begins, the woman may be "hooked" into another cycle, convinced that if only she tries harder the violence will end.

Escalation

Unless there is intervention (and a sincere commitment from the abuser to learn totally new ways of communicating in the relationship), battering relationships tend to escalate over a period of time. The battering incidents become more frequent and often increase in severity. (Battered women describe the "honeymoon stage" as being less of a "hook" in long-term battering relationships than are the enormous social and economic pressures which keep them in relationships they know are unhealthy.) Because battered women may be seeing health workers long before they turn to other services, good medical records with clear notes, and even photographs, of injuries and chronic health problems that may be related to domestic violence are essential. These can help health workers who will see the records in the future, and the battered woman herself, to see the emerging pattern.

Revictimizing the Battered Woman

Even though health workers are not good at identifying battered women, studies have found that health workers do treat battered women differently than non-battered women and that the treatment actually contributes to the consequences of battering.

Unless there is an understanding of battering, a woman who calls upon the health system regularly, with a range

Hospital Protocols Now Required

Effective January 1, 1992, all accredited hospitals are required to have protocols in place describing how they respond to battered women and how health professionals are trained on this issue. This is the ideal time for health workers and battered women's advocates to work together to make sure that protocols serve to empower battered women. There are over 1,000 programs in the U.S. specifically serving battered women. These "experts" can help a woman with the legal, safety, housing and support services she needs.

of symptoms and injuries, may be seen as a frustrating patient by health workers who pride themselves on being able to diagnose and treat specific conditions. Only 5-10 percent of battered women in emergency services are identified as such by physicians on their records. Instead, the ground-breaking work on this by Stark, Flitcraft and Frazier, found that medical records included the labels "neurotic," "hysteric," "hypochondriac" or "a well-known patient with multiple vague complaints" for one in four battered women compared to one in 50 non-battered women. One in four battered women were given pain medications and/or minor tranquilizers compared to one in ten non-battered women. This "treatment" has the same effect as paying fire fighters to *push* people back into burning homes! Medication and victimizing labels reinforce the woman's feeling that she is the problem and may contribute to depression, drug and alcohol abuse, and the high rate of suicide attempts seen as a consequence of battering.

Empowering Battered Women

Excellent resources are now available for health workers spelling out specific ways to identify and respond to battered women and to help them end the violence in their lives. Responding more appropriately to battered women does not necessarily mean more work for the healthcare provider. It means *starting* to ask about violence ("Since so many women are hurt by their partners, we ask every patient with injuries like yours whether they've ever been hit/kicked/hurt by their partner.") and documenting it, making sure safety issues are addressed for a woman before she returns to the situation that caused the mental or physical injuries, giving women information about community resources, and *stopping* treating abused women by providing only labels and tranquilizers.

Battered women must be empowered to make their *own* decisions at their *own* pace. Outside intervention, certain behaviors, or trying to leave at the "wrong" time can escalate the violence. Thirty percent of women murdered in this country are killed by the men they had loved. Most of these murders occur when women are trying to get out of a relationship. Understanding the complexities of *leaving* battering relationships is central to serving battered women's needs.

Health workers will seldom know the impact of their responses to battered women. Saying "You don't deserve to be treated like this" or "Here is a list of community resources" may be the advice that saves more lives and does more for the mental health of patients than do other more "medical" skills.

REFERENCES
A list of references is available in the original source.

"Medical Power and Control Wheel and Medical Advocacy Wheel"

by the Domestic Abuse Intervention Project, Kenosha, WI

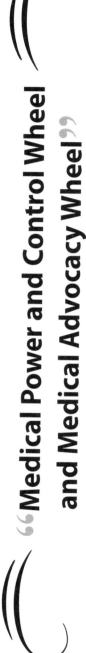

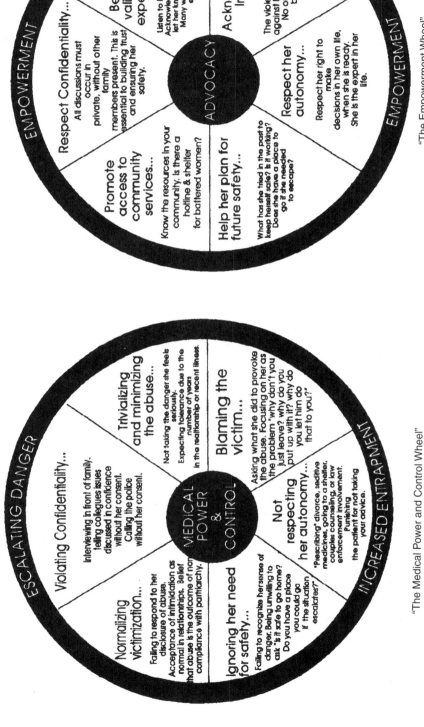

"The Empowerment Wheel"

"The Medical Power and Control Wheel"

Based on the "Power and Control Wheel" and the "Equality Wheel" by the Domestic Abuse Intervention Project. Developed by the Domestic Violence Project, Inc., 3556 7th Avenue, Kenosha, WI 53140, (414)656-8502. Reprinted by permission.

Battered Women of Color
in Public Health Care Systems
"Racism, Sexism,
and Violence"

by Beth E. Richie and Valli Kanuha

Introduction

The problems of rape, battering, and other forms of violence against women have existed throughout history. Only recently have these experiences, traditionally accepted as natural events in the course of women's lives, received significant attention as major social problems. For many years there was a tendency for both human service providers and public policy research to focus only on the individual lives of women, children, and men who are damaged or lost due to domestic violence. This narrow focus on individual victims and perpetrators involved in domestic violence rather than on an examination of the role social institutions play in the maintenance of violence against women represents one of the major gaps in our analysis of this pervasive social issue. Paradoxically, the very institutions which have been constructed for the protection and care of the public good—such as the criminal justice system, religious organizations, hospitals, and healthcare agencies—have long sanctioned disparate and unequal attention to women in society. Only through a critique of these historically patriarchal and often sexist institutions will we comprehend domestic violence as more than individual acts of violence by perpetrators against victims.

Another equally problematic gap in contemporary analysis and study of violence against women exists with regard to race and ethnicity, i.e., how individual and institutional racism affects the lives of women of color who are battered. With a few notable exceptions, there is a very little research on the ways that traditional responses of societal institutions to violence against women are complicated by racism and, therefore, how battered women of color are systematically at a disadvantage when seeking help in most domestic violence situations. The result is that battered women who are African-American, Latina, Asian/Pacific Islander, East Indian, Native-American, and members of other communities of color are vulnerable to abuse not only from their partners, but from insensitive, ineffective institutions as well.

This chapter will address an important factor which is often ignored in our understanding and analysis of domestic violence. While our increasing knowledge of battered women is usually applied in the context that "all women are vulnerable to male violence," the emphasis of this discussion will be on those differential social, economic, and cultural circumstances that render women of color, in particular, vulnerable to male violence at both individual and institutional levels. In addition, this article will focus specifically on the experiences of battered women of color within the healthcare system, including hospitals, clinics, and public health agencies. As will be described in later sections, many women of color rely significantly on public health institutions not only for ongoing preventive healthcare and crisis intervention services, but, more importantly, as a viable access point for other services and institutions, e.g., public welfare, housing assistance, legal advice, and so on. Thus the emphasis of this chapter is on the relationship between healthcare institutions and battered women of color, although similar critiques could be made about the inadequate response of other public institutions (such as religious organizations or the criminal justice system) to battered women of color. Finally, this essay will discuss some effective strategies and programs which address the unique and complex issues affecting women of color who are battered.

Reprinted from *Wings of Gauze: Women of Color and the Experience of Health and Illness,* eds. Barbara Bair and Susan E. Cayleff, Wayne State University Press, 1993 with permission of Wayne State University Press.

Balancing Our Multiple Loyalties: Special Considerations for Women of Color and Victims of Domestic Violence

In order to understand the special circumstances and tensions experienced by battered women of color it is important to understand the interface of gender inequality, sexism, and racism as they affect women both in their racial/ethnic communities and in society at large. Because of the powerful effects of a violent relationship, many battered women are required, either overtly or covertly, to balance the often conflicting needs and expectations of their batterers, their communities, and the larger society. These conflicting expectations, rules, and loyalties often compromise the strategies which are available to liberate women of color from violent relationships. This discussion will serve as a foundation for examining the compound effects of oppression which many women of color face even prior to entering the healthcare system for medical treatment of and protection from domestic violence.

Communities of color in this country have historically been devastated by discriminatory and repressive political, social, and economic policies. It is commonplace to associate high infant mortality, school drop-out rates, criminality, drug abuse, and most other indices of social dysfunction with African-American, Latino, Native-American, and other non-European ethnic groups. Even among the "model minorities," Asians and Pacific Islanders, groups of new immigrants as well as their assimilated relatives have shown increased rates of HIV and AIDS, mental health problems, and other negative co-factors which are in part attributable to their status as non-majority (nonwhite) people in the United States.

Most everyone, from historians to social scientists to politicians, whether conservative or radical, considers racism to be a significant, if not the primary, cause of this disproportionate level of social deterioration among communities of color. While the dynamics of racism have often been studied from a macro-perspective, comparing the effects of race discrimination on particular ethnic groups vis-à-vis society at large, the differential effects of racism on women versus men of color has not been given due attention. In order to adequately understand any analysis of the combined effects of racism, sexism, and battering, a consideration of gender-based tension within communities of men and women of color, separate from and related to the predominant white society, is required.

There are many stereotypes about women of color which affect not only our understanding of them as women, but particularly our analysis of and sensitivity to them with regard to domestic violence. For example, many portrayals of women of color espouse their inherent strengths as historical, matriarchal heads of households. While this stereotype of women of color as super homemakers, responsible family managers, and unselfish nurturers may be undisputed, such attributions do not mean that all (or most) women of color are therefore empowered and supported in their various family roles or have positions of leadership within their ethnic communities. Many women of color with whom we work state that they face the burden either of having to be overly competent and successful or having to avoid the too-often painful reality of becoming "just another one of those horror stories or pitiful statistics on the front page of the newspaper." For women of color who are experiencing domestic violence, the implicit community and societal expectation to be strong and continue to care for themselves and their families results in their denying not only the actual existence of battering in their lives, but the extent and nature of that abuse. For example, one Korean woman who was repeatedly punched around her head and face by her husband reported that she used cosmetics extensively each day when she went to Mass with her husband, in order to assure protection of her own, as well as her husband's, dignity among their church and neighborhood friends. When she went to work as a typist in a white business, she was especially careful not to disclose evidence of her abuse, in order to protect both herself and her husband from her co-workers' judgments that "there was something wrong with Korean people."

While public policy makers are concerned about the rapidly escalating crime rate in this country, many leaders in cities predominated by communities of color are becoming increasingly concerned about the profile of those convicted for crimes, i.e., young boys and men of color. The predominance of men of color in correctional facilities (close to 90 percent of the penal population in some cities) has polarized everyone, from scholars to community leaders to policy makers. While most mainstream legislators and public health officials are reluctant to discuss it publicly, there is a rising belief that men of color are inherently problematic and socially deviant. More progressive analysts have ascribed criminal behavior among nonwhite males to historically racist social conditions that are reinforced by criminal, legal, and penal systems which disproportionately arrest and convict men of color at least in part because of their skin color.

There are no equally concerned dialogues about how women of color continue to be victims of crime more often than white women and about the disparate treatment they receive from not only racist, but sexist social systems. An African-American woman who works with battered women as a court advocate states unequivocally that battered women of color are usually treated less respectfully by prosecutors and judges than the white women with whom she works. In addition, when this same court advocate has raised this disparity with her African-American brothers and male friends in her community, she is often derided as being "one of those white women's libbers" who has betrayed "her own" by working on a problem like domestic violence, which will further stigmatize and destroy the men of color who are charged with battering. Unfortunately, this dialectic of the comparable oppression of women and men of color has resulted in a troubling silence about the needs of women of color and led to counterproductive discussions between women and men of color about the meaning and significance of domestic violence, specifically, and sexism in general.

For a battered woman of color who experiences violence at the hands of a man of color from her own ethnic group, a complex and troublesome dynamic is established that is both enhanced and compromised by the woman's relationship to her community. She is battered by another member of her ethnic community, whose culture is vulnerable to historical misunderstanding and extinction by society at large. For the battered woman, this means that she may be discriminated against in her attempt to secure services *while at the same time* feeling protective of her batterer, who might also be unjustly treated by such social institutions as the police and the judicial system. Most battered women of color are acutely aware of how the police routinely brutalize men of color, how hospitals and social services discriminate against men of color, and the ways men of color are more readily labeled deviant than white men. In one Midwestern city, anecdotal reports from court and police monitors have shown that men of color awaiting arraignment for domestic violence charges frequently arrive in court with bruises supposedly inflicted by police officers. One Indian woman stated that when she saw her husband in court the morning after a battering incident, he looked just as bad as she did, with black eyes and bruises about his face. Feeling pity for him, she refused to testify, and upon release he told her of being beaten by police while being transported between the jail and the court house. Although the existence of police brutality is unfortunately not a new phenomenon, it is certainly compromised and complicated in the context of domestic violence, especially for men and women of color who are seeking help from this already devastating problem. For battered women of color, seeking help for the abuse

they are experiencing always requires a tenuous balance between care for and loyalty to themselves, their batterers, and their communities.

The situation is further complicated by the fact that communities of color have needed to prioritize the pressing social, economic, and health problems which have historically plagued their people and neighborhoods. Because of sexism, the particular concerns of women typically do not emerge at the top of the list. The values of family stability, community self-determination, and protection of one's racial and ethnic culture are often seen as incompatible with addressing the needs of battered women within communities of color. Most of us who have worked in the domestic violence movement are well aware of the gross misconceptions that battering is just a woman's issue or that domestic violence in communities of color is not as serious as other problems. The most dangerous consequence, for battered women of color, however, is that they are often entrapped by these misconceptions and misguided loyalties and thus remain in the confines of violent and abusive households.

While credit for a broad-based societal response to the problem of violence against women must be given to the feminist movement and its successful grassroots organizing in the mid-1970s, another process of "split loyalties" has emerged, compromising the analysis regarding battered women of color. Those women of color who identify themselves as activists, feminists, and organizers within the battered women's movement often face an additional barrier among their feminist peers when raising issues related to the particular dynamics of domestic violence and race/ethnicity. Many white feminists and the organizations they have created become very threatened when women of color, with their concomitant expanded analysis of battering and racism, have moved into leadership roles. Many women of color in the violence against women movement have challenged the long-standing belief of many white feminists that sexism is the primary, if not the only, cause of women's oppression. In a reform movement which has had such a significant impact on the values, behaviors, and subsequent policies regarding women and violence, the reluctance or inability to integrate an understanding of violence against women with other forms of oppression (such as racism, classism, ageism) in addition to sexism has been disappointing. A more significant concern, though, is the effect of limited analysis on women and children of color who are seeking refuge and safety from both hostile partners and social institutions outside the battered women's movement.

In summary, our understanding of women of color who are battered must be considered against the political, social, and cultural backdrop of their racial and ethnic communities; within the framework of institutional responses that are historically based in racism and other prejudices; and against the background of the feminist agenda, which has been primarily responsible for galvanizing all of the above to address this pervasive social issue. It is in this context that we turn to an examination of the particular influence, concerns, and barriers of the healthcare system in dealing with battered women of color.

Battered Women of Color: Health Problems and Health Care

Women who are battered are often seriously hurt; their physical and psychological injuries are life-threatening and long-lasting. In one-third of all battering incidents, a weapon is used, and 40 percent result in the need for emergency medical attention. Research suggests that one-third of all adult female suicide attempts can be associated with battering, and 25 percent of all female homicide victims die at the hands of their husbands or boyfriends. More women are injured in their homes by their spouses or male partners each year than by accidents or illnesses.

It is not surprising, therefore, that most battered women report their first attempt to seek help is from a healthcare institution, even before contacting the police. This is especially true in communities of color, where police response is likely to be sporadic, at best. Yet research indicates that of those battered women using the emergency room for acute treatment of injuries related to an abusive incident, only one in ten was identified as battered. Similar findings have been cited for women using ambulatory care settings. A random sample of women seeking health maintenance visits at neighborhood health clinics revealed that 33 percent were battered women and less than 10 percent received safety information or counseling for domestic violence. The following story of Yolanda (a pseudonym) illustrates the role of health facilities in the lives of battered women.

Yolanda is a forty-six-year old who received primary healthcare from a neighborhood health clinic. She uses the services of the walk-in clinic two or more times each month, complaining of discomfort, sleeplessness and fatigue. Yolanda never mentions that her boyfriend abuses her, but her clinic visits correspond directly with the pattern of his alcohol binges. The staff of the clinic know about her boyfriend's mistreatment, because he sometimes comes to the clinic drunk and will threaten her if she does not leave with him.

For Yolanda, the clinic symbolizes a safe, public place of refuge. From her experience, she knows it is legitimate to seek assistance when one is sick, and she trusts health authorities to take care of her needs. Health providers lose an important opportunity for intervention when they do not offer assistance to Yolanda, especially since they have clear evidence that her boyfriend is violent toward her. She, in turn, feels that the violence must be hidden and that it is a source of shame, since her healthcare providers do not acknowledge it or offer to help.

For many battered women of color, the unresponsiveness of most healthcare institutions is symbolic of the overall reality of social disenfranchisement and deterioration in poor, nonwhite communities across the United States. While lack of quality, affordable housing is a major problem for many people of color, the majority of the homeless are women of color and their children. The drug epidemic, particularly crack and heroin use, has had a significant impact on violence against women. There is growing anecdotal evidence to suggest that battered women are often forced to use drugs as part of the pattern of their abuse, yet there is a serious lack of treatment programs for women, particularly poor women with children. The spread of HIV and AIDS among many women of color has been compounded by the HIV infection rate among children of HIV-positive mothers. Many women with HIV report that negotiating for safer sex or clean needles is difficult when they are controlled by violent, coercive partners.

With regard to women and the social problems of drugs, homelessness, and AIDS, most public health officials have been quick to label women as the criminals, rather than the victims of a society that is disintegrating before our very eyes. When we add to the above the battering, rape, and psychological abuse of those same women who are homeless, drug addicted, and HIV-positive, it is clear that the healthcare system can be either a vehicle for assistance or a significant barrier for women who are seeking protection from a myriad of health and social problems.

The experience of Ana illustrates the interrelatedness that can occur between domestic violence, drug use, HIV infection, and the chronic and acute need for healthcare. Ana's husband was an injection drug user who had battered her severely throughout their ten-year marriage. He had been very ill for a period of months and had tested seropositive for HIV. Ana was already pregnant when her husband was tested, but he insisted that she carry through with the pregnancy. She was battered twice in the four months since she had gotten pregnant, and after one incident she was unable to get out of bed for two days. Her husband Daniel reportedly was concerned about the baby and took her to the emergency room of their local hospital. During the triage interview, the ER (Emergency Room) nurse noticed the tension between Ana and Daniel but was uncomfortable addressing it. The nurse later reported that she did not want to offend them by suggesting that they appeared to be having "marriage problems" because they were Hispanic, and she understood that Hispanics were embarrassed about discussing such matters with health professionals. After being admitted for observation, Ana began to complain of increased pains in her abdomen. After five days in the hospital, Ana hemorrhaged and lost her baby. At that time, she discovered that she had been tested for HIV and was seropositive. She returned home to a distraught and angry husband, who blamed the baby's death on her. She was beaten again and returned to the ER once more.

Ana's case illustrates one of the most troubling examples of the interface between healthcare and violence against women. With the longstanding lack of adequate and accessible prenatal care for poor women of color, pregnant women of color who are battered are especially vulnerable. Research indicates that 20 percent of all women who are battered experience the first incident during pregnancy. The situation for pregnant battered women is further complicated by the troubling legal trend to hold women accountable for any damage inflicted upon a fetus in utero. If a pregnant woman is battered and the fetus is harmed, she may be criminally liable for not leaving the abusive relationship. Not surprisingly, in most recent "fetal death" cases across the country, the women who are most severely punished are women of color.

As the healthcare system has labored under increased social and economical stress, specialized programs for women and for certain communities have also been curtailed. For battered women of color this trend has specific and dangerous affects. With a steady increase in immigrants from Central America, South America, and the Caribbean, battered women who do not have legal status in this country are destined to remain invisible and underserved. Because of their undocumented status and other significant barriers, (such as language and cultural differences), many battered women of color are denied assistance by the same organizations established to protect them, e.g., public welfare, legal advocacy, and health clinics. One battered women's program specifically targeted to serve Caribbean women and their children reports that battered women who must use hospital services for their injuries often have to borrow Medicaid cards from other women in order to conceal their undocumented status. Staff from this same program describe the difficulty that one undocumented woman had even getting out of the house, much less to the hospital, as her batterer was rightfully suspicious that reports of his criminal behavior would also jeopardize *his* illegal status.

Most hospital-based crisis intervention programs do not have multi-lingual or multi-cultural staff who are trained in and sensitive to the special issues of women of color. For example, reliance on translators to communicate with non-English speaking women effectively compromises the confidentiality and protection of battered women who are immigrants, from small ethnic communities, or who must use their own family members as translators to describe painful and private incidents of violence in the home. There are numerous stories of women of color receiving insensitive treatment by healthcare staff who attribute domestic violent to stereotypes such as "I've heard you Latins have hot tempers" or "Asian women are so passive, it really explains why they get beaten by their husbands."

Finally, if a battered woman of color is also a lesbian, differently abled, or from any other group that is already stigmatized, her access to quality care from health providers may be further compromised. One battered lesbian who was an African American described a physician who was continually incredulous about her claims that a "pretty girl like her" would be beaten by her female lover. In fact, she stopped going to the hospital for emergency attention, even though she had no other health insurance, because she was angry at such homophobic treatment and therefore became increasingly reluctant to use the services of that hospital.

As long as healthcare institutions continue to be the primary, and usually first, access points for battered women of color, we must require them to institute ongoing training, education, and specialized programs, and to hire culturally knowledgeable staff to address the particular needs of this special group of women.

The Response of Women of Color

Despite the philosophical and political contradictions and the practical barriers described in the previous sections, women of color have actively and creatively challenged the discriminatory, institutional practices of healthcare and crisis intervention services. Against extremely difficult economic, cultural, and political odds, battered women of color and their advocates have initiated a broad-based response to violence against women in communities of color. Aspects of this response will be summarized in the remainder of the chapter.

One of the most significant developments in response to domestic violence in communities of color has been the creation of grassroots crisis intervention services by and for women of color. The majority of these programs have been organized autonomously from white women, privileging the analysis and experience of women of color by assuming the cultural, historical, and linguistic norms of Asian/Pacific Island, Latin, African-American, Native-American and other nonwhite cultures. Typically located in neighborhoods and communities of color, these programs have a strong emphasis on community organization and public education. While many of these programs struggle for financial support and recognition from mainstream public health agencies and feminist organizations, they endure in great part because they are grounded in a community-based approach to problem solving.

The Violence Intervention Program for Latina women and their children in the community of East Harlem and the Asian Womens' Center in Chinatown are good examples of community-based programs in New York City. Refugee Women In Development (REFWID), in Washington, D. C., has a domestic violence component, as does Arco Iris, a retreat center for Native-American women and other women of color who have experienced violence in Arkansas. In Minnesota, women of color have created a statewide battered women's coalition called Black, Indian, Hispanic and Asian Women In Action (BIHA). In California, California Women Of Color Against Domestic Violence organizes and published a newsletter, "Out Loud," and women of color from seven southern states have created The Southeast Women Of Color Task Force Against Domestic Violence. Nationally, the members of the Women Of Color Task Force of the National Coalition Against Domestic Violence have provided national leadership training and technical assistance on the issues of battering and women of color, and their task force has served as a model for the development of programs for battered women of color across the country.

In addition to providing crisis intervention and emergency shelter services to battered women, these community-based programs and statewide coalitions for women of color are involved in raising the issue of battering within other contexts of social justice efforts. Representatives of grassroots battered women's programs are often in leadership roles on such issues as reproductive freedom, immigration policy, lesbian rights, criminal justice reform, homelessness, AIDS policy, and other issues that affect women of color. The National Black Women's Health Project in Atlanta is a good example of this.

Finally, in the past several years there has been a proliferation of literature on violence against women by scholars and activists who are women of color. Seal Press's New Leaf Series published Evelyn C. White's *Chain, Chain Change: For Black Women Dealing With Physical And Emotional Abuse* and Myrna Zambrano's *Mejor Sola Que Mal Acompanada.* Another good example of analysis by and for battered women of color is a publication by the Center For Domestic And Sexual Violence in Seattle, *The Speaking Profits Us: Violence Against Women Of Color,* a collection of papers edited by Mary Violet Burns. Kitchen Table, Women of Color Press in Albany, New York, has been a leader in publishing writing by women of color, addressing the issue of violence against women in the Freedom Organizing pamphlet series and in many other works.

By providing direct crisis intervention services, educating communities of color, advocating on broader feminist and social justice issues and publishing culturally relevant resources, Asian/Pacific Islanders, Latinas, Native-Americans, African Americans, Caribbeans, and other women of color have demonstrated a strong commitment to addressing violence against women. Our contributions have significantly enhanced both the conventional research on battered women and the progressive work of the battered women's movement, challenging the accepted analysis that violence against women has equivalent effects on all women. We must continue to develop community-based programs that are culturally relevant and responsive to the complexity of experiences faced by women of color, including inadequate healthcare, unemployment, homelessness, a failing educational system, and violence. Equally important, we must continue to work within our own cultures to challenge those traditions, assumptions, and values that reinforce male domination and ignore women's needs. In so doing, the struggle to end violence against women of color will include individual liberation as well as social reform. For us, the most compelling motivation for continuing this effort comes from the courage, commitment, and endurance that battered women of color have shown in their personal and collective struggles. On a daily basis they persist in defying the limits that violence, sexism, and racism impose on their lives. Our response must be to let their stories challenge and inspire us—women of color, battered women, white women, and men alike—to work actively to end individual and institutional violence against women.

NOTE

The women described in this essay are referred to anonymously or by pseudonyms to protect their safety and privacy. Their stories are both composites and individual accounts of women with whom the authors have worked.

REFERENCES

A list of references is available in the original source.

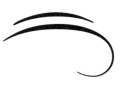

"Anishinabe Values/Social Laws Regarding Wife Battering"

from *Indigenous Woman*

In pre-reservation life, there were explicit social laws to deal with the rare occurrence of wife battering. The Ojibwe term used to identify a wife batterer is "Metattiggwa Ish" meaning "he who fights his wife always," implying that he is irrational, petty, and jealous. Once a man battered his wife, she was free to make him leave her lodge if they lived among her people. He'd leave her lodge and from then on be known as a man whose wife had broken the household because of abuse. From then on, he could never "marry" again. When a "married" woman was abused by her husband, her brothers were obligated by social law to retaliate against him by not speaking to him, beating him or even killing him. If the couple lived among the man's relatives, his parents were obligated to get her away and return her to her people.

In a situation in which a household had been broken because of abuse, it was not known as a divorced family as it is today. It was viewed as a broken household and the woman was viewed as having self-respect in leaving the destructive relationship behind. In a broken household, the sons could go with the father, the daughters with the mother.

A man who battered his wife was considered irrational and thus could no longer lead a war party, a hunt or participate in either. He could not be trusted to behave properly and thus may bring harm to the other men involved. The wife batterer could no longer own a pipe. If he somehow did, no one would smoke it with him. He was thought of as contrary to Anishinabe law and lost many privileges of life and many roles in Ojibwe society and the societies within.

A man who killed his wife was considered as not Ojibwe anymore. He had broken a primary law of Anishinabe Society, that is an Ojibwe NEVER kills another Ojibwe. He became an enemy of the people. His name would never be spoken again. He would cease to exist. The children of this household would be given to another family so they would not be known as coming from a man who did not exist, and so they would not be known as the offspring of such a person.

The People: "The Relatives Living Together"

In pre-reservation Ojibwe society beliefs such as the preceding were handed down by ALL the people to the coming generations. For a clan/group to live in unity and cooperation, it was necessary for all to live according to the same beliefs, laws, and values. When people living together do not share the same beliefs, laws and values, there will be confusion as to what is considered proper behavior; individuals will not have a foundation from which to guide their behavior.

Reservation Ojibwe Society

The perspective can be taken that the daily occurrence of wife battering among the Ojibwe people emerged as a result of the dissolution of traditional lifeways, including spirituality, the structures of government, laws, economics, relationships, values, beliefs, morals, and philosophy that were in place in the pre-reservation era, prior to the coming of the white man.

Wife battering, as we have seen, was neither accepted nor tolerated among the Anishinabe people until after the freedom to live Ojibwe was subdued. Wife battering emerged simultaneously with the disintegration of Ojibwe ways of life and the beginning use of alcohol. The behavior of the Ojibwe people under the influence of alcohol is often totally contrary to Anishinabe values. It is especially contrary to the self discipline previously necessary to the development of Ojibwe character.

There is no single philosophy among the people in today's society regarding the social illness of wife battering. Many have forgotten or DID NOT RECEIVE THE TEACHINGS of the social laws surrounding it. In the old Ojibwe society, society itself was responsible for what took place within it; today that is not so.

What is the evidence of that statement? The harmful, destructive, traumatic cycle of domestic violence that is befalling the Anishinabe Children of the Nation.

Today we have lost a lot of the traditions, values, ways of life, laws, language, teachings of the Elders, respect, humility as Anishinabe people because of the European mentality we have accepted. For the Anishinabe people to survive as a Nation, together we must turn back the pages of time. We must face reality, do an evaluation of ourselves as a people—why we were created to live in harmony with one another as Anishinabe people and to live in harmony with the Creator's creation.

Ruling the Exceptions
"Same-Sex Battering and Domestic Violence Theory"

by Gregory S. Merrill

Summary   This paper examines the challenges presented to current gender-based domestic violence theory by the existence of same-sex domestic violence. Charging that dominant theory is heterosexist and ignores the experience of battered lesbians and gay men, Island and Letellier have argued that domestic violence is not a gender issue and advocate a psychological framework that emphasizes batterer treatment. Examining the theoretical conflicts, this paper attempts to demonstrate that sociopolitical and psychological theories can be successfully integrated into a social-psychological model. Such a model, developed by Zemsky and Gilbert, Poorman, and Simmons, is explored and critiqued as an excellent beginning. By integrating psychological principles and sociological concepts, this theory explores the many dimensions of power and explains the phenomenon of domestic violence as it occurs in all relationship configurations. Suggestions for further theoretical considerations and research are made. *[Article copies available from The Haworth Document Delivery Service: 1-800-342-9678.]*

One would hope that this article could begin without the assertion and lengthy accompanying arguments that same-sex domestic violence is a serious problem. Most of the authors who have written about this phenomenon make explicit reference to the degree of resistance to accepting the frequency and severity of its occurrence. In addition to the outright refusal of the lesbian, gay, and bisexual communities to organize around this issue, current domestic violence theory contributes to denial of the problem by failing to recognize and explain same-sex domestic violence. In this paper, I will explore current theory, particularly the tension between feminist sociopolitical theory and the psychological theory proposed by gay male theorists Island and Letellier. I intend to demonstrate that the two theories are not mutually exclusive and can be meaningfully integrated into a social-psychological theory. This integrated theory, while in its early stage of development, has the potential to explain domestic violence as it occurs in all relationship configurations.

Overview of Current Feminist Sociopolitical Theory

To begin to understand the development of theory about domestic violence, we must examine the social and historical context in which it developed. Prior to the rise of the modern women's movement, the existing research and theories minimized domestic violence and, one way or another, blamed the victim. In the late 1960s and early 1970s, feminism flourishing in this country helped to change this minimization through its primary tenet, the personal is political. This tenet called upon women to examine the conditions of their lives, the roles assigned to them (and also made unavailable to them) in families, the workplace, and society in general, vis-à-vis men. Through consciousness-raising groups and efforts, women began to discover the many insidious ways by which they are made second-class citizens, subordinate to men. In particular, women who had experienced men's emotional, physical, and/or sexual abuse began to share their experiences with one another and, as a result, no longer saw battering as an individual problem. Women organized and politicized around the issue of domestic violence, defining it as a crime against women, and therefore, a women's issue.

Using the feminist lens, activists, researchers, and professionals devoted considerable energy to developing a feminist analysis of domestic violence. They determined that violence, the threat thereof, ascribed family roles, and limited economic opportunity acted together to further gender-based oppression. When looking for the root of domestic violence, feminists saw cultural misogyny and sexism. Del Martin convincingly argued that domestic violence is the logical, if brutal, extreme of sexist gender-role socialization. If a culture socializes its men to be brave, dominant, aggressive, and strong, and its women to be passive, placating, dependent, and obedient, and oppresses any attempts at androgyny or "transgendering," then that culture has effectively trained its men and women for bipolar abuser and victim roles, respectively. Men learn that it is permissible to use violence and that they are expected to be in charge of "their" women and children; women learn to accept that their role is one of a subordinate and a caretaker. According to this analysis, domestic violence is a gender-based phenomenon, a socially-based illness used as a tool of the patriarchy to keep women down.

Despite cultural sexism and the resistance of those who persist in believing that victims have some responsibility for the violence, this gender-based theory has become the most commonly accepted explanation for domestic violence among academicians, the domestic violence movement, and lay people. It has won widespread support because it coherently explains the phenomenon in a way which intuitively makes sense. While there is dissent, a substantial body of research supports feminist contentions. Coleman notes that most studies conducted about battering conclude that it is a significant problem that is almost always perpetrated by men against women.

While this theory is inarguably an important starting place, it leaves many questions unanswered and makes many experiences invisible. For example, as Island and Letellier point out, gender-based theory fails to explain why some heterosexual men batter their partners and others do not. Feminists of color also have argued legitimately that the theory does not reflect their experiences.[1]

With few exceptions, most authors have not attempted to integrate the phenomenon of same-sex partner abuse into feminist domestic violence theory. Indeed, it is not easy to do so without contributing to one of the four most popular misconceptions about same-sex partner abuse: (1) an outbreak of gay male domestic violence is logical (because all or most men are prone to violence), but lesbian domestic violence does not occur (because women are not); (2) same-sex partner abuse is not as severe as when a woman is battered by a man; (3) because the partners are of the same gender, it is mutual abuse, with each perpetrating and receiving "equally"; and (4) the perpetrator must be the "man" or the "butch" and the victim must be the "woman" or the "femme" in emulation of heterosexual relationships. Although the body of research on same-sex domestic violence is limited, Coleman, Kelly and Warshafsky, and Renzetti effectively confront and refute the above misconceptions.

Robert Geffner, editor of the *Family Violence and Sexual Assault Bulletin,* expresses a common sentiment when he makes the following statement: "We need to learn more about this [same-sex domestic] violence and be willing to modify our theories and programs to include these 'exceptions to the rule' ". Indeed, same-sex domestic violence, if viewed from the feminist lens, does seem like an exception. This is because sociopolitical theory alone does not fully or adequately explain why the same dynamic of abuse in heterosexual relationships occurs with as much frequency and severity in same-sex relationships.

Psychological Theory

Highly critical of the dominant feminist theory, Island and Letellier break with it altogether. First, they assert that it is heterosexist because it fails to acknowledge or explain the existence of same-sex partner abuse. Second, they make the controversial assertion that domestic violence is "*not* a gender issue." Island believes that sociopolitical theory has led to ineffective batterer treatment programs and that treatment must be based primarily, if not solely, on the personality and behavioral characteristics of the batterer. Sociopolitical theory, he argues, has over-focused on the experience of battered women and does not focus at all on or explain the source of the problem, that is, the psychology of perpetrators. As a result, Island and Letellier propose a gender-neutral theory of domestic violence which focuses on the psychology of the batterer. They provide batterer diagnostic criteria for the American Psychiatric Association to adopt and support its application to men and women of all sexual orientations. Essentially, Island and Letellier argue that the feminist lens should be replaced by a psychological lens and that batterers should be identified and classified by behavior, not gender.

While their objections are strong and have been controversial in the domestic violence movement, Island and Letellier have more in common with feminists than even they have acknowledged. They agree with the feminist analysis that victims are created by batterers, do not necessarily have pathology that led them to become victims, and are not necessarily in need of treatment (beyond counseling and advocacy to promote safety and to help manage the effects of the abuse). Interestingly, they also devote several pages to the discussion of masculinity as malignant, arguing that male batterers are unclear on the concept of masculinity, having equated it with violence. Finally, Island and Letellier note in the opening of their book that in heterosexual relationships where abuse is occurring, 95% of the perpetrators are male, citing statistics produced by New York's Office for Prevention of Domestic Violence. And yet, if their assertion that domestic violence is not a gender issue were true, one would assume that heterosexual domestic violence would be equally perpetrated by men and women. So, just as feminist theory alone does not fully explain same-sex domestic violence, the strictly psychological theory proposed by Island and Letellier fails to explain the disproportionate number of male perpetrators in heterosexual domestic violence.

Integrating a Social-Psychological Model

What I would like to suggest here is that domestic violence must be understood as both a social *and* a psychological phenomenon and must be examined under both lenses simultaneously in order to be completely understood. Feminist theory and psychological theory are not necessarily mutually exclusive and do not have to negate one another. In fact, if synthesized, they can enhance our vision. Viewing domestic violence through an integrated framework permits us to see that domestic violence is a gender issue; that heterosexual domestic violence is, in fact, primarily perpetrated by men against women. We also see that gender is only one of several determining social and psychological factors and that the absence of gender inequity, as in same-sex relationships, by no means precludes the possibility that battering will occur.

Zemsky, in conjunction with Gilbert, Poorman, and Simmons, proposes a social-psychological theory of lesbian battering which can be applied to heterosexual and gay male relationships as well. They separate the causation of battering into three categories: learning to abuse; having the opportunity to abuse; and choosing to abuse. The individual who abuses has first learned to abuse through a combination of three psychological processes, usually occurring in the family of origin: one, direct instruction; two, modeling or learning through observation; and three, operant conditioning, or learning by reinforcement that violence is effective and "rewarding." They also suggest that men might be especially prone to learning abuse because of sex-role socialization, but agree with Hart that women in our culture also learn and internalize relationship models that are based upon inequity.

According to Zemsky and Gilbert et al., learning to abuse does not necessarily lead individuals to enact abuse. For that to occur, they must also have the opportunity to abuse without suffering negative consequences. In other words, would-be abusive individuals must perceive that they can "get away with it." Because of the pervasiveness of cultural sexism, homophobia, racism, classism, antisemitism, ageism, and ableism, some groups are empowered with privileges at the expense of others. For the battered heterosexual woman, the cultural context of sexism and other oppressions which may affect her (such as racism in the instance of a woman of color), as enforced by friends, family members, hospital workers, mental health providers, and the criminal justice system, contribute to an environment in which her abusive partner can batter her without intervention or consequence. Likewise, homophobia, heterosexism, and other oppressions operate in the same way to isolate the battered person in a same-sex relationship, permitting the violence to continue. While the social phenomenon of prejudice does not cause battering, it does create an opportune environment that supports abusive behavior by its refusal to challenge it.

Zemsky uses an apt example to describe the roles of actual and perceived power relations in creating opportunity. She writes that it is unlikely that individuals who had learned to harass the people with whom they work would harass their supervisors because the potential consequence of being immediately fired would decrease the level of opportunity. To extend Zemsky's analysis, if these same people were the supervisors, they would, in fact, be likely to harass their employees, because they would probably believe they could get away with it. To extend this even further, while these same people may not harass their supervisors, they may harass a colleague, someone at their same level of employment. They would be particularly likely to do so if they believed the victim would be unlikely or unable to report it and/or if they believed such a report would not be taken seriously or responded to. Thus, according to this model, abuse against someone with perceived greater power and/or the perceived power to bring effective, negative consequences is unlikely to be expressed, whereas abuse against someone with perceived equal or lesser power and/or a perceived diminished capacity to bring such consequences would be a more ripe opportunity.

Lastly, Zemsky and Gilbert et al. emphasize that although the learning may have occurred and the opportunity might be present, abusive individuals make a conscious choice to abuse. Although many abusive people may not perceive it this way, they have the ability to make alternative choices (or at least to learn alternative choices) and are solely responsible for their violence.

In formulating this theory, the authors successfully integrate sociopolitical concepts and psychological principles and begin to explore their very complex relationship. For instance, the learning process they propose is explicitly psychological since it involves the individual internalizing beliefs and learning behaviors, and yet, Zemsky and Gilbert et al. acknowledge that what is internalized is most definitely shaped by social mores. Their analysis of opportunity is largely informed by feminism and an analysis of power which expands beyond gender, including racism, sexism, heterosexism, and other oppressions. They argue that the social environment, particularly the relation of power and the ability to bring consequences, impacts how the potentially abusive person behaves. And yet they posit that this is not purely sociological either, because as important as the actual power relation is, the abusers' *perception* of the power relation and their *perception* of the partner's capacity to enact consequences (which can be distorted and different from the actual) are also important in explaining battering. Zemsky and Gilbert et al. close their model by promoting a psychological healing model, emphasizing abusers' complete responsibility for their behavior.

This social-psychological theory adequately explains why men predominantly perpetrate heterosexual domestic violence and why women are less likely to perpetrate. Heterosexual men who have learned to batter live in a culture which systematically devalues, discriminates against, and exploits women. In effect, misogyny and sexism increase the opportunity for heterosexual men to batter their female partners without receiving negative consequences. As a result, it is likely that these men would choose to batter. By contrast, heterosexual women who have learned to batter are not as likely to express abuse toward their male partners because their partners generally have more perceived and actual social power and the accompanying access to punish them. Instead, a heterosexual woman who batters might choose to express her abuse toward her children, siblings, elderly parents, or others whom she perceives to have lesser or equal social power and/or a diminished capacity to enact negative consequences against her.

Social-psychological theory also explains the existence of same-sex domestic violence by acknowledging the role of homophobia and by positing that the opportunity for abuse of power can exist not only when recipients have less social power, but also when they have roughly equal social power. This phenomenon of lateral abuse is especially likely to occur in circumstances in which the potential victim is perceived to be unwilling or unlikely to report, and/or in which the abuser believes reporting will have no effect. Like their heterosexual counterparts, same-sex abusers learn to abuse. Homophobia helps to create the opportunity for abuse without consequences by isolating the victims and preventing them access to resources such as their family, appropriate social services, and the criminal justice and legal systems. As a result, battered lesbians and gay men are unlikely to seek assistance, and even if they do, are not likely to be helped. In such a climate of opportunity, it is not surprising that lesbian and gay abusive persons are as likely to express abuse toward their partners as are their heterosexual male counterparts.

The Explanatory Power of a Social-Psychological Model

One challenge to social-psychological theory is its ability to explain exceptions. How does this theory hold up if asked to explain the existence of domestic violence perpetrated against someone who has more power than the perpetrator? Specifically, how does this theory explain the occasional incidence of men who are battered by their female partners? Although most people know that a small minority of men are battered by women, this question and the challenge it poses to theory is rarely addressed. One answer might be that abusive heterosexual women only batter their partners in instances where they have or perceive themselves as having more social power, either economically, racially, or along other dimensions, and/or perceive their partners as being unwilling or unable to enact negative consequences against them.

While this explanation is plausible and remains within the framework of the theory, I believe we also need to add to our analysis a variable that is primarily psychological, the degree of severity of the batterer.[2] Those of us who work with victims and/or batterers know that some batterers will draw the line at pushing or milder forms of abuse while others will stop at nothing, the difference based largely upon their capacity for impulse control. I posit here that the more severe the degree of severity of the batterer, the more likely the batterers are to choose to abuse, regardless of the level of opportunity. For instance, a heterosexual woman who is a "severe" batterer with little impulse control might be likely to abuse her male partner, even though he has more perceived and actual power and can enact negative consequences against her. Because of the cycle of violence in which the abuse escalates over time, the degree of severity might change across time and situations, making it difficult to measure. Other complex variables which influence degree of severity and make it difficult to measure include batterers' own shifting perceptions of being powerless and of not perceiving themselves as having resolution options other than violence.[3] Future work should develop the concept of degree of batterer severity and an appropriate measure, not only because of its explanatory value, but also for its important to treatment considerstions.[4]

I also believe domestic violence theory could benefit from further analysis of power. To date, the analysis of social power, as endowed or denied on the basis of gender, race, sexual orientation, and so on has been extensively explored and is useful. By contrast, the concept of psychological or personal power, referring to a person's ability to access the social and other resources available to him or her has not been adequately explored. Just as some of my clients are physically stronger than their abusive partners and could overpower them if they chose to, some of my clients are also professional gay men who have significantly more social power, and the access it affords them, than their abusers. However, because they have been manipulated emotionally by guilt, shame, fear, attacks upon their self-esteem, a distorted sense of responsibility and other complex psychological tactics frequently employed by batterers, many have been rendered powerless to use resources that are available to them. These cases demonstrate that individuals with greater physical or social power who do not have, or have been robbed of, their sense of personal power can be dominated by an abusive person with less actual power. In other words, the experiences of same-sex domestic violence victims teach us that domestic violence is not always necessarily about the abuser having more physical or social power, but is also about their willingness to use whatever tools and tactics they may have to subordinate their partner. Further attention to this less evident type of psychological or personal power, which

is certainly related to self-esteem, will add a new, psychological dimension, strengthening the theory's ability to account for what otherwise might be considered "exceptions to the rule."

Conclusion

To conclude, this paper argues that in order for domestic violence theory to be comprehensive, it must account for both sociopolitical and psychological dynamics, and their complex, often intertwined relationship. A social-psychological model proposed by Zemsky and Gilbert et al. was discussed as an excellent starting place, and suggestions for future analysis, especially for measuring the degree of severity of the batterer and developing the concept of personal power, were made. As all theories must be tested, researchers are challenged to design tools for assessment and studies which will support or refute a social-psychological model and contribute to our understanding.

For those who strategize to stop domestic violence, the challenge is to devote ourselves to changing the social context so as to reduce the opportunities for abuse, including confronting oppressions, developing culturally-appropriate prevention and early intervention programs, and improving the legal system for all battered individuals, as well as developing a body of knowledge about the psychology of batterers that will aid individual, psychological intervention. If domestic violence is caused by both social and psychological factors, then viable solutions must address both. Finally, researchers are challenged to develop theories based upon behavior rather than upon social identity, theories which explain phenomena for every group that experiences it, not only the majority group. While these theories should not be identity-based, they also should not be blind to the very real impact of identity-based social oppression. These, indeed, are challenges to us all.

NOTES

1. A colleague of mine, Cara Page, instructed me in a feminist of color critique of domestic violence theory for which I am sincerely grateful. As Ms. Page brought to my attention, the feminist theory I have summarized here is predominately white feminist theory and does not reflect the valuable contributions of feminist of color. And yet I chose to represent it this way, exclusionary as it may be, because this is the most dominant form of the theory and the one most commonly subscribed. There is much to be gained from advocates for battered women of color and for battered lesbians and gay men of all colors working together to expand the current theoretical lens. To familiarize yourself with relevant feminist of color writings, see *Home girls: A black feminist anthology,* edited by Barbara Smith; *This bridge called my back,* edited by Cherrie

Moraga and Gloria Anzaldua; *Mejor sola que acompanada: Para la mujer golpeada: For the Latina in an abusive relationship* by Myrna Zambrano; *Chain chain change: For black woman dealing with physical and emotional abuse* by Evelyn White and others.

2. The concept *degree of severity of the batterer* assumes that batterers can be placed along a continuum of mild to severe depending upon their capacity for impulse control and the severity of violence used. This concept helps us to distinguish between batterers who have a higher degree of control over their impulses and use "milder" forms of abusive behavior and batterers who have little or no impulse control and regularly use severe, life-threatening forms of

violence. I use the words "mild" and "milder" only to provide contrast between degrees of severity, not to suggest that domestic violence in any form, mild or severe, is minor.

3. Thank you to Beth Zemsky for raising this point in her critique of this paper.

4. Further attention to this concept, while crucial, is beyond the scope of this paper and the author's current level of expertise.

REFERENCES
A list of reference is available in the original source.

Trans and Intersex Survivors of Domestic Violence
"Defining Terms, Barriers, and Responsibilities"

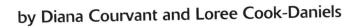

by Diana Courvant and Loree Cook-Daniels

In the early 1970's, as campaigns to raise awareness of domestic violence were first beginning in the United Kingdom and the United States, domestic violence was seen as a problem of male batterers and female survivors. Although this model still fits the vast majority of cases of domestic violence, it is no longer seen as fully describing the problem. In the 1980's, recognition spread of battering in lesbian relationships, and in the 1990's gay men awakened to battering within their own community. Therefore, over the course of the 25 years of the domestic violence survivors' movement, many communities have evolved programs to assist in meeting the needs of both male and female survivors, and developed intervention programs targeted to male and to female batterers. Within this framework, some few heterosexual men have also received survivor services.

However, even this expanded framework consistently neglects the growing class of survivors who transcend stereotypes of gender expression or physical sex. If these survivors have any interaction at all with supportive agencies, they nearly always confront staff or volunteers who lack even the necessary vocabulary to begin to un-

derstand the every day experience of these survivors. So let's begin with that vocabulary.

Defining Terms

Like the water surrounding the proverbial fish oblivious to it, all the various aspects of gender are invisible to most of us. Virtually all of us were given a *gender assignment*—boy or girl—by medical personnel at our birth, based on a visual inspection of our genitals (by using the genitals, doctors hope to match the gender assignment with the child's sex, the genetic or anatomical categories of male and female). Most of us grew into these gender assignments fairly smoothly, adopting them as our own *gender identity:* our personal view of our own gender. *Gender attribution* recognizes that what I think of myself isn't always what counts; this term refers to what someone assumes about my gender when they look at me. On the opposite side of the observer-observed dyad is *gender expression*. This is something I do (a behavior, the choice of clothing, etc.) that influences or is intended to influence another's perception of my gender. A *gender role* is the aggregate of a society's assumptions, expectations and mores for how a person of a particular gender is supposed to act. All of these terms are more likely to be heard in a therapist's office than a shelter, but knowing them can help one understand the complexities facing those who transcend stereotypes of gender expression or physical sex: those who are usually known as intersexual, transsexual, transvestite or cross-dressing, or transgendered persons.

An *intersex* or *intersexual* person has a body with external sexual characteristics typical of both male and female bodies. Nonetheless, in our society, children who are born intersexual are nearly always assigned a male or female gender role, although because of external sexual ambiguities, that assignment may not occur at birth. Intersexual children in the United States typically have their genitals surgically altered before age three to conform to gender assignment.

A *transsexual* is someone who lives full-time in the gender identity "opposite" the gender assignment they were given at birth. Currently in Western European and North American countries, transsexuals usually obtain medical intervention (hormones and surgeries) to alter their bodies to more closely conform physically to their gender identity. Some cultures have roles or institutions that allow what we would call transsexuals to live in their preferred gender identify, often without requiring them to seek medical intervention. Transsexuals may be either female-to-male (FtM) or male-to-female (MtF). They may be "post-operative" or "post-op," meaning they've had one or more surgeries to alter their body's sexual characteristics; "pre-op," meaning they have not yet had any or all such surgeries; or "non-op," a term that acknowledges that some transsexuals feel they can live out their gender identify without altering their bodies surgically.

Unlike transsexuals, *transvestites'* and *cross-dressers'* gender assignment and gender identity match. However, they occasionally wear clothes that social custom says belong to the "opposite" gender role. While crossdressed, an individual might take on a name and/or mannerisms associated with that "opposite" gender role, although this is not always the case.

Transgender is a recently-coined term whose definition is still in some flux. Some people use it to refer to people who don't fit any of the above categories but whose gender identity also won't fit into the society's two given roles of male or female. Others include transsexuals and transvestites under the transgender, or *trans,* umbrella. For the remainder of this paper, this larger definition will be used.

Trans and Intersex Survivors

In preliminary data, the Gender, Violence, and Resource Access Survey of trans and intersex individuals found 50% of respondents had been raped or assaulted by a romantic partner, though only 62% of those raped or assaulted (31% of the total sample) identified themselves as survivors of domestic violence when explicitly asked. Of those who were raped or injured, 23% (12% of the total sample) required medical attention for injuries inflicted by a romantic partner. All of those who received treatment self-identified as survivors of domestic violence when asked.

Clearly, trans and intersex survivors exist. Like other domestic violence survivors, they need the help of service agencies, including shelters, to free themselves from abusive partners and to learn to recognize future abusive relationships before the abuse becomes extreme. Unfortunately, few ever manage to access these services openly. There are many reasons why so few trans and intersex survivors are served by the community that typically aids and advocates for survivors of domestic violence. The next section will discuss these barriers.

Barriers

Despite feminist strides, ours is still not a society that supports and rewards individuals who violate gender norms. Little boys are still kept in line with phrases like, "Don't be a sissy." Little girls and particularly older girls face fierce disapproval if they behave or dress too "boyishly." This early punishment for simply expressing gender identity leaves many scars, but the experiences that lead trans and intersexual domestic violence survivors to believe that it's normal for "people like me" to live with abuse only increase in magnitude as the trans or intersex survivor matures.

Perhaps the most damaging force is the one that teaches transgender and intersexual persons that "helping" institutions are often anything but, and may actually harm them. In Washington D.C., an MtF trans woman named Tyra Hunter, the victim of an accident, was allowed to die by paramedics and emergency room staff who discovered her trans status, then decided to mock her rather than provide aid. In the central United States, an FtM trans man named Brandon Teena was raped by two men who discovered his trans status. Upon reporting the rape to the local sheriff's department, the sheriff asked Brandon, "What are you?" and refused to investigate. Brandon's rapists returned to his house to kill him and two of his friends for reporting the rape. At an annual convention of the Society for the Scientific Study of Sexuality one doctor related the case of a girl child with a large clitoris sexually mutilated by her father, who was angered at the phallic proportions of his infant daughter's clitoris. Amazingly, this doctor completed the child's mutilation by performing a clitoridectomy and was using her story to justify surgery on infants in similar situations, rather than healing the child and calling attention to her abuse. Although these stories' power is anecdotal and not statistical, they and others like them are widely known and retold among trans and intersex individuals. Because of the extreme cruelty and casual indifference of authorities and institutions exemplified in these common stories, a trans or intersex survivor may fear an unknown service institution more than a familiar abuser.

A second level of fear trans and intersex survivors face when seeking help is the possibility that their trans or intersex status, if previously hidden, might become known and expose them to more violence, as in the Brandon Teena case. Exposure might also lead to the loss of a job, as very few jurisdictions provide employment discrimination protection to trans and intersexed persons, and stories of job loss or workplace harassment upon exposure are legion.

Should a trans or intersex survivor decide to brave these risks and seek help despite them, she or he faces other barriers. Some information suggests that trans and intersex survivors have frequently been multiply abused for years or decades. Often a trans or intersex survivor has a unique body and/or a unique vulnerability to the emotional aftermath of sexual violence; either can make difficult or impossible discussing this abuse with an unfamiliar victims' advocate.

Related to this problem is the shame and self-doubt that is endemic in these communities, due to the pressures trans and intersex persons have felt from their earliest years to deny their feelings and conform to others' expectations. Adding to this shame and self-doubt is the widespread perception that trans and intersex individuals are mentally ill. This popular stigma of mental illness is furthered by the existence of Gender Identity Disorder (GID) in the DSM-IV, the guidebook to diagnosis of mental illness and personality disorders, but this perception of mental illness is independent of the DSM-IV and is often strongly felt by those completely unfamiliar with the GID diagnosis. Abusers use this shame and self-doubt against their trans and intersex victims to undermine their victims' perceptions and to convince them that no one else will want them. Combined with stories of dating violence (such as that of Chanelle Picket, an MtF trans woman who was recently murdered by a date enraged at the revelation of her trans status) these "warnings" can convince trans and intersex survivors that they are lucky just to have a partner who doesn't kill them.

Finally, two other barriers that affect some trans and intersex survivors deserve attention. One is the barrier that children present. Although every domestic violence survivor with children worries about the safety and custody of those children, the problem is much greater for trans parents, who know that because of prejudice and ignorance about trans persons, courts are extremely unlikely to grant them custody no matter how abusive the other parent is.

The other barrier is the gender segregation of survivor services. Virtually all trans survivors go through a significant period when they are in legal or medical transition. Some intersex survivors have a unique body that prevents identification with either a male or a female gender. Some trans individuals, including such notable examples as authors Kate Bornstein and Leslie Feinberg, have a gender identity and gender expression that is neither male nor female, but mixes elements of both. For all of these people, turning to a gender-segregated service agency may be inconceivable.

Barriers Specific to MtF Individuals

For those MtF individuals not raised in abusive homes, childhood social education rarely includes any information about domestic violence. An MtF child whose parents are disturbed by the child's femininity may glorify violence or minimize the child's trauma from any peer violence in an attempt to encourage behaviour deemed masculine. As an adult survivor, this may be translated into feelings of guilt for not fighting back in violent situations, reinforcing the common perspective of survivors that they are responsible for their own abuse.

The vast majority of resources for survivors of domestic violence targets women. While this benefits the few MtF individuals who have completed medical, legal and social transitions, it typically excludes the majority. Unfortunately, the few who do have resources nominally available often find themselves feared as invaders if they attempt to access women-based services. In San Francisco, one shelter that had made the decision to welcome openly trans women experienced a case where such a survivor was turned away by a shelter supervisor hired after the initial training. Other MtF survivors may refuse to seek shelter or assistance from women-centered agencies out of a respect for the fears or discomfort of non-trans and non-intersex female survivors. Others may avoid seeking help from those agencies out of low self-esteem or feelings that others will not perceive them as "real" women.

Lastly, MtF survivors battered by women often fear that their stories will not be believed. The existing dominant framework of domestic violence can make this type of violence among the most unexpected. Often it is difficult for survivors' advocates to envision this abuse even though the advocates know that the most important tools for control an abuser possesses are not physical.

Barriers Specific to FtM Individuals

Because their gender identity (and probably also their gender expression) is male, FtM individuals cannot be served by agencies that only serve women. Even if an FtM is lucky enough to be in a place where survivor services are offered to men, he may find himself facing incredulous "helpers." Although many people have heard of Christine Jorgenson or Renee Richards, few realize that FtM's exist. FtM's are so "invisible" that even professionals who are well-versed in trans issues often are surprised at the community's growing contention that there are roughly equal numbers of FtM's and MtF's. An FtM survivor may also hesitate to access services for men out of fear that the other survivors may discover his trans status and ridicule him or worse.

Many FtM's lived within the Lesbian community prior to their transition, and oftentimes their partners still identify as Lesbian and keep ties to that community. Since Lesbian communities are often tightly-interwoven and heavily involved in anti-domestic violence work, an FtM battered by a female partner may well fear that if he seeks help the battery may become public, he will not be believed and/or advocates and community members will side with his partner's version of events. This close interplay between domestic violence workers and an FtM survivor's and/or Lesbian batterer's social network may also heighten an FtM's fears that accessing services will lead to public discussion of his trans status, thus exposing him to the discrimination and violence discussed above.

Barriers Specific to Intersex Individuals

Intersex children are often subjected to multiple genital surgeries in order to ensure that outward shape matches, as closely as possible, a cultural esthetic ideal. Typically, these children are not explained the reasons for these procedures and are made to feel that they have (or, indeed, are) an embarrassing secret. Since doctors still perform these surgeries with a primary goal of preventing psychological stress in the parents, it is not surprising that these children are rarely told the truth: that doctors fear their own parents will hate their bodies enough to mutilate them. It is also not surprising that many of them feel horribly ashamed.

When these children are given reasons for these surgeries and other procedures, they are frequently told that the treatment is necessary if the child wants to be loved as an adult. This message is a brutal double-edged sword: first, it tells the child that people will love or reject them based on their body. Second, it directly states that the child is physically inadequate to be loved. The intermittent affection of honeymoon periods mixed with violent explosions may seem the most loving a relationship for which an intersex adult can hope, if raised with these expectations.

As significant as these other barriers can be, invisibility is by far the most significant barrier. Few even are aware of the existence of intersex individuals in our communities. Large, governmental helping agencies that serve tens of thousands of clients each year may never have heard the word "intersex", much less be aware of a single individual case involving an intersex survivor. This ignorance exists despite the fact that intersexuality and surgical treatment of it in infants is much more common than surgical sex reassignment in adults. When an agency is made aware of intersexuality in a survivor, it may not consider that a factor worthy of special notice or attention. This flies in the face of the motivation for surgical alteration of intersex children: doctors repeatedly state that intersex individuals are at vastly heightened risk of abuse. Even after the May, 1997 breakthrough of this issue to the pages of prominent publications such as *The New York Times* and *Newsweek,* helping agencies have not heard this message, and intersex survivors—both adults and children—are nearly always forced to heal from their abuse alone.

Defining Responsibilities

Because trans and intersex individuals are victims of abuse, and because our society is complicit in creating conditions which perpetuate this abuse, we who have dedicated ourselves to helping survivors of domestic violence must include trans and intersex survivors as a part of that mission. Although the trans and intersex communities, where organized, can provide support to these individuals, we are the ones with domestic violence expertise and should retain primary responsibility for ensuring our services are accessible and responsive to these survivors.

Including trans and intersex survivors within our current mission entails three primary responsibilities. First, we must make certain that every community has a visible place to which survivors may turn, regardless of trans or intersex status. Second, we must not revictimize trans or intersex survivors. Third, we must follow up on our own efforts or referrals in order to ensure that our efforts are positive and effective. Fulfilling these responsibilities (they are never discharged) cannot be a passive resolution. Concrete action is required. An agency can begin by taking these steps:

- At minimum, every staff member and volunteer who works with survivors must be made aware that trans and intersex survivors exist and that the agency is committed to working on their behalf. This is the first step in ensuring that the cardinal rule of domestic violence assistance is implemented for trans and intersex survivors: welcome them, and believe their stories.

- If there are any organized trans or intersex communities in your area, contact them to make sure they know you exist and are prepared to at least counsel any of their members with a domestic violence problem. If possible, establish formal or informal training and consultation procedures with these groups to share expertise and promote referrals. These groups can also help you conduct outreach campaigns to trans and intersex persons.

- If you are the sole service provider in the community, ensure at least one staff member is trained in the unique barriers that trans or intersex survivors face and is empowered to anticipate and remove your agency's barriers to sensitively serving such survivors.

- If your area has multiple providers, use or develop a coalition to determine which agencies in each community will be responsible for providing which services. In larger communities, it may even be possible to define subsections of the trans and intersex communities and assign responsibility for serving each group to a different agency, if care is taken to ensure that no one "between the cracks" is left without options. Agencies in contact with survivors can then be made aware of where survivors should be referred and what questions must be answered before a proper referral can be made.

- This coalition should also publicly identify at least one specific resource that is openly welcoming of trans or intersex survivors. This resource might be an already existing hotline, or a separate

number might be created either using regularly checked voice mail or automatic forwarding to an existing hotline or agency. Making a point of advertising the availability of this service tells frightened trans and intersex survivors that what they are experiencing is abuse and that other people feel they deserve better, a concept they may find more novel and life-changing than do many "more typical" domestic violence survivors.

- Once services are prepared to serve trans and intersex survivors, create a strategy of outreach to such survivors, including the addition of information about community resources for these survivors on written outreach materials targeting other communities.

- Finally, create a mechanism to follow up on referrals to other agencies and to make changes to coalition plans as new barriers or problems are identified.

Conclusion

Many of the barriers trans and intersex survivors face when trying to free themselves of domestic abuse are similar to those faced by all survivors: self-doubt, a belief that the known abuse is better than potential future unknown abuse, worry about the children and worry about finances. But because they have had to struggle to find pride in bodies and lives society labels "wrong" and because discrimination against them is so strong, trans and intersex survivors have many more hurdles to leap. One of these hurdles the domestic violence system itself created: a gender-segregated service system. We owe these survivors much more thought and effort to ensure that we do not either force them to stay in the hands of their abusers or revictimize them once they take that first step away.

RESOURCES

For more information about trans or intersex survivors, or for assistance in formulating policies or training staff and volunteers, contact the Survivor Project at: www .survivorproject.org

"Sexual Terrorism"

by Carole J. Sheffield

The right of men to control the female body is a cornerstone of patriarchy. It is expressed by their efforts to control pregnancy and childbirth and to define female healthcare in general. Male opposition to abortion is rooted in opposition to female autonomy. Violence and the threat of violence against females represent the need of patriarchy to deny that a woman's body is her own property and that no one should have access to it without her consent. Violence and its corollary, fear, serve to terrorize females and to maintain the patriarchal definition of woman's place.

The word *terrorism* invokes images of furtive organizations of the far right or left, whose members blow up buildings and cars, hijack airplanes, and murder innocent people in some country other than ours. But there is a different kind of terrorism, one that so pervades our culture that we have learned to live with it as though it were the natural order of things. Its targets are females—of all ages, races, and classes. It is the common characteristic of rape, wife battery, incest, pornography, harassment, and all forms of sexual violence. I call it *sexual terrorism* because it is a system by which males frighten and, by frightening, control and dominate females.

The concept of terrorism captured my attention in an "ordinary" event. One afternoon I collected my laundry and went to a nearby laundromat. The place is located in a small shopping center on a very busy highway. After I had loaded and started the machines, I became acutely aware of my environment. It was just after 6:00 p.m. and dark; the other stores were closed; the laundromat was brightly lit; and my car was the only one in the lot. Anyone passing by could readily see that I was alone and isolated. Knowing that rape is a crime of opportunity, I became terrified. I wanted to leave and find a laundromat that was busier, but my clothes were well into the wash cycle, and besides, I felt I was being "silly," "paranoid." The feeling of terror persisted, so I sat in my car, windows up, and doors locked. When the wash was completed, I dashed in, threw the clothes into the dryer, and ran back out to my car. When the clothes were dry, I tossed them recklessly into the basket and hurriedly drove away to fold them in the security of my home.

Although I was not victimized in a direct, physical way or by objective or measurable standards, I felt victimized. It was, for me, a terrifying experience. I felt controlled by an invisible force. I was angry that something as commonplace as doing laundry after a day's work jeopardized my well-being. Mostly I was angry at being unfree: a hostage of a culture that, for the most part, encourages violence against females, instructs men in the methodology of sexual violence, and provides them with ready justification for their violence. I was angry that I could be victimized by being "in the wrong place at the wrong time." The essence of terrorism is that one never knows when is the wrong time and where is the wrong place.

Following my experience at the laundromat, I talked with my students about terrorization. Women students began to open up and reveal terrors that they had kept secret because of embarrassment: fears of jogging alone, dining alone, going to the movies alone. One woman recalled feelings of terror in her adolescence when she did child care for extra money. Nothing had ever happened and she had not been afraid of anyone in particular, but she had felt a vague terror when being driven home late at night by the man of the house.

The men listened incredulously and then demanded equal time. The harder they tried the more they realized how very different—qualitatively, quantitatively, and contextually—their fears were. All agreed that, while they experience fear in a violent society, they did not experience terror; nor did they experience fear of rape or sexual mutilation. They felt more in control, either from a psychophysical sense of security that they could defend themselves or from a confidence in being able to determine wrong places and times. All the women admitted fear and anxiety when walking to their cars on the campus, especially after an evening class or activity. None of the men experience fear on campus at any time. The men could be rather specific in describing when they were afraid: in Harlem, for example, or in certain parts of downtown Paterson, New Jersey—places that have a reputation for violence. But these places could either be avoided or, if not, the men felt capable of self-protective

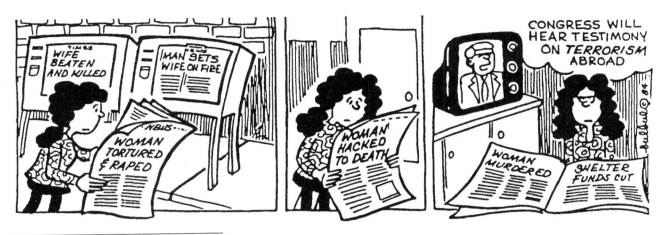

Reprinted with permission from bulbul, Feminist Connection, Madison, WI. December, 1984.

action. Above all, male students said that they *never* feared being attacked simply because they were male. They *never* feared going to a movie or to dinner alone. Their daily activities were not characterized by a concern for their physical integrity.

As I read the literature on terrorism it became clear that both sexual violence and nonviolent sexual intimidation could be better understood as terrorism. For example, although an act of rape, an unnecessary hysterectomy, and the publishing of *Playboy* magazine appear to be quite different, they are in fact more similar than dissimilar. Each is based on fear, hostility, and a need to dominate women. Rape is an act of aggression and possession, not of sexuality. Unnecessary hysterectomies are extraordinary abuses of power rooted in man's concept of woman as primarily a reproductive being and in his need to assert power over reproduction. *Playboy*, like all forms of pornography, attempts to control women through the power of definition. Male pornographers define women's sexuality for their male customers. The basis of pornography is men's fantasies about women's sexuality.

Components of Sexual Terrorism

The literature on terrorism does not provide a precise definition.[1] Mine is taken from Hacker, who says that "terrorism aims to frighten, and by frightening, to dominate and control."[2] Writers agree more readily on the characteristics and functions of terrorism than on a definition. This analysis will focus on five components to illuminate the similarities of and distinctions between sexual terrorism and political terrorism. The five components are: ideology, propaganda, indiscriminate and amoral violence, voluntary compliance, and society's perception of the terrorist and the terrorized.

An *ideology* is an integrated set of beliefs about the world that explains the way things are and provides a vision of how they ought to be. Patriarchy, meaning the "rule of the fathers," is the ideological foundation of sexism in our society. It asserts the superiority of males and the inferiority of females. It also provides the rationale for sexual terrorism. The taproot of patriarchy is the masculine/warrior ideal. Masculinity must include not only a proclivity for violence but also all those characteristics necessary for survival: aggression, control, emotional reserve, rationality, sexual potency, etc. Marc Feigen Fasteau, in *The Male Machine*, argues that "men are brought up with the idea that there ought to be some part of them, under control until released by necessity, that thrives on violence. This capacity, even affinity, for violence, lurking beneath the surface of every real man, is supposed to represent the primal untamed base of masculinity."[3]

Propaganda is the methodical dissemination of information for the purpose of promoting a particular ideology. Propaganda, by definition, is biased or even false information. Its purpose is to present one point of view on a subject and to discredit opposing points of view. Propaganda is essential to the conduct of terrorism. According to Francis Watson, in *Political Terrorism: The Threat and the Response*, "Terrorism must not be defined only in terms of violence, but also in terms of propaganda. The two are in operation together. Violence of terrorism is a coercive means for attempting to influence the thinking and actions of people. Propaganda is a persuasive means for doing the same thing."[4] The propaganda of sexual terrorism is found in all expressions of the popular culture: films, television, music, literature, advertising, pornography. The propaganda of sexual terrorism is also found in the ideas of patriarchy expressed in science, medicine, and psychology.

The third component, which is common to all forms of political terrorism, consists of "indiscriminateness, unpredictability, arbitrariness, ruthless destructiveness and amorality."[5] Indiscriminate violence and amorality are also at the heart of sexual terrorism. Every female is a potential target of violence—at any age, at any time, in any place. In her study of rape, Susan Brown-miller argues that rape is "nothing more or less than a conscious process of intimidation by which all men keep all women in a state of fear."[6] Further, as we shall see, amorality pervades sexual violence. Child molesters, incestuous fathers, wife beaters, and rapists often do not understand that they have done anything wrong. Their views are routinely shared by police officers, lawyers, and judges, and crimes of sexual violence are rarely punished in American society.

The fourth component of the theory of terrorism is "voluntary compliance." The institutionalization of a system of terror requires the development of mechanisms other than sustained violence to achieve its goals. Violence must be employed to maintain terrorism, but sustained violence can be costly and debilitating. Therefore, strategies for ensuring a significant degree of voluntary compliance must be developed. Sexual terrorism is maintained to a great extent by an elaborate system of sex-role socialization that in effect instructs men to be terrorists in the name of masculinity and women to be victims in the name of femininity.

Sexual and political terrorism differ in the final component, perception of the terrorist and the victim. In political terrorism we know who is the terrorist and who is the victim. We may condemn or condone the terrorist depending on our political views, but we sympathize with the victim. In sexual terrorism, however, we blame the victim and excuse the offender. We believe that the offender either is "sick" and therefore in need of our compassion or is acting out normal male impulses. . . .

Conclusion

Sexual terrorism is a system that functions to maintain male supremacy through actual and implied violence. Violence against the female body (rape, battery, incest, and harassment) and the perpetuation of fear of violence form the basis of patriarchal power. Both violence and fear are functional. Without the power to intimidate and to punish, the domination of women in all spheres of society—political, social, and economic—could not exist.

REFERENCES
A list of references is available in the original source.

Women's Use of Force
"Complexities and Challenges of Taking the Issue Seriously"
by Nancy Worcester

This article discusses the complexities, challenges, and urgency surrounding addressing women's use of force. The author emphasizes that women's and girls' use of force needs to be analyzed using a framework that keeps power and control central to the definition of domestic violence and identifies that violence by men and women takes place within a social, historical, and economic context in which men's and women's roles, opportunities, and social power differ. The article builds on an understanding of women's use of force in heterosexual relationships; however, a similar contextual analysis is also applied to women's use of force in teen dating relationships, lesbian relationships, and against children.

Many people are paying enormous attention to the issues of girls' and women's violence. More women are being arrested for assaulting their partners. Many domestic violence programs are making difficult decisions about whether to run "abuser" groups for arrested women or whether women arrested for fight-

"Women's Use of Force: Complexities and Challenges of Taking the Issue Seriously" by Nancy Worcester, *Violence Against Women*, Vol. 6, No. 11, November 2002.

ing back are more appropriately served by being in support groups for battered women.

The antifeminist backlash picks up on "conflict tactics"-type studies or the anti-domestic violence movement's own work to give visibility to lesbian violence in order to promote the idea that women are as violent as men. In most audiences, someone knows one man who has been hurt by an intimate partner and his story must be told. Many well-meaning professionals who have chosen to devote their lives to humanitarian service work pride themselves on publicly demonstrating that their services are equally available to men and women without the information, training, or professional support to develop an analysis of the limitations and dangers of a gender-neutral approach to antiviolence work.

This article examines some of the complexities, challenges, and urgency of reintegrating a gender analysis into violence work and addressing the issue of women using force[1] in ways that build on more than 25 years of work by some of the best thinkers and organizers addressing difficult issues within the battered women's movement. This article particularly draws on my experiences of working with the Education and Emerging Issues Committee of the Wisconsin Coalition Against Domestic Violence to encourage dialogue on the issue through a series of conference presentations, a 1-day membership meeting, think tanks, a special newsletter on this issue, and hours and hours of discussion. The article also builds on my many years of working within the battered women's movement, collaborating with others to ensure that the movement addresses challenging, cutting edge issues. I welcome the wider readership of this journal and encourage readers to explore how debates around the issue of women and girls using force can help set the agenda for the next decade of antiviolence research and activism.

Core issues of power and control and the context of violence need to be central to discussions and policies regarding domestic violence and battering and women's use of force. Violence by men or women and violence against men or women take place within a social, historical, and economic context in which men and women, in general, still play different roles, have different opportunities, and have different social power. Thus, it is important that violence is not simplistically "counted" separately from the context of societal inequalities and gender roles violence helps to keep in place. In addressing the issue of women using force, counting the violence should never be the goal so much as looking at the meaning and consequences of violence in people's lives. It is urgent that antiviolence thinkers, researchers, workers, and activists take leadership roles in taking women's use of force seriously so that information on female violence is no longer given from just antiwomen, backlash perspectives. The challenge is to take violence by women seriously without losing sight of the fact that the patterns of male and female violence within adult intimate relationships are usually very different, often happen within different contexts, and generally have very different consequences and that both the violence itself and the barriers to ending violence are related to societal inequalities.

Female violence must be taken very seriously. Female perpetrators must be held accountable. I know there are women who are violent. I have been curious about violent women ever since I read MacDonald's book *Shoot the Women First* ("The first book to tell why women are the most feared terrorists in the world," back cover), the cover of which exclaimed,

> "Shoot the women first" is the advice given to German police teams handling terrorist incidents, but is recognized as valid by anti-terrorist groups the world over. Armed men may hesitate before they shoot, women rarely do. They are more ruthless, more determined and consequently more feared than their male comrades, and make the most deadly adversaries.

I am a firm believer that many women are extremely good at whatever they decide to do, so it makes sense that if a woman "decides" violence is necessary, she might be very good at it. It also makes sense to me that when girls and women are rewarded for paying attention to what other people need and for developing good verbal and emotional skills, they could turn those areas of expertise into something that could very much hurt a loved one. Indeed, unless our society starts to give clearer, more consistent messages that will not reward or ignore violence, I think we should expect that more girls will get the message that violence is acceptable or even glamorous. I am obviously writing this article, however, because I want to inspire readers to take female violence seriously without losing sight of the general patterns in intimate partner violence (i.e., male violence keeps women from maximizing their fullest potential) that need to guide antiviolence work. We need to be careful that our curiosity about female violence, our knowledge that some women are violent and thus that some men get hurt in heterosexual relationships, and our commitment to holding abusers accountable do not get in the way of thinking through the complexities of addressing the issues of female violence.

It is time to reframe a number of issues.

Connecting and Disconnecting: Issues of Girls and Women Using Force

The question, "What about girls and women using force?" is so big. There are many answers and many more questions than answers. When the Wisconsin Coalition Against Domestic Violence Education Committee first initiated discussion on this topic, we did not want to leave out any part of the question, so we tried to address all the following questions in our first short workshop:

1. What are the experiences of domestic abuse programs with girls' and women's use of force?

2. What are the political ramifications of asking this question? How do we frame the issue to make sure we are not compromising the integrity of the battered women's movement? What are the dangers of addressing this issue?

3. Do men and women use violence in different ways? Much on the power and control wheel may look the same for male and female violence. But what about the "using male privilege" piece that supports violence against women? A lesbian batterer may use homophobia to hurt her partner, but are there similar privilege or social oppression weapons being used if a heterosexual woman is a perpetrator?

4. What are the similarities and differences of batterers' treatment for men and women? Are there different ways to hold men and women accountable for their violence? Will the same types of intervention work for abusive women and abusive men?

5. What are the similarities and differences between women as perpetrators in lesbian versus heterosexual relationships? (What are the similarities and differences between women as victims or survivors in lesbian versus heterosexual relationships?)

6. If we believe that violence against women is related to gender socialization, are we moving toward boys and men being less violent and/or girls and women being more violent? What are we doing right? What are we doing wrong?

7. Should we make these questions more central to the battered women's movement? If so, how?

8. Are there other forms of girls' and women's use of force we should be addressing? What else should we be discussing?

The fact that more than 100 people attended a workshop, which we expected to be very small (it was scheduled at the same time as many workshops by popular national speakers), demonstrated that people are eager for a chance to talk about the issues. Time ran out much too quickly, and it became obvious that each question needs weeks, not minutes, of discussion time. It was clear that one challenge for the antidomestic violence movement is making the time and creating safe spaces so that we can slowly and carefully develop our thinking about the different ways girls and women may use or are accused of using force at different ages and in different contexts.

Many of us who have worked on a range of violence against women issues have felt connected under the widest violence against women "umbrella" but have found times when we needed to specifically work on lesbian violence, sexual assault, gender harassment, elder abuse, or heterosexual domestic violence; we have done that specific work with the bigger picture of analysis of violence against women in mind. In the same way, it will be important to remember the context of sex-role socialization, societal inequalities, and violence as power and control as the questions about girls and women using force are addressed in relation to teen dating violence, gang violence, lesbian battering, child abuse, elder abuse, heterosexual domestic violence, and other issues. Unique aspects of each of these topics merit much in-depth exploration, and simultaneously, each needs to be contextualized within the broader framework of violence against and by females within a violent, patriarchal society. (Key issues related to several of these topics are introduced at the end of this article.)

Strategy: Acknowledge That Men Get Hurt by Violence

Backlash against a movement is always a sign of how successful a movement has been. No one would be talking about whether women are as violent as men if there had not been more than 25 years of organizing against violence against women; establishing shelters, anti-domestic violence programs, and support groups; working to get the criminal justice system to hold perpetrators accountable; and developing coordinated community responses to domestic violence. Quite rightly, violence against women has received much attention.

Who gets left out of attention focused on violence against women? Men and boys as victims of violence.

Acknowledging that men and boys get terribly hurt by violence may be just as important as exploring the issue of women as perpetrators of violence. It certainly helps shift the discussion in more fruitful directions. Acknowledging that men and boys are killed by violence (mostly by other men and boys) more often than are women and girls in this society may be an effective strategy for making a gender analysis more central to violence work.

Male violence not only hurts women but also disproportionately kills men, especially men of color. Of homicide victims from 1976 to 1999 in the United States, 76% were men, as were 88% of those who committed homicide. White men between the ages of 15 and 25 are more likely to be killed than White women, and Black men are more likely to be killed than Black women.[2] Male violence particularly devastates Black communities. Black women aged 15 to 24 are killed at nearly the same rate as are White men in the United States, whereas Black men are killed at a rate 8.5 times higher than are Black women or White men.

Both the battered women's movement and many parts of the wider women's (liberation) movement have done an excellent job of making connections among images of women, the socialization of women and their roles in society, and violence against women. An important next stage of working on violence prevention must be to develop a more thorough gender analysis so that the roots of violence are better understood in relation to definitions of masculinity, the socialization of men and their roles in society. Hiding the prevalence of male violence (against both men and women) contributes to the climate in which it becomes acceptable or even fashionable to ask whether women are as violent as men. For example, despite the fact that almost all the so-called school violence that hit the headlines in the 1990s has been perpetrated by (White) male youths, the media have consistently failed to note that, and one could easily get the idea that school violence is a gender-neutral problem. How many people have any idea about the disproportionate amount of violence committed by men?[3] While identifying that both men and women get hurt or killed by living in a violent society, a gender analysis also helps identify that men and women get hurt by violence in very different contexts. Men mostly get hurt by strangers, whereas women mostly get hurt by people they know and care about.[4] Women are more than five times more likely than men to be victimized by a spouse or partner, ex-partner, boyfriend, or girlfriend.

There is not a hierarchy of violence, but the ramifications for intervention, prevention, and long-term consequences are totally different for someone hurt by a stranger and someone hurt by a loved one. These are important issues to identify for anyone questioning the necessity of a gender analysis of violence. Many emergency room and criminal justice system personnel have observed that when someone (usually a man) is hurt by a stranger, they are likely to want to report the crime, to want the other person prosecuted, and to hope they will never see

that person again. In contrast, a different pattern is observed when someone (usually a woman) has lived with or loved the person who is hurting them. Reporting the abuse has different ramifications when there are shared children, dreams, identities, finances, and futures and where reporting may cause escalation of the violence. Unlike stranger violence in which men are the main victims of what is usually a one-time occurrence, intimate partner violence, with women as the primary victims, tends to be an on-going pattern of abuse of power and control. Consequently, in general, violence disrupts the lives of men and women in quite different ways.

Gender, Race, and Class

Momentarily focusing on the seriousness of how much male violence hurts men may be an effective way to reassure men that we care about anyone getting hurt by violence, it may help us get on with our presentations and our work, and it may help contextualize the fact that violence against women happens within societies that allow and support the widest range of violence. However, it is also important to recognize the limitations and dangers of this tactic.

First, it is vital to acknowledge that gender differences in homicide rates do not reflect the differences in quality of life for men and women. Many women hurt by violence get hurt every day. The woman who says, "I probably only got hurt once a year for 20 years, but I woke up every one of those other 364 days of the year wondering if that would be the day" (quote from a survivor in the video "Any Day Now," WomanReach, Inc. and the Domestic Violence Advocacy Council of Charlotte/Mecklenburg, 1991) reminds us how violence and the fear of violence affect the quality of women's lives.

Also, it is important to be careful not to leave out an analysis of how other inequalities in society are related to violence. Note that in the previous discussion of homicide victimization of Black and White people aged 15 to 24, gender analysis is meaningless unless the impact of race or racism on homicide is also examined. These figures show that Black women and White men are killed at similar rates and that the homicide rate is 4.2 times higher for Black than for White women. Black men are killed at a rate 35 times higher than are White women.

Both race and class analyses are crucial in addressing violence and understanding that the battered women's movement, the criminal justice system, and other systems have particularly failed to adequately address the needs of many battered women of color, poor women, and other women from marginalized communities. Lack of appropriate services and policies may force some women to resort to using force or other unhealthy coping strategies. In *Compelled to Crime: The Gender Entrapment of Battered Black Women,* Richie wrote,

> The extent to which some women experience this predicament [domestic violence] is directly related to the degree of stigma, isolation, and marginalization imposed by their social position. The choices are harder and the consequences are more serious for women with low incomes, women of color, lesbians, women who become pregnant at a young age, and others whose decisions, circumstances, and status violate the dominate culture's expectations or offend hegemonic images of "womanhood."
>
> Studies that have been conducted from the standpoint of battered women have been overwhelmingly concerned with the experiences of White women. . . . The aggregate effect is that while *some* battered women are safer in the 1990s than they were in the 1970s, and while we know more about *general* patterns in the population, we still have very little theoretical or empirical work that speaks to African-American battered women from low-income communities. Consequently, few anti-violence programs, criminal justice policies, or theoretical explanations are sensitive to ethnic differences or address cultural issues that give particular meaning to violence in intimate relationships for African-American or other women of color. Furthermore, those whose lives are complicated by drug use, prostitution, illegal immigrant status, low literacy, and a criminal record continue to be misunderstood, underserved, isolated, and . . . in serious physical and emotional danger. (pp. 2–12)

E. Assata Wright gives examples of well-meaning public policy having an adverse effect for women of color because no one thought through how policies like mandatory arrest might have an impact on these women's lives:

> The mandatory arrest policy is particularly problematic for Black women because . . . they are more likely to fight back and protect themselves when being abused. In cases where a woman hits her abuser, she can be arrested along with the attacker.

Many Black women and Latinas may protect the abuser from jail even if it means risking their own safety. In a 1996 report on police brutality in New York City, Amnesty International found that between 1993 and 1994 there was a "substantial" increase in the number of Blacks and Latinos who were shot or killed while in police custody. Advo-

cates point out that while women want protection from their batterers, they don't want him beaten by cops or worse, killed by them. (pp. 550–551)

Economic issues relate to battering a number of ways, such as in both the relationship between poverty and family violence and the potential loss of employment opportunities for self-sufficiency abused women arrested for assaulting their abusive partners may face. Kurz's research found that the poorest divorced women, those on welfare, experienced higher rates of violence than did any other groups of women and that the poorer the woman, the more serious the violence was that she experienced. She questions the relationship between poverty and abuse as follows:

> What is the reason for the higher levels of violence reported by low income women? Are poor women more forthcoming about the amount of violence they experience, or do more of them report the violence to the police because they have less access to other kinds of legal assistance? These are possibilities, but at this point no data answer this question. It is also possible that something about the circumstances of those living in poverty contributes to the higher rates of violence among poorer men. For example, men from lower income groups may have a stronger belief in the legitimacy of violence than other men, since they typically hold more traditional gender ideologies than other men. It is not clear, however, that lower income men actually behave in more gendered ways than do other men. Another explanation for the higher rates of violence reported by poorer women could be that lower-income men have fewer ways of controlling their partners than other men. The higher men's social class, the more ability they have to control their female partners through their greater economic resources. (pp. 136–137)

The National Clearinghouse for the Defense of Battered Women has raised awareness of the economic ramifications of battered women being arrested for and convicted of using force against abusive partners and then having a criminal record, which affects their financial situation.

> We know many women, eager to "get the case over with," accept guilty pleas without being fully appraised of the potential consequences of have a record. Might a conviction bar a woman from certain employment opportunities, public housing situations, welfare benefits, or affect her immigration status or a custody determination? We want to work with defense counsel to help them better understand the consequences of a conviction and the disparate impact on women clients

(since so many of the jobs barred by convictions are traditionally "women's work," such as child care and healthcare jobs, and because so many women, as primary caretakers for their children, are the ones to apply for public benefits and housing). (p. 8)

It is clear that researchers and practitioners need to more fully understand how gender, race, and class affect battered women's experiences and how and why they may choose to, or need to, use violence.

Domestic Violence = Woman Battering

Domestic violence is certainly not gender exclusive, but the pattern of male perpetrator and female victim reflects and is encouraged by societal power inequalities between women and men and serves to maintain gender inequality. In fact, domestic violence is an extreme example of gender inequality.

The battered women's movement was clearly built on a sophisticated understanding of how violence in intimate relationships relates to and helps perpetuate inequalities between women and men. As the movement grew more visible, as many more players became involved in providing services to victims of intimate violence, and as more funding became available, domestic violence became a hot topic and a very mainstream issue. It was no longer unusual, controversial, or even radical to work to end domestic violence. This was a very exciting phenomenon: Many more people know about and benefited from domestic violence services, and whole communities identified roles different professionals could play in recognizing and responding to domestic violence. This mainstreaming of the battered women's movement coincided with a changing environment where the work of many aspects of the women's movement became less visible and debates about "political correctness" made it much more challenging to figure out how to work on societal inequalities. Although it was no big deal that people involved in this work gradually stopped calling themselves the battered women's movement and became known as people working against domestic violence, symbolically "women" visibly got left out of the name of the movement and out of the analysis of intimate partner violence. (Throughout this article, I use both the terms *battered women's movement and domestic violence movement*). Once an issue has a gender-neutral name, it is easy to forget that it is not a gender-neutral issue.

Renzetti illustrated the dangers of a gender-neutral approach to domestic violence in relation to the criminal justice system as follows:

The police, attorneys, and judges, like the backlash writers, argue that women, like men, must be held accountable for their behavior. To them, prosecuting women who have used violence against an intimate partner represents a gender-neutral application of the law. However, by decontextualizing women's violence and scrutinizing it in terms of a male normative standard juxtaposed against stereotypes of respectable femininity, the justice system thereby treats unjustly many women who have used violence. The outcome will be—indeed, it already is—"gendered injustice." Women are increasingly being treated like men by the legal system, even though their circumstances typically are quite different. If these differential circumstances are not taken into account, the outcomes can hardly be fair. (p. 49)

With more women getting arrested for domestic violence in heterosexual relationships, it will be increasingly important to have trustworthy assessment tools that help identify when women use force in self-defense or within the context of long-term battering rather than initiate violence as power and control. The complexities of assessing who are the victims and who are the perpetrators have long been issues for discussion in relation to lesbian violence. Burk (C. Burk, personal communications, May 11, 1999, & July 14, 2000) and others have observed that unlike those working on heterosexual domestic violence, people working on lesbian intimate violence have always had to look at how any behavior can be used as power and control, how any behavior can be used as a survival tactic, and the fact that victims may well identify as abusers. There is also an important "reporting artifact" that is recognized in the violence literature: Studies show that women are more likely than men to admit they are abusive. In an article titled "Violent Women: Fact and Fantasy—Social Service Agencies Have the Responsibility to Know the Difference," Edleson stressed that accurate assessment is vital for providing different effective interventions for women who use force in different ways, for different reasons. He summarized how the Domestic Abuse Project's *Women Who Abuse in Intimate Relationships* treatment manual categorizes women who use force into the following three groups:

One group includes women who use violence in self-defense to escape or protect themselves from their partner's violence. Saunders (1986) found that this was the most frequently reported motivation for women's use of violence.

In a second group are women who have a long history of victimization at the hands of previous partners as well as during childhood. These women are described as taking a stance in life that "no one is ever going to hurt me that way again," and their violence is interpreted as an effort to decrease their own chances of victimization.

Violent women in a third group are identified as primary aggressors who use their greater physical power to control their partners. (p. 3)

Obviously, it is of the utmost importance to recognize that many women who use force are battered women who are not safe. Breaking their isolation and helping them be safer may be even more important than it is for women who do not use force because battered women's use of violence may make them even more vulnerable to their partner's aggression.

In general, the context and consequences of male and female violence within intimate relationships is different. Although studies often report that women use violence as a conflict tactic as often as men, women are the recipients of more injurious and life-threatening violence committed by intimate partners than are men. Women are also more likely than men to be killed by intimate partners.[5]

For much of the past decade, anti-domestic violence programs have been conscientiously letting their communities know that they are committed to helping both women and men in violent relationships. Although many anti-domestic violence programs do serve a few men, a committed public effort to reach out to male victims has not resulted in anti-domestic violence programs suddenly discovering they need to rethink their emphasis on serving women. In fact, no man has ever stayed in the first shelter for battered men, established in Britain in 1992 by the group Families Need Fathers. Hanusa (D. Hanusa, personal communication, November 10, 1998) and others who lead abuser groups have observed that the services needed by heterosexual men who identify themselves as abused seem to be different from those needed by abused women because safety is less of an issue and leaving the relationship is not usually associated with increased danger as it is for abused women.

In "Counseling Heterosexual Women Arrested for Domestic Violence," Hamberger and Potente concluded that domestic violence by women and men show distinctly different patterns.

First, although women are domestically violent, often at levels of severity similar to that of men, the impact of their violence is typically less than men's violence. Second, women tend to commit violence less frequently than do men, and for different reasons. Specifically, women tend to initiate physical assault motivated by a need for self-protection or retaliation of a previous assault by their partner. Men, in contrast, tend to iden-tify control or punishment as the primary motivations for assaults on their partners. (p. 59)

Saunders showed that 71% of battered women arrested for domestic violence had used violence in self-defense. Hanusa (D. Hanusa, personal communication, November 10, 1998) observed that there is a functional difference in how men and women use violence in intimate relationships: Women use it to end oppression geared toward them, whereas men use it to control someone. In 32 in-depth interviews with women court-ordered or referred to counseling because they had used violence, Dasgupta found that "the most pervasive and persistent motivation for women's use of violence is ending abuse in their own lives" (p. 217), and "when viewed in terms of motives, intentions, and consequences, these women's use of violence emerges as instrumental; that is, the incidents are directed toward the resolution of conflicts or control of immediate surroundings" (p. 210), including the fact that "many of the women became physically aggressive with their partners when their children were being abused" (p. 208).

In examining the differences between male and female violence, it may be useful to keep in mind the definition of domestic violence as an on-going pattern in which one person controls the other person and one person thus lives in fear for her or his safety. It is crucial to keep asking who is afraid and who is not safe. We need to explore much more about how men and women use emotional control. We know women can be effective at using emotional control, but whether it takes on the same level of threat to safety and whether the other person lives in constant fear may be a major difference between male and female use of emotional control. In Dasgupta's study of 32 women who had used physical violence, it was clear that even the use of violence did not equalize who was in control and who was afraid in these heterosexual relationships.

Regardless of the degree of physical force women used, none of the interviewees believed that it made their partners fearful. Neither did it control their behaviors. This perception was not without its base in reality. A group of 10 men whose female partners had been arrested on domestic abuse charges and interviewed as a part of this study also denied that their partner's violence resulted in their experiencing prolonged or significant fear for their safety. This finding is supported by studies that indicate that men in violent relationships, compared to their female counterparts, express little fear of their partners and wives. (pp. 209–210)

In addition to the research quoted throughout this article, most of the ideas and analysis in this article have grown out of on-going discussions with domestic violence service providers, abuser group facilitators, and policy makers. Everyone agrees that much better research is needed on women's use of force. Meanwhile, however, many people agree that they have observed the following different patterns in male and female violence in intimate relationships and the different consequences of male and female violence in intimate relationships:

1. Male violence is more apt to be a pattern to be repeated in subsequent relationships rather than situational in particular relationships. Adult women who are perpetrators in one relationship are less likely to become perpetrators in their next relationship. How many domestic violence programs have served several women hurt by the same man? (Talking about this phenomenon is a good way of reinforcing that most men are not violent. The high percentage of women who get hurt by domestic violence is a reflection of the same men hurting several women rather than a high percentage of men being violent.)

2. Men are more likely to physically injure their partners.

3. Women are more likely than men to be killed by intimate partners and are more likely than men to be punched, hit, burned, thrown out of a window, or strangled by intimate partners (Belluck, 1997).

4. Men have an ability to control women and children by creating an ongoing pattern whereby women and children live in fear. (How much will this situation change when more women have access to guns? In Dasgupta's interviews with women who had used force, she concluded that "only when women picked up weapons, guns, knives, and household objects did their partners become temporarily afraid," p. 210. But the interviewees also said that having used force, including weapons, led to more abusive behaviors in the future by their male partners. What are the dynamics that create an on-going pattern of fear?).

5. A different pattern in ending male and female violence in heterosexual relationships has been observed: If a woman is hurting a man, the violence usually ends when the relationship ends. If a man is hurting a woman, the violence generally escalates and becomes most dangerous when the relationship ends and in subsequent years. Therefore,

barriers to ending violence may be fundamentally different for men and women.

In the arena of sexual assault, activists working to end violence against women have been critical of the overemphasis on women learning self-defense when the real issue that needs to be addressed is stopping male violence. Ironically, with domestic violence, the issue of women fighting back is now getting increased negative attention (and more arrests), with too little attention being paid to why women need to resort to violence. Why are other strategies failing to keep women safe within their intimate relationships? Once again, the key issue of how to stop men's abuse of power and control is left out when the discussions focus on whether women should use force to protect themselves.

Violence in Lesbian Relationships

Lesbian battering includes many of the same issues as heterosexual domestic violence (power and control, fear, lack of safety) but is additionally affected by homophobia and a lack of services for victims of lesbian violence. In many communities, neither lesbian organizations nor anti-domestic violence programs have adequately addressed lesbian battering because of the fear that it could rip lesbian communities apart, dilute the issue of male violence against women, draw the "wrong" kind of attention to gay and lesbian issues, or draw the "wrong" kind of attention to a domestic violence program that may need financial support from a conservative community. Unfortunately, it is often the backlash to the violence against women movement that draws attention to lesbian domestic violence in an effort to say that women are as violent as men.

That women tend to be more likely than men to report they are violent must certainly affect studies of lesbian violence. I also wonder whether there is an additional reporting artifact in that women are more likely to identify abuse in a lesbian than in a heterosexual relationship. (Is more equality expected in a lesbian relationship so that an abuse of power and control is more easily identified?). There are extremes related to lesbian violence: It often is ignored or, in contrast, reported at quite high rates (e.g., in surveys at the Michigan Women's Music Festival, although these surveys do not use scientific sampling methods). Why these extremes? Is less known about the prevalence of lesbian violence than about heterosexual violence because of the added complexities of studying it, or are people just more honest about saying that too little is known about the prevalence or consequences of lesbian battering? As someone who teaches women's health topics to 840 university students each year, I have curiously observed that students pay much more attention to the issue of lesbian batter-ing than to other issues, such as legal discrimination against lesbians, lack of partner health insurance for les-bians, lesbian parenting, lesbian alcohol use, or lesbian menopause. Perhaps it is because the battered women's movement has been a major arena for important feminist discussion and debate during the past two decades and the issue rightly belongs here; there have not been sim-ilarly effective movements around which to organize other equally urgent lesbian issues. The good news is that because some people have made lesbian battering a visible issue, there are now some very good resources on this topic.[6]

An excellent article, "Ruling, the Exceptions: Same Sex Battering and Domestic Violence Theory" by Merrill, builds on the analysis of power and control in heterosex-ual domestic violence relationships to look at theoretical frameworks that bring together sociopolitical and psycho-logical theories to include same-sex violence. Merrill iden-tified the following three factors that make someone violent: (a) growing up learning how to be violent (obvi-ously, everyone growing up in the United States learns how to be violent, but many people choose not to act on that); (b) having an opportunity to be violent; and (c) per-sonally choosing to be violent. Merrill said that having the opportunity to be violent can be emphasized as a way to explain same-sex violence because homophobia allows someone to abuse a same-sex partner knowing that homo-phobia in the outside world will protect abusers from suf-fering negative consequences for their abusive behavior. Homophobia and heterosexism operate so that battering in same-sex relationships is ignored or not taken seriously; the perpetrators clearly get the message that our society will tolerate it. Potentially violent women in lesbian rela-tionships get the message that they will not be negatively sanctioned for being violent "in that kind of relationship." In contrast, potentially violent women in heterosexual re-lationships will get strong messages that their violence against male partners would not be socially acceptable or tolerated. Merrill concluded, "While the social phenome-non of prejudice (homophobia) does not cause lesbian or gay battering, it does create an opportune environment that supports this abusive behavior by its refusal to challenge it" (p. 15).

Lesbian battering experts have much to offer the anti-domestic violence field from their years of recognizing the complexities of identifying who are the perpetrators and who may have used force in self-defense. As anti-domestic violence programs work to develop more effec-tive assessment tools for women arrested for using force, this may be an opportunity for activists who have worked on lesbian and heterosexual battering assessment to have

more dialogue about what can be learned from each other. Clearly, all communities need to give both men and women consistent messages that violence in any re-lationship, by either partner, is not tolerated.

Women as Perpetrators of Child Abuse

Of all the areas I work in, child abuse is the area I find the most mother blaming and outright woman hating, and it is the area in which I am most concerned about the in-creasing levels of woman blaming. Society in general and child protective services in particular assign responsibil-ity for child abuse to mothers, regardless of who assaults the children or the context in which the abuse occurs.

There has now been more than a decade of organizing and education on the effects of domestic violence on children. Ironically, instead of people being better at see-ing how child abuse is an extension and predictable com-ponent of the ongoing power and control that hurts women in domestic violence, more and more battered women are being charged with child abuse because they "allowed" their children to witness domestic violence or "failed to protect" them from harm, despite the power relations that make it dangerous and impossible for many battered women to keep their children safe.

In their important article "Women and Children at Risk: A Feminist Perspective on Child Abuse," Stark and Flitcraft concluded,

> Representative sample surveys indicate that fathers may be as likely or more likely than mothers to abuse children. . . . More important, there is little doubt that if a man is involved in a relationship, he is many times more likely than a woman to abuse the children. . . . National survey data indicate that men were responsible for two-thirds of the reported incidents of child abuse in which men were present in the relationship. (p. 75)

They are careful to point out that they reach this con-clusion despite the obvious fact that women spend many more hours per day, per week with children and that many children are raised by single women.

The issues of child abuse and woman abuse are so clearly interrelated that it feels very intentional that oth-ers are not seeing or are choosing to ignore the connec-tion. Years ago, Walker, best know for her important work on battered woman syndrome, noted that if a child is being abused, the most predictable correlation is that the child's mother is also being abused. (That factor—the mother being abused—is more consistent and predictable than is any other variable, including age, income group, and geographic area.) Indeed, if the woman is abusing the child, it is even more predictable that the woman herself is being abused and that her abuse of the child is related to (or a consequence of) the ongoing power, control, and fear in her life. Walker found mothers were eight times more likely to hurt their children when they were battered than when they were safe from violence.

The example of child abuse is a model for how antiviolence activists and researchers can take the issue of women's use of force more seriously, that is, to make sure we take the context of women's violence very seriously. If women are more likely to hurt their children when they themselves are being hurt, it of course reinforces the need for ending violence against women, but it also reinforces our need to find more effective ways to communicate and collaborate with agencies and institutions that have not always seen violence against women as their issue. The Advocacy for Women and Kids in Emergencies Program at Boston Children's Hospital (Schechter & Gary) is a model that takes both child abuse and woman abuse seriously and does not leave anyone pulled between two systems or two victims. Schecter's work at the Advocacy for Women and Kids in Emergencies Program inspired others to work on the premise that if a child is being hurt, the mother may also be getting hurt and that child abuse intervention needs to be consistently done in a way that ensures the violence in a mother's life will be addressed. Different sets of advocates are available to help the child through the child protective service system, and another set of advocates helps the mother end the violence in her life. Instead of seeing a conflict between the interests of abused children and their mothers, a reframing of the issue helped this agency identify that in many cases, helping women to be safe is a very effective way to help children be safe.

Teen Dating Violence

This issue of women getting mixed messages about whether it is acceptable to initiate violence or to fight back for self-protection is particularly crucial in relation to work on girls' use of force in teen dating relationships.

An example of what is happening in teen dating violence is apparent in Molidor and Tolman's article, "Gender and Contextual Factors in Adolescent Dating Violence," which reported a study of 635 students surveyed about dating violence. The study found that male and female adolescents did not differ in overall frequency of violence in dating relationships. However, when researchers went beyond simply counting experiences of violence to looking for the context and conse-

quences of teen intimate violence, they found that adolescent girls experienced significantly higher levels of severe violence and emotional reactions to the violence than did boys.

This is an important example of an article that clarifies the difference between the amount of violence and the consequences of violence for male and female teens. But most observations of teen violence do not make that important distinction. All too often, it is simply stated that girls are pushing and shoving just as much as boys these days. How many of us have been a part of meetings where researchers indicate they know there are limitations to the usefulness of conflict tactics scales but then quickly move on to simply report the interesting data they have that girls say they are using considerable amounts of violence? Once a girl has identified herself as "using violence," how much more difficult will it be for her to identify herself as needing support and safety planning if she is in a pattern of ongoing power and control?

The American Association of University Women Educational Foundation study on sexual harassment at school reported that sexual harassment was an issue for both girls and boys but stressed that the consequences were distinctly different. Boys reported knowing they had been harassed, but they could not remember when it started. In contrast, girls could remember exactly when they were harassed and the serious consequences (i.e., hating school, skipping school, not speaking up in class) that resulted from the harassment.

There is a dangerous trend in the resources designed for teens. Concern has been expressed about the lack of antiviolence resources appropriate for young men. There is a need for resources that are male positive but clearly antiviolence, in contrast to some of the present dating violence materials that some young men feel are antimale. Unfortunately, in aiming for this newly defined "market," there is a trend toward dating violence resources showing equal levels and consequences of male and female violence. It is crucial that resources and messages are developed and disseminated that appeal to young men but do not hide the different patterns and consequences of male and female violence.

The arena of the middle school is a most urgent one in which to address the question, "What about women or girls as perpetrators?" In many ways, middle school is "no person's land: Everyone is powerless" (D. Hanusa, personal communication, November 10, 1998), but it is also the key opportunity for helping young people learn healthy ways of reclaiming their personal power and setting very high standards for themselves as to how they will perform and what they will expect from future relationships. As more and more dating violence prevention resources and messages are rightly being aimed at this age group, it is important that educators and policy makers find effective messages that do not downplay the seriousness or prevalence of male violence or present violence in intimate relationships as a gender-neutral topic.

Whenever violence in a group is first noticed, attention is wrongly paid to the fact that much of the violence is probably "mutual violence." This is what happened with the initial observations of both adult heterosexual domestic violence and lesbian violence. Then, as people were more careful about understanding the dynamics and consequences, it became apparent that most domestic violence and lesbian battering was the ongoing pattern of one person abusing power and control in all or most aspects of the relationship. Now, middle school violence is increasingly labeled *mutual abuse.* Many well-meaning educators and youth leaders describe middle schools girls as being as violent as middle school boys. What is happening here? Is there a short time in that "no person's land" when girls and boys have not yet learned their "appropriate" social roles regarding who should and should not be violent? Do they grow out of this a couple of years later when gender roles become exaggeratedly defined in high school? Is this another case in which it is dangerous not to be identifying the perpetrators (who are otherwise not held responsible or are sent to mediation)? Substantial resources need to be devoted to studying and preventing the dynamics and consequences of middle school violence.

On the other hand, if there is a real trend toward girls becoming more violent (either as perpetrators or learning that violence is the most effective way to not be controlled by someone else), it is urgent that this trend be recognized and addressed. If girls are learning that it pays to be violent, this raises important issues for the antiviolence movement. After more than 25 years of activism against violence against women, we should be reaching a point where we are starting to notice a decline in male violence. Is it possible that wider societal influences are so strong that instead of decreasing violence against women, we are seeing more young women get the message that their own violence is acceptable?

Conclusion

It is time for antiviolence researchers and activists to take the question "What about girls and women using force?" seriously. The question is useful for reframing the analysis of violence to examine more carefully how male violence hurts both women and men, although in different ways and in different contexts. We also need to find ways to take female violence seriously without taking a gender-neutral approach to violence. It is possible to simultaneously acknowledge individual female violence and show how the pattern of male violence against women reflects and perpetuates societal inequalities between men and women. We also must more carefully examine the intersection of race, class, sexuality, and gender in our antiviolence work.

The battered women's movement has been good at listening to each victim's story. Sometimes people's stories help us see general patterns that help us predict, understand, and interrupt ongoing power and control in relationships; sometimes a person's situation needs to be understood and addressed uniquely. We are fully capable of taking female violence against men seriously and serving individual men hurt by intimate partner violence without losing sight of the societal patterns of male violence hurting both men (usually as strangers) and women (usually within intimate relationships).

We can also use the question "What about female violence?" to explore other difficult issues. The gun industry, video games, and the media have been giving girls and women powerful messages about using violence. After more than 25 years of violence against women activism, is it possible that instead of diminishing or ending violence against women, we are seeing an increase in the number of girls and women who are learning that violence is an effective way to have power in a society that often limits their opportunity for healthy control in their own lives? What are we going to do about this?

Violence is a social issue. There is nothing "natural" about men being violent and women being less violent or passive. Male violence is rooted in the socialization processes our society has consistently imposed on boys and men. If there is an increase in girls and young women (and maybe even women of all ages) using force, it is a reminder that we need to start now to address socialization toward violence in new ways. The antiviolence against women movement, as with women's movements more generally, was never about making girls and women more like men. It was about building a fundamentally different, violence-free society. Asking hard questions about women's possible use of force may be an important way of remembering the social change work that still needs to be accomplished. Much work needs to be done to create a world in which girls and boys learn they can have a healthy amount of control in their own lives without controlling someone else. All communities need to give clearer, more consistent messages that neither male nor female violence is ignored or rewarded. In our work for a violence-free society, what are we doing right and what do we need to do differently? How can we use the question "What about women and girls using force?" to help set the agenda for the next decades of violence research and activism?

NOTES

1. Erin House (n.d.) has encouraged the use of the term *force* rather than *violence*, noting that

   > according to Webster's Dictionary, violence is defined as "rough or injurious physical force," "an unjust or unwarranted exertion of force and power." Thus, violence can be defined as a type of force, used unjustly, with the intention of causing injury. Force itself is descriptive of the use of physical strength to accomplish a task—but does not imply the same degree of wrong-doing or harmful intent. (p. 2)

2. In 1997, White men aged 15 to 24 were killed at the rate of 13.2 per 100,000 compared with White women aged 15 to 24, who were killed at the rate of 3.2 per 100,000 (Kumanyika, Morssink, & Nestle, 2001). Thus, White men are 4.2 times more likely to be killed than White women. Black women aged 15 to 24 are killed at nearly the same rate (13.3) as are White men in the United States. With a homicide rate of 113.3 per 100,000, Black men are killed at a rate 8.5 times higher than Black women (Kumanyika et al., 2001).

3. For example, men committed 88% of homicides in the United States between 1976 and 1999 (Fox & Zawitz, 2001b).

4. According to the National Crime Victimization Survey, in 2000, 54% of nonfatal violent crime (rape or sexual assault, robbery, and aggravated or simple assault) against men was committed by strangers and 44% was committed by intimates, other relatives, or friends or acquaintances. In contrast, 33% of nonfatal violent crime against women was committed by strangers and 66% was committed by intimates, other relatives, or friends or acquaintances (Rennison, 2001).

5. In 1999, 32.1% of female homicide victims were killed by intimates (in the cases in which the victim-offender relationship was known) compared with 3.6% of male homicide victims (Fox & Zawitz, 2001a).

6. Lesbian resource lists are available from both the Wisconsin Coalition Against Domestic Violence (phone: 608-255-0539).

REFERENCES

A list of references is available in the original source.

WORKSHEET—CHAPTER 7

Violence against Women

1. Societal Responsibility for Violence against Women

   a. How do boys and men get the message that "it's ok," "it's socially acceptable" for men to be disrespectful and abusive towards women? Give examples of ways in which boys and men are given this message. (Use examples from advertising, T.V., literature, movies, etc.)

   b. For one day, in your own life, keep track of all the situations (T.V. shows, video games, internet, cartoons, jokes, lectures, friends, language, etc.) in which violence is allowed or even encouraged.

   c. Identify ways that gender-role socialization (of both girls and boys) may play a part in violence against women.

   d. Building on the "Battered Women of Color in Public Health Care Systems: Racism, Sexism, and Violence" and "Ruling the Exceptions: Same Sex Battering and Domestic Violence Theory" articles, identify how sexism intersects with another form of oppression to explain "who has the opportunity to abuse" in this society.

2. **Many forms of violence against women.** Sexual harassment at school or work, pornography, child sexual abuse, date rape, sexual assault, battering, and elder abuse are all ways in which violence against women gets expressed. Choose any two of these forms of violence. Show ways in which those two forms of violence are similar, what they reflect about attitudes toward women, how they limit women's roles in society, and why they are mental and physical health issues.

3. **Continuum of family violence.** The continuum of family violence would look different for different women because what most hurts us is different for each of us and many hurtful actions are not listed on the continuum. Work with friends, especially survivors, to design continuums that better reflect your feelings and experiences. Be sure to add other ways abusers can control their partner, such as stalking, spreading rumors, using friends, threatening to "out" a same-sex partner, hurting a pet, hurting a child or parent, or threatening to be unfaithful.

4. Identify ways dating violence for college women is the same as and different from domestic violence for adult women. What resources are there on your campus and in your community for young women in abusive dating relationships? Who would you ask for help if a partner were controlling you?

5. Identify ways in which domestic violence in lesbian relationships is the same as and different from heterosexual domestic violence. (Think about what would be the same and different in a lesbian power and control wheel compared to the power and control wheel in this chapter.)

6. Identify some of the barriers the following women might face in trying to safely end violence in their lives:

   a poor woman _____

   an undocumented woman from another country _____

   a woman who is very ill_____

   a woman whose abuser is ill _____

   a very rich woman _____

   a doctor's wife _____

   a minister's wife _____

   a woman who is a minister _____

   a Latina woman _____

   a woman with serious disabilities _____

   an alcoholic _____

   a 40-year-old trying to get pregnant _____

7. **Health workers response to violence.** This chapter addresses the importance of health workers' response to domestic violence. Health practitioners *should* now routinely screen for domestic violence. Describe whether or not you have been screened by a health practitioner for intimate partner violence. Describe what actually happened and whether it felt appropriate to you. If you have not been screened, describe how it should have been done.

8. **Institutional response to domestic violence.** The Medical Power and Control and Medical Advocacy/ Empowerment Wheels (p. 340) were designed to help health workers identify whether their responses were hurtful/controlling or helpful. Create similar "unhelpful" vs. "helpful" wheels for another system's response to domestic violence. For example, what would the "wheels" look like for dentists, house fellows, social workers, landlords, teachers, clergy, or police?

9. **Institutional power and control.** The power and control wheel (p. 330) was designed by battered women to describe the many ways their individual abusers controlled them. Create an institutional power and control wheel to describe how institutional oppressions work to control people. Sexism as power and control would include men getting paid more than women, men using male privilege, women having major responsibilities for contraception and children, women's issues not being taken seriously. What would racism as power and control, homophobia as power and control, or ageism as power and control, include?

10. **Fear of violence.** "Sexual terrorism" powerfully captures the impact of the fear of violence in women's lives. Give examples of how the fear of violence has influenced decisions (where to live, time to leave an event, what to wear, importance of carrying a cell phone, etc.) of women you know. Do you agree or disagree that this list would look different for women and men?

FOOD, BODY IMAGE, *and* BODY MODIFICATION

Body image, keeping our bodies healthy, and how we feel about our bodies are core women's health issues. This chapter needs to be several volumes covering every inch of women's bodies from heads to toes! Think about the messages women are given about every part of the body (hair, skin, nose, eyes, breasts, lips, etc., etc.). What is needed to maximize on keeping those parts of the body healthy? What unhealthy things are women encouraged to do in order to "fit" society's ever changing definition of "attractive"?

The first articles in this chapter address body image issues from the perspective of women, food, and fat. These articles explore how social, cultural, and economic factors impact upon the basic physiological process of feeding our bodies. The relationship of women to food is as complex as any other phenomenon examined in this book.

"Nourishing Ourselves" pulls together many of the multi-layered interrelationships between women's roles as the world's food producers and how women's inferior status and internalized sexism may affect women's access to the very food they have produced. Placed within a global context, the similarities are drawn between malnutrition in poor countries/poor communities and in richer communities where societal pressure to be thin similarly deprives girls and women of the quality of diet they need for maximum mental and physical health. This leads to the ultimate question of whether the relationship to food is so different for women and men that it actually becomes a factor in determining gender differences.

The next articles concentrate on the ramifications, particularly for women, of learning to hate fatness in others and especially in ourselves. "Fatphobia" looks at one of the most prevalent, yet uncriticized, forms of prejudice in our society, and "Mental Health Issues Related to Dieting" discusses mental health consequences of this cultural obsession with trying to be thin.

"We'll Always Be Fat But Fat Can Be Fit" (first published in 1985) is an impressive example of a classic article that not only stands the test of time but actually takes on increasing significance as diet-industry propaganda continually fuels individuals, health practitioners, and government reports to buy into the ubiquitous message that "obesity is unhealthy so fat people must lose weight." Importantly, Paul Campos' *The Obesity Myth* (see the *HealthFacts* review) helps us look at the problems with that overly simplistic message by summarizing research demonstrating that the dangers of obesity have been exaggerated. Campos particularly criticizes the obsession with weight loss "by most researchers who ignore other factors that create ill health in fat people, such as sedentary lifestyle, poor diet, dieting-induced weight fluctuations (yo-yo dieting), diet drug use, poverty, lack of access to and discrimination in healthcare, and social discrimination."

Similarly, the theme of "We'll Always Be Fat but Fat Can Be Fit" was reiterated by two long-term "Health at Every Size" activists, Lynn McAfee and Pat Lyons, as they protested the Surgeon General's (December 2001) "Call to Action to Prevent and Decrease Overweight and Obesity," which put way too much emphasis on weight reduction. McAfee and Lyons (*Network News*, March/April 2002, article reprinted in the 4th edition of this book) worried that such a potentially influential government report would increase prejudice and discrimination against fat people. They emphasized that "by defining weight as the problem and 'prevention and reducing overweight and obesity' as the solution, the report ignores research over the past 40 years that has found sustaining weight loss to be nearly impossible." Nearly 20 years after the "Fat Can Be Fit" article made these points, McAfee and Lyons needed to restate:

> We believe the best approach to improving the health of Americans of all sizes is to un-couple healthy lifestyle behaviors from weight loss. Studies show considerable health benefit in increasing an individual's social support, regular exercise, and consumption of fruits, vegetables, and fiber independent of weight loss. These health benefits should be stressed.

"The Continuum of Women and Food Relationships" exercise on the worksheet is a study guide to thinking through the ambivalent relationships many women have to their bodies and their food. The next articles all examine, from different perspectives, the complicated relationships women have to food in a world that gives them strong messages about what they should look like and who is valued.

Becky Thompson has done cutting-edge work examining how race, class, and heterosexism intersect with sexism to impact body image and "eating disorders" issues. Anyone interested in "eating disorders" will benefit from reading Becky Thompson's work. She has a chapter in the highly recommended book, *Feminist Perspectives on Eating Disorders*, edited by Patricia Fallon, Melanie A. Katzman, and Susan C. Wooley. The chapter ("Making 'a Way Outa No Way'") reprinted here is from her book, *A Hunger So Wide and So Deep: American Women Speak Out on Eating Problems*. Thompson pushes us to think about "eating problems" in new, complex ways:

> These chapters show how bingeing, purging, and dieting begin as ways women numb pain and cope with violations of their bodies and how survivors of trauma use food as a logical response to injustices, given the limited alternatives available to them. The lives of the women I interviewed show why we need an expansive understanding of how trauma can be inflicted. Many of the women linked eating problems to the physical violations, and others associated them with their psychic invasions of heterosexism, poverty, acculturation, racism, and emotional abuse. Recognizing both psychic and physical invasions avoids the historical tendency to identify the body and mind as somehow disconnected entities.

In "Good Enough," third-wave feminist Megan Seely remembers that "getting my head out of the toilet bowl was the most political act I ever committed" as she shares the contradictions she felt of being both a feminist and a woman who struggled with bulimia for years. She traces the history of women being pressured to meet society's ever changing, ever narrow definition of an "ideal" body size and recognizes that "when we are obsessed with this ideal, we have little time, or confidence, for anything else—including fighting for equality."

Until quite recently, much of the research and writing on women, dieting, and "eating disorders" has been focused primarily on white middle-class women. Individual women of color have often expressed frustration that such information did not reflect their experiences and have reminded us that if studies take place at health centers "which are not trusted by women of color," women of color will be under-represented in those studies! Becky Thompson's chapter certainly puts societal inequalities at the core of understanding "eating problems." The next two articles, both by Latinas, demonstrate the importance of both looking at how cultural issues impact on body image issues and the need to remember the complexities of how that works will be different for different women. In feeling proud that she is *bien cuidadas* (well cared for) and that her Latina community has always been accepting of well cared for women, Christy Haubegger's "I'm Not Fat, I'm Latina" shares her personal reflection of what it feels like not to fit in ("Noticing that none of the magazines showed models in bathing suits with bodies like mine") but to learn to accept and like one's own body. In her "Breaking the Model," Graciela Rodriguez disputes the media image that Latinas and African-American girls aren't likely to have eating disorders as she shares her painful teenage story of trying to lose weight to be a model. In a statement that reflects too many girls and women trying to be a size or shape they weren't meant to be, she says, "I didn't end up on the cat walk, but rather, in the hospital, recovering from anorexia and bulimia."

Symbolizing that body image and body modification are about much more than just what we do or do not eat, this chapter ends with articles about cosmetic surgery and the beauty industry. The next two articles explore feminism and cosmetic surgery from different perspectives. "Extreme Makeover: Feminist Edition" looks at how the cosmetic medicine industry, now reshaping women from head to toe, in every age, race, and economic group, is deliberately co-opting feminism and feminist language. Instead of building on the feminist analysis of how cultural forces create beauty anxiety and "that cosmetic medicine exists because sexism is powerfully linked with capitalism," the industry-inspired message is of a new "activism of aesthetics" and personal *choice*, "Yet one choice goes completely unmentioned: the choice not to consider cosmetic surgery at all." In "The Pressures of Perfectionism," a young feminist, Katherine Beagle, grapples with the contradictions of having critiqued the value of women being related to their attractiveness but still wanting breast implants for herself. After researching breast implants as a National Women's Health Network intern, Beagle discovered there are many more health and safety issues with implants than most of the 250,000 women a year who have implants know. (Also see the articles related to genital surgery in Chapter 3 for additional issues related to "cosmetic" surgery.)

Issues of the health and safety of beauty products continue into the last two articles. "The Ugly Side of the Beauty Industry" shows us how little is known about the safety *or* dangers of any of the ingredients in all the personal care products we use daily, and why the cosmetic industry wants to keep it that way. Many women use ten or more products every day, but "89% of ingredients in personal care products have never been assessed for safety" and "just nine chemicals are banned from cosmetics in the U.S." And, as "The High Price of Beauty" reminds us, the dangers of cosmetic products are not just limited to the consumers who use them. This article, focusing primarily on nail salons, gives us a feel for how unregulated products in unregulated settings pose hazards to the workers. In helping us see "the toxic mix of low pay and unregulated products," Sole-Smith concludes that "there's no question that what salon workers really need is a federal law requiring the FDA (Food and Drug Administration), EPA (Environmental Protection Agency) and OSHA (Occupational Safety and Health Administration) to hold the beauty industry to a much tougher standard, and more research to pin down exactly what they're up against."

"Nourishing Ourselves"

by Nancy Worcester

What could be more ironic? Nourishing others is a fundamental part of women's lives but that very role itself limits the ability of women to take care of their own nutritional needs.

Women are the world's food producers and throughout the world, within a wide range of family units, women have responsibility for purchasing and/or preparing the daily food. Yet, both globally and within families, women are much more likely than men to be malnourished. Nearly universally, wherever there is a shortage of food or a limited supply of quality food, women's diets are inferior to men's quantitatively and qualitatively. Even when food supply is adequate or abundant, women's diets may be nutritionally inferior to men's.

It matters! At some level we all have a feel for how important a good diet is: "We are what we eat." If we feed our bodies the basic nutrients, the healthy body is amazingly clever at being able to take care of itself. An adequate diet is obviously important for *every* man, woman and child. However, both societally and individually, a terrible mistake is being made when women's diets are inferior to men's.

A woman's diet must be more "nutrient-concentrated" than a man's in order to be nutritionally adequate. Most women require considerably less energy than most men. For example, the US Food and Nutrition Board recommends an intake of 1600–2400 Calories per day for women age 23–50, compared to 2300–2700 Calories per day for the same age men. A US Food Consumption Survey showed that the average 23 year old woman consumes only two-thirds as many Calories as the average 23 year old man, 1600 compared to 2400.[1] However, women's requirements for many specific nutrients are identical or greater than men's. The ramifications for this are most serious for calcium and iron. US Food and Nutrition Board Recommended Daily Allowance (RDA)[2] for calcium is the same for men and women. The RDA of 15 mg. of iron per day for reproductive aged women is 50% higher than the 10 mg. RDA for men.

Picture a woman and a man sitting down to consume their daily nutritional needs. The man's pile of food will be 50% bigger than the woman's but in the woman's smaller pile she will need to have the same amount of calcium and 50% more iron. Each bite the woman takes must contain 50% more calcium and twice as much iron! Put another way, even if a man does not have a particularly nutrient-rich diet, he will probably be able to meet his body's needs and he will even get away with consuming quite a few empty-calorie or low-quality foods whereas a woman's diet must be of a relatively higher quality. A man's diet can be nutritionally inferior to a woman's and still be adequate for his needs. The world and millions of individuals are paying a high price for the fact that women's diets are often inferior to men's.

Sex Differential in Food Distribution and Consumption

The trend to feed boys better than girls gets established early in life. In Kashmir, girls are breastfed for only 8–10 months but boys are allowed to suckle for three years or longer.[3] In Arabic Islam, girls are breastfed for only 1–1½ years while it is common for a boy to be nursed until the age of 2–2½.[4]

A recent Italian study also showed differences in the patterns of feeding baby boys and girls—girls are breastfed less often and for shorter periods; girls are weaned an average of three months earlier than boys. Additionally, it was observed that boys were more irritable and upset before feeding but went to sleep immediately after feeding. In contrast, the girls were less aggressive in asking for food but settled down less easily after feeding.[5]

Throughout the world, men and boys get feeding priority. In many cases, men literally eat first and women and children get what food is left-over, such as in Bangladesh where the tradition of sequential feeding means adult men are served first, followed by male children, then adult women and female children. Ethiopian women and girls of all classes must prepare two meals, one for the males and a second, often containing no meat or other substantial protein, for the females.[6] Boys' better access to food based on a gender defined division of labour can get started early in life. For example, in Alor, Indonesia, very young boys are encouraged to do "masculine" work and food serves as an important incentive and reward for that work. Boys receive "masculine" meals as guests of adult men for whom they have performed some service. In contrast, young girls do less valued work like weeding and get a lower quality vegetable lunch.[7]

In whatever way a particular society works it out, there is a nearly universal pattern of men getting fed more and better. Most women recognize this pattern and can identify ways in which they feed their children and their partners better than themselves. Although this may mean nothing more serious than taking the burnt slice of toast or the least attractive piece of dessert for oneself, in times of shortage this pattern means that women are the most likely to be malnourished.

Family members may not even be aware of the sacrifices the woman is making. A British woman who fed her husband and her children even when she could not feed herself during the 1930s remembered, "Many a time I have had bread dripping [animal fat on bread] for my dinner before my husband came home and I said I had my dinner as I would not wait."[8] That pattern is becoming prevalent again as many families do not have enough food. How many women say they are on a diet when in fact they would love some of what they are serving up to their family?

Hilary Land's study of large families in Britain concluded, "It was very evident that the mother was the most likely to go without food for she was the most dependent on meals provided at home . . . It was clear that the father's needs were put first, then the children's and finally the mother's." Over half of the women had no cooked meal in the middle of the day. A quarter had no breakfast and nothing more than a sandwich for lunch. One in twelve women *never* had a cooked meal.[9]

Studies in both Britain and the US have shown that poor parents go without food in order to leave enough food for their children. A British survey found that children were generally better and more regularly fed than their parents. "Only" 15% of the children had fewer than three meals during the previous twenty-four hours in contrast to 75% of the parents having had fewer than three meals, 50% having had two meals and 25% having had only one meal in the twenty-four hour period.[10] A 1983 New York study interviewed people at various sites including emergency feeding centers, food stamp offices, health centers and community centers. When asked, "Do your children eat and sometimes you're unable to?", over one-third of all respondents answered yes and 70% of the parents interviewed at the emergency feeding sites said yes.[11] (These studies did not look for different impacts on mothers and fathers.)

The feminization of poverty means that women in singleheaded households are often the worst affected. A Northern Ireland survey of 700 lone parents found that food was the item on which economies were most likely to be made and inevitably the savings were made by the mother herself going without food.[12] An English woman living on Supplementary Benefits describes the stark "choice" between her needs and the children's:

It has to be me cutting down on what I eat. It's the only way to find the extra money you need. The rest of it, they take it before you can get your hands on it really. So it's the food. It's the only thing I can cut because I use as little heating as I can and I don't smoke.[13]

Providing food for the children is such a worry for women who are the only parent that they may actually deprive themselves more than is necessary. Marsden's study of 116 lone mothers found that they hoarded food to be able to feed the children. He observed a stress reaction to living on low income in which the caregivers economized on their own food more than the size of their income required.[14]

Efforts specifically designed to improve women's diets are not successful if programmes are not planned around the recognition that women feed their families before they feed themselves and that men tend to get the high status foods. For example, a very ambitious 86 million dollar (US dollars) World Food Programme (WFP) project set up to improve the nutrition of pregnant and nursing mothers and their young children in Pakistan has had practically no nutritional impact. The major problem with the programme was that food was rationed so that each woman would receive an individual dietary supplement of 850 Calories per day, but, of course, the women shared the extra food with their families. The average family had six people so one-sixth of the supplement, less than 150 Calories a day, did not make a significant improvement in women's diets.

The acknowledgement that women do not give themselves priority in food allocation posed new problems for evaluators of the Pakistan WFP project:

Another possibility that has been mentioned is to simply accept the realities of family structure and food habits in Pakistan and expand the rations given to the women so that they are enough to provide supplements to the entire family. Obviously, a major drawback to this approach is that the same amount of food would then supply fewer women because of the increased ration size and not nearly as many women would be drawn to the centers.[15]

Judit Katona-Apte, consultant to the World Food Programme (but apparently not terribly influential!), suggests that one way to make certain that women benefit from food aid is to provide foods which are nutritionally-rich but less desirable than traditional foods. In such situations, the high status traditional foods will be given to the men and the newer, less desirable but nutritional foods will be relegated to the members of low status in the household—the women and children![16]

The differential access to food is often exaggerated by food taboos, which have more impact on women that men. Food habits, including rituals and taboos are an integral part of defining cultures ("we" versus "others"). Food taboos serve the function of reinforcing social status differences between individuals and social groups and symbolize the place one has in society. Taboos characteristically involve the prohibition of the highest quality protein foods. Jelliffe and Jelliffe suggest that, "The reservation of the best foods for the males reflects the ancient situation where it was imperative that hunters be well fed." However, Trant's explanation seems more to the point, "Widespread prohibitions applied to women against the eating of flesh foods may have partly derived from the male wish to keep the foods for themselves."[17] Those Italian baby boys aggressively demanding their food are just perpetuating a very ancient pattern!

Overall, it seems that most permanent taboos and avoidances have little effect on the nutrition of individuals practicing them because the group's diet will have evolved so that other foods supply the nutrients found in prohibited foods. However, temporary avoidance, particularly at crucial periods of the life cycle can have grave consequences.

Such limited duration taboos particularly affect women because they occur at the most nutritionally sensitive periods. For example, hot and cold or yin and yang classifications of food are common throughout the world and are especially important in Latin America and parts of Asia. Although hot and cold and yin and yang are defined differently in diverse cultures, in all cultures practicing these classifications, the balancing concept is closely tied to women's reproductive cycles. So, however menstruation, pregnancy and lactation get defined, it will be particularly important that women avoid certain "unbalancing" foods during those times. The foods which must be avoided are often foods of high nutritional value. Some Puerto Rican women consider pregnancy to be a hot state so avoid hot foods and medications, including vitamin and iron supplements, to prevent babies from being born with a rash or red skin. Bangladeshi women must not eat meat, eggs, fish or hot curries for several days after

childbirth because those foods are believed to cause indigestion. Women are expected to eat only rice, bread, tea and cumin seed for those nutritionally-demanding post-partum days.[18]

There are two more points to consider in looking at the impact of food taboos and avoidance on women's nutrition. First, food taboos, as a cultural construct, are a part of the values of the society which are taught to people as they grow up. People learn those taboos as patterns of behavior which are right, normal, best. Other ways of doing things are viewed as wrong, misguided, or irrational. Understanding and appreciating another culture will require getting to know the food habits and vice versa. Second, sound nutritional practices can, with thought and planning, be developed and reinforced within the context of most existing food patterns.

This relates to an important theme I am introducing here which I will then weave throughout this chapter. I am suggesting that our society's fear of fat and obsession with dieting play a role in limiting women's access to optimum nutrition similarly to the way food taboos can affect women's nutrient intake in more traditional cultures. Dieting certainly has more impact on women than men, reinforces social status differences, and leaves more food for others. As a cultural phenomenon, there can be no denying that women from many parts of the world would find the notion of purposefully restricting food intake to lose weight to be "wrong" or "misguided". Imagine trying to explain the pattern of American college women who intentionally skip meals to save calories for snacking and beer drinking at parties to Western Samoan women who exaggerate the amount they eat on diet surveys because, "The more they could say they had eaten . . . the more powerful that meant the village was in being able to amass lots of food."[20,21] When we hear that many nine year old girls are already on slimming diets, we must recognize dieting to be a part of the values which our society now teaches to young women. Because much dieting is erratic behavior, "a temporary drastic measure just to take off a few pounds" (repeatedly performed!), it is more similar to temporary taboos with the potential for grave consequences than to permanent taboos for which people have learned to compensate. Just as one can eat a nutritionally adequate or even nutritionally superior vegetarian or vegan diet if one knows animal products are going to be consciously avoided or unavailable, it is certainly possible to consume nutrient-rich low calorie or weight-maintenance diets. But, that is not how the dieting taboo is usually practiced in this society.

Nutritional Consequences of Sex Differentiation

Clearly there is no way to summarize the effects of sex differentiated nutrition. Nutritional vulnerabilities vary enormously from one part of the world to another, from one region to another, and between classes in the same small community. Malnutrition, of course, is not inevitable and is totally preventable. There is enough food and land available to feed the world's population if our governments considered that to be an important priority.[22] Factors such as cultural food preferences, storage and transport facilities, the soil the food is grown in and the value placed on equal food distribution within a community will have more influence on one's chances of being malnourished than whether one is a woman or a man. But, a pattern emerges which shows that universally malnutrition is far too common and that it affects girls and women more than boys and men.

> Hunger affects whole regions and classes of people and sweeps men as well as women into its nets. It seldom happens that the male members of a family are well-fed or overfed while the females starve. The differentials are narrow, and the question is that of which sex first crosses the line between health and sickness. In general, those who skate closest to the margin of deprivation are the most powerless—the very young, the old, and, everywhere, the women.[23]

Nutritional studies do not always look for or find sex differences in nutritional deficiencies. However, when nutritional sex differences are found it is almost always in the direction of the higher occurrence being in females. *Women and Nutrition in Third World Countries*[24] summarizes hundreds of nutritional studies in poor countries and concludes:

> Calorie intake is often low among women, although a few populations show adequate intake (Mexico, Tarahumaras, Korea) or excessive (Micronesia) ones. Deficiencies in caloric intake are common, regardless of physiological status . . . where intakes are reported by income, low-income women appear to consume less than their middle and high income counterparts. Not only do women consistently eat less than men, in a number of studies, they consume, on average a smaller percentage of their recommended daily intake . . . Women often consume lower quality, vegetable protein while men receive the larger share of whatever animal protein is available . . . On the basis of quantity alone, women often consumed a smaller percentage of their protein requirements than did men.

> The adequacy of vitamin intake varies greatly by culture. Riboflavin intakes are adequate in almost every country reviewed. The adequacy of vitamin A varies considerably, while most women (except those in Singapore, Iran, and the Tarahumara Indians) are deficient in their vitamin C intakes.

> Calcium and iron are the two minerals most commonly studied and in a majority of the countries reviewed, women are seriously deficient in their intakes of both.

The particular ramifications of women's iron and calcium deficiencies will be recurring themes in this book.

Iron is vital to the oxygen-carrying capacity of the blood and muscles but iron deficiency anaemia is the most common nutrition problem in rich and poor countries and in rich and poor people. Iron is available in many foods including meats, eggs, vegetables (especially greens), cocoa powder, apricots, breads and cereals, but in light of the prevalence of iron deficiency, the United Nations Committee on Nutrition recommends that more priority be given to iron fortification and supplementation.[25]

Reproductive age women are particularly vulnerable to iron deficiency because iron lost through menstruation must be replaced and highly increased circulatory requirements of pregnancy must be supplied in addition to the body's other needs for iron. Iron deficiency anaemia's incapacitating physiological and psychological effects influence the lives of women three or four times as much as men in many parts of the world. In low income countries, about half of non-pregnant women and nearly two-thirds of pregnant women show signs of iron deficiency anaemia.[27] Bangladesh is the most extreme example where a national survey discovered abnormally low iron (measured as blood haemoglobin) levels in 95% of rural women.[28]

Serious anaemia increases the risks of difficulty and death in childbirth of these women. While the consequences of iron deficiency anaemia are usually less severe in richer countries, the debilitating condition is far too common. Anaemia was identified in 40% of pregnant women in New Mexico's Women, Infant, and Children (WIC) Program and in 33% of poor pregnant women in Minneapolis, Minnesota. Black children show consistently higher rates (often more that twice as high) of anaemia than white children, so the effects of anaemia are probably even more exaggerated for Black than white US women.[29]

The consequences of sex differentiated nutrition become most obvious at the vulnerable times just after weaning and during the childbearing years. These are the two stages of life at which the female to male sex ratios take a dive.[30]

Biologically, it seems females are stronger than males. In general, life expectancy in females is greater than that in males. More males than females are conceived (120–150 males: 100 females), seemingly to "prepare" for the male biological vulnerability. More male fetuses are spontaneously aborted or stillborn, so the male to female ratio is down to 103–105:100 at birth.[31] Fifty-four percent more males die of birth injuries, 18% more males die of congenital malformations, and males account for 54% of all infant deaths in the first year of life.

Given the apparent biological advantage of females, a fascinating exercise is to try to identify the biological versus social and political causes of sex differences in death rates. Obviously, the fact that 68% of the US deaths at age 21 are male is more related to societal messages about who should play with guns and drive fast cars than a biological difference. Whether the supposedly higher rate of coronary heart disease in middle aged men than in women is more related to different roles in society, women's higher oestrogen levels, or a difference of who gets diagnosed, is a much more complex debate. Wherever there is a higher death rate for males, there may be a combination of biological and social factors working. Higher death rates for females clearly indicate that there are social, political or economic conditions overriding the female biological advantage.

The most marked sex discrimination in nutrition occurs after disasters in which there is a food shortage. Although physiological differences between males and females suggest that figures would show an excess mortality among males, statistics which exist consistently show that it is females and especially girl children who are at highest risk.[32] In the economic disasters after flooding in West Bengal, girls under five had a 60 percent higher incidence of third-degree malnutrition than the same age boys.[33]

A number of studies in South Asia have shown dramatic differences in the food and health care available to girls and boys. Preferential treatment of boys begins at birth when the birth of a boy is almost always viewed as a splendid occasion. Attitudes to the birth of a baby girl are at best ambivalent. While explicit female infanticide is no longer commonly practiced, the withholding of food and health care resources from girls can be viewed as a modern day version of female infanticide. The end result is the same: female mortality exceeds

male mortality by as much as 50 percent in the 1–4 year age groups in rural Bangladesh.

A detailed study of six rural Bangladeshi villages pinpoints how this happens.[34] Intrafamily food distribution surveys carried out by 130 families showed that energy and protein intakes were consistently higher for males than females in all age groups.

Protein consumption in males compared to females was 14% higher in 0–4 year olds, 22% higher in 5–14 year olds, 25% higher in 15–44 year olds, and 53% higher in males over 45. Malnutrition rates reflected the intrafamily distribution pattern. Of 882 children surveyed, 14.4 percent of girls were classified as severely malnourished compared to 5.1 percent of boys.

There is usually a distinct, almost synergistic relationship between malnutrition and infection. Malnutrition severely compromises the body's ability to resist infection, and resisting or succumbing to infection increases the body's nutritional needs, thus enhancing the degree of malnutrition. The effects of malnutrition will usually be exaggerated by this malnutrition—infection—increased malnutrition cycle and malnourished children can die from normally non-lethal diseases like measles.

Surprisingly, the six village rural Bangladesh study found rates of infection among female children were consistently lower than among males, although the differences were small and statistically insignificant. (More proof of the biological strength of little girls!) The tragedy was that girls were valued so much less than boys that health resources were made available to ill boys but not to ill girls *even when transport and health care was provided for free.* Despite nearly comparable incidence levels of diarrhea, boys exceeded girls at the treatment center by 66 percent: diarrhea treatment rates averaged 135.6 per 1000 for male children in comparison to 81.9 for female children.

Studies from India show even more starkly the consistent and systematic discrimination against females in the allocation of food and health care resources. Kwashiorkor (protein-calorie malnutrition) is four to five times more common among girls than boys. Though girls were more likely to be suffering from this life-threatening form of malnutrition, boys outnumbered girls at the hospital for treatment by a ratio of 50:1. When treated, children of both sexes responded equally well, but the mortality rate was considerably higher in girls due to both a lack of food and a lack of health care.[35,36]

Male-preferential distribution of food and other resources is certainly not a phenomenon only in poor households. Excess female to male mortality in 1–4 year olds is observed even among wealthy landowning families in Bangladesh, demonstrating that competition for scarce, insufficient resources does not explain all the disparity. It is not known whether this pattern is more marked in poor families when there is simply not enough for everyone so less valued members must be "sacrificed" for the sake of others or whether it is exaggerated in wealthier families where the social role of rich women is even more inferior in comparison to the status of rich men. In Bangladesh, excess female mortality is higher in rich households some years but other years excess mortality is higher in poor families.[37]

Intergenerational Consequences of Female Malnutrition

Malnutrition in girls and women can have long term and intergenerational repercussions, because of women's reproductive role. Any nutritional deficiency, such as rickets, which interferes with the physical development of little girls can cause problems, including maternal and infant death, decades later in pregnancy and childbirth.

The most profound and long term effect of women's malnutrition is demonstrated by the link between poor maternal height and weight and low birth weight babies. Low birth weight babies, defined as weighing less than 2500 grams (five and one-half pounds) at full gestation, have a much higher mortality rate and are more susceptible to illness throughout childhood than normal weight babies. A Sri Lankan study found an average maternal height of 150 cm (4'9") for low birth weight babies and a modal maternal height of 155 cm (5'1") for well-grown babies.[38] Poor maternal height and weight can be a reflection of the mother's own intrauterine growth retardation and inadequate childhood nutrition. Healthy diets for all potential mothers from pre-conception through pregnancy can be seen as a high societal priority when one realizes that *it takes at least two generations to eliminate the effect of stunted maternal growth on future generations of women and men.*

Reversing the effect of malnutrition brings new challenges. When a basic nutritionally-adequate diet for everyone becomes a national priority, young women with a family history of malnutrition will have access to a healthy diet after their own development has been stunted. In revolutionary China, as a consequence of major improvements in food production and distribution, birth weights rose dramatically within one generation. In order to maximize on its nutritional achievements, China's health services had to be able to cope with an increased rate of complicated deliveries as there was a generation of small mothers producing relatively large babies.[39]

While the relationship of women's malnutrition to generations of limited development may be most exaggerated in the poorest countries, it is certainly also an issue for wealthier countries. Some figures will help us follow through the impact of restricted nutrition on poor women in Britain and the US but one has to be critical of categories of analysis. Not by accident, measures of social class such as wealth, income, education and job classification are seldom recorded on US records such as death certificates.[40] Britain is much better at recognizing/not hiding the importance of social class information but the information is more appropriate to men than to women. Women's social class is based on husband's occupation. Even when categorization is based on the woman's own job, as with unmarried heterosexual or lesbian women, women's jobs certainly do not sum up women's lives.[41]

In Britain, 41 percent of wives of professional men have a height of at least 165 cm (5'5") compared to only 26 percent of wives of manual workers. Similarly, in the US, women in low income families have an average height of 160.4 cm (5'3") compared to 163.4 cm (5'4") for women in higher income families.[42] Heights for US children have, on average, been increasing throughout the last century, but the average height for poor children lags behind that for nonpoor children by more than a generation. The average height of ten year olds from families above poverty level is now significantly higher than the average height of ten year olds living below poverty. (This is not a race difference, for the average height of Black children is slightly higher than that of white children of the same income.) Sweden has recently managed to eliminate growth differences between social classes and is probably the only country with this achievement.[43]

In Britain, low birth weight babies and stillbirths are nearly twice as common in poor families (social classes IV and V) as in wealthier families (classes I and II). In the US, infant mortality rate is thirty times higher in low birth weight babies than normal weight babies.[44] Infant mortality rate (IMR = the number of babies per thousand live births who die in the first year of life) is an invaluable tool for comparing the health status of groups because it is a figure which is calculated similarly all over the world and is an excellent reflection of maternal and infant nutrition, as well as general standard of living and access to preventative and curative health care. IMR is 50 percent higher for US whites living in poverty areas than for US whites living in nonpoverty areas and IMR is at least 2.5 times higher in poor than in wealthy families in the UK. The intersection of poverty and racism is obvious from national (US) figures showing IMR more than twice as high for Black babies as white babies. Blacks in poor areas have a far higher IMR than Blacks in nonpoor areas although Black IMR is higher than white IMR in both income areas.[45,46]

The potential for change with an improved standard of living, including an emphasis on nutrition and access to health care, is most striking when IMRs are compared for small geographical areas. The Physician Task Force on Hunger in America contrasts the New York City IMRs of 5.8 in the Sunset Park section of Brooklyn with the 25.6 rate for Central Harlem and the Houston, Texas IMRs of 10.0 in the Sunnyside areas versus 23.5 in the Riverside Health Center community.[47] When we see that two or four times as many babies are dying in one part of town than in another, little guessing is needed to figure out where the poor, malnourished people live in New York City or Houston.

Malnutrition: Cause and Effect on Women's Role in Society

It is women not men who are unequally distributing food within the family, giving men and boys more than their share of what is available for the household. Women depriving themselves and their daughters of life-sustaining nourishment is the ultimate example of internalized sexism. Men do not need to discriminate against women or carry out nasty plans to "keep women in their place" if women are sufficiently well socialized to their inferior role that they themselves perpetuate keeping women in inferior roles.

A profoundly intermeshing relationship exits between women's status in society and the responsibility for food production and distribution. Women's responsibility for domestic work, especially food production, is so undervalued that women internalize that low value and starve themselves literally or figuratively. Although millions of women and girls die each year as a result of malnutrition, that number is a mere fraction of the number of women and girls who cannot maximize on their full potential because of undernutrition and because their responsibilities for feeding others do not leave them food, time or energy to nourish and nurture themselves.

Women's role as food producer can actually restrict a woman's ability to feed herself and others. How often have we observed a woman who eats practically nothing herself after spending hours preparing a meal for others? How often have we seen a woman so busy serving others that she barely sits down herself? A woman's standards for feeding herself may be totally different than those she holds to for her family. For example, a (London) *Daily Mirror* survey showed that even though mothers of school-age children make sure their children have breakfast, a fifth of mothers do not take time to eat breakfast themselves.[48]

Charmian Kenner's interviews with English women who have survived times of economic hardship show how the family's dependence on mum's food can make mum so ill that she cannot feed them:

> There was a vicious circle in which sickness bred further sickness. Lacking food, women had less resistance to infections. And when a woman fell ill and especially needed better food nobody else could take over and stretch the budget. Some women did not even feel able to set aside valuable time to teach their children to help them.[49]

It is exactly the women who face the most demanding food preparation tasks who have the least time and energy for this work. The woman who can afford the latest food processor and microwave may also be able to afford to buy easy-to-cook or partially prepared nutritious foods when she is too busy to cook. The woman who has to work overtime to have money to buy beans may not be able to buy a pressure cooker to reduce cooking time. Before or after a long day, she may have to decide between spending several hours on food preparation and eating less nutritional foods.

In many agricultural communities, it is *because* women have put all their time and energy into growing and harvesting the food that they may not be able to take the final steps, often extremely time and energy consuming, of turning the raw products into an edible form so that they can feed themselves and others.

> One report speaks of African women "sitting about hungry with millet in their granaries and relish in the bush" because they were too exhausted to tackle the heavy, three-hour work of preparing the food for eating.[50]

The seasonal nature of agriculture exacerbates this. Peak periods for women's work in the fields are normally at planting, harvesting and post-harvesting processing times when the working day can average fifteen hours. This coincides with the food supply being scarcest, most expensive, least varied and least well prepared. As a consequence, it has been noted that in Gambia, pregnant women actually lose weight during the peak agricultural time and, in Thailand, there is a marked increase in miscarriages and an early termination of breastfeeding during the rice planting and harvesting seasons.[51,52]

The relationship between productivity and nutrition works in several ways. Not only does extreme work keep women from feeding themselves, but also undernutrition is clearly a factor limiting women's productivity. Intensity of work, the productive value of work activities selected, and labour time are all dimensions of productivity which have been shown to be affected by nutrition. If women are not able to maximize on their productivity, food production is limited; several studies have identified women's labour input as the critical constraint on crop production. Although the value of women's productivity is universally and consistently *not* recognized, any signs of poor performance are definitely used to prolong women's low status.

The case of Sri Lankan women tea workers illustrates the cycle whereby low status affects diet, then malnutrition perpetuates low status. Tea workers' poor social and economic position is reflected by high morbidity and maternal mortality rates. Due to poor diets and hook worm manifestation, the women also have high rates of iron deficiency anaemia (measured as low haemoglobin levels). Studies found that this iron deficiency restricted work performance; a significant relationship was found between haemoglobin levels and various treadmill tests of physiological capacity. (Iron deficiency anaemia affects work intensity by decreasing the blood's oxygen transporting capacity.) After the women were given iron supplements for one month, significantly more tea got picked! These studies were of particular interest to the Sri Lankan government because tea has been the main asset for foreign exchange and the poor nutritional status of the female labour force was seen as having far reaching socio-economic consequence. Assuming women's increasing productivity was appropriately financially rewarded, one can see where something as seemingly simple as iron supplements can be an important step to improved economic status for some women.[53,54]

This specific example suggests an even bigger question: How much does the image and reality of the malnourished woman as weak, lethargic and not maximizing on her potential become the generalized description for "women" which then justifies and perpetuates women's inferior status?

Worldwide the high incidence of iron deficiency anemia has to be seen as a major, often unrecognized, component of women's low status. We know that this one nutrition issue affects as many as 95 percent of women in some communities and has profound physiological and psychological repercussions, including impaired work capacity, lassitude, lowered resistance to infection, and increased complications of pregnancy and childbirth. The Sri Lankan tea workers' example is worth remembering as a positive example of both how easily

some consequences of iron deficiency can be reversed and the need to make sure our governments become better educated about what they have to gain from a well nourished female labour force.

A wide range of other nutrition problems also have an impact on women's status. As an illustration which has nearly universal ramifications, low Calorie diets serve as an important example of undernutrition which, for very different reasons, can interfere with women maximizing on their potential and limiting their role in society in both rich and poor countries and for both rich and poor women. It is well known that low energy intakes restrict work potential and conversely that Calorie supplementation significantly increases work intensity and capacity.[55] The body, of course, has to work equally hard at coping with the limitations of a low Calorie diet whether that restriction is imposed because of a natural disaster food shortage or the fact that someone "chooses" to diet down to a smaller size. Research from poor countries indicates that the body does have adaptation mechanisms for adjusting to *permanently* restricted food intake but the body has a particularly chaotic job adjusting to great dietary fluctuations such as erratic food supply or yo-yo dieting.

What price do individuals and society pay for women's undernutrition caused by lifelong dieting? Hilde Bruch, psychiatrist respected for her groundbreaking work on eating disorders, describes "thin fat people" as people (usually women) who routinely eat less than their bodies require in order to stay at a weight which is artificially low for themselves. Very often these women are tense, irritable and unable to pursue educational and professional goals as a direct result of their chronic undernutrition. But, if they never allowed themselves to eat properly they do not recognize the signs that these limitations are due to undereating rather than personal weaknesses. Characteristic signs of malnutrition—fatigue, listlessness, irritability, difficulties in concentration and chronic depression—often escape correct professional diagnosis because the starved appearance (and especially average weight appearance in someone meant to be heavy) is a matter for praise rather than concern by our fatphobic society. "It has become customary to prescribe tranquilizers for such people; three square meals a day would be more logical treatment, but one that is equally unacceptable to physicians and patients because they share the conviction that being slim is good and healthy in itself."[56]

Is it possible that the relationship to food is sufficiently different between women and men that it helps determine gender differences in how women and men operate in the world? What if our scientific studies which "prove" that men are superior at performing certain tasks are actually measuring men's superior ability to fulfill their nutritional requirements rather than measuring task performing abilities? How would we even begin to start to think about or "measure" such things?

Claire Etaugh and Patricia Hill have started on some fascinating research to test their theory that gender differences in eating restraint (dieting) influence previously reported gender differences in cognitive restructuring tasks. Their initial study found that gender differences were in fact eliminated on one of two tasks when men and women were matched for eating restraint. On the other task, eating-restricted females performed the task more poorly than unrestricted females, thus exaggerating the male-female difference.[57] This work certainly confirms the need for eating restraint to be a factor which must be controlled in any study which attempts to measure gender differences. This research builds on previous work which showed that many differences found between fat and thin people are actually differences between restrained eaters (dieters) and non-restrained eaters (non-dieters). Even without further research, we know that some cognitive restructuring task gender differences disappear when dieting is controlled for and we know that dieting can result in poorer performance on a range of tests. What more proof do we need that dieting can prevent women from maximizing on their potential?

Although we have started to explore how the nearly universal pattern of men and boys getting fed more and better than women and girls can play a part in perpetuating women's inferior social and economic roles, it is hard to imagine all the many subtle and unnoticed ways in which this may manifest itself.

Hamilton, Popkin and Spicer suggest that nutritional status affects one's selection of work activities. Only well-nourished workers would be expected to qualify for the higher paying jobs if they are more physically or mentally demanding. Conversely, they suggest, individuals adapt to low energy intakes by being involved in less demanding occupations.[58]

Not surprisingly, most studies concentrate on nutrition-productivity relationships in men. Much less is known about the interaction of nutrition and productivity in women and, of course, even less is known about how nutrition affects women's roles outside the paid labour force. One study reported that supplementation of women's diets improves the mother-child interactions and enhances child development by providing women with greater energy and increasing their potential capacity for physical effort and active time for interaction

with the children.[59] A study of Guatemalan peasants found that women who receive dietary supplements spent more leisure and market time in physically active tasks than women who did not receive supplements. Sixty-seven percent of the supplemented group were considered "fully active" compared to only five percent of the unsupplemented group.[60]

The long term and intergenerational costs of the malnutrition-low status relationship in girls is just starting to be recognized. It is now known that cognitive development is dependent on both adequate nutrition and intellectual stimulation. Ten year follow-up studies of children who were treated for severe protein-calorie malnutrition showed no significant difference in mental performance when compared to their siblings or controls. But, there was a strong correlation between their intellectual achievement and years of schooling. It was noted that malnourished children sometimes took a few years to recover from any mental consequences of early childhood malnutrition and that the normal curriculum might not be appropriate during that time. This finding has particular significance for girls since in many communities girls will have already been withdrawn from school before the recovery time and thus girls will be deprived of the educational opportunity even if they were lucky enough to be treated for malnutrition.[61]

Several studies have now demonstrated the crucial importance of female education as a factor contributing to lower child mortality even when family income is controlled.[62] These studies do not try to explain the complex mechanisms through which improved female education operates to reduce child mortality, but they help emphasize that women, their children, and society are deprived when women do not get to explore their educational potential.

The relationship of girls' undernutrition and girls' not being able to maximize on their mental development and educational capabilities obviously has enormous ramifications for what women can contribute to society, what women are expected or encouraged to do, and the recognition they are given for their achievements. We saw how a child's birth weight, and thus "good start in life", was influenced by the mother's height and weight which was affected by the grandmother's nutrition. We now see the vital link among childhood nutrition, female educational opportunities and child mortality. Although this may be two different ways of looking at similar information, it is also a reminder of how these social and economic factors work together and exaggerate each other.

Consequently, the low value of females can cause the mothers to feed boys better than girls so that boys are less apt to be malnourished and more likely to be capable of benefitting from, and having access to, educational opportunities. Boys will then be far more likely to be the "well-nourished workers to qualify for the higher paying, higher status, physically or mentally demanding jobs" than their undernourished sisters. In one generation, in one community, the pattern could be clear cut—the boys worked to their potential more than the girls and the boys have more status than their sisters. When the sisters have their own children, how equally will they distribute the food and will they be aware of the unequal distribution if they give more to their sons than their daughters? In the extreme Bangladesh example, women tended to deny unequal distribution except when male child preference was expressed in relation to marked food shortages or in reference to sex differentials with regard to food quality.[63]

Does this extreme but not exaggerated example give us clues to how this process may operate more subtly? Having seen that cognitive development is dependent on both adequate nutrition and intellectual stimulation and having seen gender differences disappear (in one test) when men and women were matched for eating restraint, what significance is there in the fact that many nine year old girls are now dieting? We know the physical abilities of girls and boys are pretty evenly matched until age 10–12 when social pressure discourages young women from developing their physical potential. We know that many girls excel in maths at an early age but then internalize the "girls aren't good at maths" idea by adolescence. In what ways do these messages which limit young women from maximizing on their potential now get exaggerated by the pressure on them (and their mothers) not to let themselves get fat?

A young woman's nutritional needs are among the highest of her life when she is 11–14 years: an average 100 pound girl uses up 2400 Calories a day and needs a very vitamin and mineral concentrated diet. This is also one of life's most crucial times for making educational decisions which will influence future choices. If individuals or society wish to improve the role of women in society, this is the worst possible stage for young women to start practicing their lives as "thin fat people"!

REFERENCES

1. Judith Willis, "The Gender Gap at the Dinner Table", *FDA Consumer*, June, 1984, pp. 13–17.

2. 1989 RDA

3. Mary Roodkowsky, "Underdevelopment Means Double Jeopardy for Women", *Food Monitor*, September/October 1979, pp. 8–10.

4. Lisa Leghorn and Mary Roodkowsky, *Who Really Starve? Women and World Hunger*, New York: Friendship Press 1977, p. 20.

5. Colin Spencer, "Sex, Lies and Fed by Men", *Guardian*, November 4–5, 1989, p. 11.

6. Leghorn and Roodkowsky, *op. cit.*

7. E. M. Roenberg, "Demographic Effects of Sex Differential Nutrition" in N.W. Jerome, R.F. Kandel and G.H. Pelto (ed.) *Nutritional Anthropology—Contemporary Approaches to Diet and Culture*, Redgrave Publishing Co. 1980, pp. 181–203.

8. Charmian Kenner, *No Time for Women—Exploring Women's Health in the 1930s and Today*, London: Pandora 1985, p. 8.

9. Hilary Land, "Inequalities in Large Families: More of the Same or Different?" in Robert Chester and John Peel (ed.) *Equalities and Inequalities in Family Life*, New York: Academic Press 1977, pp. 163–175.

10. Hilary Graham, *Women, Health and the Family*, Brighton, Sussex: Wheatsheaf Books 1984, pp. 120–135.

11. Ruth Sidel, *Women and Children Last—The Plight of Poor Women in Affluent America*, New York: Viking 1986, p. 149.

12. E. Evason, *Just Me and the Kids: A Study of Single Parent Families in Northern Ireland*, Belfast: EOC 1980, p. 25, quoted in Graham, *op. cit.*

13. "Food for All?" *London Food News*, no.4-Autumn 1986, p. 1.

14. D. Marsden, *Mothers Alone: Poverty and the Fatherless Family*, Harmondsworth, Middlesex: Penguin 1973, p. 43, quoted in Graham, *op.cit.*

15. Neil Gallagher, "Obstacles Curb Efforts to Improve Nutrition", *World Food Programme Journal*, no.3, July–September, 1987, pp. 19–22.

16. Judit Katona-Apte, "Women and Food Aid—A Developmental Perspective", *Food Policy*, August, 1986, pp. 216–222.

17. Paul Fieldhouse, *Food and Nutrition: Customs and Culture*, London: Croom Helm 1986, pp. 168–169.

18. *Ibid.*, pp. 41–54.

19. *Ibid.*

20. Betsy A. Lehman, "Fighting the Battle of Freshman Fat", *The Boston Globe*, September 25, 1989, pp. 23, 25.

21. Joan Price, "Food Fixations and Body Biases—An Anthropologist Analyzes American Attitudes", *Radiance*, Summer 1989, pp. 46–47.

22. See for example the excellent resources of the Institute for Food and Development Policy, 1885 Mission Street, San Francisco, CA. 94103 (USA) or Oxfam, 274 Banbury Rd., Oxford OX2-7DZ (England).

23. Kathleen Newland, *The Sisterhood of Man*, London: W.W. Norton 1979, pp. 47–52.

24. Sahni Hamilton, Barry Popkin and Deborah Spicer, *Women and Nutrition in Third World Countries*, South

Hadley, Massachusetts: Bergin and Garvey Publishers 1984, pp. 22–26.

25. United Nations Administrative Committee on Coordination—Subcommittee on Nutrition, *First Report on the World Nutrition Situation,* Rome, Italy: FAO Food Policy and Nutrition Division 1987, pp. 36–39.

26. UNICEF News Fact Sheet printed in Leghorn and Roodkowsky, *op. cit.*

27. Hamilton, Popkin and Spicer, *op. cit.* p. 55.

28. Shushum Bhatia, "Status and Survival", *World Health,* April, 1985, pp. 12–14.

29. Physician Task Force on Hunger in America, *Hunger in America—The Growing Epidemic,* Middletown, Connecticut: Wesleyan University Press 1985, pp. 119–120.

30. Newland, *op.cit.*

31. Ethel Sloane, *Biology of Women,* 2nd Edition, New York: John Wiley 1985, pp. 122–123.

32. J. P. W. Rivers, "Women and Children Last: An Essay on Sex Discrimination in Disasters", *Disasters,* 6(4), 1982, pp. 256–267.

33. Amartya Sen, "The Battle to Get Food", *New Society,* 13 October, 1983, pp. 54–57.

34. Lincoln C. Chen, Emdadul Huq and Stan D'Souza, "Sex Bias in the Family Allocation of Food and Health Care in Rural Bangladesh", *Population and Development Review,* vol. 7, no. l, March, 1981, pp. 55–70.

35. Newland, *op. cit.*

36. Bhatia, *op. cit.*

37. Chen, Huq and D'Souza, *op. cit.*

38. Priyani Soysa, "Women and Nutrition", *World Review of Nutrition and Dietetics,* vol. 52, 1987, pp. 11–12.

39. Discussions with Chinese health workers and the All China Women's Federation, March 1978 and March 1983.

40. Victor W. Sidel and Ruth Sidel, *A Healthy State—An International Perspective on the Crisis in United States Medical Care,* New York: Pantheon 1977, p. 15.

41. Jeannette Mitchell, *What Is To Be Done About Illness and Health?* Harmondsworth, Middlesex: Penguin 1984, p. 22.

42. Soysa, *op. cit.*

43. Sidel and Sidel, *op. cit.,* p. 26,

44. Physician Task Force on Hunger in America, *op. cit.,* p. 99.

45. Melanie Tervalon, "Black Women's Reproductive Rights" in Nancy Worcester and Mariamne H. Whatley (ed.) *Women's Health: Readings on Social, Economic and Political Issues,* Dubuque, Iowa: Kendall/Hunt 1988, pp. 136–137.

46. Sidel and Sidel, *op. cit.,* p.17.

47. Physician Task Force on Hunger in America, *op. cit.,* p. 109.

48. Kenner, *op. cit.,* p. 10.

49. *Ibid.,* p. 8.

50. Ester, Boserup, *Women's Role in Economic Development,* London: George Allen and Unwin 1970, p. 165 quoted in Barbara Rogers, *The Domestication of Women—Discrimination in Developing Societies,* London: Tavistock 1981, p. 155.

51. Hamilton, Popkin and Spicer, *op. cit.* p.45.

52. Ellen McLean, "World Agricultural Policy and Its Effect on Women's Health", *Health Care for Women International,* vol. 8, 1987, pp. 231–237.

53. Hamilton, Popkin and Spicer, *op. cit.,* pp. 20– 21.

54. Soysa, *op. cit.,* pp. 35–37.

55. Hamilton, Popkin and Spicer, *op. cit.*

56. Hilde Bruch, "Thin Fat People" in Jane Rachel Kaplan (ed.) *A Woman's Conflict—The Special Relationship Between Women and Food,* Englewood Cliffs, New Jersey: Prentice-Hall 1980, pp. 17–28.

57. Claire Etaugh and Patricia Hall, "Restrained Eating: Mediator of Gender Differences on Cognitive Restructuring Tasks?", *Sex Roles,* vol. 20, nos. 7/8, 1989, pp. 465–471.

58. Hamilton, Popkin and Spicer, *op. cit.*

59. *Ibid.*

60. *Ibid.*

61. Soysa, *op. cit.,* pp. 13–14.

62. Chen, Huq and D'Souza, *op. cit.*

63. *Ibid.*

"Fatphobia"

by Nancy Worcester

We learn not to like fat people, then we internalize that as anxiety of gaining weight ourselves or self-hatred if we are already overweight. Both English and American studies consistently show that excess body fat is the most stigmatized physical feature except skin color.[1,2] Fatphobia differs from racism in that being overweight is thought to be under voluntary control. Anti-fat attitudes are well established before a child reaches kindergarten. "Even at that young age, children attribute negative characteristics to the heavy physique, do not want to be like that themselves, and choose a greater 'personal space distance' between themselves and a heavy child than from other children."[3]

The animosity towards fat people is such a fundamental part of our society, that people who have consciously worked on their other prejudices have not questioned their attitudes towards body weight. People who would not think of laughing at a sexist or racist joke, ridicule and make comments about fat people without recognizing that they are simply perpetuating another set of attitudes which negatively affect a whole group of people.

The pressure to look like the "ideal" is so strong that we do not question the implications behind teaching that routinely instructs young women on how to make their bodies look "as perfect as possible". Home economics classes teach young women that horizontal stripes make one look wider, vertical stripes make one look thinner. I was so well socialized by such instruction that I still find it hard to be comfortable in horizontal stripes, unless, of course, they are strategically placed so as to make the chest look larger! Even after years of criticizing the pressure on women to look thin, instead of admiring a large woman who has the courage to wear the "wrong" stripes, I still find myself wondering, "But, doesn't she know . . . ?"

Although the prejudice against fat people affects both men and women, its impact is most exaggerated on women and their lives. Women put on body fat more easily than men for a number of social and physiological reasons. Of course, every topic in this book is a part of the explanation. The physical abilities of females and males are identical until puberty, but by that time socialization in most western cultures discourages physical fitness in young women thus encouraging weight to be put on as fat rather than as muscle. (At the age of 25, body fat content averages 14% for men and 23% for women.[4]) Although both females and males have a mixture of the sex hormones estrogens and androgens, the average female tends to have higher levels of estrogens than androgens and this influences the deposition of fat. Times of hormonal changes, adolescence, going on oral contraceptive pills, pregnancy, and menopause, are all times when some women notice that they put on fat easily.

Women are judged by appearance far more than men and a much wider range of sizes and shapes is considered attractive in men. For example, a 1982 study of the most popular North American television programs, found that of male characters, less than one-fifth were slim and more than one-quarter were plump, whereas of the female characters, over two-thirds were slim and only one-tenth were plump.[5] Women, not men, are bombarded with information that the size and shape of their bodies is central to who they are and if it is less than perfect they should be working to try to change it. Comparing the most popular of men's and women's magazines, we see that articles and advertising relating to body weight and dieting appear 17 times more often in women's magazines.[6]

At any moment in history, the ideal female figure is quite precisely defined. Studies have shown that both men and women judge women's bodies by how closely they measure up to that supposed ideal. The more a woman deviates from that 'norm', the more her appearance will adversely affect her social life, her acceptance at college, her employment, and her status.

In both England and North America, obesity is more common in working class women than in women of higher socio-economic groups. With men, the relationship of class and body weight is not so well defined.[7,8]

It seems relevant to suggest that the relationship between social class and obesity is not as simple as just the fact that poor people have less access to healthy, nonfattening foods. It is *both* poor women and men who have less access to these foods so we would expect that the relationship of class to obesity to be more consistent for both women and men. I am not convinced that differences in manual labor provide an explanation. (It has been suggested that working class men offset a tendency to obesity by doing more physical labor than middle class men. This explanation does not take into account that middle class men have more access to leisure exercise opportunities and facilities than do working class men and that working class women are also more likely to be involved in physically active jobs than middle class women.)

Is it possible that in our society a woman's body build is a factor in *determining* her socio-economic status? Nearly twenty years ago, a paper on the stigma of obesity concluded that, "Obesity, especially as far as girls is concerned, is not so much a mark of low social economic status as a condemnation to it."[9] A study of 1660 adults in Manhattan observed that overweight women compared to non-obese women are far less likely to achieve a higher socio-economic status and are much more likely to have a lower socio-economic status than their parents.[10] This relationship was not found in men. A now classical study of the late 1960's found that non-obese women were more likely to be accepted for college than obese women even though the obese and non-obese women did not differ on intellectual ability or percentage who applied for college admission.

> If obese adolescents have difficulty in attending college, a substantial proportion may experience a drop in social class, or fail to advance beyond present levels. Education, occupation, and income are social-class variables that are strongly interrelated. A vicious circle, therefore, may begin as a result of college admission discrimination, preventing the obese from rising in the social-class system.[11]

As long as women are valued and rewarded for their roles as sex objects, and the non-skinny woman is not seen as fitting this image, it is easy to see how the stigma of excess weight limits a woman's status through job discrimination, apparently less marriage to high-status men (sic!) and fewer social and economic opportunities. The discrimination against fat women should serve as a reminder to all of us that we need to change the basis upon which the worth of all women is determined by society. Tragically, instead of viewing fatphobia as *society's* prob-

lem, many women internalize the fear and intolerance of fat as their *individual* problem. Instead of trying to change the world, women end up trying to change themselves.

In this era, when inflation has assumed alarming proportions and the threat of nuclear war has become a serious danger, when violent crime is on the increase and unemployment a persistent social fact, 500 people are asked by pollsters what they fear the most in the world and 190 of them answer that their greatest fear is 'getting fat'.[12]

REFERENCES

1. S. J. Chetwynd, R. A. Stewart, and G. E. Powell, "Social Attitudes Towards the Obese Physique" in Alan Howard (ed.) *Recent Advances in Obesity Research: 1,* London: Newman Publishing 1975, pp. 223–225.

2. Susan C. Wooley and Orland W. Wooley, "Obesity and Women—I. A Closer Look at the Facts", *Women's Studies International Quarterly,* vol. 2, 1979a, pp. 69–79.

3. Orland W. Wooley, Susan C. Wooley, and Sue R. Dyrenforth, "Obesity and Women—II. A Neglected Feminist Topic", *Women's Studies International Quarterly,* vol. 2, 1979b, pp. 81–92.

4. Marion Nestle, *Nutrition in Clinical Practice,* Greenbrae, California: Jones Medical Publications 1985, p. 222.

5. Brett Silverstein, *Fed Up—The Food Forces That Make You Fat, Sick and Poor,* Boston: South End Press 1984, p. 107.

6. Silverstein, *op. cit.*

7. Wooley, 1979b, *op. cit.*

8. J. Yudkin, "Obesity and Society", *Biblthca Nutri Dieta,* vol. 26, 1978, p. 146.

9. W. J. Cahnman, "The Stigma of Obesity", *Sociological Quarterly,* vol. 9, 1968, pp. 283–299, quoted in Wooley, 1979b, *op. cit.*

10. P. B. Goldblatt, M.E. Moore, and A. J. Stunkard, "Social Factors in Obesity", *Journal of the American Medical Association,* vol. 192, 1965, pp. 1039–1044.

11. H. Canning and J. Mayer, "Obesity—Its Possible Effect on College Acceptance", *New England Journal of Medicine,* vol. 275, 1966, pp. 1172–1174.

12. *San Francisco Chronicle,* January 17, 1981, quoted in Kim Chernin, *Womansize—The Tyranny of Slenderness,* London: The Women's Press 1983, p. 23.

"Mental Health Issues Related to Dieting"

by Nancy Worcester

The assumption is that if anyone is overweight they must be trying to lose weight and if they are not trying to lose weight, they certainly should be. The slimming industry has sold us this assumption and it is time that we stop swallowing it. The dieting experience is pretty disastrous for many women. We need to be more aware of the mental hazards of slimming and figure out ways to be more supportive of women who choose not to lose weight.[1] The more that women discover that they can live in large bodies without having to torture themselves with endless slimming diets, the less pressure there will be on all women to carve themselves down to smaller sizes.

1. Women Feel Guilty If They Are Not Slimming

The most liberating gift many women can give themselves is the decision that they are not going to try to lose weight. Until that decision is made, it is tempting to put off everything else and meanwhile dislike oneself both because of the fat itself and because the fat becomes symbolic of an unfulfilled goal.

As long as someone is thinking about changing her body, she is not going to be putting energy into learning to like her body the way it is.

As long as someone is postponing accepting and liking her body, there is a tendency not to work at making that body healthy and fit. This is a part of a self-perpetuating cycle. The more 'out-of-shape' one is, the more dissatisfying (and hard!) it is to undertake even ordinary exercise, the less exercise the body has the worse it feels and fewer calories will be burned up. This, of course, contributes to the tendency to gain weight and feelings of sluggishness.

See "We'll Always Be Fat but Fat Can Be Fit"[2] which takes a positive approach to accepting one's body weight and improving both mental and physical health.

2. Dieting Makes a Person More Aware of Food

We have all heard of someone who works through lunchtime without realizing they have not eaten or the person who loses weight because they are too busy to eat regularly.

One of the primary purposes of food advertising is simply to keep food on the mind so that the consumer is aware of her appetite. Secondly, of course, advertising aims to influence which particular product is on the mind.

In much the same way, the very act of dieting works to keep food on the mind. The constant preoccupation with not overeating (or more often, not eating normally) makes food take on a new significance. Thus, paradoxically, the most unmanageable time to restrict food consumption is when one is consciously attempting to limit food intake. Can you imagine committed dieters working through a lunchtime without realizing it or being so busy that they did not eat regularly?

Old studies claimed that a difference between fat people and thin people was that fat people ate according to external cues—set meal times, attractive foods, social situation—whereas thin people ate in response to internal cues such as hunger signals. Thus, this explanation implied, thin people were less likely to eat more than their bodies needed. This work is now being reinterpreted.[3] It seems that dieting is a major factor in determining whether one responds to external or internal signals. A dieter cannot respond to internal cues saying she is hungry because dieting creates a state of almost constant hunger. The old studies simply overlooked the fact that fat people are far more likely to be dieting than thin people. Instead of looking at the differences between fat and thin people, researchers were looking at the differences between dieters (restrained eaters) and non-dieters (non-restrained eaters). Dieting makes people unable to listen to their own body signals.

Dieting may be responsible for setting up a vicious cycle which increases the need for further dieting. Once a dieter's restraint is broken, the dieter can easily move in the opposite direction and 'overeat'. Depression and anxiety are emotions likely to break a dieter's restraint. Yet, dieting itself can cause anxiety, depression, and apathy.[4]

In attempting to change food habits, we are embarking upon changing one of our most conservative behaviors, something often intricately related to our inner sense of security. Food habits are the last patterns to change even when a person is living in a new environment and living a new lifestyle, e.g., immigrant food habits often more nearly resemble the diet of the homeland than of the new country even years after settling.

Additionally, changing one's pattern of food consumption presents a uniquely arduous challenge in that one has to deal with it daily, at regular intervals throughout the day. Difficult though it is, someone who is concerned about their smoking or drinking habits may choose to give up cigarettes or alcohol. Someone concerned about their eating habits does not have the option of giving up food.

These problems are all distinctly exaggerated for a woman responsible for others. She does not have the luxury of escaping from thoughts of food. While trying to ignore her own preoccupations with food/hunger, she will need to be making grocery lists, shopping in environments filled with visions and aromas of food, preparing food, serving food to others, and then cleaning up after the meals.

Such a seemingly unappetizing task as clearing up after a meal can be an immense challenge for the dieter. Keeping food intake records for nutrition classes, my students with young children have often discovered that a high percentage of their calorie intake comes from cleaning up the children's plates. They find themselves constantly torn between their lines not to waste food and their waistlines.

A major reason why women are somewhat less successful at losing weight than men is because their domestic responsibilities are so directly contradictory to the optimum conditions for dieting. Responsibility for food preparation is the worst imaginable antidote for the diet-induced obsession with food.

3. Dieting Often Fails

Few people would encourage a loved one, a friend, or a professional client to embark upon an activity which they knew was destined for failure. Yet, knowing that most dieting fails (probably 90%–98% in the long term),

people in all types of capacities are constantly advising and cajoling each other to "try to lose some weight", to check out the newest slimming gimmick, or to try the most recent best selling diet.

While it may be an overstatement to say that it is sadistic to encourage someone else to diet, it is time to acknowledge that it is often irresponsible to influence someone else to diet. The act of encouraging dieting needs to carry with it the obligation to support the dieter practically and emotionally through the challenges of the dieting process and to nurture the dieter if the attempt to lose weight is not successful. How many people would be willing to commit themselves to something so risky and potentially demanding? There would be far less pressure on people to diet if such pressure had to be accompanied by appropriate supportive commitments.

No one likes failure in any aspect of their life. Too often failure at dieting can take on a significance unexpected and unrecognized by the dieter and her friends. Media bombardment of fictitious slimming success stories completely nullifies the fact that only one to ten percent of dieting is "successful". Therefore dieting gets experienced as "something anyone should be able to do" and is not seen as a particularly ambitious goal. Failing at such a seemingly simplistic task can be especially disheartening.

Because of all the factors which influence body weight and the unpredictable ease with which one can or cannot lose weight, body weight is one of the most difficult areas of one's life to control. But, because body image is so central to a woman's self-image and confidence and is so related to her actual experiences in the world, a woman's inability to lose weight too often becomes symbolic for her of her failure to be in control of her own life.

4. Dieting May Be "Successful"

If a woman is successful at losing weight, she will lose the advantages of being fat.

Advantages of being fat are imperceptible to most dieters. Yet having managed to lose weight, many women are shocked to discover that the expectations of a slim woman are different than those of a fat woman in this society. I have stopped being surprised by how regularly I meet women who have purposefully gained back weight because they found that "sexual attractiveness" and not being taken seriously as thin women were so problematic. *Fat Is a Feminist Issue* has been immensely popular because it explores the meaning of being fat or thin in our society and enables women to discover why they may be subconsciously choosing to stay fat.

My fat says 'screw you' to all who want me to be the perfect mom, sweetheart, maid, and whore. Take me for who I am, not for who I'm supposed to be. If you are really interested in me, you can wade through the layers and find out who *I* am.[5]

Food can be an invaluable tool for relieving tension, coping with stress, or rewarding oneself. Successful dieting inevitably means changing those food habits that one has developed over a number of years. Additionally, the stress of dieting itself may undermine even the most well established coping mechanisms. Ingenuity is necessary in providing oneself with healthy alternatives to the role that food has played in keeping life in balance.

Education against child abuse is increasingly suggesting that adults hit a pillow or eat something to relieve tension involved in some adult-child interactions. This is a questionable and simplistic approach to decreasing child abuse, but it is a reminder of the role that food can play in defusing tension which could lead to physical violence or verbal confrontation with a child or an adult. Eating, even if that means overeating, will often be the healthiest way of dealing with immediate distress. We need to be alert to the dangers of dieting blocking that outlet.

There is also an obvious problem with the inverse relationship between cigarette smoking and weight. Women have been encouraged to use cigarettes as a means of weight control since the American Tobacco Company introduced the slogan "Reach for a Lucky instead of a sweet" in 1928.[6] Probably because of the way cigarette smoking affects metabolic rate, most people gain some weight when they stop smoking. Fear of weight gain is a major reason why women are less successful than men at quitting smoking.[7] Thus, lung cancer has now surpassed breast cancer as the leading cause of death in middle-aged women (in the US).[8] Women are paying with their lives for their success in keeping off a few pounds.

5. Suicide Is Less Common in Obese

A most intriguing figure never gets explained. Hidden near the bottom of all the charts showing the differences in mortality for obese and non-obese are the figures for suicide. Suicide rates are noticeably lower in both obese men and women. If obese and non-obese committed suicide at the same rate, suicide rates for obese would be recorded as 100% of actual expected deaths. Instead, the figure is only 73% for obese women and 78% for obese men.[9]

There seems to be at least one mental health advantage of obesity that is overlooked and not understood.

REFERENCES

1. Many of the ideas in this section have grown out of discussions of *Fat Is a Feminist Issue* with students and women's groups. (Susie Orbach, *Fat Is a Feminist Issue,* London: Paddington Press, 1978.)

2. Carol Sternhell, "We'll Always Be Fat But Fat Can Be Fit", *Ms,* May, 1985, pp. 66–68 and 142–154.

3. William Bennett and Joel Gurin, *The Dieter's Dilemma,* New York: Basic Books, 1982, pp. 34–45.

4. Valerie S. Smead, "Anorexia Nervosa, Bulimarexia, and Bulimia: Labeled Pathology and the Western Female", *Women and Therapy,* vol. 2, no. 1, 1983, pp. 19–35.

5. Susie Orbach, *Fat Is a Feminist Issue,* London: Paddington Books, 1978, p. 21.

6. Bennett and Gurin, *op. cit.,* pp. 92–93.

7. Bobbie Jacobson, *The Ladykillers—Why Smoking Is a Feminist Issue,* London: Pluto Press, 1981, pp. 14–15.

8. *1986 Cancer Facts and Figures,* American Cancer Society, 90 Park Avenue, New York, N.Y. 10016.

9. Jean Mayer, "Obesity" in Robert S. Goodhart and Maurice E. Shils (ed.) Febiger Press, 1980, pp. 721–740.

We'll Always Be Fat but Fat Can Be Fit

by Carol Sternhell

Sometimes I think we've all gone crazy. Sometimes I feel like a feminist at a Right-to-Life conference, an atheist in Puritan New England, a socialist in the Reagan White House. Sometimes I fear that fat women have become our culture's last undefeated heretics, our greatest collective nightmare made all too-solid flesh. I worry—despite our new ethos of sexual freedom—that female bodies are as terrifying and repulsive as ever, as greatly in need of purification and mortification. Certainly these days, when I hear people talking about temptation and sin, guilt and shame, I know they're referring to food rather than sex. When my friend Janet calls me up and confesses "I was bad today," I don't wonder whether she committed adultery (how archaic that sounds!); I know she merely means she ate dessert. When posters quoting Mae West appeared recently on Manhattan buses ("When choosing between two evils, I always like to take the one I've never tried before"), I wasn't surprised to find her remark illustrated with a picture of two different ice cream sundaes. (As I recall, however, when Mae West talked about evil, she generally wasn't thinking of hot fudge.) Kim Chernin, in *The Obsession: Reflections on the Tyranny of Slenderness* (Harper & Row), compares the language of diet books to "The old fire-and-brimstone sermons, intended to frighten men and women away from the delights and pleasures of sexual experience of their bodies." The sins of the flesh have been redefined, but the message is the same; a tremendous fear that women's natural appetites, uncontrolled, will bring about destruction.

Everything in this world, for women, boils down to body size.

We all know the story—the ugly duckling transformed into swan after years of liquid protein, the virtuous but oppressed stepdaughter whose fairy godmother appears with a pumpkin and a lifetime membership in Weight Watchers. Our fantasies of transformation are desperate, thrilling; when women imagine changing our lives, we frequently begin with our weight. "I always feel as if real life will begin tomorrow, next week, sometime after the next diet," said one friend, a talented writer who has been cheerfully married for 12 years and a mother for five. "I know it's crazy, but I won't be happy until I lose these fifteen pounds." So far her efforts—like 98 percent of all diets—have been unsuccessful. A few years ago, when public opinion pollsters asked respondents to name their greatest fear, 38 percent said "getting fat." Even very slender women believe that their lives would be better if only they could take off five pounds, or three, or two. In a recent survey conducted for *Glamour* by Susan Wooley, an associate professor in the psychiatry department of the University of Cincinnati College of Medicine, 75 percent of the 33,000 women who replied said that they were "too fat," including, according to Wooley, "45 percent who in fact were underweight," by the conservative 1959 Metropolitan Life Insurance Company Height and Weight Table. (By the revised 1983 table, which set generally higher levels of up to 13 pounds for desirable weights, these women would be even more underweight.) Wooley, who is also codirector of the university's Eating Disorders Clinic, sees our contemporary obsession with weight in part as a perversion of feminism. "This striving for thinness is striving to have a more masculine-type body," she points out. "As we join men's worlds, we shouldn't be cashing in women's bodies. We have to reclaim the right to have female bodies and still be respected. Thinness has become the cultural symbol of competency—if we buy that symbol and foster it ourselves, that's a very self-mutilating stand to take."

Everything in this world, for women, boils down to body size.

Cinderella's unfortunate stepsisters cut off chunks of their feet in order to fit into the prince's slipper. He knew they were impostors when he saw their blood oozing insistently over the delicate glass. These days women merely wire their jaws, staple their stomachs, and cut off chunks of their intestines in their effort to win the prince. "Stomach stapling" operations—50,000 are reportedly performed each year, 80 to 95 percent of them on women—can have side effects, such as abdominal pain, severe malnutrition, nausea and vomiting, osteoporosis, brain damage, and possibly even cancer. "Weight-loss surgery, including intestinal bypass operations, has probably already killed well over a hundred times as many people as the toxic shock syndrome, and has caused more than ten times as many deaths as AIDS," notes Paul Ernsberger, a postdoctoral research fellow at Cornell University Medical College. "More Americans have died in the surgeons' War on Fat than died in the Vietnam War." Yet desperate fat women—veterans of Stillman and Atkins, Scarsdale and Beverly Hills, diet camps and amphetamines—gratefully welcome the surgeon's knife, perhaps dreaming of old fairy tales. "I sometimes wish I had cancer," said a large, pretty woman in her early twenties at a diet workshop I once attended in San Francisco. "I sometimes think I wouldn't mind dying, if only I could die thin."

Everything in this world, for women, boils down to body size.

I still remember those little girls drinking diet soda and waiting for the miracle. I was 14 years old and 145 pounds that summer, at Camp Stanley for overweight girls, but many of the campers were younger, chubby little kids who already knew their bodies were their shame. When some of us failed to lose weight even on the camp's low-calorie regime, we were put on a special plan: three scoops of cottage cheese a day and all the diet soda we could drink. I remember the hunger (I would roll my pillow up under my stomach at night, trying to fill the hollow so I could sleep), the dizziness, but also the exhilaration; I felt like a secular saint, virtuous, disembodied, utterly pure. We sat around, starving, and talked about food, food we recalled from our profligate pasts. We talked about the new lives we would inhabit in the fall, transmuted all into magical swans.

I lost 15 pounds that summer and felt quite swanlike for a while, particularly among my relatives, who often seemed to admire weight loss the way other families might esteem an Olympic medal. By Christmas, however, when a group of campers gathered for a mini-reunion, every one of us had recouped our loses, and then some. We talked about the new lives we would inhabit in the spring, after the next diet had made us swans.

After the next diet, of course, most of us were fatter than before. Not only do almost all diets fail; according to Kim Chernin, "ninety percent of those who have dieted 'successfully' gain back more than they ever lost." This is not because "overweight" people are weak-willed compulsives, unable to pull our faces out of the Haagen-Dazs. (The medical profession may still disagree, but the medical profession, remember, once advised women that our reproductive organs would shrivel if we made the

mistake of obtaining a higher education.) In fact, observes Wooley, "On the whole fat people eat no more than thin people—often women who believe they're compulsive eaters are trying to deny the need to eat at all." The one thing fat women do more than other people is diet—and continual dieting, we now know, actually causes weight gain. "Repeated starvation can encourage fatness at the same time it destroys somebody's health," explains Ernsberger. "Cutting calories turns out to be the great fattener. The body—threatened with famine—overcompensates and creates new fat cells when normal eating is resumed. The cells may even double in number, and these new fat cells are forever. The body can now store more fat—the next diet will be harder."

A decade or so after my summer at Camp Stanley, I failed at a much more ambitious diet. This time I felt like a swan humiliatingly transformed into an ugly duckling. Even worse, I felt like a criminal; I was wearing my scarlet letter for all to see. My shame was intense—but as Wooley has remarked, "If shame could cure obesity, there wouldn't be a fat woman in the world."

During this period while attending graduate school in California, I sampled a variety of weight-loss groups. Two in particular were so disturbing that they made me question for the first time my own obsession with slimness. At the first, an Overeaters Anonymous meeting in Palo Alto, a depressed group of middle-aged people—mostly large and mostly women—sat on uncomfortable chairs in a chilly church basement and acknowledged that they were helplessly controlled by food. Only the aid of their "Higher Power" could save them, they agreed. At the height of the meeting one sad, gray-haired woman got up to tell us that she "really was shit." She didn't understand why, now that she'd lost weight, her husband had left her, but she said she was sure it must be for the best because everything—of course—was part of her Higher Power's plan. She said again and again that without the guidance of her HP she was "a piece of shit," and many group members murmured that they were too.

Then, in a San Francisco workshop ironically titled "Fat Liberation"—a supposedly progressive approach to weight loss in which participants "got in touch" with their feelings about fat and food—a group of women, almost all slender (but feeling fat), sat in a circle and imagined meeting a fat person in the street. "You were huge, gigantic, obese," one women wrote, "a man or a woman, androgynous in fat. I feel uncomfortable around you, and guilty. I avoid looking at your body, I feel sorry for you, threatened—you don't have to look like that. Under the surface you have nothing. I follow you to a dark room; you go in alone and sit. I leave you sitting there in the dark. When I leave, I am happy, whistling." We then sat on the floor and told a pile of food that it couldn't scare us any more.

After this workshop I bought a new political button: "How Dare You Presume I'd Rather Be Thin?" I've never had the nerve to wear it.

Fat women are continually told to lose weight in order to improve our health—but, in fact, we are likely to damage our health while trying to lose weight. Women don't drink liquid protein, pour saccharin in our coffee, and staple our stomachs in order to be healthy; instead, women risk death in order to be thin. According to Dr. Faith Fitzgerald of the University of California at Davis, "Obesity, as we commonly use the term, may be more of an aesthetic and moral problem than one of physical health." Certainly our horrified revulsion at the sight of a fat body springs from deeper sources than a disinterested concern for that body's well-being. If it did, the billions of dollars poured into the diet industry each year would be transferred to an anti-smoking campaign.

"In general, the healthiest eaters we see are fat women," adds Susan Wooley. "Most would have to be on a starvation diet their whole lives to get them down to a weight the culture considers normal, and the physical and emotional effects of starvation are much worse than the effects of overweight."

Nevertheless, most Americans—including most medical professionals—believe that fatness and good health are antithetical. A panel convened by the National Institutes of Health recently proclaimed obesity a "killer" disease. The 14-member panel set the danger point at a level of 20 percent or more above "desirable" body weight, but said that even five to 10 pounds above recommended weights could pose increased health risks to those people susceptible to or suffering from diseases like high blood pressure, adult onset of diabetes, and some cancers. A woman of my height, five feet four, would be 20 percent overweight at about 160, 40 pounds less than I weigh. The health charge is disturbing. No one—however terrific, energetic, and attractive she may feel—wants to walk around with a "killer" disease.

According to Ernsberger, the NIH report is simply wrong. "Fatness is *not* associated with a higher death rate," he says. "In fact, in every given population examined, the thinnest people have the highest death rate." The new NIH panel "flatly contradicts" previous reports of the same data, the well-known Framingham Heart Study, he adds. "The fact is the very fattest women in Framingham had a lower death rate than women who were at their 'correct' insurance table weights." The heaviest Framingham women, ranging from 40 percent to 172 percent over the 1959 tables, had lower mortal-

ity than both underweight women and women within a few pounds of their "desirable" weight. The *lowest* death rates, Ernsberger points out, occurred in women who were between 10 percent and 30 percent over the insurance tables. About 30 controlled studies correlating mortality and weight have reported similar findings. Dr. Ancel Keys of the University of Minnesota, a cardiovascular researcher, coordinated such studies in 16 different geographical areas with an emphasis on risk factors leading to heart attacks. He concluded that "in none of the areas of this study was overweight or obesity a major risk factor for death or the incidence of coronary heart disease."

"Cancer deaths actually decrease with increasing fatness," says Ernsberger. "Only one study, the study cited in the NIH report, showed an increase in cancer rates," he adds, "while five or six that I know of show a decrease with increasing fatness." The NIH panel chose to ignore the decreased overall cancer rate in obesity, mentioning only that a single type of cancer, uterine cancer, is more common in obese women.

Wooley concurs. "A person can definitely be fat and healthy," she says. "My reading of the literature tells me that for women there's a very sizable weight range in which extra weight does *not* constitute a risk in mortality." Wooley notes that some studies have shown that women can weigh up to 200 pounds, without increased mortality risks, and even after that point, she says, being overweight may be healthier than dieting.

Many of the health problems commonly associated with fatness are probably caused by fat people's incessant pursuit of thinness, Ernsberger points out. Thus the "yo-yo syndrome"—that deadly cycle of weight loss and weight regain—may cause hypertension; diet pills can also cause high blood pressure and amphetamine psychosis; low carbohydrate diets can raise cholesterol; and liquid protein diets have led to heart disease and sudden death. "We don't know how unhealthy overweight is in and of itself because most overweight people have been doing these things," Ernsberger comments.

Furthermore, fat people receive terrible health care, partly because doctors see them as "bad patients" and partly because the overweight person herself tends to give up in despair. "We've had it drummed into our heads that the *only* route to fitness is through weight loss," explains Nancy Summer, member of the board of directors of the National Association To Aid Fat Americans (NAAFA), a nationwide fat rights organization based in New York. Summer, a dynamic blond who weighs more than 300 pounds, swims twice a week on Long Island with a group of large women. "Many of us have developed an all-or-nothing attitude. If we can't be thin, we may as well not worry about nutrition or exercise—we are going to die young anyway. I think it's time we reject that concept."

The medical evidence may be contradictory—obesity "experts" may disagree—but the message to me as a self-accepting fat woman is fairly simple. People come in lots of different sizes, and our frantic struggle to squeeze—all of us—into the thinnest 10 percent of a once-normal bell-shaped curve is driving us all crazy (and at the same time making us fatter). Self-hatred and cultural stigmatization doesn't do anyone any good; indeed, many of the diseases frequently associated with overweight are stress-related illnesses. Even, if all the other things being equal, it is "healthier" to be thin, weight-reduction programs fail 98 percent of the time, according to Chernin. Therefore I have two choices: I can be fat and unhealthy or I can be fat and healthy. I can find a new miracle diet, or I can eat sensible food (fruit and veggies, fiber, not too much fat, sugar, or salt), avoid cigarettes, and get plenty of exercise.

I'll still be fat, but fat can be fit.

The six women flash brightly colored tights and leotards, shake to a driving rock beat, smile at their reflections in shiny mirrors, bend and stretch, tap some feet. It's just another Manhattan exercise class, but here all the women look like Rubens' models, ranging in size from perhaps 150 pounds to well over 200. At the Greater Woman, "New York's first exercise studio for the large woman," clients are expected to be at least 30 pounds over their "ideal" weight—some weigh nearly 300 pounds—but the program emphasizes fitness and self-esteem rather than weight loss.

"There's a great difference between fitness and skinniness," says Mary Sams, a family psychotherapist who heads the studio. "Women are told that fat is immoral, that everyone who is overweight is out of control, consuming massive amounts of food. That's garbage."

According to Sams, the purpose of Greater Woman "is not to get people to lose weight, but to help people become fit and healthy and change their feelings about themselves. A lot of women come here wanting to get thinner," she adds, "but three weeks into the program they're thinking entirely differently." Clients are likely to lose inches rather than pounds. "Over several months, their dress sizes may go down," says Greater Woman's nutritionist, Jeannette Harris, "but they don't see a decrease on the scale." "Fitness isn't a scale measurement," agrees Sams. "Our goal is to increase lean body mass and raise the metabolic rate." In order to accomplish this, the studio has developed exercise classes specifically tailored to the needs of larger women. "The only exercise that really increases metabolic rate is aerobics," explains

Sams. "We have learned to choreograph aerobic dances that are very lively but don't involve pounding exercises, which put too much stress on the knees and back."

The class members I speak with seem genuinely enthusiastic, and sometimes amazed to find themselves moving about so vigorously. One, a psychiatric social worker who has lost 30 pounds in the last year, explains earnestly, "People don't come here to lose weight, just to feel human about their bodies."

Remember the old fairy tales, the ugly ducklings and crippled stepsisters and hungry little girls all waiting for their miracle? Well, it's not exactly the story I'd imagined, but my transformation finally took place. My chronicle has a happy ending, but it's an ending with a twist, for as Susan Wooley once remarked, "When it comes to weight, people can't accept a happy ending that leaves us different shapes and sizes. To me, a happy ending is when someone can accept her body as it is."

My fairy godmother showed up after all, but she didn't change my body: she changed my mind.

RESOURCES

Shadow on a Tightrope: Writings by Women on Fat Oppression, edited by Lisa Schoenfielder and Barb Wieser, foreword by Vivian Mayer *(Aunt Lute Book Company. Iowa City).* The best feminist collection I know of on the subject of fat. Includes much material from the original Fat Underground, a feminist fat liberation group that formed in Los Angeles in 1973.

The Obsession: Reflections on the Tyranny of Slenderness, by Kim Chernin *(Harper Colophon Book).* A subtle, well-written, and sometimes brilliant dissection of our cultures' frenzied pursuit of thinness, and its terror of female flesh.

The Dieter's Dilemma, by William Bennett, M.D., and Joel Gurin *(Basic Books).* A thoughtfully presented and scientific case against dieting as a means of weight control.

Such a Pretty Face: Being Fat in America, by Marcia Millman, with photographs by Naomi Bushman *(Norton).* A sociologist's investigation of what it is like "to live as a fat person in our society." Much of the material is drawn from interviews with fat people and from observations of organizations like NAAFA and Overeaters Anonymous.

Fat Is a Feminist Issue: A Self-Help Guide for Compulsive Eaters, by Susie Orbach *(Berkley).* Some feminists have found Orbach's discussion helpful, but it disturbs me because its emphasis is still on achieving thinness. Here fatness is seen not as a sin, but as a means of adapting to a sexist society. When women learn better ways of coping with sexism, Orbach believes, they will become slim. She also makes the mistake of confusing fatness with compulsive eating. They are two distinctly different conditions.

Big & Beautiful: How To Be Gorgeous on Your Own Grand Scale, by Ruthanne Olds *(Acropolis Books).* A fashion guide for women size 14 and up.

BBW: The World's First Fashion Magazine for the Large-Size Woman. Six-issue subscription is $13 from BBW *(Suite 214. 5535 Balboa Blvd. Encino. Calif. 91316).* A fashion magazine published six times a year. BBW stands for Big Beautiful Woman.

NAAFA—The National Association To Aid Fat Americans (P.O. Box 43. Bellerose. N.Y. 11426). The country's premier fat

rights organization, active since 1969. Call 516–352–3120 or write for information. Sponsors both political action and social events.

The Greater Woman (111 East 65 St., N.Y., N.Y. 10128; telephone: 212–737–4889). Exercise classes for the larger woman.

Book Review:
"The Obesity Myth"
by Paul Campos from *HealthFacts*

The obesity myth, according to author Paul Campos, is based on three claims: that excess weight causes illness and early death; that losing weight improves health and extends life; and that we know how to make fat people thin. The book is well armed with footnotes to support his argument that the public has gotten a skewed view of the research from the media and from obesity specialists, who are largely funded by the $50 billion a year weight loss industry.

The author is not saying that weight is entirely irrelevant to good health. (It is, he says, unhealthy to be at each extreme, morbidly obese and extremely thin.) Instead, he lays out a convincing case for how the adverse health effects of excess weight have been grossly exaggerated. Take heart disease, for example. Most cardiologists will tell you that excess weight is right up there after smoking as a major risk factor for heart attack.

Yet the nation's heart disease death rate has been steadily declining since the 1960s and continues to decline even after the upsurge in the number of overweight and obese Americans that began in the 1980s. Contrary to conventional medical wisdom, many fat people have none of the risk factors—high blood sugar levels, high blood pressure and high cholesterol—associated with illness and early death. Excess weight increases the risk of heart disease, at most, by 1-5%, says Campos, and some studies even suggest obesity is a protection against vascular disease.

By now, the extremely high failure rate of all diets is well known, and Campos, a professor of law at the University of Colorado and a syndicated columnist, reminds

us of the well publicized deaths and injuries associated with diet drugs. One popular over-the-counter weight loss drug, for example, had a now withdrawn ingredient proven to cause strokes in young women.

Still, the "get thin, live longer" message drives many people to diet and drugs with the idea that the benefits of losing weight clearly outweigh the risks. Unfortunately, numerous studies suggest otherwise. For example, The New York Times reported this in 2002: "Dr. Jules Hirsch, an obesity researcher at Rockefeller University [in New York City] provided evidence from studies conducted by others that followed thousands of people for years, keeping track of who lost weight, who kept it off, who become ill and who died. Repeatedly, investigators reported that fat people who lost weight and kept it off had more heart disease and a higher death rate than people whose weight never changed."

Campos's book is filled with references to this type of research that is largely overlooked because of its inconvenient findings. And why don't we hear about the health risks of yo-yo dieting (weight cycling)? Could it be that there are industries from—women's magazines to weight loss clinics—that would go down the tubes if word gets out? One reason why the public gets a distorted view of the adverse health effects of obesity, says Campos, is the focus on weight by most researchers who ignore other factors that create ill health in fat people, such as sedentary lifestyle, poor diet, dieting-induced weight fluctuations, diet drug use, poverty, lack of access to and discrimination in health care, and social discrimination.

New Book Review of *The Obesity Myth* by Paul Campos from *HealthFacts*, August 2004, pp. 4–5. Reprinted by permission of Maryann Napoli.

That a fat person can be healthy and physically fit has been demonstrated in the work of Steven Blair and colleagues at the Cooper Institute in Dallas, who have conducted a study of over 70,000 people and followed them for more than 20 years. Unlike other researchers who either ignore the role of physical activity or allow study participants to self-report activity levels, the Cooper Institute conducted regular treadmill testing throughout their study. Campos says that this study showed that obese, not merely overweight, people who engage in at least moderate levels of physical activity show half the death rate of sedentary people of ideal weight.

America is on the verge of an obesity-induced Type 2 diabetes epidemic, we are told, but Campos pokes holes in this contention. Here, he relies on the work of Paul Ernsberger, professor at the Case Western Reserve University School of Medicine, who is well versed in the obesity research and a critic of how the findings are portrayed to the public. "Actually, there is no hard data that says blood sugar levels are rising," according to Dr. Ernsberger, who points to telephone surveys as the source for this purported rising incidence of Type 2 diabetes. Aggressive

educational programs aimed at testing are one reason why many people report themselves as diabetics in telephone surveys, according to Dr. Ernsberger, who explained that doctors often tell people they are "borderline diabetics" or to "watch out for diabetes," and this has led some people to think they already have the condition. Not incidentally, the definition of Type 2 diabetes was changed from a fasting blood sugar of 140 to a blood sugar of 126. Overnight, millions of Americans became diabetics.

The book's parting words of advice—stop obsessing about weight. "The prosecutors in the case against fat aren't completely wrong: They've just indicted the wrong parties. Americans are too sedentary. We do eat too much junk that isn't good for us, because it's quick and cheap and easier than the alternative of spending the time and money to prepare food that is both good for us and satisfies our cravings. A rational public health policy would focus on those issues, not on weight, which isn't the problem, any more than diets and diet drugs would be the solution, even if they actually made people thin (thin people with bad health habits are no healthier than fat people with the same habits)."

"Making 'A Way Outa No Way'"

by Becky W. Thompson

Compulsive eating, bulimia, and anorexia have taken on complicated symbolic significance in late twentieth-century culture in the United States. Those suffering from eating problems invariably are thought to be young, middle- to upper-class, heterosexual white women desperately trying to mold their figures to standards created by advertisers and clothing designers. The most popular terminology used to describe these problems is "eating disorder," which suggests that some psychological frailty or inadequacy is the agent of the illness. In short, those suffering from eating problems are thought to be decadent, self-absorbed, and heavily implicated in their own troubles. Such conceptions are misguided, short-sighted, and harmful. They are built on

skewed assumptions about race, class, and sexuality that belittle the putative victims—white, middle-class, heterosexual women—while they ignore women of color, working-class women, and lesbians.

Talking with Latina, African-American, and white women—including both heterosexual and lesbian women—reveals that the origins of eating problems have little or nothing to do with vanity or obsession with appearance. In fact, eating problems begin as survival strategies—as sensible acts of self-preservation—in response to myriad injustices including racism, sexism, homophobia, classism, the stress of acculturation, and emotional, physical, and sexual abuse. The women I interviewed for this book told me stories that starkly

"Making 'A Way Outa No Way,'" from *A Hunger So Wide and So Deep* by Becky Thompson, University of Minnesota Press, 1994, pp. 1–26. Reprinted by permission.

expose how eating problems often begin as an orderly and sane response to insane circumstance.

Their candid stories about how and why they turned to food to cope requires that the reader grapple with the idea of both subtle and overt injustices regularly visited upon women. Some of the experiences the women described are of outrageous, deliberate, and sometimes brutal acts that compromised their ability to feel safe—to be comfortable and sure—in their bodies and in the world. Their experiences reveal both how they developed eating problems and how their ingenious methods of healing are nothing less than testimonies of endurance and empowerment. Their creative strategies for carrying on with their lives—often against great odds—along with their dedication to healing their minds, bodies, and spirits, give yet another face to Minnie Ransom's wise words in Toni Cade Bambara's novel *The Salt Eaters:* "Wholeness is no trifling matter."

On a concrete level, then, the book explains why eating problems are logical, creative responses to trauma, and it identifies effective methods of healing. On a political level, the book posits that bingeing, purging, and starving will continue until women's access to racial, social, sexual, and political justice is ensured. On a more philosophical level, it suggests that women who face injustice have much to teach about faith and resistance, trauma and coping, creativity and despair. My hope is that the book does justice to the experiences of the women I interviewed, reinforcing their ability to—in the words of Richard Wright—"create a sense of the hunger for life that gnaws in us all, to keep alive in our hearts a sense of the inexpressibly human."

Origins of This Book

Embedded in public and medical perceptions of health and disease are metaphors created to explain, engage with, and sometimes dismiss illness. In her creative and expansive approach to scholarship, Susan Sontag has unpacked metaphors surrounding cancer, documenting how cancer has been regarded as a disease of the psychically defeated, the inexpressive, and the repressed. As a cancer patient herself, Sontag was enraged by how much "the very reputations of this illness added to the suffering of those who have it." In her later work, Sontag expanded this framework with her illuminating insights about AIDS, detailing how metaphors about illness reveal much about current states of social disease. She is particularly interested in illness metaphors that, she believes, are used to justify authoritarian rule and militarism. She traces the origins of these militaristic metaphors back to World War I in explanations about syphilis and tuberculosis. These afflictions were de-

scribed as invasions of alien organisms to which the body responds with its own militaristic operation. While militaristic metaphors still predominate in descriptions about disease, particularly with regard to AIDS, the identity of the enemy has changed. In this shifting use of metaphors, the threat to supremacy is no longer Russia or communism; rather, it is domestic, a result of changing relations in an increasingly multicultural world. In a quintessential social constructionist analysis, Sontag roots conceptions of disease within their historical contexts, capturing public anxiety and political conflicts as they are projected onto human illness.

Like many illnesses represented in the public imagination—such as cancer and AIDS—eating problems are imbued with their own images. Among them is the image of anorexia and bulimia as transitory, self-inflicted obsessions developed by young women lost in their own worlds of fashion, scales, and calorie counting. The cost of the dedication to this idea is paid by those with eating problems, sometimes with their lives. While many know that Karen Carpenter's death was caused by anorexia, few are aware that she was only one of about 150,000 women who die of anorexia each year. More people die of anorexia in a year than died of AIDS in the Untied States from the beginning of the epidemic until the end of 1988. This comparison is not meant to minimize the tragedy of AIDS, but to uncover one of the most powerful popular assumptions about eating problems: that, although they are prevalent, they are decadent acts of self-obsession that are only in rare situations life threatening.

In 1984 I began to conduct workshops on eating problems among women and men, and, over time, I started to question this vexing portrayal along with the standard profile that has been attached to it. I soon saw that while many women fit the usual profile—white, middle and upper class, heterosexual—many did not. I began to look, largely in vain, for research about women of color and lesbians, and I resorted to incorporating any anecdotal evidence I could find. I cited, for example, Dinah Washington, the jazz singer whose untimely death resulted from a lethal combination of alcohol and diet pills; Oprah Winfrey, whose struggles with her weight have been followed by millions of television viewers; the multigenerational eating problems among African-American women in Gloria Naylor's *Linden Hills;* and poetry about anorexia by the prominent Puerto Rican writer Luz Maria Umpierre-Herrera. My friend Mary Gilfus, a social worker and sociologist who has worked in a women's prison, told me that many incarcerated women are bulimic. Other prison activists have also noted the widespread use of laxatives among women in prison. Prison policy supports the development of eating problems. Healthy food is rarely available; the meals are high in fat and starch, which makes it difficult not to gain weight. Because of severe restrictions on freedom of movement, the act of eating takes on an importance that makes incarcerated women vulnerable to bingeing. The fact that they are disproportionately African-American, Latina, poor, and working-class women raises further questions about the standard profile of women with eating problems.

My interest in women's health in general and my increasing frustration with the dearth of information on eating problems among women of color and lesbians led me to write this book. I conducted eighteen in-depth interviews with African-American, Latina, and white women with eating problems, which allowed me to scrutinize the standard profile and to develop a framework in many ways different from the one offered by the popular media and held by many researchers. Of the women I interviewed, two-thirds have had eating problems for more than half their lives—which counters the popular conception of anorexia and bulimia as transitional and temporary. The fact that the average age among the women I interviewed was thirty-three does not support the common belief that eating problems are primarily teenage problems. Several women were taught to diet, binge, and purge by older relatives—who had done so for years themselves—which suggests that eating problems may not be as historically specific as is typically thought. When eating troubles are seen as survival strategies rather than as responses to strictures about size and shape, they can be identified long before Twiggy's arrival on the fashion scene and Jane Fonda's exercise regimes.

A multiracial focus also raises questions about the adequacy of the theoretical models used to explain eating problems. The biomedical model offers important scientific research about possible physiological causes of eating problems and the physiological dangers of purging and starvation. However, this model adopts medical treatment strategies that may disempower and traumatize women, and it ignores many historical and cultural factors that influence women's eating patterns. The psychological model identifies eating problems as "multidimensional disorders" that are influenced by biological, psychological, and cultural factors. While it is useful in its exploration of effective therapeutic treatments, this model, like the biomedical one, tends to neglect women of color, lesbians, and working-class women.

A third model, offered by feminists, opened up the field of inquiry in crucial ways. With the emergence of feminist work, eating problems were rescued from the realm of individual pathology. When Susie Orbach's *Fat is a Feminist Issue* was published in 1978, its critique of dieting and self-denial and its convincing plea for understanding bingeing as a way women cope with living in a society that relegates them to second-class citizenship made it a handbook for thousands of women. This was one of many important books by therapists, sociologists, physicians, and researchers that focused on gender. The fact that most people with eating problems are women was no longer considered simply a factor in but rather integral to understanding anorexia and bulimia.

Feminist argue that patriarchy—which limits women's access to power both within and outside the family—is at the root of women's eating problems. Most women are relegated to sex-segregated jobs that pay them less well than men are paid for comparable work. What is typically referred to as the "glass ceiling" in employment is actually a euphemism for real men's bodies blocking most women's advancement. These barriers, coupled with educational systems that still steer girls away from mathematics, science, and competitive sports, help explain why adolescent girls' self-esteem declines as boys' self-esteem increases. In this context, eating problems signal women's many hungers—for recognition, achievement, and encouragement. It is no surprise that appetites and food take on metaphorical significance in a society in which women typically are responsible for food preparation and yet are taught to deny themselves ample appetites; girls are taught that the barriers they face are their own fault and therefore require individual solutions; and female socialization means caring for others, often at one's own expense.

Rightfully, feminists have raised questions about why the emphasis on dieting and thinness has become so severe. In her groundbreaking book *The Obsession: Reflections on the Tyranny of Slenderness*, Kim Chernin argues that in this historical period of women's increased struggle for economic, legal, and sexual power, one form of patriarchal backlash is defining female beauty as childlike and thin. Chernin writes, "In this age of feminist assertion men are drawn to women of childish body and mind because there is something less disturbing about the vulnerability and helplessness of a small child and something truly disturbing about the body and mind of a mature woman."

In the United States, this image is upheld by interlocking institutional powers: a multi-million-dollar weight-reducing industry in which most of the consumers are women; medical professionals who maintain the dubious assumption that fat is by definition unhealthy and ought to be eliminated; a multi-million-dollar advertising industry that promotes demeaning images of women; a job market in which women who do not fit this model of beauty face discrimination; and an insurance industry that upholds medically prescribed standards of what constitutes a healthy body size. A 1984 national poll of 33,000 women conducted by *Glamour* magazine found that the majority of women surveyed were ashamed of their stomachs, hips, and thighs—parts of the body that contribute to female shapes. The pressure to diet that many girls face from a very young age is an example of an assault aimed directly at the very parts of bodies that are decidedly female—as women throw up and out, excise or diet away breasts, hips, and buttocks. Feminists rightfully ask how different the quality of women's lives might be if the enormous energy they are taught to invest in denying themselves food were redirected toward dismantling sexism in all its many manifestations.

Feminists have also spearheaded research on the connections between eating problems and sexual abuse. In so doing, they have laid the foundation for understanding other traumatic origins of many eating problems. Identifying the functional basis of bingeing and purging helps take eating problems out of the realm of "disorder" and into the realm of coping mechanisms. As is true of feminist frameworks on the field of health in general, feminist research on eating problems has refused to diagnose them as individual psychic conflicts. Portraying them as individual "disorders" rather than as responses to physical and psychological distress is part of a historical tendency to mislabel the results of social injustices as individual pathologies. It is for this reason that some feminist theorists, including me, avoid using the term "disorder" altogether in relation to women's eating patterns, particularly since, for many women, bingeing, purging, and dieting begin as creative coping mechanisms in highly "disordered" circumstances.

Despite significant feminist contributions, scholarship typically has focused on gender to the exclusion of other analytical categories—specifically, race, sexuality, and class. This imbalance in the literature on eating problems mirrors similar exclusionary practices in much white feminist scholarship that bases its theoretical framework on a false universalism. In this way, scholarship on eating problems is not particularly behind in its lack of attention to race, sexuality, and class. Unfortunately, it mirrors health scholarship in general.

This research historically has failed to consider race a significant focus, often treating race or gender or both as "afterthoughts in analyses rather than main points of research studies." Until recently, research on cancer and alcoholism, for example, has paid little attention to African-American women, despite the fact that black women die of cancer far more frequently than white

women do. The initial nomenclature for AIDS—gay-related immunodeficiency—identified an "at risk" population that erroneously excluded women and heterosexual men. Although women of color in the United States are now the fastest-growing group infected with the HIV virus, government programs and most private agencies are still poorly equipped to respond to their health care needs.

Rethinking biased assumptions in the literature on eating problems begins with scrutinizing ideas about femininity and gender socialization. For example, the belief that women's bodily insecurities are fueled by lessons about femininity that teach women to be passive and complaint may accurately describe socialization patterns among middle- and upper-class Protestant white women, but this does not apply to many African-American and Jewish women, who are often encouraged to be assertive, self-directed, and active both within their families and publicly. Nor do passivity and dependence accurately describe lesbians and single, divorced, and widowed women who do not rely upon men for economic support and who tend to work in the paid labor market all of their lives. The notion that an institutional imperative toward thinness is a backlash against women's economic gains does speak to the advances of white middle-and upper-class women. But, as these women have been struggling to move up the occupational ladder, working-class women of all races have been striving simply to stay on the ladder—a ladder that, for them, has been horizontally rather than vertically positioned. While women of all classes and races are affected by a backlash Susan Faludi rightfully termed "the undeclared war against American women," the link some theorists draw between this backlash and augmented economic power is a race- and class-specific supposition that reinforces the association of eating problems with "achievement-oriented" business and professional women. Once again, anorexia and bulimia are rendered invisible among working-class women.

Similarly, the connection drawn between an increase in eating problems and "superwoman" expectations—as more women juggle careers and family responsibilities—accurately identifies changes in the participation of white middle-class women in the paid labor market. More middle-class white women are balancing two full-time jobs, but this double duty is not new for working- and middle-class women of color, lesbians, and single mothers. As white middle-class women have been fighting for the right to work outside the home, many black and Latina women have been fighting for the opposite: a chance to stay home with their children.

Race and class stratification breaks apart a singular reliance upon sexism as the underlying cause of eating problems. The women I interviewed linked the origins of their eating problems to many different types of trauma, many of which have received scant attention from researchers or the media. More than half of them—across race and class—were survivors of sexual abuse, which was often peppered with racism or anti-Semitism. Some women tied eating problems to a range of class factors, including poverty and stress caused by upward class mobility. Among the lesbians, some developed eating problems to cope with homophobia. Other traumas women linked to eating problems were emotional and physical abuse, often laced with racism, and witnessing abuse of siblings or parents.

The multiple traumas women link to their eating problems do not discount the important feminist analyses of the impact of sexist assaults against women's bodies and appetites. A multiracial focus, however, complicates the picture considerably. While feminists have shown how emotional, physical, and sexual abuse may lead women to binge or purge, little attention has been given to how inequalities besides sexist ones change women's eating patterns. Such a focus requires an expanded understanding of trauma that includes not only physical but also psychic injuries. In this way, trauma may include what Harriette McAdoo has termed the "mundane extreme environmental stress" of racism, injuries from poverty, incest and other sexual abuse, physical and emotional abuse, immigration, battery, heterosexism, and a variety of other socially induced injuries.

It is frightening to consider that the many extraordinary and harrowing accounts of trauma the women I interviewed identified may not, in fact, be uncommon. One African-American woman began bingeing when she was four years old because it gave her reliable comfort from the pain of sexual abuse, racism, and witnessing the battering of her mother. A white upper middle class Jewish woman attributed fasting for days on end to sexual and emotional abuse by her boyfriend. Pressed into isolation with the threat of further abuse, this woman began to think she deserved no pleasures—eating, seeing people, or even going out in the sunlight. She locked herself up in her dormitory room, sometimes even in her closet, and starved herself. A Latina woman described her body as a "shock absorber" that attracted the "world's pain," going back as far as she could remember. She ate to buffer herself from this pain. She remembered wondering at the age of five if an entire picnic table of hot dogs, hamburgers, chips, potato salad, and buns would be enough to fill her. Beset by emotional abuse and her relatives' constant criticism of her

weight, she had little chance to understand either her body or her appetite as trustworthy or safe.

Identifying the traumatic bases of many eating problems reveals the dangers of labeling a common way women cope with pain as an appearance-based disorder. One blatant example of sexism is the notion that women's foremost worries are about their appearance—a belittling stereotype that masks women's worries about paying the bills, keeping their children off the streets and in school, and building loving and egalitarian relationships. By highlighting the emphasis on slenderness, the dominant imagery about eating problems falls into the same trap of assuming that difficulties with eating reflect women's "obsession" with appearance. This misnaming fails to account for the often creative and ingenious ways that girls and women cope with multiple hardships, quite frequently with no one's help but their own.

The culture-of-thinness model has also been used, erroneously, to dismiss eating problems among women of color based on the notion that they are not interested in or affected by a culture that demands thinness. This ideology lumps into one category a stunning array of racial and ethnic groups—Japanese-Americans, Chicanas, Hopi, Puerto Ricans, Amerasians, and African-Americans, to name just a few. The tremendous cultural, religious, and historical diversity among these groups of people makes the notion that they are—as a whole—invulnerable to eating problems dubious at best.

Emphasis on thinness is certainly not universal or equally tenacious across race and ethnicity. There are aspects of African-American culture, for example, that historically have protected against a demand for very thin bodies. In addition, festivities that take place when food is being prepared and eaten are key aspects of maintaining racial identity. Many black women writers, for example, include positive images of physically large women who enjoy food, and celebrate women of varying shapes and sizes. In fact, Alice Walker's definition of "womanist" includes a woman who "loves love and food and roundness." In her poem "Song for a Thin Sister," Audre Lorde also celebrates size and rejects the notion of thinness as an ideal:

Either heard or taught
as girls   we thought
that skinny was funny
or a little bit   silly
and feeling a pull
toward the large and the colorful
I would joke you   when
you grew too thin.

But your new kind of hunger
makes me chilly   like danger
I see you forever retreating
shrinking   into a stranger
in flight
and growing up
Black   and fat
I was so sure that   skinny
was funny   or silly
but always
white.

In her poetic voice, Lorde associates "skinny" with whiteness and a culture outside her own. One African-American woman I interviewed was raised in a rural community in Arkansas that valued women of ample proportions. One Puerto Rican woman was given appetite stimulants as a child because her mother thought that skinny children looked sickly.

This ethic did not, however, stop either of them from developing eating problems. In her chronicle about eating problems, Georgiana Arnold, an African-American health educator, identifies dual and conflicting patterns about food. While eating was a joyful part of family life, fat was a topic that the family avoided:

In our home, food was a source of nourishment, a sign of love, a reward and the heart of family celebrations. It was also a source of ambivalence, guilt, shame, and conflict. Our "family fat" issues descended into the same cavern of silence that housed my father's alcoholism, gambling and willful disappearance from our lives. There was no talking about it and there were no tears.

Ironically, an ethic that celebrates food and protects against internalizing a value of thinness can work against identifying and getting help for eating problems. Furthermore, since there is no such thing as a monolithic "black community," any attempt to identify a single idea about weight, size, and food quickly breaks down.

A multiracial focus does not make the culture of thinness insignificant, but shows that its power needs to be understood in the context of other factors. For some girls, an imperative toward thinness initially has little or nothing to do with their eating problems. They link other social injustices to their eating difficulties. Furthermore, those who do internalize an emphasis on thinness also attribute other injustices to anorexia or bulimia.

By questioning the prominence of the culture-of-thinness model, I do not want to suggest that women avoid talking about their desires to be thin. Issues of appearance are essential currency for women's access to

power in this country, and thinness is a critical component. While fat men are vulnerable to ridicule and discrimination, the standards are clearly gendered: being a fat woman is a far graver "mistake" than being a fat man. For white young women, thinness may, in fact, be the most powerful marker used to judge their physical attractiveness. But for women of color, body size is only one of many factors used to judge attractiveness. For older women of any race, the approval of thinness is countered by disdain for wrinkles and an aging body. For lesbians, cashing in on the power of thinness depends upon taking care not to look too "butch." Stereotypes aimed at lesbians of color who are not thin are a stark example of what Barbara Smith termed the "simultaneity of oppression." Nedhera Landers, a black lesbian who is fat, explains:

My mere existence shows up society's lies in great relief. Being Black (and a chick) would eliminate my being fat. But since I am fat, young and childless, that must mean I'm a whore out of desperation for a man. But, since I am a lesbian and men aren't central to my life, that would eliminate my whore status. So, according to the current myths, I don't exist. When I assert my presence and insist that I am indeed fully present, I become an object of ridicule.

Ultimately, more troubling than what the reliance on the ideal of thinness reveals about health research is what it may signal about U.S. society in general: it speaks to a social inability to openly confront and deal with the results of injustice. In a country brimming with glorified images of youth, whiteness, thinness, and wealth, it makes painful sense that dissatisfaction with appearance often serves as a stand-in for topics that are still invisible.

In fact, it is hard to imagine what the world might be like if people were able to talk about trauma and the ways they cope with it with the same ease as they talk about dissatisfaction with their weight and appearance. The fact that Anita Hill was herself put on trial for testifying about sexual and racial harassment is a glaring indicator that much that we need to know about injustice and people's responses to it is still "unspeakable." The fact that more energy has been spent taking the hateful images of Public Enemy off the music racks—on the premise that the lyrics incite violence—than regulating the guns responsible for the death of thousands of young people is a glaring example of the politics of distraction. The Bush and Reagan administrations' use of the military term "vertical insertion"—a euphemism for the bombing and death of human beings—is a searing example of how language is used to hide violence and violation. In the words of Judith Herman, the "ordinary response to atrocities is to banish them from consciousness. Certain violations of the social contract are too terrible to utter aloud: this is the meaning of the word unspeakable." For a staggering number of women, atrocities done to them have been rendered unspeakable. In the place of this unuttered language are symbolic representations of their traumas—often manifested in unwanted eating patterns and supreme dissatisfaction with appetites and bodies.

Of course, not all women with eating problems have developed them to cope with trauma. The fact that 80 percent of fourth grade girls in one large study said they were on diets and that dissatisfaction with weight and size is in fact normative for women in the United States indicates the danger of such a sweeping generalization. A key distinction between periodic dieting and body disapproval and potentially life-threatening and long-term eating problems may be the history of abuse underlying them. Different exposure to trauma may distinguish a young girl who constantly worries about her weight from a woman for whom bulimia is the centerpiece of her day, a woman who occasionally uses liquid diets from a woman who, at eighty pounds, remains afraid to eat. Explicating possible distinctions like these would require examining trauma in different categories of women. This is a study yet to be done. But the experiences of the women whose lives form the basis of this book reveal that discomfort with weight, bodies, and appetite are often the metaphors girls and women use to speak about atrocities. To hear only concerns about appearance or gender inequality is to miss the complex origins of eating problems

The Politics of Invisibility

How were women of color and lesbians left out of media attention and research on eating problems in the first place, given that the stereotype of eating problems as a golden girl's disease is probably more indicative of which women have been studied than of actual prevalence? Certainly, the common reliance on studies conducted in hospitals, clinical settings, private high schools, and colleges skewed public perceptions of those most vulnerable to developing anorexia or bulimia. Basing theory on studies restricted to these locations has limited knowledge of women who are not in college, of women of color, of older women and poor women.

This skewed focus has long-term and potentially debilitating consequences. The stereotype that eating problems are "white girl" phenomena has led many highly trained professionals to either misdiagnose or ignore women of color. Maria Root explains that "social stereo-types of plump or obese Black, Latina or American Indian women may avert the therapist from examining any issues around food and body image. Similarly a thin, Japanese American woman may not be assessed for an eating disorder." When women of color are treated, their eating problems tend to be more severe as a result of delays in diagnosis. Among the women I interviewed, only two had been diagnosed bulimic or anorexic by physicians, yet all who said they were anorexic or bulimic fit the diagnostic criteria (DSM-111) for these diagnoses.

Given these realities, a more important question than *how* these groups of women have been made invisible may be *why* theorists and the media have been dedicated to stereotyped images of eating problems. The answer to this question lies in the way that ideology about black women's bodies has been invisibly inscribed onto what is professed about white women's bodies. In her work on biases in higher education curricula, Patricia Hill Collins explains, "While it may appear that the curriculum is 'Black womanless' and that African-American women have been 'excluded,' in actuality subordinated groups have been included in traditional disciplines through the groups' invisibility." Toni Morrison also offers essential tools for uncovering ideology about race and racism in literature, tools that apply well to developing race-conscious health research. In her groundbreaking essay "Unspeakable Things Unspoken: The Afro-American Presence in American Literature"—which she later expanded into the book *Playing in the Dark*—Morrison unravels the illusion that traditional literature in the United States has been "race free" or "universal," recognizing the presence of Afro-Americans, whether spoken or not, in the work of such well-known white writers as Melville, Poe, Hawthorne, Twain, Faulkner, Cather, and Hemingway, to name a few. Using Melville as a case in point, Morrison recognizes the presence of Afro-Americans and slavery in *Moby Dick*, pointing out that traditional American literature is both informed and determined by this presence. For Morrison, this analysis doubles the fascination and power of the great American writers. She warns us that "defending the Eurocentric Western posture in literature as not only 'universal' but also 'race-free' may have resulted in lobotomizing that literature, and in diminishing both the art and the artist." Avoiding future lobotomies, she writes, depends on excavating the "ghost in the machine"—the ways in which the "presence of Afro-Americans has shaped the choices, the language, the structure and the meaning of so much American literature."

Morrison's method of searching for the ghost in the machine of American literature can reveal substantial biases in research on women's mental health. This tool for theoretical excavation dredges up stereotypes of women of color, lesbians, and working-class women that not only are debilitating for these women but also ultimately backfire on white heterosexual women as well.

The portrayal of bulimia and anorexia as appearance-based disorders is rooted in a notion of femininity in which white middle- and upper-class women are presented as frivolous, obsessed with their bodies, and accepting of narrow gender roles. This representation, like the reputation of AIDS and some cancers, fuels people's tremendous shame and guilt about them. The depiction of middle-class women as vain and obsessive is intimately linked to the assumption that working-class women are the opposite: one step away from being hungry, ugly, and therefore not susceptible to eating problems. The dichotomy drawn between working-class and middle-class women reflects the biased notion that middle-class people create symbolic, abstract relations through their actions and thought while working-class people relate to the world in literal, concrete ways. Within this framework, middle- and upper-class women's eating patterns are imbued with all kinds of symbolic significance—as a way of rebelling against parents, striving for perfection, and responding to conflicting gender expectations. The logic that working-class women are exempt from eating problems, by contrast, strips away any possible symbolic significance or emotional sustenance that food may have or give in their lives. Recognizing that women may develop eating problems to cope with poverty challenges the notion that eating problems are class bound and confirms that both middle- and working-class women are quite capable of creating sophisticated and symbolic relations with food that go far beyond a biological need for calories.

Like biased notions about class, the belief that African-American women are somehow untouched by the cult of thinness is built on long-standing dichotomies—good/bad, pretty/ugly, sexually uptight/sexually loose—about white and black women. These divisions feed into an erroneous notion of black women as somehow separate from a society in which beauty standards are an integral part of the socialization of all women. The portrayal of white women as frivolous and obsessed with their appearance is linked to the presentation of black women as the opposite: as unattractive "mammies' who are incapable of being thin or who are not affected by pressures to be thin. With these multiple distortions, the fact that the dress and "look" of black youth have frequently set the standard for what constitutes style in the fashion industry is entirely unaccounted for.

In an autobiographical account, Retha Powers, an African-American woman, describes being told not to worry about her eating problems because "fat is more acceptable in the Black community." Stereotypical perceptions held by her peers and teachers of the "maternal Black woman" and the "persistent mammy-brickhouse Black Woman image" added to Powers's difficulty in finding people willing to take her problems with food seriously. The association of eating problems with "whiteness" has made some women of color unwilling to seek help. Getting help may feel like "selling out" or being treated as an oddity by friends or medical professionals. The racist underpinnings of some health care policies historically have also led some women of color to avoid seeking help out of fear of being treated in a prejudicial way. Furthermore, the historical view of black women as bodies without minds underlies their invisibility in the frame of reference; they are dismissed as incapable of developing problems that are both psychological and physical. With the dichotomy drawn between black and white women, Latinas drop out of the frame of reference altogether.

Failing to consider eating problems among lesbians reflects the unwritten but powerful belief that lesbians are not interested in or capable of being "attractive" in the dominant sense of the word. This reflects stereotypical notions of "butches" who are too ugly to care about their weight; women who have "become" lesbians because of fear of men and who have subsequently lost touch with "mainstream" society; and women who settle for women after being rejected by men. As biased notions about race reflect racial fears, so distorted ideas about sexuality reflect fears about sexuality in general, and these fears historically have been projected onto lesbians' bodies. These distortions have not only pushed attention to lesbians with eating problems out of the frame of reference, they have also rendered invisible the many ways lesbian communities have refashioned what constitutes beauty in ways that nurture multiple versions of style, glamour, and grace. It is no coincidence that much of the activism and scholarship opposing "fat oppression" has been spearheaded by lesbian feminists who astutely analyze how discrimination against fat women reflects a society hostile to women who take up space and refuse to put boundaries around their hunger for food, resources, and love.

The notion that eating problems are limited to heterosexual women has also contributed to some lesbians' secrecy. The historical association of lesbian sexuality with mental illness and deviance undercuts many lesbians' willingness to identify themselves with any stigmatizing illness. This institutional bias has been coupled with secrecy among lesbians based on the fear of being misunderstood or rejected by other lesbians. The connotation of anorexia and bulimia as problems developed by those who accept male models of beauty means that a lesbian with an eating problem is admitting to being male-centered and therefore not appropriately lesbian. In this way, linking eating problems with appearance rather than trauma has impeded lesbians' self-diagnosis.

Pioneering research on lesbians has confronted the problematic assumptions underlying their invisibility. Like the emerging research on race, this scholarship links unwanted eating patterns and internalized oppression—the process by which people from subordinated communities accept negative attitudes about themselves that are created by the dominant culture. In addition, although lesbian communities may offer women more generous versions of what constitutes health and beauty, this ethic may not be able to compete with dominant cultural beliefs about body size and weight. The scholarship on lesbians, like that on African-American women, reveals cultural methods of protection against harmful social standards previously missing in research that treated white heterosexual women as the standard.

The intricacies of race, class, and sexuality encourage us to rethink demeaning assumptions about white middle-class femininity and racist assumptions about women of color and to consider bulimia and anorexia serious responses to injustices. At their core, bulimia and anorexia are not signs of self-centered vanity and obsession with appearance but rather, at least in their initial stages, are sensible ways women cope with the difficulties in their lives. Reexamining split and oppositional images about race, class, and sexuality with a wide-angle lens reveals a single complicated frame. A multiracial focus shows that distorted notions about black, Latina, and lesbian women are embedded—both explicitly and implicitly—in notions about white heterosexual women, and that it is impossible to understand any of them without the others.

Body Consciousness

The traumatic basis of many women's eating problems can teach us much about bodies and embodiment, for trauma often disrupts an intact sense of one's body. Women's ways of using food are emblematic of a rupturing of women's embodiment, of their ability to see themselves as grounded in and connected to their bodies.

When I first began to ask women about their relationships to their bodies, I asked them to tell me about their body images, but I soon realized a basic conceptual problem in my question. By inquiring about their body "image" I was taking for granted that they imagined themselves as having bodies, an assumption that many women quickly dispelled. The notion that someone can imagine her body assumes that she considers herself to have a body. Some women do not see themselves as having bodies at all.

This painful reality is partly a consequence of oppression that has both historical and contemporary manifestations. The more than three hundred years of slavery in this country robbed African-American men and women of the right to own their own bodies. African-American women were forced into this country as pieces of property "whose purpose was to provide free labor. . . . Their roles in U.S. society were synonymous with work, labor outside of the home, and legitimized sexual victimization from the very outset." In the existential nightmare of slavery, no self was legally recognized, and therefore the body could not exist for the self either. Once slavery was abolished, all that black people had were their bodies. The legal right to own one's body, however, does not in itself ensure that one can claim this right. The legacy of slavery still informs black women's experiences of their bodies in profound ways. The portrayal of black women as mammies (women incapable of being sexual), as Sapphires (women who dominate in the family and in the bedroom), and as Jezebels (sexually promiscuous women who willingly participate in sexual exploitation) reflects the projection of white fantasies and sexuality onto black women's bodies. The idea that white women needed protection was build on seeing black women as their opposite—neither worthy of protection nor wanting to be free of sexual violation.

Debilitating and contradictory stereotypes of Latina women are among the complex and limiting messages against which Latinas have struggled. They have been viewed both as highly sexual, irrationally flamboyant temptresses and as obedient, subservient, fat, and passive—good Catholic mothers. In both their historic and contemporary versions, these stereotypes have long-lasting effects on embodiment and physical presence for Latinas. The existence of these stereotypes does not mean they are inevitably internalized. But what embodiment means for black and Latina women cannot be understood without awareness of the struggle and impact of these stereotypes on self-consciousness.

For many women, responding to social injustices directed at their bodies includes trying to escape what seems like the very location of that pain—their bodies. Pecola, a character in Toni Morrison's *The Bluest Eye*, tries to make her body disappear in response to incest, racism, and poverty:

> Letting herself breathe easy now, Pecola covered her head with the quilt. The sick feeling, which she had tried to prevent by holding in her stomach, came quickly in spite of her precaution. There surged in her the desire to heave, but as always, she knew she would not.
>
> "Please, God," she whispered into the palm of her hand. "Please make me disappear." She squeezed her eyes shut. Little parts of her body faded away. Now slowly, now with a rush. Slowly again. Her fingers went, one by one; then her arms disappeared all the way to the elbow. Her feet now. Yes, that was good. The legs all at once. It was hardest above the thighs. She had to be real still and pull. Her stomach would not go. But finally it, too, went away. Then her chest, her neck. The face was hard, too. Almost done, almost. Only her tight, tight eyes were left. They were always left.

Pecola's wish to make her body disappear dramatizes the destructive intersection of sexual abuse, racism, and poverty as no statistic can. Trying to disappear is an immediate and logical strategy to escape what Pecola came to believe caused her pain—her brown eyes and brown body. Her attempt to slip out and away from the reality of a world bent on destroying her is a vivid example of how women's embodiment is compromised. People facing these injustices cannot take for granted such a basic and elemental capacity as being able to reside comfortably in their bodies. And yet the costs of leaving one's body are monumental.

Ultimately, I put aside the concept of body image and instead thought about women's relationship to their bodies as forms of consciousness. Body consciousness is shaped by biological changes common to all women—growth spurts during childhood, puberty, menstruation, menopause, and the aging process—and by the changes of pregnancy and birthing. People are born with a self-consciousness of mind and body, with an internal body image, and a "sixth sense"—a body self-awareness and a sense of mind-body integration. It is through body consciousness that people can often sense danger, intuitively know what to do, and identify how they feel. These elemental and substantial capacities depend on residing within one's body. Embodiment that allows a person to know where his or her body stops and another's physical body begins may be at the root of a person's capacity to know him/herself as simultaneously unique and connected to the world.

Although everyone is born with a sense of embodiment, experience of it is not universal. The meanings people ascribe to their bodies and the social injustices that violate embodiment vary across gender, race, sexuality, class, religion, and nationality. Unlike the term "image," which has a psychological, individual connotation, the etymology of "consciousness" links an awareness of one's social standing directly to social conditions. Consciousness, as Karl Marx used the term, links individual people's social realities, opportunities, and perspectives to class. In a similar way, one's body consciousness is linked to one's race, gender, and sexuality. This connection more accurately captures women's complicated relationship to their bodies than is conveyed in the term "image." Representations of black and Latina women's bodies and their body consciousness are profoundly different from those of white women. Class stratification also shapes body consciousness. Poverty, for example, can significantly alter a woman's relationship to her body. Being denied the chance to own a car, a house, or even furniture can make a poor woman feel as if her body is all she has left.

Women with eating problems certainly do not have a corner on the market in terms of having difficulty residing comfortably within their bodies. As Emily Martin chronicles in her research on women's reproduction, medical and social processes of birthing, menopause, and puberty in the United States fragment women's embodiment. Feminist theorists on disability offer rich analyses of how disability changes women's embodiment. Discriminatory practices against people with disabilities—including limited access to education, employment, independent living, and sexual freedoms—are typically more restricting than actual physical conditions.

The essential issue may not be *if* women struggle to claim their bodies as their own, but rather the differing ways that embodiment is disrupted. Adrienne Rich writes:

> I know no woman—virgin, mother, lesbian, married, celibate—whether she earns her keep as a housewife, a cocktail waitress, or a scanner of brain waves—for whom her body is not a fundamental problem: its clouded meaning, its fertility, its desire, its so-called frigidity, its bloody speech, its silences, its changes and mutilations, its rapes and ripenings.

In her poetic way, Rich captures the contradictions and complexities of living in one's body.

To complicate this further, women employ a variety of survival strategies in response to violations of their bodies. The poet Wanda Coleman writes:

The price Black girls pay for not conforming to white standards of beauty is extracted in monumental amounts, breath to death. We bend our personalities, and sometimes mutilate our bodies in defense. Sometimes that bent is "bad attitude," perhaps accompanied by a hair-trigger temper, ready to go off at the mildest slight: neck-wobbling, hands to hips, boisterous, hostile, niggerish behavior.

Women may also respond to psychic and physical assaults with silent refusals to engage or show rage. They may run away from home or never leave their apartments. They may flunk out of school or hide behind books. The reasons for these coping strategies are complicated and not easily predicted—just as it is not easy to explain why some women develop eating problems and others do not.

Women with eating problems, however, offer special insights about body consciousness because they respond to trauma in particularly bodily ways. Their stories reveal how bingeing, purging, and dieting can change a woman's embodiment, and they provide vivid examples of what it means for a woman to "leave her body."

Leaving the body is a survival strategy many women use when they see no other alternatives. The sophisticated ways in which the women I talked with describe their experiences of their bodies originate in part in their having had to grapple—seriously and over the long term—with the discomfort of being in their bodies. Their stories reveal the social inequalities that whittle away at a woman's ability to identify her body as her own. They explain what it means to be in exile from one's own body, and why this is common. Their testimonies reveal why sexual abuse and racism can lead a teenager who weighs 110 pounds to see herself as fat and to consider her body the cause of her pain. Their stories also highlight the consequences of drastic weight loss and gain on a woman's sense of her body's shape and size. The average weight fluctuation among the women I talked to was seventy-four pounds. Many of the women's weight changed several times in their lives. Substantial and recurrent weight fluctuation raises complicated and painful questions about what it means to be "embodied" since a woman's possession of a significant portion of her body may be in constant flux.

The women's stories reveal that body consciousness is a highly imaginative and simultaneously concrete ability to see one's self as part of one's body and to draw upon the power generated from this embodiment. It is a concrete reality in that, regardless of one's relation to one's body, breathing, eating, sleeping, and simply being require some consciousness of one's body. But body consciousness occurs at the imaginative and symbolic level as well. In the face of debilitating stereotypes and injustices, women do struggle to claim their bodies as their own. The struggle requires being able to see one's own image of one's body rather than the images projected onto it. Consciousness both takes into account oppressive perceptions of the body and rejects what is debilitating about them.

The women's stories also reveal the often ingenious and creative strategies they develop to counter various assaults, strategies that are at the core of their journey toward self-love and empowerment. Self-love and empowerment are profoundly related to the body. Cornel West writes:

> The issue of self-regard, self-esteem, and self-respect is reflected in bodily form. . . . Toni Morrison would say, "Look you've got to love yourself not only in the abstract; you've got to love your big lips; you've got to love your flat nose; you've got to love your skin, hands, all the way down."

The women whose experiences form the basis of this book identify their injuries and their resistance with honesty and insight. In so doing, they chronicle their despair and resilience, their depression and fortitude, their ingenuity in taking care of themselves.

Methods and Ethics

Conducting life-history interviews enabled me to hear in women's own words how they interpreted the meaning of and reasons behind their eating patterns: what it feels like to turn to food for comfort, how they come to see their bodies as liabilities, and what resources have most helped them develop sane relationships with food and their bodies. They also explain why food begins as, and often remains, the drug of choice for many girls and women.

I interviewed eighteen women ranging in age from nineteen to forty-six, five of them African-American, five Latina, and eight white. All of the white women and four of the women of color are lesbian. I wanted women of color and lesbians to be at the center of my analysis since we know so little about their eating problems. A third of the women are mothers. Five are Jewish, eight are Catholic, and five are Protestant. Three of them grew up outside the United States. They represent various class backgrounds, in terms of both their families of origin and their own current situations.

The majority of the women had a combination of eating problems (at least two of the following: bulimia, compulsive eating, anorexia, extensive dieting), and the particular types often changed during their lives.

The most common problems were bingeing and extensive dieting, although half of the women were also anorexic, bulimic, or both. All had problems that were long-term and serious—for some, even life-threatening. The specific types of eating problems did not correlate with race, class, sexuality, or nationality, although the types of trauma the women associate with their unwanted eating patterns did vary with social position.

I found women willing to be interviewed by letting people know—where I work, in my neighborhood, in political and community groups—about my study. Some of the women approached me, others I asked. I typically had many conversations with them before the interviews, an important step given the secrecy, vulnerability, and fear that many people feel when they talk about eating problems and the pain underlying them.

The women and I also often discussed the origins and purpose of the study, including my personal and intellectual interest in eating problems. Like many feminist scholars, I believe that a researcher's self-disclosure counters power imbalances; people who consent to talk openly about their lives deserve the right to ask the researcher potentially personal questions as well. Self-disclosure does not eliminate power differences based on race, generation, sexual identity, or class, but our common experiences—as lesbians, as women with eating problems, as neighbors, as antiracist activists, our work-related affiliations—did serve as an initial bridge that made it easier to talk about our differences. One Latina woman asked me why a white and perhaps heterosexual woman was doing research about African-American women, Latinas, and lesbians. I explained that my research emerged from antiracist work and my frustration about the dearth of information on mental and physical health concerns of African-American and Latina women. I also talked about how relying upon friendship networks and alliances at work to find women to interview was partially based on my knowledge that women of color might understandably be skeptical of my background and motivations. Her questions about me and the study also gave us a chance to talk about the complexity of sexual identity—how lesbian identity is not necessarily apparent. This ambiguity parallels the complexity of identification for many light-skinned Latinas (such as herself).

A white woman who is a survivor of sexual abuse was quite hesitant and wanted to be sure that she could stop the interview at any time. Learning that her right as the speaker superseded my rights as the researcher influenced her eventual decision to participate. I also spoke about my own worry, as a survivor of sexual abuse and

someone who had a long-term eating problem earlier in my life, about talking about this subject with people I did not know well. In both of these situations, the women's candid questions and our discussion about methods and ethics influenced the tenor of the interview process. These conversations allowed women to talk about their fears and worries about not being understood or having to "start from the beginning all the time" in order for their story to make sense.

Tapping into friendship, work, and community networks was an effective way to find women willing to be interviewed since it allowed them to scrutinize me and the project. Many people of color have had to reckon with false generalizations and distortions put forward by white social workers who have not examined their own understanding of race. People who are willing to talk about private, painful, and power-laden issues deserve to know something about both the research and the researcher.

Clearly, the study was in no way random. I was very specific in terms of race and sexuality about who I was hoping to interview. In addition, I sought women who considered themselves to be in the process of healing, surmising that their understanding of the roots of their eating problems would be greater than that of women whose eating difficulties were at their height. I did not approach the research process as an objective observer, in part because I do not think that, for a study of this kind, "objectivity" is possible or ethical. I came to the interviews with biases: believing that the women were courageous to talk on this subject and already skeptical of the dominant imagery associated with eating problems.

During the interviews I used what Patricia Hill Collins calls "an ethic of care," which she defines as understanding that "personal expressiveness, emotions and empathy are central to the knowledge validation process." I had been conducting workshops on eating problems for several years prior to beginning the book and had been personally immersed in the topic for many years before that. From that experience, I responded to the women's stories in a way that I believe heightened their trust and therefore the integrity of the interviews. Had I approached the interviews as an objective observer, I would have been betraying myself and the women who shared their life stories with me.

Because I interviewed only a few women—who were not randomly selected—generalizations based on their experiences need to be made with caution. My point is not to confirm prevalence or even incidence but rather to examine the meaning of eating problems in these women's lives and what they have to teach us about coping, embodiment, and recovery. At the same time, I do not want to overlook the possibility that their experiences reflect a larger reality. The stakes involved in speaking openly about the traumas underlying many eating problems are high, and much injustice remains underground (only one out of ten incidences of sexual abuse is reported, for example). Perhaps the balance lies in both recognizing what makes each of the women's stories unique and understanding how their experiences reflect common injustices and methods of resistance.

Like many feminist and qualitative researchers, I approached the interviews believing that the people being interviewed, not the researcher, are the experts on their lives, that they know the best chronology, emphasis, and methods of telling about their lives. My task was to remind myself of that when I began to proceed otherwise. In some of the interviews I spoke very little, only infrequently asking for clarification. Other interviews were more like conversations, in which I followed along with questions and comments as the women talked about their lives. The ways the women told their stories mirrored the complex detours, the starts and stops, of their lives.

The multiple and textured meanings of their stories often reflected the ways they lived their lives. People often don't remember or describe their lives in a linear sequence, particularly when they're relating experiences of injustice. Judith Herman explains that people who have survived trauma often tell their stories in a "highly emotional, contradictory, and fragmented manner." In open-ended interviews the women explored subjects from more than one angle, which helped me piece together events and emotions that otherwise were too complicated or confusing for me to follow. Their stories revealed why hesitations, silences, and omissions were understandable and inevitable. Like many qualitative anthropologists and sociologists, I am not sure there is such a thing as a complete story: future experience keeps adding to and revising what the present offers. Partial truths and circuitous narratives of lived experience are often the closest approximation of the whole story available.

Body language—particularly the women's eyes—often helped me know when to move on. Typically, I waited for the woman to talk about a topic so I could use her terms rather than impose my own, so she could decide when it was all right to broach a particular subject. I deliberately did not assume a definition of eating problem or recovery, and I tried to avoid specific terms until the women used them. Humor often played a key role in their stories; laughter frequently mingled with tears.

Almost all of the interviews took place in the women's homes, which gave me vivid insights into their lives,

struggles, and dreams. An African-American woman explained that a key component of her healing was to travel to Egypt "to see the birthplace of black people prior to slavery." Her living room was a shrine: statues of Egyptian gods, portraits of Jesus with brown face and curly hair, candles, stones, and other religious instruments she had collected. Seeing her home gave me an understanding I would otherwise have been unable to grasp. A woman who linked her eating problems to poverty let me into her apartment and then bolted her door with four locks and a long metal police bar that she jammed between the door and a wall as she explained that her home had been broken into three times. She served me tea with powdered milk crystals, having run out of milk—and money—much earlier in the week. A woman who detailed the psychological abuse she suffered at the hands of her husband was forced to stop talking perhaps a dozen times as her husband came crashing into the house, screaming and yelling, interrupting her despite her pleas for privacy.

One woman explicitly requested that the interview occur outside of her home—a request that taught me a lot about language, culture, and acculturation. This young Dominican woman insisted upon meeting me in my office for the interview, which initially worried me because I associated the office with business, distance, and formality. It turned out that this was her way of seeking rather than avoiding intimacy. She lives with her parents and brothers and has never told any of her relatives about her eating problem. She has no privacy at her house, so it would have been impossible for her to talk there. Also, when she thinks about her eating problem, she thinks about it in English (even though she did not learn English until she was sixteen years old). Because she speaks Spanish at home and English at the university, the university seemed like the natural place to talk about this subject.

I transcribed my tapes of the interviews and gave copies to the women who wanted them. I had further conversations with some of the women in which they clarified ideas and made additions to the transcript. Some women said they were glad to have the transcripts but found it too hard to read them. Many said they felt exhilarated, relieved, satisfied, and glad to have told their life stories, although the costs for some were intense. One woman had a number of painful flashbacks during the interview and later told me she had left her body at some point during the interview; she had to have emergency sessions with her therapist and increase her medication for several days after the interview. Another woman had a hard time emotionally after the interview because she had remembered instances of abuse she had not previously recalled. While these two women's experiences were in the minority, they highlight the courage it takes to speak about eating problems and the traumas that often underlie them. I often felt dazed and exhausted after an interview. Sometimes I had difficulty staying fully "present," which I attributed to the pain in some of the women's stories. My reaction is yet another example of why silence about trauma—and the ways people cope with it—remains and why telling life stories is a risky endeavor.

The women's experiences that are the centerpiece of this book play a central role in each chapter. Chapter 2 examines conditions that may make girls vulnerable to developing eating problems. The women's stories offer essential clues about why many girls grow up distrusting their bodies and their appetites. Lessons they are taught about race, religion, sexuality, and ethnicity are the filters through which they learn about food and eating. Chapters 3 and 4 identify connections between eating problems and several forms of trauma—sexual abuse, racism, heterosexism, poverty, acculturation, and emotional and physical abuse. These chapters show how bingeing, purging, and dieting begin as ways women numb pain and cope with violations of their bodies and how survivors of trauma use food as a logical response to injustices, given the limited alternatives available to them. The lives of the women I interviewed show why we need an expansive understanding of how trauma can be inflicted. Many of the women linked eating problems to physical violations, and others associated them with the psychic invasions of heterosexism, poverty, acculturation, racism, and emotional abuse. Recognizing both psychic and physical invasions avoids the historical tendency to identify the body and mind as somehow disconnected entities.

The concluding chapters examine why food is women's drug of choice, how embodiment is shaped by social inequalities, and the women's healing methods. The women's stories reveal that although eating problems begin as sensible responses to various injustices, they may eventually become liabilities. Healing depends upon making the connection between trauma and eating and understanding how violations distort "body consciousness" and appetites. The healing strategies often entail recovering memories through self-help, community, religious, political, and therapy groups. Finding resources that support women financially, emotionally, and spiritually are also keys to recovery.

"Good Enough"

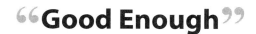

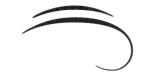

by Megan Seely

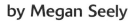

I remember reading once that "getting my head out of the toilet bowl was the most political act I ever committed"[1] and thinking—this is my life. For years I struggled with an eating disorder, bulimia, that consists of a cycle of binging and purging. I was bulimic for much of my activist life—during the grape boycott, at the same time I sat in on Bettina Aptheker's classes, and even as the president of my college NOW chapter. At my worst, I was throwing up a dozen times a day. I could throw up with no noise. I could throw up on command. I could even throw up out the car door while driving down the road. These are not braggin' rights. I was becoming more involved in the women's movement, working toward the empowerment of women and girls, and falling deeper and deeper into a pit of self-hatred.

eat·ing disor·der: *n.* any of various disorders, as anorexia nervosa or bulimia, characterized by severe disturbances in eating habits.

An·or·ex·ia ner·vo·sa: *n.* an eating disorder characterized by a fear of becoming fat, a distorted body image, and excessive dieting leading to emaciation.

Bu·lim·ia: *n.* I. Also called bu·lim·ia ner·vo·sa, a habitual disturbance in eating behavior characterized by bouts of excessive eating followed by self-induced vomiting, purging with laxatives, strenuous exercise, or fasting.

> I do not think a woman's body needs to be super thin or adorned with makeup and "sexy" clothes, yet I still have lingering issues with my body and body image in general. *Heather, 22, European American, Illinois*

I was plagued by this question: How is it possible that someone with a growing feminist consciousness can be binging and purging while remaining a staunch feminist? I was regularly talking with young women about eating disorders and media images and their harmful effects on our self-esteem, urging them to increase their empowerment and work on their sense of self—all the while feeling like a hypocrite. The more I encouraged others, the more I felt like a failure. Imposter phenomenon[2] is what it is called. It's the notion of hiding your true self from others while fearful that people will find out that you are not what you seem, that you've had them all fooled. Who was I to talk about empowerment? To criticize media images or advocate change? I threw up so much my voice was raspy. I lived on throat lozenges. And the barfing was only part of it—body obsession, working out, dieting, dieting, dieting. The saddest part was that I was more worried that someone would find me but, uncover the sham that I thought I was, than concerned for my health, my self-esteem, my self-definition, or even my life.

When I first became bulimic, I don't remember knowing if there was a label or an understanding for what I was doing to myself. I thought that I had discovered the perfect solution to my fat ass—I could eat in social settings, I could binge on my "forbidden foods," and then I could *just take care of it*. It seemed like the perfect solution; no one would have to know. But I also felt isolated by this secret. When I reluctantly went to a group session—because a friend needed me to go to support *her*—I was shocked that others did the things that I did. There was even a word for it. Bulimia. I began to understand but remained ashamed. I felt that I had a different standard to live up to. *I* was a feminist. I knew better. I was supposed to embrace my fat ass—hell, celebrate it!

Later, in hushed conversations with feminist friends, I began to note that I was not alone. They too confessed feelings of body hatred, acts of yo-yo dieting, binging and purging or self-starvation. I believe that there is a special type of pressure for self-proclaimed feminist women. We understand that nonfeminist-identified women struggle with self-image—look at our culture! Diet fads, personal trainers, and cosmetic surgery. Be-

tween 4 and 20 percent of college-age women are estimated to have an eating disorder,[3] and approximately 80 percent of fourth graders are dieting—they're nine years old![4] But feminists don't recognize themselves in those statistics—we're the ones who *know* the statistics; we're not supposed to be part of those statistics. And so we continue to harbor the secrecies of our betrayal. We fear betraying a movement that has spent so many years working to give us a better life, a better identity, a movement that has worked for decades to create an acknowledgement of, and resources for, those with eating disorders, a movement that was the first and loudest voice to critique the social pressures for women to fit the thin, white ideal and that countered the messages of advertising, film, television, and beauty pageants—in short, a movement that proudly said that women, in all their shapes, sizes, and colors, are beautiful.

I worried about writing this in a book about third-wave feminism. I worried about being this exposed. I worried that the antifeminists would use this story as an argument to prove that feminism failed. Then I realized that these fears are the same fears that kept me silent for so long. Eating disorders and body hatred are not the fault of the feminist movement; quite the contrary. The feminist movement has struggled to provide women and girls with resources and support to fight the hidden tortures within our psyches. The fact that feminist women have eating disorders is evidence of the strength of a culture that continues to send the message to women that as we are is not good enough. The culture is what needs to change, not women and not feminism.

The Flapper, Rosie the Riveter, Marilyn Monroe . . . and Me

After reading books like Mary Pipher's *Reviving Ophelia* and Laura Fraser's *Losing It* and seeing the work of documentary film makers like Jean Kilbourne, I realized that there is a correlation between the social and political power we hold as women and the projection of an ideal body size fed to us through popular culture. This emphasis is so intense that it can, and does, detract from

> The life event that turned me from just another Sassy reader into a committed, self-identified, and active activist was my own personal struggle with bulimia nervosa. I credit feminism for a large part of my successful recovery. *Sarah, 28, Irish/English, straight but open, Oregon, originally from Tennessee*

our quest for political, economic and social representation. For example, American women won the right to vote in 1920. This was a seventy-two-year battle, one that was indeed hard fought. As a result, women had more political representation and thus more social power than ever before in our modern history. But around the 1920s, who was the major fashion idol? First the "Gibson Girl," with her tall, slender frame, and then the widely popular "flapper," who was even thinner, more boyish, and without curves. And, while the flapper fashion was a response to the corset and the desire for freedom from gowns and petticoats, it also came with a requirement of whiteness, a small body size, and an emphasis on weight control. As the fashion feminist Valerie Steele writes in her book, *The Corset: A Cultural History*, "Although the traditional boned corset gradually disappeared during the 1920s, most women still wore some kind of corset, corselette, or girdle."[5] She notes that fashion magazines and advice books continued to stress exercise and diets and reinforced the fear of fat internalized by women throughout American society. Steele further writes, "the corset did not so much disappear as become internalized through diet, exercise, and [more recently] plastic surgery."[6] Additionally, as Susan Bordo, author of *Unbearable Weight: Feminism, Western Culture and the Body*, reminds us, "the flapper's freedom, as Mary McCarthy's and Dorothy Parker's short stories brilliantly reveal, was largely an illusion—as any obsessively cultivated sexual style must inevitably be."[7] Despite freedom from the corset and a growing quest for sexual equality, women began to experience a backlash. Once again, their physical beauty and worth, rather than their independence and intelligence, became paramount,. After all, let's not forget that 1921 was the year of the first Miss America Pageant, the start of the practice of formally rewarding women for their physical appearance, as opposed to establishing a scholarship program (a common defense of beauty pageants) based upon intellect and scholarly merit.

Moving forward in history, during World War II, the strong, muscular image of Rosie the Riveter took hold. This can-do image was appropriated by the government to convince women to enter the paid labor force to support the U.S. economy, industry, and war efforts while the men were away fighting. Women were told that they could do a "man's job." I should note that this effort, like Rosie herself, was largely aimed at white women, as most women of color in the United States were already working. In her study *Creating Rosie the Riveter: Class, Gender and Propaganda During World War II*, Maureen Honey writes that "[t]he woman in a nontraditional job was portrayed as valiantly leading the nation to victory. Women were provided with positive role models for entering male occupations, and the public was given a standard-bearer of home-front solidarity and protection."[8] Like Rosie, most of this imagery portrayed white, middle-class women and virtually ignored the contributions of women of color. Honey writes that "racial prejudice precluded using blacks in [heroic roles] because they were perceived by a racist culture as inferior to whites and therefore inappropriate figures of inspiration or national pride."[9] Women of color were inaccurately and unjustly left out of images of women supporting the war effort, and white women were sold the notion of nationalism and valor through their war work, along with the expectation that they would maintain their home, their family, and their femininity. After World War II, when women were essentially kicked out of the factories to make room for the returning soldiers, they returned home, and the baby boom exploded. The icon of the 1950s, Marilyn Monroe, a voluptuous size 14 or 16 by today's standards, suggested a return to femininity and the acceptance of a larger body size. Of course, Marilyn was also seen as a "dumb blonde" who doesn't ask too much, doesn't demand too much, and doesn't know too much. Marilyn's image provided for a less threatening image of white women, one that posed a smaller economic and political threat within American society.

As we moved into the 1960s, with the women's movement taking off again and women demanding equal pay, equal representation, and equal rights, the fashion icon was "Twiggie"— rail thin, white, boyish, with no curves. Chris Strodder, author of *Swingin' Chicks of the '60s*, writes that "with 31–22–32 measurements and barely 90 pounds on her 5′ 6″ frame, Twiggy in a lime-green mini and green tights represented a bold departure from the softer, rounder shapes on the 50s and early 60s."[10] Still referenced today, Twiggie and her waiflike appearance set a norm for ultrathinness.[11] Women fighting for equal rights and representation were quickly confronted with an ideal that emphasized slenderness as an ideal— an ideal for which we were, and most of us still are, expected to strive. However, within the Latina and African American communities, a fuller figure is often more the norm. As Christy Haubegger put it in her essay "I'm Not Fat, I'm Latina," "Latinas in this country live in two worlds. People who don't know us may think we're fat. At home we're called *bien cuidadas* (well cared for) . . . there is a greater 'cultural acceptance' of being overweight within Hispanic communities."[12]

Fast-forward to the twenty-first century and women have won more elected offices and thus more recognition politically than ever before and have begun to move up the corporate and union ladders, represent a greater proportion of enrolled students in colleges and universities, and so on—and yet we see "heroin chic" on the pages of our magazines and the much-talked-about "Lolliwood" and the shrinking actresses of Hollywood. "Lolliwood" refers to the image of the celebrity woman who has lost so much body mass that her head looks out of proportion to her body, making her look like a "lollipop." You see, your body can lose a great deal of mass, but your head, your cranium, will not shrink in size. One contrast to these images of heroin chic and Lolliwood are women in professional sports. With an emphasis on strength and ability, women athletes give girls a powerful alternative to look up to. With the increasing success of Title IX, we are beginning to see stronger, more positive images for young women through sports. Venus and Serena Williams, Brandy Chastain, Laila Ali, Danica Patrick, Annika Sorenstam, and Michelle Wei are just a few women in sports who present images of confident, powerful women who are comfortable in their bodies. Still, while it is true that the 1999 Women's World Cup win for the U.S. women's soccer team and the growing popularity of the WNBA have greatly impacted girls in the United States, the bigger message to women, particularly young women in the midst of adolescence, is that "thin is in." And at any cost.

Throughout history, when women have not possessed much political, economic, or social power—when we did not run for political office, when we did not demand equal pay for equal work, when we did not control our own reproductive lives, when we did not vote—then we did not determine our lives. If we are not involved, then we present little or no threat to the patriarchal power structure that supports and protects male dominance. But, as women and girls become more empowered, we confront a contradictory message about our value. We must begin to counter the notion that to be worthy is to look like the "ideal woman" delivered to us through television shows, movies, music videos, newscasts, magazine covers, and video games. And, in doing so, we begin to experience a shift in power; instead of being valued solely because of a physical image, we promote one that recognizes our other contributions. Here's the deal—when women are required—even informally—to meet an unattainable body size ideal, our energy is sucked away. Like the Barbie doll, usually even heavily promoted "role models," be they actresses or fashion models, do not naturally meet the image they project—

> I was seen as the odd ball. I was the only girl in my class who did not wear tight clothes, starve myself, and wear make-up. *Madelon, 18, bisexual, Massachusetts*

> I get in seventh grade and my mother buys me makeup. I was like what do you want me to do with this then she wanted me to start wearing high heels to church. NOT. I feel bad for my mom she tried so hard to turn me into this little prim and proper lady. I am so not that. *Serena, 26, Hispanic, straight, single mom, California.*

airbrushing, computer alteration, piece modeling, lighting, makeup, surgery, and semistarvation are all part of the process of creating an image that can sell the average woman an unattainable ideal that often looks quite natural. When we are obsessed with this ideal, we have little time, or confidence, for anything else—including fighting for equality.

Recently, in some rare cases—most notably Oprah Winfrey and Jamie Lee Curtis—our celebrities have begun to speak out about this ideal, going so far as to chronicle their transformation from their normal selves to the image we see on the cover of magazines. But the more likely story to grace our magazine racks is of the weight gains and losses of our most beautiful. Played out in the public is the accusation that eating disorders are rampant among the women on popular sitcoms and in our favorite movies—and a denial that this is the case. The media industry pits one woman against the other—on the one hand publicly condemning extreme weight loss but on the other requiring extreme thinness among actresses who appear on television and on the big screen. This added pressure, in such a public position, creates an unfair demand on, and a bit of a contradiction for, famous women. Not only are they subject to this requirement, but they are in the position of projecting this unattainable ideal. Instead of endlessly targeting famous, thin women, we should recognize that they too are pressured by the media. Why condemn a woman who is also struggling with her self-concept and body size—as well as with her job? My point is not to encourage the furthering of celebrity exaltation—certainly they have enviable lives in many ways—but rather to assert that we need to change the politics of beauty, challenge the ideal, and create more room for our diversity. We must celebrate the images of larger women in the media, and we must do so unapologetically—in other words, we must end the ubiquitous notion that if she is fat, she cannot be beautiful or that if she is fat, she is unhappy.

REFERENCES
A list of references is available in original source.

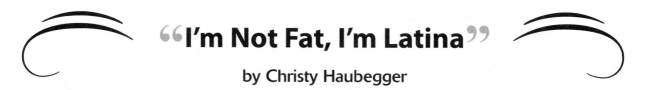

"I'm Not Fat, I'm Latina"

by Christy Haubegger

I recently read a newspaper article that reported that nearly 40 percent of Hispanic and African-American women are overweight. At least I'm in good company. Because according to even the most generous height and weight charts at the doctor's office, I'm a good 25 pounds overweight. And I'm still looking for the pantyhose chart that has me on it (according to Hanes, I don't exist). But I'm happy to report that in the Latino community, my community, I fit right in.

Latinas in this country live in two worlds. People who don't know us may think we're fat. At home, we're called *bien cuidadas* (well cared for).

I love to go dancing at Cesar's Latin Palace here in the Mission District of San Francisco. At this hot all-night salsa club, it's the curvier bodies like mine that turn heads. I'm the one on the dance floor all night while some of my thinner friends spend more time waiting along the walls. Come to think of it, I wouldn't trade my body for any of theirs.

But I didn't always feel this way. I remember being in high school and noticing that none of the magazines showed models in bathing suits with bodies like mine. Handsome movie heroes were never hoping to find a chubby damsel in distress. The fact that I had plenty of attention from Latino boys wasn't enough. Real self-esteem cannot come from male attention alone.

My turning point came a few years later. When I was in college, I made a trip to Mexico, and I brought back much more than sterling-silver bargains and colorful blankets.

I remember hiking through the awesome ruins of the Maya and the Aztecs, civilizations that created pyramids as large as the ones in Egypt. I loved walking through temple doorways whose clearance was only two inches above my head, and I realized that I must be a direct descendant of those ancient priestesses for whom those doorways had originally been built.

For the first time in my life, I was in a place where people like me were the beautiful ones. And I began to accept, and even like, the body that I have.

I know that medical experts say that Latinas are twice as likely as the rest of the population to be overweight. And yes, I know about the health problems that often accompany severe weight problems. But most of us are not in the danger zone; we're just bien cuidadas. Even the researchers who found that nearly 40 percent of us are overweight noted that there is a greater "cultural acceptance" of being overweight within Hispanic communities. But the article also commented on the cultural-acceptance factor as if it were something unfortunate, because it keeps Hispanic women from becoming healthier. I'm not so convinced that we're the ones with the problem.

If the medical experts were to try and get to the root of this so-called problem, they would probably find that it's part genetics, part enchiladas. Whether we're Cuban-American, Mexican-American, Puerto Rican or Dominican, food is a central part of Hispanic culture. While our food varies from fried plaintains to tamales, what doesn't change is its role in our lives. You feed people you care for, and so if you're well cared for, *bien cuidada,* you have been fed well.

I remember when I used to be envious of a Latina friend of mine who had always been on the skinny side. When I confided this to her a while ago, she laughed. It turns out that when she was growing up, she had always wanted to look more like me. She had trouble getting dates with Latinos in high school, the same boys that I dated. When she was little, the other kids in the neighborhood had even given her a cruel nickname: *la seca,* "the dry one." I'm glad I never had any of those problems.

Our community has always been accepting of us well-cared-for women. So why don't we feel beautiful? You only have to flip through a magazine or watch a movie to realize that beautiful for most of this country still means tall, blond and underfed. But now we know it's the magazines that are wrong. I, for one, am going to do what I can to make sure that *mis hijas,* my daughters, won't feel the way I did.

From *Essence,* December 1994. Copyright © 1994 by Christy Haubegger. Reprinted by permission of the author.

"Breaking the Model"

by Graciela (Chely) H. Rodriguez

"**A**re you a model?"
I had been walking through the metal detector at the Los Angeles airport last month when one of the attendants addressed me.

"Would a model be eating these?" I replied, pulling a huge bag of Doritos out of my purse.

I know the question was meant as a compliment, but it brought back a lot of painful memories. You see, I spent the best part of my teenage years "training to be a model . . . or just look like one." I didn't end up on the catwalk, but rather, in the hospital, recovering from anorexia and bulimia.

That's right, me—an eighteen-year-old Latina who's supposed to be immune to such things. Or so I'm told. Everyone from magazine publishers to television producers has suggested that Latina and African-American girls aren't likely to develop eating disorders, that we're less influenced by the skinny-girl images than our white peers.

But how do they explain me? I come from a traditional, hardworking Mexican family. We celebrate all the Mexican holidays, practice the Catholic religion, and, by nature, our appearance resembles that of our ancestors—prominent facial features, thick bodies and brown skin. I learned Spanish at an early age, as my parents had emigrated to California from Mazatlán, Sinaloa, when they were nineteen.

I've lived in the small town of Carpinteria, California, for my whole life. It's one of the few towns I know to be truly multicultural. My schools have always been filled with kids from all backgrounds—different ethnicities, races, religions. My own Latina identity has been just one among many—and it's never held me back. I've worked hard to fit in and be accepted.

As a young teen, I shared the dream of many girls: I wanted to be a model and an actress. Like most girls, I wanted to be popular, and more than anything that meant I had to be attractive. When I was thirteen, I was scanning a fashion magazine and saw an ad for a model search contest that was coming to Beverly Hills. I jumped at the chance and begged my parents to take me.

At first, my father was against the idea. But with a lot of pleading, I convinced my parents to make the two-hour drive one Saturday afternoon. I entered the contest with more than two thousand little girls, boys, teens and adults. There was no cost to enter, and it seemed like the chance of a lifetime. And it was easy. I just had to parade down a runway and introduce myself to a panel of judges by stating my name, my age and my interests.

Three weeks later, I got a phone call from one of the representatives, saying that I was a finalist. I wasn't one of the top *five* finalists, who were awarded money and free modeling classes. I was, however, a runner-up, which made me eligible for a partial scholarship to help cover modeling and acting lessons. My parents would only have to pay two thousand dollars, the rep told me. To this day, I'm not sure why they did it, but my parents withdrew the money from their savings. Every Saturday, we made the two-hour drive to Beverly Hills, and they waited for eight hours while I learned how to strut, pose and walk with a supermodel sashay.

On my first day, an agent named Pat took my measurements. He frowned and clucked his tongue as he scribbled my dimensions onto a clipboard-five-foot-three, 130 pounds, size seven. Then, he told me that the average model wore a size three and recommended that I drop down to that as quickly as possible.

For motivation, Pat handed me a stack of fashion magazines. He suggested I study the models in Teen and Seventeen and watch *Beverly Hills 90210* to "get an idea of what real models look like." It didn't matter that I was only thirteen years old and not even fully developed. I was expected either to lose the weight or to get lost.

I left depressed, thinking I would never look like a model because I came from a line of full-figured Mexican women. Even if I lost the weight, I would still never look like most of the girls in the magazines. I remember wishing I'd been born with blond hair, blue eyes and a small waist. I also started to think that if I got a nose job to create that perfect "button" nose, then maybe this career I really wanted could happen. Though I still had doubts whether my genetically given body could be shaped into model material, I believed that if I worked hard enough, I could succeed. As I entered junior high, my goal was not just to look like the characters on *90210*, but to *live* like them. I wanted to be popular, like the typical girl on TV. I wanted to be thin—to fit in.

I've been told that sometimes the desire for thinness is learned or reinforced at home. For me, that was true to a degree. My mother is a full-figured woman who's always been concerned about her weight. When I was younger, she used to exercise and limit her portions at mealtime. In fact, she even did some small-scale runway modeling for friends who had boutiques or clothing lines.

But my mother's example didn't spark my desire to model, even though she supported my decision. I feel the media's and society's images of women were more responsible. Like they do for so many girls, these images promised acceptance and happiness if I could only look like them.

However, my mother's habits and shaky self-image did make it easier when I began to diet and exercise obsessively at age thirteen. Early on, I discovered her diet pills and began taking them secretly. When she caught on that some were missing, she confronted me and I denied it. She didn't believe me, though, and even had the principal search my school locker. I remember thinking, "God, now people are going to know why I'm losing weight." I wanted everyone to think it was natural, and I felt like my secret had been revealed. In reality, no one else knew except for a friend (also Latina), who'd given me the idea in the first place. Soon after, I started to buy my own appetite suppressants, which I hid in my change purse.

I was eager to lose weight, and the modeling agency was happy to help. They gave me a list of "forbidden" foods, which was basically anything that didn't taste like sawdust or water. Every day, I had a salad with lemon juice or a plain baked potato, and that was it. I ate only once a day, limiting my intake to a 250-calorie maximum. After a year, my body submitted to this starvation regimen, and my appetite nearly disappeared. Although my stomach would rumble loudly in class, I learned to drink lots of water to fill it for long enough to spare me the embarrassment.

My parents noticed the dramatic change in my appearance, but they mistakenly trusted that the agency had put me on a healthy diet. Since they both worked long hours, and I was busy with extracurricular activities, they didn't have time to monitor my eating habits anyway. On the rare occasions that the family ate together, I would eat enough to escape their scrutiny, and then secretly throw it up later.

Bingeing and purging became a ritual. The same friend who introduced me to diet pills taught me that I could eat whatever I wanted and then force it back up so I wouldn't gain any weight. After a while, I didn't even have to stick my finger down my throat; I could throw up just by eating a chip. I also exercised for at least two hours a day at a local gym and at the park near my house. I was so obsessed with losing weight that I would wake up as early as 3 o'clock in the morning to run, and then jog again in the afternoon. I also enrolled in aerobics classes, and in eighth grade, I became captain of the cheerleading squad and president of the student body.

People ask me how I found the energy to do all this, especially with no food in my stomach. I can only answer that I was so driven to achieve "perfection" that it wiped out any concern I might have had for my body or my health. I would come home from school exhausted some days and flop down on my bed. But I was surrounded by pictures of teen models that I'd ripped from magazines and taped to my walls. My response was instant—one look at the wall and I'd be lacing up my Nikes and heading for the track.

But by eight o'clock, I was exhausted. Some nights, I was too tired to finish my homework, and I usually declined invitations from friends so I could stay home and work out. I wasn't the only one, though. Many of my friends—who were mostly Latina and African-American—were going through the same thing. Although there were few models who looked like us in *Teen* and *Seventeen*, we read those magazines anyway and bought into their messages. At the very least, all the girls at my junior high cared about their weight. Most of us worked out, and a lot of our conversations centered around how little we'd eaten that day. There was an unspoken competition, or at least a comparison, to see who had the most "willpower." Somehow, the quest for that power made us overlook the throbbing headaches and the gnawing hunger pangs that came with the territory of thinness.

At the modeling agency, most of the girls were also on strict diets and concerned about their bodies. In the end, going to extremes never paid off. None of us ever got any real modeling jobs. I did a couple of department store fashion shows, but that was it. It never amounted to the money my parents shelled out for my lessons.

But I did lose weight. After three years of hard work, the scales put me at one hundred pounds. In fact, I outdid myself—I dropped down to a size one. Finally, I felt okay wearing a bathing suit in public. I wore cropped tank tops and shorts all the time. There was no lack of attention or praise. People commented on how great and "healthy" I looked, and my self-esteem soared. I might not have been as "beautiful" as some models—after all, none of the models I saw on TV were Latina—but at least I was as skinny as they were.

Still, like most girls with eating disorders, I was never satisfied. In fact, I was unaware that I even had an eating disorder. All I knew was that I didn't feel "perfect" yet. My quest for the perfect body ended when a family member caught me throwing up in a restaurant bathroom. She told my parents, who took me to the hospital immediately, where I was diagnosed with anorexia and bulimia.

My family was as surprised as I was. Fortunately, I began counseling immediately. My counselor helped me to recover from my insecurity and to rebuild my self-esteem. I began to recognize that my worth was not based solely on my looks. It took me about a year to recover. I started to eat more and more and turned to healthier sources to stay in shape. I still exercised, but not nearly as much.

To this day, weight is a big issue in my life and may always be. Last night, I was watching an interview with Janet Jackson, and the thought of looking like her crept into my mind. I started to think, *God, I wish I had abs and a firm butt like hers*. I caught myself falling into an old trap. But I was able to stop myself by refocusing my thoughts on all of my good qualities and reminding myself that this was only an image.

One of the most influential things my counselor said to me was, "Chely, you are beautiful inside and out." It seems basic, yet somewhere in my quest for the perfect body, I had forgotten this. I decided never to change for anyone or try so hard to fit in. If I had had real role models—girls with round stomachs and pimples—I would probably have felt more acceptable. After all, that's what most teenage girls look like. Of course, that kind of beauty doesn't sell the way the fantasy kind does. There's a reason we're given an image that's so hard to achieve. As long as we're chasing an impossible weight, we'll always have a reason to buy more diet products, to watch *90210* and to read *Seventeen*.

I now weigh 130 pounds again, and I'm proud of my body. But I need a lot of support to maintain that. Whenever I feel bad, I remind myself, "If people don't accept me the way I am, it's their problem." I also continue to heal myself by helping others. I'm actively involved as a peer advocate, countering unrealistic images in magazines, TV shows, websites and other media that can damage girls' body image. I promote healthy eating habits and exercise and encourage girls to get involved in sports. I'm now a high school senior, and I'm still involved in cheerleading and soccer (I often find myself "counseling" younger teammates about body acceptance). I'm also active in a number of girls clubs that help me maintain my self-esteem in the face of negative body image messages.

After recovering from my eating disorder, I participated in an organization called Girls Incorporated, which helps nurture young girls to become strong, self-confident women. Girls Inc. recently awarded me ten thousand dollars toward my college tuition. I've never been prouder. It felt incredible to receive a scholarship that was based on my achievements, rather than on the way I looked.

When I talk to girls, I tell them what I've learned—that it can be okay to want to look attractive and to be concerned about body weight, but we have to understand how far to take it. Finding that balance is tricky. The influence of the media is extremely powerful. I tell my story at conferences where big-time media executives are in attendance. I challenge them to provide young people with better role models and to stop portraying girls as victims and sex objects.

Eating disorders affect girls of color, too. I'm a perfect example of a Latina who developed an eating disorder because I so badly wanted to look and be like the thin, popular girls I saw in the media. I saw very few Latina role models on TV, and if I did see any, they were in gangs, wearing bikinis or cleaning houses. I have rarely seen a Latina get acknowledged for her accomplishments rather than her large breasts. If I'd had positive Latina role models, I might never have felt ashamed to come from a full-figured line of women. I would have felt proud.

In the meantime, I've decided to become my own role model by reminding myself who I am every day. I am an eighteen-year-old Latina, a full-figured former model. I have survived an eating disorder. And I'm learning to love my body.

Extreme Makeover: Feminist Edition
"How the Pitch for Cosmetic Surgery Co-opts Feminism"

by Jennifer Cognard-Black

This spring, *Sideways* star Virginia Madsen became a spokesperson for Allergan Inc., the maker of Botox, as part of the company's latest campaign: "Keep the Wisdom. Lose the Lines." Quoted in *People* magazine, Madsen asserts that she's made "a lot of choices" to keep herself "youthful and strong": "I work out. I eat good foods. And I also get injectables."

In celebrity promos such as Madsen's, the current pop-cultural acceptance of cosmetic medicine is clear—and is borne out by the rising numbers of customers. Since 2000, the American Society of Plastic Surgeons (ASPS) reports a 48 percent increase in all cosmetic (elective) procedures, both surgical, such as breast augmentations, and minimally invasive, such as the injectable wrinkle-filler Botox.

It's debatable why cosmetic medicine has become so popular. Might it be the result of articles on "scalpel slaves" and "secret surgeries" that saturate women's magazines? Or could it be a result of makeover-focused reality TV shows that have proliferated since the 2003 debut of *Extreme Makeover*? Or perhaps it has to do with the presentation and tone of endorsements such as Madsen's.

Once considered clandestine and risky, cosmetic procedures are currently treated across a variety of media as if they were as benign and mundane as whitening your teeth. Advertisers, TV producers, publishers, PR personnel and even physicians themselves are touting it as an effortless, egalitarian way for women of all backgrounds to "enhance" their looks and "stay young."

Not only have cosmetic procedures become more acceptable, but they're being promoted in less sensationalized ways to whole new markets. Increasingly, reality TV's Cinderella tale of surgical transformation is being replaced with a smart woman's narrative of enlightened self-maintenance. While *Extreme Makeover* and its imitators shame and blame ugly-duck patients in order for

prince-surgeons to rescue them and magically unlock their inner swans through "drastic plastic" (multiple surgeries), other media sources now compliment potential customers as mature women who are smart, talented and wise. Such women are supposedly savvy enough to appreciate their own wisdom— but, then again, they should want to soften the telltale marks of how many years it took them to acquire it. "I am not using these injectables to look 25," Madsen insists. "I don't want to be 25. I just want to look like me."

Alex Kuczynski, a *New York Times* reporter and author of *Beauty Junkies* (Doubleday, 2006), calls these latest appeals "the new feminism, an activism of aesthetics." That ignores the work of feminists from Susan Faludi to Susan Bordo, who have argued for years against the global beauty industry and its misogynistic practices. Ironically, the term "feminist" has long been wielded by right-wing politicians, comedians and talk-show hosts as a pejorative label for a "masculine" woman who "lets herself go." Yet the cosmetic-surgery industry is doing exactly what the beauty industry has done for years: It's co-opting, repackaging and reselling the feminist call to empower women into what may be dubbed "consumer feminism." Under the dual slogans of possibility and choice, producers, promoters and providers are selling elective surgery as self-determination.

The cosmetic-medicine industry also appeals to the power of sisterhood. The blurb for a popular book entitled *The Smart Woman's Guide to Plastic Surgery* (McGraw-Hill, 2007) describes the author, Jean M. Loftus, as a female plastic surgeon who will offer "compassionate advice for . . . any woman considering plastic surgery." Similarly, the cover of the *Internet Guide to Cosmetic Surgery for Women* (Haworth Information Press, 2005) sports a collage of women's faces of various ethnicities, suggesting that the reader is in this with her sisters. Women with supposed insider knowledge give other women advice and support on how to revamp their faces and bodies through surgery. (Does this make them "aesthetic activists"?) The implication is that the male physician, advertiser, network producer or cosmetic-medicine mogul has been sidestepped, and women are empowering each other to be more informed consumers.

Moreover, much of the media covering cosmetic surgery centers on the idea of *choice*. Parallel to Madsen's insistence that using Botox is just another lifestyle choice with little difference from working out and eating well, *Cosmetic Surgery for Dummies* (For Dummies, 2005) promises that the reader will discover how to "decide whether surgery is right for you," "find a qualified surgeon," "set realistic expectations," "evaluate the costs," "make the surgical environment safe" and ultimately "make an informed choice." The word "choice" obviously plays on reproductive-rights connotations, so that consumers will trust that they are maintaining autonomy over their bodies. Yet one choice goes completely unmentioned: The choice not to consider cosmetic surgery at all.

It seems that this pseudo-feminist message works. A recent survey published in the British weekly magazine *Grazia*, for example, found that over half of the 1,000 women in Great Britain who were polled (average age 34) expect to have cosmetic surgery in their lifetime. And that's music to the ears of all those who benefit from women's insecurities about their looks, for cosmetic surgery is big, big business.

The ASPS reports that in 2006, there were almost twice as many cosmetic, as opposed to reconstructive, procedures. Between 2000 and 2006, the number of abdominoplasties (tummy tucks) rose 133 percent, Botox injections were up 420 percent and there was a 55 percent increase in the number of breast enlargements. Thanks to the FDA decision last fall to reapprove the use of silicone breast implants after a 14-year ban, it's likely that even more women will now consider having enlargements (since silicone is considered to look and feel more "natural" than the now-common saline implants). All in all, in 2006 nearly 11 million cosmetic procedures were performed in America, and surgeons pocketed $11.4 billion.

To ride the tide of this lucrative wave, cosmetic surgery is now being packaged and sold in conjunction with other leisure activities for "smart" women. In every major U.S. city, there are "medi-spas" offering one-stop beauty shopping, from salon treatments such as pedicures to outpatient surgical procedures, including chemical peels and injectables such as Restylane

(another face-line filler, marketed by the company Medicis). A company called Surgeon & Safari puts together medical tourism packages to South Africa that include airfare, hotel, meals, breast enlargement, a face-lift and a week at a wild-animal game reserve. And a new she's-turning-40 gift among those who can afford it—or put it on their credit card—is a Botox home party with a house-call surgeon and five to 10 friends who all receive injections.

Within such a marketplace, some cosmetic surgeons are no longer just doctors: They are vendors. Thanks to a 1982 Supreme Court ruling, all physicians may openly advertise their wares, and cosmetic surgeons have become particularly adept at working with professional marketing consultants to brand and promote their practices. Some of these doctors offer financial plans—or "beauty banks"— to their patients, with zero interest, a revolving credit line or deferred payment options. Others agree to let their patients know about various corporate promotions—such as the Restylane Awards program, which gives points to "frequent fillers."

To boost sales even further, cosmetic medical equipment and injectables are being sold to physicians who aren't even cosmetic surgeons. One Maryland college professor found that out during her annual Pap smear appointment, when her gynecologist offered to "take care of her elevens"—unknit the "teacher's frown" between her brows—with Botox.

The beauty industry has long traded on women's body angst and low self-esteem as a means of creating permanent customers. (Not that men don't have such issues, but 90 percent of all cosmetic surgery customers continue to be women.) These days, with consumers able to "choose" from among a dizzying array of procedures and providers, even the most minute areas of the female body are potential sites of worry and "intervention." Touted as cure-alls for aging and bodily dissatisfactions, surgical procedures have been developed to reduce "bra fat," to make over belly buttons, to "rejuvenate" vaginas after childbirth, or to achieve the "*Sex and the City* effect"— foot surgeries to shorten or even remove a toe in order for women to squeeze their feet into pointy shoes.

With the media's suggestion that cosmetic surgery for the discriminating consumer is almost as easy as choosing any beauty product, it's not surprising that the targeted demographic for cosmetic medical procedures has widened. Few seem immune to the sell, no matter what their income. In fact, according to an ASPS-commissioned study, more than two-thirds of those who underwent cosmetic surgery in 2005 made $60,000 or less. Easy access to credit and the declining cost of procedures have brought even the working class into the market.

While the vast majority of customers continue to be Caucasian women, "ethnic surgeries" are also on the rise. In 2006, eyelid surgery that remakes eyes from ovals to orbs was one of the top three cosmetic procedures for Asian Americans. The No. 1 procedure for African Americans was rhinoplasty to slim wide noses, and at the top of the list for Hispanics were breast implants to mold cleavage into a "standard" shape and size. As Kim Gandy, the president of the National Organization for Women, points out, "The 'standard' created for Latina and African American women's bodies was established in much the same way that standards are created for women in the U.S. and Asia—through music videos, magazines, television and movies." In other words, the media pressures every woman—regardless of class, age or ethnicity—to modify herself in order to feel "normal."

The most graphic consequences of these trends are the stretched, alien, expressionless faces worn by certain celebrities and increasing numbers of "everyday" women. There are also the disfigurements and deaths that can result from surgeries gone wrong. While the ASPS keeps no statistics on botched procedures, permanent scars, severe reactions to injectables, burst implants or deaths due to hospital-acquired infections or administration of too much anesthesia, the stories certainly exist. Indeed, Kuczynski devotes an entire chapter to "The Fatal Quest for Beauty."

But then Kuczynski ends her string of horrific examples by telling consumers to "educate themselves." Time and again, even critical assessments of cosmetic surgery conclude in this way. Rather than grapple with the hard questions of whether such surgeries should be undertaken at all, or what the cultural forces are behind the pressures to undergo cosmetic surgery, even critical voices ultimately reaffirm the industry's message: If the woman is an empowered consumer, she will be smart enough to shop safe. Ultimately, both promoters and detractors keep the question of choice to whether a woman will choose to do her homework, listen to other women and not overreach—in the words of Madsen, not try "to look 25."

At the end of *Beauty Junkies*, Kuczynski asserts that "looks are the new feminism." Yet it's feminists who have led the fight against silicone breast implants when research suggested they were dangerous. It's feminists who have pointed out that a branch of medicine formed to fix or replace broken, burned and diseased body parts has since become an industry serving often-misogynistic interests. And it's feminists who have emphatically and persistently shown that cosmetic medicine exists because sexism is powerfully linked with capitalism—keeping a woman worried about her looks in order to stay attractive, keep a job or retain self-worth. To say that a preoccupation with looks is "feminist" is a cynical misreading; feminists must instead insist that a furrowed, "wise" brow—minus the fillers—is the empowered feminist face, both old and new.

For further information on feminists challenging cosmetic surgery, visit NOW, loveyourbody.nowfoundation.org; About-Face, www.about-face.org; and the Real Women Project, www.realwomenproject.org.

"The Pressures of Perfectionism"

by Katherine Beagle

I call myself a feminist. I am preparing to graduate with a B.A. in Women's Studies from the University of California, Riverside (UCR). I believe that a woman's value should not be measured in terms of her attractiveness, sexuality, or reproductive capabilities. Nonetheless, I have wanted breast implants since I was a sophomore in college. I have simultaneously fought for women's equality and desired breast augmentation.

"Young Feminists: The Pressures of Perfectionism," by Katherine Beagle, originally published in the *Women's Health Activist*, November/December 2005, pp. 6–7, the newsletter of the National Women's Health Network (NWHN). It is reprinted with the permission of the author and the NWHN.

Like most young women, I feel the pressure to be perfect and, in our society, that means having large breasts. I see the models, actors, and dozens of women on the street with nice, curvy bodies, and I want the same. Throughout my four years in college I have listened to feminist professors lecture about women's objectification and exploited sexuality. I have read articles and written papers about women's struggles to gain equality. All the same, I fully intended to purchase a pair of perfect boobs before entering law school.

During my last year as an undergraduate, I interned for 10 weeks at the National Women's Health Network, where I researched breast implants for a special project. When I started reading about the risks involved with breast implants, I became tentative about my own intentions to go under the knife.

My initial plan had been to finance the procedure with a loan and pay it off within a couple of years. I discovered, however, that additional surgeries are often needed due to complications that include infection, rupture, extrusion, or capsular contraction (painful hardening of the breasts). I hadn't anticipated anything going wrong with my implants, but the numbers speak for themselves. About 250,000 women have breast implant surgery for augmentation each year. And studies have shown that 20-26 percent of augmentation patients receiving saline-filled implants needed additional surgery within five years of the initial procedure.[1] Health risks aside, I asked myself if it was worth risking having to pay for an additional surgery if I have a complication? Was I willing to jeopardize my education should I have to choose between law school tuition and medical bills? These were only the beginning of my worries.

The Food and Drug Administration (FDA) imposed restrictions on the availability of silicone-gel-filled breast implants in 1992, but it allowed continued general use of saline-filled implants (consisting of a silicone envelope with a saline filling). (Silicone-gel-filled implants continued to be available to some women through reconstructive surgery and clinical trials.) Manufacturers and plastic surgeons are trying to get silicone-gel-filled implants approved for general use as well, and the FDA just sent 'approvable' letters to two silicone implant manufacturers; silicone-gel-filled implants are likely to return to the market and soon be widely available.

On April 11–13, 2005, I attended the FDA Advisory Panel meeting on silicone-gel-filled implants (see the July/August *Women's Health Activist*). During the panel meeting, I met numerous women who testified that their silicone-gel-filled breast implants ruined their lives. These women suffered from various symptoms, including arthritic pains, extreme fatigue, high levels of plat-

inum in their (and their children's) bodies, and other health problems. Other women testified that they loved their silicone-gel-filled implants and had experienced no problems with them.

At this point, I had developed some serious doubts about putting a foreign object in my body when long-term studies have yet to be conducted, and have yet to prove silicone-gel-filled breast implants are safe. I assumed that they <u>were</u> safe because implants have been around for decades, and hundreds of thousands of women get them each year. I also had assumed that if the FDA approved implants, they must be safe, right?

Not necessarily. FDA approval means that the implants are "reasonably safe". After the panel meeting, I began to ask questions such as: How long do they last? What happens when silicone leaks into the body? Who will have to pay if I need multiple surgeries because of complications? How could implants affect my ability to breastfeed? Will my insurance company cover me if I have problems with the implants? It is important to ask questions and be aware of the risks and consequences involved with the procedure.

The answers I found were hardly comforting. I learned that all implants break at some point – it's just a matter of time. Newer, silicone-gel-filled implants have not been around long enough for us to know precisely how long they will last. When a saline-filled implant breaks, the saline leaks into the body and is absorbed. That is usually safe, unless the saline is non-sterile, or contaminated with a fungus or bacteria. When a silicone-gel-filled implant breaks, however, the silicone might move around the body and get stuck, making it impossible to remove. Evidence seems to suggest that implants can interfere with breast-feeding and with milk production; one study found that 39 percent of new mothers with saline-filled implants had trouble breast-feeding[2].

This is not a storybook ending; I have not completely ruled out the idea of getting implants. What I know now is that I would like to see more conclusive long-term studies that show whether implants are safe or not before I make a final decision.

I also would like women to recognize that many people (even feminists) feel the pressure to be perfect and that, when we comply with prevalent norms of beauty, we risk measuring our own value in terms of attractiveness and sexuality rather than by deeper qualities. Ultimately, I want women in our society to have worth without having to nip, cut, tuck, or enhance any parts of our bodies. The National Women's Health Network works to inform women about health issues so that we can make informed decisions about our own health, and can assist other women in doing the same. And so I stand here, still undecided about implants, but definitely more educated on the subject.

REFERENCES

1. *FDA Breast Implant Consumer Handbook—2004*. See http://www.fda.gov/cdrh/breastimplants/indexbip.html

2. Strom, S.S., Baldwin, B.J., Sigurdson, A.J., Schusterman, M.A., 'Cosmetic Saline Breast Implants: A Survey of Satisfaction, Breast-Feeding Experience.' *Cancer Screening, and Health, Plastic and Reconstructive Surgery* 1997: 100:1553–1557. See: http://www.commandtrust.org/children.shtml

"The Ugly Side of the Beauty Industry"

by Misha Warbanski

Take a look around your bathroom. The average North American woman uses 10 or more personal care products every day. From toothpaste and soap to antiperspirant and moisturizer, personal care products are made from 10,500 chemical ingredients that are as much a part of our daily routine as sitting down to breakfast. And like most things that happen before a mug of morning coffee, it's easy not to think about them too much.

But researchers and women's health activists are sounding the alarm bell about the makeup of makeup. Women and girls are particularly susceptible to exposure to certain chemicals that mimic hormone activity. Because our bodies have a greater percentage of fat in comparison to men, chemicals that are fat-soluble are more easily absorbed. Breast tissue is one such site where chemicals can accumulate.

"As more and more women are diagnosed with cancer, we have to question, where is this all coming from?" posits Carol Secter, a board member of Breast Cancer Action Montreal. With an emphasis on breast cancer prevention, Secter's group is part of a North America-wide movement to have harmful chemicals banned from personal care and household products.

Increasingly, science is pointing out that exposure to many of these chemicals—including parabens used to preserve antiperspirants and creams, and phthalates added to perfumes and nail polish—may harm our health. A 2004 study of breast tumours by Dr. Phillippa Darbre, from the University of Reading in the U.K., and published in the *Journal of Applied Toxicology*, found parabens in each of 20 samples. This led researchers to suspect that parabens, which mimic estrogen when absorbed through the skin, may play a role in the development of breast cancer. The researchers suspected the parabens came from underarm deodorants; however, they concluded that more research is needed. While parabens aren't restricted in Canada, many manufacturers are going paraben-free because of consumer demand.

Now banned in the European Union, phthalates are another common ingredient in personal care products suspected in a variety of health problems from liver malfunction to low testosterone levels and low sperm counts in men. In 2002, researchers in Chicago tested 72 brand-name cosmetics and found that 52 contained phthalates, a compound that helps cosmetics stay put without smudging. Phthalates are also used to make perfumes and soaps. Scientists suspect the absorption of cosmetics through the skin could explain why young women in one study had 20 times the level of phthalates in their body compared to young men.

Seventy years ago, the first cosmetics law in the U.S. banned the use of coal tar dye in mascara after the ingredient was found to cause blindness. Today, the accumulation of chemicals found in personal care products may affect men and women's offspring. In August 2005, researchers, including University of Rochester epidemiologist Shanna Swan, published the first study to examine prenatal exposure to phthalates. The study found that the development of the genitals of boys whose mothers had high levels of phthalates in their bodies was less complete compared to those exposed to lower levels. Swan believes phthalate exposure may be contributing to increasing rates of male infertility and testicular cancer.

In response to a growing concern about the risks associated with personal care products, Health Canada now requires personal care product manufactures to list product ingredients by the end of the year. The department also maintains a hotlist of already restricted and banned chemicals. The hotlist was expanded in 2003 from less than 100 to almost 500 after reviewing some chemicals that are restricted in the E.U. However, no independent testing is done prior to a new product hitting the shelves in Canada—manufacturers are only required to submit a list of product ingredients. This is just one reason critics are demanding that the precautionary principle be imposed on Canada's $3.5-billion personal care industry.

"There is no review to ensure the list on the label is accurate," says Madeleine Bird, a researcher at McGill University's Centre for Research and Teaching on Women.

Bird cites a Danish study on parabens that discovered that contents listed on a product's label were different from the makeup of the product, which sometimes had much higher concentrations. "Some check and balance is needed," adds Bird.

However, health activists say harmful chemicals shouldn't be there, period. Formaldehyde, benzene and lead are associated with not only cancer, but endometriosis, birth defects and developmental disabilities in children. Coal tars used in hair dye have long been associated with liver cancer. Petroleum distillates, a suspected human carcinogen banned in the E.U., are still in use in North America.

According to the Washington-based Environmental Working Group, 89 percent of ingredients in personal care products have never been assessed for safety. Breast Cancer Action Montreal figures Canada would be roughly similar, as ingredients were grandfathered into use in Canada without being tested for safety. Under the 1999 Environmental Protection Act, Health Canada and Environment Canada are reviewing more than 23,000 chemicals that were never tested for safety.

Until recently, the contents of personal care products have been a mystery. While the Canadian government requires food manufacturers to list ingredients on packaging, cosmetics and personal care products have historically been exempt. Last November, Canada caught up with the United States and European Union and will require the contents of personal care products to be labelled by the end of the year. Retail outlets and manufacturers were given a year's grace to sell off unlabelled products. Still, Dr. Samuel Epstein, coauthor of *The Safe Shopper's Bible* and head of the Cancer Prevention Coalition, has said that the labelling will be meaningless to anyone without a pharmacology degree.

Secter agrees. "I don't want to go shopping for my body products, my cosmetics, with a chemical dictionary telling me this one's okay, this one's not. I want to be able to walk in and buy it off the shelf with the understanding that it's safe."

In Europe, Secter would be better protected. The European Union bans more than 1,100 chemicals from personal care products because they may cause cancer, birth defects or reproductive problems. In stark contrast, just nine chemicals are banned from cosmetics in the United States; Canada follows U.S. standards. Women in California won a recent victory with the passage of the Safe Cosmetics Act, which takes effect later this year. The law compels manufacturers to disclose product ingredients if they are on state or federal lists of chemicals associated with cancer and birth defects. Importantly, California's bill also contains provisions designed to protect the safety of nail-salon and cosmetology workers who handle solvents, chemical solutions and glues.

In the rest of North America, governments remain slow to regulate, so activists and consumers are taking the matter into their own hands, using the power of the pocketbook to pressure companies to change their formulas.

"Information is something that can be very empowering," says Bird, who completed her degree in women's studies and is now working to raise awareness about chemicals so that individuals can reduce their own exposure, seek out alternatives and demand change.

Abby Lippman, a professor of epidemiology at McGill University, says the answer for her is simple: "If you can't say it, don't wear it." Although not using cosmetics may seem like a simple answer, Lippman doesn't expect most women will suddenly stop using them.

"I don't want to make women who are wearing makeup sound like victims when they're making a conscious decision," says Lippman, who is also a member of Breast Cancer Action Montreal. "But when they make a conscious decision, I want them to be able to be aware of what they're putting on their bodies, and I want them to have access to the safest products. We need good choices, not just an array of some worse than others."

Deciding which products are safest can be a time-consuming task. Designed to make those decisions easier, the Environmental Working Group's Skin Deep report created a searchable database of personal care products and ingredients. The Working Group's information looks at American brands and formulas, most of which are sold in Canada. The group created fact sheets that identify which chemicals and which companies to avoid. Revlon, Estée Lauder, Avon, L'Oreal and Johnson & Johnson are ranked in the group's top 20 of concern. Chanel cosmetics are not tested on animals, but the group gives them the number two rating of brands to avoid, citing a lack of safety data available for the ingredients used. In 2006, The Body Shop announced it would phase out the use of phthalates from its products and packaging, but the company still uses parabens, which are not among the 37 top ingredients of top concern on Skin Deep's list.

With its custom shopping list feature, Skin Deep provides consumers with information to enable them to choose the safest products. The website offers suggestions on where to find that elusive non-toxic lipstick or deodorant and lists over 300 companies that either don't use harmful chemicals or have pledged to eliminate ingredients related to cancer, birth anomalies or hormonal disruption within three years. Companies like The Body Shop, Burt's Bees and Afterglow Cosmetics have signed

on. However, the industry's major players such as Avon, Estee Lauder, L'Oreal, Revlon and Proctor and Gamble, are notably absent.

According to the Environmental Working Group cosmetics report, hair colour, nail polish and nail treatments contain some of the most toxic chemicals. One product in particular, OPI natural nail strengthener, received the highest hazard rating of all 14,100 products in the database. The company's nail polish and nail treatments contain toluene, formaldehyde and dibutyl phthalate—three of the top ingredients of concern.

Of particular concern are products aimed at black consumers that promise lighter skin and straighter hair. Not only do these products impose a white standard of beauty that is harmful, but many hair relaxers and skin lighteners contain ingredients linked to cancer, early puberty and other ailments. For example, hydroquinone, a skin whitener, is deemed a carcinogen by the E.U. While not permitted in Canada in cosmetics, hydroquinone is available in products classified as drugs in Canada. Black women under 40 have a higher breast cancer incidence compared to white women of

---

What's In Your Bathroom?

If personal care ingredients are not listed, you can request content information from the manufacturer. Check the Environmental Working Group's Campaign for Safe Cosmetics report *Skin Deep* to get details on specific ingredients and to find safer products. Hotlisted ingredients in Canada may be subject to limitations in their concentration or can still turn up in products categorized as drugs, like antiperspirant and anti-dandruff shampoos.

These are some ingredients you may want to avoid:

Lead Acetate Found in some hair dye, and cleansers, lead acetate is hotlisted in Canada and banned in the E.U. Lead acetate is a reproductive and developmental toxin.

Formaldehyde Found in some nail products, antibacterial soaps and foundations, formaldehyde is a carcinogen restricted in Canada.

Toluene Found in some nail polish and hardeners. It is suspected of being a reproductive or developmental toxin. One form, Toluene-2,4-diamine, is prohibited in Canada.

Parabens A class of preservatives commonly found in moisturizers, deodorants and many personal care products. Methlyparaben, butlyparaben, isobutylparaben and propylparaben are classed as endocrine disruptors in *Skin Deep*.

Petroleum Distillates Found in mascara, perfume, lipstick and foundation, petroleum distillates are a suspected carcinogen.

Coal Tar Found in dark hair dyes and anti-dandruff shampoo, coal tars are carcinogenic and permitted in hair dyes in Canada when accompanied by a warning.

Dibutyl Phthalate Found in nail products. All phthalates are banned in the E.U., but not restricted in Canada. Dibutyl phthalate is an endocrine disruptor and suspected to reproductive toxin.

Source: Environmental Working Group Campaign for Safe Cosmetics

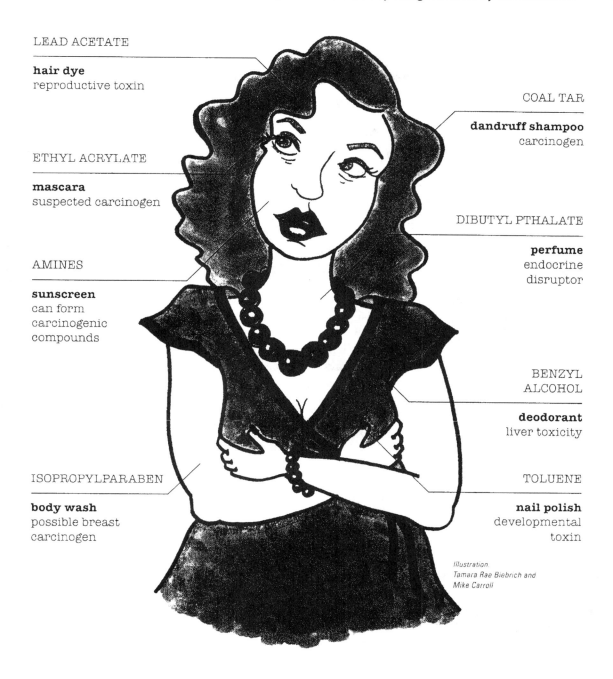

LEAD ACETATE

hair dye
reproductive toxin

ETHYL ACRYLATE

mascara
suspected carcinogen

AMINES

sunscreen
can form
carcinogenic
compounds

ISOPROPYLPARABEN

body wash
possible breast
carcinogen

COAL TAR

dandruff shampoo
carcinogen

DIBUTYL PTHALATE

perfume
endocrine
disruptor

BENZYL
ALCOHOL

deodorant
liver toxicity

TOLUENE

nail polish
developmental
toxin

*Illustration.
Tamara Rae Biebrich and
Mike Carroll*

a similar age, and studies have noted that many of these products are used starting in childhood, prolonging exposure.

The cosmetics industry says it can regulate itself and lobbies for fewer, not more, regulations. Organizations like Breast Cancer Action Montreal aren't waiting for industry to change its practices voluntarily. That's why the organization has launched letter-writing campaigns to four cosmetics companies—Unilever, Johnson & Johnson, Avon and Estée Lauder—the big names that have been stubborn about changing their ingredients. Until we can get all toxic ingredients banned from per-sonal care products, a generous application of consumer pressure may be our best bet.

Online Resources

The Environmental Working Group's Skin Deep Report:
www.ewg.org/reports/skindeep2

Campaign for Safe Cosmetics:
www.safecosmetics.org

Cosmetic Ingredient Hotlist:
www.hc-sc.gc.ca/cps-spc/person/cosmet/hotlist-liste
_e.htm

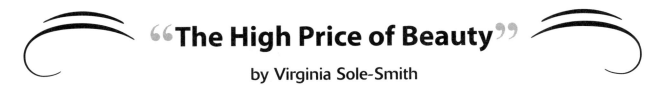

"The High Price of Beauty"

by Virginia Sole-Smith

Tomi Tran works as a nail technician in Raleigh, North Carolina. She pays around $100 per week to rent a booth in a hair salon, buys all her polishes and supplies and finds her own clients, often giving free manicures at local malls and distributing fliers to drum up business. It's hard work, but Tran, 22, says it's heaven compared with her last salon job.

"It was basically a sweatshop," she explains. "I would feel lightheaded and get terrible headaches from the smell of the chemicals, and I was working around sixty-four hours a week, usually with no lunch breaks." The final straw came when Tran became sick with a stomach virus but her boss told her she would lose her job if she didn't come to work. "She told me I had to work, but I could rest in the back in between customers," she says. Tran decided to quit and risk going into business for herself so she could choose her own hours and avoid the acrylic nail products that made her so sick.

Tara Horton, 37, of Sanger, California, wishes she had dropped out of beauty school. "Out of the eleven of us training to do nails, one woman had a baby that was stillborn at eight months, and another was born all messed up with his bowels and intestinal tract on the outside of his body," she says. "I remember thinking that's a pretty high failure rate." Horton began working in salons and later lost two babies herself and was diagnosed with non-Hodgkins lymphoma. "You just don't go from being a nonsmoking, healthy, active person to dying of cancer without asking why," she says. "Now, I realize, we were standing over those chemicals all day long."

Stories like Tran's and Horton's have become rampant as the nail salon industry has exploded in the past ten years, with the number of nail technicians in America jumping 374 percent to more than 380,000 nationwide, with women making up 96 percent of the industry workforce. But "no one is really looking at these folks," says Alexandra Gorman, director of science and research for Women's Voices for the Earth, an environmental justice organization in Missoula, Montana, who co-wrote its March report called *Glossed Over: Health Hazards With Toxic Exposure in Nail Salons.* "There's a major lack of studies, so these women are going to work and having symptoms, but the authorities are telling them they're fine."

In fact, the cosmetology industry uses more than 10,000 chemicals in its products, 89 percent of which have not been evaluated for safety, according to the non-profit Campaign for Safe Cosmetics, which corrals available evidence in its *Skin Deep* database (cosmeticsdatabase.com). The polishes, acrylics and other products used in nail salons contain some twenty chemicals flagged as having "potential symptoms and health effects" by the Environmental Protection Agency. The list includes solvents like acetone, which may cause central nervous system depression, and ethyl methacrylate, linked to eye, skin and respiratory tract irritation. It also highlights chemicals banned by the European Union and since removed by international brands like OPI, Sally Hansen and Revlon. Those include formalin, which may cause asthma-like respiratory problems and cancer in high or prolonged doses, and toluene, a solvent with the potential to cause dizziness, headaches and liver and kidney damage. Perhaps most contentious of all is dibutyl phthalate, a plasticizer that makes nail polish more flexible. It has been linked to eye and upper respiratory system irritation and may be toxic to the reproductive system.

"Most kinds of house paint are less toxic than what you find in nail polish," says Cora Roelofs, ScD, an assistant professor at the University of Massachusetts, Lowell, whose research has documented acute health problems like skin irritations and asthma among nail salon workers in the Boston area. "Yet we still know very little about more serious health effects, nor do we understand how these chemicals interact with each other in the salon environment."

It's the lack of knowledge about nail polish's potential reproductive toxicity that's most chilling for advocates and salon workers. "We're seeing a substantial number of folks from the beauty industry who are concerned about whether they can work during their pregnancies," says John Meyer, MD, an assistant professor in the Division of Occupational and Environmental Medicine at the University of Connecticut Health Center. He responds to queries on a risk line run by the Connecticut Department of Health and estimates that the center receives seventy to 140 calls a year from concerned work-

---

"The High Price of Beauty," by Virginia Sole-Smith, *The Nation,* October 8, 2007, pp. 21–23. Reprinted with permission. For subscription information, call 1-800-333-8536. Portions of each week's Nation magazine can be accessed at http://www.thenation.com.

ers or their physicians. An analysis of a California occupational health hot line found that manicurists and cosmetologists were the third-largest occupational sector to call with pregnancy-related inquiries.

"Just because we don't know something is dangerous doesn't mean it's safe," says Mark Cullen, MD, director of Occupational and Environmental Medicine at Yale University School of Medicine. "These are a class of chemicals where the data is incomplete but the concern is real." Studies show that when laboratory workers are exposed to similar solvents without proper ventilation, there is a small but increased risk for miscarriages and birth defects similar to fetal alcohol syndrome, explains Dr. Meyer. Meanwhile, most research on phthalates comes from animal studies, making it difficult to predict human response.

But this lack of data allows the industry to dismiss health issues out of hand. "There are no risks to these products if you use them safely," says Doug Schoon, vice president of science and technology for Creative Nail Design, a leading manufacturer of professional nail products. "It's a misconception to say these products haven't been studied. They've been looked at by the leading experts in the world and found to be safe."

By "leading experts in the world," Schoon means the Cosmetic Ingredient Review, which he describes as "famous for being fair and honest." The CIR is a panel of scientists funded by the industry's Cosmetic, Fragrance and Toiletry Association (CFTA) who assess the safety of ingredients used in cosmetics. They're quick to distance themselves from the manufacturers: "The industry gets the privilege of paying to support us, but that's pretty much it," says Alan Andersen, PhD, the board's director and scientific coordinator. "I think it's actually quite an unfair leap to suggest that there is any influence. Our situation closely parallels the situation at the FDA, where companies pay user fees for safety assessments of medical devices. Would you say the industry is controlling the FDA?"

Well, you might. "The CIR has this weird semi-deputized status with the FDA," explains Mark Schapiro, author of *Exposed: The Toxic Chemistry of Everyday Products and What's at Stake for American Power*. "The FDA doesn't have the manpower to do their own safety assessments, so they rely on the CIR for all their data." Indeed, an FDA spokesman who preferred not to be named is quick to give the CIR his blessing: "They're really good about being objective; I've never seen any bias. The system does work, though it might feel a little bit weak to consumers."

"A little bit weak" is putting it mildly. Even if the CIR "doesn't hesitate to tell a company if an ingredient is unsafe," as the FDA spokesman claims, that company

is on the honor system to heed its advice—the panel has no authority to restrict the use of a product. It's clear the industry has a seat at the table. After all, it's their table; CFTA and CIR share office space and support staff in Washington. "When I attended the CIR's assessment of dibutyl phthalate, the room was full of PR folks and a CFTA lobbyist dominated the meeting," says Bryony Schwan, a founding member of Campaign for Safe Cosmetics. "He was sitting there doing calculations on the back of a napkin, dismissing any data that conflicted with his point of view."

The numbers tell the rest of the story. While the European Union's Cosmetics Directive has banned some 1,200 chemicals, the FDA has restricted only nine for use in cosmetics. "The EU appears to have more authority," admits the FDA spokesman. "The burden of the FDA is that we must demonstrate an ingredient is harmful as used before we can ban it." The CIR has concluded that it has insufficient data on the safety of an additional 119 chemicals but balks at the idea of regulating them per the precautionary principle. "Ours is a risk assessment approach, and it requires data," says the CIR's Andersen.

When it comes to nail salons, the FDA is quick to point out that any health risks presented by a hazardous working environment are out of its jurisdiction—even if the hazards are posed by cosmetics. This responsibility is shared between the Environmental Protection Agency (EPA), which regulates indoor air quality, and the Occupational Safety and Health Administration (OSHA), which sets permissible exposure limits for all the chemicals nail salon workers use.

The EPA first took an interest in nail salons when Asian community groups around Houston approached its regional office with concerns. The Region 6 office published *A Guide to Protect the Health of Nail Salon Workers and Their Working Environment* in May 2004, which outraged the industry. "It's a ridiculous piece of garbage," Schoon said of the brochure. "The EPA was very embarrassed and pulled it off their website." Region 6's Nail Salon Project was transferred to the DC office, and in March a revised manual, *Protecting the Health of Nail Salon Workers*, appeared. This time, "we involved all the stakeholders," says Clive Davies, coordinator of the project, including Schoon and the Nail Manufacturers' Council, another industry association.

Their influence is palpable. The 2004 manual stated, "Nail salon products may contain many potentially harmful chemicals that can be a major cause of occupational asthma as well as other health and environmental concerns." The updated version takes a different stance: "Products that nail salon workers use are critical to performing high-quality services, and indeed, without them, these services would not be possible." It later adds a caveat: "If proper care is not taken, overexposure may occur and could result in adverse health effects, such as skin irritation, allergic reaction, or serious eye injury."

Perhaps the biggest drawback of the updated manual is that the EPA evaluates a chemical's health risks based on whether it exceeds OSHA's permissible exposure limits, developed for industrial settings. As Dr. Meyer notes, "These standards are designed to prevent acute problems like neurological intoxication or respiratory difficulty that develop soon after a large dose. They aren't set up to assess cancer and chronic disease which develop from long-term, low-dose exposure." Many of the standards also haven't changed since OSHA first set limits in 1968, when the populations it studied were mostly male. "They don't take into account female reproductive health issues," says Meyer.

The one thing scientists, advocates, industry and government agencies agree on is that more education about "best practices" is crucial to avoiding, or at least minimizing, health problems. But it's a stopgap measure, passing the buck to the technicians—who have the least control over the situation. "Education only goes so far," says Meyer. "It shouldn't be incumbent on the workers to be their own protectors."

Especially because making "best practices" happen in the real world is a complicated process for this workforce, whose average salary is less than $17,000 per year; many rent booths or work on commission, meaning traditional workers' rights laws don't protect them. About 40 percent of nail technicians are Vietnamese immigrants, many of whom don't speak much English and earn as little as $50 for an eight- to ten-hour day.

In California, where 80 percent of the state's 80,000 technicians are Vietnamese, advocates are working on filling the research and education gaps through a coalition of nonprofits called the California Healthy Nail Salons Collaborative. They plan to publish the first baseline study of nail salon workers' health. Community advocate Lenh Tsan makes weekly visits to hundreds of salons in the Bay Area, toting a rolling suitcase filled with rubber gloves, face masks and incense to test air circulation, and collecting reports of eye infections, skin rashes, asthma, headaches, nausea and dizziness. She encourages workers and owners to come together to improve conditions, but it's slow going. "There's a lot of fear," Tsan says. "It takes several visits before they get comfortable enough to tell us what's going on."

"My community is suffering silent," says C.M. Nguyen, 47, a Vietnamese immigrant and salon worker Tsan recruited to help. "They have lots of concerns, but they don't like me to speak out." Tsan thinks the problem is partly cultural: "In Asian culture, you're taught to be very respectful of hierarchy," she explains. "It's hard for these women to speak up. So if your boss doesn't care about chemicals and safety, why should you?"

It's also just plain bad for business. Owners and workers alike are concerned about how customers will respond to nail technicians wearing carbon filter masks and gloves, as well as the expense of installing better ventilation systems. And the industry's huge growth makes for cutthroat competition. In Oakland, eleven nail salons crowd into a five-block stretch of Grand Avenue. "I'm trying to get everyone around here to agree to raise their prices by $2, but I don't know if they'll do it," says Jeannie, a 23-year-old nail technician who runs one of the salons with her mother. They both suffer constant allergies and want to switch from generic products to safer, more expensive brands of polish and acrylic. But long work days and relentless worries about making the rent on their salon make it hard to find time or money for changes.

Non-Vietnamese salons feel the pressure too. Horton says that when she quit, her co-workers didn't want to hear it: "They like their salons, they like their gossip, they're in denial about what's going on." What many US workers do get fired up about are the "discount chop shops" stealing their business. "The technicians that are going to get sick are those girls who are normally of Oriental background. They are not well trained, they don't get the education and they have very poor work habits," says Long Island-based Debbie Doerlamm, who runs beautytech.com. Nguyen isn't surprised: "It's like a cold war between us."

The Collaborative's biggest victory is the Safe Cosmetics Act, passed by the California State Assembly in 2005 after a handful of salon workers testified—as beauty industry lobbyists passed out bags of free makeup. The law, which went into effect January 1, is the first of its kind and requires manufacturers to disclose all potentially harmful product ingredients to the state health department. The State of Washington is considering a similar bill, and advocates hope the state-by-state approach will inspire more companies to voluntarily reformulate all their products. But there's no question that what salon workers really need is a federal law requiring the FDA, EPA and OSHA to hold the beauty industry to a much tougher standard, and more scientific research to pin down exactly what they're up against. Until then, a handful of hard-to-impose "best practices" is the only protection we can offer these workers, who didn't realize that painting nails would mean putting their health on the line.

WORKSHEET—CHAPTER 8

Food, Body Image, and Body Modification

PART I: **Body Image /Body Modifications: Products and Procedures**

1. *Your* **personal care products.** Pull out all the containers for the products (make-up, shampoo, deodorant, lotions, etc.) you use regularly. Make a list of all the ingredients on the labels. Using information in "The Ugly Side of the Beauty Industry" and the on-line resources listed in that article, what do you know about the safety or hazards of the ingredients in *your* products?

2. Draw a map of a woman's body. Going from head to toe, identify messages women get about "attractive" vs. "unattractive" versions of this body part, what women are encouraged to do to make that part "attractive," and what products and procedures get marketed to "improve" that part of the body.

3. For each product and procedure you mentioned for question 2, identify whether there are health advantages or health hazards for the products and procedures women are encouraged to use.

4. For each product or procedure you mentioned for question 2, based on "The High Price of Beauty," think of health issues for the workers who help produce or use the products and procedures.

PART II: The Continuum of Women and Food Relationships

This study guide is designed to help us see the similarities among a wide range of behaviors that get labeled as "eating disorders" and very related patterns which do not get labeled as "eating disorders."

The so-called "eating disorders" feel less threatening to us if we can view them as extreme cases that have nothing to do with us. However, even if we look at how common the extremes are, we must already face the fact that "eating disorders" are very much a part of our lives.

It may be more helpful to understanding the ambivalent relationship many women (in most western countries) have to their bodies and their food if we look at a wide range of eating patterns as a part of a continuum. If anorexia, bulimia, and compulsive eating are seen as exaggerated manifestations of dieting, we may be better able to understand both how our society encourages "eating disorders" and the unnaturalness and unhealthiness of most dieting.

1. Make a list (collect examples from magazines, T.V., conversations, jokes) of messages women get about what they should look like. Make a list (collect examples from magazines, T.V., conversations, on-street advertising) of messages women get about delicious food available to them to eat or prepare.
   What is contradictory about these messages? How do women internalize these confused messages?

2. Read the definitions for all the "eating problems" (pp. 436). Look for similarities between the different patterns. Be creative! Think of a way to show the similarities between different patterns by connecting them with overlapping circles or lines. You may want to photocopy the words for eating problems and do a "cut and paste" job. You may want to use several different colors to identify themes that keep occurring.

3. Reread definition #9 for "unnatural relationship to food and eating." Do you think this description of women for a body image study reflects *all* women or is it peculiar only to women concerned with body image? Can you think of ten women you know who are not concerned about body image? Can you think of ten women you know who are not very conscious of food/weight/exercise issues?

4. Based on your own experiences and the articles by Becky Thompson, Christy Haubegger, and Graciela Rodriguez, describe how you think body image issues are the same and different for white women and women of color.

5. Describe how you think race, class, and heterosexism impact on body image issues.

6. Many girls and women are pressured to be thinner than they are genetically meant to be. Based on the articles in this chapter and your own observations, identify some of the consequences of this for individual women and society.

The Continuum of Women and Food Relationships

Starving[16]   Large for years[15]

Anorexia[1]   Subgroup of   Weight   Up and down dieters[14]
                     weight preoccupied[2] preoccupied[3]

Anorexia-like symptoms[4]   Compulsive eater[13]

Chronic anorexia[5]   Dieter
                                                         ex-"normal eater"[12]

Recovered anorexic[6]   Bulimorexic[8]

                                                         Thin fat people[11]

Ex-anorexic difficulties resolved[7]   Used to living on
                                                        semi-starvation diet[10]

                              Unnatural relationship
                              to food and eating[9]

1. **Anorexia**—Try to avoid eating as far as possible. Often have a distorted view of their bodies seeing themselves as grotesque and enormous instead of thin. Tend to be extremely close mouthed about their eating but observe others closely. (Orbach, 1984, p.30)

2. **Sub-group of weight pre-occupied women.** This group scored high or higher than the anorexia nervosa group on all Eating Disorder Inventory (EDI) subscales. (The EDI is designed to assess the cognitive and behavioral dimensions characteristic of anorexia and to differentiate between patients with anorexia and those without the disorder.) "It is likely that at the very least, they suffer from a subclinical variant of the disorder." (Garner, 1984, pp.255–266.)

3. **Weight preoccupied women.** This group was compared to women with anorexia by the EDI (see 2). Weight preoccupied women and anorexic women were comparable on body dissatisfaction, bulimia, perfectionism, and maturity fears subscales. The EDI subscales which best differentiated weight preoccupied women from anorexics were ineffectiveness and interreceptive awareness. (Garner, 1984, pp. 255–266)

4. **Women with anorexia-like symptoms.** College women who scored high on Garner and Garfinkel's Eating Attitudes Test. This group was similar to the anorexia group in the proportion of subjects reporting binge eating and self-induced vomiting. This group did not show distress on a psychiatric symptom checklist. "These findings indicate that food and weight preoccupations common in anorexia nervosa do occur on a continuum, but the milder expression was not associated with psychosocial impairment." (Thompson and Schwartz, 1982, quoted in Garner, 1984)

5. **Chronic anorexia.** An anorexic makes a partial recovery, gains enough weight to keep her alive but maintains it at an artificially low level, sometimes for years. Her life continues to be utterly dominated by the desire to avoid food. (Lawrence, 1984, p. 108)

6. **Recovered anorexic.** Sizeable proportion of ex-anorexics are able to live creative and independent lives but still retain some elements of their preoccupation with food and weight. (Lawrence, 1984, p. 108)

7. **Ex-anorexic difficulties resolved.** "The woman is no longer vulnerable to further anorexic episodes and *is no more neurotic about food than anyone else.*" (Lawrence, 1984, p. 109)

8. **Bulimorexic.** Women often of average size, but weekly, daily, sometimes hourly, they binge on substantial amounts of food which they bring up. Very few feel comfortable talking about their way of coping. Feel purging after gorging is the only way to stay slim. (Orbach, 1984, p. 30) Estimated 15–20% of USA college women have bulimia. Only 44% sought professional help. (Potts, 1984, pp. 32–35)

9. **Unnatural relationship to food and eating.** For body image study, "I sought subjects with no history of psychiatric illness or eating disorder. It immediately became clear that it is a rare woman in this culture who is not eating disordered or who does not experience herself as struggling with food and weight issues. Of 114 women screened for this study 109 reported an unnatural relationship to food and eating. Of those selected as subjects—whose weights all fell within the normal range—only 1 woman was not actively waging a war against fat. This astonishing statistic suggests that weight and eating issues are inseparable from body image struggles in today's woman." "Although describing themselves as eating disordered . . . most women reported eating patterns typical of the culture as a whole, patterns that in men would never be labeled as pathological. These women are for the most part suffering not from eating disorders but from labeling disorders." (Hutchinson, 1982, p.61)

10. **Used to living on semi-starvation diet.** Having grown up with the concept that thinness is identical with beauty and attractiveness … these women have grown used to living on a semi-starvation diet, never eating more than their bony figures show. Never having permitted themselves to eat adequately, they are unaware of how much their tension, bad disposition, irritability, even inability to pursue educational and professional goals is the direct result of chronic undernutrition. (Bruch, 1980, p. 19)

11. **Thin fat people.** People who stay reduced but who cannot relax. They seem as preoccupied with weight and dieting after they have become slim as before. (Bruch, 1980, p. 18)

12. "**Diets** turn 'normal eaters' into people who are afraid of food." (Orbach, 1984, p. 29)

13. Compulsive eating means eating without regard to physical cues signalling hunger or satisfaction. Feels out of control about what she eats. (Orbach, 1984, p. 29)

14. Women who go up and down the scale (maximum of 60 lbs), diet from time to time and binge irregularly. Open about talking about food problems. Feel that things would be better for them if they were thin. "The largest group of women." (Orbach, 1984, p. 30)

15. Women who have been large for years, who feel themselves to be fat, but are despairing about ever being able to lose weight. Experience their eating as chaotic. Discuss the topic openly. Feel things would be a lot better if they were slim. (Orbach)

16. Both starvation and dieting may produce many of the behaviors associated with anorexia. Both obese humans and starving organisms demonstrate thrifty metabolism, heightened preference for sweets and inhibition of satiety mechanisms. (Smead, 1983)

REFERENCES

Bruch, H., "Thin Fat People" in Kaplan, J. R. (ed) *A Woman's Conflict: The Special Relationship Between Women and Food,* Prentice Hall, New York, 1980.

Garner, D. M., Olmstead, M. P., Polivy, J., and Garfinkel, P. E., "Comparison Between Weight-Preoccupied Women and Anorexia Nervosa", *Psychosomatic Medicine,* Vol. 46, No. 3, 1984, pp. 255–266.

Hutchinson, M. G., "Transforming Body Image: Your Body, Friend or Foe?", *Women and Therapy,* Vol. 1, No. 3, 1982, pp. 59–67.

Lawrence, M., *The Anorexic Experience,* Women's Press, London, 1984.

Orbach, S., *Fat Is a Feminist Issue 2,* Hamlyn Paperback, London, 1984.

Potts, N. L., "Eating Disorders—The Secret Pattern of Binge/Purge", *American Journal of Nursing,* Vol. 84, No. 1, 1984, pp. 32–35.

Smead, V. S., "Anorexia Nervosa. Bulimarexia, and Bulimia: Labeled Pathology and the Western Female" , *Women and Therapy,* Vol. 2, No. 1, 1983, pp. 19–35.

SEXUALITY

Sexuality can be a very important part of women's mental and physical health. The other way around, problems with mental or physical health often manifest themselves in women not being able to maximize their sexual health and enjoyment. This chapter explores how social and cultural definitions of sexuality can be either positive or detrimental to emotional and physical health. The male-centered emphasis on vaginal intercourse as the "real thing" limits or invalidates the experiences and preferences of many women. The question of who defines sexuality, and whether those definitions encourage or limit women's enjoyment of sexuality and ability to be sexually healthy, will be central to this chapter.

"Education for Sexual Intimacy and Agency," written specifically for this book by Susan K. Pastor, opens the chapter with an excellent analysis of many of the key contemporary sexuality issues in the U.S. The author focuses attention on ways in which inadequate and inappropriate sexuality education contributes to reinforcing problematic views of sexuality, particularly by teaching that sex is only about reproduction:

> Schools also teach that sex is reproduction. . . . Public outcry about the scientific inaccuracies and negative outcomes of abstinence only curricula, while entirely legitimate, misses an important point. It is possible to add substantial information on contraception and an arsenal of facts about sexually transmitted infections to the facts of conception, leaving the definition of sex as reproduction unchanged. Teaching sex as reproduction contributes to the idea that a normal girl would not be interested in sex for its own sake and a normal boy always would.

This article provides much of the information about sexuality that is so often lacking in education—even at the college level. It also introduces many of the major themes of this chapter.

The Advocates for Youth fact sheets reinforce the arguments made in Pastor's article. Compared to adolescents in several European countries, U.S. adolescents have alarmingly high rates of pregnancy, birth, abortion, HIV infection, and other STIs. Both "The Lessons Learned" section of the first fact sheet and the second fact sheet on "Effective Sex Education" outline clearly the directions for change that could greatly benefit the sexual health of adolescents—and people of all ages—in the U.S. (Note that Ronna Popkin's article in Chapter 4 also addresses some of the problems that arise from the way sexuality education is taught in the U.S.)

"Exposed at Last: The Truth about Your Clitoris" adds to the discussion of the clitoris introduced in Pastor's article. Although textbooks have often defined the clitoris as the "key" to female sexuality (the term "clitoris" is derived from the Greek work for key), they have also hidden it and presented it as very small, described as pea-sized. Jennifer Johnson's article notes that "the clitoris was more accurately described in some 19th century anatomy texts, but then it was mysteriously shrunk into a mere speck on the anatomical map." When the clitoris is more fully and accurately described as homologous (arising from the same structure) to the penis (see Pastor's article in this chapter and Sloane's *Biology of Women* for details of the sex differentiation of the embryo), many things about female anatomy and sexual response make more sense. As we read this article, we should once again ask ourselves whether different potential areas of research would be considered "scientifically interesting" and studied if more scientific decision-makers were women.

"How Being a Good Girl Can Be Bad for Girls," by Deborah Tolman and Tracy Higgins, gives both a societal overview and three specific adolescent girls' experiences of how "women's sexuality is frequently suspect in our culture, particularly when it is expressed outside the bounds of monogamous heterosexual marriage." In the same way that we have seen healthy women defined as passive and dependent (see "Mental Health Issues," Chapter 6), "good" women are sexually defined as "passive and threatened sexual objects" with no sexual desire. Tolman and Higgins point out that "When women act as sexual agents, expressing their own sexual desire rather than serving as objects of men's desire, they are portrayed as threatening, deviant, and bad." This article looks at all the no-win situations this puts girls and women in as they are held responsible for sexual gate-keeping. Within this framework, girls/women do not have permission to discover, express, or enjoy their own sexual desire, but are too often held culturally or legally responsible for not stopping rape. The authors discuss how such good girl/bad girl dynamics can be resisted, and encourage feminists "to analyze the complexity of living in women's bodies within a culture that divides girls and women within themselves and against each other."

The provocative article, "The Orgasm Gap," pushes us to recognize the cultural construction of sexuality, the price women pay for this, the enormous possibilities for "making sex an act of shared, mutual pleasure" and why that must be a core component of work toward gender equality:

> Seventy-five percent of men have orgasm in partner sex on a regular basis, but only 29 percent of women do . . . Women are not inherently less orgasmic than men. In fact, women are physically capable of multiple orgasms, and most women who masturbate reach orgasm without fail. Women who have sex with a female partner come 83 percent of the time. Clearly, the problem lies not with women themselves, but in the way *heterosexuals* have sex.

The New View Manifesto and the brochure for the New View Campaign are responses to the ways women's sexual problems have been defined as "dysfunctions," using a medical model that ignores the social and cultural realities of women's lives, such as those raised in this chapter. The authors argue that:

> A corrective approach is desperately needed. We propose a new and more useful classification of women's sexual problems, one that gives appropriate priority to individual distress and inhibition arising within a broader framework of cultural and relational factors. . . . We call for research and services driven not by commercial interests, but by women's own needs and sexual realities.

Continuing the focus on the importance of "women's own needs and sexual realities," June Jordan's classic essay, "The New Politics of Sexuality," asserts the important points that freedom is indivisible, that the politics of sexuality are not the province of "special interest" groups, and that bisexuality gives an important perspective on the complexity of sexuality.

The next three articles in this chapter work together to demonstrate the urgency for both individual health practitioners and the health system as a whole to learn to serve more appropriately *all* their patients regardless of patients' sexual identity or practices. Society's homophobia and heterosexism are very much reflected in the medical system's homophobia and heterosexism. Fear and shame are recurring themes in stories of lesbian, bisexual, gay, and trans people's experiences with the health system. Studies have consistently shown that a major health issue for lesbians is that they do not take care of regular routine health care, such as gynecological exams, because of actual or feared poor interactions with homophobic or heterosexist providers. Dr. Jennifer Potter's "Do Ask, Do Tell" relates her own story of moving from being a frightened suicidal young lesbian:

> Many lesbians and gay men find it difficult to avoid internalizing some of these (society's) homophobic attitudes. As a consequence, shame and fear are common emotions, and we are more likely to be isolated, engage in risky behaviors, suffer from stress-related health conditions, or from substance abuse, depression, and attempted suicide.

to being a proud, out lesbian, physician, and educator. "For Better Lesbian Health, Fewer Barriers" is a good follow-up to Potter's article, as Leah Thayer discusses a program, "Removing the Barriers," which "aims to build the cultural competence of health care providers while creating systematic changes that help lesbians feel safe and comfortable disclosing their sexual orientation in health care settings." Note the additional section "Removing More Barriers," which discusses a clinic started by the Feminist Women's Health Center in Atlanta to address the unmet needs of trans men (FtM), for gynecological and other routine healthcare.

Dr. Charles Moser's very practical, very explicit chapter, "Health Care Without Shame—Some Background for the Practitioner" comes from his book *Health Care Without Shame—A Handbook for the Sexually Diverse and Their Caregivers* (published by Greenery Press but now apparently out of print), which we recommend that every health practitioner read. Refer back to "Trans Health Criis: For Us It's Life or Death," in Chapter 2. Think about how much more appropriate and humane Leslie Feinberg's experiences with the health system would have been if healthcare providers, including front desk staff, had followed the suggestions in "Health Care Without Shame."

The question of who defines women's sexuality is next explored in terms of issues of disability. Social attitudes about women's sexuality are also extremely problematic in their impact on women with disabilities. In "Forbidden Fruit," Anne Finger examines the strong prejudice against people with disabilities in our society—the beliefs that they should neither be sexual nor have children.

We close this sexuality chapter with the important classic, "The Need for Intimacy." We could have placed this article in the chapter on ageing, as we had in earlier editions, but we have decided that the issues raised are too important to be marginalized as an issue only for older, widowed women. Clearly, opportunities for healthy intimacy are crucial at *every* stage of people's lives: "No matter what our age, we each need intimacy in our lives—at least one other person with whom we can share both pleasure and pain." In keeping with the other questions explored in this chapter, it seems imperative to ask how the cultural definitions of sexuality limit people's opportunities for intimacy, especially for people who are not in a "socially sanctioned couple" and what we can (collectively) do to change this. The reader is asked to synthesize points made in both "The Need for Intimacy" article and "Myth 4: Women Want Intimacy; Men Want Sex" in "The Orgasm Gap" to come up with a comprehensive statement acknowledging the roles that both intimacy and orgasms could play in both women's and men's lives.

"Education for Sexual Intimacy and Agency"

by Susan K. Pastor

Introduction: The Problem

When "sex" is defined for young children by parents, it is in terms of how babies are made. Schools also teach that sex is reproduction. Even where abstinence-only or abstinence-based curricula are used, this definition of sex is underscored. Public outcry about the scientific inaccuracies in and negative outcomes of abstinence-only curricula, while entirely legitimate, misses an important point. It is possible to add substantial information on contraception and an arsenal of facts about sexually transmitted infections to the fact of conception, leaving the definition of sex as reproduction unchanged. Teaching sex as reproduction contributes to the idea that a normal girl would not be interested in sex for its own sake and a normal boy always would. Erections and ejaculation are standard topics in school puberty education in fourth or fifth grade, but sex appears to be only about periods for girls. How would anyone know girls can become aroused? How would a girl realize her wetness is normal? No one learns the physical signs of female arousal. This silence supports beliefs held by many people, including some scientists, that the sexual double standard is "natural" and women are "wired" for monogamy. According to a neuroscientist writing in *Men's Health*, women mainly desire a good provider for their offspring (Amen and Bodegraven 2004).

A more viable explanation for the persistence of the sexual double standard today is that we teach it, in part by initially constructing female pleasure as irrelevant to partner sex, defined as heterosexual intercourse. One pamphlet produced by the federal government and used in elementary schools depicts a female figure with no external "parts" at all. A uterus, fallopian tubes and ovaries are shown, with an upper vagina leading nowhere. (Department of Health and Human Services 1981). Seeking extra-curricular materials will not help. The latest editions of the best-selling books on puberty, the "*What's Happening to My Body?*" books, include two chapters dedicated to the internal reproductive organs and menstruation for girls, while two chapters in the boys' book address the physiology of desire (Madaras 2007a;2007b). The chapter on "Erections, Sperm and Ejaculation" is followed by another on "Spontaneous Erections, Orgasms, Masturbation and Wet Dreams". In the entire book for girls, three paragraphs are devoted to female arousal and orgasm (Madaras 2007a:83). This topic is equally neglected in the boys' book. Both books discuss the clitoris and female orgasm only in connection with masturbation and give as much attention to the hymen as to the clitoris (Madaras 2007a:74–48; 2007b:172–173). In discussing intercourse, however, the books do mention that "fluid comes out of the vaginal walls when a female is sexually excited" (2007a:14; 2007b:12), so there is some indication that female sexual arousal is possible.

The author probably means to be complete, but what she chooses to emphasize is foundational to a pattern that continues into adult life. Female pleasure is so unnecessary in heterosexual encounters that popular writer John Gray counseled one married woman to have "fast food" sex with her husband, even though these encounters did not last long enough for her to become aroused. In the deal Gray negotiates, the man gets to have sex, but promises not to require his wife to pretend she enjoys it. This husband later reported that his wife did "lie there like a dead log" and "he didn't mind at all" (Gray 1995:80). Gray directs heterosexual couples to incorporate "quickies" into their sex lives, pointing out that the woman benefits in part by not having to fake interest and pleasure (ibid:141).

Gray's problem-solving is consistent with one use of medical and scientific authority since the development of gynecology, which has been to render women physically capable of satisfying men's desire for heterosexual intercourse. In the 19th century, the "father of modern gynecology" used anesthesia to accomplish this with patients experiencing vaginismus, a condition involving muscle spasms that make vaginal penetration impossible. Once these women were under anesthesia, their husbands could have intercourse with them (Kapsalis 1997:47). If you think no one has this kind of attitude

---

today, consider the comments of sex therapist Drew Pinsky, M.D., in an interview with *O: The Oprah Magazine*. To illustrate men's lack of interest in an eager and knowledgeable female partner, Pinsky was quoted as saying "Now if a guy had slept with Claudia Shiffer, it wouldn't matter what the hell she did. She could have been dead and he'd be overjoyed" (Brody 2003).

Certainly Dr. Drew doesn't mean to suggest that men should be having sex with female corpses, but his comments reflect the history of sexual interaction between men and women as something considerably less than mutually satisfying. Dr. Drew's words also project that history onto the present and future, suggesting that male lack of regard for female pleasure (or even willing participation) is normal. Women's greater interest in "cuddling" and emotional closeness becomes normative too. Gray suggests that women can barter for cuddling by providing the "quickies" their male partners desire (Gray 1995:141). Commentators such as Pinsky and Gray most likely have good intentions and mean to smooth relations between the sexes. It is just that the usual formulas for smooth relations appear to be based mainly on women's accommodation of what everyone understands as men's greater need for sex—including sex that is not especially . . . relational.

Education and socialization also help explain the "orgasm gap" to which Douglas and Douglas (1997) refer, in which men are more likely to have an orgasm as a result of heterosexual partner sex, usually intercourse, than women are. These authors draw on data reported in *The Social Organization of Sex* (Laumann et al 1994:114). This same study reports that women have orgasms much more reliably from solo sex (ibid:82). Unless we see this part of the picture, we may fall back on the myth that women are just less sexual and harder to arouse than men. A male partner would have to know he was missing something and seek out information about female bodies and pleasure. Among the 40 young men I interviewed in the mid-1990s, no one had learned more than sex as reproduction. Nevertheless, almost every man thought he had learned everything necessary. Only one said he would have liked to know something about pleasing a female partner.

Suggesting that men ask female partners what is pleasurable does not entirely solve the problem. Before puberty, girls have more knowledge of boys' genitals than of their own (Bem 1989), and less direct experience of touching themselves—since they don't have to hold themselves to urinate. Today the female genitalia have a name, but it is the wrong name. To call the female genitalia "vagina" instead of "vulva" is to render the other structures invisible and/or irrelevant. Add these circumstances to the official teaching only of reproduction and

periods and some women might find "What should I do?" and "What do you like?" to be challenging questions. Growing up, girls hear mostly silence on female sexual anatomy and female pleasure. A now well-established literature in the social sciences has documented the confusion and inequality to which that silence leads (see for examples Tolman 2002 and Fine 1988). Based on the usual version of puberty and sex education, women in general will not be more knowledgeable about female pleasure than men in general, and neither will be encouraged to seek out more information. The usual version of knowledge is constructed as what there is to know (Pastor, undated).

At the same time, heterosexual girls in search of sexual agency may find it in pleasing boyfriends. Masters and colleagues quote a 17-year-old who seems to appreciate her capacity in this area. When her boyfriend wants sex but she isn't in the mood, she reports relying on oral sex: "I don't even have to take my clothes off and I can still get the job done" (Masters, Johnson and Kolodny 1994:445). The authors offer this quote as evidence for the casual attitude toward oral sex among young people, not to call attention to the young woman's sense of obligation to produce her partner's pleasure when she herself has no interest in sex. Nevertheless, the possibility that she takes pleasure in the control this strategy gives her, or in pleasing her boyfriend should not be overlooked.

Toward a More Egalitarian Understanding of Sexuality

What counts as knowledge about sex has been skewed toward what points to gender difference and justifies gender inequality. Certainly sex roles in reproducing are different. Yet beyond penises entering vaginas and ejaculating to make babies are biological facts that suggest more erotic possibilities for both partner and solo sex. This is definitely not to say that there is no erotic potential for penises and vaginas together. However, the exclusive focus on sex as reproduction through childhood and into adolescence limits both men's and women's spectra of erotic imagination and experience. The first president of the Sexuality Information and Education Council of the United States (SIECUS), Dr. Mary Calderone, believed that our failure to understand sexual response apart from reproduction, together with taboos against children's masturbation, explained the high rates of sexual dysfunction in American society. She argued that sexual response is a capacity that develops beginning at birth, and which our beliefs and practices impair (Calderone 1983). Since 1998, urologists and other professionals have hastened to define and treat "female sexual dysfunction" as a medical condition including lack of desire, impairment of arousal and difficulty with or inability to reach orgasm (anorgasmia). Lenore Tiefer has been foremost among feminist scholars criticizing this medicalization of sexuality and calling for more attention to cultural attitudes toward sexuality, women's early experiences and the conditions of women's intimate relationships (Tiefer 2001).

Embryonic Sex Differentiation

The belief that women and men are so sexually different by nature begins to unravel if one starts at the beginning. Before the sixth to eighth week of development, the genital and reproductive structures of human embryos are identical—regardless of male (xy) chromosomes and programming for male development or female chromosomes (xx). Testicles and ovaries develop from the same initially undifferentiated gonad and all embryos have a "genital tubercle", which will become either a penis or a clitoris. These structures will be approximately the same size, except that most of the clitoris lies below the skin and so is not visible. Similarly, the "labio-scrotal" folds in all embryos will fuse in normal male development, becoming the scrotum. In females, the labio-scrotal folds become the labia majora, or outer labia. The tissue that becomes the labia minora, or inner labia in females will form the underside of the penis in males (see Sloane 2002:145–151 for a thorough explanation).

Women's bodies also have a structure analogous to the prostate gland in men. *A New View of a Woman's Body* calls this structure the urethral sponge, because its spongy tissue surrounds, cushions and protects the urethra (Federation of Feminist Women's Health Centers 1991). Like the prostate gland, the urethral sponge produces a clear fluid and a protease, prostate specific antigen, or PSA. While it was previously believed that only male bodies produce PSA, it has now been identified in the vaginas of women, independent of sexual activity with men (Sundahl 2003). It is reasonable to say, therefore, that the structure that becomes the prostate gland in males becomes the urethral sponge in females. These facts explain female potential for ejaculation.

When this structure is finally recognized in medicine, it is likely to be called the "female prostate". The term has been in use in the sexology literature for some time, and reflects that this part of the anatomy is the same structurally in women and men (see Zaviacic and Whipple 1993). In terms of erotic significance, the urethral sponge is the anatomical structure to which the term "G-spot" refers. The prostate has erotic potential in men as well.

Perhaps the puberty education version of embryonic sex differentiation would be: "Girl parts and boy parts start out exactly the same and come from the same structures. These structures do different things when it comes to reproduction, but they respond similarly to sexual stimulation." Ejaculation could be explained in connection with the prostate gland. Some students in my classes have indicated that they did learn about embryonic sex differentiation in biology, while for others the information is new. However, very little biology education or sex education links similar morphology to erotic potential—even at the college level. Embryonic sex differentiation is therefore constructed as irrelevant to information about sexuality, although this knowledge is becoming somewhat more widespread as awareness of the conditions that lead to intersexuality increases (see Preves 2003).

Female Sexual Anatomy

The lack of information about female anatomy disadvantages girls as they begin to explore sexually. A girl who does not know her own anatomy cannot direct a partner. A girl who is self-conscious as to whether her genitalia are normal is less likely to enjoy exploring. Boys are also affected. Because of the stereotype that boys want sex and should initiate, they will be expected to know what to do with a female partner—though they have no more knowledge. The college students I interviewed consistently reported that they had learned "the basics" about sex, meaning only that penises enter vaginas. The following information points to ways in which the "basics" are in great need of expansion.

Labia Puberty education assures boys that normal penises come in a range of sizes and shapes, although such assurances don't dispel anxiety. Men's anxiety about size is well-recognized and the subject of much email spam. Reassurance for women on the normal variation in labia has generally been absent—that is, until cosmetic surgery on the labia began growing in popularity (see Woods 2007). In anatomical drawings, labia are always of uniform size and hairless. They are often hairless in pornographic representations too. Anyone who has seen the range of sizes and shapes of labia knows that some are very pronounced. Sometimes the inner labia protrude and are larger than the outer labia. Labiaplasty reduces the inner labia and makes them more symmetrical. Failure to teach girls about normal variation makes them more likely to become customers for genital cosmetic surgery.

Perhaps the increasing number of labiaplasties performed has encouraged women's magazines to reassure their readers about genital variation, although such articles may also serve to call attention to labiaplasty as an option. Recent articles in *Seventeen* (Brodman-Grimm 2005), *Cosmopolitan* (Perron 2004) and *Redbook* (Graham and Lister 2003) tackled this subject. *Redbook* readers even learned that it is normal for there to be color variations in the labia of the same woman. The photographs in *Femalia*, edited by Joani Blank, are an excellent representation of normal variation. The *"What's Happening to My Body" Book for Girls* includes five drawings showing variation, described by a few lines of text. While this is a start, there are approximately six pages devoted to reassuring boys about penis shape and size in the boys' book (Madaras 2007a:74–75; 2007b:47–54).

Clitoris   Most girls probably cannot identify all the structures of the external genitalia, much less the normal variation. Most girls probably do not know that the clitoris is really as big as a penis. In terms of the visible parts of the clitoris, there is variability in how much of the shaft is visible and the extent to which the hood covers the glans. Examples of these variations can be seen in the photographs in *Femalia*. The high concentration of nerve endings in the glans make it the most erotically charged part of a woman's body. All of the structures of the clitoris under the skin are made up of erectile tissue and respond to stimulation. The spongiest and most erotically sensitive tissues, after the glans, are the "bulbs", which are located on either side of the vaginal opening, and the perineal sponge, which underlies the perineum. The legs, or crura, angling away from the front of the body are also made up of erectile tissue, though they are not as spongy as the bulbs and perineal sponge. *A New View of a Woman's Body* provides several different views of the entire clitoris.

Urinary Opening and Urethral Sponge   The area between the inner labia, officially called the vestibule, contains the urinary opening. A woman spreading her inner labia and looking at this area with a mirror might be able to see the urinary opening above the vaginal opening—how far above varies. As the photographs in *Femalia* demonstrate, the opening is quite visible in some women. Other women may not be able to identify the opening at all. This range is normal. Whether visible or not, the opening is surrounded by the urethral sponge, or female prostate. The existence of this structure is not acknowledged in mainstream medical literature as of this writing. It is also not acknowledged in the *"What's Happening to My Body"* books. Girls are told experts disagree as to whether there is a G-spot and that ejaculate might really be urine (Madaras 2007a:83). Boys are assured that "females don't ejaculate when they have an orgasm" (2007b:173).

Milan Zaviacic has documented variance in the shape of the urethral sponge/female prostate. While the bulk of the structure is usually felt on the lower anterior wall of the vagina, some women may identify the structure deeper in the vagina, and some women may have a variation in which the tissue is more evenly spread—no bulky part can be felt. Therefore, instructing women to find their G-spot as though every woman would find it the same way and experience the same sensations may lead some only to frustration (Sundahl 2003:31–34). This is true also with regard to ejaculation. Now that ejaculation in women is becoming acknowledged, some particular experience of it need not come to define the success or failure of women's sexual expression.

Ejaculation   The best understanding available at this time suggests that all women have the anatomy to ejaculate, whether ejaculation is experienced or not. Glands within the urethral sponge produce a clear fluid in varying amounts from a few drops to as much as a cup or a cup and a half. *A New View of a Woman's Body* calls these the "paraurethral glands" but they are referred to as "Skene's glands" in medical literature, where their fluid-producing function is not necessarily acknowledged. It appears that ejaculation can occur with or without orgasm. It is probable that the ejaculate can seep through the vaginal wall (Sundahl 2003:34) and be experienced as lubrication. Ejaculate is not urine but it may contain some of the same compounds. It is not clear whether these compounds would normally be present in ejaculate or suggest, for example, that the pelvic floor muscles are not strong enough to seal off urine from the bladder. A woman who ejaculates in noticeable amounts and does not know about ejaculation may think she is incontinent (Boston Women's Health Book Collective 2005:197).

Vagina   Just inside the vagina, along each wall, are glands which *A New View of a Woman's Body* calls the vulvo-vaginal glands, and which are called Bartholin's glands in the medical literature. The extent to which a woman can feel these glands varies. In some women, it may be relatively easy to feel them as small, rounded bumps under the vaginal wall. A woman who does not know that these structures are normal may become alarmed when she feels them. The vulvo-vaginal glands are thought to produce a small amount of lubrication, which is generally considered to be insignificant.

The depth of the vagina also varies. A woman who has always believed she cannot use tampons because they won't go in, or they fall out, may be able to use shorter tampons. The protrusion of the cervix into the vagina creates a space called a fornix to the front, back and sides. The space between the cervix and the frontal wall of the vagina, toward the bladder, is the anterior fornix. Some researchers suggest that a triangular space in this area is the real location to which Grafenberg pointed in his documentation of an erotically sensitive area inside the vagina. The G-spot is named after him. Since understanding of the G-spot has now settled on the urethral sponge, the sensitive location within the anterior fornix has been named the "T-zone" (Wilhite 2005). Testimonies from women point to erotic sensitivity in this area, but as yet no systematic research has been published. The space between the cervix and the back wall of the vagina, toward the rectum, is the posterior fornix. The proximity of the posterior fornix to the rectum becomes significant when the erotic potential of anal penetration is considered. The best-selling puberty books do not describe erotic sensitivity within the vagina or acknowledge the erotic potential of the anus.

Erotic Response

The physiology of erotic response points to similarity between women and men. The two main processes of vasocongestion and mytonia are central to arousal and orgasm in both. Vasocongestion is the process in which new blood is drawn to spongy erectile tissue, such as the clitoris and the penis, causing the tissues to swell. Sensitivity to touch increases as the tissues become engorged. Vasocongestion is likely related to vaginal lubrication, though vaginal lubrication is not a well-understood process. It has been suggested that the cells in the vaginal walls secrete lubrication; based on an understanding of vasocongestion, a more specific understanding is plausible as well. The very spongy tissues of the bulbs of clitoris and the perineal sponge surround the lower vagina on both sides and across the bottom. As new blood fills those tissues, clear fluid may be pushed out of the old blood in the capillaries and through the permeable vaginal walls. *Our Bodies, Ourselves* attributes vaginal lubrication to "increased blood circulation" (Boston Women's Health Book Collective 2005:194; see also Sloane 2002:173). Any physical condition or medication that interferes with circulation can impair vasocongestion.

The second process is myotonia. Myotonia is the medical term for muscular contractions. Orgasmic response is characterized by muscle contractions in both women and men. Different orgasms can involve a different number of contractions. In women, the muscles that make up the outer third of the vaginal wall contract, producing throbbing sensations. The uterus, also a muscle, contracts. (Sloane 2002:175). Weak pelvic floor muscles can impair orgasmic response.

In addition to the similarity of erotic response, some structures with erotic potential are undifferentiated in women and men. Erotic sensitivity of the nipples and anus is present in both. The following discussion is organized around the best explanations available at this time for the potential erotic response of particular structures to stimulation. There is an important caveat to this discussion. Erotic potential is not the same as erotic experience. Potential does not define experience. Hysterectomy is a good example. From a biological perspective, there are a number of reasons why this surgery could reduce sexual functioning. Yet many women report improved sexual functioning. Most women reporting sexual problems post-hysterectomy have been those who enjoyed good sexual functioning before (Maas, Weijenborg and Kuile 2003). What is erotic may be based on what we *believe* will be erotic in some cases and on factors beyond biology.

Knowledge of erotic potential should not be used to conclude that any person *should* welcome or enjoy any particular form of stimulation. There appears to be individual variation in the sensitivity of particular structures and certainly there is variation in what people enjoy. While this discussion suggests ways in which stimulation of particular structures may trigger orgasm, it is important to note that some feminist writing on sexuality has criticized such a focus, with good reason. Erotic sensations do not reduce to orgasm and the range of erotic practices should not be reduced to the production of orgasm (Tiefer 2001). The term "orgasm" encompasses a range of physical sensation, intensity and emotion; orgasms may feel different based on the structure around which stimulation is centered. Sundahl suggests that physical and emotional sensations of orgasms centered around the clitoris, urethral sponge and deeper in the vagina may feel different from one another because different neural pathways are involved. Two different major nerves connect the female genital and reproductive anatomy to the brain (Sundahl 2003:46–47).

Most discussions of arousal and orgasm are based on the stage model of human sexual response—excitement, plateau, orgasm, and resolution, toward which feminist writers have also directed incisive criticism (Tiefer 1995). There are ample opportunities for individuals to learn about the model and decide for themselves whether it is useful (e.g. Sloane 2002:172–178). There are also ample opportunities to match the information provided here with information on safe sex practices widely available elsewhere. Finally, existing knowledge about erotic potential should not be seen as expressing the limits of that potential. For example, women with spinal cord injuries who have lost feeling in the pelvic area can develop erotic responses in other parts of the body (Whipple, Gerdes and Komisaruk 1996).

Clitoris The high concentration of nerve endings in the glans of the clitoris account for its erotic sensitivity. Women's experiences of and preference for certain types of clitoral stimulation vary. Some women find direct stimulation of the glans uncomfortable and too intense. Direct stimulation of the glans can lead to orgasm, but the erectile tissue of the bulbs and perineal sponge are sensitive as well. This explains why some women might prefer stimulation of a larger area of the vulva. A woman might reach orgasm through this stimulation without directly touching the glans. The bulbs of the clitoris and the perineal sponge are in close proximity to the vaginal opening and lower vagina. Shallow vaginal penetration could stimulate those structures and may partly explain a woman's pleasure in vaginal penetration.

Urethral Sponge Women also report variance in enjoyment of stimulation of the urethral sponge. While some women find the sensation highly erotic, others find it uncomfortable or unpleasant. Stimulation of the urethral sponge can also produce a sensation that feels like the urge to urinate (Boston Women's Health Collective 2005:197). This structure can be stimulated from the inside, through vaginal penetration, or outside, from pressure to the area below the glans of the clitoris and above the vaginal opening. Orgasm centered around stimulation of this structure can occur with ejaculation or without noticeable ejaculation, as with any orgasm. Ejaculation can also occur without orgasm.

In men, the prostate can similarly be stimulated externally by pressure to the area between the scrotum and the anus; it can also be stimulated internally through anal penetration angled toward the front of the body. As with women, some men enjoy the sensations, while others do not. Often for men the erotic potential of the prostate will remain unknown. If it is known, exploration of this potential may be considered inappropriate for heterosexual men. This is one of the ways in which the equation of sex with reproduction limits erotic expression. If "normal" sex is heterosexual intercourse, then sexual practices without the potential for reproductive outcomes can always be constructed as deviant, no matter who practices them. People can be made to experience shame and guilt in connection with their desires. One semester a vocal group of women in my advanced course on Women and Sexuality insisted that only gay men would desire anal penetration. As long as there remains a stigma attached to homosexuality, that stigma will also work to limit the erotic experience of heterosexuals.

Nipples Some women and some men report pleasure from stimulation of the nipples, while others indicate that the nipples are not particularly sensitive. The nipples are made up of erectile tissue. Nipple stimulation can lead to erection in men and arousal in women. Some women can reach orgasm from nipple stimulation alone. Nipples are one anatomical location that can become highly charged erotically in women whose spinal cord injuries prevent sensation below the area of the injury. The pleasurable sensations can extend to breastfeeding an infant for some women. While many people might be shocked at the idea of the mother's pleasure in breastfeeding, the physiological reasons for that pleasure are clear, and clearly normal. Nipple stimulation can trigger release of the hormone oxytocin, which leads to uterine contractions (remember that the uterus contracts during orgasm). The limited knowledge of female anatomy and the physiology of erotic pleasure has had tragic consequences in some lives. One mother lost her child to the foster care system for nearly a year, because her call inquiring about the pleasurable sensations she was feeling during nursing was transferred to a rape crisis center, where staff contacted a sexual abuse hotline, instead of the La Leche League (Blum 1999:96–97).

Vagina and Vaginal Penetration Studies have shown that most women do not achieve orgasm reliably from vaginal penetration by a male partner. In reports collected from women by Shere Hite beginning in the 1970s, about 30 percent could reach orgasm regularly in this way (Hite 1993:35). Groundbreaking feminist work on women's sexuality, such as "The Myth of the Vaginal Orgasm" (Koedt 1996) focused on the experience of most women and pointed to the centrality of clitoral stimulation for women's orgasm. This made sense. It was important to counter the assertion of medical and scientific authorities that the hallmark of a woman's sexual maturity and normalcy was the ability to have an orgasm as a result of heterosexual intercourse. By this standard, two-thirds of women were sexually immature or abnormal. But what of women in that last third, who reported regular orgasms as a result of vaginal penetration?

There is erotic potential in vaginal penetration, and it does not make one a dupe of the patriarchy to say so. *The Whole Lesbian Sex Book* devotes an entire chapter to vaginal penetration (Newman 2004). Perhaps there is now enough known about female anatomy to leave behind the need to pinpoint the epicenters of orgasms. Penetration can stimulate the clitoris and/or the urethral sponge, and potentially produce orgasm in this way. It makes sense that sensation will vary with the angle and depth of penetration. Deeper penetration angled to the anterior fornix may stimulate the T-zone, under which lies a concentration of nerves (Wilhite 2005), and lead to orgasm. Deeper penetration can also lead to orgasm through direct, rhythmic pressure on the cervix, triggering contraction of the uterus. In one study, women with spinal cord injuries were able to feel orgasms they experienced as a result of cervical stimulation, although they could not feel the stimulation itself (Whipple, Gerdes and Komisaruk 1996).

Anus and Anal Penetration   Nerve endings in the anus, although not concentrated to the extent of the nerve endings on the glans of the clitoris, account for its erotic sensitivity in both women and men. In women, the close proximity of the anus to the underlying perineal sponge may also account for the pleasure associated with touching and shallow penetration. This stimulation can lead to orgasm, as can deeper penetration. Depending on the angle and the depth, deeper penetration into the rectum will bring a finger, penis or sex toy close to the cervix, as the posterior fornix is adjacent to the rectum. Based on available research, anatomy and women's individual accounts of pleasure, it is likely that—as with vaginal penetration—the rhythmic pressure on the cervix, though less direct, could trigger uterine contractions and orgasm. In men, anal penetration can also lead to orgasm, including through internal stimulation of the prostate. Joannides provides a number of individual perspectives related to anal stimulation and penetration (2004:365–380), and *The Whole Lesbian Sex Book* includes a chapter devoted to anal penetration (Newman 2004).

Conclusion   Left to our own desires and inventiveness, some men and some women might be interested in sex all the time, and others might be interested rarely. We are not usually left to our own desires and inventiveness though. Beginning in childhood, lessons about sexuality profoundly shape our experience of sexuality and limit our potential. This was *exactly* the point of formal sex education, from its inception in the early 20th century. The first advocates of sex education in public schools wanted to teach only enough to blunt young people's curiosity, and they were quite clear that the only redeeming aspect of sex was reproduction (Strong 1972). Rury (1987) identifies the way in which educators sought to repress female sexuality in particular. If we know this history, it is perhaps not so surprising that this trend continues today. What we teach still channels behavior and experience into gendered patterns, which many people believe are only natural. We even warp biology to make it fit social expectations of males who naturally want sex and females who naturally don't. Young people are misled to think that only males have "male" hormones and only females have "female" hormones (Whatley 1985).

Some current advocates of comprehensive sexuality education believe that sexuality education was better before the abstinence-only education movement achieved popularity. In truth, only information about contraception

and sexually transmitted diseases was more thorough (McKay 1999; Sears 1992). Attempts to implement the comprehensive sexuality education curriculum developed by the SIECUS have been rare. This curriculum, now in its third edition, includes developmentally appropriate messages about pleasure and sexual anatomy, including the clitoris, from kindergarten on and acknowledges individuals who are intersexed (Sexuality Information and Education Council of the United States 2004).

Finding educational resources for young people that do not reduce sex to reproduction is challenging. An important exception is Joani Blank's *A Kid's First Book about Sexuality*, which seems to be directed at five to 11-year-olds. The idea that sex should be taught only as reproduction is so ingrained that some students in my classes have insisted that sharing this resource with a young person would be child abuse. Why should we not validate children's knowledge that touching certain parts of the anatomy produces particular feelings and explain cultural views about when touching is appropriate, as Calderone (1983) suggests? Teaching about sex only as reproduction is at best a distortion of reality and at worst a lie. Much of the time people engaging in sexual behavior are not trying to reproduce.

This is not to say that everyone would need or want the all information in this article. "If you had your way, sex would be boring," one student in Women and Sexuality said. His point has become increasingly compelling over time. Official language and knowledge have a limiting, circumscribing quality. It is hard to know what amount of knowledge is needed to address ignorance, heal shame or guilt and preserve a space for imagination, discovery and empowerment in individual practices. An enlightened culture would seek to find that amount, even knowing that the recipe could not be exactly the same for everyone. Schools and government are more likely to resist the conversations this process would require than to facilitate them, but we can look to ourselves to broaden the scope and veracity of sexual knowledge at the grassroots.

I am deeply indebted to the Women's Studies Program at the University of Wisconsin-Madison for the many opportunities to teach classes in which the insights from my research could be shared. I am also deeply indebted to the students in my Women's Studies classes since 2001. Special thanks to students in Women and Sexuality for engaging, challenging and extending those insights. Your work has made this article possible.

References

Amen, Daniel G. and Amy Jo Bodegraven. 2004. Sex on the Brain. *Men's Health* 19(10, December):157–164.

Beland, Nikki. 1998. Does He Think You're a Labia Loser? *Cosmopolitan* 225(5):150.

Bem, Sandra Lipsitz. 1989. Genital knowledge and gender constancy in preschool children. *Child Development* 60(3): 649–662.

Blank, Joani. 1993. *Femalia*. San Francisco, CA: Down There Press.

Blank, Joani. 1983. *A Kid's First Book About Sexuality*. San Francisco, CA: Yes Press.

Blum, Linda M. 1999. *At The Breast: Ideologies of Breastfeeding and Motherhood in the Contemporary United States*. Boston: Beacon Press.

Boston Women's Health Book Collective. 2005. *Our Bodies, Ourselves*. New York: Touchstone.

Brodman-Grimm, Karen. Your Body Questions Answered. 2005. *Seventeen* 64(4):100.

Brody, Liz. 2004. How Sex is Like Pizza . . . and Other Startling Features of the Male Mind. *O: The Oprah Magazine* 5(6):190–193.

Calderone, Mary S. 1983. Above and Beyond Politics: The Sexual Socialization of Children. Pp. 131–137 in Vance, Carole S. (Ed.), *Pleasure and Danger: Exploring Female Sexuality*. London: Pandora.

Department of Health and Human Services. 1981. *Changes—Sex and You*. Publication Number HSA 81-5648. Washington D.C.: United States Government Printing Office.

Douglas, Marcia and Lisa Douglas. 1997. *Are We Having Fun Yet?* New York: Hyperion

Federation of Feminist Women's Health Centers. 1991. *A New View of a Woman's Body*. Los Angeles, CA: Feminist Health Press.

Fine, Michelle. 1988. Sexuality, Schooling and Adolescent Females: The Missing Discourse of Desire. *Harvard Educational Review* 58:29–53.

Graham, Janis and Pamela Lister. 2003. Her Most Secret Sex Question. *Redbook* 200(1):62.

Gray, John. 1995. *Mars and Venus in the Bedroom*. New York: HarperCollins.

Hite, Shere. 1993. *Women as Revolutionary Agents of Change: The Hite Reports 1972–1993*. London:Bloomsbury.

Joannides, Paul. 2004. *Guide to Getting It On*. Waldfort, OR:Goofy Foot Press.

Kapsalis, Terri. 1997. *Public Privates: Performing Gynecology from Both Ends of the Speculum*. Durham, NC: Duke University Press.

Koedt, Annette. 1996. The Myth of the Vaginal Orgasm. Pp. 111–116 in Jackson, Stevi and Sue Scott (Eds.) *Feminism and Sexuality*. New York: Columbia.

Laumann, Edward O., John H. Gagnon, Robert T. Michael, and Stuart Michaels. 1994. *The Social Organization of Sexuality*. Chicago: Univ. of Chicago.

Maas, Cornelis P., Philomeen Th. M. Weijenborg and Moniek M. Ter Kuile. 2003. The Effect of Hysterectomy on Sexual Functioning. *Annual Review of Sex Research* 14:83–114.

Madaras, Lynda. 2007a. *"What's Happening to My Body?" Book for Girls*. New York: Newmarket Press.

Madaras, Lynda. 2007b. *"What's Happening to My Body?" Book for Boys*. New York: Newmarket Press.

Masters, William H., Virginia E. Johnson and Robert Kolodny. 1994. *Heterosexuality*. New York: HarperCollins.

McKay, Alexander. 1999. *Sexual Ideology and Schooling: Towards Democratic Sexuality Education*. Albany, NY: State University of New York Press.

Newman, Felice. 2004. *The Whole Lesbian Sex Book* (Second Edition). San Francisco, CA: Cleis Press.

Pastor, Susan K. Unpublished Research. Learning the Basics: The Social Construction of Knowledge about Sexuality. Madison, WI.

Perron, Celeste. 2004. My Labia Are Long and Uneven—Am I a Freak? *Cosmopolitan* 237(5):158.

Preves, Sharon E. 2003. Intersex and Identity: The Contested Self. New Brunswisck, NJ: Rutgers University Press.

Rury, John L. 1987. 'We Teach the Girl Repression, the Boy Expression': Sexuality, Sex Equity and Education in Historical Perspective. *Peabody Journal of Education* 64(4, Fall):44–58.

Sears, James T. 1992. Dilemmas and Possibilities of Sexuality Education: Reproducing the Body Politic. Pp. 5–33 in Sears, James T. (Ed.), *Sexuality and the Curriculum: The Politics and Practices of Sexuality Education*. New York: Teachers College Press.

Sexuality Information and Education Council of the United States National Guidelines Task Force 2004. *Guidelines for Comprehensive Sexuality Education Kindergarten Through 12th Grade*. New York: Sexuality Information and Education Council of the United States.

Sloane, Ethel. 2002. *Biology of Women* (Fourth Edition). Albany, NY: Delmar/Thomson Learning.

Strong, Bryan. 1972. Ideas of the Early Sex Education Movement in America, 1890–1920. *History of Education Quarterly*. Summer: 129–161.

Sundahl, Deborah. 2003. *Female Ejaculation and the G-spot*. Alameda, CA: Hunter House.

Tiefer, Lenore. 2001. Arriving at a 'New View' of Women's Sexual Problems: Background, Theory and Activism. Pp. 63–98 in Kaschak, Ellyn and Lenore Tiefer (Eds.) *A New View of Women's Sexual Problems*. New York: Haworth.

Tiefer, Lenore. 1995. *Sex Is Not a Natural Act and Other Essays*. Boulder, CO: Westview. Pp. 41–58, Historical, Scientific, Clinical and Feminist Criticism of the Human Sexual Response Cycla Model.

Tolman, Deborah. 2002. *Dilemmas of Desire*. Cambridge, MA: Harvard University Press.

Whatley, Mariamne H. 1985. Male and Female Hormones: Misinterpretations of Biology in School Health and Sex Education. Pp. 67–88 in Sapiro, Virginia (Ed.) *Women, Biology and Public Policy*. Newbury Park, CA: Sage Publications.

Whipple, Beverly, Carolyn A. Gerdes and Barry R. Komisaruk. 1996. Sexual Response to Self-Stimulation in Women with Complete Spinal Cord Injury. *The Journal of Sex Research* 33(3):231–241.

Wilhite, Myrtle. 2005. T-zone and G-spot. (Pamphlet) Madison, WI: A Woman's Touch Sexuality Resource Center.

Woods, Stacey Grenrock. 2007. Sex. *Esquire* 148(5):78.

Zaviacic, Milan and Beverly Whipple. 1993. Update on the Female Prostate and the Phenomenon of Female Ejaculation. *Journal of Sex Research* 30(2):148–151.

"Adolescent Sexual Health in Europe and the U.S.— Why the Difference?"

by Advocates for Youth

Regularly since 1998, Advocates for Youth has sponsored study tours to France, Germany, and the Netherlands to explore why adolescent sexual health outcomes are more positive in these European countries than in the United States.

Rights. Respect. Responsibility.®   The study tour participants—policy makers, researchers, youth serving professionals, foundation officers, and youth—have found that this trilogy of values underpins a social philosophy regarding adolescent sexual health in France, Germany, and the Netherlands. Each of the three nations

has an unwritten social contract with youth: "We'll respect your right to act responsibly and give you the tools you need to avoid unintended pregnancy and sexually transmitted infections, including HIV."

In France, Germany, and the Netherlands, two things create greater, easier access to sexual health information and services for *all* people, including teens. They are: (1) societal openness and comfort in dealing with sexuality, including teen sexuality; and (2) *pragmatic* governmental policies. The result—better sexual health outcomes for French, German, and Dutch teens when compared to U.S. teens.

Adolescent Pregnancy, Birth, and Abortion Rates in Europe Outshine Those in the United States*

Pregnancy

The United States' **teen pregnancy rate** is over five times that of the Netherlands, over four times that of Germany, and over three times that of France.[1,2,3]

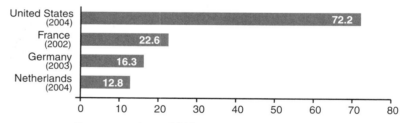

Pregnancy rate per 1,000 women ages 15 to 19, latest year available

Birth

U.S. teens account for about 71 percent of all teenage births occurring in all developed countries.[4] The United States' **teen birth rate** is nearly nine times higher than the Netherlands', four and a half times higher than France's, and over four times higher than Germany's.[1,3,5]

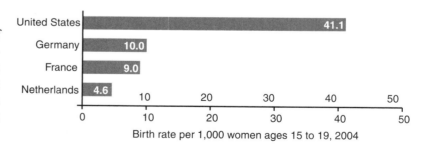

Birth rate per 1,000 women ages 15 to 19, 2004

Abortion

In the United States, the **teen abortion rate** is more than twice that of Germany and nearly twice that of the Netherlands.[3,6,7]

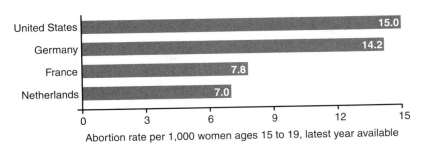

Abortion rate per 1,000 women ages 15 to 19, latest year available

U.S. HIV/STI Rates Also Compare Poorly

HIV

The proportion of the United States' adolescent and adult population that has been diagnosed with HIV or AIDS is six times greater than in Germany, three times greater than in the Netherlands, and one and a half times greater than in France.[8,9]

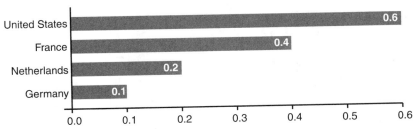

Proportion of the total adolescent and adult population of the country diagnosed with HIV or AIDS

Syphilis

Among teens, syphilis rates are more than 70 percent higher in the United States than in the Netherlands.[10,11,12]

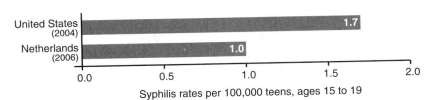

Syphilis rates per 100,000 teens, ages 15 to 19

Gonorrhea

Gonorrhea is the second most commonly reported infectious disease in the United States, and the U.S, adolescent rate is 28 times greater than teen rates in the Netherlands.[10,11,12]

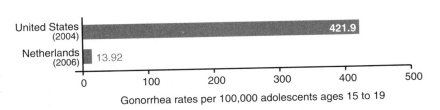

Gonorrhea rates per 100,000 adolescents ages 15 to 19

Chlamydia

Chlamydia infection is more than 15 times more common among U.S. teens than Dutch teens.[10,11,12]

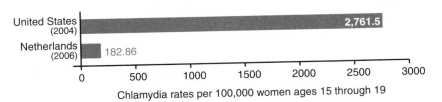

Chlamydia rates per 100,000 women ages 15 through 19

Contraceptive Use at Most Recent Sexual Intercourse

Although U.S. teens report using contraception (usually either birth control pills or condoms or both) far more often than their peers of previous decades, U.S. teens still use contraception or condoms much less consistently than their peers in Europe. When measuring use of highly effective hormonal contraception, condoms, or both, researchers found that German, French, and Dutch youth were significantly more likely to be well protected at most recent sex than were their U.S. peers.[13,14,15,16]

Implementing the Model: Potential Impact on Adolescent Sexual Health in the U.S.

If society in the United States were to become more comfortable with sexuality and *if* governmental policies were to create greater and easier access to sexual health information and services, *then* US. teens' sexual health outcomes would improve markedly. Imagine that the United States' teen pregnancy, birth, and abortion rates would improve to match those of the Netherlands, Germany, and France. Improved *rates* would mean large reductions in the *numbers* of pregnancies, births, and abortions to US. teens each year.

Percent of sexually active 15 year old youth reporting use of contraception at most recent sex.

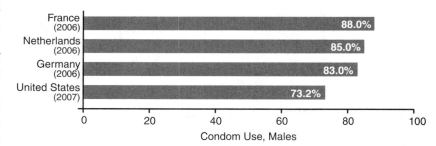

Condom Use, Males

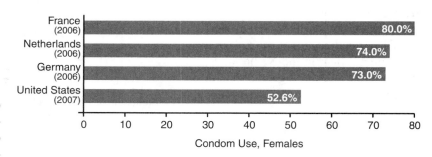

Condom Use, Females

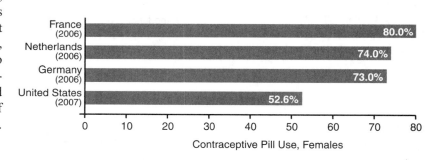

Contraceptive Pill Use, Females

If U.S. Rates equaled those in:	The number of U.S. teen pregnancies would be reduced by:	The number of U.S. teen births would be reduced by:	The number of U.S. teen abortions would be reduced by:
France	515,000	333,000	8,000
Germany	581,000	323,000	83,000
Netherlands	617,000	379,000	75,000

If the U.S. birth rates in 2004 equaled those in:	U.S. annual public savings in 2004 would have equaled:
France	$476,190,000
Germany	$461,890,000
Netherlands	$541,970,000

It has been estimated that the public costs associated with teen birth in the United States were at least **$9.1 billion** in 2004, an annual average cost of $1,430 per child born to a teen mother.[17]

Therefore, if the U.S. could reduce its teen birth rate to equal that of France, Germany or the Netherlands, it would save significantly on public funds expended to support families begun by a teen birth.

The Lessons Learned: A Model to Improve Adolescent Sexual Health in the United States

So, if Dutch, German, and French teens have better sexual health outcomes than U.S. teens, what's the secret? Is there a 'silver bullet' solution for the United States that will reduce the following statistics?

- *Nine million* new cases of sexually transmitted infections among 15- to 24-year-old. youth;[18]
- *Five thousand* new HIV infections among 13- to 24-year-old youth;[19]
- Estimated *750,000* pregnancies among U.S. teens;
- *125,000* abortions among U.S. teens; and
- *435,000* births among 15- to 19-year-old women.[20]

Unfortunately, there is no single, 'silver bullet' solution! Yet, the United States can use the experience of people in the Netherlands, Germany, and France to guide its efforts to improve adolescents' sexual health. The United States can achieve social and cultural consensus that sexuality is a normal and healthy part of being human and of being a teen. It can do this by using the lessons learned from the European study tours.

- Adults in France, Germany, and the Netherlands view young people as assets, not as problems. Adults value and respect adolescents and expect teens to act responsibly. Governments strongly support education and economic self-sufficiency for youth.
- Research is the basis for public health policies to reduce unintended pregnancies, abortions, and sexually transmitted infections, including HIV. Political and religious interest groups have little influence on public health policy.
- A national desire to reduce the number of abortions and to prevent sexually transmitted infections, including HIV, provides the major impetus in each country for ensuring easy access to contraception and condoms, consistent sex education, and widespread public education campaigns.
- Governments support massive, consistent, long-term public education campaigns, through the Internet, television, films, radio, billboards, discos, pharmacies, and health care providers. Media is a respected partner in these campaigns. Campaigns are direct and humorous and focus on both safety and pleasure.
- Youth have convenient access to free or low-cost contraception through national health insurance.

- Sex education is not necessarily a separate curriculum and is usually integrated across school subjects and at all grade levels. Educators provide accurate and complete information in response to students' questions.
- Families have open, honest, consistent discussions with teens about sexuality and support the role of educators and health care providers in making sexual health information and services available to teens.
- Adults see intimate sexual relationships as normal and natural for older adolescents, a positive component of emotionally healthy maturation. At the same time, young people believe it is 'stupid and irresponsible' to have sex without protection. Youth rely on the maxim, 'safer sex or no sex.'
- Society weighs the morality of sexual behavior through an individual ethic that includes the values of responsibility, respect, tolerance, and equity.
- France, Germany, and the Netherlands struggle to address issues around cultural diversity, especially in regard to immigrant populations whose values related to gender and sexuality differ from those of the majority culture.

Rights. Respect. Responsibility.® A National Campaign to Improve Adolescent Sexual Health

In October 2001, Advocates for Youth launched a long-term campaign—*Rights. Respect. Responsibility.*®—based on the lessons learned from the European study tours. The Campaign works to shift the current U.S. societal paradigm of adolescent sexuality away from a negative emphasis on fear and ignorance and towards an acceptance of sexuality of healthy and normal and a view of adolescents as valuable and important.

- Adolescents have the right to balanced, accurate, and realistic sex education, confidential and affordable health services, and a secure stake in the future.
- Youth deserve respect. Today they are often perceived as part of 'the problem'. Valuing young people means they are part of the solution to societal issues and participate in developing programs and policies that affect their well-being.
- Society has the responsibility to provide young people with the tools they need to safeguard their sexual health and young people have the

responsibility to protect themselves from too early childbearing and sexually transmitted infections, including HIV

Advocates develops and disseminates campaign materials for specific audiences, such as the entertainment industry and news media professionals, policy makers, youth-serving professionals, parents, and youth activists. Advocates will continue its thought-provoking European study tours. Advocates will also collaborate with key national and statewide organizations to promote

Rights. Respect. Responsibility.® through Campaign materials, workshops, presentations, and technical assistance. For additional information on the Campaign or to become a partner in this important initiative, contact Advocates for Youth at 202.419.3420 or visit www.advocatesforyouth.org

REFERENCES
A list of references is available in the original source at www.advocatesforyouth.org.

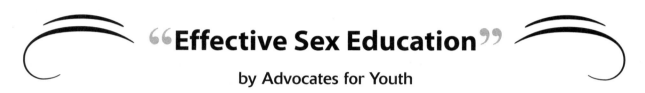

"Effective Sex Education"
by Advocates for Youth

Each year, U.S. teens experience as many as 850,000 pregnancies, and youth under age 25 experience about 9.1 million sexually transmitted infections (STIs).[1,2] By age 18, 70 percent of U.S. females and 62 percent of U.S. males have initiated vaginal sex.[3] Comprehensive sex education is effective at assisting young people to make healthy decisions about sex and to adopt healthy sexual behaviors.[4,5,6,7] No abstinence-only-until-marriage program has been shown to help teens delay the initiation of sex or to protect themselves when they do initiate sex.[8,9,10,11] Yet, the U.S. government has spent over one billion dollars supporting abstinence-only-until-marriage programs.[12] Although the U.S. government ignores it, adolescents have a fundamental human right to accurate and comprehensive sexual health information.[8,11]

Comprehensive Sex Education Is Effective, Does Not Promote Sexual Risks

- Research has identified highly effective sex education and HIV prevention programs that affect multiple behaviors and/or achieve positive health impacts. Behavioral outcomes have included delaying the initiation of sex as well as reducing the frequency of sex, the number of new partners, and the incidence of unprotected sex, and/or increasing the use of condoms and contraception among sexually active participants.[4,5,6,7] Long-term impacts have included lower STI and/or pregnancy rates.[4,5,6,7]

- No highly effective sex education or HIV prevention education program is eligible for federal funding because mandates prohibit educating youth about the benefits of condoms and contraception.[13]

- Evaluations of comprehensive sex education and HIV/STI prevention programs show that they *do not* increase rates of sexual initiation, *do not* lower the age at which youth initiate sex, and *do not* increase the frequency of sex or the number of sex partners among sexually active youth.[4,5,6,7,14,15]

- Between 1991 and 2004, the U.S. teen birth rate fell from 62 to 41 births per 1,000 female teens.[16,17] Some experts attribute 75 percent of the decline to increased contraceptive use and 25 percent to delayed initiation of sex.[18] Others credit increased contraceptive use and delayed initiation of sex about equally.[19] Regardless, contraceptive use has been critical to reducing teenage pregnancy.

Abstinence-Only Programs Are Dangerous, Ineffective, and Inaccurate

- The Society for Adolescent Medicine recently declared that "abstinence-only programs threaten fundamental human rights to health, information, and life."[8,11]

- According to Columbia University researchers, virginity pledge programs increase pledge-takers' risk for STIs and pregnancy. The study concluded that 88 percent of pledge-takers initiated sex prior to marriage even though some delayed sex for a while. Rates of STIs among pledge-takers and non-pledgers were similar, even though pledge-takers initiated sex later. Pledge-takers were less likely to seek STI testing and less likely to use contraception when they did have sex.[20,21]

- Evaluations of the effectiveness of state-funded abstinence-only-until-marriage programs found no delay in first sex. In fact, of six evaluations that assessed short-term changes in behavior, three found no changes, two found *increased* sexual activity from pre- to post-test, and one showed mixed results. Five evaluations looked for but found *no* long-term impact in reducing teens' sexual activity.[9]

- Analysis of data from the Youth Risk Behavior surveys found that sexual activity among high school youth declined significantly from 1991 to 1997, prior to large-scale funding of abstinence-only-until-marriage programs, but changed little from 1999 to 2003, with federal funding of such programs.[22]

- Analysis of federally funded abstinence-only curricula found that over 80 percent of curricula supported by the U.S. Department of Health & Human Services contained false, misleading, or distorted information about reproductive health. Specifically, they conveyed:
  - False information about the effectiveness of contraceptives;
  - False information about the risks of abortion;
  - Religious beliefs as scientific fact;
  - Stereotypes about boys and girls as scientific fact; and
  - Medical and scientific errors of fact.[23]

Medical Organizations, Parents, and the Public Support Comprehensive Sex Education

- The American Academy of Pediatrics, American College of Obstetricians & Gynecologists, American Medical Association, American Public Health Association, Institute of Medicine, and Society for Adolescent Medicine, among others, support comprehensive sex education, including education about *both* abstinence *and also* contraception and condoms.[1,10,11,24,25]

- In one study, most American adults supported sex education that includes information about both abstinence and also contraception and condoms. In fact, 89 percent believed that it is important for young people to have information about contraception and prevention of STIs and that sex education should focus on how to avoid unintended pregnancy and STIs, including HIV.[26]

- In another recent survey, 94 percent of adults and 93 percent of parents said that sex education should cover contraception. Only 15 percent of Americans wanted abstinence-only education taught in the classroom.[27]

Characteristics of Effective Sex Education

Experts have identified critical characteristics of highly effective sex education and HIV/STI prevention education programs. Such programs:

1. Offer age- and culturally appropriate sexual health information in a safe environment for participants;
2. Are developed in cooperation with members of the target community, especially young people;
3. Assist youth to clarify their individual, family, and community values;
4. Assist youth to develop skills in communication, refusal, and negotiation;
5. Provide medically accurate information about both abstinence and also contraception, including condoms;
6. Have clear goals for preventing HIV, other STIs, and/or teen pregnancy;
7. Focus on specific health behaviors related to the goals, with clear messages about these behaviors;
8. Address psychosocial risk and protective factors with activities to change each targeted risk and to promote each protective factor;
9. Respect community values and respond to community needs;
10. Rely on participatory teaching methods, implemented by trained educators and using all the activities as designed.[4,5,6,7,10,14,]

REFERENCES
A list of references is available in the original source. See www.advocatesforyouth.org

Exposed at Last
"The Truth about Your Clitoris"

by Jennifer Johnson

"At a witch trial in 1593, the investigating lawyer (a married man) apparently discovered a clitoris for the first time; he identified it as a devil's teat, sure proof of the witch's guilt. It was 'a little lump of flesh, in a manner sticking out as if it had been a teat, to the length of half an inch,' which the gaoler, 'perceiving at the first sight there of, meant not to disclose, because it was adjoining to so secret a place which was not decent to be seen. Yet in the end, not willing to conceal so strange a matter,' he showed it to various bystanders. The witch was convicted."

from The Vagina Monologues *by Eve Ensler [Villard].*

Pick up almost any medical, anatomy or biology text and you'll find something missing: the greater part of the clitoris.

The clitoris is like an iceberg; only the tip is visible on the outside, its larger mass is under the surface. The visible tip is the glans, or head of the organ. While modern medical science books stop there, the clitoris actually continues under the pelvic bone, then turns down to surround the vagina from above and on either side. The structure forms a dense pyramid of tissue, well-supplied with nerve and vascular network, and is comparable in size to the penis. Like the male organ, the clitoris is flaccid when unaroused and erect when aroused.

And yet, even in the most ponderous, detailed texts, the clitoris is described as a "vestigial organ," or "pea-sized." The diagrams typically show a diagram of a spread-legged female, with a little bulb arrowed "clitoris." The internal diagrams show her reproductive organs, but the bulk of the clitoris—the shaft (body), legs (crura), and bulbs—are missing. Next to the illustration showing the female sex organ as a bump usually appears a drawing of the male sex organ on an extremely well-hung man. Even *Gray's Anatomy*—the authoritative text of biologists—doesn't accurately depict the clitoris.

As a biologist, I first discovered this while doing an anatomical study (dissection) on a human subject. I was shocked to discover that the clitoris was far larger than I had been taught. I could not understand how such a basic—not to mention crucial—piece of biological information had been neglected. I searched textbooks, con-

sulted doctors and professors and found all of them unaware of the actual size of the clitoris.

Of course, I was not the only student of science to discover this. When Helen O'Connell became curious about why the female sex organ was "glossed over" in the texts, she made it her business to take a closer look when she became a doctor. Now a surgeon at the Royal Melbourne Hospital in Australia, she and her colleagues have been dissecting and measuring the clitoris; her

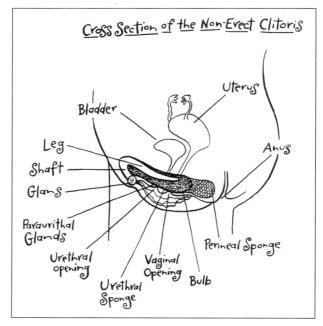

Illustration: Noreen Stevens

findings were reported in a recent article in *New Scientist.* "Sometimes the whole structure is drawn as a dot," says Dr. O'Connell. In fact, the legs of the clitoris, called the crura, are five to nine centimeters long, extending from the body (shaft) of the clitoris and filling the space between its legs are two bulbs, one on either side of the vaginal cavity. Contrary to the belief that the urethra and clitoris are entirely separate, the clitoris actually encompasses the urethra. Dr. O'Connell believes the clitoris squeezes the urethra shut during sex, reducing the entry of bacteria.

Drawing a more accurate picture of the female sexual anatomy explains a few things. It helps explain why some women are not having orgasms, since women must first be erect before they can reach orgasm. It may also explain why Viagra appears to work for women even though it's not supposed to—suggesting that women may be impotent for the same physiological reasons as men. It also explains why women frequently report that their sex lives were damaged following some types of pelvic surgery—the nerves to the clitoris, and sometimes the organ itself, can be damaged or severed during surgery. It also sheds light on the controversy of the clitoral vs. vaginal orgasm that was debated a few years ago.

When seen as an entire complex organ, there is room for a wide range of experiences. Some women experience orgasm through stimulation of the outer glans of the clitoris; at other times they may experience a different orgasm when combined with penetration. An orgasm reached through external stimulation may feel quite different. For many women, orgasm is intense and relatively easy to reach with digital or oral contact because this is the most direct way to stimulate the large pudendal nerve which runs straight down into the tip of the clitoris (the glans). What has been referred to as "the vaginal orgasm" is a vaginal-induced orgasm, brought on by stimulating the clitoris indirectly through the vaginal walls. (Of course, it's common to add some direct pudendal stimulation on the outside.)

Then there is the G-spot. Part of the vaginal wall clinically known as the urethral sponge, the G-spot can be found by exploring the roof of the vagina. It's about a knuckle-length in—from one and a half to three inches inside. The easiest way to find it is to have your partner crook a finger or two and reach toward the belly button. The size varies from half an inch to 1.5 inches. When unaroused, it feels like the back of the roof of your mouth. If your partner presses up on this spot and you feel like you have to urinate, they've found it. When it is stroked, it will puff out and feel like a marshmallow.

While there are many differences between male and female sexual responses, there are unmistakably many

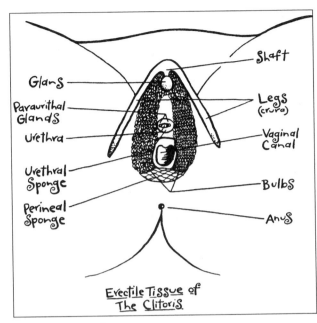

Erectile Tissue of The Clitoris

Illustration: Noreen Stevens

similarities. When the clitoris is engorged and erect, endorphins are released and induce a 'high.' The long bands of the crura become hard and flare out along the pubic bones. Vaginal blood vessels widen and fill with blood and the perineal sponge thickens. The uterus balloons forward, the tubes and ovaries swell. The broad ligament tightens, pulling up the uterus and causing the vagina to enlarge. The neck of the cervix is flexible, like an accordion, and during orgasm, the cervix moves forward and down, dipping its head in the seminal pool if a male partner has ejaculated. As well, ejaculation fluid squirts from the woman's paraurithal glands, located on either side of the urethra. This may come as news to women who haven't had a female sexual partner and therefore may not have experienced a female ejaculation first hand. The ejaculate may be a small amount and not noticeable, or it may be a copious amount that 'soaks the sheets.'

The size of the clitoris is actually not a new 'discovery' but the revealing of a secret. The clitoris was more accurately described in some 19th century anatomy texts, but then it was mysteriously shrunk into a mere speck on the anatomical map. The French, however, have been more accurately depicting the clitoris since before the turn of the century.

While doing research for this article, I contacted many sex-related organizations, including the famous Kinsey Institute, the British Association for Sexual and Marital Therapy, even the German Society for Sex Research. None had accurate information on the clitoris, and most did not believe that the clitoris is larger and more complex than medical texts indicate. In bookstores, I found current sexology books that didn't have more than a paragraph on the clitoris, some only a few lines, many did not have "clitoris" indexed at all! Even the famous British 'feminist' scientist Desmond Morris's new book, *The Human Sexes,* contains no indexed references for clitoris. Without exception, every sex book gave 'penis' all kinds of room—entire sections, chapters and references.

What does it all mean? Dr. Jennifer Berman, director of the Women's Sexual Health Clinic at Boston University, predicts that knowing the proper female anatomy will lead to research in this area of female function and dysfunction, which she says has been "grossly neglected."

In an article published with her colleagues in *The Journal of Urology* in June 1998, Dr. O'Connell and her colleagues wrote, "Since the studies of Masters and Johnson, there has been surprisingly little investigation of basic female sexual anatomy or physiology." The article describes the intricate connection between the urethra and the clitoris and says that surgeons should be made aware of the damage that can be done to the organ during urethral surgery. O'Connell says anatomy texts should be changed to accurately depict the clitoris and perineal anatomy. She is now mapping the nerves to the pelvic region innervating the female sex organ.

"They were mapped in men a decade ago," says O'Connell, "but they've never been mapped in women."

It does beg the question doesn't it? Why not? One anthropologist I spoke to explained that the size of the clitoris may have been overlooked because "the size of the male phallus" is a symbol of power; admitting women have the same size organ would be like admitting they are equally powerful. Indeed.

Sex psychologist Dr. Micheal Bailey doesn't buy into the patriarchal conspiracy theory. "There's been very little scientific interest in female sexuality," he insists. Then adds, "It's possible *we* didn't look."

 # "How Being a Good Girl Can Be Bad for Girls"

by Deborah L. Tolman and Tracy E. Higgins

Women's sexuality is frequently suspect in our culture, particularly when it is expressed outside the bounds of monogamous heterosexual marriage. This suspicion is reflected in the dominant cultural accounts of women's sexuality, which posit good, decent, and normal women as passive and threatened sexual objects. When women act as sexual agents, expressing their own sexual desire rather than serving as the objects of men's desire, they are often portrayed as threatening, deviant, and bad. Missing is any affirmative account of women's sexual desire. Yet, even while women's sexuality is denied or problematized, the culture and the law tend to assign to women the responsibility for regulating heterosexual sex by resisting male aggression. Defined as natural, urgent, and aggressive, male sexuality is bounded, both in law and in culture, by the limits of women's consent. Women who wish to avoid the consequences of being labeled "bad" are expected to define the boundaries of sexual behavior, outlined by men's desire, and to ignore or deny their own sexual desire as a guide to their choices.

The cultural anxiety precipitated by unbounded female sexuality is perhaps most apparent with regard to adolescent girls. Coming under scrutiny from across the political spectrum, girls' sexuality has been deemed threatening either to girls themselves (potentially resulting in rape, sexually transmitted diseases, unwanted pregnancy), or to society (as evidenced by the single mother, school dropout, welfare dependent). Although none of these issues is limited to teenage girls, all frequently arise in that context because of society's sense of entitlement, or, indeed, obligation, to regulate teen sexuality. Accordingly, the cultural and legal sanctions on teenage girls' sexuality convey a simple message: good girls are not sexual; girls who are sexual are either (1) bad girls, if they have been active, desiring sexual agents or (2) good girls, who have been passively victimized by boys' raging hormones. Buttressed by the real concerns that girls themselves have about pregnancy, AIDS, and parental as well as peer disapproval, the good-girl/bad-girl dichotomy organizes sexuality for young women. This cultural story may increase girls' vulnerability to sexual coercion and psychological distress and disable them from effectively seeking legal protection.

The Cultural Story of Girls' Sexuality in the Media and in Law

Sexually assertive girls are making the news. A disturbed mother of a teenage boy wrote to Ann Landers, complaining of the behavior of teenage girls who had telephoned him, leaving sexually suggestive messages. After publishing the letter, Landers received twenty thousand responses and noted, "If I'm hearing about it from so many places, then I worry about what's going on out there. . . . What this says to me is that a good many young girls really are out of control. Their hormones are raging and they have not had adequate supervision" (qtd. in Yoffe 1991). What were these girls doing? Calling boys, asking them out, threatening to buy them gifts, and to "make love to [them] all night." In the *Newsweek* story, "Girls Who Go Too Far," in which the writer described this Ann Landers column, such girls were referred to as "obsessed," "confused," "emotionally disturbed," "bizarre," "abused," "troubled." Parents described the girls' behavior as "bewilder[ing]" or even "frighten[ing]" to boys. A similar, more recent story in the *Orlando Sentinel* noted that "girls today have few qualms about asking a boy out—and they have no qualms about calling a boy on the telephone" (Shrieves 1993). Describing late-night telephone calls from girls to their teenage sons, the adults interviewed characterized the situation as "frustrating" and "shocking" and suggested that "parents should be paying more attention to what their daughters are doing." Girls' behavior, including "suggestive notes stuck to a boy's locker or even outright propositions," was deemed "obsessive."

In contrast, media accounts of boys' sexuality tend to reflect what Wendy Hollway has called the "discourse of male sexual drive," wherein male sexuality is portrayed as natural, relentless, and demanding attention, an urge

that boys and men cannot help or control (Hollway 1984). Media coverage of the so-called Spur Posse in Lakewood, California, reflects this discourse. Members of the Spur Posse, a group of popular white high school boys in a middle-class California suburb, competed with one another using a point system for their sexual "conquests" (Smolowe 1993). When girls eventually complained, several boys were charged with crimes ranging from sexual molestation to rape. Although many criticized the incident as an example of unchecked adolescent sexuality, others excused or even defended the boys' behavior. One father explained, "Nothing my boy did was anything any red-blooded American boy wouldn't do at his age." Their mother commented, "What can you do? It's a testosterone thing."

A comparison of the different boundaries of acceptable sexual behavior for girls and boys illustrates the force of the cultural assumption of female passivity and male aggression. Although the Spur Posse incident was covered as a troubling example of male sexuality out of control, the point at which adolescent sexual aggression becomes suspect is strikingly different for girls and boys. For girls, it's phone calls; for boys, it's rape. The girls' suggestive phone calling is described as shocking to the parents and even threatening to the sons, not because the desire expressed was unusual in the realm of teen sexuality, but because the agents were girls and the objects were boys. In the Spur Posse incident, the possibility of girls' sexual agency or desire shifted responsibility from the boys' aggression to the girls' failure to resist. For some observers, whether or not the boys in the Spur Posse were considered to have acted inappropriately depended upon an assessment of the sexual conduct of the girls involved. If the girls were shown to have expressed any sexual agency, their desire was treated by some as excusing and justifying the boys' treatment of them as objects or points to be collected. As one mother, invoking cultural shorthand put it, "Those girls are trash." The boys' behavior was excused as natural, "a testosterone thing," and the girls were deemed culpable for their failure to control the boys' behavior.

Through these cultural stories, girls are simultaneously taught that they are valued in terms of their sexual desirability and that their own desire makes them vulnerable. If they are economically privileged and white, they become vulnerable because desiring (read "bad") girls lose credibility and protection from male aggression. If they are poor and/or of color, or bisexual or lesbian, they are assumed to be bad, as refracted through the lenses of racism, classism, and homophobia that anchor the cultural story (Tolman forthcoming). While in some communities girls' and women's sexuality is acknowledged and more accepted (Omolade 1983), the force of cultural stories permeating the dominant culturel presses upon all girls. This constant pressure often inflames the desire of marginalized girls to be thought of as good, moral, and normal, status denied them by mainstream standards.[1] Moreover, all girls' vulnerability is compounded by the extraordinary license given to adolescent boys regarding the urgency of their sexuality. Perhaps more than any other group of men, teenage boys are assumed to be least in control of their sexuality. The responsibility for making sexual choices, therefore, falls to their partners, usually teenage girls, yet these "choices" are to be enacted through passivity rather than agency. Girls who attain good girlhood are at constant risk of becoming bad girls if they fail in their obligation to regulate their own sexual behavior and that of their partners. It is during adolescence, then, that girls are both most responsible for sexual decision making and most penalized for acting on their own sexual desires. It is also during adolescence that girls are socialized into cultural stories about being sexual and being women (Brown and Gilligan 1992; Tolman 1994a and 1994b).

The power of these cultural norms to mediate the interpretation of teen sexuality is perhaps most vividly revealed in the comments of those who would defend "aggressive" girls. Teenage girls interviewed in the *Sentinel* story explained their peers' behavior in terms of girls giving boys what the boys wanted. One suggested that "sometimes girls, in order to get certain guys, will do anything the guy wants. And that includes sex." That would include propositioning a boy "[I]f that's what she thinks *he wants*." The girl's actions are reinterpreted in terms of satisfying the boy's desire rather than her own. Explaining away the possibility of the girls' sexual desire, one counselor suggested that the girls may not really be "sex-crazed." Rather, they are probably simply "desperate for a relationship" (Shrieves 1993). Describing the girls as trading sex for relationships, the counselor reinterprets their actions in a manner that is consistent with the cultural story of male aggression and female responsibility, which is devoid of female desire. The girl gives the boy what he (inevitably or naturally) wants, negotiating her need only for a relationship by managing his drive for sexual pleasure.

The contrasting media coverage of teenage girls' and teenage boys' sexuality stands as one manifestation of a broader cultural message about gendered norms of sexual behavior. Feminists have documented and discussed this message as a theme present throughout literature, law, film, advertising, and general sources of cultural wisdom on sexuality such as self-help books, advice columns, and

medical treatises. The story of male aggression and female responsibility suffuses the culture and operates to regulate human sexuality on conscious and subconscious levels in a gender-specific way. By discouraging women's sexual agency and men's sexual responsibility, these cultural norms undermine communication and encourage coercion and violence. This effect is perhaps nowhere more clear than in the legal regulation of sexuality through rape statutes and the media coverage of rape trials.

Premised on the notion of male sexual aggression and irresponsibility, the law of rape incorporates cultural norms that place upon the woman the burden of regulating sexual activity and, at the same time, penalize her for acting as a sexual subject (Henderson 1992). In so doing, the law of rape incorporates both sides of the good girl/bad girl dynamic. The good girl's attempt to exercise her responsibility to regulate male sexuality is encoded in the requirement of nonconsent to sexual intercourse. Proof of nonconsent, however, frequently depends upon establishing an absence of desire. To be a victimized good girl and therefore entitled to protection, a girl or woman must both resist *and* lack desire. A desiring bad girl, on the other hand, is often deemed deserving of the consequences of her desire.

In cases of nonstranger (acquaintance) rape, rape trials frequently hinge upon whether nonconsent is established, a standard which, as feminists have noted, takes little account of women's sexuality. As Carol Smart has argued, the consent/nonconsent dyad fails to capture the complexity of a woman's experience (Smart 1989). A woman may seek and initiate physical intimacy, which may be an expression of her own sexual desire, while not consenting to intercourse. Nevertheless, by imposing the consent/nonconsent interpretive framework, rape law renders a woman's expression of any desire immediately suspect. Expression of desire that leads to intimacy and ultimately submission to unwanted sex falls on the side of consent. As the "trashy" girls who were the victims of the Spur Posse illustrate, to want anything is to consent to everything. The woman has, in effect, sacrificed her right to refuse intercourse by the expression of her own sexual desire. Or, more precisely, the expression of her desire undermines the credibility of her refusal. Evidence that the rape victim initiated sexual interaction at any level operates to undermine her story at every stage of the process—police disbelieve her account, prosecutors refuse to press the case, and juries refuse to convict. At trial, the issue of consent may be indistinguishable from the question of whether the woman experienced pleasure. Thus, within rape law, a woman's behavior as a sexual subject shifts power to the aggressor, thereby maintaining the power hierarchy of the traditional story of male aggression and female submission. As in pulp romance, to desire is to surrender.

The centrality of the absence of female desire to the definition of rape cuts across racial lines, albeit in complicated ways. As African American feminists have pointed out, rape and race are historically interwoven in a way that divides the experiences of women of color from white women (i.e., Collins 1990 and Harris 1990; see also Caraway 1991). Nevertheless, whatever the woman's race, the absence of female desire stands as a prerequisite to the identification of a sexual act as rape. The difference emerges as a product of the interlocking elements of the cultural story about women's sexuality which segregate white women and women of color. For example, a key element in the cultural story about women's sexuality is that African American women are sexually voracious, thereby making them unrapable—as distinguished from white women, who are asexual and thus in a constant state of rapability. The absence-of-desire standard is still applied to women of color but presumed impossible to meet. Conversely, when white women accuse African American men of raping them, the required absence of female desire is simply presumed.

If, under ordinary rape law, expression of female sexual desire takes women and girls outside the protection of the law, rendering them unrapable, statutory rape law defines female sexuality as outside the law in a different way. By criminalizing all intercourse with minors, statutory rape laws literally outlaw girls' expression of their own sexuality.[2] In terms of female sexual desire, statutory rape laws represent a complete mirroring of rape law regulating men's access to adult women—with statutory rape, absence of desire is presumed. Instead of rendering a woman unrapable or fully accessible to men, the law simply makes young women's expression of sexual desire illegal.

Both rape law and statutory rape law reinforce cultural norms of female sexuality be penalizing female sexual desire. The coverage of rape in the media, in turn, frequently heightens the focus on the sexuality of the victim, casting her as either good (innocent) or bad (desiring). For example, in the coverage of the Mike Tyson rape trial, the media referred repeatedly to the fact that Desiree Washington taught Sunday school, as though that fact were necessary to rebut the possibility that she invited the attack by acting on her own sexual desire. In an even more extreme case, the mentally disabled adolescent girl who was raped by a group of teenage boys in her Glen Ridge, New Jersey, neighborhood was portrayed both by her lawyers and by the media as largely asexual. To establish nonconsent, the prosecution argued explicitly that she was incapable of knowing or expressing her sexuality.[3] Although she was not sexually inexperienced, this strategy rendered her sexually innocent. Coverage of these two trials stands in sharp contrast to another highly publicized rape trial at the time, that of William Kennedy Smith, in which the media revealed not only the victim's name but her sexual history and her driving record. Much was made in the media of the victim's sexual history and her apparent willingness to accompany Smith home that night. Her desire to engage in flirtation and foreplay meant that her alleged refusal of intercourse could never be sufficiently credible to convict. Smith was acquitted.

As illustrated by the coverage of rape trials, the media and the law interact to reinforce the cultural story of male aggression and female passivity, reinforcing the good girl/bad girl distinction. With the suffusion of this story throughout our culture, girls and women come to understand the norms of acceptable sexual behavior—that good girls are those who are sexually innocent, meaning without sexual desire, although not necessarily without sexual experience. These girls are sexual objects, not subjects, charged with defending the boundaries of their own sexual activity by resisting male aggression. In contrast, bad girls are girls who express their desire, acting as sexual subjects on their own behalf. They are assertive girls, "girls who go too far." Vilified by the media and the culture more broadly as deviant and threatening, these girls are rendered far less likely than good girls to be able to invoke the protection of rape laws and are thus made doubly vulnerable.

Problem of Desire for Adolescent Girls

In this section, we turn to the voices of adolescent young women speaking about their experiences. We rely on a feminist method of analyzing interviews to understand how cultural stories about girls' sexuality may create vulnerability for girls rather than protect them from it.[4] This method takes women as authorities on their own experiences. We listen to what they say and how they say it so that our role as interpreters of their words is clear; that is, we do not claim the authority to say what they are saying but convey how we understand the stories they tell, given our perspective on these issues. We have drawn two case studies from a psychological study of adolescent girls' experience of desire (Tolman 1994a and 1994b),[5] and one from the legal literature. We selected the cases from the study because each of these girls chose to speak about a sexual experience with a boy who was not her boyfriend. Although each associated her experience with sexual violence, the two girls differ profoundly in their understanding of these experiences and also in their critical perspective on gender relations, the cultural story about male and female sexuality, and the good girl/bad girl dynamic. In Jenny's case, a lack of a critical perspective on these issues disables her from feeling outraged or empowered to act on her own behalf. For Pauline, such a perspective appears to enhance her sense of entitlement and ability to act. Through this contrast, we demonstrate how being a good girl can be bad for girls and, conversely, how challenging the terms of the good girl/bad girl dichotomy can be enabling. Finally, we selected the case of Sharon from the legal literature to underscore our point that denying desire in the name of good girlhood can diminish girls' ability to garner protection under the law.

Jenny: When Bad Things Happen to Good Girls

Sixteen-year-old Jenny, who lives in a suburb of a large city, looks like the quintessential good girl. She is white, has long, straight, blond hair framing a lightly freckled, fair face. She is slim, dressed fashionably yet unassumingly. She sits with her legs tensely crossed; she is polite and cooperative and smiles often. Like many girls in this study, throughout the interview Jenny describes how she lives her life by trying to stay carefully within the boundaries of good girl. She and her mother are "very close," and it is very important to her to be "nice" and a "good friend"—even if it means silencing her own displeasure or dissent in relationships.[6] Complying with conventional norms of femininity, Jenny explains that she has never experienced feelings she calls sexual desire: "I actually really don't think I've ever like, wanted anything, like sexually that bad. I mean I don't think I've ever been like sexually deprived or like saying, oh I need sex now or anything, I've never really felt that way before, so, I don't know. I don't really think that there's anything that I would, I mean want." Given Jenny's concern about and success at being a good girl in other domains of her life, it is not surprising that she does not report feeling desire. Having a "silent body" is a psychological response to the belief that good girls are not sexual (Tolman 1994a).

The vulnerability of this silence in her life is tangible in the narrative she tells about the first time she had sexual intercourse, which occurred just prior to our interview. This experience was not what she had hoped it would be:

> We got alone together, and we started just basically fooling around and not doing many things. And then he asked me if I would have sex with him, and I said, well I didn't think I, I mean I said I wanted to wait, 'cause I didn't want to. I mean I like him, but I don't like him so, and I mean he sorta pushed it on me, but it wasn't like I absolutely said no, don't, I—it was sort of a weird experience. I just, I sort of let it happen to me and never like really said no, I don't want to do this. I mean I said no, but I never, I mean I never stopped him from doing anything. . . . I guess maybe I wanted to get it over with, I guess . . . I don't know. I, I just, I mean I could've said no, I guess and I could've pushed him off or whatever 'cause he, I mean, he wasn't, he's not the type of person who would like rape me or whatever, I mean, well I don't think he's that way at all. . . . I was always like, well I want to wait, and I want to be in a relationship with someone who I really like, and I want it to be a special moment and everything, and then it just sort of like happened so quickly, and it happened with someone who I didn't like and who I didn't want a relationship with and who didn't want a relationship with me, and it was just sort of, I don't, I don't know, I regret it. . . . I wish I had just said no. I mean I could've, and I did for once but then I just let it go. And I wish that I had stood up for myself and really just like stood up and said no, I don't want to do this. I'm not ready or I want it to be a different experience. I mean I could've told him exactly how I felt. . . . I don't know why I didn't.

In this story, Jenny is unsure about how to understand her first experience with sexual intercourse. In listening to her, we, too, are unsure. When she begins this story, Jenny knows that she did not want to have sexual intercourse with this boy, although she did want to "fool around." She, in fact, said "no" when the boy asked her if she would have sex with him. There is a clarity to her no that she substantiates with a set of compelling reasons for not wanting to have sex with this boy: she "wanted to wait," she didn't "like him" or "want a relationship with him." After the fact, she is again clear that she did not want to have sex with this boy. She "regrets it." But we notice that this clarity gives way to a sense of confusion that colors Jenny's voice and gains momentum as her narrative, itself an interplay of description and assessment, unfolds. Cleaving to the convention that girls are ultimately responsible for boys' sexual behavior, she attempts to make sense of the fact that this boy behaved as though she had not said no. Assuming responsibility, Jenny suggests that she had "never stopped him from doing anything," implying, perhaps, that she had not meant the no that she had said.

Jenny's suggestion that she might have said *no* and meant *yes* raises a troubling issue for feminists who have rallied around the claim that "no means no." Although "no means no" is effective as an educational or political slogan or perhaps even as a legal norm, such norms protect girls only at the margin. Within the broader context of adolescent sexuality, girls' no must be credible both to girls and to their partners. Yet the cultural story that good girls do not have sexual desire undermines the credibility of their no, not only to others but also to themselves. When girls cannot say yes, no (or silence) is their only alternative and must express the range of their choices. Some have suggested that girls can ameliorate the problem by simply taking responsibility for communicating their desire (e.g., Roiphe 1993). This answer falls short and, in fact, leaves girls in the lurch by failing to account for the cultural sanctions on girls' expression of their sexuality. Leaving those sanctions unaddressed, so-called power feminists reinforce the assignment of responsibility to girls for sexual decision making without criticizing the constraints under which such decisions are made.

Jenny struggles within those constraints as she attempts to take seriously the possibility that she may have wanted to have sex with the boy despite having said no; the possibility that her no meant yes. Yet her reflection, "I guess maybe I wanted to get it over with, I guess" is literally buttressed by doubt. While this statement stands as a potential explanation of why she had sex even though she said no, Jenny herself does not sound convinced. The explanation sounds even less plausible when compared to the clarity of her elaborated and unambiguous statements about why she did not want to have sex. She explains, "I want to be in a relationship with someone who I really like, and I want it to be a special moment and everything."

As her story progresses, we hear Jenny's confusion about what she wanted intensify. This confusion seems to undermine Jenny's knowledge that she had actually said no to this boy. Eventually, Jenny seems to forget that she ever said no at all. Despite having just explained that she had not wanted to have sex with this boy and had told him so, Jenny starts to speak as if she had not said no. "I said no" becomes "I sort of let it happen to me and never like, really said no, I don't want to do this." She progressively undoes her knowledge that she articulated her wish not to have sex. "I mean I could've said no, I guess, and I could've pushed him off or whatever," finally becomes "I wish I had just said no." Thus, when this boy behaved as though Jenny had not said no, Jenny loses track of her knowledge and her voice, becoming confused not only about what she wanted but also about what she said.

The conditions Jenny gives for an appropriate sexual encounter—"a special relationship," someone she "really like[s]"—resonate with the cultural story that girls' sexuality is about relationships and not desire. Because the encounter she describes did not meet these conditions, she decided that she did not want to have sex and told the boy no. Yet these conditions did not supply an adequate framework for Jenny either to make a clear decision and insist that it be respected, or, if it was not respected, to identify the incident as one of violation. In this context, it is significant that Jenny makes no reference to her own sexual desire. It is only later in the interview, in response to a direct question, that Jenny reports that she "hadn't felt desire for the person I was with." She notes, however, that this absence of desire does not distinguish this encounter from any other: "I've never like had sexual feelings to want to do something or anything." We wonder whether, in the moment, Jenny was not able to hold onto her knowledge that she did not want to have sex because her own desire has never been available as a guide to her choices. We suggest that not feeling desire is one way to cope with the good girl/bad girl dichotomy. Were Jenny not subject to the good girl standard that prevents her from attending to her own sexual feelings, perhaps she would feel desire in some situations, and her lack of sexual desire could operate as a clear signal to her, perhaps leaving her less vulnerable to such confusion.

The consequences of Jenny's confusion include physical and psychological vulnerability. Her difficulty in holding on to her no and insisting that her no be respected leaves her physically vulnerable to sexual encounters that she does not in any clear way want. Jenny's confusion makes her vulnerable psychologically as well. By discounting her own thoughts and feelings, she risks becoming dissociated from her own experience and from reality. Such dissociation makes it difficult for Jenny to be able to know and name sexual exploitation. Accustomed to being the object of someone else's sexual desire, not considering that her own sexual desire might be relevant or significant, Jenny pastes over the complexity of what did, in fact, happen with the phrase "it just sort of like happened." This "cover story" symbolizes and sustains Jenny's vulnerability in a culture that leaves out her sexual desire.

At the same time, Jenny's suggestion that "it just sort of like happened" keeps another story at bay, a story of a girl whose spoken wish was not heeded, who was coerced. Was Jenny raped? Jenny herself brings the word "rape" into her story: "I mean I could've said no, I guess and I could've pushed him off or whatever 'cause he, I mean, he wasn't, he's not the type of person who would like rape me, or whatever. I mean, well I don't think he's that way at all." She seems to wonder whether this experience might somehow be connected to rape. She may associate this experience with rape because the word signifies something about what it felt like for her, a violation. Although she stopped saying no and apparently assented nonverbally to the act, this sexual experience was not related to any feeling of yes on Jenny's part. Jenny's experience of having passively consented and of having been violated suggests the disjuncture between consent and desire in women's experience, a disjuncture that likely heightens Jenny's confusion over how to interpret what happened to her. Such confusion prevents Jenny from speaking clearly in the first instance about her desire and from later interpreting what happened in a way that acknowledges her own resistance.

Nonetheless Jenny is an astute observer of the social landscape of adolescent heterosexual relationships. She identifies some imbalances in how girls and boys behave and in how they are treated by others in response to their behavior. Later in the interview, she notes that "whenever like a girl and a guy do something and people find out, it's always the girl that messed up or, I mean, maybe the guy messed up, but the guys like get praise for it [laughing] and the girl's sort of like called, either a slut or something, or just like has a bad reputation. Which is sort of [laughing] awful." Jenny believes that "it is just as much the guy's fault as it is the girl's fault. . . . It's just like the guys and the girls make fun of the girls but no one makes fun of the guys [laughing]." What Jenny needs is an analytic framework that links the inequities she observes to cultural stories about sexuality. She suspects, but does not know, that these stories operate in a way that creates gendered power differences. Identifying the good girl/bad girl divide, Jenny tries without success to make sense of the contradiction she observes, that both girls and guys may be at "fault" in sexual situations like hers, but only girls are chastised. We notice that she does not say what she thinks about this contradiction. When she is asked directly, her constant confusion about gender relations is audible: "I really don't know."

Sharon: The Slippery Slope off Good Girlhood

The legal vulnerability created when girls become confused about their own desire is illustrated by the testimony of Sharon, the victim in the U.S. Supreme Court's statutory rape case *Michael M.* v. *Sonoma County.* In her portion of the trial transcript reproduced in the Supreme Court's opinion, Sharon, who, like Jenny, is sixteen and white, is being questioned by the defendant's lawyer about whether she wanted to have sex with the defendant, a boy who was not her boyfriend. Ordinary rape law requires that she make a clear claim that she did not

want to have sex with the defendant in order to gain legal recourse. The confusion that emerges as she testifies not only renders the case problematic under ordinary rape law but also calls into question the legitimacy of the statutory rape prosecution. The lawyer's questions about Sharon's desire subtly garner the good girl/bad girl dynamic as part of a strategy to undermine the credibility of her claim that she did not want to have sexual intercourse. In the face of these questions, Sharon appears to lose her clarity about the exact parameters of her desire:

Q: Now, after you met the defendant, what happened?

A: We walked down to the railroad tracks.

Q: What happened at the railroad tracks?

A: We were drinking at the railroad tracks and we walked over to this bus and he started kissing me and stuff, and I was kissing him back, too, at first. Then I was telling him to stop—

Q: Yes.

A: —and I was telling him to slow down and stop. He said, "Ok, Ok." But then he just kept doing it. He just kept doing it and then my sister and two other guys came over to where we were and my sister told me to get up and come home. And then I didn't. . . . We were laying there and we were kissing each other, and then he asked me if I wanted to walk with him over to the park. We walked over to the park, and then we sat down on a bench, and then he started kissing me again, and we were laying on the bench. And he told me to take my pants off. I said "No," and I was trying to get up and he hit me back down on the bench, and then I just said to myself, "Forget it," and I let him do what he wanted to do and he took my pants off and he was telling me to put my legs around him and stuff.

Q: Did you have sexual intercourse with the defendant?

A: Yeah.

Q: Did you go off with [the defendant] away from the others?

A: Yeah.

Q: Why did you do that?

A: I don't know. I guess I wanted to. (Michael M. *v.* Sonoma County 450 U.S. 464 [1980]: 483–488)

Sharon begins by speaking clearly about what she did and did not want to do with the boy. She wanted to kiss him back, she wanted him to slow down and stop, and she also wanted to walk over to the park with him. However, when the sexual interaction turned from kissing or "fooling around" to "tak[ing] off [her] pants," she said "no," unequivocally and clearly and "tri[ed] to get up." We hear that her desire had specific contours: while she had wanted to "fool around," she did not want to have sexual intercourse. Nevertheless, like Jenny, she stopped saying no and "let him do what he wanted to do." In so doing, she may have given her consent legally although not emotionally or psychologically.

Initially Sharon maintains clarity about the limits of her desire. Confusion creeps into her previously straightforward account, however, as she is asked about her motives for having gone to the park with the defendant. Implicit in the lawyer's question "[why] did you go off with [the defendant] away from the others?" is the unspoken condemnation of the actions of a bad girl, the conditional phrase *"unless you wanted to have sexual intercourse with him?"* So understood, the question is really about her desire. Having been asked to speak about her own desire, Sharon loses the clarity of her earlier explanation. She seems to suspect (along with the lawyer) that there is an inconsistency between having wanted to go to the park and having not wanted to have sex with the boy.

Confronted with the threat of bad girl status, Sharon retreats from the earlier articulation of her desire. Following on the heels of an unequivocal account that portrays the parameters of her desire, Sharon's statement of ambivalence makes her seem confused and uncertain. By responding that she does not know what she wanted, that she "guess[es]" that she "wanted to," Sharon undermines the credibility of her previous testimony. As a witness, Sharon becomes trapped within the good girl/bad girl dichotomy. Her admission of her desire to go to the park with the boy undermines the credibility of her claim that she was coerced. At this point, her reiteration of her direct statement that she wanted to go to the park coupled with her retreat from that statement render her testimony unreliable. Her mistake, as she seems to realize, was to relinquish good girl status by confessing her desire.

Paulina: Empowerment through Rejecting the Good Girl/Bad Girl Dichotomy

Paulina, a white girl who lives in an urban environment, tells stories that offer a counterpoint to Jenny's. Seventeen-year-old Paulina looks like the other adolescent girls in this study: long, dark hair frames her pretty, open face; stylish jeans and sweater clothe a slim figure. Despite

her appearance, Paulina does not sound like the other girls: having immigrated from Eastern Europe several years prior to the interview, Paulina speaks with a strong accent. It is the content of her narrative, however, that distinguishes her from most other study participants. Like Jenny, Paulina is also a competent consumer of cultural stories about girls and sexuality, and can recite them without a moment's hesitation:

> They expect the woman to be pure, I mean, she has to be holy and everything, and it's okay for a guy to have any feelings or anything, and the girl has to be this little virgin who is obedient to the men. . . . usually a guy makes the first move, not the girl, or the girl's not supposed to do it, the girl's supposed to sit there going, no, no you can't. I can't do that. . . . I mean the guy expects the girl to be a sweet little virgin when he marries her, and then he can be running around with ten other women, but when he's getting married to her, she's not supposed to have any relationship with anybody else.[7]

Paulina echoes Jenny's observation about how the label "slut" is—and is not—used: "Guys, they just like to brag about girls. Oh she does this, and she's a slut because she slept with this guy, and with this guy, but they don't say that about guys. It's okay for them to do it, but when a girl sleeps with two guys it's wrong, she shouldn't do that, she automatically becomes a slut."

In contrast to Jenny's ambivalence and uncertainty, Paulina has strong opinions about the sexual double standard: "I just don't agree with it. . . . I just don't think so." A sense of entitlement, accompanied by outrage, suffuses her well-articulated view of female sexual agency: "Woman can do whatever they want to, why shouldn't they? . . . . I think that women have the same feelings as men do, I mean, I think it's okay to express them too. . . . I mean, they have the same feelings, they're human, why should they like keep away from them?" While Jenny seems unable to make sense of this inequity, Paulina grounds her dissension in an analysis linking gender and power: "I think males are kind of dominant, and they feel that they have the power to do whatever they want, that the woman should give in to them." Paulina also parts from Jenny in her detailed knowledge about her own sexual desire.

Perhaps not coincidentally, Paulina speaks of this embodied experience with an ease that reflects and underscores her belief that girls' sexual desire is normal or, in her words, "natural": "I feel really hot, like, my temperature is really hot. . . . I felt like a rush of blood like pumping to my heart, my heart would really beat fast, and it's just, everything are combined, you're extremely aware of every touch, and everything, everything together . . . you have all those feelings of want." Paulina is clear that this desire can guide her choices and that it should be respected: "To me if you have like a partner that you're close to, then it's okay. And if you feel comfortable with it, 'cause if you don't, then you shouldn't do it. You just don't want to." Thus, Paulina grounds her sexual decisions in her own feelings and beliefs—she can identify and is able to account for the presence and absence of her own desire. As a result, Paulina appears to be less vulnerable to becoming confused about what she feels and what she has said.

Like Jenny, Paulina has had a "bad" sexual experience with a boy whom she thought of as a friend. In the interview, she describes a time when this male friend tried to force her to have sex with him:

> There was one experience, the guy wanted to have sexual intercourse and I didn't. I didn't have sex with him. He, he like pulled me over to the couch, and I just kept on fighting. . . . I was just like begging him to like not to do anything, and like, I really did not have like much choice. Because I had my hands behind me. And he just like kept on touching me, and I was just like, just get off me. He goes, you know that you want to, and I said no I don't. Get off me, I hate you. . . . So he's like, well, I'll let you go if you're gonna kiss me. So I kissed him, and I'm like well I can go now. And he was like no. But um, the phone rang later on, I said I have to answer this, it's my mother. . . . So he let me answer the phone. So. And it was my friend and I just said, oh can you come over? And, since I'm Polish I spoke Polish, so I'm like oh just come over, come over as soon as you can.

Ultimately, when her friend arrived, she was able to convince the boy to leave.

Paulina's assailant attacked her both physically and psychologically, telling her, "You know that you want to." However, because Paulina had a clear understanding of her sexual feelings, she is able to speak clearly about not feeling sexual desire. In response to his coaxing, Paulina's retort is direct and unequivocal: "No, I don't. Get off me. I hate you." Unlike Jenny and Sharon, Paulina does not become confused: she has no doubt in her mind about the parameters of her own sexual feelings; she did not want any sexual interaction with this young man. Her sense of entitlement to her feelings and choices empowers her to resist the attack.

It must be emphasized that Paulina was very lucky in this situation. She was able to think clearly and take advantage of an opportunity—her friend's phone call—to protect herself from being raped. The critical point is not that she was able to avoid assault in this case, but that she was clear about the threat of violence. Had Paulina not escaped attack, it seems likely that she would have maintained her clarity about her own actions and desires, a clarity that would enable her to claim the protection the law offers.

Conclusion

In listening to three adolescent girls voice experiences with their own sexuality, we hear both how the good girl/bad girl dynamic becomes embodied and embedded in girls' psyches and relationships and how it can be resisted. We suggest that Paulina's ability to know her desire and know its absence, in contrast to Jenny's "silent body" and Sharon's confusion, is linked to her critical consciousness about how male power and dominance underpin the good girl/bad girl dichotomy. Because she rejects a cultural story about her sexuality that makes her own desire dangerous, we think she is less vulnerable to the confusion that Sharon and Jenny voice and more empowered to know and to speak with clarity about her sexual interactions and the social landscape of gendered relationships.

The voices of these three girls living (with) the good girl/bad girl dynamic suggest the necessity of what Michelle Fine terms an affirmative discourse of desire (Fine 1988) for adolescent girls. Such a discourse must recognize, reveal, and then reject the good girl/bad girl categories as patriarchal strategies that keep girls and women from the power of their own bodies and their bonds with one another. It should center on all girls' entitlement to their sexuality, rather than focus solely on the threat of lost status and respect or diminished safety. With the words and analysis to interrupt the good girl/bad girl dynamic, girls and women can identify and critique cultural stories that impair them psychologically and under the law.

The task for feminists, then, is to help adolescent girls and women to analyze the complexity of living in women's bodies within a culture that divides girls and women within themselves and against each other. It is true that the threat of sexual violence against girls and women, as well as social isolation, is real and constant, effectively keeping girls' and women's bodies and psyches filled with fear, rendering sexual desire difficult and dangerous. Yet it is also true that girls and women at this moment in history can feel profound pleasure and desire and should be entitled to rely on their own feelings as an important aspect of sexual choices. By holding the contradiction of pleasure and danger, girls and women can expose and loosen the tight weave seamlessly worked by the good girl/bad girl dynamic in society and in their individual lives.

Notes

1. Some young women are able to resist such norms by anchoring their sexual self-concept in their culture of origin (Robinson and Ward 1991).

2. Although the modern reinterpretation of the purpose of statutory rape laws is that such legislation is designed to prevent teen pregnancy, the historical justification was the protection of female virtue. For example, in 1895, the California Supreme Court explained:

    The obvious purpose of [the statutory rape law] is the protection of society by protecting from violation the virtue of young unsophisticated girls. . . . It is the insidious approach and vile tampering with their persons that primarily undermines the virtue of young girls, and eventually destroys it; and the prevention of this, as much as the principal act, must undoubtedly have been the intent of the legislature. (People *v.* Verdegreen, 106 Cal. 211, 214–215, 39 P. 607, 607–609 [1895]

    In 1964, the same court explained that "an unwise disposition of her sexual favor is deemed to do harm both to herself and the social mores by which the community's conduct patterns are established. Hence the law of statutory rape intervenes in an effort to avoid such a disposition" (People *v.* Hernandez, 61 Cal. 2d 531, 393 P. 2d 674 [1964]).

    As Professor Fran Olsen has argued, although the boy's conduct is punished by criminal sanction, it is the girl who is denied the capacity to consent. Under gender-specific statutory rape laws, the boy may legally have intercourse with women who are over the age of consent (Olsen, 1984).

3. The prosecution's strategy to portray the victim as asexual was controversial among advocates for people with mental disabilities. (See Houppert 1993, citing Leslie Walker-Hirsch, president of the American Association on Mental Retardation's special interest group on sexual and social concerns). Nevertheless, in this, as in many other rape trials, the surest means of establishing lack of consent was to establish the sexual innocence of the victim.

4. This method adopts the psychodynamic concept of the layered psyche in interpreting girls' and women's narratives in individual interviews conducted by women (Brown et al. 1991). Importing this clinical construct into empirical research is not by fiat a feminist act. But requiring the interpreter to focus actively on her own subjectivity and theoretical framework in the act of interpretation subverts the tendency in psychology of an authoritative, expert "voice over" of a girl or woman's words. This psychological method, called the Listening Guide, enables an exploration of ways in which internalized oppression may operate to constrain what a girl or woman says, thinks, or knows, and how she may resist such oppressions. This method asks us to consider what is not said as well as what is said and how power differences embedded in the brief research relationship may circulate through the narrative. The method obligates the interpreter to ask herself persistently how a woman's structural position in society or individual relational history may contribute to layered ways of understanding her voice—what she says, where she falters, when she is silent. The use of this method yields multiple interpretations of women's narratives by highlighting different voices or perspectives audible in a single story. Using this method means creating a dialectic between the way one girl or woman speaks and how another woman, from a distinctly feminist point of view, hears her story.

5. The study was designed to fill in a gap in the psychological literature on adolescent girls' sexuality: how girls experience their own sexual feelings, particularly their bodies. This feminist question challenged the belief that girls' sexuality is essentially a response to boys' sexual feelings and began to flesh out how sexual desire is a part of adolescent girls' lives. For her dissertation, Tolman interviewed a random sample of thirty girls from two different social contexts: they were juniors, aged fifteen to eighteen, at a suburban and an urban public high school. These girls were black, Hispanic, and white and represented a range of religious backgrounds, sexual experiences, and ethnicities. The interviews often had a conversational tone because the feminist approach used emphasizes listening to girls, in contrast to the traditional procedure of strict adherence to a preset questionnaire. Overall these girls reported that their own desire was a dilemma for them because they were not supposed to experience sexual feelings but, in fact, did. For more on this study see Tolman 1994a, 1994b, and forthcoming. The analyses of this data have focused on class rather than race differences, due to the demographics of the sample. Both qualitative and quantitative analyses revealed similarities across class, such as in the proportion of girls who reported an absence of or confusion about desire and those who reported an awareness of their own desire, and significant class differences in the association of desire with vulnerability and pleasure. Urban girls' narratives were more likely to be about vulnerability and not about pleasure, while suburban girls' narratives were more likely to be about pleasure rather than vulnerability.

6. Brown and Gilligan 1992 and Jack 1991 describe these qualities of the "tyranny of nice and kind" and the tendency to silence or sacrifice the self's disruptive feelings as characteristic of girls' and women's descriptions of their relationships.

7. Paulina's responses have been reported previously in Tolman 1994b.

References

Brown, Lynn, and Carol Gilligan. 1992. *Meeting at the Cross-roads.* Cambridge, MA: Harvard University Press.

Brown, Lynn, Elizabeth Debold, Mark Tappan, and Carol Gilligan. 1991. "Reading Narratives of Conflict for Self and Moral Voice: A Relational Method." In *Handbook of Moral Behavior and Development: Theory, Research and Application,* ed. William Kurtines and Jacob Gewirtz. Hillsdale, NJ: Lawrence Erlbaum.

Caraway, Nancie. 1991. *Segregated Sisterhood.* Knoxville: University of Tennessee Press.

Collins, Patricia Hill. 1990. *Black Feminist Thought.* New York: Routledge.

Fine, Michelle. 1988. "Sexuality, Schooling, and Adolescent Females: The Missing Discourse of Desire." *Harvard Educational Review* 58 (10: 29–53).

Harris, Angela. 1990. "Race and Essentialism in Feminist Legal Theory." *Stanford Law Review* 42: 581–592.

Henderson, Lynne. 1992. "Rape and Responsibility." *Law and Philosophy* 11 (1–2): 127–128.

Hollway, Wendy. 1984. "Women's Power in Heterosexual Sex." *Women's Studies International Forum* 7 (1): 63–68.

Houppert, Karen. 1993. "The Glen Ridge Rape Draws to a Close." *Village Voice* (March 16): 29–33.

Jack, Dana. 1991. *Silencing the Sell.* Cambridge, MA: Harvard University Press.

Michael M. v. Sonoma County, 450 U.S. 464 (1980).

Olsen, Frances. 1984. "Statutory Rape: A Feminist Critique of Rights Analysis." *Texas Law Review* 63: 387.

Omadale, Barbara, 1983. "Hearts of Darkness." In *Powers of Desire: The Politics of Sexuality,* ed. Ann Snitow, Christine Stansell, and Sharon Thompson. New York: Monthly Review Press.

Robinson, Tracy and Janie Ward. 1991. "A Belief in Self Far Greater than Anyone's Disbelief: Cultivating Resistance Among African American Female Adolescents." In *Women, Girls, and Psychotherapy: Reframing Resistance,* ed. Carol Gilligan, Annie Rogers, and Deborah Tolman. New York: Haworth Press.

Roiphe, Katie: 1993. *The Morning After: Sex, Fear, and Feminism on Campus.* Boston: Little, Brown.

Shrieves, Linda. 1993. "The Bold New World of Boy Chasing." *Orlando Sentinel* (22 December): E1.

Smart, Carole. 1989. *Feminism and the Power of the Law.* New York: Routledge.

Smolowe, Jill. 1993. "Sex with a Scorecard." *Time* (5 April):41.

Tolman, Deborah. Forthcoming. "Adolescent Girls' Sexuality: Debunking the Myth of the Urban Girl." In *Urban Adolescent Girls: Resisting Stereotypes,* ed. Bonnie Leadbetter and Niobe Way. New York: New York University Press.

———. 1994a. "Daring to Desire; Culture and the Bodies of Adolescent Girls." In *Sexual Cultures: Adolescents, Communities and the Construction of Identity,* ed. Janice Irvine. Philadelphia: Temple University Press.

———.1994b. "Doing Desire: Adolescent Girls' Struggle for/with Sexuality." *Gender and Society* 8(3): 324–342.

Yoffe, Emily. 1991. "Girls Who Go Too Far." *Newsweek* (22 July): 58.

 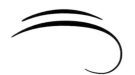

"The Orgasm Gap"

by Marcia Douglass and Lisa Douglass

Nikki and Joe lie naked in their bed, kissing in passionate embrace. As they caress one another, Nikki slowly glides her hand down Joe's chest and abdomen to his penis. She delights in the way it responds to her touch and savors its warm, firm feel in her hand. Joe reaches between Nikki's legs and slides his finger into her vagina. Nikki tilts her hips so that his fingertip meets her clitoris. She closes her eyes to focus on the rush of excitement his touch sends through her genitals. As Joe rubs her clitoris and kisses her neck, shoulder, and nipples, Nikki's pleasure borders on orgasm.

After a few minutes on this erotic edge, Nikki begins to worry that Joe wants to move on. She gets up, straddles him, and together they roll on a condom. Nikki massages on some lubrication then slips Joe's penis into her vagina. She caresses his penis inside her, alternately tightening and releasing her vaginal muscles. As Joe's excitement builds, Nikki senses that her own arousal is not keeping pace. The intensity of her pleasure dissipates, and she feels her orgasm slipping away. Nikki does not want to deny Joe his pleasure, so they flip over. Joe thrusts rhythmically and deeply inside her, then quickly comes. Nikki is disappointed that she has not had an orgasm, but as they rest in each other's arms, she takes pleasure in their intimacy.

For Nikki, as for most women, orgasm in sex is like a mirage: It appears on the horizon one minute, like a delicious glass of water to a thirsty traveler. But the next minute—poof!—it is gone. Sometimes, especially when she is on top during intercourse, Nikki comes, too. But at other times, she fakes orgasm. (Actually, she just lets Joe believe she has come.) Occasionally, when Joe asks, Nikki tells him, "It felt great! Really, it's OK. I love just being close to you." These are words that Joe has never uttered. He never has to: Like most men, Joe always has an orgasm when he has sex. As Joe begins to snore in satisfied slumber, Nikki lies awake trying to convince herself that it really was good for her, too.

Most men would not see the point of sex if their orgasms were so elusive. Yet Nikki and millions of other heterosexual women put up with unsatisfying sex on a regular basis, and the sexual culture—the way people in our society define sex—seems undisturbed by this fact. Both women and men expect sex to be a physically satisfying experience, but for many women it is not. Although sex virtually always includes *his* orgasm, hers is optional—nice, but not necessary.

The orgasm gap disrupts the pleasure of sex for both Nikki and Joe. When Joe comes but Nikki does not, they both feel frustrated or somehow deficient. Nikki thinks it is her mood. *I just could not let go tonight.* Sometimes she blames how she looks. *If I could just lose ten pounds.* Joe feels he has not "performed" adequately. *Maybe if I had lasted longer. Maybe if my penis were bigger.* Nikki and Joe tell themselves that orgasm is always harder for *women to achieve. Women just do not come as easily as men.*

What Nikki and Joe never blame is the *way* they have sex. For them, sex is synonymous with intercourse. They never have sex that does not include it. Intercourse gives Joe direct genital stimulation and virtually ensures his orgasm. Nikki loves the way intercourse feels, too, but most of the time it does not lead to her orgasm.

Nikki knows that she comes every time she masturbates by massaging her clitoris. But in partner sex, she never touches herself there. Joe pays her clitoris some attention during foreplay, but the stimulation he gives her usually stops short of orgasm. When they move to intercourse, the clitoris is all but forgotten. Nikki enjoys the feeling of Joe's penis inside her, but because penetration bypasses the clitoris, it does not make her come. Sometimes Nikki is tempted to ask Joe to keep his fingers on her clitoris a little longer or to give her cunnilingus. But having an orgasm from manual or oral sex is seen as inferior somehow. Both Nikki and Joe have learned that orgasm should come from intercourse. So they cut foreplay short and begin penetration, even though it is likely to mean that sex will soon culminate in his, but not her, orgasm.

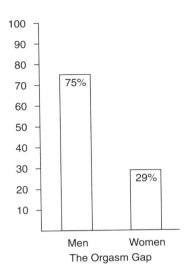

The Orgasm Gap

The orgasm gap between women and men is not just an individual problem. Nikki's experience of hit-or-miss orgasm is typical of sex for heterosexual women in the United States today. Seventy-five percent of men have orgasm in partner sex on a regular basis, but only 29 percent of women do. Two-thirds of women have orgasms only sometimes or not at all. It is difficult to imagine men accepting sex that excluded their orgasm. Yet because women have learned to accept this double standard, the orgasm gap has hardly budged over decades of social change—the sexual revolution of the 1960s, the women's movement of the 1970s, the antisex backlash in the era of AIDS in the 1980s, and into the sexual quandary of the 1990s. The 29/75 gap continues today in a social environment that appears to be more open than ever about sex. Intimate details of sexual activity are now discussed in safer sex instruction, on television and radio talk shows, and explicit sex acts are regularly portrayed in the popular media. But the orgasm gap is rarely discussed. It is simply accepted as the way sex is.

The orgasm gap between women and men is not restricted to any particular group of people. It crosses all lines of income, race, and ethnicity. It exists not only in every region of the United States but in every society around the world. Its near universality is not, however, proof that the orgasm gap is inevitable. Women are not inherently less orgasmic than men. In fact, women are physically capable of multiple orgasms, and most women who masturbate reach orgasm without fail. Women who have sex with a female partner come 83 percent of the time. Clearly, the problem lies not with women themselves, but in the way *heterosexuals* have sex.

Most people attribute the orgasm gap to biology and ignore the fact that people learn to have sex and to have orgasms according to the beliefs of their particular

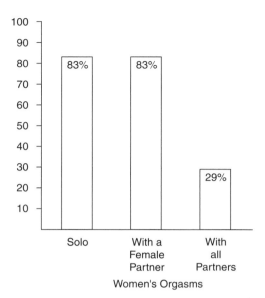

Women's Orgasms

culture. In the United States, people believe that there is a difference in hormones that makes men want and need sex more than women. They believe that it is natural fact that men reach their sexual peak at age eighteen, while most women's sexuality surges at thirty-five. They believe that women have a harder time having orgasms than men as a result of some evolutionary master plan of nature, when the real culprit is the way women and men are taught to have sex. It usually takes a woman decades before she figures out that the model of sex she was taught was wrong: It leaves out her orgasm.

Other people, including many sex experts, attribute the orgasm gap to women's psychology. In this view, women do not have orgasms because they have psychological hang-ups about sex. If women can just learn to relax in sex, they will have orgasms. But even the most carefree and uninhibited woman will not have an orgasm unless she gets the appropriate stimulation. Yet the sexual culture defines sex in such a way that women and men either never learn to use or are discouraged from using the kind of stimulation that works.

At the start of a new millennium, most young women face the same confusing path toward orgasm their mothers and grandmothers encountered. They must make their way through a morass of inconsistent messages about sex. The most damaging of these is that sex is essentially intercourse and every other kind of sexual activity is not the real thing, even when they are more likely to give women orgasms. The sex = intercourse message leaves a woman to flounder through a long series of unsatisfactory sexual encounters before she finally figures out that clitoral stimulation, not intercourse alone, will bring her to orgasm. Although the role of the clitoris in

women's orgasm is mentioned in sex manuals and sex education texts, a woman can easily miss this important fact. Most women eventually discover the clitoris-orgasm connection. But then they face the higher hurdle of making this knowledge mesh with the way their partner (and the sexual culture) expects them to have sex.

The information a woman receives about orgasm is often so garbled and contradictory that she gives up trying to have one. Orgasm should come from intercourse, she is told, yet for most women it never does. Orgasm comes from clitoral stimulation, she reads, but a woman should nevertheless try to come from intercourse. Don't worry if you have never had an orgasm or only have them sometimes, she hears. Sex is so much more than orgasm: It is romance, sensuality, emotional intimacy, and above all, an expression of love.

But love is not enough to make sex good. And bad sex can interfere with love. An intimate relationship cannot thrive and grow where the physical pleasures of sex are as unequal as they are between Nikki and Joe. Some women settle for orgasms that happen now and then, and they focus their energies on romance and intimacy. But for women who find sex more frustrating than pleasurable, more embarrassing than ecstatic, and more of a duty than an opportunity, not having orgasm takes them further away from a loved partner, not closer. When the man has an orgasm but the woman does not, sex is not only less fun, but a gap can develop between two lovers in which doubt, anger, and blame begin to fester. Some women just stop having sex. One woman told us, "I faked it for over twelve years. And then it got to a point where I felt turned off to sex altogether. I didn't even want to deal with it because I wasn't getting anything out of it."

Men suffer from the orgasm gap, too. They have learned that it is up to them to "give" their partner an orgasm with their penis. If she does not come, they feel that it is a failure of either their own sexual prowess or a result of their partner's "frigidity." A man may tell a woman that she just needs to let go. The woman, too, believes that the problem is all in her head. They both accept the sexual culture's explanation that women's psychological hang-ups are the main cause of the orgasm gap. Yet the fault actually lies with a sexual culture that defines sex as intercourse.

Some women manage to defy the sexual culture and learn to have satisfying orgasmic sex. Some stumble upon orgasm by chance or luck. Others make a conscious effort to cultivate their sexuality. Of the women who regularly experience orgasm, some have one orgasm, some have multiple orgasms (more than one orgasm in a sexual session), and some ejaculate, a sexual pleasure most women never even learn about. Because sex is more often alluded to than honestly and openly discussed, women in our society have little chance of growing sexually unless they question the sexual culture and determine to cultivate their sexuality on their own.

There is little social support for women who challenge the sexual status quo. Even though women talk to each other about their periods, their relationships, and other intimate subjects, what they do in sex is a topic even the closest friends fear to broach. Women never take the opportunity to learn from other women about orgasm. Nor do most women talk frankly with their male partners about safer sex, much less better sex.

Nikki and Joe have never talked about what they actually do in bed. Neither of them has ever stopped to think about how they might do things differently because, in spite of their orgasm gap, they consider their sex life to be pretty good. They are equally interested in having sex, they enjoy foreplay, and when they have intercourse, it lasts longer than the national average of two and a half minutes. Yet, at some level, both of them know that sex between them could be so much better if Nikki had an orgasm, too.

Although primarily a problem for straight women, the orgasm gap also affects lesbians, bisexual women, and all men who care about gender equality and who like good sex. When the sexual culture focuses on what gives men pleasure in sex with a woman, all other sexual activities and everyone who is not a heterosexual male gets short sexual shrift. All women are pushed to the margins of sex defined as intercourse—lesbians do not have "real" sex, bisexual women "play around" with women until a man comes along, and straight women are expected to get pleasure from the same things that please men. If the sexual culture considers women's pleasure at all, it is only insofar as it fits into a model for sex designed to satisfy men.

Is Orgasm Important?

I don't think orgasms are the be-all, end-all, but I sure as hell wouldn't want to live without them.

—*Betty Dodson*

Most men never question the importance of orgasm—it is simply their sexual right. Many women cannot say whether or not orgasm is important, however, because they have never had one. A woman who does insist on having an orgasm may be accused of being too unromantic, too male, or too demanding. Yet no man ever has to justify his desire for orgasm. The goal of sex for women in contrast, is supposed to be intimacy, not or-

gasm. Yet orgasmic sex improves intimacy. When only one partner's orgasm is important, even necessary, while the other partner's is ignored or denied, true intimacy is impossible.

The Sexual Culture

The orgasm gap can be bridged only by changing the way women and men have sex. Changing the way people have sex means changing the sexual culture and confronting the assumptions upon which it is based. The first assumption is that sex is natural and that people are driven by hormones and genital urges. A person is thought to have a "sex drive" that motivates sexual behavior. Yet, as Leonore Tiefer's recent book proclaims in its title, *Sex Is Not a Natural Act*. Everyone who has ever had sex knows that it involves not only the body, but the mind and spirit. They know that it occurs in the context of complex relations with other people. Furthermore, sex is learned. And it is carried out according to the standards of a particular culture. Although sex takes place in and through the body, it is not governed by people's hormones or gonads. Sex is a social act to its very core, including in the way we define the body and sex itself.

Recognizing that sex is learned, people can act to change it. Until now, women have learned to have sex in ways that favor male pleasure, but they can unlearn those ways and invent new ones that foster more equal and satisfying sex.

To make sex as good for her as it is for him, Nikki and Joe need to examine each layer of their sexual activity to look at what they do and why. This means talking about sex. Already, sex is a popular topic of public discussion, but in the age of AIDS, the talk sometimes gets reduced to a debate about whether to "just say no" or to "do it, do it, do it," without ever asking what are we doing when we "do it"? Why are we doing it? For pleasure? Out of obligation? To demonstrate love? For all of these reasons? And why is one way of having sex considered right, and another considered wrong? The sexual culture promotes intercourse between a woman and a man as something that should "come naturally." But if intercourse "comes naturally," why is only one partner coming?

Recognizing that sex is not natural, but rather a product of culture, opens up exciting possibilities for change. Reinventing sex is a radical project that involves more than just trying new positions or buying a sex toy (although these can definitely add to the fun). Changing the way we have sex requires thinking in profoundly different ways about the body, about power relations between women and men, and about sex itself. It means developing a new language to talk about sex in more equal terms. By imagining a new sexuality, women and men will do much more than enhance their own enjoyment. Making sex an act of shared, mutual pleasure is an essential part of creating true gender equality.

Four Myths

In order to begin rethinking sex, it is useful to first consider several taken-for-granted assumptions or myths that are the foundation of the sexual culture.

Myth #1: Women = Sex

In our society, the body of a woman—a young, beautiful, revealingly dressed woman—is the symbol for sex. More precisely, certain parts of a woman's body stand for sex because they are a turn-on for heterosexual men. A woman's breast and buttocks are probably the prime icons of sex, but long legs, high heels, big hair, and a round, red mouth are also widespread cultural symbols that set up the sexual equation. The woman, like the car, the beer, or the magazine her body advertises, is an object of desire. A sexy woman is an item of consumption, and man is her consumer.

Equating sex with an idealized female image puts real women in a sexual no-person's land. The vast majority of women neither meet the criteria of what is sexy nor fit the profile of the consumer. Most women know that our sexual culture does not have them in mind when, for example, a magazine article entitled "Sex" is illustrated by a nineteen-year-old blonde in a Wonder-bra, garter belt, and spike heels.

Every woman knows what it is to struggle with what one friend calls "the body thing." Women learn from the time they are young to treat their own bodies as perpetual improvement projects as they strive to emulate an externally imposed image of what is sexy. A woman's growth as a sexual person is compromised by the goal of looking sexy on the outside, and eventually a woman becomes estranged from what her body feels on the inside.

One woman told us that from the time she was a teenager, she felt she was expected to look *sexy* but never to be or feel *sexual*. She often dressed in provocative ways. "But if I went beyond a certain point," she says, "my father would call me awful names. I never had it right, and I still don't." A woman is made to feel like a performer on a tightrope who walks a fine line imposed by the demands of the audience below—an audience that eggs her on while simultaneously criticizing her as shameless for performing in the first place. Despite its perils, this performance is one that many women feel compelled to carry out.

In a sexual culture that equates sex with the female body, a woman is told that she deserves sexual pleasure only if she looks attractive. Many women get great satisfaction from dressing up, but focusing on being attractive on the outside can interfere with sexual satisfaction within. A woman may never cultivate or respond to her own feelings or desires because she develops her sexuality based on the way others see, touch, and treat her.

The sexual culture's emphasis on a woman's exterior makes it difficult for her to develop a healthy sexual self. In reinventing sex, women can turn the focus of sex to their own experience of their bodies. They can have sex on their own terms, a privilege most men take for granted. Instead of handing her sexuality over to others, a woman controls and possesses it herself. She can enjoy orgasm when and if she wants to—she is neither pressured into coming to boost her partner's ego, nor denied orgasm because of neglect. When women reinvent sex, a woman will not earn good sex because she fits a sexy physical ideal. Instead, she will deserve good sex because she is a human being.

Myth #2: Sex = Intercourse

When heterosexuals refer to "sex," they usually mean vaginal intercourse. Whether euphemism ("the sex act"), slang ("getting laid"), or profanity ("fucking"), most words for *sex* are actually words for *intercourse*. Even many women get in the habit of thinking of intercourse as the only *real* sex. A woman recently told us that she likes to use a vibrator to have an orgasm before she has "sex." Apparently, sex does not begin until a penis gets into the act.

Vaginal penetration by the penis is the defining act of sex for most heterosexuals. A recent survey found that 95 percent of heterosexuals usually or always have intercourse when they have sex. Other sexual activities, such as manual and oral sex, sometimes serve only as either a warm-up for intercourse or an imitation of it. French kissing and finger penetration are sometimes performed to mimic it more than for their own intrinsic pleasures. Even though intercourse is the way women are least likely to come, the sexual culture places the greatest value on orgasm that results from intercourse. Clitoral stimulation is overlooked in favor of penetration, and the stereotype is that women want a man who is "long, hard, and can go all night long." Even many vibrators are shaped like a penis because it is assumed that a man's source of pleasure—the penis—should also sexually satisfy a woman.

Vaginal penetration is a rite of passage in our sexual culture. It is the only sex act that can validate marriage. (Lesbians are not granted any comparable rite to validate a partnership.) It is a testament to the crucial meaning of intercourse that a woman can engage in masturbation or in manual, oral, or anal sex with a partner and have an orgasm, perhaps multiple orgasms, but she is still a "virgin" if her vagina has not been penetrated by a penis. A woman's virginity is something *only* a man's penis—and not his hands or mouth, much less the woman herself, or another woman—has the power to take away.

To "go all the way" means arriving at the ultimate destination: vaginal penetration. For most men, intercourse is the last stop on the sex train. His orgasm announces to the woman that the trip is over. Intercourse is where she should get off, too. But it leaves most women idling on the tracks, their engines still running.

It is little wonder that men come easily during vaginal penetration. Intercourse brings a man to orgasm because the male counterpart of the clitoris lies within the penis, and the penis is surrounded on all sides by massaging vaginal walls. A woman's clitoris lies mostly within her body separate from the vagina. Her clitoris is mostly untouched by intercourse. Only the exposed tip and clitoral shaft receive some stimulation from the tugs and strokes of the man's penis or from intermittent pressure from his pelvis. For some women, this is sufficient for orgasm, especially if they are "on top." Most of the time, however, expecting intercourse alone to result in a woman's orgasm is comparable to expecting Joe to be satisfied by a massage of his testicles. It feels good, but the longer Nikki does it, the more likely he is to feel annoyed than to have an orgasm.

The low rate of orgasm for women is correlated with the high rate of intercourse-oriented sex. Intercourse simply does not give enough direct stimulation to the clitoris for orgasm to occur in most women. The penis and the clitoris pass one another like ships in the night, but only the penis makes it to port. Yet amidst multiple messages that it is the high point of sex, a woman battles a lingering feeling that she *should* be able to achieve orgasm during coitus.

A woman gets caught in a catch-22. Sex consists of intercourse, which does not make her come. Oral and manual sex do make her come, but they are seen as remedial or even "deviant" forms of sex. Oral sex is only a rare offering and manual sex is confined to foreplay, if done at all.

To some, intercourse may seem an imperative of nature. The vagina and the penis appear destined for each other, or rather, the vagina is made for the penis. The penis slips so easily into the vagina, like a sword into its sheath. Indeed, vagina *means* sheath. Its very name implies that the vagina has no sexual identity of its own but only becomes a sexual organ when the penis enters it.

The act of intercourse reflects the larger cultural notion that sex is something that men do *to* women. Even women's active role in reproduction is made to seem passive. The penis in intercourse is likened to a plow that prepares the soil and presses the seed into a receptive earth. Because of its role in reproduction, intercourse is seen as the natural way to have sex. People often point to other animals: Birds "do it," bees "do it," and so do cats and dogs. Sexual intercourse is indeed the typical and optimal means for egg to meet sperm in humans. But people engage in sex for conception only a few times in their lives. Above all, they have sex for pleasure. And as anyone who masturbates knows, the most fun one can have in sex, hands down, is orgasm.

Myth #3: Women and Men Are Different and Unequal

Perhaps the most influential myth of our sexual culture is that women and men are opposite sexes. But rather than opposite and equal, men are taken as the norm, and women the deviation. Women are both men's opposites and their inferiors. The apparently greater size of men's genitals is sometimes read as evidence of their more powerful sex drive, while women's seemingly smaller genitals reflect a lesser interest in sex. Seen as inferior in so many ways, it is not surprising that women tend to come out "on the bottom" in sex.

The myth that women are sexually inferior to men is supported by three beliefs: (1) that women have a lesser sex drive than men; (2) that women do not need orgasm as men do; and (3) that women have lesser genitals than men.

Women Have a Lesser Sex Drive Than Men   The sex drive is not considered the result of social conditioning or experience but as an inborn or natural gender trait. In our sexual culture, it is believed that "female hormones" (actually, the excess of female and shortage of male hormones, especially testosterone) make women less sexual. Yet hormones and other biological processes used as evidence of sex difference are always interpreted according to the terms of the culture. Women's lower levels of testosterone are said to explain why women initiate sex less often than men, but this ignores how women get decades of training to please others and are told they are "bad" if they act on their own sexual desires. Women can be so busy responding to desires of men and the sexual culture that they hardly get a chance to cultivate their own. Women's capacity for multiple orgasms, for example, rarely gets nurtured, while the qualities that contribute to men's pleasure—beauty and sexual acquiescence—are rewarded and emphasized.

The notion of a natural sex drive helps to validate men's sexual priority. It is believed that women simply never experience the same urge to have sex "right now" that men do. Indeed, some men blame their uncontrollable sex drive when they pressure women for sex ("You got me so turned on"). It explains why men visit prostitutes or cheat on their wives or girlfriends ("Men have sexual needs"). It is even used to absolve the man and blame the woman for her own rape ("He was so turned on by her, he couldn't stop"). It seems that men simply cannot help themselves when sex goes into overdrive. For a woman to express a strong sex drive, in contrast, is seen as unnatural, even immoral. A woman who expresses an urgent desire for sex risks being seen as a "slut."

That our society considers sex a "drive" at all renders it a force beyond human control. It supports the notion that there is little an individual can do to control nature's engine. But neither men's so-called sex drive nor women's apparent indifference to sex is the product of biology and hormones, for sex unfolds in a social context. In a society that organizes sex around achieving men's orgasm and that caters to men's sexual pleasure in countless other ways, it is not surprising that a woman might show less interest in sex. But it is not because they are born that way. When sex lacks the clitoral stimulation that most women enjoy to orgasm, it becomes a self-fulfilling prophecy that women are the less sexual half of the population. Yet when men have orgasms and women do not, the difference is treated as the playing out of the distinct sexual natures of females and males, rather than as the result of sex socialization by gender and the sexual culture's definition of sex as intercourse to the man's orgasm.

Women Do Not Need Orgasm as Men Do Orgasm is practically a medical Rx for a man. If he becomes sexually aroused and does not reach orgasm and ejaculate, it is said he will suffer "blue balls." The man's visually obvious erection makes penetration (or, as many women well know, a hand job or a blow job) seem imperative. Even though a woman also experiences the equivalent of an erection, our sexual culture neither names nor recognizes this event. A woman is not described as suffering from "blue clit" if her sexual arousal does not culminate in orgasm—even though the frustration of sex that ends before orgasm is a much more common experience for women than it is for men.

To acknowledge that women need orgasms as much as men do is to suggest that women and men are much more alike sexually than different. This idea challenges the sexual culture because it implies that women are capable of and deserve pleasure no less than men.

> There are very few absolute sex differences and . . . without complete social equality we cannot know for sure what they are.
> —Anne Fausto Sterling, *Myths of Gender*

Women Have Lesser Genitals Than Men The sexual culture focuses on the towering erection of the man's penis while it ignores the fact that the erectile tissues of a woman's clitoris and bulbs are the same size and also respond to stimulation. The organs of both sexes expand and become firm during sexual arousal, yet the event that is so significant in men, erection, is not even acknowledged in women.

The sexual culture defines erection as a purely male phenomenon and spotlights vaginal "wetness" in women. Vaginal lubrication is interpreted as a sign of female readiness for penetration (and the man's pleasure). It ignores how a woman's genitals become erect in the same process of blood engorgement and muscle tension that a man experiences.

Our sexual culture evaluates genitals based not on how people experience pleasure, but on how well they fit into a model of sex that features the penis in a starring role. When the stage is set for sex, the man's large, assertive organ appears at center stage and the vagina plays the part of its accommodating sidekick. The woman's clitoris acts only as a puny, uncredited extra who barely emerges from the wings.

Myth #4: Women Want Intimacy; Men Want Sex

An extension of the myth of gender difference is the belief that women and men want different things when they have sex: Women want decor (wine and candlelight), while men want hard core (genital sex and orgasm). Men want to penetrate and come; women want to cuddle and talk. Intimacy and genital sex are presented as opposite and irreconcilable goals. Women complain of not getting enough intimacy and attention, while men complain of not getting enough "sex." Women and men have indeed been taught to eat different halves of the sexual pie. But even after she gets her slice of closeness, and he gets his serving of orgasm, they both may be left feeling hungry. Perhaps the reason men get sex less often than they want is because women are not sexually satisfied. And women who are sexually unsatisfied turn their interests elsewhere. Susan Quilliam, who surveyed British women on sex, suggests that women may focus on intimacy to compensate for the lack of orgasms. A woman who reg-

Your (Society's) Sexual IQ Test

1. What sexual activity is most likely to bring a woman to orgasm?
   a. intercourse
   b. clitoral stimulation
   c. sex with a partner she loves
2. What shape does the female clitoris most resemble?
   a. a four-inch wishbone
   b. a pea
   c. a miniature penis
3. When is sex between a woman and a man usually considered over?
   a. when the woman has an orgasm
   b. when each partner is sexually satisfied
   c. when the man ejaculates
4. What is the most common sign that a woman is having an orgasm?
   a. her pelvic muscle contracts
   b. her chest flushes red
   c. she moans
5. Some women ejaculate a fluid in sex that is chemically closest to
   a. urine
   b. vaginal secretions
   c. prostatic fluid similar to men's

6. What is the average duration of heterosexual vaginal intercourse?
   a. one hour
   b. two to three minutes
   c. fifteen minutes
7. Who can masturbate to orgasm faster?
   a. men
   b. women
   c. women and men can be equally fast
8. Only some women have a G spot.
   T
   F
9. A woman's vagina always lubricates or gets "wet" when she is sexually excited.
   T
   F
10. When sexually excited, women experience the same engorgement and increased muscle tension that is known as "erection" in men.
    T
    F

ANSWERS AT THE END OF THE READING.

ularly has sex without orgasms would indeed begin to think that pleasure must lie elsewhere.

With the mantra "Women want intimacy and men want sex," sexuality splits into two parts, each assigned to one gender. Author and relationship guru John Gray goes even further. He argues in his books *Men Are from Mars, Women Are from Venus* and *Mars and Venus in the Bedroom* that, when it comes to relationships and sex, women and men are from different planets. This view is popular because it reassures heterosexual couples that there is nothing wrong with them. If they feel alienated from their partner, it is because she or he truly is an alien. Gray's view encourages people to believe that the problems between women and men are a result of innate differences that cannot be changed. Gray completely ignores how the sexual culture teaches women to focus on intimacy and men to focus on sex. By characterizing women as an emotional "planet" and men as a sexual "planet," he dresses up the sexual culture's oldest stereotypes in New Age garb. In bed, the two planets remain separated by the orgasm gap.

Rather than assigning intimacy to women and sex to men, sex could be better for everyone if it included both experiences. The last time we looked, women and men both lived on Earth, a planet located midway between Venus and Mars. Here on Earth, both women and men are capable of enjoying intimacy along with orgasmic sex. In fact, instead of conflicting, the two pleasures enhance one another. Orgasmic sex and intimacy are part of a single continuum of sexual, emotional, mental, and physical expression. When women reinvent sex, both women and men will have equal access to all the fruits in the same garden of earthly delights.

What Women (Do Not) Want

What do women want, Freud asked. The old fool, the charlatan. He knew what women wanted. They wanted nothing. Nothing was good enough. Everyone knew that.

—A Woman Reflecting on Sex
in Carol Shields's Novel, *The Stone Diaries*

In this book, we gather together ideas and resources women can use to reinvent sex. We focus on the body and begin by rethinking women's bodies and sexuality; but a similar process for men is also needed. By considering the pleasures and desires women and men share, both can work together to debunk the myths and develop alternative, more inclusive, and more equal attitudes and activities that will make sex not just male fun, but mutual fun.

In Orgasm Denial

Reinventing sex requires that women recognize the problems of the sexual culture. Yet many women are in denial about the orgasm gap. Some ignore the problem because they have great, orgasmic sex with their partners. They say they feel no need to rethink sex, thank you very much. "Is there a problem?" asked one twentysomething college graduate who told us she has three orgasms every time she has sex. Some thirty-, forty- and fiftysomething urban professional women ask us: "Didn't we already do this in the 1970s?" And our mother tells us that she and all her World War II–generation friends figured out orgasmic sex without a hitch.

The key phrase here is "figured out." Many of these women just stumbled upon orgasm by accident or they were lucky enough to have a knowledgeable partner. Others became orgasmic in solo sex by violating the taboo against masturbation. All of them figured out how to enjoy sex not through the sexual culture, but *in spite of it.* One by one, each woman had to reinvent the sexual wheel.

There are other women, however, who are either unable or not inspired to make this effort. In a sexual culture in denial about women's orgasms, it can take a substantial effort to make partner sex satisfying. Since women's pleasure is not a topic either among women, in sex education, or even in the media, only a woman who goes out of her way to learn about sex is likely to become orgasmic. The silence surrounding female sexuality hurts even orgasmic women because it fails to acknowledge or give authority to their experiences of sex. A woman who comes with oral sex, for example, may enjoy sex less because she is wondering, "Am I coming the 'right' way?" A woman who has orgasms now and then may lack the information, opportunity, and encouragement to ask why sex is not always orgasmic. She may prefer to keep the peace rather than stir up trouble, especially when the solution challenges not only her taken-for-granted assumptions about sex, but also her relations with men.

Many women are aware of the orgasm gap but prefer not to confront it. We know women who have been married for decades, with grown children and sexually satisfied husbands, who have never had an orgasm. When they have sex they focus on the man's pleasure. Some have orgasms when they masturbate, but have not mustered the courage or developed the communication skills to talk to their partner about making orgasm a mutual part of sex together. A few have partners who refuse to change they way they have sex. For these women, orgasm looms as a rather daunting challenge rather than being something they look forward to enjoying.

Attaining orgasmic sex is sometimes so bewildering that, when a woman finally does have orgasms regularly with a partner, she may confuse what she feels with love. Or, she may stay in a relationship because she is afraid she will not find another partner who "gives" her orgasms. Good sex may enhance love, and love often enhances sex, but they are not the same thing.

Some feminists and sex therapists fear that encouraging women to strive for orgasm only adds to the women's feelings of sexual inadequacy. But in the name of protecting women's feelings, this view may inadvertently make orgasm all the more elusive for women. It implies that it is a woman's own fault that she does not have orgasms, rather than the fault of the way sex is defined. Others downplay the importance of orgasm because they believe that to celebrate orgasm is to succumb to male values. In a more female-oriented sexuality, they suggest, sensual pleasures such as caressing, kissing, and holding would supersede genital sex and orgasm. Women can enjoy what a special 1995 issue of *Ms.* magazine referred to as "hot unscripted sex," that is, "whatever turns you on."

Widening women's options for sexual pleasure is important, but to dismiss orgasm is to throw out the baby with the bathwater. This view also falls into the gender-stereotyped orgasm-versus-intimacy trap. Leaving women's physical pleasure vaguely defined as "whatever" makes it more likely that women's natural capacity for orgasm will remain undeveloped. A woman can always choose *not* to come, but it only truly becomes a choice for her when orgasm becomes a readily available option.

Dismantling the Sex Machine

Most observers of the 1960s now agree that the sexual revolution was a boon for sex—that is, if you were a heterosexual male. Many women expected that all the commotion would revolutionize sex for them, too. Some of them believed that by simply having *more* sex, with *more* partners, in *more* intercourse positions, or *more* days of the week, sex would become as good for them as it seemed to be for men. But more sex did not necessarily mean better sex for women, because the balance of pleasure did not change. Even when oral sex came into fashion, and more men were willing to give women cunnilingus (oral sex on a woman) than ever before, rates of fellatio (oral sex on a man) rose, too, and always remained higher. The so-called sexual revolution failed women because it did not change sex in the fundamental ways necessary to make it more *equal* fun. Ultimately, the revolution only revved up the existing sex machine. It oiled the gears, when what was needed was to dismantle the engine, melt down the parts, and completely rebuild sex from the inside out of women's experience. This has not yet happened and, as a result, at the turn of a new century, many women are still stuck in the missionary position wondering, "Did the sexual revolution come yet? . . . because I haven't!"

It is now time to rethink sex in fundamental ways. Feminists and lesbian, gay, and bisexual activists of recent decades form the vanguard of a contemporary rethinking that promises a *real* revolution in sex. Like the little girl in the village crowd who announced that the emperor had no clothes, these groups are revealing the secret that women habitually keep to themselves: Sex as it is currently defined does not satisfy women.

Crucial ingredients for reinventing sex have been contributed by people such as Shere Hite, who published a study reporting what thousands of women themselves said about sex. *The Hite Report: A Nationwide Study of Female Sexuality* was a highly controversial book that revealed the discrepancy between what women were supposed to experience in sex and what they actually felt. Critics found fault with its lack of statistical method (even though the gist of Hite's findings has been borne out by other, more "scientific" studies). Some bristled at its radical views of both sex and society. But many women found that what Hite was saying rang true to their own experience. The sexual culture was not ready to hear that sex (essentially, intercourse) was not as satisfying for women as it was for men.

Out of the grass-roots women's health movement came a new view of women's bodies. Organized through community clinics and epitomized by books such as The Boston Women's Health Book Collective's *Our Bodies, Ourselves,* first published in 1969, this movement encouraged women to take charge of their own health, including their sexual health, and to resist the alienating messages of the media and the medical establishment that treated women as either objects *for* or imperfect versions *of* men. By advocating that each woman learn to examine her own cervix and breasts and to take responsibility for her own sexual pleasure, the movement helped women to gain a greater measure of control over their bodies and lives.

The rethinking of female sexual well-being continues with books such as *A New View of a Woman's Body,* by a collective known as the Federation of Feminist Women's Health Centers, which replaces the male model of sex with one based on women's own experiences, observations, and self-examinations.

Lesbians and bisexual women are among the feminists who have challenged many facets of women's role in the sexual culture. With their critique of what Adrienne Rich called compulsory heterosexuality, activists in the lesbian, gay, bisexual, and transgender movement have helped imagine a new sexual culture for both themselves and others. Their work has made it easier for young women to avoid settling into sexual roles and ways of having sex that do not have women's best interest in mind. In their assertion that "we are here," lesbians, bisexual women and men, gay men, and transgendered people have forced the whole society to question traditional assumptions about sex and sexual categories. Bisexual visibility has put flesh on sex researcher Alfred Kinsey's view of sexual orientation as a continuum by suggesting that sexuality is more fluid and open than the categories of "heterosexual" or "homosexual" allow. Mainstream popular culture now acclaims gender-bending performers, such as the androgynous k.d. lang and flamboyant drag queen Ru Paul, who undermine the sexual culture's insistence that "femininity" and "masculinity" are inherent to people who have the genitals of women and men respectively. Books such as Martine Rothblatt's *The Apartheid of Sex,* Leslie Feinberg's *Transgender Warriors,* appearances by transsexuals on TV talk shows, and public writings by feminist scientists such as biologist Anne Fausto-Sterling (who asserts that there are five sexes at least) have created greater awareness that neither the genitals nor gender come in two neatly separated types.

The impact of these challenges on the sexual culture has been heightened by the AIDS epidemic. The need for a conscious and radical change in the way people engage in sex has rarely been more urgent than it is today when the questions are no longer simply whether to say yes or no. The questions people now face confront the very purpose and definition of sex. What is sex? Why have sex? Who is sex for? These questions force everyone to scrutinize and rethink the most taken-for-granted and fundamental aspects of sex. They unsettle sexual complacency and prepare the ground for reinventing sex for women's pleasure.

A clear alternative framework for sex has yet to be established, but it is in the process of emerging. Women are at the vanguard of this change, one that will transform not only how people have sex, but how the genitals themselves are envisioned.

It's the Clitoris, Stupid

Reinventing sex for women and men starts with outing the clitoris. The clitoris is absent from most talk about sex, especially compared to its high-profile acquaintance and alleged counterpart, the penis. References to the penis so often go without mention of its orgasm-producing counterpart in women that it sometimes seems as if the sexual culture had undergone a clitoridectomy. The vagina gets far more attention than the clitoris, and not just because it is the pathway to the uterus and conception. The vagina matters because it provides pleasure to the penis. The clitoris sometimes receives perfunctory attention as a prelude to intercourse, but that stimulation is usually neither sufficient nor appropriate for setting off a woman's orgasm.

Given its low profile, it is not surprising that the location, size, and behavior of the clitoris is a mystery for some men. One woman told us that she has considered pinning up a picture over her bed with a diagram of her genitals with arrows pointing to her clitoris and a label "Touch here."

Even men who earnestly search out the clitoris in order to pleasure their partner often have trouble finding or keeping track of it. Others have difficulty staying with it long enough to allow the woman to come, or they are not sure how to stimulate it to their partner's satisfaction. When men realize that they have a clitoris too (which, as we will show, is inside their penis), they may be better able to appreciate why it is worth finding on a woman.

Women themselves may often be unable to instruct their partner because their own familiarity with female anatomy is limited. Many women avoid touching their genitals, and few are on the same first-name basis with their own clitoris that they are with their partner's penis. Boys grow up hearing jokes and stories about the exploits of the penis, but girls hear the word clitoris so infrequently that many are not even sure where the accent falls (clí-to-ris and cli-tor´-is are both acceptable). A boy often learns from other boys what his penis can do, but a girl rarely talks about her clitoris with other girls and few get acquainted with it on their own. Indeed a woman can reach adulthood without even being aware that she has a clitoris. If a girl discovers clitoral pleasure, she often does so only by accident. The exact location of the good feeling between her legs remains a mystery to her.

Contributing to the clitoris's anonymity are sex education texts that portray it as a tiny organ that "hides" beneath its hood when erect, invoking the stereotype that women are sexually shy. Even when the sexual culture does acknowledge the clitoris, it cuts the organ down to a smaller size. Few women or men are aware that the clitoris is not a pea-sized penis, but is more than four inches long and extends inside the body.

It was decades ago that laboratory studies confirmed millions of women's own experience that the clitoris was the trigger for orgasm. Every sexologist from Hite to Masters and Johnson to Dr. Ruth has made it clear that the clitoris is the place to stimulate a woman to orgasm. Yet the sexual culture's focus on intercourse continues undeterred. Freud's contention that women who came only via clitoral stimulation suffered from a "sexual dysfunction" still infects how people talk about sex, and there is a lingering sentiment that the "vaginal orgasm" should be a mature woman's goal.

Other misconceptions haunt the clitoris as well. Updated sex manuals such as *Sex: A Man's Guide* by Stefan Bechtel, Laurence Roy Stains, and the editors of Men's Health Books and *Mind-blowing Sex in the Real World: Hot Tips for Doing It in the Age of Anxiety* by Sari Locker describe the woman's clitoris as "the only organ designed solely for pleasure." But even their inaccurate hyperbole (since men have this sensitive organ, too) does not raise the clitoris to the stature of the penis. Sex remains focused on penis-in-vagina intercourse, often to the exclusion of the kinds of sexual activity that directly stimulate the clitoris. In women's magazines, for example, articles on sex dutifully mention the importance of clitoral stimulation for women's orgasm, but rather than encouraging women to stimulate the clitoris directly, they frequently end up advising women to get on top in intercourse and hope for the best.

There are signs that the clitoris is beginning to get noticed. Many sex educators, activists, and researchers are trying to bring the clitoris out into public discussion. Humor books such as Holly Hughes's *Clit Notes* put the word on the front table of some bookstores and woman-friendly sex outlets such as Good Vibrations and Eve's Garden advertise vibrators and other sex toys in mainstream magazines. But in a sexual culture either afraid or disinclined to examine women's genitals too closely, there are still millions of women and men who remain unaware of the clitoris's orgasmic power.

It's the G Spot, Too

In 1982, a book called *The G Spot* by Alice Kahn Ladas, Beverly Whipple, and John D. Perry brought attention to another source of female sexual pleasure at a spot that can be reached through the vagina a few inches inside on the front wall. With the book, women familiar with pleasurable sensations from that area finally had their experience validated. But some feminists believed that the G spot was just a craze or a fad. Worst of all, it seemed to revive

Freud's notion of the vaginal orgasm. Many women never even bothered to look for the G spot because they considered it a hoax, while others saw it as just one more sexual goal women were expected to achieve. Despite the controversy, the book helped women who were willing to explore to find their G spot. (Using the fingers works better than searching with their partner's penis.) A woman we know in her forties who never read the earlier book only found her G spot recently after reading Chapter 6 of this book. "I can't believe I've been having sex all these years and didn't know about this!" she told us.

Some researchers hypothesize that the G spot is the female prostate gland, similar to the male prostate gland. Men's prostate gland is also sexually sensitive and can be stimulated along the front anal wall, while the woman's G spot can be stimulated along the front vaginal wall. (Women can get "prostate" cancer, too, although it is less common and usually not life-threatening.) Although it is stimulated through the vagina, the G spot surrounds the urethra. Stimulating the G spot with the fingers, what we call G spotting, creates pleasurable feelings and can lead to orgasm.

G spotting also makes some women ejaculate. Like male ejaculation, female ejaculation is a pleasurable sexual experience in which fluid spurts out of the urethra. Yet women who ejaculate are often told they are "urinating." If they look female ejaculation up in books, they will find either no reference to it at all or contradictory opinions about what it is and doubts about whether it occurs. Those who have experienced or observed female ejaculation know that it occurs, and that ejaculate does not smell or look like urine. It is thought to be prostatic fluid similar to male ejaculate without the sperm. But debate persists among researchers about where it comes from and why only some women ejaculate.

The current sexual culture takes little account of either female ejaculation or the G spot because they do not fit into the existing framework for female sexuality. The current model of sex also keeps the clitoris a secret, depriving women of the information they need to enjoy orgasm. All of these secrets and misconceptions can be cleared away by reinventing sex from the inside of women's own experiences of pleasure.

Sex Transformed

Reinventing sex requires a new framework for understanding the body and sexual activity. Because the sexual culture has focused on men, and even sees women's bodies in terms of male (and, only secondarily, female) pleasure, women currently lack the concepts and words with which to talk about their sexuality. Women have neither names for genital parts nor words to describe the sexual techniques that make sex orgasmic. New words and a new language for sex will allow women to talk with and learn from one another. A new vocabulary will help women to communicate with a partner and will fundamentally change how women and men have sex.

Some new terms for *women's genitals* we develop in this book include:

- **Orgasmic Crescent.** This is our term for the crescent-shaped area that is women's pleasure center. The orgasmic crescent begins at the clitoris and extends back across the opening of the urethra (another sexual area) and up inside the vagina behind the pubic bone to the G spot. The labia swell when a woman is erect. Stimulating all the areas along the orgasmic crescent at the same time can give a woman a powerful orgasm. Some women also ejaculate.

- **Cligeva (cli-GEE-va).** This is our name for women's genitals as a whole. No word now exists that includes all of women's sexual parts. The word combines the most important sexual parts for women's pleasure. The word combines the first syllable of each sexual part—the clitoris, the G spot, and the vagina. The final "a" also refers to the anus, an often overlooked site of pleasure. The word also has the advantage of listing the parts in the order in which many women like to be genitally stimulated.

We also use new words for *sexual techniques* that focus on women's pleasure including:

- **Manual Sex.** Many people use their hands in partner sex to great effect, yet they rarely use the name for it, manual sex. Manual sex is a widely practiced and highly pleasurable sexual art that has been trivialized as "foreplay" or "petting." As one of the most direct routes to orgasm for women, it deserves being promoted to a category of sex on a par with intercourse and oral sex.

- **Clittage (cli-TAZH).** This is our word for the most basic kind of manual sex—manual stimulation of the clitoris. It combines clitoris and massage. Clittage or clitoral massage is the most common way women reach orgasm, yet this sexual act has no name. Fingers—one's own or a partner's—can provide orgasmic pleasure at any time, including during intercourse or in a mutually orgasmic quickie. Clittage can also be effectively performed with a vibrator.

Your (Society's) Sexual IQ Test Answers

1. b

Most women reach orgasm from direct clitoral stimulation, not from vaginal intercourse. Women who have orgasms during intercourse are probably doing so primarily because of clitoral stimulation, either from indirect pressure or from direct manual stimulation. While feelings of love certainly can enhance sexual pleasure, love does not provide the genital stimulation needed for orgasm.

2. a

The shape of the entire clitoris resembles a four-inch wishbone. It extends from the external and visible pea-sized tip, up the shaft and into the body. The legs of the clitoris inside the body split off like those of a wishbone onto either side of the vaginal walls. Men also have a clitoris inside the penis that is the same size as women's (relative to body size), but its legs are shorter. The tip of the man's clitoris cannot be touched directly because it lies underneath the head of the penis. The tip of the woman's clitoris is usually compared to the whole penis, but this is like comparing a part to a whole. The more accurate comparison is between the entire female and the entire male clitoris, from tip to legs.

3. c

Sex between a woman and a man is usually considered over when the man ejaculates (it is assumed he has had an orgasm, too). The woman's orgasm (and certainly not her ejaculation) is not a required part of sex as currently defined.

4. a

The pelvic muscle (specifically the PC or pubococcygeus muscle) usually contracts during orgasm in both women and men. Masters and Johnson observed a red flush on some women's chests during orgasm, but most women do not experience or observe this. A woman and a man can tell when a woman is having an orgasm by the buildup of her erection, her PC muscle contractions, and the subsequent release of muscle tension and blood in her genitals.

Many men expect women to make the same synthesized moans during orgasm that women perform in pornographic movies and on records. Instead, when her attention is truly riveted on the pleasure in her body, a woman may let out a scream or make no sound at all. There is no standard performance for orgasm.

5. c

It is not known what percentage of women ejaculate. It is possible that all women ejaculate but the amount of fluid is very small, so they are not aware of it. All women have a prostate gland or G spot and a urethra and therefore all are potentially capable of ejaculating. Yet because the sexual culture rarely acknowledges female ejaculation, most neither find their G spot nor learn how to ejaculate. Women who do ejaculate are sometimes told they are urinating and some women stifle their ejaculations. Others mistake the fluid as an abundance of vaginal juices. But female ejaculate comes out of the urethra, just as it does in men, and is a watery fluid chemically similar to prostatic fluid in men.

6. b

Vaginal intercourse lasts an average of two to three minutes. The average length of the whole sexual encounter is typically just fifteen minutes. Sex that begins with the man's erection and ends when he comes rarely lasts more than an hour.

7. c

It takes women and men about the same amount of time—about four to five minutes, on average—to reach orgasm. When women take longer to come than men or do not come at all, it is usually because they are not getting adequate clitoral stimulation.

8. F

Most body parts are not optional. If some women have a G spot, it is likely that all women do. Many women have never looked for their G spot because they are either unaware of it or doubt it exists. Rather than asking whether or not all women have a G spot, women should be asking why it remains a mystery instead of being treated as a pleasurable fact of a woman's sexual experience.

9. F

Some women get wet when they are sexually excited, yet all women are made to feel that vaginal lubrication is a measure of their sexual "responsiveness." Vaginal wetness is not always an accurate way to evaluate a woman's state of arousal. The more useful indicator in both women and men is the genital engorgement and muscle tension that occurs with erection.

10. T

When a woman is aroused, her genitals, including the clitoris and G spot, engorge with blood and the PC muscle becomes taut. This same process is called an *erection* in men. Women's genital erections have so far gone ignored and unnamed.

- **G Spotting.** Another kind of manual sex involves stroking the G spot with the fingers. G spotting can also be done with a dildo or performed by a man with his erect penis.

- **Forget Foreplay.** In a sexual culture that includes women's pleasure, "foreplay" will disappear. Instead of being treated as a prelude to sex, the manual and oral sex that now make up foreplay would become the central features of sex.

- **Ladies First.** This rule of orgasmic etiquette appears in many sex manuals but is frequently ignored in practice. Ladies first reminds a man that woman's orgasm (at least her first one) ideally comes before intercourse and always before the man ejaculates. This ensures a woman of orgasm every time she has sex with a man.

- **Mutual Erection.** The genitals of both women and men become erect when sexually aroused. Even though women's genitals become engorged (and therefore erect), women's erections have been ignored. Erection is as conducive to a woman's orgasm as it is to a man's. Similarly, a woman's erection is as essential for intercourse as a man's penis. Vaginal penetration is far more pleasurable for a woman when she is erect. Mutual erection makes intercourse an orgasmic experience for *both* partners.

New words and concepts for sex will enable women to bridge the orgasm gap. Sex will not longer take place solely on men's terms. Instead, it will unfold according to a new sexuality that is equally oriented toward women's pleasure.

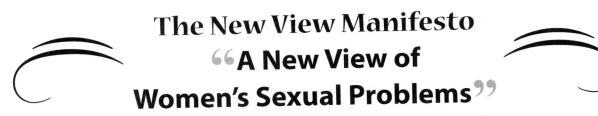

The New View Manifesto
"A New View of Women's Sexual Problems"

by The Working Group on A New View of Women's Sexual Problems[1]

Introduction: Beyond the Medical Model of Sexuality

In recent years, publicity about new treatments for men's erection problems has focused attention on women's sexuality and provoked a competitive commercial hunt for "the female Viagra." But women's sexual problems differ from men's in basic ways which are not being examined or addressed. We believe that a fundamental barrier to understanding women's sexuality is the medical classification scheme in current use, developed by the American Psychiatric Association (APA) for its *Diagnostic and Statistical Manual of Disorders (DSM)* in 1980, and revised in 1987 and 1994.[2] It divides (both men's and) women's sexual problems into four categories of sexual "dysfunction": sexual desire disorders, sexual arousal disorders, orgasmic disorders, and sexual pain disorders.

These "dysfunctions" are disturbances in an assumed universal physiological sexual response pattern ("normal function") originally described by Masters and Johnson in the 1960s.[3] This universal pattern begins, in theory, with sexual drive, and proceeds sequentially through the stages of desire, arousal, and orgasm.

In recent decades, the shortcomings of the framework, as it applies to women, have been amply documented.[4] The three most serious distortions produced by a framework that reduces sexual problems to disorders of physiological function, comparable to breathing or digestive disorders, are:

1. A false notion of sexual equivalency between men and women. Because the early researchers emphasized similarities in men's and women's physiological responses during sexual activities,

they concluded that sexual disorders must also be similar. Few investigators asked women to describe their experiences from their own points of view. When such studies were done, it became apparent that women and men differ in many crucial ways. Women's accounts do not fit neatly into the Masters and Johnson model; for example, women generally do not separate "desire" from "arousal," women care less about physical than subjective arousal, and women's sexual complaints frequently focus on "difficulties" that are absent from the *DSM*.[5]

Furthermore, an emphasis on genital and physiological similarities between men and women ignores the implications of inequalities related to gender, social class, ethnicity, sexual orientation, etc. Social, political, and economic conditions, including widespread sexual violence, limit women's access to sexual health, pleasure, and satisfaction in many parts of the world. Women's social environments thus can prevent the expression of biological capacities, a reality entirely ignored by the strictly physiological framing of sexual dysfunctions.

2. The erasure of the relational context of sexuality. The American Psychiatric Association's *DSM* approach bypasses relational aspects of women's sexuality, which often lie at the root of sexual satisfactions and problems—e.g., desires for intimacy, wishes to please a partner, or, in some cases, wishes to avoid offending, losing, or angering a partner. The *DSM* takes an exclusively individual approach to sex, and assumes that if the sexual parts work, there is no problem; and if the parts don't work, there is a problem. But many women do not define their sexual difficulties this way. The *DSM*'s reduction of "normal sexual function" to physiology implies, incorrectly, that one can measure and treat genital and physical difficulties without regard to the relationship in which sex occurs.

3. The levelling of differences among women. All women are not the same, and their sexual needs, satisfactions, and problems do not fit neatly into categories of desire, arousal, orgasm, or pain. Women differ in their values, approaches to sexuality, social and cultural backgrounds, and current situations, and these differences cannot be smoothed over into an identical notion of "dysfunction"—or an identical, one-size-fits-all treatment.

Because there are no magic bullets for the sociocultural, political, psychological, social or relational bases of women's sexual problems, pharmaceutical companies are supporting research and public relations programs focused on fixing the body, especially the genitals. The infusion of industry funding into sex research and the incessant media publicity about "breakthrough" treatments have put physical problems in the spotlight and isolated them from broader contexts. Factors that are far more often sources of women's sexual complaints—relational and cultural conflicts, for example, or sexual ignorance or fear—are downplayed and dismissed. Lumped into the catchall category of "psychogenic causes," such factors go unstudied and unaddressed. Women with these problems are being excluded from clinical trials on new drugs, and yet, if current marketing patterns with men are indicative, such drugs will be aggressively advertised for all women's sexual dissatisfactions.

A corrective approach is desperately needed. We propose a new and more useful classification of women's sexual problems, one that gives appropriate priority to individual distress and inhibition arising within a broader framework of cultural and relational factors. We challenge the cultural assumptions embedded in the *DSM* and the reductionist research and marketing program of the pharmaceutical industry. We call for research and services driven not by commercial interests, but by women's own needs and sexual realities.

Sexual Health and Sexual Rights: International Views

To move away from the *DSM*'s genital and mechanical blueprint of women's sexual problems, we turned for guidance to international documents. In 1974, the World Health Organization held a unique conference on the training needs for sexual health workers. The report noted: "A growing body of knowledge indicates that problems in human sexuality are more pervasive and more important to the well-being and health of individuals in many cultures than has previously been recognized." The report emphasized the importance of taking a positive approach to human sexuality and the enhancement of relationships. It offered a broad definition of "sexual health" as "the integration of the somatic, emotional, intellectual, and social aspects of sexual being."[6]

In 1999, the World Association of Sexology, meeting in Hong Kong, adopted a Declaration of Sexual Rights.[7] "In order to assure that human beings and societies develop healthy sexuality," the Declaration stated, "the following sexual rights must be recognized, promoted, respected, and defended":

- The right to sexual freedom, excluding all forms of sexual coercion, exploitation and abuse;
- The right to sexual autonomy and safety of the sexual body;
- The right to sexual pleasure, which is a source of physical, psychological, intellectual and spiritual well-being;
- The right to sexual information . . . generated through unencumbered yet scientifically ethical inquiry;
- The right to comprehensive sexuality education;
- The right to sexual health care, which should be available for prevention and treatment of all sexual concerns, problems, and disorders.

Women's Sexual Problems: A New Classification

Sexual problems, which The Working Group on A New View of Women's Sexual Problems defines as discontent or dissatisfaction with any emotional, physical, or relational aspect of sexual experience, may arise in one or more of the following interrelated aspects of women's sexual lives.

I. SEXUAL PROBLEMS DUE TO SOCIOCULTURAL, POLITICAL, OR ECONOMIC FACTORS

A. Ignorance and anxiety due to inadequate sex education, lack of access to health services, or other social constraints:
  1. Lack of vocabulary to describe subjective or physical experience.
  2. Lack of information about human sexual biology and life-stage changes.
  3. Lack of information about how gender roles influence men's and women's sexual expectations, beliefs, and behaviors.
  4. Inadequate access to information and services for contraception and abortion, STD prevention and treatment, sexual trauma, and domestic violence.
B. Sexual avoidance or distress due to perceived inability to meet cultural norms regarding correct or ideal sexuality, including:
  1. Anxiety or shame about one's body, sexual attractiveness, or sexual responses.
  2. Confusion or shame about one's sexual orientation or identity, or about sexual fantasies and desires.
C. Inhibitions due to conflict between the sexual norms of one's subculture or culture of origin and those of the dominant culture.

D. Lack of interest, fatigue, or lack of time due to family and work obligations.

II. SEXUAL PROBLEMS RELATING TO PARTNER AND RELATIONSHIP

A. Inhibition, avoidance, or distress arising from betrayal, dislike, or fear of partner, partner's abuse or couple's unequal power, or arising from partner's negative patterns of communication.
B. Discrepancies in desire for sexual activity or in preferences for various sexual activities.
C. Ignorance or inhibition about communicating preferences or initiating, pacing, or shaping sexual activities.
D. Loss of sexual interest and reciprocity as a result of conflicts over commonplace issues such as money, schedules, or relatives, or resulting from traumatic experiences, e.g., infertility or the death of a child.
E. Inhibitions in arousal or spontaneity due to partner's health status or sexual problems.

III. SEXUAL PROBLEMS DUE TO PSYCHOLOGICAL FACTORS

A. Sexual aversion, mistrust, or inhibition of sexual pleasure due to:
  1. Past experiences of physical, sexual, or emotional abuse.
  2. General personality problems with attachment, rejection, co-operation, or entitlement.
  3. Depression or anxiety.
B. Sexual inhibition due to fear of sexual acts or of their possible consequences, e.g., pain during intercourse, pregnancy, sexually transmitted disease, loss of partner, loss of reputation.

IV. SEXUAL PROBLEMS DUE TO MEDICAL FACTORS

Pain or lack of physical response during sexual activity despite a supportive and safe interpersonal situation, adequate sexual knowledge, and positive sexual attitudes. Such problems can arise from:
A. Numerous local or systemic medical conditions affecting neurological, neurovascular, circulatory, endocrine or other systems of the body;
B. Pregnancy, sexually transmitted diseases, or other sex-related conditions.
C. Side effects of many drugs, medications, or medical treatments.
D. Iatrogenic conditions.

Conclusion

This document is designed for researchers desiring to investigate women's sexual problems, for educators teaching about women and sexuality, for medical and nonmedical clinicians planning to help women with their sexual lives, and for a public that needs a framework for understanding a rapidly changing and centrally important area of life.

For further information, see the web site www.fsd-alert.org

REFERENCES
A list of references is available in the original source. See www.fsd-alert.org

---

New View Campaign
(www.fsd-alert.org)
An educational campaign about the dangers of medicalizing sex

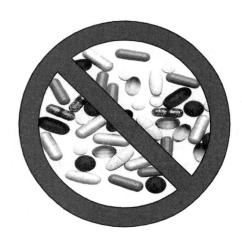

Sex for *your* pleasure or *their* profit?

Sexual fulfillment can't be found in a pill, patch, cream, spray or herbal concoction. Reducing female sexuality to genital functioning is *not* progress. What do women need for good sex lives?
- Accurate information
- Good sex partners
- Sexual safety
- Freedom from media pressure
- Health and energy
- Informed and unbiased healthcare

A New View of Women's Sexual Problems

There is no single definition of sexual satisfaction or what is "normal." Sex is interpersonal and changes over time.

Sexual dissatisfaction results from:
- Physical, sexual and/or emotional harassment or abuse
- Fatigue or stress because of work, family, money or health problems
- Worries about pregnancy, pain, STDs or loss of reputation
- An unsatisfactory relationship, lack of sexual self-knowledge, insecure feelings (about self or partner) or social pressure

The Medical Model distorts women's sexual problems.

In the medical model women are expected to have the same ("normal") amount of sex, fantasy and desire or else they are diagnosed with "female sexual dysfunction" (FSD).

This mistaken medical model:
- Defines satisfaction as "proper" genital functioning
- Minimizes the impact of relationship quality, feelings and learning on sex
- Leads to unnecessary medical tests
- Results in prescribing hormones and drugs of questionable safety
- Ignores sexual individuality and cultural variations
- Is promoted by Big Pharma overtly and covertly

New View Campaign Projects
(see www.fsd-alert.org)
- Resources
  - Books
  - Special journal issues
  - Training manual
  - Continuing ed. courses
  - Ongoing online listserv discussion.
- Special Projects
  - Textbook reviews
  - Activist activities
  - Collaboration with documentaries about Big Pharma
- New View Conferences 2002, 2005, 2009 (in planning)
- Drug Company monitoring and FDA testimony
- Information for media
- Coalitions with:
  - Health activist groups
  - Sex ed groups
  - Public health conflict of interest groups

Support our work:
(see www.fsd-alert.org)
- Endorse the New View Manifesto
- Buy books through our website
- Join our listserv
- Co-sponsor our conferences
- Send a tax deductible donation for our work:
  - New View Campaign
    163 Third Ave., #183
    New York, NY 10003

What You Can Do
- Get your sex information from noncommercial sources. Don't believe ads.
- Support public sexuality education for children, teens and adults.
- Don't substitute pills for sexual comfort and knowledge.
- Be suspicious about simple drug or herb solutions for sexual problems.
- Know about the side effects of any drugs you use.
- Encourage women's health activism through nonprofit groups.
- Advocate reforms for affordable healthcare.
- Believe that women are entitled to sexual pleasure – whatever way they want it.

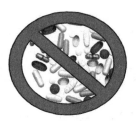

For more information, visit our website at:
www.fsd-alert.org
or contact:
Leonore Tiefer, Ph.D.
Campaign Coordinator
ltiefer@mindspring.com
Tel: 212-533-2774

A New Politics of Sexuality

by June Jordan

As a young worried mother, I remember turning to Dr. Benjamin Spock's *Common Sense Book of Baby and Child Care* just about as often as I'd pick up the telephone. He was God. I was ignorant but striving to be good: a good Mother. And so it was there, in that bestseller pocketbook of do's and don't's, that I came upon this doozie of a guideline: Do not wear miniskirts or other provocative clothing because that will upset your child, especially if your child happens to be a boy. If you give your offspring "cause" to think of you as a sexual being, he will, at the least, become disturbed; you will derail the equilibrium of his notions about your possible identity and meaning in the world.

It had never occurred to me that anyone, especially my son, might look upon me as an asexual being. I had never supposed that "asexual" was some kind of positive designation I should, so to speak, lust after. I was pretty surprised by Dr. Spock. However, I was also, by habit, a creature of obedience. For a couple of weeks I actually experimented with lusterless colors and dowdy tops and bottoms, self-consciously hoping thereby to prove myself as a lusterless and dowdy and, therefore, excellent female parent.

Years would have to pass before I could recognize the familiar, by then, absurdity of a man setting himself up as the expert on a subject that presupposed women as the primary objects for his patriarchal discourse—on motherhood, no less! Years passed before I came to perceive the perversity of dominant power assumed by men, and the perversity of self-determining power ceded to men by women.

A lot of years went by before I understood the dynamics of what anyone could summarize as the Politics of Sexuality.

I believe the Politics of Sexuality is the most ancient and probably the most profound arena for human conflict. Increasingly, it seems clear to me that deeper and more pervasive than any other oppression, than any other bitterly contested human domain, is the oppression of sexuality, the exploitation of the human domain of sexuality for power.

When I say sexuality, I mean gender: I mean male subjugation of human beings because they are female. When I say sexuality, I mean heterosexual institutionalization of rights and privileges denied to homosexual men and women. When I say sexuality I mean gay or lesbian contempt for bisexual modes of human relationship.

The Politics of Sexuality therefore subsumes all of the different ways in which some of us seek to dictate to others of us what we should do, what we should desire, what we should dream about, and how we should behave ourselves, generally, on the planet. From China to Iran, from Nigeria to Czechoslovakia, from Chile to California, the politics of sexuality—enforced by traditions of state-sanctioned violence plus religion and the law—reduces to male domination of women, heterosexist tyranny, and, among those of us who are in any case deemed despicable or deviant by the powerful, we find intolerance for those who choose a different, a more complicated—for example, an interracial or bisexual—mode of rebellion and freedom.

We must move out from the shadows of our collective subjugation—as people of color/as women/as gay/as lesbian/as bisexual human beings.

• • •

I can voice my ideas without hesitation or fear because I am speaking, finally, about myself. I am black and I am female and I am a mother and I am bisexual and I am a nationalist and I am an anti-nationalist. And I mean to be fully and freely all that I am!

Conversely, I do not accept that any white or black or Chinese man—I do not accept that, for instance, Dr. Spock—should presume to tell me, or any other woman, how to mother a child. He has no right. He is not a mother. My child is not his child. And, likewise, I do not accept that anyone—any woman or any man who is not inextricably part of the subject he or she dares to address—should attempt to tell any of us, the objects of her or his presumptuous discourse, what we should do or what we should not do.

Recently, I have come upon gratuitous and appalling pseudoliberal pronouncements on sexuality. Too often, these utterances fall out of the mouths of men and women who first disclaim any sentiment remotely related to homophobia, but who then proceed to issue outrageous opinions like the following.

That it is blasphemous to compare the oppression of gay, lesbian, or bisexual people to the oppression, say, of black people, or of the Palestinians.

That the bottom line about gay or lesbian or bisexual identity is that you can conceal it whenever necessary and, so, therefore, why don't you do just that? Why don't you keep your deviant sexuality in the closet and let the rest of us—we who suffer oppression for reasons of our ineradicable and always visible components of our personhood such as race or gender—get on with our more necessary, our more beleaguered struggle to survive?

Well, number one: I believe I have worked as hard as I could, and then harder than that, on behalf of equality and justice for African-Americans, for the Palestinian people, and for people of color everywhere.

And no, I do not believe it is blasphemous to compare oppressions of sexuality to oppressions of race and ethnicity: Freedom is indivisible or it is nothing at all besides sloganeering and temporary, short-sighted, and short-lived advancement for a few. Freedom is indivisible, and either we are working for freedom or you are working for the sake of your self-interests and I am working for mine.

If you can finally go to the bathroom, wherever you find one, if you can finally order a cup of coffee and drink it wherever coffee is available, but you cannot follow your heart—you cannot respect the response of your own honest body in the world—then how much of what kind of freedom does any one of us possess?

Or, conversely, if your heart and your honest body can be controlled by the state, or controlled by community taboo, are you not then, and in that case, no more than a slave ruled by outside force?

What tyranny could exceed a tyranny that dictates to the human heart, and that attempts to dictate the public career of an honest human body?

Freedom is indivisible; the Politics of Sexuality is not some optional "special-interest" concern for serious, progressive folk.

And, on another level, let me assure you: If every single gay or lesbian or bisexual man or woman active on the Left of American politics decided to stay home, there would be *no* Left left.

• • •

One of the things I want to propose is that we act on that reality: that we insistently demand reciprocal respect and concern from those who cheerfully depend

upon our brains and our energies for their, and our, effective impact on the political landscape.

Last spring, at Berkeley, some students asked me to speak at a rally against racism. And I did. There were 400 or 500 people massed on Sproul Plaza, standing together against that evil. And, on the next day, on that same Plaza, there was a rally for bisexual and gay and lesbian rights, and students asked me to speak at that rally. And I did. There were fewer than seventy-five people stranded, pitiful, on that public space. And I said then what I say today: That was disgraceful! There should have been just one rally. One rally: Freedom is indivisible.

As for the second, nefarious pronouncement on sexuality that now enjoys mass-media currency: the idiot notion of keeping yourself in the closet—that is very much the same thing as the suggestion that black folks and Asian-Americans and Mexican-Americans should assimilate and become as "white" as possible—in our walk/talk/music/food/values—or else. Or else? Or else we should, deservedly, perish.

Sure enough, we have plenty of exposure to white everything so why would we opt to remain our African/Asian/Mexican selves? The answer is that suicide is absolute, and if you think you will survive by hiding who you really are, you are sadly misled: There is no such thing as partial or intermittent suicide. You can only survive if you—who you really are—do survive.

Likewise, we who are not men and we who are not heterosexual—we, sure enough, have plenty of exposure to male-dominated/heterosexist this and that.

But a struggle to survive cannot lead to suicide: Suicide is the opposite of survival. And so we must not conceal/assimilate/ integrate into the would-be dominant culture and political system that despises us. Our survival requires that we alter our environment so that we can live and so that we can hold each other's hands and so that we can kiss each other on the streets, and in the daylight of our existence, without terror and without violent and sometimes fatal reactions from the busybodies of America.

Finally, I need to speak on bisexuality. I do believe that the analogy is interracial or multiracial identity. I do believe that the analogy for bisexuality is a multicultural, multi-ethnic, multiracial world view. Bisexuality follows from such a perspective and leads to it, as well.

Just as there are many men and women in the United States whose parents have given them more than one racial, more than one ethnic identity and cultural heritage to honor; and just as these men and women must deny no given part of themselves except at the risk of self-deception and the insanities that must issue from that; and just as these men and women embody the principle of equality among races and ethnic communities; and just as these men and women falter and anguish and choose and then falter again and then anguish and then choose yet again how they will honor the irreducible complexity of their God-given human being—even so, there are many men and women, especially young men and women, who seek to embrace the complexity of their total, always-changing social and political circumstance.

They seek to embrace our increasing global complexity on the basis of the heart and on the basis of an honest human body. Not according to ideology. Not according to group pressure. Not according to anybody's concept of "correct."

This is a New Politics of Sexuality. And even as I despair of identity politics—because identity is given and principles of justice/equality/freedom cut across given gender and given racial definitions of being, and because I will call you my brother, I will call you my sister, on the basis of what you *do* for justice, what you *do* for equality, what you *do* for freedom and *not* on the basis of who you are, even so I look with ad-

miration and respect upon the new, bisexual politics of sexuality.

This emerging movement politicizes the so-called middle ground: Bisexuality invalidates either/or formulation, either/or analysis. Bisexuality means I am free and I am as likely to want and to love a woman as I am likely to want and to love a man, and what about that? Isn't that what freedom implies?

If you are free you are not predictable and you are not controllable. To my mind, that is the keenly positive, politicizing significance of bisexual affirmation:

To insist upon complexity, to insist upon the validity of all of the components of social/sexual complexity, to insist upon the equal validity of all of the components of social/sexual complexity.

This seems to me a unifying, 1990s mandate for revolutionary Americans planning to make it into the Twenty-first Century on the basis of the heart, on the basis of an honest human body, consecrated to every struggle for justice, every struggle for equality, every struggle for freedom.

"Do Ask, Do Tell"

by Jennifer E. Potter

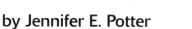

As a consequence of bias and ignorance within the medical profession, lesbians and gay men frequently receive suboptimal health care. Knowledge of each patient's sexual orientation and behaviors is critical for the development of a productive therapeutic relationship, accurate risk assessment, and the provision of pertinent preventive counseling. However, clinicians often forget to ask about this information, and many lesbians and gay men are reticent to reveal the truth. I present vignettes from my personal experiences as a lesbian patient and doctor to illustrate the importance of creating an environment in which such disclosure can occur and to portray the challenges and rewards of coming out as a gay physician.

I juggle many hats in my life: mother, partner, doctor, and educator. Like all my female colleagues, my experiences as a daughter, sister, patient, and student have influenced my approach to each of these roles. But I am also lesbian, and this fact has shaped my life profoundly. It underlies my decision to become a primary care doctor; select women's health as an area of clinical expertise; and commit myself especially to improving

the lives of lesbians, gay men, and people from other minority groups.

It is a challenge to be lesbian in our society. People assume that a young woman is straight, will marry, can get pregnant if she is sexually active, and will have children. This progression is "normal." Anything else is different and may be perceived as abnormal, wrong, or bad. Historical and continuing records of harassment, as-

"Do Ask, Do Tell," by Jennifer E. Potter, MD, *Annals of Internal Medicine*, 2002; 137: 341–343. Reprinted by permission of the American College of Physicians - American Society of Internal Medicine.

saults, and homicides against lesbians and gay men abound. The medical profession itself has viewed homosexuality as a disorder; aversion techniques, hormone administration, shock treatment, castration, and even lobotomy have been used as purported "treatments".[1] I feel fortunate that I have never been the target of clearly overt actions because of my sexual orientation.

Insidious effects of prejudice affect my life deeply, however. Imagine how it feels to hear yet another gay joke or to open the paper to confront yet another antigay news story. Examples include the U.S. military's "don't ask, don't tell" policy, repeated referenda that limit the civil rights of lesbians and gay men (even compared with other minority groups), and the opposition of many religious organizations. Many lesbians and gay men find it difficult to avoid internalizing some of these homophobic attitudes. As a consequence, shame and fear are common emotions, and we are more likely to be isolated; engage in risky behaviors; suffer from stress-related health conditions, substance abuse, or depression; and attempt suicide.[2]

Finding help is not easy. It is hard to trust other people, even health professionals, when one anticipates disapproval. Doctors share the same biases as the rest of society and are frequently ignorant about lesbian and gay health issues. I have often been disappointed with the medical care I have received; several examples from my experience as a lesbian patient are illustrative.

As a teenager, I reacted to the emergence of attraction to other girls with a jumble of conflicting feelings: excitement, fear, fascination, and horror. When I tried to broach the topic cautiously with my family doctor, he laughed and said, "Don't worry about that; it's just a phase a lot of girls go through." He meant to reassure me, but his comment trivialized and dismissed me instead. An important opportunity was missed to explore and validate my feelings.

By age 15, I was overwhelmed and isolated and made a suicidal gesture that might have had grave consequences. The psychiatrist to whom I was referred believed that same-sex attraction was a sign of stunted psychological development. His attitude perpetuated my notion that something was wrong with me; I stifled exploration of my identity during 2 ensuing years of therapy. I eventually found the support I needed when I met a lesbian couple who listened to me, encouraged me to be myself, and demonstrated that it was possible both to be lesbian and to pursue the goals I wanted in life— a committed relationship, a family, diverse friends, and a deeply challenging and rewarding career.

In college, I consulted a physician for evaluation of vaginal symptoms. She asked if I was sexually active (yes), whether I was using contraception (no), and whether I was trying to conceive (no). Before I had a chance to explain, she began to talk about birth control options and the importance of using condoms to prevent sexually transmitted diseases. At that point, I was too embarrassed to reveal my lesbianism. I never did ask the question that was on my mind ("Could I infect my lover?") and left, uncomfortable, with an absurd prescription for the pill. Her immediate assumption that I was straight and my reticence to reveal the truth prevented the development of a productive doctor–patient relationship and resulted in inappropriate care.

Later in life, when I disclosed my lesbianism to a new internist, she told me that my risk for cervical cancer was so low that I did not need to have regular Papanicolaou smears. This advice was incorrect. She assumed that my sexual relationships were exclusively lesbian and that the chief cause of cervical cancer, human papillomavirus, cannot be transmitted by woman-to-woman sexual contact. However, sexual identity cannot be equated with sexual behavior. Some lesbians are celibate, many have male partners, and some have partners of both sexes. Moreover, emerging evidence suggests that several genital infections can be acquired during lesbian sexual activity.[3] A detailed sexual history is necessary to understand the situation of each patient, ascertain risks for sexually transmitted diseases, and provide pertinent medical counseling.

As a result of my experiences with doctors who did not know how to communicate effectively, I became interested in ways to break down barriers that prevent gay and other minority patients from obtaining good care. I joined a lesbian and gay speaker's bureau and told my story to students at local high schools, colleges, and medical schools. I believe I helped to enlighten others and demolish some stereotypes. Then, after considering teaching, nursing, psychology, and medicine, I decided that my best course of action was to become a physician.

The medical establishment was an inhospitable place for gay trainees in the 1980s. As recommended by my premedical advisor, I concealed my lesbianism during the medical school application process; I question whether I would have received my "Welcome to the Harvard family" letter if I had been more forthright. Once a trainee, I faced all the challenges that every medical student and resident encounters: trying to master a huge body of knowledge, accepting the enormous responsibility of caring for people, learning to function with aplomb in emergency situations, and competing with others for advancement. In addition, I had to cope with tacit and overt advice that my lesbianism would be tolerated only as long as I kept quiet about it.

Ambivalence about being open is a problem that heterosexual persons can barely comprehend. It arises because of a continuing lack of acceptance of gays by most of the population and the fact that homosexuality is invisible, unlike the minority status of people with different skin color or language. As a consequence, disclosure is a choice left to each gay person.

On the face of it, maintaining silence makes almost everyone happy. I can interact with others without fear of prejudice, and people are spared the discomfort of responding to a sensitive proclamation. But invisibility has many downsides. Self-respect is difficult to preserve when one lies by omission. Silence implies acceptance that, as a member of a minority group, I have nothing valuable to contribute—that I am a "minus." If I selectively omit mention of involvement in activities that could identify me as gay, I cannot highlight all of my accomplishments. If I attend professional social gatherings alone, I miss the opportunity to introduce my partner of 23 years, show our example of a long-term relationship, and provide everyone with a chance to build acceptance.

Secrecy leads to isolation. Whenever I encounter new and unfamiliar situations, I am tempted to watch, wait, and figure out the lay of the land before revealing my lesbianism. Although this strategy feels safe, it produces loneliness. A subculture of lesbians and gay men exists through which clandestine identification takes place. But when secrecy is the paramount mode of operation, people are reluctant to gather together because of guilt by association. Silence limits opportunities for friendship, support, and professional collaboration not only with other lesbians and gay men but also with sympathetic people from the mainstream who share my values and goals.

Secrecy also requires an enormous expenditure of energy. Staying "in the closet" is not a passive process; constant vigilance is required to steer conversations away from personal issues. Of course, people sometimes ask directly whether I am in a relationship. If I deny that I am involved, I enter a vicious cycle of deception. If I admit to having a partner but try to conceal her sex, I have to take great care to avoid the pronouns "she" and "her" in subsequent discussion. Such behavior wastes a great deal of energy that could be channeled productively.

When I remain silent, people make assumptions about me that can be very awkward, especially if they later realize that their beliefs were wrong. When I started to practice medicine, many of my colleagues assumed that I was single because I did not talk about a boyfriend or husband or wear a wedding ring. Some concluded that I was an "old maid by choice"—a woman who had subjugated family to career. Others assumed that I was available, so I had to decline advances. When I became pregnant, nearly everyone assumed that I was married. In a particularly embarrassing moment, the chief of a major service told me in a public forum that he thought he knew my husband!

I have gradually learned that it is advantageous to be open about my sexual orientation. Disclosure is empowering: It allows me to be myself, integrate my public and private lives, voice my opinions, celebrate all of my achievements, and work passionately to increase tolerance and acceptance. I know that I deserve respect and recognize that I serve as an important role model.

Coming out is a process that never ends. Every time I meet someone new, I must decide if, how, and when I will reveal my sexual orientation. I find it simplest to be candid with colleagues from the start, but this approach can be awkward with patients, because it is considered inappropriate to mention intimate personal details in the context of a professional relationship. However, every doctor–patient interaction is built on trust, and I believe strongly that I have an obligation to be honest. Patients often ask me personal questions about my family and how I balance home life and career. Up-front disclosure of my sexual orientation avoids embarrassing people who might otherwise assume that I am straight and ask about my "marriage" or "husband" and allows patients who feel uncomfortable having a lesbian as their physician to choose a different doctor.

In general, I try to communicate who I am nonverbally, by displaying pictures of my family and having gay-friendly posters and health literature in my office. I developed and use an intake form that is inclusive of alternative lifestyles and avoids the designations "single," "married," "divorced," and "widowed." My name is listed in a lesbian and gay health guide, I give talks to lay audiences on lesbian and gay health issues, and I volunteer free health screening for lesbians and other minority groups in the community. I have also developed and teach a curriculum on lesbian and gay health to medical students and residents as well as to peers at continuing medical education conferences. When I am asked directly about my private life, I answer truthfully.

Reactions to my openness have been mixed, but my experiences coming out as a lesbian health professional have been rewarding overall. When I decided to coordinate a lesbian and gay student group in medical school, I had to identify myself to the administration in order to apply for funding and take the risk of being seen posting notices about group activities. Some flyers were defaced, presumably by other medical students, and I once saw one being removed by a dean. I tried to channel my anger into eloquence and gave a talk to my classmates. Although a few ignored me subsequently and one student began to pray for me every morning before class began, the posters were no longer disturbed and attendance at group-sponsored educational events increased.

Later, as a resident in the early AIDS era, I encountered numerous examples of homophobia in the hospital. There were many antigay jokes; some implied that gay men were getting what they deserved. Some of my peers refused to shake hands with gay patients or put on gowns and gloves before entering their rooms. My coming out stopped the jokes, at least in my presence, and seemed to result in more humane behavior toward people with AIDS-related illnesses.

Over the years, I have received a few lectures on the ills of homosexuality and even a letter stating that people like me should not be permitted to become doctors. However, several gay patients have told me that my visibility enabled them to find me and finally receive the understanding and support they craved. My openness has also allowed gay medical students and residents to identify me as a role model and mentor, and many of my straight colleagues and patients have thanked me for the opportunity to examine their assumptions and biases about gay people.

Somewhat to my surprise, my openness has not harmed my clinical practice. On the contrary, I have many referrals from medical colleagues and hospital administrators who want me to care for their wives and daughters, and I was recognized by *Boston Magazine* as a top internist for women in the February 2001 issue. Coming out has also afforded me some novel professional opportunities. I believe that my openness during an era of emphasis on cultural competence was a factor in my appointment to the Beth Israel Deaconess Hospital Board of Trustees. Likewise, my willingness to speak out has resulted in invitations to participate in a panel discussion on lesbian and gay health at the Massachu-setts Department of Public Health and to serve on an advisory board to the American Cancer Society.

Despite these successes, much work still needs to be done. In recent years, Harvard Medical School has taken steps to diversify the racial and ethnic composition of its student body and to increase tolerance and acceptance of its gay community by sponsoring town meeting discussions. However, few minority faculty members have been promoted to leadership positions, and consequently, many of my values and those of minority colleagues remain poorly represented. I strive to promote further institutional change by being visible and voicing my questions and concerns.

A professor at my institution once warned that it is a mistake to "ghetto-ize" one's career in women's health. I take issue with this statement. I believe that my work is not only legitimate but of critical value. My talents include an instinctive ability to understand and empower patients from highly diverse backgrounds and a gift for changing the attitudes and behaviors of medical students and doctors. My work requires courage and resilience, and I believe that the outcomes are as important as the results of basic science research and clinical trials. Challenging clinicians' stereotypes and increasing the sensitivity with which they communicate with people from different cultures will benefit all of their present and future patients. I am proud to be a lesbian physician and educator.

REFERENCES

1. Miller N. Out of the Past: Gay and Lesbian History from 1869 to the Present. New York: Vintage Books; 1995.

2. Dean L, Meyer IH, Robinson K, Sell RL, Sember R, Silenzio VMB, et al. Lesbian, gay, bisexual, and transgender health: findings and concerns. Journal of the Gay and Lesbian Medical Association. 2000;4:101–51.

3. Diamant AL, Lever J, Schuster M. Lesbians' sexual activities and efforts to reduce risks for sexually transmitted diseases. Journal of the Gay and Lesbian Medical Association. 2000;4:41–8.

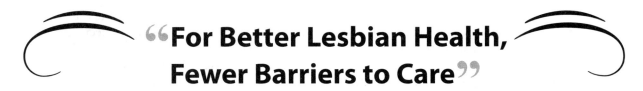

"For Better Lesbian Health, Fewer Barriers to Care"

by Leah Thayer

An innovative partnership aims to close a dangerous gap between the health concerns of lesbians and the knowledge and/or perceptions that health providers have of those concerns. Removing the Barriers™ to Accessing Health Care for Lesbians (RTB), developed by The Mautner Project for Lesbian Health with the support of the U.S. Centers for Disease Control and Prevention (CDC), aims to build the cultural competence of health care providers while creating systemic changes that help lesbians feel safe and comfortable disclosing their sexual orientation in health care settings.

"Even with the significant societal changes taking place today, lesbians often face daunting barriers to obtaining quality health care," according to Kathleen De-Bold, executive director of The Mautner Project. She cited a growing body of research identifying numerous barriers—institutional, cultural, financial and personal—that cause many lesbians to avoid or delay medical care, making them more vulnerable to disease and poor health outcomes.

Launched in 2002, RTB has reached some 1,000 providers through trainings held with local organizations, medical schools, hospitals and clinics, said De-Bold. In March, new CDC funding enabled RTB's expansion into the National Breast and Cervical Cancer Early Detection Program (BCCEDP), which helps low-income, uninsured and underserved women access breast and cervical cancer screening. By "training the trainers" at 140 BCCEDPs nationwide, the goal is to create an echo effect that reaches a far wider audience than Mautner staff could reach personally.

RTB training can be as brief as a lunchtime presentation or as intensive as a two-day program. Nurses, social workers, physicians and administrators who attend receive continuing medical credits and continuing education units. The program targets non-medical staff as well. "In the health care system, you spend a lot more time with staff than you actually do with doctors or nurses—people doing intake and filing your insurance papers," noted DeBold. "From the minute you walk in, you need

to know it's a safe and accepting place that lets you be honest about who you are."

Demolishing the Myths

In 2000, the U.S. Department of Health and Human Services released its health action plan for the next decade. Healthy People 2010 broke new ground by, for the first time, identifying sexual orientation as a marker of health disparities. For women who partner with women, these disparities stem from a variety of factors, many of them interrelated. For instance:

- In a 1999 study of second-year medical students, 25 percent believed homosexuality to be "immoral and dangerous to the institution of the family."[1] An earlier survey of lesbian, gay, bisexual and transgendered (LGBT) physicians found that 67 percent knew of an LGBT patient who received substandard care or was denied care due to his or her sexual orientation.[2] Many lesbians have had negative encounters with the health care system including derogatory comments, voyeurism and undue roughness in physical examinations.

- In a 2002 survey by Witeck-Combs Communications and Harris Interactive, only 55 percent of lesbians had disclosed their sexual orientation to their doctor or health care provider. As acknowledged by the American Medical Association, ". . . unrecognized homosexuality by the physician or the patients' reluctance to report his or her sexual orientation can lead to failure to screen, diagnose or treat important medical problems."[3]

- Many lesbians exhibit greater risk factors for common health problems, often due to the stress of living in a homophobic society. They are significantly more likely to be heavy drinkers, obese, or current or previous smokers; to have never had a mammogram; to have waited longer since their last Pap smear; and to eat fewer fruits and vegetables daily.[4] Lesbians overall are also more likely

"For Better Lesbian Health, Fewer Barriers to Care," by Leah Thayer, originally published in the *Women's Health Activist*, May/June 2004, pp. 6–7, the newsletter of the National Women's Health Network (NWHN). It is reprinted with the permission of the author and the NWHN.

Removing More Barriers

Transgendered men—women who identify and express themselves as men—face even more barriers to quality health care than lesbians. "Southern Comfort," a critically acclaimed documentary released in 2001, explored the consequences of medical discrimination through the story of Robert Eads, a 52-year-old FtM (female-to-male) transsexual who had undergone a partial sex change several years before and was dying of cervical and ovarian cancer. Eads' sex-reassignment doctor had decided that a hysterectomy wasn't necessary, since Eads had been through menopause. Once his cancer was diagnosed, more than 20 doctors had refused to treat him, saying his presence in their offices would upset their female patients.

Inspired in part by Eads' story, the Feminist Women's Health Center in Atlanta (FWHC) a few years ago launched a clinic to provide FtM individuals with gynecological exams, Pap smears and other routine health care. The clinic is a collaborative effort with an annual conference in Atlanta (also called Southern Comfort) that draws transgendered people from all over the South. Janelle Yamarick, FWHC's community

services director, said the care is provided by the same doctors, nurses and counselors that already work with FWHC clients. "We have done some training for our staff, but our health care approach has always been a nonjudgmental and respectful approach that is also about empowering individuals in their health care decisions," said Yamarick.

Even so, the relative rarity of FtM transgendered people means "the practice of medicine, as far as we can ascertain, has much less research" into this population, and therefore there is limited information for practitioners to base their protocols upon, noted Yamarick. FWHC is building its own institutional knowledge by retaining staff who have been involved with the clinic since its start and by sending staff to workshops at Southern Comfort. In addition, a doctor from FWHC, in consult with several outside practitioners, created a protocol for testosterone prescriptions.

Feminist Women's Health Care Center: www .atlfwhc.org. Southern Comfort conference: www.sccatl.org.

to be uninsured (largely because of spousal benefits, which lesbians rarely have), diminishing their likelihood of receiving preventive care or catching disease early.

In an interactive format that includes videos, readings and role playing, RTB sets out to demolish the myths, judgment-making and inaccurate information that can diminish the quality of care for lesbians. Heterosexism— the presumption that someone is heterosexual—is especially prevalent in the health care arena, noted DeBold. For instance, intake forms whose only options are single, married and divorced may signal to lesbians that the practice is not comfortable with their sexuality, preventing them from listing their partners as emergency contacts or bringing their partners along for important visits. This presumption also can keep providers from asking questions that can reveal health problems. A lesbian whose intake form says she is single, for instance, is less likely to be evaluated for domestic violence.

RTB also targets inaccurate information, such as many providers' persistent belief that lesbians don't need Pap smears or other screening tests. Finally, a "toolkit for quality care" helps providers use better language, create more inclusive intake forms and respect patient confidentiality. Lesbians have lost their jobs, lost custody of their children and been discharged from the military due to confidentiality breaches by health providers, according to DeBold.

Initial feedback from RTB training has been overwhelmingly positive. The Survey Evaluation and Research Laboratory at Virginia Commonwealth University found that RTB significantly changed providers' knowledge, attitudes and behaviors toward lesbian clients. "We've gotten really wonderful feedback because the bottom line is that health care providers want to help you," said DeBold. In this age of managed care and shrinking reimbursements, there are also indirect benefits of having better rapport with patients. These include higher retention and referrals, noted DeBold, along with fewer unnecessary tests, reduced liability risks and greater likelihood of catching diseases early.

REFERENCES

1. Klamen DL, Grossman LS, Kopacz DR. "Medical student homophobia." *Journal of Homosexuality* 1999; 37(1): 53–63.

2. Schatz B, O'Hanlan K. "Anti-gay discrimination in medicine: results of a national survey of lesbian, gay and bisexual physicians." *Journal of the Gay and Lesbian Medical Association* 1994; May.

3. Report 8 of the Council on Scientific Affairs [I-94]. "Health needs of gay men and lesbians in the United States." *Journal of the American Medical Association* 1996; 275: 1354–1359.

4. Valanis BG, Bowen DJ, Bassford T, Whitlock E, Charney P., Carter R. "Sexual orientation and health." *Archives of Family Medicine 2000*; Sept/Oct.

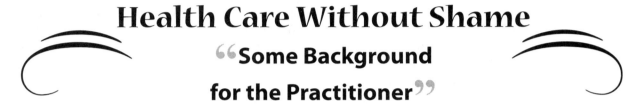

Health Care Without Shame
"Some Background for the Practitioner"

by Charles Moser

(This chapter is adapted from an article which first appeared in *San Francisco Medicine,* Nov./Dec. 1998, pp. 23–26.)

Physicians and other health care practitioners have just begun to address the special health and lifestyle issues of the gay, lesbian or bisexual patient. However, the medical concerns of other sexual minorities (including transgendered patients, patients with multiple sexual partners, sex workers, and patients involved in S/M and other "kinky" sexual behaviors) have received little to no attention. This chapter will, I hope, be a starting point for physicians and other health care professionals who wish to address the health concerns and needs of sexual minority patients.

The first question to answer for yourself is whether or not you really wish to treat such patients. Some physicians are unable to overcome their own issues about alternative sexual behaviors and should refer these patients. Even if you're a member of one sexual minority community, you may not be able to nonjudgmentally treat any or all sexual minority patients.

Just because you choose to refer these patients does not relieve you of the responsibility of learning at least the basics of how to care for them. I do not, and unfortunately never will, speak Japanese, so it is reasonable for me to refer new patients who only speak Japanese to a Japanese-speaking physician. Nevertheless, I have had to take care of such patients. I try to employ translators (both Japanese speakers who work in the hospital and family members). I have learned something of Japanese culture. The hospitals where I work have devised "Asian diets" (comfort food is important when you are sick) and have made other accommodations. Physicians confronted with sexual lifestyles with which they are not comfortable need to take similar actions: seek out experts and attempt to make accommodations for patient comfort.

If you decide that sexual minority patients will be a significant aspect of your practice, here are some recommendations on how to treat them effectively and respectfully.

Who They Are vs. What They Do   In treating such patients, you must distinguish between identity and behavior—a task which is not as simple as it seems. Individuals may choose to define their sexuality with a label, but their actual behavior may be very different. Medical risk is related to a patient's behavior, heredity or environment, not his or her identity. It does not matter medically whether a male patient identifies as gay, but it does matter if he has sex with men. Additionally, anal sex with a man opens him up to a different type of medical risk than anal sex with a dildo-wielding woman.

Nevertheless, identity is also an issue. A woman who self-defines as a lesbian is often subjected to a variety of stresses that a heterosexual-identified woman is not, without regard to her behavior. There are social stresses regarding partner choice ("Will my partner be allowed to visit into the MICU? What will happen when my co-workers meet my lover?"). There are also genuine physical dangers—rape, assault and even homicide—associated with being gay, lesbian, a sex worker, an S/M practitioner, or transgendered, as the crime sheet in any city can attest.

Sexual identity and behavior are both fluid. There are people who defined themselves first as gay, then straight, then bisexual. It can be hard to imagine, but there are people who are not quite sure which gender they are, people who are frustrated when no one will acknowledge their chosen gender, and people who find any gender at all intolerable. Is a woman who is happily married, but secretly desires sexual contact with other women, a lesbian or bisexual or even heterosexual? Does that orientation change if she begins an affair with another woman, if she leaves her husband, or even if she becomes celibate? There are no simple answers. Just remember that because someone identifies with one sexual orientation, it does not necessarily define their actual behavior. Acceptance of this fluidity is the first step in providing nonjudgmental health care and not alienating your patient.

Your sense of a patient's probable identity may not match up with the patient's own self-identification; you're not a mind-reader, and appearances can be deceptive. Be aware that many people, when faced with a question about someone's sexual identity, tend to categorize people into the less societally accepted roles. For example, a heterosexual man who has sex with a man is assumed to be a closeted gay, but a homosexual man who has sex with a woman is not assumed to be a closeted straight.

No Assumptions Associating certain medical problems with specific sexual minorities acts to stigmatize that minority. We all know that unprotected anal coitus is a risk factor for HIV transmission, but it may surprise some that more heterosexuals take part in anal coitus than homosexuals. The point is: talk with *all* your patients about anal safer sex practices. The assumption that you can choose whom to advise on this issue will unfortunately be proved wrong too often.

Just as an aside, anal sexuality is an area often forgotten in our medical school education. Possibly the best piece of advice you can give to patients interested in exploring anal sex is to make sure anything inserted into the anus has a flange to prevent it from being lost in the rectum. A second safety technique, which should *also* be included, is attaching a string to the device to allow for retrieval if the flange fails to prevent the object from being lost in the rectum. Discussions of how to prevent colonic perforations (smooth soft toys, exceedingly short fingernails, quick referral for bleeding) should also be emphasized, in addition to safer sex advice. Information about sexually transmitted diseases (STDs) that can be transmitted by anal sex and oral/anal contact should also be reviewed.

How Does Your Office Appear to the Sexual Minority Patient? Your prospective patient's first contacts with your practice are your office staff and your forms. Patient information sheets routinely ask questions that may seem simple and routine to you, but are really quite difficult. Prospective transgendered patients must choose between male and female; S/M practitioners must choose between listing their spouse or their S/M mistress as their emergency contact. How will the new doctor respond to a newly married gay couple? A new patient will judge your paperwork, before ever finding out how accepting you are.

Your office staff can also be the cause of a misunderstanding. The odd look from your receptionist . . . the nurse who does not understand the need for a male doctor to have a chaperon when examining a female-to-male transsexual . . . the medical assistant who shudders when seeing nipple rings . . . the bookkeeper who refuses to explain a charge on the bill to the patient's significant other . . . all these can represent genuine obstacles to health care for the sexual minority patient.

The somewhat unfriendly form or staff can all lead to a hostile or fearful patient. It is probably a good idea to read over your patient materials to make sure they are not inadvertently offensive. A frank discussion with your office staff, letting them know that you welcome sexual minority patients into your practice and will not tolerate any disrespect, can also be useful. Be especially aware of the staff member who is tolerant of most sexualities, but frightened or upset by a particular sexual lifestyle or behavior; perhaps some education on your part can help allay this person's qualms.

Your Own First Impression A physician who is not knowledgeable or respectful about sexual minority practices often reveals that ignorance in the initial history and physical. To avoid a bad first impression, consider some better ways of asking questions, whether you're asking them during the initial interview or on your forms:

Rather than ask "marital status?"

Ask "Are you single, married, divorced, separated, or partnered?" The next question is "With whom do you live?"

Rather than "What form of birth control do you use?"

Ask "Do you use birth control?" If the patient says yes, ask "What methods do you use?" If the patient says no, then ask "Do you need birth control?" (If you ask the second question first, you will overlook the patient who is relying on the rhythm method.)

Rather than "Do you have any sexual problems?"

Ask, "Do you have any sexual concerns?" Then follow up with more detailed questions: there is research to indicate that the general question alone will not uncover sexual dysfunctions. You have to ask about each specific dysfunction: for example, do you have difficulty having an orgasm, getting an erection, maintaining an erection, with pain during sex, orgasm too soon, lubricate enough or long enough, do you desire sex? Also, referring to sexual "concerns" allows the patient to bring up concerns other than dysfunctions.

Rather than "With how many partners do you have sex?"

Ask, "Are you currently having sex with anyone?" If the patient says "no," you can ask "Is that a problem for you?" If the patient says "yes," you can ask "Do you have more than one partner?"

Rather than "Who beat you up?"

Ask, "How did you get those marks/bruises/welts?"

Rather than "What is your sexual orientation?"

Ask, "Do you have sex with men, women or both?"

Finish the sex-oriented part of the interview with, "Do you engage in any sexual activities about which you have health questions?"

Respecting Patients' Identity and Relationships

It seems only courteous to refer to patients as they request. Nevertheless, it can be difficult to remember to refer to your budding, but balding, male-to-female (MtF) transsexual patient as a "she"—to write "Frank" on the prescription, but refer to her as "Francesca." It can be hard to remember to do a pap smear on Dick, your female-to-male (FtM) transgendered patient.

I hope that you already include the patient's significant other in major decisions if that is the patient's desire, despite the relationship's legal status. Sometimes it is difficult to ferret out the relationships that are important to your patient. Your patient may have a wife and a master, or two significant others. It is appropriate and desirable to ask the patient who they would like present.

Dealing with the Mistrustful Patient

Many sexual minority patients mistrust traditional medicine. Some of this mistrust is understandable: many alternative sexual behaviors are also psychiatric diagnoses, and in some cases may be illegal; many patients have had less than pleasant interactions with non-accepting physicians. Reliance on alternative medicine and folk remedies, and avoidance of traditional medicine, are common. Sexual minority patients tend not to take care of health care maintenance or even simple problems. So when they finally seek medical care, there can be serious medical concerns.

For similar reasons, many sexual minority patients also mistrust mental health professionals—so a suggestion that your patient see a psychiatrist or psychotherapist may be greeted with skepticism or hostility, particularly if the patient believes that you are suggesting such therapy to "cure" the patient's sexual behavior.

I hope it goes without saying that consensual and satisfying sexual behaviors among adults that do not interfere with the patient's functioning do not need curing. Nevertheless, depression, personality disorders, stress and other psychiatric problems are at least as likely among sexual minorities as the general population. Due to the stresses of living a non-traditional lifestyle, some emotional difficulties may be more common. Illicit drug fads within (and outside) the various sexual minority communities may lead to psychiatric and medical problems. Sensitive physicians are able to assure their patients that they are recommending mental health treatment because of the psychiatric problem and not because of the sexual behavior.

Sexual minority patients are concerned, often with cause, that health care providers will pathologize them because of their sexual identity or behaviors. You will have better success with these patients if you can assure them truthfully that you do not consider their sexuality to be, in and of itself, a problem.

Forbidden Fruit

by Anne Finger

Before she became a paraplegic, Los Angeles resident DeVonna Cervantes liked to dye her pubic hair 'fun colours'—turquoise, purple, jet black. After DeVonna became disabled, a beautician friend of hers came to the rehabilitation unit and, as a Christmas present, dyed DeVonna's pubic hair a hot pink.

But there's no such thing as 'private parts' in a rehab hospital. Soon the staff, who'd seen her dye job when they were catheterizing her, sent the staff psychiatrist around to see her. Cervantes says that he told her: 'I know it is very hard to accept that you have lost your sexuality but you don't need to draw attention to it this way.' Cervantes spent the remainder of the 50-minute session arguing with him, and, in perhaps the only true medical miracle I've ever heard of, convinced him that he was wrong—that this was normal behaviour for her.

Cervantes' story not only illustrates woeful ignorance on the part of a 'medical expert'; equating genital sensation with sexuality. But it shows clearly a disabled woman's determination to define her own sexuality.

Sadly, it's not just medical experts who are guilty of ignoring the reproductive and sexual rights and needs of people with disabilities. The movements for sexual and reproductive freedom have paid little attention to disability issues. And the abortion rights movement has sometimes crudely exploited fears about 'defective fetuses' as a reason to keep abortion legal.

Because the initial focus of the women's movement was set by women who were overwhelmingly non-disabled (as well as young, white, and middle-class), the agenda of reproductive rights has tended to focus on the right to abortion as the central issue. Yet for disabled women, the right to bear and rear children is more at risk. Zoe Washburn, in her poem, 'Hannah', grieves the child she wanted to have and the abortion she was coerced into: '. . . so she went to the doctor, and let him suck Hannah out with a vacuum cleaner. . . . The family stroked her hair when she cried and cried because her belly was empty and Hannah was not only dead, but never born. They looked at her strange crippled-up body and thought to themselves, thank God that's over.'

Yet the disability rights movement has certainly not put sexual rights at the forefront of its agenda. Sexuality is often the source of our deepest oppression; it is also often the source of our deepest pain. It's easier for us to talk about—and formulate strategies for changing—discrimination in employment, education, and housing than to talk about our exclusion from sexuality and reproduction. Also, although it is changing, the disability rights movement in the US has tended to focus its energies on lobbying legislators and creating an image of 'the able disabled'.

Barbara Waxman and I once published an article in *Disability Rag* about the US Supreme Court's decision that states could outlaw 'unnatural' sex acts, pointing out the effect it could have on disabled people—especially those who were unable to have 'standard' intercourse. The *Rag* then received a letter asking how 'the handicapped' could ever be expected to be accepted as 'normal' when we espoused such disgusting ideas.

Because reproduction is seen as a 'women's issue', it is often relegated to the back burner. Yet it is crucial that the disability-rights movement starts to deal with it. Perhaps the most chilling situation exists in China where a number of provinces ban marriages between people with developmental and other disabilities unless the parties have been sterilized. In Gansu Province more than 5,000 people have been sterilized since 1988. Officials in Szechuan province stated: 'Couples who have serious hereditary diseases including psychosis, mental deficiency and deformity must not be allowed to bear children'. When disabled women are found to be pregnant, they are sometimes subjected to forced abortions. But despite widespread criticism of China's population policies, there was almost no public outcry following these revelations.

Even in the absence of outright bans on reproduction, the attitude that disabled people should not have children is common. Disabled women and men are still sometimes subject to forced and coerced sterilizations—including hysterectomies performed without medical justification but to prevent the 'bother' of menstruation.

Los Angeles newscaster Bree Walker has a genetically transmitted disability, ectrodactyly, which results in fused bones in her hands and feet. Pregnant with her second child, last year, she found her pregnancy the subject of a call-in radio show. Broadcaster Jane Norris informed listeners in a shocked and mournful tone of voice that Bree's child had a 50-percent chance of being born with the same disability. 'Is it fair to bring a child into the world knowing there's two strikes against it at birth? . . . Is it socially responsible?' When a caller objected that it was no one else's business, Norris argued, 'It's everybody's business.' And many callers agreed with Norris's viewpoint. One horrified caller said, 'It's not just her hands—it's her feet, too. She has to [dramatic pause] wear orthopaedic shoes.'

The attitude that disabled people should not have children is certainly linked with the notion that we should not even be sexual. Yet, as with society's silence about the sexuality of children, this attitude exists alongside widespread sexual abuse. Some authorities estimate that people with disabilities are twice as likely to be victims of rape and other forms of sexual abuse as the general population. While the story of rape and sexual abuse of disabled people must be told and while we must find ways to end it, the current focus on sexual exploitation of disabled people can itself become oppressive.

As Barbara Faye Waxman, the former Disability Project Director for Los Angeles Planned Parenthood states, 'The message for disabled kids is that their sexuality will be realized through their sexual victimization. . . . I don't see an idea that good things can happen, like pleasure, intimacy, like a greater understanding of ourselves, a love of our bodies.' Waxman sees a 'double whammy' effect for disabled people, for whom there are few, if any, positive models of sexuality, and virtually no social expectation that they will become sexual beings.

The attitude that we are and should be asexual seems to exist across a broad range of cultures. Ralf Hotchkiss, famous for developing wheelchairs in Third World countries, has travelled widely in Latin America and Asia. He says that while attitudes vary 'from culture to culture, from subculture to subculture,' he sees nearly everywhere he travels, 'extreme irritation [on the part of disabled people] at the stereotypical assumptions that people . . . make about their sexuality, their lack of it.' He also noted: 'In Latin American countries once they hear I'm married, the next question is always, "How old are your kids?" '

Some of these prejudices are enshrined in law. In the US, 'marital disincentives' remain a significant barrier. To explain this Byzantine system briefly: benefits (including government-funded health care) are greatly reduced and sometimes even eliminated when a disabled person marries. Tom Fambro writes of his own difficulties with the system: 'I am a 46-year-old black man with cerebral palsy. A number of years ago I met a young lady who was sexually attracted to me (a real miracle).' Fambro learned, however, that he would lose his income support and, most crucially, his medical benefits, if he married. 'People told us that we should just live together . . . but because both of us were born-again Christians that was unthinkable. . . . The Social Security Administration has the idea that disabled people are not to fall in love, get married, have sex or have a life of our own. Instead, we are to be sexual eunuchs. They are full of shit.'

Institutions—whether traditional hospitals or euphemistically named 'homes', 'schools', or newer community care facilities—often out-and-out forbid sexual contact for their residents. Or they may outlaw gay and lesbian relationships, while allowing heterosexual ones. Disabled lesbians and gays may also find that their sexual orientation is presumed to occur by default. Restriction of access to sexual information occurs on both a legal and a social plane. The US Library of Congress, a primary source of material for blind and other print-handicapped people, was instructed by Congress in 1985 to no longer make *Playboy* available in braille or on tape. And relay services, which provide telecommunication between deaf and hearing people have sometimes refused to translate sexually explicit speech. In her poem, 'Seeing', blind poet Mary McGinnis writes of a woman being watched by sighted men while bathing nude:

> . . . the guys sitting at the edge of the pond
> looked at her, but she couldn't see them . . .
> and whose skin, hair, shirts and belts
> would remain unknown to her
> because she couldn't go up to them
> and say, now fair is fair, let me touch the places
> on your bodies you try to hide,
> it's my turn—don't draw back or sit on
> your hands, let me count your rings, your scars,
> the hairs coming from your nose. . . .

I have quoted poets several times in this piece; many disability-rights activists now see that while we need changes in laws and policies, the formation of culture is a key part of winning our freedom. Disabled writers and artists are shaping work that is often powerful in both its rage and its affirmation.

In Cheryl Marie Wade's 'side and belly', she writes:

> He is wilty muscle sack and sharp bones fitting
> my gnarlypaws. I am soft cellulite and green eyes

of middle-age memory. We are side and belly trading dreams and fantasies of able-bodied former and not real selves: high-heel booted dancers making love from black rooftops and naked dim doorways. . . . Contradictions in the starry night of wars within and being not quite whole together and whole. Together in sighs we say yes broken and fire and yes singing.

The Need for Intimacy

by Jane Porcino

How long has it been since someone touched me? Twenty years? Twenty years I've been a widow, respected, smiled at, but never touched. Never held so close that loneliness was blotted out. . . . Oh, God, I'm so lonely.

These poignant words from the poem "Minnie Remembers," by Donna Swanson, reflect one of our deepest fears about aging. No matter what our age, we each need intimacy in our lives—at least one other person with whom we can share both pleasure and pain. We hunger for someone who will accept us as delightfully different. This other person can be female or male, young or old.

Research demonstrates that babies who never are held or touched suffer psychologically and may actually wither and die. This also is true as we grow older. And yet, an increasing number of women over 65 live alone, without partners, many of them deprived of any expression of intimacy.

One reality we will face as we grow older female is that there are more women than men; we are likely to find ourselves without a male partner. In the beginning decades of this century, there were equal numbers of women and men over the age of 65. Today, there are almost 150 older women for every 100 men. Divorce after 25 to 30 years of marriage is becoming commonplace, and the average age for a widow is only 56. Complicating all of this is the fact that men who are widowed or divorced in mid- or late-life quickly remarry, most often to younger women. There are nine bridegrooms to every bride over the age 65. Not only is remarriage rare for older women, but there are few social opportunities for close relationships with men. As a result, almost half of all older women live alone—many of them lonely. One woman stated the problem well when she wrote to me:

One thing unites us all—babies, adults, and grandmothers—our need for response from some living creature. Of course, tender loving care would be better, but we can survive without that luxury. What we cannot do without is some kind of reciprocal sharing of life experiences.

Are millions of us doomed to loneliness in old age? Not if we are willing to plan now for our later years, and not just let them happen to us. First, it is important to strengthen and nurture our friendships with women—indeed, glory in them. Fortunately, we were encouraged to develop close female friendships, to share trust and confidences, and to express our feelings to one another. Many of us, even many married women whose relationships with their husbands lack intimacy, presently share much of our social life with women. We seek out environments in which we can express our innermost thoughts. The coffeeklatch, PTA-days have evolved to rap groups, consciousness-raising meetings, and professional networking (the "old girls' club").

Collective living is one way to counter loneliness in our later years. Small groups of us can join together to share living space, incomes, companionship, thoughts, and tasks in a supportive environment. Women are successfully doing this throughout the country. There is a great deal that we can do together that we cannot do alone.

The seeking of intimacy could be encouraged even within nursing homes. My own mother lived out her last years in such a facility, where she developed a close friendship with another woman. They shared all the details of their daily lives, and yet to the end, these two proper women called each other "Mrs.," and rarely touched. The friendship was so deep that when one died, the other followed in a few months.

A prevailing fear of homosexuality among many heterosexual older women may prevent them from acknowledging their human need for intimacy. Some women have shared sexual intimacy with other women most of their adult years. Even women who prefer heterosexuality are moving toward intimacy with women in their later years because of the limited choices available to them. Only a few women may find sexual gratification in their female relationships. But they will find many other kinds of intimacy. Women I know say that they enjoy the companionship of other women; many say they have no desire at all to make the accommodations that would be necessary to form new heterosexual relationships. Two wrote the following to me:

I am blessed with a few special women friendships. They are nonsexual, greatly sharing, mutually supportive "conversational love affairs."

I've a whole circle of supportive, nutritive, loving women friends. I talk over life circumstances, problems and interests with them very openly, receive a great deal of support from them, and give the same. We often have just fun together. I love them and they love me. These friendships have been the most stable thing in my life.

The upcoming generation of elderly women (those now in their late 30s and 40s—the baby-boom generation) are more open to exploring different ways to be intimate. Those of us presently in our middle or late years can learn from them. Although we have been socialized to seek only one significant other, perhaps our search should be for a few such people in our lives—people to have fun with, to share our pleasure and pain, and to give us the physical touching we need.

Love has the potential for deepening as we age. We have years of experience behind us, and now we have the time. Sensuous grandmothers abound—women like Lena Horne, Mary Calderone, and Ingrid Bergman, whose vibrant way of being in the world draws people to them. Our only limit may be a weak imagination.

WORKSHEET—CHAPTER 9

Sexuality

This worksheet needs to be optional. It asks personal questions that no one should be *required* to answer.

1. **Sexual orientation/identity.** Society, parents, and friends give very clear messages about whom one should relate to sexually, how, and when! We are all aware that we are "breaking the rules" if we are sexually involved with someone of the "wrong" age, the "wrong" color, the "wrong" social status, the "wrong" religion, or the "wrong" sex. Heterosexism is so prevalent that most heterosexuals never think about why they relate sexually to the opposite sex. Imagine a mother asking her 18-year-old daughter to explain why she is going out with men instead of women. But most lesbians and bisexuals have had to think through, question, and explain their choices.

   Answer the following questions for yourself and a friend who would identify their sexual identity or situation as different from yours. (If you prefer not to answer these questions yourself, interview two people with different identities and compare their answers.)

   a. Briefly describe your present lifestyle and your sexual identity.

   b. Describe how you made this choice about your sexuality. Was it a gradual evolution or a sudden awareness? Has your sexuality changed or stayed the same since your first sexual identity? What factors have influenced this?

   c. Do you have a sexual partner or partners now? Would your sexual identity be the same if you did not have a partner/partners?

   d. In what specific ways do you consciously work towards a balance of power in your relationships? How equal are your relationships sexually?

   e. How does your sexual relationship(s)/identity affect your relationships with friends, both men and women, with whom you are not having a sexual relationships?

   f. How does your sexuality affect your choices regarding having children/being a parent?

g. The women's movement has emphasized that "the personal is political": the decisions we make in our personal lives and the way we live our lives are political issues. How do you see "the personal is political" relating to sexuality, sexual identity, and sexual choices?

h. Do you feel there is such a thing as "heterosexual privilege"? If so, how does this affect your life?

2. After reading "Do Ask, Do Tell," "Health Care Without Shame," "For Better Lesbian Health, Fewer Barriers to Care," and "Trans Health Crisis" (Chapter 2), think about your recent visits to health settings. Think about the illustrations on the walls and brochures, the forms you were asked to fill out, and questions you were asked in person. Were the setting and interaction designed to be equally comfortable for heterosexual, bisexual, gay, lesbian, and trans people? If yes, describe how this was accomplished. If no, give specific recommendations for how your healthcare setting could be made more welcoming for a diversity of patients.

3. After reading "The Need for Intimacy," give suggestions for how our society could make it easier for people of all ages to have opportunities for healthy intimacy.

4. Synthesize points made in both "The Need for Intimacy" article and "Myth 4: Women want intimacy; men want sex" in "The Orgasm Gap" to come up with a comprehensive statement acknowledging the roles that both intimacy and orgasms could play in both women's and men's lives.

Kegel Exercises

The pubococcygeus (P.C.) muscles support the walls of the vagina, the urethra, and rectum. Good, strong P.C. muscles can be important for childbirth, and for preventing stress incontinence (loss of urine when coughing or sneezing), and can enhance sexual enjoyment. Kegel exercises (developed by Dr. Arnold Kegel) are designed to strengthen the P.C. muscles. Unlike most exercises, no special clothes, gyms, and the like are required. These exercises can be done anywhere and no one else will even know you are doing them.

1. Find your P.C. muscles. When you are urinating, stop the flow of urine in midstream. The muscles you are feeling are your P.C. muscles, the muscles you want to strengthen.

2. Examples of Kegel exercises:

Flicks: Do a series of contractions as rapidly as possible. It has been suggested that one does this in time to the car's turn signals.

Squeeze and hold for as long as possible, trying to work up to holding for 8–10 seconds.

Take a slow, deep breath, squeezing the P.C. muscles as you are breathing in. Pretend you are slowly drawing something into your vagina. Imagine you are lifting weights in your vagina!

REPRODUCTIVE JUSTICE,* FERTILITY, *and* INFERTILITY

*Loretta Ross, a long-time women's health activist, uses the term "reproductive rights" in connection with the more white-dominated movements that have focused very much on abortion and contraceptive issues, and the terms "reproductive freedom" and/or "reproductive justice" for the organizations, with women of color leadership, that have worked on a much wider range of issues related to women's reproductive lives.

Real reproductive rights would mean that a woman is able to choose when, whether, and under what conditions to have children, how many children to have, and to assume that she and her children would survive (and thrive) during pregnancy, childbirth, and the post-partum periods. What kind of health system would truly allow *all* women to have healthy babies, healthy children, and healthy families? What other societal changes need to happen for women to be able to make their own "choices" not to have children or to have the number of children they want?

Too often the media, and sometimes even the movements themselves, have promoted the image that the struggle for reproductive rights is completely about abortion and contraceptive issues. Certainly access to affordable, safe contraception, with affordable, safe abortion as a back-up, is an essential part of women being able to control their bodies and their lives, but many other issues are also part of the bigger picture of what reproductive rights and reproductive justice*/reproductive freedom* really mean.

Identifying the need, framework, and organizing for "reproductive justice" (also called "reproductive freedom") has probably been the most inclusive, exciting, radical, cutting-edge women's health work being done at this turn of the century. Loretta Ross identifies:

> that reproductive justice—the complete physical, mental, spiritual, political, economic, and social well-being of women and girls—will be achieved when women and girls have the economic, social, and political power and resources to make healthy decisions about our bodies, sexuality, and reproduction for ourselves, our families, and our communities in all areas of our lives.

At its most basic, "reproductive justice can be described as reproductive rights embedded in a human rights and social justice framework used to counter all forms of population control that deny women's human rights." A number of articles in this chapter reflect current thinking about reproductive justice and the work by specific women of color organizations that led up to this analysis.

Loretta Ross's stimulating and thought-provoking "The Color of Choice: White Supremacy and Reproductive Justice" provides the essential history and framework for understanding why and how the call for reproductive justice has become core to today's feminist women's health movement thinking and organizing. (As a critique of population control is key to reproductive justice, we have also included the "10 Reasons to Rethink 'Overpopulation'" fact sheet. We recognize that many students moved by the reproductive justice framework feel conflicted by what they have heard about "overpopulation." We think this fact sheet will help!)

"The Political Context for Women of Color Organizing" analyzes the history of reproductive rights organizing very specifically through the lenses of race and class and demonstrates both the role of women of color in mainstream movements and in developing their own organizations. Equally important, this chapter is here to introduce students to the book the chapter is from, *Undivided Rights: Women of Color Organize for Reproductive Justice* (2004), by Jael Silliman, Marlene Gerber Fried, Loretta Ross, and Elena R. Gutiérrez. Every women's health student is encouraged to use this invaluable unique resource for discovering key women's health issues, grassroots organizations, and national organizations for Latina, African-American, Native American, and Asian-Pacific Islander American women.

The articles here, "Latina Agenda for Reproductive Justice," "For Native Women Reproductive Rights Mean . . . ," and "Reclaiming Choice, Broadening the Movement" (in Chapter 2) provide examples of specific ways Latinas, Native American women, and Asian-Pacific Americans are organizing for reproductive justice.

The "politics of information"—that is, questioning who has access to scientifically accurate and personally empowering information, and making such information available to all women—is a vital issue of women's health activism. The next articles explore specific "politics of contraceptive information" issues.

"Contraceptive Jelly on Toast and Other Unintended Consequences of Sexuality Education" is included here to stimulate a discussion of the folklore and contemporary legends we hear about contraception (and other women's health issues) and what we can learn about people's misinformation, anxieties, and fears by analyzing such stories. From my (Mariamne Whatley) perspective as a health educator and my sister's (Elissa Henken) perspective as a folklorist, "One of the clear messages sexuality educators should get from these stories is that education about contraceptives needs to be specific, concrete, and as literal as possible."

The next article is a reminder of crucial information that women are *not* getting. The seemingly apolitical article from the *FDA Consumer*, " 'The Pill' May Not Mix Well with Other Drugs," raises very worrying questions about the politics of information when the reader realizes that very basic information (available in a classic 1987 article) with life-changing ramifications, such as "certain drugs may decrease the effectiveness of your contraceptive or your contraceptive may alter the way your body responds to other medications," is still not available to most women choosing to use the contraceptive pill more than thirty years later.

Another example of the life-saving contraceptive information that women need to know is given in the short articles, "Using YouTube, Public Citizen Warns of Unsafe Birth Control" and "Public Citizen: Newer Birth Control Pills Put Women at Unneeded Risk." (Public Citizen is an example of a national advocacy group fighting for safe products and consumer information.) An important part of women's health activism is finding the resources we trust to keep us up to date on such urgent matters as contraceptive warnings. For example, the National Women's Health Network's web-site (www.nwhn.org) was one of the first places where women heard that the contraceptive patch delivered much higher amounts of estrogen into a woman's body than it was supposed to. Similarly, the *Our Bodies Ourselves* website (www.ourbodiesourselves.org) is always an excellent source for the breaking news related to women's health.

What do women know about the contraceptive *choices* they are making? Are they making *choices* if they don't even know there are important scientific questions to be asking? As long-time women's health educators, we are surprised at three conflicting patterns we see in 2009: (1) "Hormonal contraception is on the rise. Never before have so many young women ingested synthetic hormones for such long periods of time, starting at such a young age." (Wallace) (2) There is a greater need for protection against sexually transmitted infections (STIs) to be incorporated into most people's sexual activities, and (3) Fewer young women seem to be aware of any controversies about the long term safety of hormonal contraception. In "Acquiescence in the Contraceptive Marketplace," Claudine Isles Wallace describes the social pressure most young women feel from their partners, health practitioners, and the wider community to be on hormonal contraception. She explores the many factors that come together to encourage the use of synthetic hormones and discourage other forms of protection against pregnancy or STIs. Even as a young woman very concerned about the safety of hormonal contraceptives, she finds it "extraordinarily difficult" to switch to a "less dependable and sexy" contraceptive method.

"Acquiescence in the Contraceptive Marketplace," should be read in conjunction with Ronna Popkin's "A Dangerous Combination: Direct-to-Consumer Advertising: Abstinence-Only Education, and Young Women." (See Chapter 4.) In addition to issues raised in the "Acquiescence" article, Popkin's articles emphasizes how the power of advertising and the lack of comprehensive sexuality education contribute to the social climate that pushes hormonal contraception. Complementing that, Wallace's article concludes by exploring the *internal* pressure women feel to choose synthetic hormones: "As young women, we are socialized to please those around us, even when that means suspending our own needs and fears." Also, see "To Bleed or Not to Bleed: New Options in the Birth Control Arsenal" (in Chapter 5) to understand how women, in a society that doesn't value menstruation, are now being pushed to simultaneously use hormonal contraception and to not have (regular) periods.

Readings in the beginning of this chapter explore important distinctions in progressive movements between "reproductive rights" and "reproductive justice" agendas. It is equally important that women's health students are aware of debates on the *other* ("Right" wing) side of reproductive issues. While everyone is aware of specific battles over whether abortion should or should not be legal and under which conditions, "Next Target: Birth Control" informs us that we should also be paying attention to the fact that some anti-abortion groups are increasingly organizing against many or all forms of birth control. We have already seen examples of this happening as legislators tried to restrict university health services from dispensing some forms of birth control, pressure was put on the FDA to put inappropriate warnings on condoms, and a range of activities have worked to restrict access to Plan B emergency contraception. Young adults today have grown up with a "contraceptive mentality"—the assumption that people are able to prevent pregnancies if they choose to. "Next Target: Birth Control" reminds us that we should not take the "contraceptive mentality" for granted, but instead must work to make sure that good contraceptives are available.

Such activism in fighting for the availability of Plan B, is the story Stephanie Sequin shares in her "Confessions of a Radical Feminist: Sex, Drugs and the Department of Homeland Security." Following the previous article that showed "social conservatives" increasingly limiting contraceptive choices, Stephanie reminds us how the political climate caused much delay and inappropriate restrictions on American women's access to Plan B, even when that product was easily available to women in at least 38 other countries and the FDA Advisory Committee (the group of scientists given responsibility for evaluating the safety of products) had voted to make Plan B available over the counter, without prescription. As exciting as the title of her article is Stephanie's sense of accomplishment from her taste of activism, having sat in at the FDA:

> We *can* change our world by organizing, by shouting our experiences from the rooftops, and by showing up on the doorsteps of those in power. We hold more cards than we think. In August of 2006, the FDA made the morning-after pill available without prescription to women eighteen and older. A victory for feminist organizing!

What about contraceptives for *men*? An important political question is "why are 'reproductive rights' so much seen as issues for *women?*" If we lived in a more egalitarian society or if men shared equally in the responsibility for childcare, how would that affect *all* reproductive rights and health issues? Why has almost all of reproductive research focused on finding ways to interfere with a woman's body to prevent pregnancy or understanding how a pregnant woman's environment affects fetal health? Is it fair that women have to bear the burden of nearly all the health risks associated with contraception? If safe, reliable contraceptives were available for men, how many women would trust their partners with responsibility for contraception in their heterosexual relationships? Do you think more male contraceptives would be developed and available if more women had the power to help determine reproductive health research priorities?

Our history of looking for good articles on male contraception for this book is symbolic of the lack of progress on this topic! We were pleased to find the 1992 article "Eight New Nonhormonal Contraceptive Methods for Men" promising that "with eight new methods in the wings, men and women don't need to wait any longer" (for male contraception.) Through the 2nd and 3rd editions of our book, we saw much interest in these male methods. But, by the 4th edition of our book, when still no one had heard or seen any of these methods, we ironically added the "classic" symbol to the "old" article promising new methods. By then, the information from the 1992 article that felt most poignant was that "Funding agencies have found reasons not to fund research on male contraception . . . (and) Simple methods with low profit margins have received . . . less support. With funding levels so low, even supportive researchers couldn't accomplish much." We aren't sure we are really updating things when we add the *new* article, "Beyond Condoms: Years in the Making, Male Hormonal Contraceptives May Finally Be on Track." Although the title sounds promising, and we do get updated on the state of the research, the conclusions sound too familiar: A male birth control drug will not be on market in this decade. "At the end of a large, three-year European study, researchers decided the combination tested . . . was not likely to be acceptable for 'widespread daily use.'" "Wyeth Pharmaceuticals announced it is discontinuing its entire research program for new male and female contraceptive drugs. Financial pressures, scientific difficulties, and even an unknown market for male contraception were among the factors that contributed to the decision." Or put most directly by Diana Blithe, Program Director of NIH's male contraceptive development, "Pharmaceutical companies have not chosen to pursue this aggressively. Male birth control is both an untapped and untested market and many drug companies prefer to follow less risky avenues of research."

The next set of fact sheets and article answer some of the most asked questions about surgical and medical (RU-486) abortion. The Abortion Access Project's fact sheets update us on "Who Has Abortions" and the "Shortage of Abortion Providers." "The Side Effects, Risks and Complications of Medical Abortion" chapter from the Australian book, *RU-486: The Abortion Pill,* provides important factual information that most American women never see. Accurate scientific information is essential for women making any decision about health issues. However, because of the political issues surrounding RU-486, any problems with it have too often been sensationalized rather than thoughtfully covered. This was particularly the media response to four deaths (between September 2003 and June 2005) following medical abortions. In "Side Effects, Risks and Complications," Caroline deCosta, Professor of Obstetrics and Gynecology at James Cook University School of Medicine, explains that the deaths were caused by a bacterial infection, *Clostridium sordelli (Cl sordelli),* and that "neither the drugs nor the techniques were the cause of the infection . . . It is very possible that if these women had undergone surgical abortion or if their pregnancies had proceeded to term, *Cl sordelli* infection would still have occurred." and that "Long before medical abortion was practiced in the US, fatal infections from *Cl sordelli* were reported following normal childbirth, caesarean section, gynecology surgery, bowel surgery and orthopaedic (bone) operations." Of course, those procedures are not controversial so no media coverage was given to those deaths. DeCosta's chapter is valuable for clarifying factors that might help a woman choose a surgical abortion over RU-486 or factors (such as prophylactic antibiotic use) that might decrease infection risks. The chapter ends with an interesting comparison of risks: "The overall risk of death associated with medical abortion is less than 1 in 10,000 woman and is very similar to the risk of death from surgical abortion . . . Such figures can be compared to the chances of a woman dying from proceeding to a full-term pregnancy, which in developed countries is around 10 per 10,000 women."

Working against the backlash to the reproductive rights that we have won often takes so much of our energy that we do not take time to discuss controversial and contradictory issues about abortion with other reproductive rights activists. The next article, "The Bad Baby Blues—Reproductive Technology and the Threat to Diversity," should be thought-provoking enough to stimulate some healthy debates among friends or students who usually simply pride themselves on being "prochoice." This article asks us to remember that real choice must include the choice to have a child with disabilities, and to look at how oppressive societal attitudes about disability impact on pregnant women facing prenatal screening. We might ask ourselves what the role of prenatal screening would be in a society where many of the societal "handicaps" of disability had been eliminated or minimized. What would it mean if there were more social supports for people with disabilities so that individual families could more easily "choose" to have a child with disabilities?

Connie S. Chan's "Reproductive Issues Are Essential Survival Issues for Asian-American Communities" describes how she, as a middle-class, educated, bi-lingual Asian-American, was unaware of the reproductive health issues of poor, non-English speaking immigrant women, and what she learned as a translator. This article is a reminder of how easy it is not to understand what reproductive rights mean to another woman or group of women; it begs us to think through the ramifications for poor women when healthcare benefits are not available to them because of their immigrant status or because Medicaid benefits will not cover abortion. At its most provocative level, this article asks us to think about the many ways the health system and society have failed a woman and her children when abortion becomes the only "choice" for basic survival.

In working for a broader definition of reproductive justice that includes women being able to have as many children as they choose, we need to have an analysis of how the issue of infertility has been medicalized. High-tech medicine certainly promises exciting possibilities for offering some women with infertility the possibility of producing a baby. In many cities, it is now routine to offer in vitro fertilization, bypassing blocked fallopian tubes, to many heterosexual women who happen to have an extra $5000 to $10,000 to try it. But, health activists have questioned who benefits, who makes money, and who is determining priorities in the rapidly growing field of infertility technology? Why is all the research emphasis on finding expensive highly technological solutions instead of looking at ways to prevent infertility (safer contraceptive methods, safer work and living environments) that could benefit far more people? Which women do and do not have access to infertility investigations and infertility treatments, and should it be a goal to make these resources equally available to all women? Anne Woollett's moving personal diary (now a "classic" from a book by Pfeffer and Woollett) serves to remind us that there is much more to infertility than sophisticated medical technology: how does the healthcare system respond to many of the key issues of the experiences of infertility (including the tests and treatments) that are related to self-image, sexuality, relationships, and dreams for the future? Anne Woollett and Naomi Pfeffer have written an update to their 1983 book, especially for our book. Their update answers many of the questions of students who read Anne's diary, ask how the field of infertility has changed since the early 1980s, and want to know what happened to the authors after they wrote *The Experience of Infertility,* one of the first books to explore personal feelings about infertility. Both Dr. Anne Woollett and Dr. Naomi Pfeffer have been visible, much published women's health lecturers, working in London universities. In their update, they describe how infertility technology has changed since 1983 but how many of the personal and social issues remain the same. Finally, Anne moves us to share in her thinking of herself now as "childless" rather than "infertile" and trying to disentangle what it means to be a "mother" and to be a "woman."

Similar to Woollett and Pfeffer's "update" to their infertility book, Elizabeth Ruth's 2008 infertility article, "The Colour of Loss," lets us know all the latest products and procedures offered to, or forced upon, women trying to conceive. As a women's health researcher/writer who very much wants to be a mother, Ruth eloquently sets her own experiences in the wider contexts of women's relationships with modern medicine and society's expectations of women as mothers:

> Women who take fertility drugs feel like we're making decisions largely in the dark, leaping at fate, hoping to land softly, babe in arms. We feel uniquely unsuccessful when the drugs don't bring the desired result, and overexposed as we share personal information with myriad professionals who use terms like "poor egg quality," "incompetent uterus," and the present-day scarlet letters, "advanced maternal age." We make martyrs of ourselves, but no one notices because the very cultural definition of motherhood is tangled up in martyrdom.

Ruth's insights as a lesbian and as a critical thinker make her ask provocative questions about homophobia in the healthcare system and the medicalization of infertility.

> A free-choice analysis of the present-day fertility model is short-sighted and stops at easy, non-threatening questions about over-medication and equal access. It doesn't extend to an institutional critique of the industry, which would look at how profit-driven motives might

be guiding or defining (in)fertility . . . We ought to be challenging how the fertility machine participates in—or prevents—the creation of non-traditional families, and we must demand an honest examination of the relationship between pharmaceuticals and fertility doctors.

A few more questions about who does and doesn't benefit from infertility technology are answered in "Grade A: The Market for a Yale Woman's Eggs." This story about a college woman *hoping* to be selected to earn $25,000 for donating eggs, is described as personally unsettling for the "candidate." We think the article may also be unsettling for readers who reflect on Patricia Hill Collins's ("Will the 'Real' Mother Please Stand Up? The Logic of Eugenics and American National Family Planning" from *Revisioning Women, Health, and Healing*, which was reprinted in the 4th edition of this book.) analysis of "real" mothers:

> New reproductive technologies are emerging as central to reorganizing the experiences of all women with motherhood. Working with longstanding patterns of race and social class in the United States, these technological advances fragment the meaning of motherhood. The proliferation of reproductive technologies . . . has allowed the splitting of motherhood into three categories: genetic, gestational, and social motherhood. Genetic mothers are those who contribute the genetic material to another human being. Gestational mothers are those who carry the developing fetus in utero until birth. Social mothers care for children actually born. Traditional views of motherhood forwarded by the traditional family ideal present one middle-class white woman as fulfilling all three functions, assisted by domestic servants. But new reproductive technologies have made it possible for women to specialize in one of these mothering categories.

From the other side of the equation, choosing the sperm from a sperm bank for inseminations, "Father Knows Baste" is the story of one woman's decision to become a single mother by choice.

The Color of Choice:
"White Supremacy
and Reproductive Justice"

by Loretta J. Ross[1]

[T]he regulation of reproduction and the exploitation of women's bodies and labor is both a tool and a result of systems of oppression based on race, class, gender, sexuality, ability, age and immigration status.[2]

It is impossible to understand the resistance of women of color to the reproductive politics of both the Right and the Left without first comprehending how the system of white supremacy constructs different destinies for each ethnic population of the United States through targeted, yet diffuse, policies of population control. Even a cursory examination of the reproductive politics dominating today's headlines—such as debates on abortion and welfare—reveals that some women are encouraged to have more children while others are discouraged. Why are some women glorified as mothers while others have their motherhood rights contested? Why are there obstacles for women who seek abortions while our society neglects mothers and children already here? As we move toward "designer babies" made possible by advances in assisted reproductive technologies, does anyone truly believe that all women will have an equal right to benefit from these "new reproductive choices," that children of all races will be promoted, or that vulnerable women will not be exploited?

Women of color reproductive justice activists oppose all political rationales, social theories, and genetic justifications for reproductive oppression against communities of color, whether through blatant policies of sterilization abuse or through the coercive use of dangerous contraceptives. Instead, women of color activists demand "reproductive justice," which requires the protection of women's human rights to achieve the physical, mental, spiritual, political, economic and social well-being of women and girls.[3] Reproductive justice goes far beyond the demand to eliminate racial disparities in reproductive health services, and beyond the right-to-privacy-based claims to legal abortion made by the pro-choice movement and dictated and limited by the U.S. Supreme Court. A reproductive justice analysis addresses the fact that progressive issues are divided, isolating advocacy for abortion from other social justice issues relevant to the lives of every woman. In the words of SisterSong president Toni Bond, "We have to reconnect women's health and bodies with the rest of their lives."[4] In short, reproductive justice can be described as reproductive rights embedded in a human rights and social justice framework used to counter all forms of population control that deny women's human rights.

White Supremacy and Population Control on the Right, and Left

Population control is necessary to maintain the normal operation of US commercial interests around the world. Without our trying to help these countries with their economic and social development, the world would rebel against the strong US commercial presence.[5]

Although the United States does not currently have an explicit population control policy, population control ideologies march from the margins to the mainstream of reproductive politics and inform policies promoted by the Right and the Left. Fears of being numerically and politically overwhelmed by people of color bleach meaning from any alternative interpretations of the constellation of population control policies that restrict immigration by people of color, encourage sterilization and contraceptive abuse of people of color, and incarcerate upwards of 2 million people, the vast majority of whom are people of color.

The expanded definition of white supremacy as I use it in this essay is an interlocking system of racism, patriarchy, homophobia, ultranationalism, xenophobia, anti-Semitism, and religious fundamentalism that creates a complex matrix of oppressions faced by people of color in the United States. As a tenacious ideology in practice, it is evidenced on both the Right and the Left—in the Far Right, the Religious Right, paleoconservatives, neoconservatives, neoliberals, and liberals. Abby Ferber, a researcher on the intersection of race, gender, and white supremacy, writes that "defining white supremacy as extremist in its racism often has the result of absolving the mainstream population of its racism, portraying white supremacists as the racist fringe in contrast to some non-racist majority."[6]

White supremacy not only defines the character of debates on reproductive politics but it also explains and predicts the borders of the debate. In other words, what Americans think as a society about women of color and population control is determined and informed by their relationship to white supremacy as an ideology, and these beliefs affect the country's reproductive politics. Both conservatives and liberals enforce a reproductive hierarchy of privatization and punishment that targets the fertility, motherhood, and liberty of women of color.

Population control policies are externally imposed by governments, corporations, or private agencies to control—by increasing or limiting—population growth and behavior, usually by controlling women's reproduction and fertility. All national population policies, even those developed for purportedly benign reasons, put women's empowerment at risk. Forms of population control include immigration restrictions, selective population movement or dispersal, incarceration, and various forms of discrimination, as well as more blatant manifestations, such as cases in which pregnant illegal immigrants and incarcerated women are forced to have abortions. According to a 1996 study by Human Rights Watch, abuses of incarcerated women not only include denial of adequate health care, but pressure to seek an abortion, particularly if the woman is impregnated by a prison guard.[7]

Meanwhile, impediments are placed in the way of women who voluntarily choose to terminate their pregnancies. The only logic that explains this apparent moral inconsistency is one that examines precisely who is subjected to which treatment and who is affected by which reproductive policy at which time in history. Women of color have little trouble distinguishing between those who are encouraged to have more children and those who are not, and understanding which social, political, and economic forces influence these determinations.

Population control policies are by no means exclusively a twentieth-century phenomenon. During the Roman Empire, the state was concerned with a falling birthrate among married upper-class couples. As has been the case for elite classes throughout history, procreation was seen as a duty to society. Emperor Augustus consequently enacted laws containing positive and negative incentives to reproduction, promoting at least three children per couple and discouraging childlessness.[8] Augustus probably knew that the falling birthrate was not a result of abstention among Roman men and women, but rather of contraceptive and abortifacient use by Roman women to control their fertility. Through legislation, he asserted the state's interest in compelling citizens to have more children for the good of society.[9] Because no ancient Roman texts offer the perspectives of women on this issue, it is difficult to ascertain what women thought of this territorial assertion of male privilege over their private lives. However, the Roman birthrate continued to decline despite the emperor's orders, suggesting that Roman women probably did what most women have done throughout the ages: make the decisions that make sense for them and refuse to allow men to control their fertility. As historian Rickie Solinger points out, "The history of reproductive politics will always be in part a record of women controlling their reproductive capacity, no matter what the law says, and by those acts reshaping the law."[10]

Despite the Roman failure to impose the state's will on individual human reproductive behavior, many governments today have refused to recognize the virtual impossibility of regulating human reproductive behavior through national population policies. China and Romania have instituted population control measures with catastrophic results. Even governments seeking to achieve their population objectives through more benign policies, such as offering financial incentives for women to have children, can only report negligible results. Despite government and moralistic pronouncements, women perceive their reproductive decisions as private, like their periods and other health concerns. Even when the law, the church, or their partners oppose their decisions, they tend to make the decision about whether or not to use birth control or abortion, or to parent, for themselves.

This lived reality has not stopped lawmakers from trying to assert control oven women's reproduction. Who gets targeted for positive, pronatalist policies encouraging childbirth versus negative, antinatalist policies that discourage childbirth is determined by powerful elites, informed by prejudices based on race, class, sexual identity, and immigration status. Policies that restrict abortion access, distort sex and sexuality education, impose parental notification requirements for minors, allow husbands to veto options for abortion, and limit use of emergency and regular contraception all conspire to limit access to fertility control to white women, especially young white women. Meanwhile, women of color face intimidating obstacles to making reproductive choices, including forced contraception, sterilization abuse, and, in the case of poor women and women of color on social assistance, welfare family caps. These population control policies have both domestic and international dimensions, which are rarely linked in the minds of those who believe that the struggle is principally about abortion.

Internationally, the fertility rate of women of color is the primary preoccupation of those determined to impose population controls on developing countries. According to the United Nations, in 2000, more than one hundred countries worldwide had large "youth bulges"—people aged fifteen to twenty-nine accounted for more than 40% of all adults. All of these extremely youthful countries are in the developing world, where fertility rates are highest, and most are in sub-Saharan Africa and the Middle East. Many of the young people who make up these "youth bulges" face dismal prospects because of deliberate underdevelopment. Over the past decade, youth unemployment rates have risen to more than double the over-all global unemployment rate. In the absence of a secure livelihood, many experts believe that discontented youth may resort to violence or turn to insurgent organizations as sources of social mobility and self-esteem. Recent studies show that countries with large youth bulges were roughly two and a half times more likely to experience an outbreak of civil conflict than countries below this benchmark.[11]

To respond to these alarming trends, many on the Right and the Left want to restrict the growth of developing world populations, and in this context, "family planning" becomes a tool to fight terrorism and civil unrest. Some on the Left want to increase access to family planning, economic development, and education as a way to curb population growth, even if achieved through the coercive use of contraceptives and sterilization. Some on the Right prefer military interventions and economic domination to achieve population control.

The Bush administration's family planning and HIV/AIDS policies are also having the impact of serving as tools of population control in the Global South. The US government's "ABC program" (A is for abstinence, B is for being faithful, and C for condom use) is purportedly designed to reduce the spread of HIV/AIDS. Critics of the policy point out that the ABC approach offers no option for girls or women coerced into sex, for married women who are trying to get pregnant yet have unfaithful husbands, or for victims of rape and incest who have no control over when and under what conditions they will be forced to engage in sexual activity. As a result, instead of decreasing the spread of HIV/AIDS, some suspect the ABC policy of actually increasing the ravages of the disease. In combination with the US government's failure to provide funding for and access to vital medications for individuals infected with HIV, the effects are deadly.

Meanwhile, right-wing policies that appear to be pronatalist—such as the Global Gag Rule which prohibits clinics in developing countries that receive USAID funds from discussing abortion—are, in fact, achieving the opposite result. Catering to its radical antiabortion base, the Bush administration has withdrawn funds from programs for family planning for women around the world, withholding $136 million in funding for the United Nations Population Fund (UNFPA) since 2002. This money could have prevented at least 1.5 million induced abortions, 9,400 maternal deaths, and 154,000 infant and child deaths.[12] In September 2005, the U.S. State Department announced that it was denying funding to UNFPA for the fourth year.

One might ask why staunch conservatives are opposed to family planning in developing countries when family planning so clearly limits population growth and reduces the need for abortions. One of the leading causes of death for women in developing countries is maternal mortality—death from childbirth. The UN estimated a worldwide total of 529,000 maternal deaths in the year 2000, with less than 1% of deaths occurring in developed nations.[13] Women of color cannot help but observe that family planning is not nearly as efficient in reducing populations of color as factors such as maternal mortality, infant mortality, and AIDS. We are also not oblivious to the wealth of natural resources like oil, gold, and diamonds in the lands where these populations are shrinking—after all, a depopulated land cannot protect itself.

Overt and covert population control polices are also at play on the domestic front. In October 2005, former secretary of education William Bennett declared on his radio talk show that if "you wanted to reduce crime . . . if that were your sole purpose, you could abort every Black baby in this country, and your crime rate would go down." While Bennett conceded that aborting all African American babies "would be an impossible, ridiculous, and morally reprehensible thing to do," he still maintained that "the crime rate would go down."

Bennett is merely echoing widespread perceptions by many radical and moderate conservatives in the United States who directly link social ills with the fertility of women of color. The Heritage Foundation, a right-wing think tank influential in the national debates on reproductive politics, offers the following analysis: "Far more important than residual material hardship is behavioral poverty: a breakdown in the values and conduct that lead to the formation of healthy families, stable personalities, and self-sufficiency. This includes eroded work ethic and dependency, lack of educational aspiration and achievement, inability or unwillingness to control one's children, *increased single parenthood and illegitimacy* [emphasis added], criminal activity, and drug and alcohol abuse."[14]

This mainstream white supremacist worldview is based on the notion that people are poor because of behaviors, not because they are born into poverty. In reality, according to Zillah Eisenstein, "poverty is tied to family structures in crisis. Poverty is tied to the unavailability of contraceptives and reproductive rights. Poverty is tied to teenage pregnancy. Poverty is tied to women's wages that are always statistically lower than men's. Poverty is tied to the lack of day care for women who must work. Poverty is tied to insufficient health care for women. Poverty is tied to the lack of access to job training and education."[15]

It would be logical to assume that people who claim to value all human life from the moment of conception would fiercely support programs that help disadvantaged children and parents. Sadly, this is not the case. Surveys show that, on average, people who are strongly opposed to abortion are also more likely to define themselves as political conservatives who do not support domestic programs for poor families, single mothers, people of color, and immigrants.[16] They are also opposed to overseas development assistance in general, and to specific programs for improving women's and children's health, reducing domestic violence, helping women become more economically self-sufficient, and lowering infant mortality.[17]

Perspectives from the Left are hardly more reassuring to women of color. Is Bennett, a member of the Heritage Foundation, any worse than an environmentalist who claims that the world is overpopulated and drastic measures must be taken to address this catastrophe? Betsy Hartmann writes about the "greening of hate," or blaming environmental degradation, urban sprawl, and diminishing natural resources on poor populations of color. This is a widely accepted set of racist myths promoted by many in the environmental movement, which is moving rather alarmingly to the right as it absorbs ideas and personnel from the white supremacist movement, including organizations such as the Aryan Women's League.[18]

The reality is that 20% of the world's population controls 80% of the global wealth. In other words, it is not the population growth of the developing world that is depleting the world's resources, but the overconsumption of these resources by the richest countries in the world. The real fear of many in the population control movement is that the developing world will become true competitors for the earth's resources and demand local control over their natural wealth of oil and minerals. Rather than perceiving overconsumption by Americans, agricultural mismanagement, and the military-industrial complex as the main sources of environmental degradation, many U.S. environmentalists maintain that the fertility of poor women is the root of environmental evil, and cast women of color, immigrant women, and women of the Global South as the perpetrators, rather than the victims, of environmental degradation.[19] This myth promotes alarmist fears about overpopulation, and leads to genocidal conclusions such as those reached by writers for *Earth First! Journal* who said, "The AIDS virus may be Gaia's tailor-made answer to human overpopulation," and that famine should take its natural course to stem overpopulation.[20]

Population control groups on the Left will often claim that they are concerned with eliminating gender and economic inequalities, racism, and colonialism, but since these organizations address these issues through a problematic paradigm, inevitably their efforts are directed toward reducing population growth of all peoples in theory and of people of color in reality.[21] In fact, these efforts are embedded within the context of a dominant neoliberal agenda which trumps women's health and empowerment. And some prochoice feminists have supported the neoliberal projects of "privatization, commodification, and deregulation of public health services that . . . have led to diminished access and increasing mortality and morbidity of women who constitute the most vulnerable groups in both developing and developed countries."[27]

Similarly, the prochoice movement, largely directed by middle-class white women, is oblivious to the role of white supremacy in restricting reproductive options for all women, and, as a result, often inadvertently colludes with it. For instance, a study published in 2001 in the *Quarterly Journal of Economics* by John J. Donohue III, a professor of law at Stanford University, and Steven D. Levitt, a professor of economics at the University of Chicago, claimed that the 1973 legalization of abortion prevented the birth of unwanted children who were likely to have become criminals. Of course, the authors state that these children would have been born to poor women of color. They also disingenuously and incorrectly assert that "women who have abortions are those most at risk to give birth to children who would engage in criminal activity"[23] and conclude that the drop in crime rates approximately eighteen years after the *Roe v. Wade* decision was a consequence of legal abortion. Despite the quickly revealed flaws in their research, some prochoice advocates continue to tout their findings as justification for keeping abortion legal, adopting a position similar to Mr. Bennett's.[24]

Indeed, the prochoice movement's failure to understand the intersection between race, class, and gender led leaders of the movement to try their own "Southern Strategy" in the 1980s. Central to this strategy was an appeal to conservative voters who did not share concerns about women's rights, but who were hostile to the federal government and its public encroachment on individual choice and privacy. Some voters with conservative sympathies were pruned from the antiabortion movement for a while, uneasily joining the ranks of the prochoice movement in an admittedly unstable alliance based on "states' rights" segregationist tendencies.[25] Not surprisingly, on questions of abortion policy—whether the government should spend tax money on abortions for poor women or whether teenagers should have to obtain parental consent for abortions—the alliance fell apart. And this appeal to conservative, libertarian Southern voters drove an even deeper wedge in the pro-choice movement, divorcing it from its original base of progressive white women and alienating women of color.

Meanwhile, the Right pursued its population control policies targeting communities of color both overtly and indirectly. Family planning initiatives in the Deep South in the 1950s encouraged women of color (predominantly African American women) to use contraceptives and sterilizations to reduce the growth of our populations, while obstacles were simultaneously placed in the paths of white women seeking access to these same services. A Louisiana judge, Leander Perez, was quoted as saying, "The best way to hate a nigger is to hate him before he is born."[26] This astonishingly frank outburst represented the sentiments of many racists during this period, although the more temperate ones disavowed gutter epithets.

For example, conservative politicians like Strom Thurmond supported family planning in the 1960s when it was used as a racialized form of population control, aimed at limiting Black voter strength in African American communities.[27] When it was presented as a race-directed strategy to reduce their Black populations, North Carolina and South Carolina became the first states to include family planning in their state budgets in the 1950s. One center in Louisiana reported that in its first year of operation, 96% of its clients were Black.

The proportion of white clients never rose above 15%.[28] Generally speaking, family planning associated with women of color was most frequently supported; but support quickly evaporated when it was associated with white women.

Increased federal spending on contraception coincided with the urban unrest and rise of a militant Civil Rights movement in the late 1960s. In 1969, President Nixon asked Congress to establish a five-year plan for providing family planning services to "all those who want them but cannot afford them."[29] However, the rationale behind the proposed policy was to prevent population increases among Blacks—this would make governance of the world in general, and inner cities in particular, difficult. Reflecting concerns strikingly similar to those driving U.S. population policies overseas, Nixon pointed to statistics that showed a "bulge" in the number of Black Americans between the ages of five and nine. This group of youngsters who would soon enter their teens— "an age group with problems that can create social turbulence"— was 25% larger than ten years before.[30] This scarcely disguised race- and class-based appeal for population control persuaded many Republicans to support family planning.

Today the U.S. government's less obvious—but no less effective—approach of promoting policies overseas that contribute to high maternal mortality rates and devastation as a result of HIV/AIDS was also recently revealed to have a counterpart on the domestic front. Images of chaos and death as Hurricane Katrina's floodwaters engulfed Black neighborhoods shocked many Americans. But according to Jean Hardisty, a researcher on white supremacy in America, these pictures of poor New Orleans residents, many of them Black women and their children, revealed some essential truths:

> Much of the white public will never understand that those images were more than the result of neglected enforcement of civil rights laws, or the "failure" of the poor to rise above race and class. They were images of structural racism. In one of the poorest cities in the country (with 28% of New Orleanians living in poverty—over two times the national poverty rate), the poor were white as well as African American. But, the vast majority (84%) of the poor were Black. This is not an accident. It is the result of white supremacy that is so imbedded in US society that it has become part of the social structure. Structural racism is not only a failure to serve people equally across race, culture and ethnic origin within private and government entities (as well as "third sector" institutions, such as the print, radio and TV

media and Hollywood). It is also the predictable consequence of legislation at the federal, state, and local level.[31]

This racial illiteracy on the part of white people is part of the hegemonic power of whiteness. Through a historical mythology, white supremacy has a vested interest in denying what is most obvious: the privileged position of whiteness. For most people who are described as white, since race is believed to be "something" that shapes the lives of people of color, they often fail to recognize the ways in which their own lives and our public policies are shaped by race. Structural or institutionalized racism is not merely a matter of individual attitudes, but the result of centuries of subordination and objectification that reinforce population control policies.

Politicians have continuously used policies of population control to conquer this land, produce an enslaved workforce, enshrine racial inequities, and preserve traditional power relations. For just as long, women of color have challenged race-based reproductive politics, including the forced removal of our children; the racialization and destruction of the welfare system; the callousness of the foster care system that breaks up our families; and the use of the state to criminalize our pregnancies and our children. These become an interlocked set of public policies which Dorothy Roberts calls 'reproductive punishment.' She observes that the "system's racial disparity also reinforces negative stereotypes about . . . people's incapacity to govern themselves and need for state supervision."[32]

Reproductive politics are about who decides "whether, when, and which woman can reproduce legitimately and *also* the struggles over which women have the right to be mothers of the children they bear."[33] Entire communities can be monitored and regulated by controlling how, when, and how many children a woman can have and keep. This is particularly true for women on Native American reservations, incarcerated women, immigrant women, and poor women across the board, whose reproductive behavior is policed by an adroit series of popular racist myths, fierce state regulation, and eugenicist control. The use of the "choice" framework in the arena of abortion, as Rhonda Copelon points outs, underwrites "the conservative idea that the personal is separate from the political, and that the larger social structure has no impact on [or responsibility for] private, individual choice."[34]

For the past thirty years, women of color have urged the mainstream movement to seriously and consistently support government funding for abortions for poor women. The 1977 Hyde Amendment prohibited the use of taxpayer funds to pay for abortions for women whose health care is dependent on the federal government, and it affects women on Medicaid, women in the military and the Peace Corps, and indigenous women who primarily rely on the Indian Health Service for their medical care. Yet despite its obvious targeting of poor women of color, prochoice groups have not made repealing the Hyde Amendment a priority because polling data has indicated that the majority of Americans do not want taxpayer money used to pay for abortions.

When the Freedom of Choice Act was proposed by prochoice groups in 1993, it retained the provisions of the Hyde Amendment. According to Andrea Smith, one NARAL Pro-Choice America (formerly known as the National Abortion Rights Action League) petition in favor of the act stated that, "the Freedom of Choice Act (FOCA) will secure the original vision of *Roe v. Wade*, giving *all* women reproductive freedom and securing that right for future generations [emphasis added].[35] As Smith wryly points out, apparently poor women and indigenous women did not qualify as "women" in the eyes of the writers of this petition.

In a 1973 editorial, the National Council of Negro Women pointed out the link between civil rights activism and reproductive oppression that mitigated the concept of choice for oppressed communities:

> The key words are "if she chooses." Bitter experience has taught the Black woman that the administration of justice in this country is not colorblind. Black women on welfare have been forced to accept sterilization in exchange for a continuation of relief benefits and others have been sterilized without their knowledge or consent. A young pregnant woman recently arrested for civil rights activities in North Carolina was convicted and told that her punishment would be to have a forced abortion. We must be ever vigilant that what appears on the surface to be a step forward, does not in fact become yet another fetter or method of enslavement.[36]

Yet currently the hard-core Right has begun to demand the political disenfranchisement of people receiving public assistance. For example, in 2005 a law was proposed in Georgia that would have required voters to have driver's licenses or other forms of state identification to vote; right-wing proponents complained that the bill didn't go far enough, and that the vote should be taken away from welfare recipients.[37] And while linking political enfranchisement to population control is blatantly coercive and antidemocratic, it has not been unusual in the United States. In 1960, when the city of New Orleans was ordered to desegregate its schools, local officials responded by criminalizing the second pregnancies of women on public assistance; after they were threatened with imprisonment and welfare fraud, many of these African American women and children disappeared from the welfare rolls.[38] The Right is often blatant in its determination to restrict the fertility of women of color, and thus control our communities. They endlessly proffer an array of schemes and justifications for intruding on the personal decisions of women of color and for witholding the social supports necessary to make healthy reproductive decisions.

On the other hand, in its singular focus on maintaining the legal right to abortion, the prochoice movement often ignores the intersectional matrix of race, gender, sovereignty, class and immigration status that complicates debates on reproductive politics in the United States for women of color. The movement is *not* the personal property of middle-class white women, but without a frank acknowledgement of white supremacist practices in the past and the present, women of color will not be convinced that mainstream prochoice activists and organizations are committed to empowering women of color to make decisions about our fertility, or to reorienting the movement to include the experiences of *all* women.

Mobilizing for Reproductive Justice

Prior to the 1980s, women of color reproductive health activists organized primarily against sterilization abuse and teen pregnancy, yet many were involved in early activities to legalize abortion because of the disparate impact illegal abortion had in African American, Puerto Rican, and Mexican communities. Most women of color refrained from joining mainstream pro-choice organizations, preferring instead to organize autonomous women of color organizations that were more directly responsive to the needs of their communities. The rapid growth of women of color reproductive health organizations in the 1980s and 1990s helped build the organizational strength (in relative terms) to generate an analysis and a new movement in the twenty-first century.

This was a period of explosive autonomous organizing.[39] Women of color searched for a conceptual framework that would convey our twinned values—the right to have and not to have a child—as well as the myriad ways our rights to be mothers and parent our children are constantly threatened. We believed these values and concerns separated us from the liberal pro-choice movement in the United States, which was preoccupied with privacy rights and maintaining the legality of abortion. We were also skeptical about leaders in the pro-choice movement who seemed more interested in population restrictions than women's empowerment. Some promoted dangerous contraceptives and coercive sterilizations, and were mostly silent about economic inequalities

and power imbalances between the developed and the developing worlds. Progressive women of color felt closest to the radical wing of the women's movement that articulated demands for abortion access amd shared our class analysis, and even closer to radical feminists who demanded an end to sterilization and contraceptive abuse. Yet we lacked a framework that aligned reproductive rights with social justice in an intersectional way, bridging the multiple domestic and global movements to which we belonged.

We found an answer in the global women's health movement through the voices of women from the Global South. By forming small but significant delegations, women of color from the United States participated in all of the international conferences and significant events of the global feminist movement. A significant milestone was the International Conference on Population and Development in 1994 in Cairo, Egypt. In Cairo, women of color witnessed how women in other countries were successfully using a human rights framework in their advocacy for reproductive health and sexual rights.

Shortly after the Cairo conference, drawing on the perspectives of women of color engaged in both domestic and international activism, women of color in the United States coined the term "reproductive justice." In particular, we made the link between poverty and the denial of women's human rights, and critiqued how shared opposition to fundamentalists and misogynists strengthened a problematic alliance between feminists and the population control establishment.

The first step toward implementing a reproductive justice framework in our work was taken two months after the September Cairo conference. A group of African American women (some of whom became cofounders of the SisterSong Women of Color Reproductive Health Collective) spontaneously organized an informal Black Women's Caucus at a national pro-choice conference sponsored in 1994 by the Illinois Pro-Choice Alliance in Chicago. We were attempting to "Bring Cairo Home" by adapting agreements from the Cairo program of action to a US-specific context. In the immediate future, we were very concerned that the Clinton administration's health care reform proposals were ominously silent about abortion rights, which appeared to renege on the promises the Administration made at Cairo. Even without a structured organization, we mobilized for a national signature ad in the *Washington Post* to express our concerns, raising twenty-seven thousand dollars and collecting six hundred signatures from African American women to place the ad in the *Post*. After debating and rejecting the choice framework in our deliberations, we called ourselves Women of African Descent for Reproductive Justice. We defined reproductive justice, at that time as "reproductive health integrated into social justice," bespeaking our perception that reproductive health is a social justice issue for women of color because healthcare reform without a reproductive health component would do more harm than good for women of color. Three years later, using human rights as a unifying framework and reproductive justice as a central organizing concept, the SisterSong Women of Color Reproductive Health Collective was formed in 1997 by autonomous women of color organizations.

SisterSong maintains that reproductive justice—the complete physical, mental, spiritual, political, economic, and social well-being of women and girls—will be achieved when women and girls have the economic, social, and political power and resources to make healthy decisions about our bodies, sexuality, and reproduction for ourselves, our families, and our communities in all areas of our lives. For this to become a reality, we need to make change on the individual, community, institutional, and societal levels to end all forms of oppression, including forces that deprive us of self-determination and control over our bodies, and limit our reproductive choices to achieve undivided justice.[40]

An instructive example of how the reproductive justice framework employed by SisterSong has influenced the mainstream movement is the organizing story behind the March for Women's Lives in Washington, D.C., on April 25, 2004. The march, which mobilized 1.15 million participants, was the largest demonstration in US history. Originally organized to protest antiwoman policies (such as the badly named Partial Birth Abortion Ban Act) and to call attention to the delicate pro-choice majority on the Supreme Court, it also exposed fissures in the pro-choice movement that have not been fully analyzed.

Mobilizing for the march uncovered cleavages on the Left. The event's original title, the "March for Freedom of Choice," reflected a traditional focus on a privacy-based abortion rights framework established by the Supreme Court. At the same time, the dominant issue on the American Left was the illegal war against Iraq, not abortion politics. Tens of millions of people had marched around the globe to protest Bush's invasion in February 2003. As the initial organizing for the march progressed in 2003, it became clear that targeted supporters would not turn out in sufficient numbers if the march focused solely on the right to legal abortion and the need to protect the Supreme Court. Abortion isolated from other social justice issues would not work.

Ultimately, in order to broaden the appeal of the march and mobilize the entire spectrum of social justice activists in the United States, organizers sought a strategic framework that could connect various sectors of US social justice movements. They approached SisterSong in the fall of 2003, asking for endorsement of and participation in the march. SisterSong pushed back, expressing problems with the march title and the then all-white decision-makers on the steering committee. SisterSong demanded that women of color organizations be added to the highest decision-making body, and counteroffered with its own "reproductive justice" framework. (The original March organizers were the Feminist Majority Foundation, the National Organization for Women, Planned Parenthood Federation of America, and NARAL Pro-Choice America. Eventually, the National Latina Institute for Reproductive Health, the Black Women's Health Imperative and the American Civil Liberties Union were added to the march steering committee.) Reproductive justice was a viable way to mobilize broader support for the march. It also had the potential to revitalize an admittedly disheartened pro-choice movement. The central question was: were pro-choice leaders ready and willing to finally respect the leadership and vision of women of color?

Through the leadership of Alice Cohan, the march director, the March for Freedom of Choice was renamed in the fall of 2003, and women of color organizations were added to the steering committee. Using the intersectional, multi-issue approach fundamental to the reproductive justice framework, march organizers reached out to women of color, civil rights organizations, labor, youth, antiwar groups, anti-globalization activists, environmentalists, immigrants' rights organizations, and many, many others.

The success of the march was a testament to the power of reproductive justice as a framework to mobilize and unite diverse sectors of the social justice movement to support women's human rights in the United States and abroad. Just as importantly, it also showed how women of color have to take on the Right and the Left when asserting control over our bodies, our communities, and our destinies.

> I am not wrong: Wrong is not my name
> My name is my own my own my own
> and I can't tell you who in the hell set things up like
>   this
> but I can tell you that from now on my resistance
> my simple and daily and nightly self-determination
> may very well cost you your life.
>
> —June Jordan

NOTES
A list of end notes is available in the original source.

10 Reasons to Rethink 'Overpopulation'

by the Population and Development Program at Hampshire College

Fears of overpopulation are pervasive in American society. From an early age we are taught that population pressure is responsible for poverty, hunger, environmental degradation and even political insecurity. Conventional wisdom, however, is not always wise. It is important to rethink 'overpopulation' in relation to the following:

1 NUMBERS

The population 'explosion' is over.

Although world population is still growing and is expected to reach 9 billion by the year 2050, the era of rapid growth is over. With increasing education, urbanization, and women's work outside the home, birth rates have fallen in almost every part of the world and now average 2.7 births per woman. The UN projects that world population will eventually stabilize, falling to 8.3 billion in 2175.

2 POVERTY

The focus on population masks the complex causes of poverty and inequality.

A narrow focus on human numbers obscures the way different economic and political systems operate to perpetuate poverty and inequality. It places the blame on the people with the least amount of resources and power rather than on corrupt governments and rich elites. In the late 1990s, the 225 people who comprise the 'ultra-rich' had a combined wealth of over US $1 trillion, equivalent to the annual income of the poorest 47% of the world's people.

3 HUNGER

Hunger is not the result of 'too many mouths' to feed.

Global food production has consistently outpaced population growth. People go hungry because they do not have the land on which to grow food or the money with which to buy it. In Brazil, one percent of the land owners control almost half of the country's arable land. The U.S. is the largest food producer in the world, yet more than one in ten American households are either experiencing hunger or are at the risk of it.

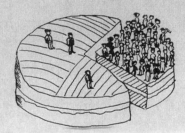

4 ENVIRONMENT

Population growth is not the driving force behind environmental degradation.

Blaming environmental degradation on overpopulation lets the real culprits off the hook. The richest fifth of the world's people consume 66 times as many resources as the poorest fifth. The U.S. is the largest emitter of greenhouse gases responsible for global warming. Militaries worldwide are major agents of environmental destruction. War ravages natural landscapes and military toxins pollute land, air and water. Focusing on population blinds us to the positive role many poor people play in protecting the environment, such as preserving plant biodiversity.

5 POLITICAL INSTABILITY

Population pressure is not a root cause of political insecurity and conflict.

Blaming population pressure for instability takes the onus off powerful actors and political choices. Especially since 9/11, conflict in the Middle East has been linked to a 'youth bulge' of too many young men whose numbers supposedly make them prone to violence. Missing from this simple picture is how oil politics, the Israeli-Palestinian conflict, and the Bush administration's war on Iraq are causing unrest in the region.

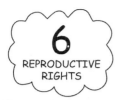

Population control targets women's fertility and restricts reproductive rights.

All women should have access to high quality, voluntary reproductive health services, including safe birth control and abortion. In contrast, population control programs try to drive down birth rates through coercive social policies and the aggressive promotion of sterilization or long-acting contraceptives that can threaten women's health. In India, a number of states punish poor parents who have more than two children by denying them access to government assistance, employment and election to public office. In China, the one-child policy is still enforced through forced sterilizations and abortions.

Population control programs have a negative effect on basic health care.

Under pressure from international population agencies, many poor countries made population control a higher priority than primary health care from the 1970s on. Reducing fertility was considered more important than preventing and treating debilitating diseases like malaria, improving maternal and child health, and addressing malnutrition. This not only took a tragic toll on human life, but left countries without the public health infrastructure needed to face new threats like HIV/AIDS. The World Bank and International Monetary Fund have further undermined primary health care by forcing countries to cut and/ or privatize health services, putting them out of the reach of poor people.

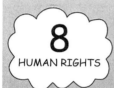

Population alarmism encourages apocalyptic thinking that legitimizes human rights abuses.

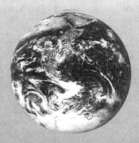

Dire predictions of population-induced mass famine and environmental collapse have long been popular in the U.S. Population funding appeals still play on such fears even though they have not been borne out in reality. Fear does more than sell, however. It convinces many otherwise well-meaning people that it is morally justified to curtail the basic human and reproductive rights of poor people in order to save ourselves and the planet from doom. This sense of emergency leads to an elitist moral relativism, in which 'we' know best and 'our' rights are more worthy than 'theirs.' Politically, it legitimizes authoritarianism.

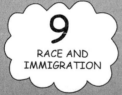

Threatening images of overpopulation reinforce racial and ethnic stereotypes and scapegoat immigrants and other vulnerable communities.

Negative media images of starving African babies, poor, pregnant women of color, and hordes of dangerous Third World men drive home the message that 'those people' outnumber 'us.' Fear of overpopulation in the Third World often translates into fear of increasing immigration to the West, and thereby people of color becoming the majority. Eugenics programs and punitive welfare policies have subjected African Americans and other marginalized communities to sterilization and contraceptive abuse because of racist assumptions that their fertility is out of control. Even though women on welfare have on average fewer than two children, the image of the overbreeding 'welfare queen' remains firmly fixed in the white imagination.

Conventional views of overpopulation stand in the way of greater global understanding and solidarity.

In order to solve the world's pressing economic, political and environmental problems, we need more global understanding and solidarity, not less. Fears of overpopulation are deeply divisive and harmful. Population control programs distort family planning and diminish human rights. In order to protect and advance reproductive rights in a hostile climate, we urgently need to work together across borders of gender, race, class and nationality. Rethinking population helps open the way.

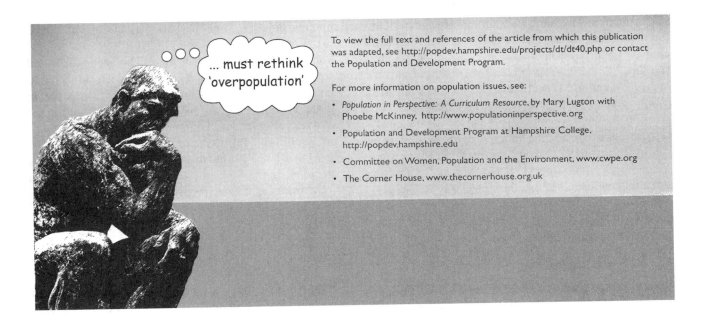

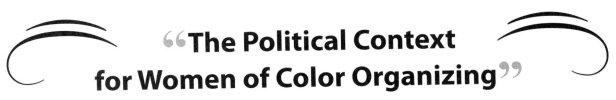

"The Political Context for Women of Color Organizing"

from *Undivided Rights: Women of Color Organize for Reproductive Justice*

This chapter outlines the multiple political contexts within which women of color have organized for reproductive rights. The first section charts the rise of a fierce anti-abortion movement, its role in the re-grouping of the Right, and subsequent efforts to control women's reproduction. While these forces threatened the reproductive rights of all women, women of color were often special targets. The second section sketches the various responses by three sectors of the women's movement, including the mainstream pro-choice, repro-ductive rights, and women's health movements. We see how each movement's response to the attack on women's reproductive freedom was framed by the ability, or in-ability, to meaningfully incorporate class and race into its organizing. With the anti-abortion movement and white women's responses to it as backdrop, the third sec-tion places the strategies and actions of women of color—organizing on their own behalf—in the fore-ground.

The Anti-Abortion Movement and the New Right

In the US, the Catholic Church has always opposed the government's support of birth control. In 1966, to explic-itly condemn government support of contraception, it formed the National Conference of Catholic Bishops after the Supreme Court legalized contraception for mar-ried couples.[1] However, it was *Roe v. Wade*, the landmark 1973 Supreme Court decision legalizing abortion, that galvanized religiously motivated opponents of reproduc-tive freedom and abortion into a "Right to Life" politi-cal movement.[2] In November 1973, the first edition of the National Right to Life Committee's newsletter issued

---

a call to action: "We must work for the passage of a constitutional Human Life Amendment," signaling the beginning of an orchestrated campaign to re-criminalize abortion.[3] Since *Roe*, abortion opponents have pursued multiple legal and illegal strategies—even employing deadly violence—to undermine abortion rights. The growing anti-abortion movement had important legislative successes in restricting abortion rights. Its first major victory came in 1977 when Congress passed the Hyde Amendment prohibiting Medicaid funding for abortion at the federal level. Most of the states followed suit.[4]

The anti-abortion movement was becoming a more powerful political force in the late 1970s as part of a larger conservative mobilization. Incensed by the loss of the Vietnam War, the success of the civil rights movement in dismantling segregation, and the gains of the women's and gay rights movements, conservatives wanted to win back the White House from Democratic president Jimmy Carter. In the 1980 presidential election, the Republican Party courted the emerging anti-abortion, anti-gay rights, and anti-Equal Rights Amendment constituencies that came to be known as the New Right.[5]

Weaving together anti-gay and anti-abortion strands into a perversely labeled pro-family agenda, Republicans called for a return to traditional sex roles and patriarchal family structures. With this as the centerpiece of a broader conservative agenda, they were successful in mobilizing evangelical and fundamentalist Christians and thereby revitalizing the Republican Party. Jerry Falwell founded the "Moral Majority" in 1979, proclaiming the organization to represent the real majority in America. This and other New Right organizations brought Christian fundamentalists and Catholics into a coalition that helped to elect Republican Ronald Reagan as president in 1980.[6] In turn, his election bolstered the anti-abortion movement and enabled conservative Republicans to rapidly mobilize a legal and political backlash against feminism and civil rights.

President Reagan appointed staunch anti-feminists in virtually every social policy-making position, and he moved quickly against abortion rights. In 1981, he supported a Human Life Amendment to the US Constitution that would legally recognize fetuses as persons and subordinate women's rights to fetal rights. When this effort proved too politically divisive,[7] even among opponents of abortion, Reagan's administration opted for federal legislation that would have bypassed the onerous constitutional amendment process. Though both efforts failed, they bolstered subsequent attempts to elevate the legal status of the fetus. At the state legislative level, abortion foes pushed for restrictive legislation to control the behaviors of pregnant women which they claimed were

endangering the "unborn," such as the use of illegal drugs and alcohol consumption. By 1999, an estimated 200 women in more than 30 states had been prosecuted for "fetal abuse."[8] Women have even been subjected to court orders forcing them to have cesarean births, and in 2004, a woman in Utah who delayed her C-section for two weeks was accused of murder when one of her twins was stillborn.[9] Professor of politics Jean Shroedel argues that many of the post–*Roe v. Wade* abortion cases decided by the Supreme Court have shifted concern away from the woman toward the fetus.[10] The most high-profile and significant development thus far came in April 2004, when President Bush signed the Unborn Victim of Violence Act which, for the first time, accords legal status to the fetus throughout pregnancy.[11]

During the early 1980s, Operation Rescue and its affiliates around the country mobilized thousands of eager participants in a strategy of civil disobedience.[12] Anti-abortion activists staged prayer vigils and sit-ins and blockaded entrances at family planning clinics. The success of Operation Rescue's tactics was evident in 1988 during the Democratic National Convention in Atlanta, when anti-abortion movement groups targeted local clinics in an effort to shut them down. Over 1,000 protesters were arrested, and thousands more were involved in the actions. While the clinics remained open during the "Siege of Atlanta," abortion providers were under daily attack, and the women who worked at the clinics, as well as the women who sought their services, had to cross a blockade of protesters.[13]

For this work, Operation Rescue claimed the mantle of the civil rights movement,[14] provoking the response of 14 veterans of the civil rights movement who issued a statement, "Civil Rights and Reproductive Rights," at a 1989 press conference, expressing their resentment at the theft of civil rights imagery:

> The adoption of the tactic of civil disobedience is their right, but the appropriation of the moral imperative of the civil rights movement is all wrong. The civil rights struggle sought to extend constitutional rights to all Americans and have those rights enforced. Today's anti-abortionists, quite to the contrary, are attempting, in the Operation Rescue protests, to deny American women their constitutional right to freedom of choice. They want the constitution rewritten.[15]

Women of color were not taken in by the poorly disguised anti-abortion-as-civil-rights rhetoric. For the most part, they knew that the waves of primarily white (male) protesters were not seeking to save their babies, and that their real targets were young white women—who happened to be obtaining more than 70 percent of the abortions in the United States at that time.[16] Dázon Dixon Diallo, who worked at the Feminist Women's Health Center in Atlanta, described a client's resistance to the protestors' messages,

> The [young, black] client I was protecting seemed to handle the pleas to "save her baby from these murderers" very well—she realized that these people just didn't understand or care about her. But when a young-looking, blonde and blue-eyed man screamed charges at her that the Rev. Martin Luther King Jr. would "turn over in his grave for what she was doing" and that she was "contributing to the genocide of African Americans," she broke. She stopped, stared him in his eyes with tears in hers, then quietly and coolly said, "You're a white boy, and you don't give a damn thing about me, who I am, or what I do."[17]

Despite intense organizing, only a small number of people of color joined the anti-abortion movement. However, those who did, such as Dr. Mildred Jefferson, were vocal and prominently displayed. Jefferson was the first prominent woman of color to speak out publicly against abortion; she served as chairperson of the board of the National Right to Life Committee and she provided congressional testimony in 1974 in favor of a constitutional amendment that would protect fetal life. A few African American women who had experienced sterilization abuse were also recruited by the anti-abortion movement and gained national attention when they formed Blacks for Life. In 2003, sociologist Louis Prisock found it difficult to determine the number of African American anti-choice organizations, but he reports indications that their numbers are rising.[18]

Not all opponents of abortion embraced nonviolence. During this same period of time, anti-abortion terrorism developed,[19] and throughout the 1980s and 90s there was an escalation of violence against abortion clinics and clinic personnel, especially abortion providers. The tactics they used were borrowed from the far Right white supremacist movement and included bombings, arson, and kidnappings. By 1990, 80 percent of clinics had experienced some serious form of violence or harassment. Throughout the 1990s, these threats and attacks became routine. To date, there have been seven murders at abortion clinics, and clinics must now devote considerable portions of their budgets to security.

Violence and harassment have contributed to decreasing abortion access. These tactics are part of a long-term anti-choice strategy whose ultimate goal is outlawing abortion entirely. Legislation and judicial actions are also key to this strategy. Consequently, the anti-abortion battle in the courts has raged continuously since *Roe* with mixed success. In 1981 the Supreme Court upheld the Hyde Amendment.[20] Then, in 1989, with the decision in *Webster v. Reproductive Health Services*, the Court upheld the right of states to restrict abortion in a range of ways that had previously been deemed inconsistent with *Roe*.[21] In his dissent, Justice Blackmun, author of the *Roe* decision, articulated the fear that *Webster* augured the end of abortion rights.

> Thus, "not with a bang, but a whimper," the plurality discards a landmark case of the last generation, and casts into darkness the hopes and visions of every woman in this country who had come to believe that the Constitution guaranteed her the right to exercise some control over her unique ability to bear children . . . For today, at least, the law of abortion stands undisturbed. For today, at least, the law of abortion stands undisturbed. For today, the women of this Nation still retain the liberty to control their destinies. But the signs are evident and very ominous, and a chill wind blows.[22]

Following closely behind *Webster*, in 1990 the Supreme Court upheld restrictions on minors' rights to abortion in *Hodgson v. Minnesota*, which seriously curtailed abortion rights for young women under 18 years old. Again in 1992, in *Planned Parenthood v. Casey*, the Court further chipped away at abortion rights.[23] The assault on abortion rights abated somewhat at the federal level after Clinton's election in 1992 but reignited under the 2000 Bush administration. Meanwhile, state-level attacks have been persistent for over 25 years. The net result has been significant erosion in access to abortion, which has the most adverse impact on low-income women, young women, and women of color.

Responses to the Anti-Abortion Movement
Stopping Water with a Rake

Three parts of the feminist movement—the pro-choice, reproductive rights, and women's health movements—responded with significantly different approaches to the anti-abortion movement and the rise of the New Right. This section offers a glimpse into the differences and gives insight into the questions of inclusion raised in the first chapter. Although women of color were active in all three movements, the majority was primarily white and middle class. This section also details the evolution of and need for race- and ethnic-based organizing by women of color.

The Mainstream Pro-Choice Movement

While the legalization of abortion mobilized opponents, it demobilized the majority of pro-choice advocates. Because the ability to find and finance abortion services was not a problem for middle-class white feminists, it appeared to them that with *Roe*, the battle for abortion rights had been won. Thus in 1977, when Congress passed the Hyde Amendment prohibiting federal funding for abortions, the leading women's organizations that had rallied for *Roe* did not marshal a large-scale response. This issue was of primary importance to women of color, who are disproportionately low-income. Thus, this was a divisive and watershed moment for the pro-choice movement. It could have confronted the overt white supremacy of the Right's agenda and its own internal racism, had it made overturning Hyde and fighting for public funding a priority. By not doing so, it seemed to women of color that the pro-choice movement was not concerned with their rights.

As we have seen, between *Roe* and Reagan, a full-blown and multi-faceted war on abortion rights had been launched in the courts and in the streets. Finally, with the looming threat of an anti-abortion constitutional amendment, a visible pro-choice movement re-emerged in 1981. However, the pro-choice response was defensive and its mission narrow. Pro-choice activists framed their politics in terms of choice and privacy, instead of using the language of women's rights and autonomy. "Abortion" itself was replaced by the more neutral appeal to defend the "legal right to choose." Their focus was on creating a winnable strategy to defend the legal right to abortion, not to secure access.

Journalist William Saletan argues that mainstream pro-choice groups made a considered decision to recast their demands in an effort to broaden their base. Believing that most voters did not care about women's rights, they framed the issue in terms of intrusions by big government, a fundamentally conservative approach. In 1984, working with political strategists whose experience was in electoral politics in the Democratic Party, National Abortion Reproductive Rights Action League (NARAL), Planned Parenthood, and others conducted a national poll to determine what messages would be effective with conservative voters and could drive a wedge into the conservative opposition. They found that many voters, hostile to welfare and taxes, opposed both banning and paying for abortions. There was a clear racial divide: Blacks were in favor of funding, albeit by a narrow margin, while whites were overwhelmingly opposed.[24] Saletan starkly articulates the possible courses of action: "Confronted by this latent coalition of pro-life, anti-government, anti-tax, anti-welfare, and anti-black voters, abortion rights activists had two choices. They could declare war against all of these constituencies in the name of a broad liberal agenda. Or they could divide the coalition and isolate pro-lifers by seducing the other constituencies."[25] To woo voters who routinely opposed government interference in social issues,[26] they chose the latter and put a libertarian spin on it. Abortion restrictions were criticized as encroachments by big government on tradition, family, and property.

This approach was partially successful, at least temporarily. It split the opposition by bringing pro-family, anti-government voters into the pro-choice electoral coalition. However, adopting privacy as the rubric for long-term pro-choice organizing backfired politically. It undercut demands for public access to abortion that had characterized the feminist struggle for legalization in the 1960s and 70s.[27] It also played into the hands of conservatives who were denouncing "big government," thus reinforcing the federal government's position, under the 1977 Hyde Amendment, that it had no obligation to pay for women's private decisions to have abortions. Saletan argues that the pro-choice movement created a "mutant version of abortion rights as a viable alternative to the feminist, egalitarian version originally envisioned by pro-choice activists."[28] He further notes that the limited definition of abortion rights made it possible to be pro-choice *and* to accept restrictions such as parental involvement laws and bans on public funding of abortion.

It is important to acknowledge that within the mainstream, there were other dissenting voices. For example, the American Civil Liberties Union (ACLU) and the National Organization for Women (NOW) consistently kept a feminist women's rights approach that incorporated a breadth of issues and strategies.[29] NOW also believed in the importance of large, visible mobilizations. For example, on April 9, 1986, NOW organized the first national march for abortion rights, the March to Save Women's Lives. Exceeding the organizers' expectations, more than 600,000 demonstrators participated in what was at that time the largest women's march in U.S. history. This was also a turning point in the age composition of the pro-choice movement—half the participants were young women who came of age in a country where abortion had always been legal. As we shall see later in the chapter, NOW, along with a handful of other organizations, made efforts—with varying degrees of success—to reach out to women of color. The organization was also an early opponent of welfare reform.

However, the broader and more radical approach did not prevail. Instead, the narrowly gauged conservative strategies and messages came to dominate the mainstream pro-choice movement. It did not address access to abortion or the larger context of reproductive health care and left out a central element of the reproductive rights agenda of women of color: the right to have children. While this framing brought moderate and conservative voters to abortion rights,[30] it was at the expense of dividing feminists, alienating poor women, women of color, more radical white activists, and those from the holistic women's health movement.[31]

We think that this strategy was a mistake in the long run, and that it was predicated on a misreading of the organizing tactics employed by the opposition. The Right created single-issue organizations for tactical purposes, but never lost sight of its multi-issue agenda. Thus it could achieve an important degree of unified action despite internal tensions on specific issues. In this way, people with strong feelings about a specific issue were brought into a broader conservative movement.

In contrast, the single-issue approach of the pro-choice movement did not create a broader politics or lead to building an enduring progressive coalition. Instead, activists with a broader perspective were driven away and created their own organizations outside the mainstream pro-choice groups. Some moved from choice to reproductive rights; others focused on access to and information about reproductive health services; and women of color began mobilizing for a new reproductive rights agenda. The following sections explore these various approaches.

The Reproductive Rights Movement

The pro-choice movement's failure to mount significant opposition to the Hyde Amendment and its refusal to join women of color in connecting sterilization abuse to abortion rights mobilized white abortion rights advocates who had broader politics and different political roots. Activists who came from the progressive movements of the 1960s—civil rights, the New Left, the antiwar and the women's liberation movements—insisted on keeping abortion rights within a feminist framework, which emphasized sexual freedom and highlighted how race and class shape reproductive choice. These activists criticized the mainstream pro-choice movement for being too middle-class focused, for lacking an emphasis on access, and for being too defensive and conservative. They were also critical of the preoccupation with electoral politics. They formed grassroots groups and feminist clinics, articulated broader messages, and promoted radical and direct-action strategies. Their goal was to mobilize the large numbers of people who would not be attracted to the mainstream's politics.

One of the first and largest organizations to embrace a reproductive rights agenda was the Committee for Abortion Rights and Against Sterilization Abuse (CARASA). The organization was formed in 1977 by women who had been involved in the civil rights and anti-Vietnam War movements in the 1960s and 70s. CARASA distinguished itself from the major national organizations, specifically NARAL and Planned Parenthood, whose abortion rights efforts were focused primarily on lobbying, legislative work, direct mail, and education through the media. CARASA saw a need for other forms of activism: "While this work is necessary at the present time, exclusively focusing on it ignores the importance of grassroots organizing and education—going directly into neighborhoods, workplaces, schools, churches and the streets, where the Right-to-Life Movement has organized, in order to create a truly popular movement for reproductive freedom and not just a lobby of experts."[32] CARASA saw the mainstream pro-choice organizations as narrow at best and, at worst, as taking positions that undermined the reproductive freedom of many women. In this regard, they specifically cited hostility to regulations regarding sterilization abuse and the use of population control arguments for abortion rights. Following the lead of women of color, CARASA placed opposition to sterilization abuse on a par with support for abortion rights.

In 1979, CARASA co-founded the Reproductive Rights National Network (R2N2), an umbrella organization for national and grassroots groups that situated abortion rights within a broader social justice and anti-racist context. R2N2's membership was varied; affiliates included feminist health clinics, women's caucuses of national Left organizations, and unaffiliated local activist organizations. They defined themselves as reproductive rights activists to distinguish their perspective from the single-issue politics of the pro-choice movement. R2N2 also espoused the critique of population control and "choice" that had been articulated by women of color. It emphasized access to abortion services and funds, arguing that without access, abortion rights would not be realized for low-income women and women of color.

R2N2 was an eager ally for the newly emerging women of color reproductive rights organizations. However, while R2N2 saw the link between women's oppression and ending racism, it was not always successful in putting its politics into practice, nor was it equipped to deal with racism within its organizations. Thus, in 1981, national R2N2 split and ultimately dissolved over disputes about whether to make fighting racism within the organization its top priority. There was a painful struggle which pitted opposition to the anti-abortion offensives against internal anti-racist work. This polarization itself is evidence of the inability of many white women to overcome the racial divide. As activists and scholars of color have noted, at that time even the more radical wings of the women's movement did not consistently or meaningfully integrate race, class, and gender oppression into their agendas.

The Women's Health Movement

While there was some overlap in membership and in politics, the women's health movement developed outside and alongside the pro-choice and reproductive rights movements. Beginning in 1969, when abortion was still illegal in most states and reproductive health care was in the hands of the mostly male health care establishment, many feminists mobilized "to wrest back some control over their sexuality, their reproductive lives, and their health from their doctors, and particularly their obstetrician gynecologists."[33] This was a largely decentralized movement of grassroots organizations. Historian Sandra Morgen's description of its beginnings captures this well: "In different sites, through different means, across the country, women began to take their health care into their own hands."[34] Women's health activism took several forms, which included disseminating information, advocating new ways of providing services, promoting Self-Help, patient advocacy, community organizing and counseling services, providing safe illegal abortions, and in many communities, establishing feminist clinics.[35]

The post-*Roe* assault against abortion rights had a severe impact on women's clinics and health advocacy groups. Many had received financial support from federal or state programs. Thus the specific restrictions on abortion (such as the Hyde Amendment and similar laws at the state level), the overall cuts in social spending for programs and services for poor women, and the anti-abortion violence all took their toll. Organizations and clinics faced constant financial pressures. They were forced to lay off staff and cut programs. Ultimately, many had to close or were bought out by mainstream providers. Then, in the 1980s, HIV/AIDS brought new actors and issues, reinvigorating women's health activism.

Though the women's health movement was grounded in local grassroots activism, advocates sought to consolidate its influence on Capitol Hill. In 1975, the National Women's Health Lobby was founded in Wash-

ington, D.C. Later renamed the National Women's Health Network (NWHN), the organization was established "to monitor Federal health agencies and ensure that the voice of a national women's health movement would be heard on Capitol Hill."[36] The network was a key player in the women's health movement in general and was particularly important to women of color, emphasizing organizational support for activists of color from the outset. When several women of color were brought onto the NWHN board at once, their presence and voting power were maximized. The diverse NWHN board membership also enabled the white women and women of color to learn from and support one another. Longtime network board member and program committee chair Judy Norsigian observed, "We developed relationships by making ourselves available for advice, counsel, and information. We provided ongoing support through these more informal yet sustained contacts. The idea was to be there when you were needed."[37] The network encouraged women of color to establish their own organizations.

The women's health movement developed a critique of mainstream health care, which incorporated racism and classism as well as sexism. This movement provided an important home and support network for women of color activists, many of whom worked in clinics or other feminist health advocacy organizations. However, like the reproductive rights movement, the women's health movement was a site of struggle around differences of race, ethnicity, class, and sexual orientation. In clinic settings these were not abstract debates, but intense disagreements, especially over specific issues such as mission, development and location of services, and hiring and firing.[38]

As we have seen, the politics of race and class permeated all three responses to the political threats posed by the rise of the New Right and the anti-abortion movement. These forces set the context within which women of color organized for reproductive rights.

Organizing by Women of Color

Although the National Black Women's Health Project (NBWHP), formed in 1984, was the first women of color reproductive health organization to be created and remained the only national women of color group until the late 1980s, many of the individuals and organizations of women of color featured in this study became active in pro-choice organizing in the 1970s and early 80s. They were alarmed by the thinly veiled white supremacist agenda of the New Right and the rise of the anti-abortion movement.

Women of color organizing for reproductive rights have always needed to respond simultaneously to state-imposed policies aimed at controlling their fertility and to social justice movements that neglected their reproductive health concerns. Loretta Ross sets out the various strategies used by women of color:

> Sometimes we work with predominantly white organizations that marginalize issues of race and class, and privilege abortion rights over other issues of reproductive justice . . . Some of us work with people of color organizations that marginalize gender and class issues, and where women's reproductive health issues are tangential to struggles against racism . . . Some women of color work with anti-poverty organizations that sometimes neglect race and gender issues altogether, assuming that class issues subsume concerns about reproductive health.[39]

This section outlines a few of the ways in which women of color organized for reproductive justice.

Working with Mainstream Pro-Choice Organizations

By the mid-1980s, several activist women of color had been recruited to positions of leadership in the large mainstream pro-choice groups. In 1978, Faye Wattleton became the first African American to head the Planned Parenthood Federation of America, a position she held for 14 years until 1992. Luz Alvarez Martínez joined the national NARAL board and called for greater representation of women of color in the organization. Emily Tynes was NARAL's first African American director of communications (1983–1988); Judy Logan-White and Faith Evans (an African American woman and man) created the Women of Color Partnership Program as part of the Religious Coalition for Abortion Rights (RCAR) in 1984.[40] Loretta Ross became the first director of Women of Color Programs at NOW (1985–1989), a post that had previously been called the "minority rights" staff position.

These activists were able to accomplish significant outreach to women of color through and in coalition with mainstream organizations. In 1986, women of color at RCAR, NOW, NARAL, and Planned Parenthood began organizing local and regional forums for women of color about reproductive rights.[41] These gatherings provided the opportunity for activists of color to meet together—often for the first time—to discuss how to move their reproductive health concerns to the national level.

On the heels of these synergy-building gatherings and one year after the historic 1986 NOW-sponsored pro-choice march, Loretta Ross organized the first National Conference on Women of Color and Reproductive Rights, held at Howard University. Despite the fact that women of color had been active and in the leadership of NOW from its inception, they were also skeptical of NOW.[42] Ross intended for the conference to build a bridge between women of color and NOW. She reached out to women of color she knew from other movements, including violence against women, teen pregnancy, and anti-poverty organizations, to involve them in reproductive rights activism. She states, "It was the first conference in history that brought women from the feminist, civil rights, and black National movements together to promote reproductive freedom."[43] Casting a wide net was necessary since, despite the fact that they were pro-choice, relatively few women of color activists would have responded to a narrow call.

In addition to Ross, this trailblazing conference was coordinated by women of color working at pro-choice organizations, including Planned Parenthood, NARAL, and RCAR, who were responding to the concerns of women of color who felt their perspectives and leadership were not adequately advanced by the pro-choice movement. As a result, at the conference women of color, not the white leaders of sponsoring organizations, were prominently featured. Of the more than 400 women of color who attended the conference, two-thirds were African Americans—with a sizable delegation from the NBWHP, by then a three-year old organization. Participants came together across identity groups to talk about the reproductive health issues in their different communities. Many of the women of color active in the movement today met for the first time at that conference, and went on to build long-term networks and relationships which spurred future activism.

The conference was a place for women of color to articulate their own agendas, and it demonstrated that they would mobilize for reproductive justice if race and class dimensions were prioritized. While the explicit purpose of the conference was to mobilize more women of color to participate in the pro-choice movement, the women who came also advanced a critique of that movement.[44]

Two years later, the impending Supreme Court decision in *Webster v. Reproductive Health Services* (1989) catalyzed other organizing activities by women of color. Seeking to limit the public provision of abortion services, *Webster* posed a severe threat to low-income women and women of color. A national conference called "In Defense of *Roe*" was organized in April of 1989 by the Women of Color Partnership Program of RCAR and Lynn Paltrow of the ACLU's Reproductive Freedom Project. Women of color, community organizers, and women of faith came together to strategize against the anticipated state-level attacks on *Roe v. Wade* that would follow *Webster*.

The meeting identified two priorities: a national reproductive rights organization for women of color and the development of local coalitions. It inspired women of color to engage in reproductive rights organizing across the country. For example, the meeting marked the first time that Asian and Pacific Islander women from different cultures came together to discuss reproductive rights issues. They wrote a collective statement stressing their diverse perspectives and common purpose: "This is a historic moment for us. Recognizing the tradition of family and community, including alternative lifestyles, we, as Asian Pacific American women, underscore the importance of a reproductive health agenda for our communities."[45]

Patricia Camp, state coordinator of the Illinois affiliate of the national RCAR, said, "Being able to make a movement of our own, which deals with reproductive health issues in our own way and from our own perspective is the most valuable service that this conference provided."[46] Inspired and angered by what she learned at the conference, Migdalia Rivera, consultant to the Hispanic Health Council of Hartford, Connecticut, took information about the potential impact of anti-choice public policies on poor Latinas back to her community and energized activists.[47]

The "In Defense of *Roe*" conference was planned to coincide with the second National March for Women's Lives organized by NOW. While more than 100 organizations of women of color had endorsed the first march, Sharon Parker of the National Institute for Women of Color described their actual presence as "drowning in a sea of white." In striking contrast to the 1986 march, in 1989 women of color took steps to make their presence highly visible. With Parker's assistance—further aided by the NBWHP sending 13 bus loads of women to the Washington, D.C., march—a delegation of 5,000 women of color rallied behind one giant banner, "Women of Color for Reproductive Rights." Following the march, Reverend Yvonne Delk, director of the Office of Church in Society of the United Church of Christ, issued a call to action:

We are women who have been and continue to be discriminated against in employment, locked into stereotyped roles, sexually exploited, politically subdivided, trivialized and domesticated by those who would deny us the right to control our bodies and our lives. What we say and do today has long reaching implications, not only for the women of color in this nation and for women of color throughout the globe, but it is our legacy to the generations of women who are yet unborn.[48]

In May 1989, one month after the *Webster* decision, Donna Brazile of the National Political Congress of Black Women and Loretta Ross of NOW organized African American Women for Reproductive Freedom, a new coalition of high-profile women. They published *We Remember: African American Women for Reproductive Freedom*, written by Marcia Gillespie, then an editor of *Ms. Magazine*. The statement was a way to elevate African American women's voices in the public debate about abortion. Gillespie wrote:

This freedom—to choose and to exercise our choices—is what we've fought and died for. Brought here in chains, worked like mules, bred like beasts, whipped one day, sold the next . . . Somebody said that we were less than human and not fit for freedom. Somebody said we were like children and could not be trusted to think for ourselves . . . Somebody said that black women could be raped, held in concubinage, forced to bear children year in and year out, but often not raise them. Oh yes, we have known how painful it is to be without choice in this land.[49]

We Remember was a profound articulation of the connection between reproductive justice and the struggle for racial justice. The *We Remember* campaign was overwhelmingly successful. In six brief months, more than 250,000 copies of the brochure were reprinted and distributed across the country, through mailings, at conferences, and at events organized by women of color. Faye Wattleton[50] of Planned Parenthood and Kate Michelman of NARAL provided the funding and agreed not to put their organizational logos on the brochure so that the focus would remain on women of color. The coalition's impassioned statement represented an important national collaboration between autonomous African American women's organizations that were not necessarily focused on abortion access and black women who worked in mainstream pro-choice organizations.

Women of Color Working for Social Justice Organizations

Historically, civil rights, environmental, and immigrant rights groups have not included reproductive rights in their agendas. Nevertheless, women of color participating in reproductive rights organizations have consistently looked for ways to work with groups that focus on economic and racial justice. Reproductive rights activists have joined in coalitions with the NAACP, Asian Pacific Environmental Network, American Indian Movement, and Mexican American Legal Defense Fund and drawn attention to reproductive rights in the context of these struggles.

In addition to bringing reproductive rights to social justice organizations, the search for allies has also led women of color to build coalitions that bring a wide range of groups to the service of reproductive justice. For example, the 1993 Campaign for Abortion and Reproductive Equity (CARE), organized by the NBWHP, brought over 300 civil rights, labor, and pro-choice organizations together in an effort to overturn the Hyde Amendment and restore federal Medicaid funding for abortion. While many of these groups were not interested in supporting abortion rights per se, they were concerned about equity and responded to the call to challenge discrimination and support racial and economic justice.[51]

Reproductive rights activists faced other challenges in trying to work with economic justice organizations. Although many of the organizations that work on poverty, homeless advocacy, and welfare reform are led by women of color, ironically, these groups have sometimes neglected race and gender issues. Because some groups are financially dependent on the Catholic Church, openly expressing their support for reproductive rights would jeopardize their funding.

Organizations and groups working on HIV/AIDS and violence against women have also been important allies for reproductive rights activists of color. Because problems such as HIV/AIDS and domestic violence are widespread in their communities, women of color have had more success recently in bringing these issues out in the open—after encountering initial silence and resistance. Through responding to the direct service needs of the communities, serving battered women and people with HIV/AIDS, they linked together advocacy and service delivery. Churches in particular have focused on helping women and children through direct services such as providing meals and shelter. Through these services, bridges were built between churches and other community institutions that had been reluctant to address feminist and gay and lesbian issues and advocates from these movements.

National Coalitions of Women of Color

Since the late 1980s, there have been four major national collaborations among women of color. Several of the founders of the eight organizations included in our case studies played leading roles in these efforts, met each other through these activities, and formed alliances that strengthened them as leaders. By 1992, there were national women of color organizations, but they were frus-

trated by their inability to be fully respected partners in the pro-choice movement. In order to have a greater impact on both the mainstream movement and U.S. domestic policy, in 1992 six organizations launched the Women of Color Coalition for Reproductive Health Rights (WOCCRHR): Asians and Pacific Islanders for Choice, National Black Women's Health Project, National Latina Health Organization, Latina Roundtable on Health and Reproductive Rights, National Coalition of 100 Black Women, and Native American Women's Health and Education Resource Center. WOCCRHR represented the first effort to build a national women of color reproductive health coalition.

The most immediate challenge for WOCCRHR was to determine the role it would play in the third national March for Women's Lives organized by NOW in 1992, given that the women of color organizations had not been included in the planning. Despite excluding them from the leadership, march organizers expected women of color to mobilize their constituencies to attend. Ultimately WOCCRHR decided to support the 1992 NOW march, but published a statement objecting to the fact that they were not included in the organizing process. A memo from the NBWHP circulated with WOCCRHR's statement clearly states the problem:

> The NBWHP has joined with a number of women of color reproductive rights organizations to protest NOW's process (or lack of process) for the inclusion of women of color in the scheduled April 5 March for Reproductive Freedom . . . We do not want people to stay away, especially women of color. These issues affect us and we need to be seen and heard in support of reproductive freedom. However, we must also speak out regarding NOW's practices involving the lack of inclusion of all the women of color reproductive rights groups.[52]

The coalition's response was an unprecedented challenge from women of color to NOW and the other major pro-choice organizations regarding their politics of exclusion. NOW's practice in march planning had been to invite to the decision-making table only those people who were able to commit significant financial resources to organizing multi-million-dollar marches. This process ensured that women with power stayed in power and marginalized women of color.

Two years following NOW's third March for Women's Lives, the founders of WOCCRHR organized again in order to have an impact on the September 1994 United Nations International Conference on Population and Development (ICPD) in Cairo, Egypt. As part of the US delegation to the Cairo conference, WOCCRHR delegates and other women of color within the larger delegation, in a first joint effort, established the U.S. Women of Color Delegation Project. The project members authored a "Statement on Poverty, Development, and Population Activities," which they presented at an ICPD workshop. The introduction outlines the reasons for their intervention:

> Much of what is known of US policies is developed mostly by white, upper and middle class Americans. This document reflects a people of color perspective on issues of population as they interact with institutional policies of racism, political oppression, and classism and gender bias to entrench poverty and "underdevelopment" within our society.[53]

The delegation's statement connected the lack of reproductive freedom for poor and marginalized women in the U.S. many of whom are women of color, with that of women in developing countries. It made clear that many women in the US did not enjoy reproductive rights.

Through these efforts, WOCCRHR brought the situation of women of color in the United States to the attention of the international community and created enduring friendships and alliances. Upon returning from Cairo, they decided to join ranks a third time to bring women of color to the United Nations Fourth World Conference on Women in Beijing, China in September 1995. The US Women of Color Beijing coalition provided information, leadership training, and strategic planning for women of color to participate effectively in the Beijing conference.

After the Cairo and Beijing conferences, the women in WOCCRHR found that funding was unavailable for them to continue their working relationships once they returned home. This was largely because funding for international "population" activities is separated from funding for domestic reproductive rights work within foundations. Nevertheless, their participation in these international events produced significant shifts in their thinking about how to frame the demand for reproductive freedom for women of color in the United States. By attending the conference, they connected their local and national struggles to the global movements against poverty and for women's rights. They returned home determined to forge ahead in building a national movement of women of color for reproductive health that would, for the first time, incorporate the global human rights framework into their activism.

The fourth coalition effort came in 1997 when the SisterSong Women of Color Reproductive Health Collective was formed.[54] The Collective included 16 organizations representing four communities of women of color: African American, Asian American and Pacific Islander, Latina, and Indigenous. SisterSong's original mission was advocacy for the reproductive and sexual health needs of women of color. Its strategy has been to mobilize at the grassroots level while also developing a public policy agenda.[55]

The groups involved in SisterSong address a wide range of reproductive health issues, including HIV/AIDS services, midwifery, services for incarcerated women, health screenings, abortion and contraceptive advocacy, clinical research, teen pregnancy programs, cancer screenings, drug and alcohol treatment programs, and programs for the treatment and prevention of sexually transmitted diseases. This inclusive range of programs illustrates the scope and depth of the organizing work on reproductive and sexual health issues done by women of color from Puerto Rico to Hawaii. SisterSong sponsored its first national conference on women of color and reproductive health and sexual rights issues in November 2003 at Spelman College in Atlanta. More than 600 people, mostly women of color, participated in this event, marking a new era of reproductive justice organizing by women of color. Most recently, the collective organized women of color to participate in the April 2004 March for Women's Lives under the banner "Women of Color for Reproductive Justice."

These coalitions have taken essential steps in building a movement of women of color for reproductive justice. The threats to reproductive rights and women's health continue unabated. As always, the effects from erosions in access to care and services fall disproportionately on women of color.

NOTES
A list of endnotes is available in the original source.

"Latina Agenda for Reproductive Justice"

by Angela Hooton

Latinas are facing a reproductive health care crisis in the United States: over 41 percent of Latinas are uninsured and almost one-third lack a regular health care provider. In addition, immigrant Latinas are being systematically shut out of the public health system and, as a result, face even greater barriers to reproductive health care.

Limited access to basic reproductive health care services has forced many Latinas to forgo or delay essential preventative screenings. As a result, Latinas suffer from many preventable conditions. For example, their HIV/AIDS infection rate is six times higher than the rate among non-Hispanic Caucasian women, and Latinas have higher rates of syphilis, gonorrhea, and chlamydia than Caucasian women. As a result of inadequate screening, Mexican-American and Puerto Rican women's cervical cancer rates are approximately twice that of Caucasian women. Although Latinas have lower rates of breast cancer than Caucasian and African American women, breast cancer is the leading cause of cancer-related deaths among Latinas. The five-year survival rate for non-Hispanic Caucasian women with breast cancer is 85 percent, compared to 76 percent for Latinas.

Many of the reproductive health disparities that plague Latinas can be attributed to low health insurance rates. Yet, other barriers, including language and poverty, also inhibit their ability to achieve positive reproductive health outcomes and to exercise their reproductive rights. For example, the poverty rate among Latinos was 22.5 percent in 2003, compared to 8.2 percent for Caucasians. According to recent Census reports, about 28 percent of Latinas speak English either poorly or not at all. It is not surprising, since interpretive services are not always available, that many Latinas report that they have difficulty communicating with their health care providers.

Latinas' high poverty rates, coupled with restrictive reproductive health policies, affect their childbearing decisions and impede their ability to freely choose between parenting and abortion. Increased restrictions on access to abortion and the dearth of public funding for abortion force many low-income Latinas to make serious sacrifices in order to obtain abortions. In fact, Rosie Jimenez, a Latina college student who was unable to pay for a legal abortion, was the first woman documented to have died from an illegal, back-alley abortion after the 1977 Hyde Amendment restricted federal funding of the procedure.

At the same time, Latinas faced barriers—including widespread and coercive sterilization practices—that have restricted them from bearing children. Coercive and punitive policies are proliferating in the U.S. and disproportionately affect women of color, including Latinas. These policies include caps on the amount of welfare support a woman receives when she has additional children, court-mandated use of contraceptives such as Norplant, and cuts in Medicaid-funded services for pregnant immigrants. All of these policies have had a disproportionate impact on low-income women of color, including Latinas. While their tactics vary, these policies seek to remove control of reproductive health decisions from women, thereby violating the fundamental human right to self-determination and undermining Latinas' health and well-being.

The National Latina Institute for Reproductive Health (NLIRH)'s mission is to address these issues and to safeguard the fundamental human right to reproductive health care for Latinas, their families, and their communities. NLIRH understands that the fight for reproductive health and rights is inextricably linked to the struggle for social justice. There can be no reproductive justice for Latinas without racial equality, without quality health care, without educational opportunities, without immigration reform, and without affordable child care options.

NLIRH has created a model national policy agenda to address the broad range of reproductive health challenges Latinas face today. The *National Latina Agenda for Reproductive Justice* has several priority areas: increasing access to affordable health care; ensuring the availability of culturally and linguistically competent

"Latina Agenda for Reproductive Justice," by Angela Hooton, originally published in the *Women's Health Activist*, September/October 2005, pp. 10 & 14, the newsletter of the National Women's Health Network (NWHN). It is reprinted with the permission of the author and the NWHN.

health care services; expanding family planning options; promoting comprehensive sexuality education; protecting reproductive rights; and developing accurate and unbiased research on Latina health status. We hope that the *Agenda* will not only serve as a useful tool for improving Latina reproductive health, but also contribute to national efforts to broaden and diversify the reproductive rights movement.

NLIRH focuses on three specific policy campaigns. First, we work to expand Latinas' access to and knowledge of Emergency Contraception (EC). NLIRH believes that EC can play an important role in reducing Latinas' unwanted pregnancies and enabling them to exercise greater reproductive choice. Latinas who do not have access to a health care provider will benefit greatly if EC is available without prescription—provided it is affordable and women know about the method. We are working with our activists to expand EC access at the state and national levels. We are also supporting state legislation that requires emergency rooms to provide EC to sexual assault survivors and allows pharmacists to dispense EC without an advance prescription. On the national level, we are advocating for the FDA to make EC available over-the-counter (OTC) and for state Medicaid programs to continue to cover EC if it becomes an OTC product.

Our second campaign is aimed at improving the reproductive health status of Latina immigrants. NLIRH recognizes that many Latina immigrants lack access to prenatal care and other basic reproductive health care services. Further, there is a growing trend to provide health care for pregnant immigrants by covering the fetus rather than the woman. We believe that Latinas have a right to health care regardless of their immigration status. For this reason, NLIRH advocates for state and federal policies to expand health care coverage (especially family planning and prenatal care services) for Latina immigrants. Specifically, we are fighting to pass the 'Immigrant Children's Health Improvement Act', which would allow states to use federal Medicaid and S-CHIP funding to provide health care to legal immigrant children and pregnant women. Under current law, these groups are barred from these programs unless they have lived in the United States for over five years. Although states can choose to cover immigrant women and children through state Medicaid funds, budget constraints and pressure from anti-immigrant legislators has resulted in many states electing not to cover this vulnerable population.

Third, NLIRH is dedicated to ensuring that all Latinas have access to reproductive health care services through viable public funding sources. Through public education and advocacy efforts, we advocate that Congress increase Title X's family planning funds, protect Medicaid funds from threatened budgetary cuts, and eliminate the Hyde Amendment that restricts federal funding of abortions.

NLIRH does not work in a vacuum. We collaborate with Latina leaders across the country and provide a Leadership Training series to ensure that our national policy agenda and grassroots campaigns remain relevant and reflect the reality of Latinas' lives. If you are interested in joining NLIRH in our advocacy and community mobilization efforts, or want a copy of the *National Latina Agenda for Reproductive Justice* please visit our website at www.latinainstitute.org.

For Native Women Reproductive Rights Mean . . .

by Native Women for Reproductive Rights Coalition

1. The right to knowledge and education for all family members concerning sexuality and reproduction that is age, culture and gender appropriate.

2. The right to all reproductive alternatives and the right to choose the size of our families.

3. The right to affordable health care, including safe deliveries within our communities.

4. The right to access safe, free, and/or affordable abortions, regardless of age, with confidentiality and free pre and post counseling.

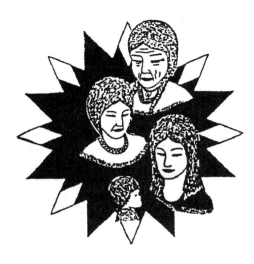

8. The right to programs to reduce the rate of infant mortality and high risk pregnancies.

9. The right to culturally specific comprehensive chemical dependency prenatal programs, including, but not limited to, prevention of Fetal Alcohol Syndrome and Effects.

10. The right to stop coerced sterilization.

11. The right to a forum for cultural/spiritual development, culturally-oriented health care, and the right to live as Native women.

12. The right to be fully informed about, and to consent to any forms of medical treatment.

13. The right to determine who are members of our Nations.

14. The right to continuous, consistent and quality health care for Native People.

15. The right to reproductive rights and support for women with disabilities.

16. The right to parent our children in a non-sexist, non-racist environment.

In order to accomplish the foregoing stated rights, the Native Women for Reproductive Rights will create coalitions and alliances to network with other groups.

5. The right to active involvement in the development and implementation of policies concerning reproductive issues, to include, but not limited to, pharmaceuticals and technology.

6. The right to include domestic violence, sexual assault and AIDS as reproductive rights issues.

7. The right to programs which meet the nutritional needs of women and families.

"Contraceptive Jelly on Toast and Other Unintended Consequences of Sexuality Education"

by Mariamne H. Whatley and Elissa R. Henken

A doctor reported that he had fitted a 23-year-old woman with a diaphragm. When she returned to the doctor for a check-up, the doctor noticed a purple stain on the center of the diaphragm. When he asked the woman about it, she told him it was a stain from the jelly she used with it. He asked her what brand she was using and she answered, "Smucker's grape jelly."

A first reaction to this story is usually laughter at the punch line, followed by disbelief about this being a "true" story, and amazement that, if it is true, anyone could make such a ridiculous mistake. On one level, many of the stories in this chapter can be read as focusing on the ignorance of the client/patient, but another more useful reading is that the education/health care practitioner was at fault for presenting information in ways that facilitated misunderstandings. There are many ways, which will be explored throughout this book, in which folklore can help sexuality and health educators in their practice. This chapter focuses on one potential role of folklore—to point out the nature of errors, whether they have actually occurred or not, that can be made in educational processes. The following stories focus on attempts at contraception, so the consequences of the misunderstandings are serious—unplanned pregnancies. While the ungainly attempts are often presented humorously in the story, the results are often devastating for the woman (and man) involved. The opening story and the one following were reported by a student who heard them on her father's AutoDigest tapes of an obstetrics/gynecology conference. It is important to note that even though these stories were collected from a seemingly reliable source, they have all the earmarks of contemporary legends.

> A doctor reported that another woman had been using a diaphragm, but had immediately become pregnant. When he examined the diaphragm, he found the center was cut out. Because there had been no center when she had been fitted for the diaphragm, she cut it out of hers.

A similar story was published in the journal *Hospital Pharmacy* in 1987. A student nurse reported that she had been teaching new mothers about child care and contraception:

> After giving one of the lectures on contraception, a fifteen-year-old, who had received no prenatal care, reacted in astonishment to what I said about how contraceptive jellies should be used. After explaining how the jellies needed to be applied vaginally prior to intercourse, the mother realized for the first time how she had become pregnant. She had purchased a contraceptive jelly from a retail pharmacy and routinely had been placing it on her toast at breakfast! She said that she had received no instruction on how the jelly was supposed to be used and just thought that jellies were for toast—not for intravaginal use. (Cohen, 1987, p. 956)

Although this version was reported in 1987, the story is very persistent and made a big comeback ten years later. A reader wrote to advice columnist Ann Landers (Landers, 1997):

> It seems a woman has filed suit against a small mom-and-pop pharmacy because she purchased a tube of contraceptive jelly, spread it on a piece of toast and ate it. She then had unprotected sex, believing she was "safe" and became pregnant.

The contraceptive came with instructions, but the woman says the pharmacist should have put a specific warning on the box saying it wasn't effective if eaten. She is asking for a half million dollars, even though she is quoted as saying, "Who has time to sit around reading directions these days, especially when you're sexually aroused?"

One contributor to *FoafTale* News reported that this story of oral use of contraceptive jelly was circulating widely in May and June, 1997, through the media and Internet (Hiscock, 1998). The same contributor also reported an e-mail of a first-person narrative by a public health nurse that had been forwarded to him. When a pregnant woman is asked by the nurse about her contraceptive practices, the woman shows the nurse "vaginal foaming pills (about the size of a Necco wafer). She said, 'I've been taking them just like the doctor told me—every time I have sex I take one. They're hard to swallow but I manage'" (Hiscock, 1998, p. 17). Describing the pills as resembling a specific candy does help explain some of the confusion; however, these may be more accurately described as about the size of a thumb joint and about one-half inch thick.

Another story, told as a legend or a joke, relates that a woman became pregnant after the birth control pill kept rolling out of her vagina. This is the reverse of the jelly on toast story, for in this case a woman uses vaginally what should be taken orally. Actually, hormones are well absorbed vaginally, so the vagina could work as a delivery site for birth control pills, though it would certainly not be recommended. A story reportedly told by someone working in a pharmacy also illustrates another misunderstanding of how oral contraceptives work:

> A woman kept coming in to get her birth control pills at a point where she ought to be only halfway through with them. The pharmacy workers finally got suspicious and asked her if she was taking one a day like she was supposed to and she replied, "Yes, and so is my husband."

One student reported watching a documentary on television in which young teenagers discussed sex:

> Some of the girls said they knew of other girls who would steal one birth control pill from a sister's pack. They would take the pill before having sex and think they were protected from becoming pregnant.

There are also similar condom stories. For example, one student reported that after a nurse demonstrated how to put a condom on, using her hand as a model, a couple used it by carefully covering the man's hand. This mistake was discovered after the woman became pregnant. As far as we know there have been no similar mishaps after the popular demonstrations of condom strength and elasticity that involve the educator's pulling a condom on over his or her head.

Rather than focusing on the likelihood that any of these incidents could really have happened or on the lack of understanding by the people involved of reproductive anatomy, health educators should reflect on what these examples say about contraceptive education in clinical and other settings. Many of these stories are examples of what Greenberg (1985) has named "iatrogenic health education disease," the condition in which health education has made learners less healthy. Certainly, health education that results in a woman eating contraceptive jelly and becoming pregnant would fit this definition. In the diaphragm stories, it is clear that careful and thorough explanations, with more realistic assumptions about the common understandings of terms such as jelly, could have prevented these mistakes. A description of the function of the spermicidal jelly would have made it clear both that grape jelly would be ineffective and that the jelly would need to be placed vaginally or in the diaphragm, not on toast. Even a brief explanation of the way a diaphragm works would have prevented a woman from assuming that a fitting ring was the model for an effective contraceptive. One of the clear messages sexuality educators should get from these stories is that education about contraceptives needs to be specific, concrete, and as literal as possible. If a woman were actually handed a tube of spermicide, shown how to apply it to a diaphragm (not a fitting ring), and helped to insert it vaginally (in a class, this can be done on a plastic model, though in clinical settings, the woman should get a chance to insert it in herself to gain assurance that it is in correctly), it is unlikely that any of the above errors could be made. An explanation of how to use the vaginal tablet, rather than "Use one just before sex," would be much more effective. Because these are sold over the counter, however, a purchaser would not have to see a health care practitioner, who might give some instructions and explanations. As the Ann Landers story points out, people do not always read instructions, due to low literacy, not being able to read English, too small print, assuming they know what to do, or just being in a hurry. Most people would agree that the purported lawsuit against the pharmacy is inappropriate, but it is a strong reminder to pharmacists about their potential role in health education. Explanations of how oral contraceptives work in a woman's body should certainly keep anyone from assuming that a man should take them along with his partner or that a woman should just take one

before intercourse. While a model of a penis is not necessary for a condom demonstration, it is important to note that the banana, or whatever item is used, does represent a penis. Even if the previous examples are rare or even totally apocryphal, other problems could be prevented by this concrete approach. For example, a demonstration may prevent the mishap of applying so much spermicide that the compressed diaphragm flies out of the woman's fingers. In all areas of health and sexuality education, the same rules apply: be specific and concrete, with appropriate visuals and hands-on demonstrations.

Language is also very important. For example, for some people the term "contraceptive" is so closely associated with oral contraceptives (the Pill) that referring to any contraceptive may connote oral use, a meaning reinforced by such terms as jelly, cream, and tablet. Another story, recounted by a folklorist, while clearly in the joke genre, also reveals an important point about language:

> By the way, I recall from my adolescent years a story about condoms. A couple wishing to avoid pregnancy was told by their doctor to use them. A few months later they returned and told the doctor that pregnancy had occurred even though they had used condoms. When the doctor asked, "Did you follow the directions on the package?" the husband replied, "It said 'place on organ,' but we don't have an organ so we put them on the piano."

This joke/story probably served as a means for young adolescent boys to check out their own and others' knowledge about condoms and "organs," but is unlikely to have been accepted as a true story. However, it is a reminder that we can never make assumptions about the vocabulary of learners, either their knowledge of technical terms or their use of certain slang or euphemisms. It is important to make sure everyone is talking about the same thing. Often health educators will ask students to list all the words they can think of for penis or vagina or other relevant terms. Once the list is generated, they can then suggest that everyone use the same specific term (usually the correct medical or anatomical term, but in some cases it may work better to use the most common slang term). In any case, it would be clear what an individual meant when using a certain term. If an educator is unclear about what a slang word means, it is better to ask than to try to appear cool and knowledgeable, while actually being wrong. For example, in parts of the South, *cock* refers to female rather than male genitalia (Cassidy, 1985). Slang terms are very specific culturally and historically. By using the term "cool" above, we were assuming a certain common understanding of a term that, in fact, may be very out of fashion with certain age groups or meaningless for certain cultural groups. It is better to ask them to clarify a term or to say, "I think it means this but I'm not sure, so let me know if I'm wrong." They will.

Health care practitioners who complain about "non-compliance" may be neglecting their own failures to provide the kind of information that would help someone follow through on a prescription or recommendation. By collecting folklore such as these legends and using them to analyze failures of educational practice, health educators may create much more effective communication.

"The Pill" May Not Mix Well with Other Drugs

by Judith Willis

young newlywed had been taking birth control pills several months in the early 1970s when she developed a bladder infection. She consulted her doctor, who prescribed an antibiotic. The infection cleared up quickly. But nine months later she gave birth to her first child.

Today, with proper communication between physician and patient, the inadvertent pregnancy in this mythical example would be far less likely to occur. Many interactions between oral contraceptives (OC's) containing both estrogen and progestogen and other drugs are now well-known and included in both the physician and patient labeling of the pill.

Such interactions can not only diminish the contraceptive's effectiveness, but also increase or decrease the potency of the other drug. Both those who take oral contraceptives and those who don't may find it interesting to look at what is known about the how and why of such OC-drug interactions.

Some drugs decrease contraceptive effectiveness apparently because they increase the metabolism of the contraceptives. This means that the liver breaks down the hormones in the contraceptive faster, and they are eliminated from the body more quickly. Thus, the levels of estrogen and progestogen are reduced, sometimes so much that they no longer suppress ovulation. Breakthrough bleeding is often a symptom of this reduced effectiveness. This type of interaction is of even more concern with the very-

low-dose contraceptives, since the level of hormones they contain is already low.

The first drug with which that type of OC interaction was reported was rifampicin, used to treat tuberculosis. In the early 1970s, medical journals reported breakthrough bleeding and contraceptive failure in OC users taking rifampicin. Alerted to this effect with one drug, physicians over the next few years noted the possibility of this type of decreased effectiveness with many different drugs. They include:

- antibiotics such as isoniazid, ampicillin, neomycin, penicillin V, tetracycline, chloramphenicol, sulfonamides, nitrofurantoin, and griseofulvin,
- barbiturates,
- anticonvulsants such as phenytoin and primidone, and
- the anti-inflammatory phenylbutazone.

Also, some analgesics, tranquilizers and anti-migraine preparations may have this type of interaction. OC users taking such drugs are advised *to use an additional form of contraception until they discontinue therapy with the second drug.*

When it comes to the other side of the coin—OC's affecting the potency of other drugs—knowledge about such interactions is more limited. But again, the how and why seem to be tied to the way the drug is metabolized; that is, changed into a form that can be eliminated from the body.

Some drugs are metabolized in the liver primarily by oxidation, and thus are excreted through the kidneys rather than the bowels. These drugs appear to be metabolized more slowly in OC users, according to research by a group of scientists headed by Darrell Abernathy, M.D., Ph.D., and reported in the April 1, 1982, *New England Journal of Medicine*. The researchers reported that long-term use of low-dose estrogen-containing OC's may cause diazepam (Valium), a benzodiazepine anti-anxiety drug, to stay in the body longer. This means that OC users may require lower dosages of diazepam and other drugs that are metabolized in the same way. However, since not all people metabolize drugs in the same way, the patient should be monitored by her physician to see if the dose should be adjusted. Other drugs that may stay in the body longer because of OC's include: other benzodiazepines such as chlordiazepoxide (Librium); hydrocortisone; antipyrine; phenothiazines; and some tricyclic antidepressants.

In contrast, some drugs that are excreted mainly through the bowels (and at times partly through the kidneys) may be eliminated more quickly in OC users. Even though the metabolism of some benzodiazepines may be slowed by OC's, there are other benzodiazepines (such as lorazepam, oxazepam and tamazepam) whose metabolism may be enhanced, so they may be excreted more quickly in women taking birth control pills. However, information on exactly how such drugs interact with OC's is scarce. In an article in the September 1982 issue of *Obstetrics & Gynecology,* Abernathy reported that, in women using low-dose OC's containing estrogen for more than three months, acetaminophen (Tylenol) was eliminated more quickly than in non-OC users. The authors theorized that this increase in the speed at which the drug is eliminated from the body might offer some protection against liver toxicity in cases of acetaminophen overdose.

But OC users taking only the recommended dosages of acetaminophen might need a higher dosage than non-OC users. Again, because response to medication is so individual and because different combinations and dosages of estrogen and progestogen may have different effects, OC users should consult their physicians about any deviation from recommended dosages.

OC users taking other drugs may need to have the dosage monitored and possibly adjusted for a variety of reasons. Some epileptics may need a change in the dosage of an anticonvulsant drug they are taking, depending on the type of OC they're using. But other women taking the same combination may not need the dosage changed. The exact reason for this "iffiness" is not known, but it may be because OC-related changes in fluid retention could influence the frequency of seizures.

Because of these difficulties, many doctors recommend that women taking anticonvulsants rely on another contraceptive than birth control pills.

A similar recommendation is often made for diabetics, because OC's may cause blood sugar levels to rise. If a diabetic does take birth control pills, she should be closely monitored to see if there needs to be a change in her diabetes medication.

Hypertension can be a problem in women on birth control pills, and elevated blood pressure has been known to occur in women not hypertensive before taking OC's. To complicate matters further, some of the medications used to control high blood pressure do not work the same way in those on The Pill as in non-OC users. In particular, the blood pressure drug guanethidine often does not adequately control hypertension in OC users. OC users taking blood pressure drugs need to be more carefully monitored.

In addition to interactions with drugs, OC's may also interact with certain vitamins. Labeling for birth control pills notes that OC users may have disturbances in the metabolism of tryptophan, an amino acid. Although such a disturbance is not considered cause for undue concern, it may result in a deficiency of pyridoxine (vitamin B6). Whether that is a cause for concern is not known. Also, in rare cases, megaloblastic anemia, a certain type of anemia due to insufficient pyridoxine, has been reported in OC users. In addition, levels of folic acid—one of the B vitamins—may be lower in women on The Pill.

Preliminary studies have shown that vitamin C may increase the bio-availability of estrogens. This means that women using birth control pills who take large doses of vitamin C may be risking increased side effects from the pill's estrogen. For this reason, some experts suggest that OC users take no more than 1,000 milligrams of vitamin C daily.

Some laboratory test results can be altered by OC use. The pathologist or other lab personnel should be informed when a woman undergoing lab tests is taking birth control pills so that this can be taken into consideration when evaluating the tests. Tests that are altered by OC use include those measuring: liver function, coagulation (clotting), thyroid function, blood triglycerides and phospholipid (fats) concentrations, serum folate, glucose tolerance, and plasma levels of some trace minerals.

In most young, healthy women, the effects of taking other drugs while using oral contraceptives are no cause for alarm and should not keep women who can benefit from the contraceptive effectiveness of OC's from taking them. The effects of OC-drug interactions may vary greatly from woman to woman. Yet women should be aware of the possibility of such interactions and tell their doctor if they are taking birth control pills so that other therapy can be properly coordinated.

"Using YouTube, Public Citizen Warns of Unsafe Birth Control"

by Royelen Lee Boykie

In recent weeks, Public Citizen has jumped into a completely new realm: reaching out to citizens—mostly young citizens—via video posted on the Internet.

In January, Public Citizen's Health Research Group decided to launch a campaign to highlight the dangers of third-generation birth control pills (*see story, page 13*). The group wanted to reach out to as many young women as possible to warn them against taking these pills, which increase a woman's risk for blood clots, although older birth control pills do not have such side effects.

So Health Research Group staffers, along with others at Public Citizen, produced a video featuring six young women discussing their thoughts about birth control pills and warning about the dangers of the third-generation pills.

On Feb. 6, Public Citizen posted the video on YouTube .com, an online site where anyone can post and see videos. Public Citizen posted a link to the video from a new Web site it launched, www.not.mypill.org.

This Web site is interactive. Not only can people read the information that Public Citizen has posted, but they can submit their own videos about why the issue is important to them. They also can use the site to send a letter to the FDA, saying they want only the safest birth control options.

Since its launch, the video and www.notmypill.org have been visited thousands of times from people around the world. More than 7,000 people have urged the FDA to ban the drug as a result of this campaign.

All this is just a beginning. Public Citizen is now exploring how to cultivate this technology to encourage civic action. It is likely that more Public Citizen videos will be posted on sites such as YouTube in the coming months.

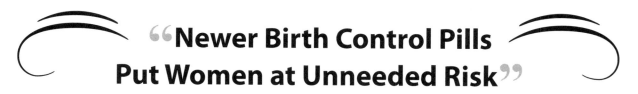

"Newer Birth Control Pills Put Women at Unneeded Risk"

by Kate Resnevic

A newer generation of birth control pill places hundreds of thousands of women each year at an increased risk of developing life-threatening blood clots, so Public Citizen is urging the Food and Drug Administration (FDA) to ban this form of birth control.

Public Citizen's Health Research Group petitioned the FDA on Feb. 6, asking the agency to ban third-generation birth control pills—the newest of the three forms of birth control pills on the market. Third-generation pills double a woman's risk of developing blood clots compared to second-generation birth control pills.

"Women are at an increased risk of blood clots when using any type of oral contraceptives that combine hormones, but third-generation birth control pills double that risk without preventing pregnancy any more effectively than older pills," said Dr. Sidney Wolfe, health group director. Wolfe co-wrote the petition with Jay Parkinson, M.D., MPH, and Sylvia Park, M.D., MPH, both research analysts for Public Citizen. Another co-author was Frits Rosendaal, M.D., of Leiden University in the Netherlands, who has published hundreds of papers and conducted ongoing studies of blood clots, particularly in connection with oral contraceptives.

Third-generation birth control pills, which contain the drug desogestrel, were developed in the 1980s in an unsuccessful attempt to create an oral contraceptive with fewer side effects (such as acne and unwanted hair growth) than the two previous versions. More than 7.5 million prescriptions for third-generation oral contraceptives were filled in the United States from November 2005 to October 2006.

Instead of using the latest generation of birth control, Public Citizen recommends that women use second-generation oral contraceptives (containing norgestrel, levonorgestrel, norgestimate or norethindrone), which provide the same protection against pregnancy but do not come with an added risk of blood clots.

Health Risk Nothing New

The first time researchers discovered that there were risks associated with third-generation birth control pills was in December 1995, when three independent studies showing these dangers appeared in *The Lancet*, a highly respected medical journal. The studies concluded that these contraceptives were associated with about twice the risk

---

Dangerous Birth Control

These third generation birth control pills contain desogestrel. Third generation pills increase a woman's risk for developing clots compared to second generation pills.

- Desogestrel with Ethinyl Estradiol
- Desogen
- Mircette
- Velivet
- Apri-28
- Kariva
- Ortho-Cept
- Reclipsen
- Cyclessa

Source: Public Citizen's Research Group

---

of blood clots compared to second-generation pills. Since then, many additional studies have confirmed this elevated risk.

The manufacturers of third-generation pills have essentially acknowledged the increased risks of blood clots by including a warning about the risk on the labels of all third-generation birth control pills.

Blood clots typically form in a patient's legs and can travel through the veins and block blood flow at another location. Blood clots that travel to the lungs can be fatal.

"The FDA has known for more than 10 years that these oral contraceptives were more dangerous but has allowed them to stay on the market," Wolfe said. "The risk is unacceptable. The agency should immediately take these drugs off the market."

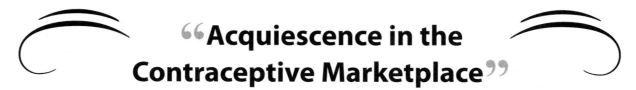

"Acquiescence in the Contraceptive Marketplace"

by Claudine Isles Wallace

I came of age in the era of hormonal contraception. I, and almost everyone I know, have taken oral contraceptives for close to my entire sexual life.

Many of my friends were prescribed the Pill from the time of their first periods to alleviate debilitating cramps and nausea. Birth control pills are accepted as a modern convenience for women, one that emboldens us in our sexuality and provides a sense of control over our own fertility.

Young women enter into our sexuality overwhelmed by social influences that promote hormonal contraception. Our mothers take us to Planned Parenthood to secure a future of choice and freedoms they themselves may not have enjoyed. Partners encourage us to "go on the Pill," complaining that condoms inhibit spontaneity and sensation. Commercials promise that the Pill will give us clear skin. Friends compliment our bigger breasts. Doctors counsel us in the Pill's efficacy and assure us of its safety.

In spite of these encouragements, I've always had reservations about taking the Pill. I remember reading in *Our Bodies, Ourselves* that synthetic hormones would affect every organ in my body. I recall my mother, full of worry and protest, cautioning me about the health risks caused by first-generation Pills in the 1960's. I remember reading the patient information insert in my first packet of Pills, struggling to reassure myself that the new version had lower doses of hormones and must, therefore, be safer. Wariness grew inside me but did not offset the convenience and protection that oral contraceptives provide.

In the U.S., the Pill is the most common contraceptive method used by women in their 20's; over 1 million teenagers rely on it every day.[1] Many women stay on the Pill for significant lengths of time. When I began my internship at the NWHN, I had been on the Pill for almost 5 years. I had long since stopped thinking about my morning ritual, too preoccupied with the more vivid and pressing concerns of being young and broke in New York City. But somewhere in the many hours of health research at NWHN, between trying to understand the pathology of breast cancer and answering women's questions about hormone replacement therapy—my concerns about the Pill returned with a quiet panic.

The more I read about oral contraceptives, the less I seemed to know. I learned that most hormones have no "normal" level. Even if such a level could be estimated, our hormones fluctuate considerably throughout the life cycle, the days of the month, and even the hours of the day. What is known is that the hormones used in oral contraceptives are much more potent than those naturally occurring in our bodies. Moreover, the estrogen in second-generation pills, while administered in lower doses, is twice as potent as that contained in the first-generation of Pills.

Synthetic hormones manipulate certain processes in our bodies with both expected and unexpected outcomes. While some studies have examined links between using oral contraceptives and the subsequent development of cancer, each study has produced results and recommendations different from the next. Amidst this scientific uncertainty, hormonal contraception is on the rise. Never before have so many young women ingested synthetic hormones for such long periods of time, starting at such young ages.

The medical community, family planning community, and greater consumer public have all embraced hormonal contraception. The debate over its long-term safety is minimal and generally relegated to certain pockets of activist and scientific communities. Given the mass acceptance of synthetic hormones, the commercial market has little incentive to develop non-hormonal alternatives for women.

In the past 25 years, only two significant non-hormonal contraceptive options have been developed and are still available today: the cervical cap and the female

"Young Feminists: Acquiescence in the Contraceptive Marketplace," by Claudine Isles Wallace, originally published in the *Women's Health Activist*, March/April 2005, pp. 6–7, the newsletter of the National Women's Health Network (NWHN). It is reprinted with the permission of the author and the NWHN.

condom. The cervical cap is essentially a British version of the diaphragm, operating on the same barrier principle and requiring the use of spermicide. The U.S. allows only one active ingredient to be used in spermicide—nonoxynol-9. Unfortunately, many women are allergic to nonoxynol-9, making the cap undesirable for much of the female population. The highly touted female condom emerged in the early 90's and was marketed as a prophylactic that gave women greater control. Yet, female condoms are more expensive than male condoms, offer less protection against sexually transmitted infections, and can be more disruptive of sexual sensation.

Neither the cervical cap nor the female condom has proven very popular among American women, for whom the most widely used methods are tubal ligation, male condoms, and the Pill. For women under 34, particularly those in monogamous relationships, hormonal contraceptives are the primary choice.

We have fallen into a vicious cycle. There is a shortage of creative ingenuity in developing more effective and marketable non-hormonal contraceptives. Newly introduced products, however, are not popular and do not generate profitable sales. Thus, manufacturers have no incentive for increased creativity. Meanwhile, the market for synthetic hormones keeps expanding; at each doctor's visit women are invited to try a new medium for hormone distribution. The patch, the ring, and the shot are all enthusiastically recommended and promoted through free samples.

We may find that continued hormonal contraception use from puberty through menopause is safe for women without certain risk factors. If this proves true, the Pill will be heralded as the most effective and convenient form of birth control ever invented. But if we discover that long-term use leads to negative hormonal outcomes, it will be a devastating continuation of my generation's intimate relationship with cancer. We will shift from nursing our mothers and beloved aunts to caring for our friends, our cousins, and ourselves.

As young women, we are socialized to please those around us, even when it means suspending our own needs and fears. Resisting a trend that your partner, medical advisor, and broader community believe in is extraordinarily difficult—especially when it also means using a contraceptive method that is less dependable and sexy. This holds true even for women who are wary of synthetic hormones.

Compliance will not provide us with any true security, however. We need to expand the dialogue surrounding birth control in our culture and demand efficacious choices that do not rely on synthetic hormones. Hanging in the balance of uncertainty is a familiar place for women's health. We must learn from the women before us that silence rarely equals protection.

REFERENCE

The Alan Guttmacher Institute (AGI). *Contraceptive Use, Facts in Brief.* New York: AGI, 2004.

"Next Target: Birth Control"

by Barbara Miner

The basement office in the Milwaukee suburb of Brookfield could be mistaken for an H&R Block franchise. But it is actually the headquarters of Pro-Life Wisconsin, which proclaims that birth control is murder.

On a recent afternoon, Pro-Life Wisconsin's Legislative Director Matt Sande talked for several hours, meticulously explaining the group's views. Embracing "the

embryonic person" and denouncing "chemical abortion," he wants to ban all hormonal birth control.

This would include not just emergency contraception but the pill, the IUD, the patch, and the shot. He wouldn't outlaw condoms and barrier methods, but he is uncomfortable with the attitudes they promote.

"There are some in the pro-life community who will say we can oppose abortion but we don't need to take a position on birth control. That's pure folly," says Sande, a graduate of the University of Notre Dame, the father of three young children, and part of that young breed of hard-core conservatives who came of age under Ronald Reagan and Newt Gingrich.

Pro-Life Wisconsin is one of several dozen groups affiliated with the Virginia-based American Life League, which is in the forefront of the fight against birth control.

Heading up the American Life League is Judie Brown. Back in 1976, Brown was a staff member at the National Right to Life Committee. Then, as now, it was the most well known of the groups opposing a woman's right to choose. But over the years, Brown became increasingly uncomfortable with the group's refusal to oppose birth control and with its acceptance of abortion in cases of rape and saving the life of the mother.

"As a Catholic, I just couldn't stay there," Brown says.

In 1979, Brown left to help found the American Life League. "Pro-lifers must see the connection between contraception and abortion," Brown argues. "And we must talk about it, point it out, and teach others the truth."

For hardliners like Sande and Brown, this is the next battle of the anti-abortion movement. And they are nudging that movement—and the Republican Party—even further to the right, opposing "the contraceptive mentality," as their leaders put it.

They argue that hormonal birth control might, in rare instances, act on a fertilized egg to prevent implantation in the womb. Thus, in their religiously based view, birth control would be acting as an "abortifacient."

Birth control pills generally work by preventing ovulation, and emergency contraception is little more than highly concentrated doses of the pill. (According to the Alan Guttmacher Institute, 98 percent of American women between fifteen and forty-four who have had sexual intercourse have used contraceptives.)

The American Medical Association defines pregnancy as beginning with the fertilized egg's implantation in the womb, not with the union of an egg and sperm.

The anti-abortion American Association of Pro Life Obstetricians and Gynecologists says it is impossible to argue definitively that oral contraceptives are "abortifacients" that prevent implantation, and it calls upon its members to "agree to disagree."

But the American Life League doesn't go along with that. It has 300,000 families and more than sixty associated groups nationwide that share its uncompromising views.

One of the most influential is Pharmacists for Life International, which is spearheading efforts to exempt pharmacists from dispensing birth control prescriptions. Karen Brauer, who was fired by a Kmart pharmacy in Ohio in 1996 for refusing to fill a birth control prescription, leads this web-based group, which says it has 1,600 members. In a 2001 appearance on *The O'Reilly Factor* on Fox News, Brauer admitted she lied to the patient and told her the pharmacy did not have the medicine on hand.

Brown's American Life League also founded the Crusade for the Defense of Our Catholic Church, which gained notoriety during the 2004 elections with its calls for U.S. bishops to refuse communion to politicians supporting the right to abortion.

The crusade's aggressive stance has been unpopular with many Catholics, including many Catholic bishops.

Of the 272 Catholic bishops in the United States, the league lists only thirteen who would deny communion to Catholic public figures who support the right to choose. (Many Catholics are unaware that church teaching considers all contraception "intrinsically evil," and many bishops downplay the church's stance against birth control. At the same time, the church actively opposes legislation mandating increased access to emergency contraception in hospital emergency rooms and requiring that health insurance plans cover contraceptives.)

While Brown's statements might seem to put her on the fringe, the Vatican has rewarded her loyalty. She is one of four Americans participating in the Pontifical Academy for Life, an international group dealing with ethical questions. She was appointed by the late Pope John Paul II seven years ago.

Brown says efforts are under way to develop a more unified position among anti-abortion forces on contraception. Last spring, for instance, about thirty anti-abortion activists met informally in Chicago to discuss their public stance—which groups would openly oppose contraception, which wouldn't, and why.

"It's the first time we have actually approached the subject, all of us, sitting down together at the table," Brown says.

The meeting was organized by Joe Scheidler of the Chicago-based Pro-Life Action League. Described by Pat Buchanan as the Green Beret of the anti-abortion movement, Scheidler is perhaps most well known for his role in the 1980s in promoting disruptive demonstrations outside medical clinics providing abortion.

Scheidler, who plans to have another meeting of anti-abortion forces in the early months of 2006, believes the efforts are a watershed and will push more groups to directly take on birth control.

"At our pro-life meetings, there's not much of a discussion on contraception, except as they are abortifacients," Scheidler said in an interview. "And we all agree on that pretty much. But we're going beyond that to the whole concept of the contraceptive mentality."

This opposition to the "contraceptive mentality" comes through in the recent effort by social conservatives to undermine the use of condoms on the grounds that they promote promiscuity and bad health practices. Condoms are used by about 20 percent of those practicing contraception, according to the Guttmacher Institute, and they have been a powerful tool in the fight against sexually transmitted diseases such as HIV/AIDS.

Under pressure from social conservatives, the FDA recently proposed new warning labels for condoms, saying they "greatly reduce, but do not eliminate" the risk of some sexually transmitted diseases. Many health advocates fear the new warnings will confuse people and cause them to stop using them—a potentially ominous development.

Scheidler notes that the Pro-Life Action League itself has not yet formally taken a position against birth control.

"Until we get this thing settled among other groups, we don't want to get out ahead," he explains.

Not many of the other leading anti-abortion groups want to get out ahead, either. Brown, when asked which other groups are most willing to take on birth control, mentions the Virginia-based Human Life International, a Catholic group, and the Catholic bishops. She says Concerned Women for America and Focus on the Family have been very active in opposing emergency contraception but that "they don't have a position on the pill."

Concerned Women for America was founded in 1979 by Beverly LaHaye, wife of Tim LaHaye, best-selling author and co-founder of the Moral Majority. It has about 500,000 supporters and describes itself as "the nation's largest public policy women's organization."

Wendy Wright, executive vice president of the group, says it does not oppose birth control or emergency contraception per se. "We approach the problem . . . as one of women's health and safety," she says. Wright argues, though, that emergency contraception is an "abortifacient," and information on the group's website reflects a similar view.

Focus on the Family—considered the largest international religious-right group in the United States, with a multimedia empire that includes its own campus and zip code in Colorado Springs—has also prominently opposed emergency contraception because it says it acts as an "abortifacient."

It is clear, however, that the group finds itself in a quandary over oral contraceptives in general.

A lengthy statement from founder Dr. James Dobson distinguishes between various types of birth control pills, outlining which are acceptable and which are not. The statement then notes that after two years of extended deliberation and prayer, the group "has not been able to reach a consensus" on whether the most commonly prescribed birth control pills are abortifacients. Dobson ends by calling on the anti-abortion movement to respect that groups may hold "differing opinions" on the use of oral contraceptives.

For its part, the Christian Coalition—founded in 1989 by Pat Robertson and describing itself as "America's leading grassroots organization defending our Godly heritage"— does not have articles on its website discussing emergency contraception or birth control.

"We are not, how can I say this, it is not one of our big issues, not like some of these other people," says Michelle Combs, a spokesperson for the group. "We have a female president, and we're not going to come out and tell women they cannot use birth control. I don't see us doing that." Perhaps realizing she had said too much, Combs then put any further comment off the record.

The Eagle Forum, founded in 1972 by Phyllis Schlafly, is likewise cautious about attacking birth control. John Schlafly, Phyllis's son and an Eagle Forum spokesperson, said: "We have not had anything to say, except we have spoken out about making that product [emergency contraception] an over-the-counter item because it is dangerous to young teenage girls," he said.

And what of the National Right to Life Committee with over 3,000 chapters in all fifty states?

Founded in 1971 by the Catholic bishops as an arm of their Family Life office, it spun off two years later as a single issue, nonsectarian, and secular organization. Focused on lobbying and legislative work, the group is most active on abortion, stem cell, and end-of-life issues. Its mission statement explicitly notes that it does not take a position on contraception.

The organization refused to respond to almost a dozen e-mails and phone calls other than to send a brief statement noting, in part: "The National Right to Life Committee (NRLC) is opposed to abortion, infanticide, euthanasia, and assisted suicide. NRLC takes no position on the prevention of the uniting of sperm and egg."

For now, it's difficult to know how the attack on birth control will play out. A key, unanswered question is whether more moderate conservatives will challenge extremist positions on birth control.

The issue has become so touchy that President Bush refuses to say whether he supports birth control. Bush's silence led to a letter last October 24 from thirty-two members of the House asking him to clarify his position.

"It's truly amazing that in the twenty-first century, the leader of the free world will not affirm his support for birth control," says Representative Carolyn Maloney, Democrat of New York, who organized the letter.

In the meantime, grassroots activists such as Judie Brown and Matt Sande continue their work, comforted by a belief in their moral superiority.

"We are a Christian organization, and we are trying to spread the truth with a capital T," says Sande. "Jesus Christ is the way, the truth, and the life. It is our charge to spread the truth on these issues. And every day we have people coming over to our side."

Confessions of a Radical Feminist
"Sex, Drugs, and the Department of Homeland Security"

by Stephanie Seguin

The morning-after pill was only a myth to me until one night at a French sidewalk bar. I was an exchange student hanging out with friends on a warm night in Avignon. A summer theater festival was on and the streets were teeming with strolling musicians and avant-garde theater troupes promoting plays. From our curbside table we watched people going by and smelled the lavender breeze drifting through the town.

Out of the crowd, two men on bicycles emerged and made their way toward our table. Huge black letters spelled AIDES ("help") across their shirts. Table by table, they peddled something from their baskets. People grabbed anxiously for their mystery goods. As they neared our table, we saw they were handing out condoms and packets of pills. They introduced themselves as city employees and gave us the official condom of France (complete with a picture of the Eiffel Tower) and a little packet containing some aspirin. The guys at the table made lewd comments about draping the official condom of France over their own Eiffel Towers and we marveled at the thoughtfulness of a country that provides protection from STDs *and* defense against our hangovers the next day.

The following morning, I told my host mother, Josette, about the condom and aspirin, shuffling through my things to show her the goods. She wiped her hands on her apron, studied the pills, and then laughed in that tone of hers that oozed, *Silly American*. She struggled for the words and looked at me with a smile. They were, as she put it, "not-baby" pills.

I stared at the packet. My plain old "aspirin" were in fact something much better. Back in the United States, this pill was a ladies'-bathroom legend: the "morning-after pill." The few women I knew who had actually gotten it had had to scale mountains and convince an overlord that they were deserving of this magic little pill. Yet here it was, right in my hand—and it had been *delivered* to me, in a bar, by government workers on bikes.

Since then, every time I have a misstep with a condom or I forget to take my birth control pill, my mind turns to that night in France—and how easy it was. How the fairy godfathers of pregnancy prevention rolled right up and handed me the morning-after pill as I finished my beer. What I wouldn't have given for those "magic beans" after countless high school mishaps that left me terrified and crying alone in my bathroom, trying to figure out how to hide the pregnancy test from my parents.

Every woman knows no birth control method is 100 percent reliable. Whether you're using rhythm or the pill, there's always a chance you'll end up crouched over a plastic stick waiting for that little pink line. I'd tried the pill and hated it. I blew up like a balloon and suffered the cruelest joke of a side effect: no sex drive. Wasn't the whole reason I was on the pill so I could have sex? If I didn't want to have sex, I'd skip the thirty dollars a month and just spend the weekend with a bag of Oreos and Matt Damon movies. After college, I stopped taking the pill and relied on condoms. I got my sex drive back, but still had to deal with the occasional condom mishap.

One such mishap occurred after I was married and my husband and I came home a little frisky and a lot drunk. Neither of us was ready for children, so we kept a barrel o' condoms next to the bed. Afterward, I noticed he wasn't doing the usual drill of cleanup and disposal. "Um, where's the condom?" I asked. He looked at me as if I had posed an interesting question that somehow hadn't occurred to him. He shrugged, glanced around, and answered, "I don't know, maybe it's still inside you." I looked at him like he was insane and wondered if we had somehow skipped the all-important step couples are supposed to take when they are trying not to get pregnant. I immediately set my inebriated mind to the task of figuring out how to get a morning-after pill. Could I call my doctor in the morning? I didn't think she'd be in the office, and even if she was, good old-fashioned embarrassment barred me from explaining to her, at seven o'clock on a Saturday morning, that I didn't know what had happened to the condom. I shut my eyes and prayed to the "not-baby" goddess. Luckily, my prayers were answered. I thought of France. Why should I have to rely on luck when there was a perfectly safe solution out there? I wanted to have the morning-after pill in my house, in my medicine cabinet, in my PEZ dispenser—anywhere I could actually get to it.[1]

A couple of years ago, I sat in a humid meeting room in Florida. My arms were sticky on the board table as I met with other members of Gainesville Women's Liberation. Alex, a member who had recently moved to New York, was visiting. She told us that the drug company that makes the morning-after pill had applied to the Food and Drug Administration (FDA) for over-the-counter status. "This is the opportunity to make our fight national," Alex said.

The following December, the FDA's advisory panel was scheduled to have a hearing about Plan B (the morning-after pill). Our group piled into two vans and drove fourteen hours to Washington, D.C. Women from other feminist groups, such as the Redstockings from New York, met us there. The panel of experts needed to hear about the effect this was having on our lives.

I spoke to the panel about the times I couldn't get my hands on the morning-after pill. Other women told of similar difficulties. It wasn't fair that all of us were scrambling to keep from getting pregnant while women in thirty-eight other countries (like France) could trot down to their local drugstore and get those wonderful magic beans along with their shampoo—no waiting, hoping, praying, or calling a doctor after hours.

The advisory panel voted overwhelmingly (23–4) that the morning-after pill should be available without a prescription; one panelist said it was safer than aspirin. In the following weeks, we waited for the FDA to announce the decision. We regrouped our forces in Florida to strategize. We didn't want to merely sit on our hands and wait.

We devised a plan. Margaret Sanger had broken the law by giving out birth control information when it was illegal. Following in her footsteps, we would publicly give out morning-after pills, defying the prescription requirement. We developed a pledge women could sign, saying that if they had a morning-after pill and a friend needed it they'd pass it on, even though it's illegal to do so.

We had our first "pill-passing" the morning after Valentine's Day. Even with thirty women and three weeks' time, the pills proved somewhat difficult to get. But we hoped that would change.

A week later, the FDA postponed its decision (the first of *many* postponements).

Meanwhile, more than seventy health groups, including the American Medical Association and the American College of Obstetricians and Gynecologists, continued to assert what they'd been saying for years—that the morning-after pill did not require a doctor's prescription. We pushed on with our own campaign, handing out pills in Florida, New York, and Washington, D.C. Thousands of women from all over the country continued signing our pledge to do the same.

High-level FDA officials were ignoring women, scientists, health groups, and their own advisors, all of whom said Plan B should be available over the counter. We knew we'd have to show up on their doorstep to make them listen. We would sit down and block access to the FDA, just like they were blocking *our* access to birth control.

In January 2005, we again made the fourteen-hour trek in borrowed cars and rented vans to the headquarters of the FDA in Rockville, Maryland, just outside of D.C. We timed our visit to two weeks prior to the date when the FDA was scheduled to make a final decision. The troops from New York met us there. We gathered in a parking lot down the street with our supporters.

We spoke our minds to a horde of news cameras and marched to the entrance with our crowd of supporters in tow. A pack of officers from the Department of Homeland Security scrambled to make a wedge between the entry doors and the swarm of angry women heading toward them. Nine of us lined up to face the wall of cops. We demanded to meet with the head of the FDA and said we would not leave until Plan B was available over the counter. I was excited, nervous, and proud.

Holding hands, we stretched out like paper dolls and sat down on the cold cement. We spanned the length of the entryway, blocking all access in and out. We stayed there nearly half an hour while news cameras crowded us to get their close-ups and a mob of women cheered us on. I was in the middle of the sit-down line and saw when two officers picked up the first of us and dragged her away. My heart was full of admiration for her courage. I took a deep breath to fight back the tears. We were actually doing it: We had organized that throng of shouting women who filled the sidewalk with signs and banners. We were having a sit-in at the FDA headquarters and demanding that women not be denied access to birth control and, ultimately, control over our lives.

I watched the cops pick up the second woman and the third, each cop grabbing an armpit and heaving us up one by one to carry us to the armored car. As I watched the eighth woman being dragged away, I braced myself to get hauled across fifty feet of ice-cold pavement.

All nine of us were handcuffed, stuffed in a police truck, and charged with disorderly conduct. The cheering crowd was still across the parking lot after they released us. We made a big step forward for women's liberation that day. We let the people in power know that we mean business, and that we won't stop until we win.

We *can* change our world by organizing, by shouting our experiences from the rooftops, and by showing up on the doorsteps of those in power. We hold more cards than we think. In August of 2006, the FDA made the morning-after pill available without prescription to women eighteen and older. A victory for feminist organizing! But only a partial victory because it traps Plan B behind the counter, forcing all women to show an ID for birth control and leaving younger women to try to scrape up a prescription. It's a step in the right direction, but if the FDA has its way, it will be the *final* step.

Now more than ever, we've got to keep fighting for full over-the-counter access for all women. If George Bush and his cronies who are responsible for strangling the FDA knew that every woman in the United States belonged to a feminist group, they'd be shaking in their boardrooms.

Then again, considering their recent decision, it looks like they already are.

Eight New Nonhormonal Contraceptive Methods for Men

by Elaine Lissner

Can you think of a male contraceptive other than the condom and vasectomy? Probably not, and for good reason: though more than eight new methods exist, some of them ready to use, none have been publicized. The methods range from simpler, safer, less surgical vasectomy to ancient "folk" methods which have performed well under scientific scrutiny. They are:

#1 No-scalpel Vasectomy According to Dr. Douglas Huber, recent medical director of the Association for Voluntary Surgical Contraception, "The no-scalpel vasectomy technique is the way all vasectomies should be done. If a vasectomy can be accomplished with this minimal surgery, then any surgeon doing more surgery should justify why more is necessary."

No-scalpel vasectomy, which has been performed for 4-8 million men in China and more than 1500 men in the rest of the world, involves gently poking and stretching a small opening in the scrotal skin rather than cutting the skin. Each vas deferens (sperm duct) is then blocked just as in a standard vasectomy. No-scalpel vasectomies bleed less and heal faster than standard vasectomies;

they also eliminate the need for stitches. A list of U.S. physicians who perform no-scalpel vasectomy can be obtained from the Association for Voluntary Surgical Contraception at (212) 561-8000.

#2 Permanent Contraception by Injection

In this experimental method, an injection of chemicals is used to close off the vas deferens, rather than cutting it surgically.

#3 Potentially Reversible Contraception by Injectible vas Deferens Plug

Tests in China in over 512,000 men have shown a 98% effectiveness rate, and all the men who have had their plugs removed for at least a year have regained fertility. Encouraged by these results, the World Health Organization recently started tests in ten men. Continued success will reportedly lead to a trial in 3500 men around the world (and availability in some parts of the world within two years).

#4 Potentially Reversible Contraception by Surgically Implanted vas Deferens Plug

Here, a soft silicone plug, or "Shug," is implanted in the vas deferens in an operation similar to vasectomy. The Shug's main advantage over injectible plugs is its two-plugs-in-one design, which gives it the potential to be more leak-free. Any sperm which leak past the first plug are likely to stay in the space between the plugs rather than continuing on their course. Currently being studied on men in the Chicago area, the Shug is proceeding slowly but steadily.

#5 Temporary Injectible Contraception

The interior of the vas deferens is coated with a sperm-killing solution that keeps its effects for up to five years and can be reversed before then with a simple injection. Fertility can be restored at any time. This method has been completely safe and effective in ten years of animal trials. Human trials are beginning in India, but testing in the United States is stalled partly because the necessary polymer has not been sent to the National Institutes of Health.

#6 Wet Heat Method

The deleterious effect of heat on male fertility has been known since the time of Hippocrates. Much as aspirin was "discovered" in the 1800s from a bark that Native Americans had long been accustomed to chewing to relieve pain, heat methods are now being "discovered" as a new form of male contraception. In this method, the testes are bathed in hot water every night for three weeks. Effectiveness goes up with increased temperature (hot tub temperature is not enough). At the recommended temperature, 116 degrees Fahrenheit, forty-five minutes per day provides contraceptive effect for six months. Although 116 degrees may sound very hot, one man has reported that this temperature is actually more comfortable on the testes than on any other part of the body.

Heat methods should be used in conjunction with sperm count checks (unless, for example, the heat method is just being used to enhance another method such as condoms or diaphragms). Sperm count can be checked easily at a doctor's or urologist's office.

#7 Artificial Cryptorchidism ("Jockey Method")

Special jockey shorts are worn during the day to hold the testes inside the inguinal canal (the same tube to which the testes retract naturally during cold or dangerous conditions.) This raises the testes to body temperature, thereby achieving the heat effect. Men appear to be about equally divided between those who find it a strange feeling and those who wouldn't mind it. Some men have expressed concern that this method would cause "jock itch," but this problem has not arisen for volunteers.

#8 Ultrasound Method

Ultra-short sound waves (the same type used by physical therapists to heal injuries) are applied to the testes for ten minutes once every six months, efficiently achieving the heat effect. Ultrasound should be used only after knowing all the details, as it may also be a permanent method in much greater doses.

All of these methods are nonhormonal (and thus not as prone to complicated side effects). Two of the methods (artificial cryptorchidism and wet heat) require little or no doctor intervention and could be put to use almost immediately. In addition to providing self-determination to men, any of these methods would improve the health, economic status and survival rates of women in countries (including the United States) where inadequate medical care makes many female methods unsafe or unavailable.

Do you wonder why you've never heard of these? In addition to the hurdles which face all contraceptive development, research bias has played a large part. In the past, funding agencies have found reasons not to fund research on male contraceptives, such as claiming that men are not committed to contraception (even though vasectomy makes up 12% of the world's contraceptive use) and that new male methods shouldn't be developed because they don't prevent the spread of HIV (even though new female methods such as Norplant don't either). Simple methods with low profit-margins have received even less support. With funding levels

If You Want to Use These Methods

The only methods which are "ready to go" are wet heat, artificial cryptorchidism and no-scalpel vasectomy.

No-scalpel Vasectomy is a small improvement on vasectomy. However, if you or someone you know is considering a vasectomy, this is the way to do it. To get a list of physicians who perform no-scalpel vasectomies, call the Association for Voluntary Surgical Contraception's general number at (212)561-8000. No-scalpel vasectomy is even safer and less invasive than the already safe vasectomy procedure.

Wet Heat method and Artificial Cryptorchidism ("Jockey Method") are in some sense ready to use—if you are willing to be your own researcher, method user, doctor and critical thinker all rolled into one. Neither of these methods is in widespread use or well-known to doctors. Hopefully, in the near future men will be able to go to their doctors for an ultrasound treatment or for a "do's and don'ts" manual for using the other heat methods. However, until that time men and women who use these methods must take full responsibility for reading up,

knowing what they're doing and making a fully informed choice.

If you are interested, start by reading the original paper, **"Frontiers in Nonhormonal Male Contraceptive Research."** Then go to a medical library and photocopy all the references in that citation on heat methods in general and the specific method you're interested in. Be certain to read the Kandeel and Swerdloff paper, even though it is very technical. **Contact the Male Contraception Information Project if you need more information.**

If you decide to use the wet heat method you'll have to experiment a bit to find a way to keep the water hot. Be creative. For example, modified old-style baby bottle warmers might work. If you come up with a good idea, let us know so we can pass it on. Regarding the use of hot tubs, you should know that it would take hours of hot-tubbing every day to produce contraceptive effect. That is why the wet heat method involves testes-only bathing at higher temperatures.

—Elaine Lissner
Male Contraception Information Project

so low, even supportive researchers couldn't accomplish much.

According to a 1990 committee convened by the Institute of Medicine/National Research Council, "Unless immediate steps are taken to change public policy, the choice of contraceptives in the United States in the next century will not differ appreciably from what it is today." However, many researchers and policymakers believe men don't care about contraception.

How can this be changed? Read up on the subject and make it one of your priorities, since research will increase only when public pressure is strong enough to provide incentive. Think about these methods, talk about them, and share this article with a friend. Bias is already fading, and with eight new methods in the wings, men and women don't need to wait any longer.

Beyond Condoms
"Years in the Making, Male Hormonal Contraceptives May Finally Be on Track"

by Regina Nuzzo

Four offspring is plenty for 37-year-old Glen Magdaleno of Los Angeles. "Children are grand, but they're a bit of a hassle too," he says. "I love my kids, but I just can't have any more and still be a good parent."

Not only would Magdaleno, a nursing attendant in a hospital orthopedic ward, be happy to share contraceptive responsibility with his wife, he'd also like for all men to have options beyond condoms, withdrawal or a vasectomy. To those ends, he recently volunteered at Harbor-UCLA Medical Center to test one of several male birth control drugs being developed around the world.

Every morning during the monthlong study, Magdaleno smeared hormone-laced gel over his upper body. The experimental drug was designed to penetrate his skin, enter his bloodstream and trick his body into shutting down testicular functioning—a reward he considers well worth the bit of acne he encountered. "At first I was worried about my libido and other side effects, but then I got excited about the idea of making love without the consequences," he says.

If widespread, Magdaleno's enthusiasm would bode well for drug developers. Forty years after the introduction of the female birth control pill—and despite sluggish progress in recent years—researchers are still optimistic about the ultimate feasibility of a male contraceptive.

Drugs now in development all use hormonal methods similar to those used in many female contraceptives. Small studies have found their delivery—a combination of implants, injections and gels—to be generally safe, reversible and effective in lowering sperm counts.

Now researchers are fine-tuning the methods to make them convenient enough for men to use consistently. And several studies are planned or underway in the United States, Europe and Asia to look at the real-life effectiveness of male hormonal methods in couples using no other protection during sex.

That's not to say a male birth control drug will hit the market in the next five or even 10 years. And the first product isn't likely to be a daily pill.

A man's reproductive system is even trickier to tame than a woman's. "Theoretically, all it takes to impregnate is one sperm," says Dr. Christina Wang, a professor and program director at the Los Angeles Biomedical Research Institute at Harbor-UCLA Medical Center. Every day, men churn out tens of millions of sperm. Women, however, produce a single egg once a month. "It's much more difficult to suppress sperm production," Wang says. "And you have to suppress it every single day."

Male hormonal methods work by adding testosterone or other male hormones to the bloodstream. The brain senses these extra hormones and, to keep the reproductive system in balance, sends chemical signals to shut down the testes, Wang says. This halts production of sperm cells. It also blocks normal production of testosterone—responsible for male characteristics throughout the body, from facial hair to sex drive—but the added male hormones serve to take up the slack.

Men can still ejaculate with suppressed sperm levels, but the hope is that they would be functionally infertile. Contraceptive researchers aim to reduce sperm counts from a normal average of 20 million to 200 million sperm per milliliter of semen to 1 million sperm per milliliter—or even lower, says Dr. John Amory, a professor of medicine at the University of Washington who has been studying a testosterone gel. Studies suggest that lowering the sperm count that much could result in a contraceptive that's as much as 99% effective.

Researchers have found they can boost the sperm-suppressing effects of the added male hormones by also administering progestin, a type of hormone used in female birth control pills and found naturally in small amounts in men. The progestin reinforces the chemical messages that shut down the testes.

Sperm production can then be suppressed with even less testosterone, which helps avoid some of the hormone's side effects. Researchers are most worried about testosterone's tendency to decrease levels of heart-healthy HDL cholesterol, which they've seen in some clinical trials, as well as possibly contributing to prostate cancer, which would require longer trials to study.

In the short term, testosterone's side effects can be similar to those of steroid use, including mood changes, lean muscle weight gain, acne breakouts and a temporary shrinking of the testes—the latter being a response to decreased sperm volume, Amory says.

The need for high doses of testosterone makes a male birth control pill tough to formulate, Wang says. Drops or spikes in hormonal levels can trigger sperm production, so a steady delivery method is crucial. Unlike estrogen, however, testosterone doesn't work well in a daily pill. The hormone tends to immediately break down in the liver.

To bypass this route, researchers are instead experimenting with ways to administer hormones directly into the bloodstream—including a combination of slow-release implants, long-lasting injections or daily gels.

Researchers in China are wrapping up the largest of these trials, a two-year efficacy study of approximately 1,000 volunteers, says Kirsten Vogelsong, a scientist at the World Health Organization, which sponsored the trial. The men received monthly testosterone shots and began having otherwise unprotected sex with their partners after researchers verified a drop in sperm count. Preliminary results suggest that most men remained infertile during the injection regimen, Vogelsong says, but a full report is expected sometime next year.

Also, the World Health Organization will help sponsor a smaller injection trial in Europe and Asia next year. Researchers plan to give 400 men bimonthly shots of testosterone and progestin at nine sites and follow them and their partners for a year, says Doug Colvard, associate director of CONRAD, a nonprofit reproductive health organization in Virginia.

A small study in Seattle suggests that testosterone might also be effective when applied onto the skin. Thirty-eight volunteers used a daily testosterone gel in addition to slow-release progestin implants, according to a report published by Amory and his colleagues in September. In 90% of the men, sperm counts dropped to infertile levels within six months, Amory says. Most of these levels returned to normal soon after the trial ended.

To continue this work, Amory and Wang are conducting a new gel-only trial in Seattle and Los Angeles. Vol-

unteers like Magdaleno apply separate progestin and testosterone gels daily, and researchers monitor their sperm count over the course of a few weeks. The researchers hope to enroll 140 volunteers and publish results after the trial concludes next spring.

For men who dislike daily routines, once-a-year surgery might be more attractive. The Population Council, a nonprofit international research organization in New York, is working on a slow-release implant of a powerful testosterone derivative, says Dr. Regine Sitruk-Ware, executive director of product research and development. This compound—administered through four small plastic rods that release hormones for up to a year—could spare the prostate from long-term side effects, she says. In initial tests in Europe, South America and Los Angeles over the last five years, the drug blocked sperm production completely in 72 out of 87 volunteers. Researchers are now tinkering with the rubber material used in the implant and hope to test a new single-rod implant in clinical trials within a couple of years.

Still, questions about the scientific mechanisms remain. Puzzlingly, men of Asian descent seem to respond more quickly and completely to male hormones than do non-Asians, Amory says. And some men in all hormonal studies are simply "non-responders," remaining fertile after standard treatments. "This is a real problem for drug companies," he says. "We don't have the same problem with women." He hopes that larger clinical trials will tease out slight differences in biology, which could then guide development of other methods.

Even if a drug proves effective, however, it still needs to be convenient. At the end of a large, three-year European study, researchers decided the combination tested—yearly progestin implants with testosterone injections every three months—was not likely to be acceptable for "widespread everyday use," according to a joint press release by the study's sponsors, Schering AG of Germany and Organon of the Netherlands. Although both companies say they remain individually committed to bringing a male hormonal contraceptive to the market, they don't plan to continue with further trials of this drug combination.

Also in September, Wyeth Pharmaceuticals in Madison, N.J., announced it was discontinuing its entire research program for new male and female contraceptive drugs. Financial pressures, scientific difficulties and an unknown market for male contraception were among the factors that contributed to the decision, says Gerald Burr, a spokesman for the company's research and development program.

Indeed, most research in the United States is being done by nonprofit, academic or government organizations, says Diana Blithe, program director of male contraceptive development at the National Institute of Child Health and Human Development at the National Institutes of Health.

"Pharmaceutical companies have not chosen to pursue this aggressively," she says. Male birth control is "both an untapped and untested market," and many drug companies prefer to follow less risky avenues of research, she says.

Still, Glen Magdaleno is hoping a good birth control will be available for his sons, ages 7 and 9, by the time they're old enough to need it. "This could be a great thing for my boys," he says. "I'd be more than happy to make them take it."

A survey of 9,000 men in nine countries, published in 2005 in the journal Human Reproduction, found that 55% were willing to use male hormonal contraceptives. Only 21% were unwilling. Of those countries:

- At 29%, Indonesia had the smallest percentage of men willing to use hormonal contraceptives.

- At 71%, Spain had the largest percentage willing to use such methods.

Of all the countries, including Germany, France, Sweden, Argentina, Brazil and Mexico, the United States ranked sixth on the greatest-acceptance list, with 49% of men in this country willing to use hormonal contraceptives. Among men who would use a hormonal method:

- 23% would prefer an annual implant.

- 22% would choose a daily pill.

- And 12% would choose a monthly injection.

Men who were willing to use hormonal methods were more likely to have higher education levels, report a higher income, have no religious objections, live in a metropolitan area and be willing to undergo a vasectomy.

Kirsten Thompson, director of the Male Contraception Coalition, says the demand for new male contraception is clear. "Every week I get e-mails from men asking where they can get access to experimental products they read about."

Would women trust them?

An earlier survey, published in 2000 in the journal of Human Reproduction, found support for a male contraceptive among 1,900 women attending family planning clinics in Scotland, China and South Africa.

More than 65% said responsibility for contraception fell too much on women.

More than 90% of Scottish and South African women considered the "male pill" a good idea, while 71% of women in Hong Kong and 87% of women in Shanghai thought it was a good idea.

2% said they would not trust their partner to use male hormonal contraceptive.

"You have to think of this in terms of couples in a stable relationship, where for some reason perhaps the woman can't take oral contraceptives," says Diana Blithe, program director of male contraceptive development at the National Institute of Child Health and Human Development. "In this country, 17% of men undergo vasectomies, which is much more drastic than hormonal methods. I think the market is there."

 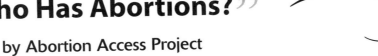

"Who Has Abortions?"

by Abortion Access Project

- 50% of American women have experienced an unintended pregnancy, and at current rates 35% will have had an abortion by the age of 45.[1]
- A broad cross section of U.S. women have abortions:[2]
  - 56% of women having abortions are in their 20s
  - 61% have one or more children

  - 67% have never married
  - 57% are economically disadvantaged
  - 88% live in a metropolitan area
  - 78% report a religious affiliation
- 52% of U.S. women obtaining abortions are younger than 25: Women aged 20–24 obtain 33% of all abortions, and teenagers obtain 19%.[3]

"Fact Sheet: Who Has Abortions?" March 2007 Abortion Access Project, www.abortionaccess.org. Reprinted by permission.

- Of the women obtaining abortions in 2000:
  - 57% of women have some college education
  - 88% were from metropolitan areas
  - 57% were low income
  - 66% had never been married

- Of women obtaining abortions, 41% were non-Hispanic white, 32% were non-Hispanic black, 20% were Hispanic, 6% Asian or Pacific Islander, and 1% Native American[4]

- Over 60% of abortions are among women who have previously birthed one or more children.[5]

- Women who obtain abortions represent every religious affiliation. 13% of abortion patients describe themselves as born-again or Evangelical Christians; while 22% of U.S. women are Catholic, 27% of abortion patients say they are Catholics.[6]

Sources

1. Henshaw, SK. Unintended pregnancy in the United States, *Family Planning Perspectives*, 1998, 30(1):24–29 & 46; and AGI, State facts about abortion: Texas, http://www.guttmacher.org, accessed Feb. 16, 2006.

2. An Overview of Abortion in the United States. June 2005. Accessed on March 13, 2007 from http://guttmacher.com.

3. Jones, RK, Darroch, JE and Henshaw, SK. Patterns in the socioeconomic characteristics of women obtaining abortions in 2000–2001, *Perspectives on Sexual and Reproductive Health*, 2002, 34(5):226–235.

4. Ibid.

5. Jones, RK, Darroch, JE and Henshaw, SK. Patterns in the socioeconomic characteristics of women obtaining abortions in 2000–2001, *Perspectives on Sexual and Reproductive Health*, 2002, 34(5):226–235.

6. Ibid.

 # "Shortage of Abortion Providers"

by Abortion Access Project

- In 2000, there were a little over 1,800 abortion providers in the United States, an 11% decrease since 1996.[1]

- In 2001 5,801 hospitals were recorded in the United States, however, only 600 were identified as providing abortions.[2]

- 34% of women live in counties which lack facilities that provide even one abortion a year.[3]

- 25% percent of patients travel between 50 and 100 miles to obtain abortion services, 8% travel more than 100 miles.[4]

- Almost every state has a policy explicitly allowing health care professionals or institutions to refuse to provide or participate in abortion, contraceptive services or sterilization services.[5]

- 44 states have "physician only" provisions in their abortion laws which prevent qualified practitioners such as nurse-midwives, nurse practitioners, and physician assistants from performing abortions.[6]

- 74% of all family practice chief residents receive no training in first-trimester abortion.[7]

- 58% of all physicians who provide abortions are over the age of 50. Younger physicians replacing them in the field of women's health, have little direct experience with the consequences of illegal abortions and the public health benefits of ensuring that safe abortions remain available.[8]

- Refusal clauses in each state allow providers to deny abortion care if against their moral or religious beliefs. This clause limits women's access to honest information and medical care, making it virtually impossible for some women to access abortion services altogether.[9]

Sources

1. S.K. Henshaw, "Abortion Incidence and Services in the United States, 2000," *Perspectives on Sexual and Reproductive Health*, 35:1, Jan/Feb 2003.

2. Guttmacher Institute. Facts in Brief: Induced Abortion. January, 2003.

3. S.K. Henshaw, "Abortion Incidence and Services in the United States, 2000," *Perspectives on Sexual and Reproductive Health*, 35:1, Jan/Feb 2003.

4. S.K. Henshaw, "The Accessibility of Abortion Services in the United States, 2001," *Perspectives on Sexual and Reproductive Health*, 2003, 35:1: 16–24.

5. Ibid.

6. Strategies for Expanding Abortion Access: The Role of Physician Assistants, Nurse Practitioners, and Nurse-Midwives in Providing Abortions. *Symposium Report*. Washington, DC: National Abortion Federation, 1997.

7. J.E. Steinauer, "Training Family Practice Residents in Abortion and Other Reproductive Health Care: A Nationwide Survey." *Family Planning Perspectives*, 29(5), 222–7, 1997.

8. Ibid.

9. "Access to Abortion", NARAL:ProChoice America and NARAL Pro Choice America Foundation, February 2007.

"The Side Effects, Risks, and Complications of Medical Abortion"

by Caroline de Costa

It is now 26 years since RU-486 was first used by women. In that time a huge number of trials and studies have been conducted in many parts of the world, and comprehensive records have been kept of the use of the drug. Most recent studies have been conducted by workers and institutions quite independent of the drug's manufacturers and marketers. There is thus a very large body of good evidence to tell us exactly what mifepristone does and does not do, its side effects, and the risks faced by women using it.

Medical abortion by definition involves the expulsion from the uterus of what doctors call the products of conception—the embryo or fetus, the placenta and membranes. This is the same process as occurs with natural miscarriage. It of necessity involves some vaginal bleeding and some lower abdominal pain—the pain is due to the contractions of the uterus brought about by prostaglandins, both the misoprostol used for the procedure and naturally-occurring prostaglandins.

When medical abortion is performed early (up to 63 days—nine weeks) the pain prior to and during the passing of the products of conception is usually reported by women as similar to menstrual cramps and is controlled by analgesics (painkillers) such as codeine/paracetamol compounds. Once the process is complete the pain should ease off. Occasionally a woman undergoing early medical abortion may need stronger, narcotic pain relief. Narcotics are also often indicated for later medical abortion when the pains are more on the scale of the contractions of labour. Bleeding is also found by most women having an early medical abortion to be similar to a heavy period, or, if they have previously experienced a miscarriage, to the bleeding they experienced then. Bleeding tails off over a number of days following the abortion process itself, as it does following a natural miscarriage or normal childbirth. Most studies show an average of around nine days of bleeding, the amount of bleeding lessening with each day. Some women will have heavier bleeding at the time of the abortion, studies showing a range of around 2–5%. Some of these women will respond to one of the drugs usually used in obstetric and midwifery practice for bleeding following normal childbirth: oxytocin or ergometrine. These drugs need to be given by injection. Alternatively, a woman may be given a a further dose of misoprostol, which has a similar effect. About 1–2% of women will need to have the abortion completed by surgical means in order to stop the bleeding. A very small number of women— around one in 500 to one in 1,000—will need a blood transfusion.

Women undergoing a late medical abortion have a higher incidence of heavier bleeding. Some of these women will also not deliver the placenta at the time the fetus is passed. This condition of retained placenta requires that the placenta be removed by a doctor under an anaesthetic. The condition also occurs after normal childbirth. For this reason, and because women undergoing later abortion may require narcotics, and certainly require good psychological support from trained nursing staff, late medical abortions should take place in hospitals or suitable clinics.

RU-486 itself has very few side effects. Misoprostol may cause diarrhoea, nausea and vomiting. Diarrhoea has been reported in 14% of women and nausea and vomiting in up to 40% when misoprostol has been taken orally but the incidence of these side effects is much less when the misoprostol is given intravaginally as is now the current method. Misoprostol may also cause dizziness, headache, shivering and occasionally a slight fever. Most women who experience these symptoms report them as tolerable.

Up to 1% of women may not respond to the drugs. The pregnancy may continue and remain in the uterus, or it may have been interrupted but not expelled. Where a pregnancy continues there is a risk of abnormalities in the fetus if the pregnancy continues to term. These are due to the effects of misoprostol rather than of mifepristone. The abnormalities include defects of the face and limbs. There have been a very few reported cases of women changing their minds about abortion after taking the mifepristone but before taking the misoprostol. In these cases and where the pregnancy has continued to full-term there have been rare reports of abnormalities, although there have also been reports of normal infants. Women need to be informed of these facts before consenting to medical abortion and they need to be offered surgical abortion if medical abortion fails.

As already mentioned it is essential that doctors providing medical abortion make absolutely sure that the pregnancy is not ectopic, meaning that it is developing somewhere outside the cavity of the uterus, usually in one or other of the fallopian tubes. Mifepristone/misoprostol is currently contraindicated in ectopic pregnancy

which must be treated either with surgery or with the drug methotrexate. There has been one case in the US where a woman died following an attempt at medical abortion, when the attending doctor had failed to detect that the pregnancy was ectopic, in the fallopian tube; the pregnancy subsequently ruptured with fatal results. Although this is not directly attributable to the drugs involved in the abortion it was certainly attributable to faulty technique on the doctor's part. In most clinics vaginal ultrasound is used to confirm that the pregnancy is in the uterus (and also that the duration of the pregnancy is within the prescribed period for early medical abortion, that is, less than nine weeks.) All RU486 sold in the US now carries a 'Black Box' warning on the packaging alerting doctors to the importance of confirming that a pregnancy is not ectopic.

Care should also be taken in providing medical abortions to women with a history of heart disease especially those who are heavy smokers. One death has been reported in the US in a woman of 44, with a previous history of heart disease, diabetes and obesity; this woman had a myocardial infarct (heart attack.) She was of course a woman at high risk in any case, if she continued with the pregnancy, however surgical abortion and care in hospital might have been more appropriate for her.

Infection involving the cavity of the uterus (endometritis) has been reported in between 0.9% and 2.7% of women undergoing medical abortion. This is most likely when some pregnancy tissue remains in the uterus. Such infections are caused by bacteria normally living in the woman's lower bowel. These bacteria migrate via the vagina into the open cavity of the uterus and multiply there. There is a similar incidence of infection like this associated with natural miscarriage and after surgical abortion. The infection will declare itself with some lower abdominal pain and vaginal discharge and will need to be treated adequately with antibiotics to prevent spread to the fallopian tubes and the uterus itself (pelvic inflammatory disease) which may lead to subsequent infertility or ectopic pregnancy. In some cases there will need to be a D&C (a surgical procedure to remove tissue from the uterus) as well. Infections such as these usually respond completely when promptly treated with antibiotics.

Opinion is divided as to whether women undergoing medical abortion should have antibiotics prophylactically—meaning at the time of the procedure or soon after, to prevent infection. At the moment the FDA does not recommend this and it is not part of the guidelines of the RCOG. However in 2006 Dr Baulieu, (the 'godfather' of medical abortion) published an article in the

New England Journal of Medicine recommending that antibiotics be used routinely and certainly some practitioners do this. Further research is needed in this area.

Another, very rare infection has been associated with medical abortion in North America. Between September 2003 and June 2005 there were four cases of this infection following medical abortion, all of which were fatal. All these cases occurred in the United States and all in California. In 2001 there was one case of the same infection following a medical abortion with RU486 in Canada. That case was also fatal. The U.S. FDA carried out an extensive investigation of all the Californian cases in order to determine whether either of the drugs used for medical abortion, or the techniques of medical abortion, could be linked in any way to the deaths. Their conclusion was that neither the drugs nor the techniques were the cause of the infection and although they have now included on their website a further Black Box warning about infection following medical abortion, and the need for women to seek emergency care if they develop symptoms, they have seen no reason to advise women against medical abortion using the mifepristone/misoprostol combination.

The bacteria that caused the infection have been identified as *Clostridium sordellii* (*Cl sordellii*). Other related bacteria more commonly cause infections in humans but *Cl sordellii* is rare. Many kinds of Clostridia may live in the human bowel without causing infection—this is known as colonisation. In people who undergo surgery there can be migration of bacteria from the bowel to the area operated upon, with the development of infection. Long before medical abortion was practiced in the U.S. fatal infections from *Cl sordellii* were reported following normal childbirth, caesarean section, gynaecological surgery, bowel surgery and orthopaedic (bone) operations. Like other related bacteria *Cl sordellii* brings about damage and death by producing a powerful toxin which circulates in the bloodstream causing heart and kidney failure. There is not usually a high fever in people infected. Initial symptoms include weakness, nausea, vomiting, abdominal pain and diarrhoea. Rapid overwhelming infection can follow with very low blood pressure, a rapid pulse and very high levels of red and white blood cells appearing in the bloodstream, and despite intensive care death rapidly supervenes. There have been no reported cases of fatal *Cl sordellii* infection following surgery in Australia or indeed anywhere else in the world outside of North America.

All the American women who died lived within the same region of California. All had taken 200 mg of mifepristone orally and had 400µgm misoprostol inserted vaginally by themselves. In all of them the abortion process was complete—autopsies did not show any retained pregnancy tissue in the uterus that might have predisposed to infection. The FDA tested samples of both drugs from the batches supplied to the women and found no contamination with the bacteria. It was concluded that since the factor linking the women was residence in the particular region it was the occurrence of *Cl sordellii* in the area, with the probable colonisation of the bowels of these women, rather than the fact of medical abortion per se that had brought about the deaths. It was very possible that if these women had undergone surgical abortion or if their pregnancies had proceeded to term, *Cl sordellii* infection would still have occurred. Nevertheless the FDA ordered the additional 'Black Box' warning to be included in all packets of mifepristone sold in the US, to include information about the symptoms of the illness and advice to women that if they had any of these symptoms, or felt otherwise unwell, they should report without delay to a doctor or emergency department. In addition the manufacturers of mifepristone in the US, Danco Laboratories, sent every emergency department doctor and abortion provider in the U.S. information about *Cl sordellii* infection.

Because mifepristone also acts to block cortisol receptors (see Chapter 8), some scientists have suggested that it may suppress the natural immune responses to infection, allowing bacteria to overwhelm the various systems of the body. However other scientists have pointed out that if this were the case it would be expected that all sorts of serious infections would have been reported, not just *Cl sordellii*—and this has not happened. Fortunately there have been no further deaths reported from this infection following medical abortion in North America since 2005 so it seems that the extra vigilance practiced has been rewarded and hopefully this will continue.

The overall risk of death associated with medical abortion is less than 1 in 100,000 women and is very similar to the risk of death from surgical abortion. These are the figures from the United Kingdom. It would seem that figures in the US are very similar but because of the uncertainty of how many women have actually used mifepristone the exact rate is difficult to calculate. Such figures can be compared with the chances of a woman dying from proceeding to a full-term pregnancy, which in developed countries is around 10 per 100,000 women. This however is not a very meaningful comparison for a woman trying to make a decision for herself about unwanted pregnancy.

The longterm effects of mifepristone have been studied in patients who have taken the drug for a number of years for conditions such as meningioma. No longterm changes in liver or kidney function have been found. There has been some thickening of the endometrium, the lining of the womb, in women who have taken the drug for a long period of time. Changes like these need to be followed carefully in such patients to avoid the possible development of cancer in the endometrium.

The risks and complications of medical abortion using methotrexate/misoprostol combinations are similar to those of mifepristone/misoprostol regimens—most of the side effects are due to misoprostol. Methotrexate has a risk of causing abnormalities in the fetus if an unsuccessful abortion proceeds to term, and women taking this drug need to be fully informed about this risk. There have been no reports of *Clostridium sordellii* or other such fatal infections in association with methotrexate-induced medical abortion. Misoprostol-only regimens will have the side effects and risks already described for misoprostol.

The Bad Baby Blues
"Reproductive Technology and the Threat to Diversity"

by Lisa Blumberg

The public discourse we need has been stalled—even in the disability community—because when people discuss the implication of the new reproductive technology at all, they tend to do so within the framework of their views on abortion. Yet these issues transcend the abortion controversy.

It was my feminist leanings superimposed on my disability orientation that fueled my interest in the implications of reproductive technology. In 1980, a woman I worked with who was pregnant told me she was having amniocentesis. "I really don't want the test," she said. "I don't know what I'm supposed to do if there is a problem. I don't want to make a decision about having the child." When I asked why she was having it, she said, "I'm 37, and my doctor told me every expectant mother over 35 needs to have it. He wouldn't feel comfortable if I refused."

I just said "good luck" (as is usually the case, the test, revealed nothing) without telling her that her doctor's stance made me uncomfortable. Until then, I thought that whether to have prenatal tests was a decision that prospective parents made for themselves, based on their own attitudes on pregnancy, disability, family life and a host of other things. Without being able to articulate why, I thought it was dangerous for a doctor to impose an obligation on a woman to learn beforehand whether her child might be disabled.

A few years later, I was a watching a news story on the merits of a predictive test for spina bifida. A woman explaining why she had gotten an abortion after test results had been positive said, "I defy any woman, no matter how much she wants a child, to continue a pregnancy after they show her a picture of a deformed baby and tell her that 'this is going to be yours.'"

I thought about that woman a lot. What concerned me was not so much the choice she made as the approach of her medical advisors. What a baby with an untreated medical problem looks like does not indicate what a person with a disability can become. Was it fair to urge people to make such a profound decision as to whether to bring a particular type of child into world on the basis of such a firsthand visceral response?

I started seeing articles in news magazines suggesting that if prenatal testing were used widely and women were then "willing" to abort fetuses found to be "defective," the incidence of children with certain types of disabilities could be significantly reduced.

The word "willing" always jumped out at me. Amniocentesis had originally been touted as a way to expand pregnant women's options, but now it seemed that women were expected to use the knowledge that could be gained by prenatal testing in a way that satisfied others.

In the past decade, prenatal testing has become a multi-billion dollar industry, with hundred of conditions now capable of pre-birth detection. Screening methods, some invasive and some not, are constantly evolving. Ultrasound, which used to just measure fetal growth and position, is giving way to targeted ultrasound which can zero in on a specific body part of the fetus such as the face. In most cases (but by no means in all) when a fetus is diagnosed as having a permanent disability, the pregnancy is terminated.

It is amazing that there has been scant public debate about this revolutionary new technology that allows us for the first time in all of human history to ascertain certain medical facts before one is even a person. Nothing that earlier generations dealt with during pregnancy was in any way comparable. In what varying ways can we react as individuals? How should we react as a society? What are legitimate public health goals? Can we view all people as equals and still feel that it is important to identify some traits prenatally? These are some of the questions that we must start addressing or else we could find ourselves drifting toward a society where there is little tolerance for either physical diversity or diversity in decision-making.

Disability activists need to be aggressive in initiating and framing the debate because our interests, along with those of women, are the most directly involved.

There are differences between ordinary abortion and selective abortion. Most abortion occurs because the pregnancy is unexpected and the prospect of parenthood itself is creating a crisis for the woman. Selective abortion, which constitutes a tiny fraction of all abortions, occurs when the pregnancy is planned but the fetus is perceived as having undesirable characteristics. In other words, selective abortion involves judgments about people. Indeed, women who abort due to fetal "defect" are often urged to get pregnant again quickly.

Almost everyone, regardless of how pro-choice they are, has views on where a moral line should be drawn in selective abortion. Where the difference in opinion arises is the positioning of that line. Many feminists express misgivings over abortion based on sex. Most medical ethnicists would oppose abortion based on eye color. The idea that a couple who share an inherited trait such as some types of deafness might want to end a pregnancy involving a fetus that did not have the same gene and "try again" out of the belief that their family will work better if all members have the same characteristics is controversial even in the disability community.

Without suggesting there should be restrictions on abortion, it is legitimate for disability activists to question the general public consensus that fetal disability is one of the "best" reasons for abortion—right up there with rape or incest and what right-to-lifers call "hard cases." It is not inevitable that prenatal diagnosis must change a wanted future baby into a "defective" fetus about which a decision must be made. As Adrienne Asch, a professor at Wellesley College has written, "suppose Down syndrome, cystic fibrosis or spina bifida were depicted not as an incalculable, irreparable tragedy but as a fact of being human? Would we abort because of those conditions or seek to limit their adverse impact on life?"

The disability rights movement in the quarter century it has been in existence has been successful on some nuts-and-bolts access issues. Important civil rights laws have been passed. However, basic attitudes towards disability really have not changed. It is a premise of the movement that a person with a disability is limited more by society's prejudices than by the practical difficulties that may be created by the disability. Unfortunately, by and large, nondisabled people don't believe it. Most people, to the extent they must think about disability at all adhere to the medical model of disability. Under the medical model, a person's disability is seen to be the cause and sum of that person's problems, with the paramount question therefore being whether the impairment can be alleviated.

Nowhere is the medical model more entrenched than with medical professionals. And it is medical professionals, and in particular genetic counselors, who help prospective parents evaluate their options after prenatal diagnosis.

The role of genetic counselors is to give prospective parents advice about how their child's expected condition can affect people—so the parents can make an informed decision regarding whether to continue the pregnancy. Genetic counseling is intended to be "nondirective," and most counselors do refrain from telling their clients what their decision should actually be. However, when counselors provide prospective parents with merely a list of deficits their future child may have (or may not have, since the same diagnostic label can reflect itself in different individuals in widely disparate ways), they are only telling half of the story. The other half is how people cope with these limitations and what other factors may influence their lives.

Perhaps the most serious limitation of genetic counseling is that counselors rarely offer clients the opportunity to meet persons with disabilities similar to those their child might have or to talk with parents of disabled children. Indeed, some genetic counselors resist the idea out of the belief that this would increase the discomfort of their clients. Yet clients who did not want to accept the offer could just say so. We can and must urge that the sources of information people have access to within the genetic counseling process be broadened.

Persons affected by disability are the most qualified to provide insight on the lifestyle concerns that prospective parents will have after prenatal diagnosis. We cannot tell others what they can personally cope with, but we can tell them how it is for us—and we can share with them our individuality and the range of our views. We can suggest that it is alright to embark on an endeavor which sometimes may be hard, which may make one an outsider and where there are few signposts. We can point out that it is OK to do the unusual thing.

On a more general social level, consideration also needs to be given to how the emphasis on prenatal testing and the perceived need to make decisions after diagnosis affect people's relations with one another. A prominent newspaper columnist once described the reactions she got to her veto of her doctor's age-based recommendation that she have amniocentesis. She chose to forego the option of termination in the unlikely event the fetus was disabled, she said, because of the children she already had. She did not know how she could find the words to explain to them a decision not to have a child who might use a wheelchair or always need special guidance, she said, and still affirm for them her view that differences in people should be accepted.

She pointed out that this was not a snap judgment but something she had reflected upon at length. However, she said, people she thought knew her well dismissed her desire to contemplate older motherhood without prenatal tests with an "Oh, it must be because you're Catholic." She is, in fact, pro-choice.

The woman had hit upon something important. In an open letter to genetic counselors published in a professional journal, one woman described the aftermath for her family of a decision to end a pregnancy involving a fetus with Down syndrome. Her school-aged children disturbed by their parents' grief, asked what was so bad about this type of disability.

Their father, said the letter writer, then had to instruct the children on the realities of life with a "handicapped child"—or at least what he thought the realities were. He asked them to imagine what it would be like to be trying to cross a street and always get confused about whether red meant "go" or green meant "go."

Later, when the children were asked to write down their feelings about what had happened, the older one told how sad it had been, and said "the only good thing is not having a child like that in our family." One wonders how children specifically encouraged to see disability as an all-encompassing burden both for the person who has it and for others will interact with the people with noticeable disabilities that they will most certainly meet in life.

Genetic counselors should be urged to help parents who do decide to abort after prenatal diagnosis to find "disability neutral" ways to talk about their decision with children—discussions which focus on the limitations or competing priorities of the family, rather than on assumptions about the potential of people with disabilities.

Reproductive technology can be divisive. It can reinforce prejudices.

There is another side of prenatal testing though. At a conference designed to start a dialogue between disability rights activists and the medical community, I listened as a parent recounted how, after her first child died from Tay-Sachs, she chose to have Tay-Sachs screening in her subsequent pregnancies. All she wanted was children who would live, she said; and eventually she had them. She told us, "I was given an option which I would not otherwise have had—the option to have a family." Another woman with a family history of cystic fibrosis had a predictive test when she was pregnant because, if her child were affected, she wanted to get on a particular doctor's roster right away. There are people who do want the tests, and people who have benefitted from them.

However, it is one thing to acknowledge a couple's right to make a personal and private decision to use prenatal testing based on their own unique circumstances, it is quite another thing for there to be a general expectation that every pregnant woman over 35 will go on defect alert.

What scares me is not the individual decisions people make—although I may disagree with some of these decisions—but the fact that society has latched onto the new reproductive technology as a lead weapon in a simplistic war against "birth defects." It is chilling to read decisions in wrongful birth and wrongful life suits where judges opine that avoiding the births of disabled children is a social good. It is equally chilling to hear public health analysts debate whether the abortion rate of "defective fetuses" will be high enough to make state-sponsored prenatal programs cost effective and efficacious. The legislature of at least one state (Alabama, in a law first passed in the late 1970s) has declared it to be state policy "to encourage the prevention of birth defects and mental retardation through education, genetic counseling and amniocentesis . . ."(Section 22-lOA-l of the Alabama statutes).

How easily ignored is the ethical imperative placed on genetic counselors to be nondirective! And how easily blurred is the critical distinction between preventing persons from *having* disabilities and preventing persons *with* disabilities! Most frightening in my view, though, are the articles in legal and medical journals suggesting that carrying a disabled fetus to term constitutes "fetal abuse" on the part of the woman.

Ruth Hubbard, professor emeritus of Biology at Harvard, has written, "my problems with amniocentesis stem mostly from my concern about how it creates eugenic thinking. We act as if we can look at a gene and say 'Ah-ha, this gene causes this . . . disability' when in fact the interactions between the gene and environment are enormously complex. It moves our focus from the environmental causes of disabilities—which are terrifying and increasing daily—to individual genetic ones." This misplaced focus will not only result in individuals acquiring disabilities unnecessarily: it will undermine the status of people with disabilities, regardless of the origins of their disabilities, and of women.

The new reproductive technology represents a boon for some and terror for others.

It is startlingly new but it invokes feelings that are age-old. I believe that the public discourse that we need has been stalled—even in the disability community—because when people discuss the implication of the new reproductive technology at all, they tend to do so within the framework of their views on abortion. Yet these issues transcend the abortion controversy, even as they cut across both sides of that debate. Somehow, we must begin to think more creatively and learn to meld together different world views. It is only then that we will have the hope of solving the conundrums created by the new reproductive technology in ways that will respect the individuality of us all.

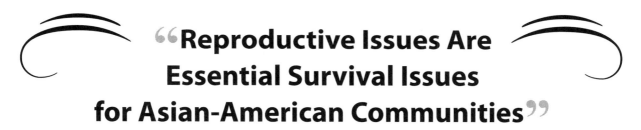

"Reproductive Issues Are Essential Survival Issues for Asian-American Communities"

by Connie S. Chan

When the Asian-American communities in the U.S. list their priorities for political action and organizing, several issues concerning basic survival are usually included: access to bi-lingual education, housing, health, and child care, among others. Yet the essential survival issue of access to reproductive counseling, education, and abortion is frequently missing. Why are reproductive issues perceived as unimportant to the Asian-American communities? I think there are several reasons—ignorance, classism, sexism, and language barriers. Of course, these issues are interrelated, and I'll try to make the connections between them.

First, let me state that I am not an "expert" on the topic of reproductive issues in Asian-American communities, but that I have some firsthand experiences which have given me some insight into the problems. Several years ago, I was a staff psychologist at a local community health center serving the greater Boston Asian population. Most of our patients were recent immigrants from China, Vietnam, Cambodia, Laos, and Hong Kong. Almost all of these new immigrants understood little or no English. With few resources (financial or otherwise) many newcomers struggled to make sense of life in America and to survive in whatever fashion they could.

At the health center, the staff tried to help by providing information and advocacy in getting through our confusing system. I thought we did a pretty good job until I found out that neither our health education department nor our ob/gyn department provided *any* counseling or information about birth control or abortion services. The medical department had interpreted our federal funding regulations as prohibiting not only the performance of abortions on-site, but prohibiting the dissemination of information which might lead to, or help patients to obtain an abortion.

Needless to say, as a feminist and as an activist, I was horrified. When I found out that pregnant women who inquired about abortions were given only a name of a white, English speaking ob/gyn doctor and sent out alone, this practice seemed morally and ethically neglectful. One of the nurse-midwives agreed with me and suggested that I could serve as an interpreter/advocate for pregnant women who needed to have abortions or at least wanted to discuss the option with the English-speaking ob/gyn doctor. The only catch was that I would have to do it on my own time, that I could not claim any affiliation with the health center, and that I could not suggest follow-up care at the health center.

Not fully knowing the nature of what I was volunteering for, I agreed to interpret and advocate for Cantonese-speaking pregnant women at their appointments with the obstetrician. It turned out that over the course of three years I interpreted during at least a hundred abortions for Asian immigrant women who spoke no English. After the first few abortions, the obstetrician realized how essential it was to have an interpreter present, and began to require that all non-English speaking women have an interpreter during the abortion procedure.

As a middle-class, educated, bi-lingual Asian-American woman, I was aware of the importance of having the choice to have an abortion, and the necessity to fight for the right to choose for myself, but I had been unaware of how the right to have an abortion is also a right to survival in this country if you are a poor, uneducated, non-English speaking immigrant.

The women I interpreted for were for the most part not young. Nor were they single. They ranged in age from 25–45, with a majority in their late twenties and early thirties. Almost all of the women were married and had two or more children. Some had as many as five or six children. They needed to have an abortion because they had been unlucky enough to have gotten pregnant after arriving in this country. Their families were barely surviving on the low wages that many new immigrant workers earned as restaurant workers, garment factory workers, or as domestic help.

Almost all of the women worked full-time: the ones who had young children left them with older retired family members or did piecework at home; those with older children worked in the factories or hotels. Without fail, each woman would tell me that each needed to have an abortion because her family could not afford another mouth to feed, that they could not afford to lose her salary contribution, not even for a few months, to care for an infant. In some ways, one could not even say that these women were *choosing* to have abortions. The choice had already been made for them and it was a choice of basic survival for the members of their family unit.

Kai was one of the women for whom I interpreted. A 35-year old mother of four children, ages 2 to 7, she and her husband emigrated to the U.S. from Vietnam. They had no choice in their immigration either, they were refugees whose village had been destroyed, and felt fortunate to escape with their lives and all four of their children. Life in the U.S. was difficult, but they were scraping by, living with another family in a small apartment where their entire family slept in one room. Their hope was that their children would receive an education and make it in American society: They lived with the day-to-day hope of that deferred dream for the next generation.

When Kai found out that she was pregnant she felt desperate. Because she and her husband love children and live for their children, they wanted desperately to keep the child, this one that would be born in America and be an American citizen from birth. Yet they sadly realized that they could not afford another child, they could not survive on just one salary, they could not feed another one. Their commitment was to the children they already had, and keeping their family together.

When I accompanied Kai to her abortion, she was saddened, but resigned to what she had to do. The $300 that she brought to the clinic represented almost a month of wages for her, she had borrowed the money from family and friends. She would pay it back, she said, by working weekends for the next ten weeks. Her major regret was that she would not be able to buy any new clothes for her children this year because of this unexpected expense.

Kai spoke very little English. She did not understand why she had to go to a white American doctor for her abortion, instead of receiving services from her Asian doctor at the health center. She had no understanding, really, of reproductive rights issues, of *Roe v. Wade,* or why there were demonstrators waving pictures of fetuses and yelling at her as we entered the clinic. Mercifully, she did not understand the questions they shouted at her in English, and she did not ask me what they said, remarking only that they (the protestors) seemed very angry at someone. She felt sure, I think, that they were not angry at *her.* She had done nothing to provoke anyone's anger. She was merely trying to survive in this country under this country's rules.

It is a moral crime and an injustice that Kai could not receive counseling in her language by her doctors at the Asian neighborhood health center. It is an injustice that she had to borrow $300 to pay for her own abortion, because her Medicaid benefits did not pay for it. It is a grave injustice that she had to have me, a stranger, interpreting for her during her abortion because her own doctor could not perform the procedure at her clinic. Again, it was not a matter of choice for her to abort her pregnancy, but a matter of basic survival.

Kai will probably never attend a march or rally for choice. She will not sign any petitions. She might not even vote. But it is for her and the countless thousands of immigrant women like her that we need to continue the struggle for reproductive rights. Within the Asian American community, the immigrant women who are most affected by the lack of access to abortions have the least power. They do not speak English, they do not demand equal access to health care; their needs are easily overlooked.

Thus it is up to us who are bi-lingual, those of us who can speak English and who can speak to these issues, to do so. We need to insure that the issue of reproductive rights is an essential one in the Asian American political agenda. It is not a woman's issue; it is a community issue.

We must speak for the Kais, for their children, for their right to survive as a family. We must, as activists, make the connection between the issues of oppression based upon gender, race, national origin, sexual orientation, class or language. We can, and must lead the Asian American community to recognize the importance of the essential issue of reproductive rights for the community's survival.

Discovering That You Are Infertile
One Woman's Experience

by Naomi Pfeffer and Anne Woollett

'Well,' they said, 'If you're going to have a baby you should start soon. You're not getting any younger you know.'

It took me a long time to decide that I wanted a child. I started thinking about it perhaps four years ago. I thought about it. I talked to other women. I listened to other women, to mothers and women without children. I found out about childcare arrangements. I thought about my job and how having a child would influence my work. I talked to the man I live with about a child and the effects one might have on our lives and on our relationship. We thought about when would be a good time to have a child. A baby born in the spring or summer would fit in well with my work.

April 1978   I put my cap away.

August 1978   We go away on holiday.

September 1978   Period two days late and breasts feel very tender. Are they normally tender just before my period? I become much more sensitive to my body. I live inside myself, my centre of gravity seems to be somewhere inside my uterus. I feel full, preoccupied, pleased that I might be pregnant. Then blood. No pregnancy. No baby. Perhaps next month.

1 October 1978   Perhaps next month.

30 October 1978   Blood, period, perhaps next month.

Why am I not getting pregnant? I begin to ask questions about my body. I've been taking my temperature for several months and I know that I am ovulating. How long does it normally take to get pregnant? I had assumed it could take up to six months and we have been trying for that time.

People reassure me. Sometimes it takes a long time. I'm given advice, information, details about how other people did it. I'm consoled, never mind, you'll make it. I'm trying to grapple with the idea that perhaps I won't make it. That idea creeps into my mind and I want to discuss it. But it's not something people are willing to

Reprinted with permission from *The Experience of Infertility* by Naomi Pfeffer and Anne Woollett, Virago Press, London, England, 1983.

discuss. A friend gets pregnant. It didn't take her long. She gets bigger. We discuss home confinements, epidurals, baby clothes, names. The world seems to be full of pregnant women, in the streets, holding babies, pushing prams. I'm surrounded by pregnant women. I read up on conception and find that infertility tests begin with an examination of the man's sperm.

4 December 1978   A friend, a nurse, arranges for us to have a sperm test. She provides us with the plastic container in its brown box, complete with instructions. 'The sperm must be produced by masturbation and reach the laboratory within four hours.' So today, the alarm goes off, I get up and make a cup of tea while Paul produces the specimen (how quickly we get into the jargon) and we rush it up the road to my friend who takes it to the lab at work.

The same friend arranges for us to attend the fertility clinic attached to the birth control clinic where she works. This is the same clinic I have been attending for years. The appointment is for after Christmas. We hope that I get pregnant over Christmas so that we won't need to keep the appointment. In the meantime I read up on infertility investigations.

5 January 1979   Our first appointment. Our medical histories are taken and we are both examined physically. We are seen by the consultant separately and then he talks to us together. 'Yes, everything seems quite normal.' But we are told that the sperm count is not terribly high, about thirty million, but high enough. Conception is possible with lowish sperm counts. Paul is told to give up his Y-fronts and to wear boxer shorts. This may increase the sperm count. I'm told that from my charts it looks as though I'm ovulating. I'm to continue taking my temperature but I must use the official forms rather than bits of graph paper. We are told that the next step is the post-coital test for which I am to make an appointment after my next period has started.

In some ways I feel quite elated after this first appointment. Our problem has been recognized and something is being done for us. We go straight to Marks and Spencers to buy the shorts, feeling that things had started, that we had acquired some kind of control.

7 January 1979   Period begins. I start my new temperature chart on the official form and ring the hospital to make an appointment for a post-coital test. At this particular clinic post-coital tests are done only on Tuesday mornings.

16 January 1979   First post-coital test. Attending the clinic is a depressing experience. A feeling of heaviness comes over me as I get closer to the clinic. I walk past the Family Planning clinic which I've attended for many years, down the corridor, past the row of women waiting their turn, to the door marked 'Subfertility Clinic'. I am redefined. I am now infertile, a woman with a problem. I announce my arrival, show my card with my new number on it. When I was fertile I was E34976. Now that I'm infertile, I'm 4032.

I wait my turn, sitting by myself, getting lower and lower, trying to fight the tears, and the feelings of self-pity. It is my turn. I go in and undress, and lie on the couch as instructed. A doctor, a woman, not the one we'd seen previously, inserts a speculum and then using a long rubber tube takes a sample of my cervical mucus. While I get dressed, she goes over to the other side of the room to examine my mucus under a microscope. 'I don't like this at all,' she says. I panic. What have I done? Hadn't we followed the instructions? I feel like a naughty child and I start to cry. The tears stream down my face and they continue unabated for the rest of my appointment. It transpires that what she doesn't like is the way the sperm and the mucus are getting along. There aren't enough sperm and they don't seem to be surviving well in my mucus. The doctor suggests that Paul sprays his testicles twice a day with cold water using one of those small indoor plant sprays. I don't know how he will take to that. If this spraying is such a good idea, then why hadn't the doctor suggested it on our first visit when Paul was there. That way at least he'd have been told directly. Now it was up to me to tell him. I'd brought his sperm to them and now I was taking bad news back home. My mucus didn't meet with her approval either. It was described on my form as 'tacky.' I am given a prescription for some oestrogen tablets and told to come back next month for another post-coital test.

There are lots of questions I want to ask. But the tears are still streaming down my face and I feel far too distraught to ask them. So I fumble around for my coat and bag and leave, while the doctor talks into her tape recorder about my case.

The force of my feelings and my inability to cope with them surprises me. During the next month I think a great deal about what happened and how I might cope in the future.

8 February 1979   Period starts. I feel depressed. I've got to go back to the clinic again. I ring up to make an appointment. Tuesdays arrive this cycle either on day eight or day fifteen of my cycle. The nurse thinks that I should go for the earlier date. I take the oestrogen tablets in preparation for the appointment.

16 February 1979   Second post-coital test. This time I feel much stronger. When the doctor appears and calls my name my stomach turns over. I force it back into place and I follow her into the room. I try to attend very carefully to what she does. Both the procedure and the doctor are the same as before. 'Well, the mucus is better, but the sperm are much the same as before.' She writes this down. I confess that Paul has refused to spray his testicles. The doctor points out that this is quite important as the present emphasis is to get the balance right between my mucus and his sperm. She suggests that I douche myself with a solution of bicarbonate of soda just before intercourse during the fertile days. This may make my vagina more conducive to the survival of Paul's sperm. I tell her that I am puzzled. Should I take the oestrogen tablets for my mucus to coincide with my clinic appointments or around ovulation as the two days are a week apart? Am I undergoing tests or treatment? The doctor says that, as she has an empty slot the following Tuesday, I can return for another post-coital so she can check the sperm and the mucus nearer to ovulation and after I have been using the douche. When she'd got the mucus right, she'd move on to other things, in particular, on to checking whether my tubes were unblocked. I'm even more puzzled. Why bother spending months checking my mucus if we then discover that my tubes are blocked? Why is only one test done at a time? I suppose I'd expected the investigation to be more like an MOT, where your car is given a whole range of tests at one go, and so you know what's wrong fairly rapidly. I tell the doctor how depressed I feel and that I'm worried that the investigations might destroy the relationship into which the child would be born. But any talk of emotions is brushed aside with the comment that some people feel quite heartened to think that treatment is being offered and that some couples are willing to go to the most elaborate extremes to have a child. I take the hint and shut up.

The clinic nurse shows me how to use the douche. She is much more cheery and tries to boost me by telling me how successful the doctor is at getting women pregnant.

The visit is over. The tension gradually subsides. At least this time I didn't collapse and I did manage to ask most of my questions. Now I have to go home with my collection of bits and pieces, instructions and information and prepare us for the next appointment.

I tell Paul what the doctor said about spraying his testicles, that he must do it to improve motility. He refuses. She made it clear that this is the next step in the pro-

ceedings. If he's not prepared to do it then we've reached a stalemate. Will they be prepared to continue the investigations if he's uncooperative? I feel cross with him. I've had to go to the clinic, go through the humiliating examinations and face the doctor and now he won't do his share. Later he agrees to try. Our sex life has taken on new elements: Paul sprays his balls twice a day; just before intercourse I pop into the bathroom and spend five minutes with the douche.

20 February 1979   Third post-coital test. My mucus has remained good and the number of sperm has improved but their motility is still low. The doctor suggests I continue with the current regime of tablets, douche and spray. We now move on to other things: an X-ray of my Fallopian tubes. A form is filled in and I am told to ring the hospital's X-ray department when my next period arrives to make an appointment for day ten of my cycle. Via me, Paul is advised to see the semenologist, in six weeks' time.

26 February 1979   My fertile period is over and so the rites can cease for a while till next month. I can stop gently bullying Paul for a while, and relax. My friend has had her baby and I go to see it. I feel very thrilled for her. But after the excitement wears off I feel very sad. If I'd got pregnant quickly my baby would be almost due. I realize how much I'd stopped thinking about children and babies. My goal now is conception.

13 March 1979   Period starts. It is about three days late and I'd just begun to feel really hopeful. Yesterday I'd had moments of discomfort; and stomach ache but I'd ignored them till I saw the blood today. I feel weak and tearful. All the strength I thought I'd acquired just seems to have drained away. The discomfort serves as a reminder of my failure. So much for menstruation as a sign of femininity and the potential for motherhood. All it signifies to me is my failure.

21 March 1979   To the hospital for an HSG (X-ray of my Fallopian tubes). I had rung them beforehand to find out how long it would take and whether I would feel well enough to go back to work afterwards. I'm nervous so I've asked my friend to come with me. In the X-ray department, I undress completely and put all my clothes into a brown paper bag and cover myself with one of the hospital's green overalls. I'm shown into the X-ray room and told to sit on a long table with the equipment all around and above it. The doctor and radiographer, both men, arrive. My friend who is a nurse and works at the hospital is allowed to stay. The doctor tells me what will happen. I can watch the proceedings on a TV screen. The insertion of the dye may feel like a period pain. He inserts the dye. It is very painful and the pain gets worse. I pass out. When I come round the doctor shows me the X-ray. I try to concentrate but I can't take in what he's saying. The left tube appears to be clear but my right tube has gone into spasm. I fear there may never be a baby. I am put on to a trolley and wheeled into the corridor where I lie in pain for some time. Gradually the pain begins to ease and I am able to get dressed. My friend finds a taxi, takes me home and puts me to bed with a hot water bottle. By the evening I feel better.

The investigations seem to be taking so long. A day does not pass by without my thinking about them and my infertility. I feel I must go on with the tests, and all the pain they cause, because I need to know if I will ever be able to have a child, and because there is no other source of help for my infertility to which I can turn.

19 April 1979 Appointment with the semenologist. The appointment is at 3:40 and so at 2:30 Paul produced his sperm sample into the little plastic container provided by the hospital. We then rush to the hospital, clutching the sample. The doctor looks at some of the sperm under the microscope and sends the rest to the lab for a sperm count. He thinks that the count and motility are increased, but this will be confirmed by the laboratory test. That's it basically. It's heartening to think there's an improvement. The spraying must be working so Paul will continue with that. We fix another appointment with the semenologist to see whether the improvement has continued.

26 April 1979 I'm in contact with children who have German measles so I have a blood test to see whether I am immune to German measles.

1 May 1979 Appointment at the Infertility Clinic to hear the results of the HSG. The doctor tells me the same tale as I was told in the X-ray room. One tube is definitely clear but the result is uncertain for the other. This tube may be blocked or it might be a technical problem which made it difficult for the dye to get through. My agony is reduced to a technical hitch. If I have not conceived in three months time, I am to have a laparoscopy. This will involve a short stay in hospital. The waiting list is long so she will put my name down on it the next time I see her, in three months' time. Why do I have to wait till then? Why can't my name be put on the list now? Meanwhile, the doctor suggests I try an insemination cap. I am to return to the clinic in two days to be

shown how to use it. I am to use it in the middle of the cycle and then come back to her with it in place to see if I am using it properly and to check whether it's improving the sperms' chances of survival. This calls for another new element in our sex life: I take the oestrogen tablets around the time of ovulation; then before 'intercourse' I am to spend five minutes in the bathroom with the douche after which I am to insert the insemination cap. Meanwhile Paul is masturbating into the hospital's plastic pot, with his balls nicely chilled twice daily. I am then to syringe his sperm into the tube which dangles from the insemination cap. What erotic excitement!

3 May 1979 To the hospital to learn how to use the insemination cap. It's a bit fiddly and difficult to get into place.

19 May 1979 Fourth post-coital but with insemination cap in place. The results seem exactly the same as for the test we had in February. Mucus is okay, sperm count is fine, but the motility is low. The insemination cap has not made any difference so the doctor doesn't think it's worth continuing with it. I indicate my relief at that news. We are sent back to the semenologist for a sperm-mucus compatibility test to see if my mucus is killing off Paul's sperm.

12 June 1979 Second appointment with semenologist. We go together with a sperm sample in a little container. The semenologist examines it and pronounces his approval of both the count and motility. We then persuade him to do the sperm-mucus compatibility test which is the reason we came to see him. He seems happy with the result. I feel totally confused. One doctor says the motility is low. Another says it's fine. One tells me to douche. The other says that it's unnecessary. How am I to deal with this lack of consensus? The only response seems to be to feel cheerful. At least someone has said we're okay. I may not be pregnant but any ray of hope is to be appreciated.

1 August 1979 Appointment to see the consultant. He puts me on the list for a laparoscopy. I should have an appointment within six months. It's just a question of waiting. And because my cycle is somewhat irregular, he decides to put me on an ovulation-inducing drug. I am given one month's supply. Am I to go back each month for another prescription?

10 August 1979 We go on holiday. It is the second holiday we've taken since trying to get pregnant. Events like this remind me of time passing.

On our return from holiday, we decide to buy a house. We had been thinking for some time about where we were going to live. The flat was a bit small for a child. We had no garden and getting up and down the stairs would not have been easy with a small baby. When we first started trying to conceive, our plan had been to move out soon after the baby's birth. But as the months passed with no signs of a baby, we put this plan to one side. It just did not seem possible to make any decisions about where we were to live until we knew more about whether we were likely to have a baby. How much longer could we go on delaying plans and decisions because one day there might be a baby? So many aspects of our lives were becoming controlled by our frustrated attempts to become parents. We went ahead and bought a house. It is a large house—one that gives us plenty of space for us and for children.

15 October 1979 Receive a card from the hospital telling me to fix the date for a laparoscopy in the second half of my next cycle.

7 November 1979 I enter hospital for a laparoscopy the next afternoon. I have never been in hospital before and I am nervous. It is much jollier than I expected. There are thirteen women in the ward and we quickly discover who we all are. Six of us are to be operated on tomorrow. As we have all come in for different operations, we each have different anxieties, but we are great company for one another, laughing and joking together. I realize how much more pleasant it is to have other women around you while going through tests, someone to share the worries and the news. There are two other women on the ward who are having problems in conceiving. It is good to talk to them, to compare notes about the tests and their reactions to infertility. I realize that I did not know anyone who had been through the investigations or who is infertile. While a lot of women have been very kind and listened to my tales of tests and anguish, none of them have been through similar experiences or had similar feelings. This is the first time I've spoken to women who've said, 'Yes, they did that to me,' or 'Yes, I felt like that too'. I see that I've become very careful about the people I get close to. I am only relating to close friends and relatives who know about my problem. I feel very vulnerable about stepping outside of that group into the great beyond of those who don't know.

9 November 1979 The doctor comes round to tell us all about the results of our operations. He confirms that I am ovulating and that my tubes, ovaries and uterus are okay. So I am proclaimed fit and told to report back to the consultant in six weeks' time.

I feel now as though I have done the rounds. A series of tests have revealed little that was seriously wrong with either Paul or myself. I imagined that at the next appointment I would be told that medical science had its way with us and that now it was up to us to go away, to forget the hassles we had been through, to relax and conceive.

24 November 1979 Period starts.

22 December 1979 It comes again. Another Christmas passes and I'm not pregnant.

4 January 1980 Appointment to see the consultant. This is the anniversary of my first appointment at the Infertility Clinic. The consultant looks at the report of my laparoscopy, reads all the notes and thinks. He suggests a blood test to check my progesterone level. This is fixed for 13 January as it has to be done late in my cycle. I'm also told to make an appointment for a fifth post-coital test to check that everything is still all right there.

13 January 1980 I have a blood sample taken for the progesterone test. I delay making the appointment for a fifth post-coital.

2 February 1980 We move into our new house. It requires a lot of work which the builders have started. At first I organize the rooms around a child. One room is to be a nursery. Later that same room becomes my study.

8 May 1980 I make an appointment for a post-coital test.

20 May 1980 Fifth post-coital test. I have taken the oestrogen tablets for the first time in months. I had a hard job finding them. When I arrive at the clinic, I feel that I need to explain to the nurse why I hadn't come sooner. The doctor, however, either doesn't notice or doesn't ask about the long delay. So I say nothing. I take off my knickers. I get on the couch. It's all so familiar, I feel positively light-headed. A seasoned traveller. The result seems the same as ever. The sperm are there but not very motile. So one year and a half later, we are back where we started. The results of the progesterone test are not too encouraging. I am ovulating, but not very well. To improve my ovulation, I am given Clomid as well as oestrogen tablets. I am also sent off to have a blood test to see if I have antibodies to sperm.

I go away feeling fed-up. It seems as if a whole lot of new problems are coming up—low progesterone, sperm antibodies. If they are significant factors, why were they not looked for months ago. I've had a number of blood tests. Why hadn't these been included then? And I don't understand why the motility of Paul's sperm is a matter of differing opinions. If it is a significant factor in our infertility then why put me on Clomid? We seem to be going round in circles, backtracking over ground that I thought we'd explored. I feel like a detective story, with the doctors sniffing round for clues, going over old suspects as well as checking on esoteric possibilities. Nevertheless, I take the Clomid in my next cycle as well as the oestrogen tablets.

20 June 1980 I feel very ill.

4 July 1980 Period starts. It's fourteen days since I felt so ill so I feel sure that it was due to the Clomid. Why hadn't I been warned of the side-effects? Also, how am I to know if the Clomid is working? No tests are being done to check on my defective progesterone levels. I am depressed.

31 July 1980 Period starts. I've run out of oestrogen tablets. The hospital no longer dispenses them so I have to go to my GP. Since I moved, I haven't found a new GP. By the time I work all this out, it's too late to take Clomid this cycle.

This summer is the third since we tried to conceive. We work on the house. I find out through my friend at the hospital that the test showed that I do not have antibodies to Paul's sperm. It dawns on me that I have decided by default not to continue with the Clomid or with the tests. I feel uneasy about giving up the investigations. Having gone so far it seems silly not to continue. The next test might be the one which gives me the answer. They might just find something that works for me. But then I remember what the tests were like and I feel loathe to go back to the hospital and try again.

I feel the key question is changing slowly. I am asking less why am I infertile. Instead, I am thinking about how to reconcile myself with my infertility, and how I can move forward into a life in which children may not have a central role. I feel that this is where I prefer to put my energies, and that continuing with the tests will interfere with this. So I do not go back to the clinic.

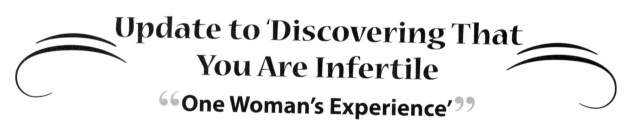

Update to 'Discovering That You Are Infertile

"One Woman's Experience"

by Anne Woollett and Naomi Pfeffer

"**D**iscovering that You Are Infertile" was written some years ago. In a number of respects infertility, its impact for women and their reproductive decisions have changed considerably. Treatment options have increased, so that while many of the investigations mentioned in the diary continue to be part of their experiences, the decisions infertile men and women now commonly make include those which relate to the new techniques of assisted conception, such as IVF and surrogacy (Franklin, 1997).

These techniques are complex and expensive and so are available only to those who can afford the costs of treatment and associated drugs, travel and accommodation. In the US, they are rarely covered by health insurance (King and Meyer, 1997). These techniques of assisted conception are seen as producing new treatment opportunities (and career and financial opportunities for medical and scientific staff). The first child conceived by IVF was born in 1978 and we have, as yet, little evidence about the effects and long term psychological development of children conceived in these ways (McMahon and Ungerer, 1998). There is now more recognition of the emotional and psychological costs of treatment for women and partners (Sandelowski, 1993), but there is still little discussion about and research into the effects on the long term health of women of IVF and especially drugs employed to stimulate ovulation (Klein and Rowland, 1989).

The techniques of assisted conception have opened up treatment options and fertility choices for some women and their partners. However, these treatments still have a low success rate, and hence result in the birth of a live baby for only a minority of infertile couples (Pfeffer, 1993). For many women, therefore, coming to terms with infertility and finding ways of relating to others as infertile/ childless women remains as much of an issue as when this diary was written (Franklin, 1997).

The new techniques of assisted conception have changed considerably the ways in which infertility is represented and written about. There is now more discussion of infertility in professional accounts (medical, bioethical, psychological, sociological) and in popular culture. These suggest that while women may find it easier to recognize infertility as a 'problem', many women still experience a strong desire to become mothers and motherhood is viewed as a central, 'normal', and expected role for women (Phoenix, Woollett and Lloyd, 1991; Morrell, 1994). As Mardy Ireland (1993) argues, within this framework infertility continues to be construed as a shock, a loss, and as a lack of reproductive choice. A different representation of infertile women (but not infertile men) has emerged in the debates about the ethics of the new techniques. Women prepared to become mothers by means of these unconventional routes are said to threaten the stability of the nuclear family. Yet, ironically, it is the nuclear family which many of these women are seeking to create.

However, in spite of greater public recognition, there are still many unasked and unanswered questions about infertility. One concerns the diversity of women's lives, their social and economic situations, and ideas about motherhood and mothering (Collins, 1994) hence how they view infertility and being childless (Woollett, 1996). Another concerns the ways in which women's ideas about infertility change over time. The diary points to some ways in which one woman's thinking about infertility changed over time: from concerns about being a mother and how motherhood would fit into her life and relationships, to concerns about her body, why she was not getting pregnant, what 'the problem' was, and about the swings in her mood during her menstrual cycle. Since writing that diary, Anne's thinking about infertility has changed considerably. She decided to step off what felt like an emotionally draining and isolating roundabout of infertility investigations. This meant thinking of herself not so much as 'infertile' as 'childless' (Woollett, 1996). Professionally she became more interested in how women resist representations of themselves as 'mad', 'sad' or 'desperate'. Drawing on research such as that of Morell (1994) and Ireland (1993) she began to think about the identities, activities and ways in which childless women relate to others, and to disentangle what it means to be a 'mother' and to be a 'woman'.

REFERENCES

Collins, P. H. (1994) Shifting The Centre: Race, Class and Feminist Theorizing about Motherhood. In E. N. Glenn, G. Chang, and L. R. Forcey (eds) Mothering: Ideology, Experience and Agency. New York. Routledge.

Franklin, S. (1997) Embodied Progress: A Cultural Account of Assisted Conception. London. Routledge.

Ireland, M. S. (1993) Reconceiving Women: Separating Motherhood from Female Identity. New York. The Guilford Press.

King, L. and Meyer, M. M. (1997) The politics of reproductive benefits: US insurance cover of contraceptive and infertility treatments. Gender and Society, 11, 3–30.

McMahon, C. A. and Ungerer, J. A. (1998) Parenting and infant development following conception by reproductive technology. In C. A. Niven and A. Walker (eds) Current Issues in Infancy and Parenthood. Oxford. Butterworth Heinemann.

Morell, C. (1994) Unwomanly Conduct: The Challenge of Intentional Childlessness. London. Routledge.

Pfeffer, N. (1993) The Stork and The Syringe: A Political History of Reproductive Medicine. Cambridge. Polity.

Phoenix, A., Woollett, A. and Lloyd, E. (eds) (1991) Motherhood: Meanings, Practices and Ideologies. London. Sage.

Sandelowski, M. (1993). With Child In Mind: Studies of the Personal Encounter with Infertility. Philadelphia. University of Pennsylvania Press.

Woollett, A. (1996) Infertility: From 'Inside/Out' to 'Outside/In.' Feminism Psychology, 6, 74–78.

"The Colour of Loss"

by Elizabeth Ruth

I know something of missed opportunities, stunted and miswoven cells, futures undone. I know relentless, raging optimisms, babies not yet wished into being. Yes, I know all too well these trying, trying times that so many face, because, for almost five years, my partner and I have watched younger women with buoyant, hopeful energy push double strollers through fertility clinic doors and flip the pages of glossy magazines while we wait for blood draws and ultrasounds, and a successful pregnancy. We've celebrated friends and family as they gave birth to their second children, while we experienced miscarriages and continued trying for our first. They are everywhere, the fresh, naive faces. They don't look haggard, weary, defeated. How I've hated them for their blind privilege, and especially for their optimism. Not being able to bear a child will break your heart, but hopes raised and dashed, month after month, will bleed all joy from living.

Flesh of my flesh,
Blood of my blood, who will I be without you?
Who would I have been if you'd stayed?

More than a decade ago, at the University of Toronto, I concentrated my graduate studies in the areas of women's reproductive and mental health, researched the history of various cutting-edge drug treatments and pored over recommendations made by the Royal Commission on New Reproductive and Genetic Technologies. I wrote papers on the ethics of anonymous sperm and egg donation and argued, from a feminist point of view, for regulation. I investigated potential long-term side effects of pills like Clomid, both on women who took them and on the offspring produced. I learned that very little research had been done in the area. There are still no long-term studies—which is why doctors are able to tell me, with great assurance, that there's no link between the fertility drugs so many of us now swallow and inject, and the cancers all women fear.

So, when I decided, on my 35th birthday, to have a child, I wasn't naive about the history of the Western medical model responding to women's health. I knew other drugs deemed safe had later been proven dangerous and taken off the market. I believed our bodies, es-

pecially our hormonal bodies, are routinely perceived and treated as defective, or in need of control and management, and that childbirth itself has become a state of emergency in North America, with sections and early interventions fast becoming the norm. I also expected that, because I was old, reproductively speaking, and because my partner was a woman, I'd find myself in a doctor's office. At the very least, I had a sperm access issue. What I couldn't envision then, and swore I'd never do, was to give over control of my body. Of course, that's exactly what I ended up doing.

I conceived without drugs on our first attempt, using frozen sperm from an anonymous donor. I was optimistic, with no visible stress in my life. I knew it wouldn't be long before I was pregnant. The procedure was a simple, non-invasive insemination (sperm deposited in the vagina, at the opening of the cervix) and not, as it would be for years subsequently, the highly touted, invasive and more expensive intrauterine insemination (IUI). I was certain I was pregnant within hours, though people told me it wasn't possible to know so soon. Two weeks later, the pregnancy was confirmed with a blood test. Unfortunately, I miscarried at eight weeks. Despite reassurances to the contrary, I wondered whether my hypothyroidism was a factor.

My thyroid, previously regulated with a prescription medication, had spiralled out of control the instant I became pregnant. I searched for answers online, in bookstores, and at the library as to why this might've been and how to prevent it happening again. Though I can never know for certain what caused that miscarriage, the doctor doubted it was my thyroid. (Another fertility doctor was adamant that it probably *had* been the cause.) What exactly is the relationship between hypothyroidism and miscarriage? I still don't know. I was told to grieve and move on, because miscarriage is common, and an easy first conception is a sign of fertility. I tried for another year without success.

That first doctor had many lesbian patients, yet her receptionist routinely asked for my husband's health card number. The doctor, a walking infomercial who answered our questions before we had a chance to finish asking them, never spent more than 10 minutes with us.

She told us she wouldn't speak with my partner, as I was the patient, so that's how it was for almost a year—both of us at morning ultrasounds and blood draws (10 days per month), both at scheduled information appointments, and both at two monthly inseminations—but only one of us invisible. I only understood this to be discriminatory after a straight couple I knew began seeing the same doctor and, though they were also using anonymous donor sperm, the male partner in that couple was actively involved in conversations and decision-making. That first doctor was a gynecologist and reproductive specialist, but not an endocrinologist, which is the reason I finally left. I was willing to put up with discrimination because I wasn't sure the situation would be different at another clinic, and finding a new doctor meant being on a waiting list for months.

My second fertility doctor, reportedly one of the best in city, was extensively renovating his multimillion-dollar Toronto clinic while we dug ourselves deeper into debt, stepped through plaster dust and suffered summers in the attic waiting room without air conditioning. My thousand dollars a month for two inseminations wouldn't buy the leather chair I sat on while I waited. This specialist recommended fertility drugs to us on my first visit because of my age, he said, and because I was a lesbian, not because any tests showed me to be infertile. "Fertility drugs will save time," he told us. He looked me up and down. "My guess is you'll respond best to injectables."

His plan was the usual—to have me inject gonadotropins and carpet-bomb my uterus with multiple eggs each cycle, thereby increasing the likelihood of conception with our frozen sperm. I wondered whether his reputation and his stats (and, perhaps, research funding) were dependent upon high success rates. Would I lower those success rates if I took too long to conceive? If I took a natural amount of time to conceive? So I said no to fertility drugs. For two more long years I said no.

Definitions of infertility have shifted dramatically in the past decade, arguably since drugs have been more accessible. Whereas once a woman would be referred to a specialist after two years of unsuccessfully trying with her male partner, now many doctors refer after one year, and increasingly after only six months of consecutive attempts. Why? Have women's bodies changed? Or, perhaps our eggs are a new cash crop?

Refusing drugs was not easy. I secretly wondered if I shouldn't give in, if I wasn't denying myself because of ideological principles, and overinflating the potential unknown risks. It was harder to say no when most of my friends, many of them lesbian, had said yes without similar reservations. My partner was becoming anxious about our mounting debt. It was also a monthly struggle with the doctor, who, at each insemination, while he sat with his face between my legs and deposited sperm into my uterus, would remind me of how low my chances of conceiving were without drugs. He'd remind me of how relatively ineffective frozen sperm was, compared with fresh, despite the fact that we had no access to fresh—he said he would not treat us with a known donor. Once, he told me that my becoming pregnant a second time would be the equivalent of winning the lottery.

We tried to find a doctor who would allow us to do IUIs with a known donor's sperm, but we were plainly told, by three, that they weren't legally permitted to have a known donor's sperm washed and inseminated in me. Was it, as one specialist claimed, because if I contracted an STI the clinic would be liable? Or, as another claimed, because they worried our known donor might be gay, and gay men are not allowed to donate sperm? The third specialist told me bluntly that it was because I was a lesbian and he wasn't comfortable. We pointed out that heterosexual patients could also contract STIs and that I should have an equal right to the donor of my choice. Those conversations left my partner and I frustrated, confused and angry, but apparently powerless, since doctors' hands were tied because of legislation. For anyone to be willing to wash and inseminate me with this better, fresher sperm of a known donor, they'd have to be convinced I was in a sexual relationship with that donor. In other words, I'd have to lie. I've known of lesbian couples who've done this, at great cost to their personal relationships, their anxiety levels and their senses of self.

Interestingly, The Assisted Human Reproduction Act and Health Canada are clear that no distinction is to be made between semen from a known donor (including men who are not a patient's sexual partner) and semen from anonymous donors. Further, according to Dr. Leah Steele and Dr. H Strotmann, in their May 2006 article for *Canadian Family Physician*, doctors shouldn't use fresh semen in their offices, and "any physician planning therapeutic donor insemination is legally obliged to use semen that's been cryo preserved for six months." What we initially thought was denial of service to us because of paternalistic legal barriers was, in fact, something more subtle and insidious. Our doctors weren't willing to bend the rules for us, but they'd routinely do so for their heterosexual clients, and hide their bias behind a misleading veil of legality. Meanwhile, we continued to purchase frozen sperm each month, at a cost of $500 per sample, plus $150 to the specialist and a $50 delivery charge to the cryobank.

Watching friends conceive through the same clinics and with the same doctors was difficult, but knowing that some had an edge on us because they were straight was infuriating. We learned that by not doing IVF (in vitro fertilization) we were moving through a second-rate treatment model. Had I wanted to, IVF was not something we could have afforded. The costs are staggering, ranging from between $6,000 to $10,000 per cycle. But the odds are better. With IVF, a woman receives gonadotropin injections to stimulate her follicles to produce multiple eggs, which are then surgically retrieved from her body, fertilized in a laboratory and reimplanted in that same woman—or in another woman. Our friends used their relatives' cashed-in RRSPs to do IVF with frozen sperm and, afterwards, told us the attention they received as IVF patients was better than when just doing intrauterine inseminations; they'd felt like a priority. We never felt like anyone's priority. In fact, we felt like a nuisance. Those friends conceived on their second IVF attempt, after years of doing exactly what we were still stuck doing.

One of the many mornings when I was at the clinic to cycle monitor (psycho monitor I call it), I met a patient who was also a GP. We broke the unwritten code of silence in the waiting room and exchanged details about our treatments. By this point, I'd grown desperate and had, against my own judgment, agreed to three cycles of fertility drugs. My partner's insurance plan offered partial coverage for a limited number of attempts. The GP-patient told me that in her private practice, because of anecdotal research, she advises women not to take gonadotropin injections or Clomid, even for the recommended period of less than six months, but that she had been taking Clomid for eight months and was terrified of what she was doing to her body. Most of all, she was fearful of what she was willing to do. Like me, she'd entered the process with a bottom line that was continually shifting, so she no longer trusted herself to be able to stop. Would she end up with ovarian cancer in 10 years? Would it all be worth it if she conceived?

Clomiphene, a.k.a. Clomid and Serophene, is a relatively inexpensive drug (about $60 per month) taken from day four or five of your cycle through to near ovulation. It's meant to promote regular ovulation. Injectable gonadotropins are synthetic or (originally) distilled from menopausal women's urine, and they push your body to mature multiple eggs. They cost us, on average, $1,700 per month. Both classes of drugs have common side effects compromising the likelihood of conception: thinning of cervical fluids in the case of Clomid and ovarian hyperstimulation syndrome in the case of injectables.

Why are there no long-term studies? Who benefits from not tracking such information? Would being fully informed stop women from taking fertility drugs? Probably

not. But it would guide our decision-making, as more of us might decide against drug treatments altogether, or disentangle from them earlier. Knowing the actual risks to long-term health would, at the very least, make our consent to treatment legitimate. What does yes really mean in a system where saying no feels impossible?

There are known short-term side effects of the drugs (read the packaging). On injectables, I experienced headaches, skin rashes, racing heart, chest pain, numbness in my toes, anxiety and ovaries hyperstimulated to many times their natural size, making it dangerous for me to do physical activity (like riding my bicycle), lest they rupture. Each week, after a pregnancy test would come back negative and my hormones would drop from artificially high to normal again, acute depression would set in. I skipped months of cycles after each round, waiting for my ovaries to return to normal size. On Clomid, I had a steady migraine, weight gain and anxiety. All of this is routine. And the treatments are unsuccessful just as often as they are successful. Even with technology, the doctor is, at best, guessing what dose of drug might produce the desired number of follicles in a given woman.

Women who take fertility drugs feel like we're making decisions largely in the dark, leaping at fate, hoping to land softly, babe in arms. We feel uniquely unsuccessful when the drugs don't bring the desired result, and overexposed as we share personal information with myriad professionals who use terms like "poor egg quality," "incompetent uterus" and the present-day scarlet letters, "advanced maternal age." We make martyrs of ourselves, but no one notices because the very cultural definition of motherhood is tangled up in martyrdom.

After all, fertility has always been a life-and-death matter—women have been dying for their children for centuries, or been expected to do so. In some parts of the world, women still die in childbirth or because of related complications. But in wealthy nations, like ours, where "choice" can be purchased on VISA or paid for in cash, the notion of dying to be mom isn't something doctors or patients are willing to acknowledge.

We can't, because admitting that we are, in effect, guinea pigs in a field with less than scientific diagnostics and treatments, and maybe putting our lives in danger, might mean stopping. Doctors can't admit to undocumented risks without calling their purpose into question.

After another year and thousands of dollars more debt, I walked away from the second doctor, too. I came to see that the stress and treatment were anathema to my well-being. It became clear one day, as my partner and I waited almost half an hour for the doctor to perform the intrauterine insemination. Our sperm was thawed and we began to panic—after 20 minutes of being exposed to air, frozen sperm begins to die. My partner found the doctor and asked him to please hurry. He waved her off. Again, five minutes later, my partner went to fetch him. This time he came with the nurse, but was obviously angry. He ignored my greeting and briskly told me to lie down. I was already undressed, my feet in the stirrups. As he threaded the catheter through my cervix, an unpleasant, if not painful experience, he raised his voice and reprimanded us: "You people think you know best. If I tell you the sperm is fine, it's fine. This'll never work if you don't trust me. You ask too many questions. Next month I'll prepare cue cards and hold them up so I don't have to keep repeating myself!"

I should've kicked him in the face, but of course I was desperate to get the sperm into me as quickly as possible. When it was done, I stared at the beige ceiling I'd stared at for so long and knew I couldn't harm myself in this way any longer. Perhaps it was my lack of belief in the drugs and biomedical model, but I would never succeed at a clinic. Leaving was scary, too, for it meant being willing to risk the unknown, believing more in my intuition about my body being healthy than in "expert" advice. Possibly, it meant never becoming pregnant.

I sought out an experienced traditional Chinese doctor who performed acupuncture on me several times a month and reminded me at each hour-and-a-half-long visit that there was nothing fundamentally wrong with me, that I was still young enough, healthy enough and deserving enough to become somebody's mother. Each time I left her office, I felt more at home in my own skin, like myself again. More than three years of paying doctors to tell me I was defective, show me statistics on rates of pregnancy for my age group and push drugs as the only hope for success produced no pregnancy. Three months within a traditional Chinese model, and I was pregnant for the second time.

North American boomers who saw the advantages of the pill were weaned on the nebulous concept of freedom of reproductive choice, and that limited perspective has filtered down to us, their children. You'd think that having greater reproductive options (assuming you can pay) would be easy. But, of course, it's not.

Having choice means bearing the burden of responsibility for our yeses and our nos and that's a heavy burden to carry when the outcome is so profound. In fact, it requires superhuman strength to say no to drugs, or exploratory surgery, or even daily ultrasounds, without feeling you're potentially closing off your option of having children, without doubting yourself and being judged as treatment-resistant. So what if there are side effects? Our second doctor told me that if I wanted to be a mother

badly enough, I'd take a second mortgage on our home and increase my odds by doing IVF. I was a new homeowner who barely scraped into the market. (We ultimately sold the house.) What about women who don't own homes or can't even pay their rent? What about people who can't imagine doing what we did: maxing out credit cards and overdraft? What about the more logical option of having both my partner and I try, thereby doubling our monthly egg pool and odds, without drugs?

I met a young lesbian couple on Pride Day one year, pushing a double stroller. They'd tried to conceive without technology, when, perhaps out of frustration, or because of the financial stress of paying for anonymous sperm, they'd agreed to gonadotropin injections. "Whatever happens to you," one mother told me, "don't do it." Their twins had been born premature and one baby needed several emergency surgeries because part of his intestine was sitting outside his body. He'd have lingering health problems as an adult. The couple was drained, emotionally and financially, and had spent their first year as new parents separate, each caring for one baby, both worried for their gravely ill newborn.

"But it worked out," I said. "I mean those are the chances all parents take, right?"

"Maybe," said the other mother. "We love the boys. . . ." She spoke with the honesty of a stranger and the raw wisdom that only comes from surviving a trauma. "But we wouldn't do it again if we knew." I smiled politely, envying them their children, despite their arduous journey. I dismissed it as an unusual case, exceptional, and made their situation rare. But stress on prospective parents' relationships, massive debt, pregnancy and delivery complications, high rates of multiple births, lack of social support for same-sex parents trying to have a family, lack of support in general for all people within the fertility machine—these are the norm.

A free-choice analysis of the present-day fertility model is short-sighted and stops at easy, non-threatening questions about over-medication and equal access. It doesn't extend to an institutional critique of the industry, which would look at how profit-driven motives might be guiding or defining (in)fertility. There have been other feminist critiques of the new reproductive and genetic technologies before now, but what's new today is that lesbians and single women of all sexual orientations—those who need access to safe sperm, women who are not by any objective measure infertile—are using these technologies in great numbers. As a result, more women in Canada are being referred to fertility clinics and undergoing drug treatments when they've failed to conceive fast enough. We ought to be challenging how the fertility machine participates in—or prevents—the creation of non-traditional families, and we must demand an honest examination of the relationship between pharmaceuticals and fertility doctors. We might even want to talk about the social construction of infertility itself. What frightens me most isn't the actual drug treatments, though they may indeed prove dangerous, but the culture of uncritical thinking and denial in which we willingly submit to them.

Yet, women are not passive, ignorant, dupes. We're simply pressed to keep trying under our doctor's hand by our own deep desires, pushed on by those who want us to be happy, or by a medically driven society that believes in taking drugs the way other people, in less secular times, believed in God. We're just plain frightened at the prospect of never being anyone's mother. Above all, we become disembodied through the process of being poked and prodded, and treated under the assumption that we're defective. We stop believing in our bodies, and eventually stop listening to them and begin following directions. Sometimes we forget that our bodies, that *we*, are there at all. After a time, we see with blinkers, registering only the minority of women for whom the drugs work, holding them up as beacons of hope. We search out those in clinics and on television with whom we might identify, and all the while we're tempted, painfully tempted, by that candy dangling before us—a baby, a healthy baby, our baby.

It is possible to have too many choices.

I know the denial, minimization and myopia that are required when on a mission to conceive. My partner and I know the repeated disappointment, anguish over what life might look like if pregnancy never happens, and how these fears cause you to begin to welcome the drugs despite risks, to welcome anything that brings a baby, so hey—even twins begin to sound great. After all, two babies are better than none. We patients grow into this mindset because we must contort, intellectually and emotionally, to fit a model of treatment that's inflexible, pathologically negative and refuses to see us in holistic terms. Should we hear only the stories of those who succeed? Are *they* not perhaps the most biased, the least likely to question their treatments? Don't they just need to get on with the business of parenting?

I don't wish to demonize individual women who opt for fertility drugs, or argue against the existence of actual infertility, but I want to remind us all that, in our brave new world, the interpretation of infertility and the need for fertility treatments is always political. We must think critically. Are the drugs dangerous? Are there alternatives, such as acupuncture, that could be explored first? Are queers in a uniquely vulnerable position within the system, and if so, how is that being played out? But most significantly, is the model for treatment itself gen-

erating or exacerbating the very problem it purports to rectify? Can infertility or subfertility be an iatrogenic disorder? In other words, can childlessness result from the inherent stress and negativity of Western infertility treatments?

I conceived the first time when I'd not yet become embroiled in the medicalization of my own fertility, when I was making the decisions, had no debt or stress, and before I came to believe my body was too old and defective to bear a child. I conceived the second time only when I disentangled from the medical model, took back control of my body and the process, and was therefore able to trust both. Finding an encouraging, supportive, traditional Chinese doctor who engaged with my questions and fears made a difference. She didn't dismiss me as irrational or uneducated, because the model she works from teaches that there *is* a connection between the mind and body, and that the body is something to be respected, not only corrected. Instead of statistics and percentages, she offered stories of success. She also told me openly that I might never become, or stay, pregnant.

Despite all that's happened, I still find myself alone by the blue-note light of the Alberta moon listening to k.d. lang sing "Helpless" while I write this and miscarry, for a second time. My thyroid, once more shocked into overdrive by pregnancy, failed to respond to aggressive treatment. Again, doctors tell me it probably had nothing to do with the miscarriage, but this time I don't believe them. I think of the incredible debt I've accumulated paying for something I once swallowed for free, the books I might've written all these years, the trips my partner and I might've taken had every penny not been going towards buying sperm and paying for inseminations. I think of other undiscovered dreams, secondary for so long, that never had a chance to materialize. And I think it's time to stop. Yes, there comes a final, terrible point of clarity for any woman trying in vain to have a child, where the choice that matters most becomes the choice between the life before us now and the life we so desperately imagine creating.

Again, I wonder what sins I've committed to draw such bad luck my way? I see my future laid out before me, and that future may be too quiet, free of obligation. Perhaps there'll be no new love. I'm alone tonight but I'm only one of many childless mothers watching cradles rock empty, seemingly banished for no reason from the club that is motherhood. This is all I know: Reproductive technology offers queers options we couldn't have dreamed decades ago, but we're not the intended or desired recipients. And, there is no meant to be. Babies are random gifts from gods, as well as measured reproductive science, bestowed upon the undeserving just as often (though it seems to me now, more often) as the deserving. Trying to become pregnant for a long time is like swimming in molasses, a dark curse that grows more powerful with each negative pregnancy test, each appointment, invasive procedure or injection. So while a tiny beam of light fades from me tonight, a clawing, crystalline sense of frustration also fades. The struggling and trying and hoping and waiting feels as though it's finally coming to an end. Even the world beyond my keyboard seems to be slipping away. In some senses it's a

relief. Yet, tomorrow I'll pick up the phone and call my partner, who's at home in Toronto, naive and still hopeful, and I'll read her this story I don't want to tell. My story. Our story. And I'll ask:

If red is the colour of love, what colour is loss? A year after this article was written, my partner and I are thrilled to be expecting a baby in December. Ignoring the advice of three fertility doctors, my partner conceived without fertility drugs.

Grade A
"The Market
for a Yale Woman's Eggs"

by Jessica Cohen

When a Yale undergraduate explored becoming an egg donor for a wealthy couple willing to pay top dollar to the right candidate, she didn't realize how unsettling the process of candidacy would prove to be

Early in the spring of last year a classified ad ran for two weeks in the *Yale Daily News*: "EGG DONOR NEEDED." The couple that placed the ad was picky, and for that reason was offering $25,000 for an egg from the right donor.

As a child I had a book called *"Where Did I Come From?"* It offered a full biological explanation, in cartoons, to answer those awkward questions that curious tots ask. But the book is now out of date. Replacing it is, for example, *Mommy, Did I Grow in Your Tummy?: Where Some Babies Come From,* which explains the myriad ways that children of the twenty-first century may have entered their families, including egg donation, surrogacy, in vitro fertilization, and adoption. When conception doesn't occur in the natural way, it becomes very complicated. Once all possible parties have been accounted for—egg donor, sperm donor, surrogate mother, paying couple—as many as five people can be involved in conceiving and carrying a child. No wonder a new book is necessary.

The would-be parents' decision to advertise in the *News*—and to offer a five-figure compensation—immediately suggested that they were in the market for an egg of

a certain rarefied type. Beyond their desire for an Ivy League donor, they wanted a young woman over five feet five, of Jewish heritage, athletic, with minimum combined SAT score of 1500, and attractive. I was curious—and I fit all the criteria except the SAT score. So I e-mailed Michelle and David (not their real names) and asked for more information about the process and how much the SAT minimum really meant to them. Then I waited for a reply.

Donating an egg is neither simple nor painless. Following an intensive screening and selection process the donor endures a few weeks of invasive medical procedures. First the donor and the woman who will carry the child must coordinate their menstrual cycles. Typically the donor and the recipient take birth-control pills, followed by shots of a synthetic hormone such as Lupron; the combination suppresses ovulation and puts their cycles in sync. After altering her cycle the donor must enhance her egg supply with fertility drugs in the same way an infertile woman does when trying to conceive. Shots of a fertility hormone are administered for seven to eleven days, to stimulate the production of an abnormally large number of egg-containing follicles. During this time the donor must have her blood tested every other day so that doctors can monitor her hormone levels, and she must come in for periodic ultrasounds. Thirty-six hours before retrieval day a shot of hCG, human chorionic gonadotropin, is administered to prepare the eggs for release, so that they will be ready for harvest.

The actual retrieval is done while the donor is under anesthesia. The tool is a needle, and the product, on average, is ten to twenty eggs. Doctors take that many because "not all eggs will be good," according to Surrogate Mothers Online, an informational Web site designed and maintained by experienced egg donors and surrogate mothers, "Some will be immature and some overripe."

Lisa, one of the hosts on Surrogate Mothers Online and an experienced egg donor, described the process as a "rewarding" experience. When she explained that once in a while something can go wrong, I braced myself for the fine print. On very rare occasions, she wrote, hyperstimulation of the ovaries can occur, and the donor must be hospitalized until the ovaries return to normal. In even rarer cases the ovaries rupture, resulting in permanent infertility or possibly even death. "I must stress that this is very rare," Lisa assured prospective donors. "I had two very wonderful experiences . . . The second [time] I stayed awake to help the doctor count how many eggs he retrieved."

David responded to my e-mail a few hours after I'd sent it. He told me nothing about himself, and only briefly alluded to the many questions I had asked about the egg-donation process. He spent the bulk of the e-mail describing a cartoon, and then requested photos of me. The cartoon was a scene with a "couple that is just getting married, he a nerd and she a beauty," he wrote. "They are kvelling about how wonderful their offspring will be with his brains and her looks." He went on to describe the punch line: the next panel showed a nerdy-looking baby thinking empty thoughts. The following paragraph was more direct. David let me know that he and his wife were flexible on most criteria but that Michelle was "a real Nazi" about "donor looks and donor health history."

This seemed to be a commentary of some sort on the couple's situation and how plans might go awry, but the message was impossible to pin down. I thanked him for the e-mail, asked where to send my pictures, and repeated by original questions about egg donation and their criteria.

In a subsequent e-mail David promised to return my photos, so I sent him dorm-room pictures, the kind that every college student has lying around. Now they assumed a new level of importance. I would soon learn what this anonymous couple, somewhere in the United States, thought about my genetic material as displayed in these photographs.

Infertility is not a modern problem, but has created a modern industry. Ten percent of American couples are infertile, and many seek treatment from the $2-billion-a-year infertility industry. The approximately 370 fertility clinics across the United States help prospective parents to sift through their options. I sympathize with women who cannot use their own eggs to have children. The discovery must be a sober awakening for those who have always dreamed of raising a family. When would-be parents face this problem, however, their options depend greatly on their income. All over the world most women who can't have children must simply accept the fact and adopt, or find other roles in society. But especially here in the United States wealth can enable such couples to have a child of their own and to determine how closely that child will resemble the one they might have had—or the one they dream of having.

The Web site of Egg Donation, Inc., a program based in California, contains a database listing approximately 300 potential donors. In order to access the list interested parties must call the company and request the user ID and the password for the month. Once I'd given the receptionist my name and address, she told me the password: "colorful." I hung up and entered the database. Potential parents can search for a variety of features, narrowing the pool as much as they like according to ethnic origin, religion of birth, state of residence, hair color, eye color, height, and weight. I typed in the physical and religious characteristics that Michelle and David were looking for and found four potential donors. None of them had a college degree.

The standard compensation for donating an egg to Egg Donation is $3,500 to $5,000, and additional funds are offered to donors who have advanced degrees or are of Asian, African-American, or Jewish descent. Couples searching for an egg at Egg Donation can be picky, but not as picky as couples advertising in the *Yale Daily News*. Should couples be able to pay a premium on an open market for their idea of the perfect egg? Maybe a modern-day Social Darwinist would say yes. Modern success is measured largely in financial terms, so why shouldn't the most successful couples, eager to pay more, have access to the most expensive eggs? Of course, as David illustrated in his first e-mail, input does not always translate perfectly into output—the donor's desirable characteristics may never actually be manifested in the child.

If couples choose not to find their eggs through an agency, they must do so independently. An Internet search turned up a few sites like Surrogate Mothers Online, where would-be donors and parents can post classified ads. More than 500 classifieds were posted on the site: a whole marketplace, an eBay for genetic material.

"Hi! My name is Kimberly," one of the ads read. "I am 24 years old, 5'11" with blonde hair and green eyes. I previously donated eggs and the couple was blessed with BIG twin boys! The doctor told me I have perky ovaries! . . . The doctor told me I had the most perfect eggs he had ever seen." The Web site provided links to photographs of Kimberly and an e-mail address. Would-be parents on the site offered "competitive" rates, generally from $5,000 to $10,000 for donors who fit their specifications.

About a week after I sent my pictures to David and Michelle, I received a third e-mail: "Got the pictures. You look perfect. I can't say this with any authority. That is my wife's department." I thought back to the first e-mail, where he'd written, "She's been known to disregard a young woman based on cheekbones, hair, nose, you name it." He then shifted the focus. "My department is the SAT scores. Can you tell me more about your academic performance? What are you taking at Yale? What high school did you attend?"

The whole thing seemed like a joke. I dutifully answered his questions, explaining that I was from a no-name high school in the Midwest, I couldn't do math or science, and my academic performance was, well, average; I couldn't help feeling a bit disconcerted by his particular interest in my SAT score.

Michelle and David now had my educational data as well as my photos. They were examining my credentials and trying to imagine their child. If I was accepted, a harvest of my eggs would be fertilized by the semen of the author of the disturbing e-mails I had received. A few embryos would be implanted; the remaining, if there were any, would be frozen; and then I would be out of the picture forever.

The modern embryo has been frozen, stolen, aborted, researched, and delivered weeks early, along with five or six instant siblings. The summer of 2001 was full of embryo news, and the first big story was President Bush's deliberation on stem-cell research. The embryos available for genetic research include those frozen by fertility clinics for later use by couples attempting in vitro fertilization.

Embryos took the spotlight again when Helen Beasley, a surrogate mother from Shrewsbury, England, decided to sue a San Francisco couple for parental rights to the twin fetuses she was carrying. The couple and Beasley had agreed that they would pay her $20,000 to carry one child created from a donated egg and the father's sperm. The agreement also called for selective reduction—the abortion of any additional embryos. Beasley claimed that there had been a verbal agreement that such reduction would occur by the twelfth week. The problem arose when Beasley, who had discovered she was carrying twins, was told to abort one, but the arrangements for the reduction weren't made until the thirteenth week. Fearing for her own health and objecting to the abortion of such a highly developed fetus, she refused. At that time she was suing for the right to put the babies up for adoption. She was also seeking the remainder of the financial compensation specified in the contract. The couple did not want the children, and yet had the rights to the genetic material; Beasley was simply a vessel. The case is only one of a multitude invited by modern fertility processes. On August 15, 2001, *The New York Times* reported that the New Jersey Supreme Court had upheld a woman's rights to the embryos that she and her ex-husband had created and frozen six years before. A strange case for child-custody lawyers.

Nearly ten years ago, at the University of California at Irvine's Center for Reproductive Health, doctors took the leftover frozen embryos from previous clients and gave them without consent to other couples and to research centers. Discovery of the scam resulted in more than thirty prosecutions: a group of children had biological parents who hadn't consented to their existence and active parents who had been given stolen goods. Who can say whether throwing the embryos away would have been any better?

Even if Michelle and David liked my data, I knew I'd have a long way to go before becoming an actual donor. The application on Egg Donation's Web site is twelve pages long—longer than Yale's entrance application. The first two pages cover the basics: appearance, name, address, age, and other mundane details. After that I was asked if I'd ever filed for bankruptcy or ever had counseling, if I drank, what my goals in life were, what two of my favorite books were, what my paternal grandfather's height and weight were, what hobbies I had, what kind of relationship I would want to have with the parents and child, and so forth. A few fill-in-the-blanks were thrown in at the end: "I feel strongly about __. I am sorry I did not __. In ten years I want to be __." Not even my closest friends knew all these things about me. If Egg Donation, offering about a fifth what Michelle and David were offering, wanted all this information, what might Michelle and David want?

Michelle and David were certainly trying hard. On one classified-ad site I came across a request that was strangely familiar: "Loving family seeks exceptional egg donor with 1500 SAT, great looks, good family health history, Jewish heritage and athletic. Height 5'4"–5'9", Age 18–29. We will pay EXTREMELY well and will take care of all expenses. Hope to hear from you." The e-mail address was David and Michelle's familiar AOL account. Theirs was the most demanding classified on the site, but also the only one that offered to pay "EX-TREMELY well."

I kept dreaming about all the things I could do with $25,000. I had gone into the correspondence on a whim. But soon, despite David's casual tone and the optimistic attitude of all the classifieds and information I read, I realized that this process was something I didn't want to be a part of. I understand the desire for a child who will resemble and fit in with the family. But once a couple starts choosing a few characteristics, shooting for perfection is too easy—especially if they can afford it. The money might have changed my life for a while, but it would have led to the creation of a child encumbered with too many expectations.

After I'd brooded about these matters, I received the shortest e-mail of the correspondence. The verdict on my pictures was in: "I showed the pictures to [my wife] this AM. Personally, I think you look great. She said ho-hum."

David said he might reconsider, and that he was going to keep one of my pictures. That was it. No good-bye, no thanks for my willingness to be, in effect, the biological mother of their child. I guess I didn't fit their design; my genes weren't the right material for their *chef d'oeuvre*. So I was rejected as a donor. I keep imagining the day when David and Michelle's child asks where he or she came from. David will describe how hard they both worked on the whole thing, how many pictures they looked at, and how much money they spent. The child will turn to them and say, "Ho-hum."

"Father Knows Baste"

by Tamar Abrams

"**D**A" was Hannah's first and favorite sound. When she said it, at nine months old in the pediatrician's waiting room, another mother told me she must be thinking of her daddy. Frankly, I doubt it. Hannah's daddy has a number, not a name. He is 741, an anonymous Los Angeles law student who, in 1992, was paid about $50 to produce the sperm that helped create my beautiful daughter.

I arrived at the decision to become a single mother by choice fairly quickly and without a great deal of angst. My twenties and early thirties were spent focusing on my career, and I prided myself on my independence. A series of boyfriends came and went, leading my father to declare, when I was only 28, that I was too picky with men and would likely never find one I could settle down with.

He was smarter than I thought. One day I woke up and realized that I was 34 and alone. I lived in a condo that I owned in Washington, D.C. I had no houseplants, no pets, nothing that required constant care and nurturing. My job for Planned Parenthood entailed nonstop travel. It was exciting and exhilarating, but I was painfully aware of my abandoned childhood plan to marry and have at least four children.

Weeks of soul-searching led me to the conclusion that I could live without regret if I never was a wife, but I couldn't be happy if I were never a mother. And that's how, in August of 1991, I ended up in the offices of Dr. Belinda Marascalco, then with Columbia Hospital for women in Washington, D.C. She offered no lectures on the inadequacies of single motherhood, no judgments. I realized as she spoke how little I knew of the reproductive process and how much I would have to learn. I also realized how committed I was to bearing and mothering a child.

I left the clinic with a list of donors from California Cryobank—a Los Angeles-based sperm bank—and a sense of tremendous anticipation. California Cryobank was one of two choices available to me; the other sperm bank was in Louisiana. I stuck with the California Cryobank because it has an excellent reputation for screening donors, and because I liked the idea of my East Coast baby-to-be having some California blood in her or him.

In those days, you would begin by looking through a donor book of more than 100 listings. Each listing gave the basics—blood type, ethnic origin, hair color and texture, height and weight, educational background, general medical history, family history, and some essay questions. Once you found a few you were interested in, you could request a more comprehensive 20-page listing that included medical histories going back several generations. Today the process has been brought into the 21st century: you can peruse the lists online, listen to an audio tape of the donor, ask Cryobank staff to find a donor who looks like a family member and even ask a panel to rank the attractiveness of your chosen donor.

But back then, it was just me and a few pieces of paper. I combed the listings, not sure what I was looking for. Finally, I decided that I wanted a donor who could give the child all the physical characteristics I could not—long legs, a tall, slender body, and good eyesight. I screened out anyone with a relative who had died of cancer or other possibly genetic diseases. I didn't care about religion or hair color, although I admit that SAT scores were marginally significant. One donor was eliminated because he listed tuna casserole as his favorite food.

Over the course of the next six months, I attempted to conceive twice a month with four different donors. I did this with the help of Dr. Marascalco, a basal body thermometer and monthly parties. The parties involved my girlfriends—and the occasional red-faced male—who would listen as I read donor information sheets, and vote on their choice for Donor of the Month. Fueled by wine and the upbeat mood of the parties, we had a blast and I always ended up with a donor.

Once I had determined that ovulation had just occurred, I would race over to the clinic for my insemination. The room was clinical, the procedure involved a syringe and about ten seconds of the doctor's time—but it was a magical time for me. I would lie in the room for half an hour afterwards, visualizing conception. It was peaceful and invariably hopeful.

In December, however, my most fertile day happened to fall on the day of Columbia Hospital's holiday party. As a result, the doctor wasn't going to be available to do the insemination. Instead, arrangements were made for me to visit the clinic between 8:30 and 9 that morning to pick up a vial of my donor's sperm to take home. The woman working in the andrology lab showed me where the specimens were stored and even put a tiny bit of the sperm under a microscope so I could see all the activity. She seemed happy to have the company and cheerfully explained the do-it-yourself insemination. I should have paid more attention.

Placing the vial in my bra to keep it warm, I pushed the D.C. speed limit and reached my Capitol Hill home in record time. In the kitchen, I successfully emptied the vial into the syringe I was given—but I lost most of the sperm

down the sink while trying to tap out any air bubbles. Literally, $150 and a lot of hope went down the drain.

Like failing to become pregnant in more conventional ways, failing with donor insemination is accompanied by disappointment and fear that infertility is one's lot in life. At the time, one of my friends commented that the process of trying to conceive was no fun my way. I disputed that. While it wasn't soft lights and Luther Vandross ballads, there was an element of fun and anticipation. Several times during the six months it took me to conceive, I would spend an hour or more in the fertility center's conference room poring over lists of donors. Sometimes nurses on their lunch breaks would help me. It was a bit like shopping—starting out with a good idea of what you want, but finding yourself distracted by the unexpected.

The search ended and the journey began on March 8, 1992—my father's birthday—when my darling daughter was conceived. By this time I had begun to lose patience with the process. To speed things along, I had been taking Clomid, a fertility drug. And in the end, the donor wasn't even chosen by my friends or by me—he was selected by a nurse at the fertility center who said he was a "sure thing." And so I was matched with 741. The Prince of Fertility. Mr. Super Sperm Count. He was no slouch in other departments, either: green eyes, curly red hair, a law student who scored 1400 on his SATs.

His essay-question responses looked like he was in a hurry to complete the form, but he did manage to write about himself: "fun-loving, active, patient, athletic, enjoy life, hard-working, driven, intellectually stimulated." He's someone I think I would have liked knowing.

On March 8, 741's defrosted sperm registered a 4-plus on the fertility scale—the highest possible rating. Those little guys were ready to party. Thanks to Clomid, I had produced five eggs just waiting for the music to begin.

By this time, I had spent about $2,000 of my own money, six months of my life and a great deal of time praying. But in the end, it was worth every penny and every second. On December 1, 1992 at 3:38 a.m., the lovely Hannah Lily Abrams was born into the world by emergency C-section. Through the haze of drugs and fatigue, I looked at this tiny, puffy child and knew with certainty that this was the greatest accomplishment of my life. The lack of a husband in no way diminished the pride and joy of that moment. We were now a family.

More than nine years later, I can still recall the moment of my daughter's birth. Sometimes she's even willing to cuddle in my arms while I tell her the story of her conception and birth, though more often she rolls her eyes and runs off to ride her bike. This story is hers now, not mine. But I protect it and cherish it until she's ready to take it from me.

Hannah's life is indistinguishable from that of her friends. She's a Brownie knocking on doors to sell Girl Scout cookies. She's a child who has had the same best friend since they met in Montessori school seven years ago. Our house is filled with light and toys and books and videos and, increasingly, CDs of Britney, the Backstreet Boys, and a few Broadway musicals. For the Brownies' Father/Daughter Snowflake Ball in February, Hannah donned a burgundy velvet-and-taffeta gown, and beamed as her beloved grandpa slid a corsage onto her wrist.

My child has grown up knowing the story of how she came to be. I began telling her about it while she was still too young to understand, because I wanted the words to be familiar to her. We never talked about "father" or "daddy," but about "donor" instead. This led to the time, when she was two, that she told her friends that her father was a "doughnut." But familiarity doesn't ease the way entirely.

When Hannah was three and we were driving somewhere in the dark, she suddenly announced that she knew who her father really was. Despite the frequency with which she stated eternal truths while riding in the back seat of the car, I was shocked. As calmly as I could, I asked who her father really was and she replied, "Peter Pan." It made sense to me—eternally youthful, wearing green tights, able to fly, and of course living somewhere far away in Never Neverland. She stuck with that story for several months.

At four, she began crying in the tub and exclaimed fiercely, "But I want a daddy! All my friends have one!" It was a moment I had anticipated and dreaded in equal measure. I said the first thing that came to mind, "I'm so sorry you don't have a daddy. I know you want one." Later, following the advice of a much wiser single mom, I asked Hannah what she would do if she had a Daddy. She thought long and hard and said, "I don't know. Just stuff."

That conversation has evolved over the years. It was punctuated by her request at the age of six to know more about the donor. In a nod toward full disclosure, I sat beside her on the couch and handed her the long form donor profile. She was excited to read it and full of self-discovery. "He likes math like I do!" she yelled. "He likes music too." She read each page carefully and then announced she wanted to call him . . . immediately.

We both wept as I explained that we couldn't call him, that he was deliberately anonymous to us. But she could write him a letter that would be delivered to him when she turned 18. That was perhaps the hardest day of this journey for me. She was so bitterly disappointed and all the positive reasons that I chose to have her on my own could not, in that moment, compensate for the obvious negatives. I cried long after she stopped.

To Hannah's credit, though, she has handled her difference with grace and dignity. When her preschool friends would ask why there was no daddy in her home, she would state in a matter-of-fact-tone, "I don't have one. I have a mommy and a grandma and a grandpa and an aunt and a cat." To those who challenged her by pointing out that everyone has a father, she would reply, "I don't."

As she gets older, Hannah seems almost bored by the fact that she is the child of a single mother. Perhaps it's because she's puzzling through larger issues—why she has to practice the violin so often, why boys can excite and repel her at the same moment, why she can't be a famous actress right now. I am relieved that embarrassment and shame are not the legacies of her unusual beginning.

Hannah tells her story to friends patiently and slowly. She starts by saying, "My mom really wanted to have a baby but didn't have a husband. So she found a nice doctor who got her some seeds . . ." I've received a few calls from parents who were not happy that their children were getting this explanation, but it seems reasonable to me.

More unexpected have been the reactions of men to my method of having a child. I didn't begin dating again until about a year ago. It wasn't from lack of interest, but more a lack of time and energy. As Hannah gets older, she needs my time a little less. And I've found myself missing the intimacy and love of a mature relationship. Most of the men I've gone out with have been divorced fathers. So their assumption is universally that Hannah's dad is lurking somewhere in the background.

I never introduce the topic of donor insemination, but am always ready to discuss it if a man asks where Hannah's father is or when I got my divorce. I assumed initially that men would be disgusted by the idea of donor insemination or threatened by my assertiveness in having a child on my own. I was wrong. They have all been fascinated and even delighted. It means that there is no bitter divorce in my past, no shared custody, no complications. And they seem to admire my courage in doing it my way. One man said he was attracted to me because I never chose the conventional path to getting what I wanted in life. Who knew?

But there are complications with having a child through donor insemination that are unique to the process. For example, during the time that Hannah's donor was actively "giving," he may have fathered several dozen children. We have met and formed a relationship with one of them. Sam is three years younger than Hannah and lives in New York. I told her about him when she was five and she has since claimed him as a "half-brother." They exchange letters and photos that show some remarkable physical similarities. Last summer we spent the day together in Manhattan. The two children walked down Ninth Avenue, huddled together under an umbrella and talking in conspiratorial terms. We have claimed Sam and his mom as family.

So many of Hannah's friends are adopted or the children of divorced parents or even the children of single mothers by choice that it barely registers anymore that she has only one parent. I'm not naïve enough to expect that it won't become a much bigger issue for Hannah as she cruises into adolescence. I'm as prepared as I can be. And I'm entirely comfortable with the choices I made that led to her birth. No regrets.

I'm also very careful to speak respectfully of marriage when Hannah is around. I have never wanted her to infer that I became a single mom because of some deep-seated animosity toward men or marriage. She announced when she was four or five, "Mom, I hope you don't mind, but I think I'd like to be married before I have children." I was thrilled!

I still hold out hope that one day I may marry. But I'm not desperate for it. I've discovered that my journey is a circuitous one, filled with happiness and drama. When I first came to the conclusion that being a mother was important, I was realistic enough to know that there would be moments of great loneliness and loss and rigorous hurdles. I know now that I had no idea of the depth and breadth of the joy I would experience with my child, or the sometimes haunting loneliness. I had only the slightest inkling of the patience, fortitude, and humor that parenting requires—even when one is part of a couple. The requirements are doubled when you're doing it on your own.

Sometimes I meet women who are considering becoming single mothers by choice. I tell them there are no bad motivations for making that choice. Reproduction is inherently a selfish act, no matter how many people are involved. But those single mothers who seem to be the happiest have thought through the ramifications of their decision. They look beyond the sweet-smelling infant to the cranky toddler and the demanding fifth grader and the impossible adolescent. They understand that dating will be difficult and saving money is a pipe dream. They know that in achieving one dream, they are also letting go of another.

It has been ten years since I made one of the most important decisions of my life. The theme of these years has been gratitude. Every night since my lovely daughter was born, I wash up and get ready for bed. Just before I turn out the light, I quietly sneak into Hannah's room. Standing by her bed, I rearrange any covers she's kicked off. I check that the room temperature is appropriate. I bend low over her sleeping body and ensure that I see her chest rising and falling. I kiss my fingertip and lay it on her cheek. And then I thank God, Columbia Hospital for Women, the donor, my parents, and the universe for giving to me the child I once dreamed of. Only then can I sleep.

WORKSHEET—CHAPTER 10

Reproductive Justice, Fertility, and Infertility

1. **Contraceptive choice.** Three situations are described below. Make a list of all possible contraceptives that are options in the situations and briefly comment on the pros and cons for each contraceptive option. Be sure to include the widest range of contraceptives, and specifically comment on how the choice of contraception will be affected by or impact on protection against sexually transmitted infections.

Linda and Larry

Linda and Larry are 22. They have been married for one year and want a family someday. Linda feels it is very important that she does not get pregnant while she is supporting both of them because Larry (a scientist) is unemployed. Because of their shared religious beliefs, Larry is not happy about Linda using birth control and both feel very strongly against abortion. Linda does not feel comfortable about her own body and does not have much understanding of the menstrual cycle or the process of fertilization.

Betsy and Bob

Betsy and Bob are 22. They have been married for one year and want a family someday, but want to wait until they are older. Betsy and Bob are working towards equality in their relationship, so both are working half time and going to school half time. Although Betsy and Bob hope to prevent an unplanned pregnancy, they have the money and views that would permit abortion as a back-up to failed contraception. Both Betsy and Bob feel comfortable with their bodies and both recently got A's in a women's health course.

Susie and Sam

Susie and Sam are 22. Susie identifies as bisexual. She is mostly sexually active with women, but once in awhile she is still sexually active with her old boyfriend, Sam. Both Susie and Sam are responsible and well informed about sexual relationships. Both Susie and Sam feel strongly that their infrequent sexual encounters should not result in a pregnancy.

2. **Contraceptive mentality.** "Next Target: Birth Control" warns us about organizations trying to restrict access to some or many forms of birth control. Identify ways that you think the availability of modern contraceptives and the "contraceptive mentality" (the assumption that people are able to prevent pregnancies if they choose) have been related to the improving status of women in our society. How would your life be different if contraceptives were no longer available?

3. **Activism.** "Confessions of a Radical Feminist" describes one woman's activism to pressure the FDA to make the morning-after pill available. List forms of activism that you or people you know have done. If you haven't yet done activism, can you think of a form of activism you might be involved in, and the issues you care enough about to "fight for"?

4. **Reproductive justice.** We get used to thinking about ways a woman can control her fertility to limit the number of children she has. As reflected in the articles in this chapter, true reproductive freedom means being able to have as many or few children as desired. List a wide range of factors that would enable women to have as *many* children as they wish. (What would be the factors to enable men to have as many children as they wish?)

5. Identify ways in which reproductive justice and being valued by society are closely related issues. List specific examples of how a lack of reproductive justice is related to racism, homophobia, ageism, poverty, and other issues.

6. After reading "The Bad Baby Blues," identify some of the ramifications of routine prenatal genetic testing.

   a. Give a reason why a woman might choose to have prenatal genetic testing even if she knew she would not choose to have an abortion.

   b. What could our society do to make it easier for women, couples, and families to choose to have a child with a disability?

7. After reading "Contraceptive Jelly on Toast and Other Unintended Consequences of Sexuality Education," identify an example of folklore (joke, belief, or urban legend) you have heard about sexuality, contraception, or pregnancy. What is the point of the story and how does it reflect social values, misinformation, or people's anxieties?

CHILDBIRTH *and* LACTATION

Many of the problems in the relationship between women and the healthcare system are clearly visible in the area of childbearing. The paternalism, the reliance on technology, and the performance of unnecessary surgery characterizing certain aspects of the medical profession in the U.S. are all evident. On a positive note, this is also an area in which organized movements by women have had a major impact in improving care for women and their babies, and increasing their options. It is an area of continuing struggle, in which apparent victories may actually weaken the movement for new fundamental changes. For example, in some cases, "birthing centers" are merely hospital rooms decorated to look like home, with families allowed to be present for the birth, sometimes with a nurse midwife attending, but with the same medical interventions and little change in who makes the decisions. Such birthing centers may "pacify" some women who would otherwise push for major changes.

As with organizing around any women's health issue, activists for increasing choices for women during pregnancy and childbirth have had to take into account the ways different women benefit from different choices. For example, many women have worked to increase the availability of home births, but this is certainly not an option for homeless women or women in other difficult living situations. Similarly, many women have worked to have husbands, boyfriends, and female partners present during childbirth, but this now routine practice may not be appropriate for a battered woman because battering often begins or escalates during pregnancy. A theme of this book is the importance of activism to make information and choices available so women can empower themselves and have more control over the decisions affecting their health. However, as we read critiques of the medicalization of childbirth, we must remember that at a time when childbirth killed many women, women wanted more, not less, intervention, and medicalization, along with improved hygiene and a better understanding of disease processes, played an important role in making childbirth safer for women and their babies. Also, it is important to remember that consumer lawsuits are a driving force pushing healthcare providers to "over" medicalize childbirth, and that not all women are equally enthusiastic about being involved in medical decision-making.

Doris Haire's classic paper, The Cultural Warping of Childbirth," was first published in the *International Childbirth Education Association News* in 1972. It was a very influential article, comparing the experience and outcomes of childbirth in the U.S. with that of other countries. It identified common pathologically oriented practices throughout the pregnancy and postpartum period that "served to warp and distort the childbearing experience in the United States." The specific issues defined in this paper became many of the key issues around which childbirth activists organized for the next 30 plus years.

Although childbirth remains one of the most medicalized areas of women's lives, midwives offer an alternative, though not as accessible in the U.S. as supporters would like. The question raised in the title of the article "Routine Midwifery Care: Why Not Here?" is an important one. Leah Hyder points out that "the majority of healthy women in Europe use professionally trained midwives," and compares that to the barriers midwifery encounters in the U.S. The two fact sheets, "Overview of Maternity Care in the U.S." and "Ideals vs Reality in U.S. Births," provide information that demonstrates the benefits of midwifery and shows that routine maternity care in the U.S. is not working.

This can be seen in the facts that the U.S. has extremely high rates of Caesareans, extremely high infant mortality, and high maternal mortality.

These latter two measures, infant mortality rates (IMR) and maternal mortality (MM), provide useful ways to evaluate the health of a nation. As Deborah Maine points out in "How Do Socioeconomic Factors Affect Disparities in Maternal Mortality?" these two measures may be affected by socioeconomic factors in different ways, with the U.S. being relatively better off than many countries in the latter (MM) compared to the former (IMR), where its ranking in the world is poor for a "developed" nation. While there have been major decreases in maternal mortality in the U.S., there are still major disparities as, for example, African American women have much higher MM than white women. Understanding the factors affecting MM can help reduce the gaps among groups by improving health for all.

One of the issues related to pregnancy that is often overlooked is that of miscarriage; those who experience this loss often do not receive the support they need. "Understanding Distress in the Aftermath of Miscarriage" provides useful information about reactions by the woman, her partner, and society to miscarriage, and how these relate to support and treatment. Another psychological dimension to childbirth that remains insufficiently studied and understood is postpartum depression. Leslie Tam presents a summary of risk factors and possible interventions.

The remaining three articles in this chapter focus on issues related to breast feeding, which is an important factor in infant health and, along with other benefits to the mother, reduces risk of breast cancer. "Formula for Profit" explores the marketing of infant formula and how that reduces breast feeding and directly affects the health of infants. Sandra Steingraber's article is written from her perspective as a biologist, cancer activist, woman with a history of cancer, and a mother. As a strong advocate for breast feeding, she identifies the need for environmental policies that will protect milk from contamination by such potentially harmful substances as dioxin. The Precautionary Principle she invokes is one that has become central to discussions of environmental health (also discussed in Chapter 13, particularly in relation to breast cancer). This principle holds that proof of harm is not necessary before we can act to prevent harm, or, in other words, if there is evidence pointing in the direction that a chemical is toxic or carcinogenic, we do not need definitive proof before controlling or banning its use. The last article also addresses the connections among the environment, breast feeding, and health, linking environmental and reproductive justice, by focusing on the experiences and work of Katsi Cook, a Mohawk woman activist. The Mother's Milk Project (MMP), which she started, "asserted that the Native children are at greater risk from *not* being breast fed than from environmental contaminants, and worked to re-establish breast feeding in the community. . . ." At the same time as promoting breast feeding, the MMP helped women reduce the risk of contamination of their breast milk by advising them to avoid eating fish, a staple of their diets, from contaminated waters. Being unable to both continue their traditional diet *and* safely breast feed their children helped lead many Native people involved with MMP to activism to create a healthier environment.

The Cultural Warping of Childbirth

by Doris Haire

While Sweden and the Netherlands compete for the honor of having the lowest incidence of infant deaths per one thousand live births, the United States continues to find itself outranked by fourteen other developed countries.[1] A spokesman for the National Foundation March of Dimes recently stated that according to the most recent data, the United States leads all developed countries in the rate of infant deaths due to birth injury and respiratory distress such as postnatal asphyxia and atelectasis. According to the National Association for Retarded Children there are now six million retarded children and adults in the United States with a predicted annual increase of over 100,000 a year. The number of children and adults with behavioral difficulties or perceptual dysfunction resulting from minimal brain damage is an ever growing challenge to society and to the economy.

While it may be easier on the conscience to blame such numbing facts solely on socioeconomic factors and birth defects, recent research makes it evident that obstetrical medication can play a role in our staggering incidence of neurological impairment. It may be convenient to blame our relatively poor infant outcome on a lack of facilities or inadequate government funding, but it is obvious from the research being carried out that we could effect an immediate improvement in infant outcome by changing the pattern of obstetrical care in the United States. It is time that we take a good look at the overall experience of childbirth in this country and begin to recognize how our culture has warped this experience for the majority of American mothers and their newborn infants.

As an officer of the International Childbirth Education Association, I have visited hundreds of maternity hospitals throughout the world—in Great Britain, Western Europe, Russia, Asia, Australia, New Zealand, the South Pacific, the Americas, and Africa. During my visits I was privileged to observe obstetric techniques and procedures and to interview physicians, professional midwives, and parents in the various countries. My companion on many of my visits was Dorothea Lang, C.N.M. (Certified Nurse-Midwife), Director of Nurse-Midwifery for New York City. Miss Lang's experience as both a nurse-midwife and a former head nurse of the labor and delivery unit of the New York–Cornell Medical Center made her a particularly well-qualified observer and companion. As we traveled from country to country certain patterns of care soon became evident. For one, in those countries that enjoy an incidence of infant mortality and birth trauma significantly lower than that of the United States, highly trained professional midwives are an important source of obstetrical care and family planning services for normal women, whether the births take place in the hospital or in the home. In these countries the expertise of the physician is called upon only when the expectant mother is ill during pregnancy, or when labor or birth is anticipated to be, or is found to be, abnormal. Under this system, the high-risk mother—the one who is most likely to bear an impaired or stillborn child—has a better opportunity to obtain in-depth medical attention than is possible under our existing American system of obstetrical care where the obstetrician is also called upon to play the role of midwife.

Deprivation, birth defects, prematurity, and low birth weight are not unique to the United States. While it is tempting to blame our comparatively high incidence of infant mortality solely on a lack of available prenatal care and on socioeconomic factors, our observations indicate that, comparatively, the prenatal care we offer most clinic patients in the United States is not grossly inferior to that available in other developed countries. Furthermore, the diet and standard of living in many countries which have a lower incidence of infant mortality than ours would be considered inadequate by American standards.

As an example, when one compares the availability of prenatal care, the incidence of premature births, the average diet of various economic groups, and the equipment available to aid in newborn-infant survival in two such diverse countries as the United States and Japan, there are no major differences between the two countries. The differences lie in (a) our frequent use of prenatal and obstetrical medication, (b) our pathologically oriented management of pregnancy, labor, birth, and postpartum, and (c) the predominance of artificial feeding in the United States, in contrast to Japan.

If present statistics follow the trend of recent years, an infant born in the United States is more than four times more likely to die in the first day of life than an infant born in Japan. But a survival of the birth process should not be our singular goal. For every American newborn infant who dies there are likely to be several who are neurologically damaged.

Unfortunately, the American tendency to warp the birth experience, distorting it into a pathological event rather than a physiological one for the normal childbearing woman, is no longer peculiar to just the United States. In my visits to hospitals in various countries I was distressed to find that some physicians, anxious to impress their colleagues with their "Americanized" techniques, have unfortunately adopted many of our obstetrical practices without stopping to question their scientific or social merit.

Few American babies are born today as nature intended them to be.

It is not unlikely that unnecessary alterations in the normal fetal environment may play a role in the incidence of neurological impairment and infant mortality in the United States. Infant resuscitation, other than routine suctioning, is rarely needed in countries such as Sweden, the Netherlands, and Japan, where the skillful psychological management of labor usually precludes the need for obstetrical medication. In contrast, in those European countries, such as Belgium, where the overall pattern of obstetrical care is similar to our own, the incidence of infant mortality also approaches our own.

Obviously there will always be medical indications which dictate the use of various obstetrical procedures, but to apply the following American practices and procedures routinely to the vast majority of mothers who are capable of giving birth without complication is to create added stress which is not in the best interests of either the mother or her newborn infant.

Let us take a close look at some of our common obstetrical practices from early pregnancy to postpartum which have served to warp and distort the childbearing experience in the United States. While not all of the practices below affect infant mortality, it is equally apparent that they do not contribute to the reduction of infant morbidity or mortality and therefore should be reevaluated.

Withholding Information on the Disadvantages of Obstetrical Medication   Ignorance of the possible hazards of obstetrical medication appears to encourage the misuse and abuse of obstetrical medication, for in those countries where mothers are not told routinely of the possible disadvantages of obstetrical medication to themselves or to their babies the use of such medication is on the increase.

There is no research or evidence which indicates that mothers will be emotionally damaged if they are advised, prior to birth, that obstetrical medication may be to the disadvantage of their newborn infants.

Requiring All Normal Women to Give Birth in the Hospital   While ICEA does not encourage home births, there is ample evidence in the Netherlands and in Chicago (Chicago Maternity Center) to demonstrate that normal women who have received adequate prenatal care can safely give birth at home if a proper system is developed for home deliveries. Over half of the mothers in the Netherlands give birth at home with the assistance of a professional midwife and a maternity aide. The comparatively low incidence of infant deaths and birth trauma in the Netherlands, a country of diverse ethnic composition and intermarriage, is evidence of the comparative safety of a properly developed home delivery service.

Dutch obstetricians point out that when the labor of a normal woman is unhurried and allowed to progress normally, unexpected emergencies rarely occur. They also point out that the small risk involved in a Dutch home delivery is more than offset by the increased hazards resulting from the use of obstetrical medication and obstetrical tampering which are more likely to occur in a hospital environment, especially in countries where professionals have had little or no exposure to normal labor and birth in a home environment during their training.

Elective Induction of Labor   The elective induction of labor (where there is no clear medical indication) appears to be an American idiosyncrasy which is frowned upon in other developed countries.

The elective induction of labor has been found almost to double the incidence of fetomaternal transfusion and its attendant hazards.[2] But perhaps the least appreciated problem of elective induction is the fact that the abrupt onset of artificially induced labor tends to make it extremely difficult for even the well-prepared mother to tolerate the discomfort of the intensified contractions without the aid of obstetrical medication. When the onset of labor occurs spontaneously, the normal, gradual increase in contraction length and intensity appears to provoke in the mother an accompanying tolerance for discomfort or pain.

Since the British Perinatal Hazards Study found no increase in perinatal mortality or impairment of learning ability at age seven among full-term infants unless gestation had extended beyond forty-one weeks,[3] there would appear to be no medical justification for subjecting a mother or her baby to the possible hazards of elective induction in order to terminate the pregnancy prior to forty-one weeks' gestation.

Separating the Mother from Familial Support During Labor and Birth

Research indicates that fear adversely affects uterine motility and blood flow,[4] and yet many American mothers are routinely separated from a family member or close friend at this time of emotional crisis.

In most developed countries, other than the United States and the Eastern European countries, mothers are encouraged to walk about or to sit and chat with a family member or supportive person in what is called an "early labor lounge." This lounge is usually located near but outside the labor-delivery area in order to provide a more relaxed atmosphere during much of labor. The mother is taken to the labor-delivery area to be checked periodically, then allowed to return to the labor lounge for as long as she likes or until her membranes have ruptured.

Confining the Normal Laboring Woman to Bed

In virtually all countries except the United States, a woman in labor is routinely encouraged to walk about during labor for as long as she wishes or until her membranes have ruptured. Such activity is considered to facilitate labor by distracting the mother's attention from the discomfort or pain of her contractions and to encourage a more rapid engagement of the fetal head. In America, where drugs are frequently administered either orally or parenterally to laboring mothers, such ambulation is discouraged—not only for the patient's safety but also to avoid possible legal complications in the event of an accident.

Shaving the Birth Area

Research involving 7,600 mothers has demonstrated that the practice of shaving the perineum and pubis does not reduce the incidence of infection. In fact, the incidence of infection was slightly higher among those mothers who were shaved.[5] Yet this procedure, which tends to create apprehension in laboring women, is still carried out routinely in most American hospitals. Clipping the perineal or pudendal hair closely with surgical scissors is far less disturbing to the mother and is less likely to result in infection caused by razor abrasions.

Professional Dependence on Technology and Pharmacological Methods of Pain Relief

Most of the world's mothers receive little or no drugs during pregnancy, labor, or birth. The constant emotional support provided the laboring woman in other countries by the nurse-midwife, and often by her husband, appears greatly to improve the mother's tolerance for discomfort. In contrast, the American labor room nurse is frequently assigned to look after several women in labor, all or most of whom have had no preparation to cope with the discomfort or pain of childbearing. Under the circumstances, drugs, rather than skillful emotional support, are employed to relieve the mother's apprehension and discomfort (and perhaps to assuage the harried labor attendant's feeling of inadequacy).

Routine Electronic Fetal Monitoring

The wisdom of depending on an experienced nurse using a stethoscope to monitor accurately the effects of obstetrical medication on the well-being of the fetus has been demonstrated by Haverkamp.[6] No one knows the long-term or delayed consequences of ultrasonic fetal monitoring on subsequent human development. The fact that some electronic fetal monitoring devices require that a mother's membranes be ruptured and the electrode be screwed into the skin of the fetal scalp creates hazards of its own. Current research indicates that obstetrical management which reduces the need for such monitoring is advisable.

Chemical Stimulation of Labor

Oxytocic agents are frequently administered to American mothers in order to intensify artificially the frequency or the strength of the mother's contractions, as a means of shortening the mother's labor. While chemical stimulation is sometimes medically indicated, often it is undertaken to satisfy the American propensity for efficiency and speed. Hon suggests that the overenthusiastic use of oxytocic stimulants sometimes results in alterations in the normal fetal heart rate.[7] Fields points out that the possible hazards inherent in elective induction are also possible in artificially stimulated labor unless the mother and fetus are carefully monitored.[8]

Shortening the phases of normal labor when there is no sign of fetal distress has not been shown to improve infant outcome. Little is known of the long-term effects of artificially stimulating labor contractions. During a contraction the unborn child normally receives less oxygen. The gradual buildup of intensity, which occurs when the onset of labor is allowed to occur spontaneously and to proceed without chemical stimulation, appears likely to be a protective mechanism that is best left unaltered unless there is a clear medical indication for the artificial stimulation of labor.

Delaying Birth until the Physician Arrives   Because of the increased likelihood of resultant brain damage to the infant the practice of delaying birth by anesthesia or physical restraint until the physician arrives to deliver the infant is frowned upon in most countries. Yet the practice still occurs occasionally in the United States and in countries where hospital-assigned midwives do not routinely manage the labor and delivery of normal mothers.

Requiring the Mother to Assume the Lithotomy Position for Birth   There is gathering scientific evidence that the unphysiological lithotomy position (back flat, with knees drawn up and spread wide apart by "stirrups"), which is preferred by most American physicians because it is more convenient for the *accoucheur,* tends to alter the normal fetal environment and obstruct the normal process of childbearing, making spontaneous birth more difficult or impossible.

The lithotomy and dorsal positions tend to:

1. Adversely affect the mother's blood pressure, cardiac return, and pulmonary ventilation.[9]

2. Decrease the normal intensity of the contractions.[10]

3. Inhibit the mother's voluntary efforts to push her baby out spontaneously[11] which, in turn, increases the need for fundal pressure or forceps and increases the traction necessary for a forceps extraction.

4. Inhibit the spontaneous expulsion of the placenta[12] which, in turn, increases the need for cord traction, forced expression, or manual removal of the placenta[13]—procedures which significantly increase the incidence of fetomaternal hemorrhage.[14]

5. Increase the need for episiotomy because of the increased tension on the pelvic floor and the stretching of the perineal tissue.[15]

Australian, Russian, and American research bears out the clinical experience of European physicians and midwives—that when mothers are supported to a semisitting position for birth, with their feet supported by the lower section of the labor-delivery bed, mothers tend to push more effectively, appear to need less pain relief, are more likely to want to be conscious for birth, and are less likely to need an episiotomy.[16]

The increased efficiency of the semisitting position, combined with a minimum use of medication for birth, is evidenced by the fact that the combined use of both forceps and the vacuum extractor rarely exceeds 4 percent to 5 percent of all births in the Netherlands, as compared to an incidence of 65 percent in many American hospitals. (Cesarean section occurs in approximately 1.5 percent of all Dutch births.)

The Routine Use of Regional or General Anesthesia for Delivery   In light of the current shortage of qualified anesthetists and anesthesiologists and the frequent scientific papers now being published on the possible hazards resulting from the use of regional and general anesthesia, it would seem prudent to make every effort to prepare the mother physically and mentally to cope with the sensations and discomfort of birth in order to avoid the use of such medicaments. Regional and general anesthesia not only tend adversely to affect fetal environment pharmacologically, which has been discussed previously herein, but their use also increases the need for obstetrical intervention in the normal process of birth, since both types of anesthesia tend to prolong labor.[17] Johnson points out that epidural and spinal anesthesia significantly increase the incidence of midforceps delivery and its attendant hazards.[18] Pudendal block anesthesia not only tends to interfere with the mother's ability effectively to push her baby down the birth canal due to the blocking of the afferent path of the pushing reflex, but also appears to interfere with the mother's normal protective reflexes, thus making "an explosive" birth and perineal damage more likely to occur.

The Routine Use of Forceps for Delivery   There is no scientific justification for the routine application of forceps for delivery.[19] The incidence of delivery by forceps and vacuum extractor, combined, rarely rises above 5 percent in countries where mothers actively participate in the births of their babies. In contrast, as mentioned previously, the incidence of forceps extraction frequently rises to as high as 65 percent in some American hospitals.

Routine Episiotomy   There is no research or evidence to indicate that routine episiotomy (a surgical incision to enlarge the vaginal orifice) reduces the incidence of pelvic relaxation (structural damage to the pelvic floor musculature) in the mother. Nor is there any research or evidence that routine episiotomy reduces neurological impairment in the child who has shown no signs of fetal distress or that the procedure helps to maintain subsequent male or female sexual response.

The incidence of pelvic floor relaxation appears to be on the decline throughout the world, even in those countries where episiotomy is still comparatively rare. The contention that the modern washing machine has been more effective in reducing pelvic relaxation among American mothers than has routine episiotomy is given some credence by the fact that in areas of the United States where life is still hard for the woman pelvic relaxation appears in white women who have never borne children.

In developed countries where episiotomy is comparatively rare the physiotherapist is considered an important member of the obstetrical team—before as well as after birth. The physiotherapist is responsible for seeing that each mother begins exercises the day following birth which will help to restore the normal elasticity and tone of the mother's perineal and abdominal muscles. In countries where every effort is made to avoid the need for an episiotomy, interviews with both parents and professionals indicate that an intact perineum which is strengthened by postpartum exercises is more apt to result in both male and female sexual satisfaction than is a perineum that has been incised and reconstructed.

Why then, is there such an emotional attachment among professionals to routine episiotomy? A prominent European professor of obstetrics and gynecology recently made the following comment on the American penchant for routine episiotomy, "Since all the physician can really do to affect the course of childbirth for the 95 percent of mothers who are capable of giving birth without complication is to offer the mother pharmacological relief from discomfort or pain and to perform an episiotomy, there is probably an unconscious tendency for many professionals to see these practices as indispensable."

Interviews with obstetrician-gynecologists in many countries indicate that they tend to agree that a superficial, first degree tear is less traumatic to the perineal tissue than an incision which requires several sutures for reconstruction. There is no research which would indicate otherwise.

Early Clamping or "Milking" of the Umbilical Cord

Several years ago De Marsh stated that the placental blood normally belongs to the infant and his or her failure to get this blood is equivalent to submitting him or her to a rather severe hemorrhage. Despite the fact that placental transfusion normally occurs in every corner of the world without adverse consequences, there is still a great effort in the United States and Canada to deprecate the practice. One must read the literature carefully to find that placental transfusion has not been demonstrated to increase the incidence of morbidity or mortality in the placentally transfused infant.[20]

Delaying the First Breast-feeding

The common American practice of routinely delaying the time of the first breast-feeding has not been shown to be in the best interest of either the conscious mother or her newborn infant. Clinical experience with the early feeding of newborn infants has shown this practice to be safe.[21] If the mother feels well enough and the infant is capable of suckling while they are still in the delivery room then it would seem more cautious, in the event of tracheo-esophageal abnormality, to permit the infant to suckle for the first time under the watchful eye of the physician or nurse-midwife rather than delay the feeding for several hours when the expertise of the professional may not be immediately available.

In light of the many protective antibodies contained in colostrum it would seem likely that the earlier the infant's intake of species specific colostrum, the sooner the antibodies can be accrued by the infant.

Offering Water and Formula to the Breast-fed Newborn Infant

The common American practice of giving water or formula to a newborn infant prior to the first breast-feeding or as a supplement during the first days of life has not been shown to be in the best interests of the infant. There are now indications that these practices may, in fact, be harmful. Glucose water, once the standby in every American hospital, has now been designated a potential hazard if aspirated by the newborn infant, yet it is still used in many American hospitals.

Restricting Newborn Infants to a Four-hour Feeding Schedule and Withholding Nightime Feedings

Although widely spaced infant feedings may be more convenient for hospital personnel, the practice of feeding a newborn infant only every four hours and not permitting the infant to breast-feed at all during the night cannot be justified on any scientific grounds. Such a regimen restricts the suckling stimulation necessary to bring about the normally rapid onset and adequate production of the mother's milk. In countries where custom permits the infant to suckle immediately after birth and on demand from that time, first-time mothers frequently begin to produce breast milk for their babies within twenty-four hours after birth. In contrast, in countries where hospital routines prevent normal demand feeding from birth, mothers frequently do not produce breast milk for their babies until the third day following birth.

Overdistention of the breast or engorgement is a hospital acquired condition which does not occur to any comparable degree in cultures where mothers are permitted to breast-feed their babies on demand from birth.[22]

Preventing Early Father-child Contact   Permitting fathers to hold their newborn infants immediately following birth and during the postpartum hospital stay has not been shown by research or clinical experience to increase the incidence of infection among newborns, even when those infants are returned to a regular or central nursery. Yet only in the Eastern European countries is the father permitted less involvement in the immediate postpartum period than in the United States.

Research has consistently confirmed the fact that the greatest sources of infection to the newborn infant are the nursery and nursery personnel.[23] One has only to observe a mother holding her newborn infant against her bathrobe, which has probably been exposed to abundant hospital-borne bacteria, to realize the fallacy of preventing a father from holding his baby during the hospital stay.

Restricting Intermittent Rooming-in to Specific Room Requirements   Throughout the world great effort is made to keep mothers and babies together in the hospital, no matter how inconvenient the accommodations. There is no research or evidence which indicates that intermittent rooming-in should be restricted to private rooms or to rooms which have a sink, or which provide at least eighty square feet for mother and baby. Such requirements are based on conjecture and not on controlled evaluation.

Restricting Sibling Visitation   The common American practice of prohibiting toddlers and children from visiting their mothers during the hospital stay is an emotional hardship on both the mothers and their children and is unsupported by scientific research or evidence. Experience in other countries and in several hospitals here in the United States suggests that where sibling visitation is permitted, a short explanation as to the importance of not bringing suspect illnesses into the hospital seems to be effective in controlling infection.

Summary

As mentioned previously, most of the practices discussed above have developed not from a lack of concern for the well-being of the mother and baby but from a lack of awareness as to the problems which can arise from each progressive digression from the normal childbearing ex-

perience. Like a snowball rolling down hill, as one unphysiological practice is employed, for one reason or another, another frequently becomes necessary to counteract some of the disadvantages, large or small, inherent in the previous procedure.

The higher incidence of fetal, neonatal, and maternal deaths occurring in our large urban hospitals, as opposed to our smaller community hospitals,[24] is undoubtedly due, in part, to the greater proportion of high-risk mothers in the urban areas. But we in the United States must stop looking for scapegoats and face up to the fact that by individualizing the care offered to maternity patients, much can be done immediately to improve infant outcome without the slightest outlay of capital.

There is currently an increasing emphasis on consolidating maternity facilities. However, we in ICEA do not see the consolidation of community obstetrical facilities as being always in the best interest of the vast majority of mothers who are capable of giving birth without complications. There should, of course, be centers where those mothers who have had no prenatal care or who are anticipated to be obstetrical risks can be properly cared for. But to insist that every healthy mother must go to a major maternity facility which is unnecessary for her needs and inconvenient for her family, and where she is very apt to be "lost in the crowd," will only spur the growing trend in the United States toward professionally unattended home births.

Throughout the United States the current inclination of many expectant parents is to seek out, to "shop around" for the type of physician and hospital they feel they need in order to have the type of childbearing experience they want. They not only want a doctor who will support them in their efforts to have a prepared, natural birth, with a minimum of or no medication; they also want a hospital which offers education for childbearing and a supportive family-centered atmosphere. These expectant mothers appreciate the availability of such facilities as an early labor lounge, a dual purpose labor-delivery room, a mother-baby recovery room, and a children's visiting room if they have older children. But most of all they want a supportive atmosphere in which they can share the childbearing experience to the extent that they desire, and one which makes an effort to meet the individual needs of the mother, the father, and their newborn baby as they form their family bonds during the hospital stay.

NOTES

1. H. Chase, "Ranking Countries by Infant Mortality Rates," Public Health Reports 84 (1969): 19–27; M. Wegman, "Annual Summary of Vital Statistics—1969," *Pediatrics* 47 (1971): 461–64.

2. A. Beer, "Fetal Erythrocytes in Maternal Circulation of 155 Rh-Negative Women," *Obstet. & Gynec.* 34 (1969): 143–50.

3. N. Butler, "A National Long-Term Study of Perinatal Hazards," Sixth World Congress of the Federation of International Gynecology & Obstetrics, 1970.

4. J. Kelly, "Effect of Fear Upon Uterine Motility," *Am. J. Obstet. & Gynec.* 83 (1962): 576–81.

5. R. Burchell, "Predelivery Removal of Pubic Hair," *Obstet. & Gynec.* 24 (1964): 272–73; H. Kantor et al., "Value of Shaving the Pudendal-Perineal Area in Delivery Preparation," *Obstet. & Gynec.*[25] (1965) 509–12.

6. Haverkamp, A. D., Thompson, H. E., McFee, J. G. et al., "The Evaluation of Continuous Fetal-Heart Monitoring for High Risk Pregnancies." *Am. J. Obstet. & Gynec.* 125, no. 3 (June 1, 1926): 310–20.

7. E. Hon, "Direct Monitoring of the Fetal Heart," *Hospital Practice* (September 1970): 91–97.

8. H. Fields, "Complications of Elective Induction" *Obstet. & Gynec.* 15 (1960): 476–80; H. Fields, "Induction of Labor: Methods, Hazards, Complications, and Contraindications," *Hospital Topics* (December 1968): 63–68.

9. C. Flowers, *Obstetric Analgesia and Anesthesia* (New York: Hoeber, Harper & Row, 1967); L. S. James, "The Effects of Pain Relief for Labor and Delivery on the Fetus and Newborn," *Anesthesiology* 21 (1960): 405–30; A. Blankfield, "The Optimum Position for Childbirth," *Med. J. Australia 2* (1965): 666–68.

10. Blankfield, "The Optimum Position for Childbirth"; F. H. Howard, "Delivery in the Physiologic Position," *Obstet. & Gynec.* 11 (1958): 318–22; I. Gritsiuk, "Position in Labor," *Ob-Gyn Observer* (September 1968).

11. Blankfield, "The Optimum Position for Childbirth"; Howard, "Delivery in the Physiologic Position"; N. Newton and

M. Newton "The Propped Position for the Second Stage of Labor," *Obstet. & Gynec.* 15 (1960): 28–34.

12. Newton and Newton, "The Propped Position for the Second Stage of Labor."

13. M. Botha, "The Management of the Umbilical Cord in Labour," *s. Afr. J. Obstet.* 6, no. 2 (1968): 30–33.

14. Beer, "Fetal Erythrocytes in Maternal Circulation of 155 Rh-Negative Women."

15. Blankfield, "The Optimum Position for Childbirth."

16. Ibid.; Newton and Newton, "The Propped Position for the Second Stage of Labor."

17. L. Hellman and J. Pritchard, *Williams Obstetrics,* 14th ed. (New York: Appleton-Century-Crofts, 1971).

18. W. Johnson, "Regionals Can Prolong Labor," *Medical World News,* October 15, 1971.

19. Butler, "A National Long-Term Study of Perinatal Hazards."

20. S. Saigal et al., "Placental Transfusion and Hyperbilirubinemia in the Premature," *Pediatrics* 49 (1972): 406–19.

21. H. Eppink, "Time of Initial Breast Feeding Surveyed in Michigan Hospitals," *Hospital Topics* (June 1968): 116–17.

22. M. Newton and N. Newton, "Postpartum Engorgement of the Breast," *Am. J. Obstet. & Gynec.* 61 (1951): 664–67.

23. H. Gezon et al., "Some Controversial Aspects in the Epidemiology of Hospital Nursery Staphylococcal Infections," *Amer. J. of Public Health* 50 (1960): 473–84; R. Ravenholt and G. LaVeck, "Staphylococcal Disease—An Obstetric, Pediatric & Community Problem," *Amer. J. of Public Health* 46 (1956): 1287–96.

24. E. Bishop, "The National Study of Maternity Care." *Obstet. & Gynec.* (1971): 745–50.

Routine Midwifery Care
"Why Not Here?"

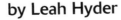

by Leah Hyder

In our ever-changing fast paced system of health care delivery, many women feel that they receive little personal attention, especially during pregnancy and childbirth. Into this breach step midwives, who have a long history of providing women with holistic care during pregnancy and childbirth. Despite the high quality of care that midwives provide to expectant mothers, American women have few opportunities to use the services of midwives and to have those services covered by their health insurance plans. Clearly, midwifery in the Untied States faces more barriers than most other countries.

From *Network News,* July/August 1998 by Leah Hyder. Copyright © 1998 by National Women's Health Network. Reprinted by permission.

Certified Nurse-Midwives (CNMs)—CNMS are Registered Nurses (RNs) who complete training to become certified in nurse-midwifery by the American College of Nurse-Midwives (ACNM). In the U.S., CNMs care for 5% of all births and 95% of all births delivered by midwives.

Certified Midwives (CMs)—CMs are not registered nurses, but are accredited by the ACNM and have graduated from an ACNM accredited midwifery school.

Certified Professional Midwives (CPMs)—Midwives who are certified by the North American Registry of Midwives (NARM).

Licensed Midwife—A legal term denoting state-licensed direct-entry midwives.

Direct-Entry Midwives—Direct-entry midwives have completed a formal midwifery education program or are licensed to practice in their state or local jurisdiction or are certified by a local or state organization.

Birth Attendants—Birth attendants assist the primary birth attendant, usually a CNM or physician. This term is also used by some non-CNM midwives who practice in states where midwifery is illegal unless practiced by a CNM or a physician.

Granny and Lay Midwives—Granny and lay midwives are other types of midwives which have existed in the U.S. but that are virtually nonexistent today. Midwives historically called lay or professional midwives often call themselves traditional or independent midwives today.

Midwifery Is Welcomed in Europe

The United States is lagging behind other nations of the world in fully integrating midwifery into its health care system. While midwives deliver only 6% of the approximately 220,000 babies in the United States each year, midwives in other countries attend up to 80% of their countries' births. Barriers against and support for midwifery vary from country to country.

The majority of healthy women in Europe use professionally-trained midwives. Most European countries have passed laws regulating midwives and publicly support midwifery schools and professional organizations. Most midwives in Europe work for governmental health services.

Austria, Sweden, the United Kingdom (UK), and particularly the Netherlands possess sound systems of midwifery. In Austria, the law requires that a midwife be present at every birth. In Sweden, midwives provide more than 80% of prenatal care and family planning services. Midwives in the UK attend 70% of all births and also provide the vast majority of care to women who want home births. They also provide a high proportion of care between pregnancies. The midwives in England are independent practitioners, responsible for the full spectrum of care for healthy women. The Netherlands is the only industrialized country where the majority of women have home births.

Midwifery in the Developing World

Midwifery is also prevalent in developing countries, though standards of practice are not at the same level as European nations. Developing countries often use lay midwives to complement the sparse distribution of physicians. Often, the only training midwives have is observation of relatives and physicians. In most third-world countries, the care midwives provide includes treatments which reflect cultural practices such as fasting, prayers, herbal medicines, and sacrifices to appease gods.

Further, midwives in developing countries face unique challenges, such as lack of information about and access to proper sanitation measures, illiteracy, scarcity of training programs and the means to attend them, and the lack of financial resources to sustain their own practice. Often, even where physicians are available, women prefer midwives because of economic and sociocultural reasons.

Midwifery in the United States

Barriers to midwifery care in the United States are numerous and imposing. They include physician opposition, public perception of midwives as substandard, state and federal regulations, the current economic and political environment, lack of training programs, strife between midwifery groups, lack of access to malpractice insurance, and lack of acceptance among third-party payers, including Medicaid.

Physician Opposition

Although some physicians encourage midwifery, others adamantly oppose it. While Ob-Gyns are specialists trained in interventions which are sometimes necessary in complicated or high-risk pregnancies, midwives' training emphasizes skills which help women have healthy outcomes with as little intervention as possible. A common perception is that women are safer in a hospital, with a doctor. In fact, studies show that both mothers and babies are safer with midwives. Births attended by certified Nurse-Midwives (CNMs) produce fewer cesarean sections, infant abrasions, complications, perineal lacerations, postpartum hemorrhage, and vacuum- or forceps-assisted deliveries than physicians. CNMs also cost approximately $1000 less than physicians per birth and most develop a strong relationship with the mother. Is it any wonder that many physicians oppose midwives? Midwives treat normal pregnancies as the natural processes that they are. Midwives need to fight this physician opposition and medicalization, as well as the accompanying public perceptions.

Regulatory Barriers

Often regulations pose another barrier to midwifery care. Laws governing midwifery care vary from state to state and often do not comply to the national standards of practice set by the American College of Nurse-Midwives (ACNM). Laws that require midwives to practice in hospitals or be supervised by a physician limit the midwives' scope of practice. This often means that women in rural areas who, without such restricting laws, would have convenient access to local midwives must instead travel for miles to reach a hospital or physician. In addition, the Joint Commission on Accreditation of Health Care Organizations (JCAHCO), a regulatory organization overseeing activities of most healthcare organizations in the United States, requires that physical examinations of women be done only by physicians. Because eligibility requirements for health care providers to have hospital privileges often include completing physical examinations, which non-physicians cannot do per JCAHCO standards, midwives would not be allowed to practice in a hospital.

Economic Woes

Midwives face economic barriers as well. Although they do similar work, midwives are paid thousands of dollars less per year than physicians. Medicare reimburses CNMs up to 65% of the physician fee schedule which means that physicians earn over 1/3 more than nurse-midwives for the same services. Many third-party payers adopted this payment policy, making the injustice more widespread. In this session of Congress, U.S. Rep. Edolphus Towns (D-NY) is proposing "The Certified Nurse-Midwives Medicare Services Act" to increase this reimbursement to 95%, which although progressive, fails to address the similar needs of midwives who are not CNMs. Additionally, many free-standing birth centers receive no coverage in numerous state and federal Medicaid programs at all. Midwives also disproportionately render care to underserved populations who often do not have insurance and can not pay out of pocket for services.

Access to Liability Insurance

Midwives often lack available and affordable malpractice insurance. This is a primary impediment to maternity care by midwives. As a result of the liability insurance crisis of the 1980s, many Ob-Gyns and midwives left practice because they could not find adequate malpractice insurance. Most CNMs now obtain insurance from their employers, the ACNM, or from local insurance companies. Some problems with obtaining malpractice insurance include its increasing cost, restrictions related to the place of birth, and medical management of pregnancy and childbirth as the accepted standard.

Dearth of Education Programs

Access to midwife education and training is challenging. Midwifery programs across the U.S. are filled to capacity due to the demand for midwives, which is greater than the supply. One reason so few schools educate midwives is lack of funding. Additionally, the U.S. is still very physician-oriented. But because the public demand for physicians is higher than it is for midwives, funding for the training of physicians receives more attention than that for midwives. As women increasingly use midwifery services, leverage may be created for funding of midwifery programs.

Barriers to U.S. Subpopulations

Barriers to midwifery care exist for subpopulations of the general public in the U.S. as well. Historically, poor, rural, Hispanic, African-American, and Native-American women have used midwives the most frequently. This prevalence was often due to the cost of care, exclusion by white hospitals, and transportation problems. Because of these factors of inequality, these women often felt that they were given inferior care when treated by a midwife. Midwives have fought this perception of the quality of their care.

Building Bridges in U.S. Midwifery

Although midwives currently face these political barriers, various groups are working for change. The American College of Nurse-Midwives (ACNM) is a professional organization for CNMs. It speaks for its membership on issues affecting education, practice, recognition, and reimbursement. A second professional group, MANA (the Midwives Alliance of North America), welcomes and hopes to unite all midwives, including both lay and certified midwives. While MANA focuses on direct-entry midwives, their agenda includes all midwives.

Although some tension among the groups exists, different groups have taken measures to unify all midwives. The Bridge Club is an organization of the nurse-midwives who want to unify the ACNM and MANA, which sometimes have conflicting views. The Midwifery Communication and Accountability Project (MCAP) of Boston, Massachusetts, has midwives work together on the community level to raise money for policy issues, hoping that working together towards a common goal would help unify the midwives. MANA welcomes all midwives and encourages dialogue among the groups. Despite their varying educational backgrounds, all midwives have much in common and many realize that working together to promote the causes of midwifery will help them all as well as the women they serve.

Future Prospects of Midwifery in the United States

While some third-party payers are apprehensive about using midwives because of liability issues, other third-party payers utilize midwives because of their cost-effectiveness. It remains to be seen whether the trend in third-party payers will be to utilize midwives in the name of cost efficiency or not to utilize them because of their liability. As more women demand midwifery services and the professional reputation of midwives grows, more third party payers may utilize midwives.

The barriers to midwifery in the U.S. are substantial, but midwives constantly work to lessen them. Yet we can look to European countries for a good model and to show us areas in which we could improve to make midwifery affordable, accessible, and acceptable in the U.S.

To learn more about midwifery or its advocacy, contact the ACNM at (202) 728-9860, the Massachusetts Friends of Midwives at (508) 369-1468, or MANA at (931) 964-2589.

I would like to thank Doris Haire, Linda Holmes, and Carol Sakala for their input into this article.

Leah Hyder was a summer Network intern.

REFERENCES

A list of references is available in the original source.

The American College of Nurse-Midwives at www.acnm.org or the Midwives Alliance of North America at http://mana.org

"Overview of Maternity Care in the U.S."

by Carolyn Keefe

With four million births each year[1] and three-quarters of American women becoming mothers, maternity care affects large numbers of women. It is also big business. The United States has the highest per capita spending on health care in the world, with care for mothers and newborns combined as the fourth largest category of hospital expenses,[2] and childbirth as the most common reason for the hospitalization of women in the United States.

Women are subjected to an ever-increasing array of interventions and technologies, many of which are highly invasive, with little or no evidence of their effectiveness. In fact, the medical evidence shows that the routine use of unnecessary interventions put mothers and babies at risk. Medical interventions are also expensive and often used not for the benefit of women and babies, but for the convenience or legal protection of doctors and hospitals.

All of this would be acceptable if we had better outcomes to show for it. Unfortunately, our outcomes are not nearly as good as those of developed countries that rely more heavily on midwifery care. Some of the clear problems with our maternity care system include:

• A high infant mortality rate compared to other developed countries—27th in the world.[3] Infant mortality rates are higher for African American, Latina and Native American babies—with the rate for African American babies twice that of white babies.[4]

- A maternal mortality rate that has not improved in 20 years—15th in the world.[5] Maternal mortality is higher for women of color than for white women, nearly 4 times higher for African American women.[6]

- A cesarean birth rate of 24.4%—among the highest in the world. Cesarean birth rates are highest for African American women, followed by white women, Latina women, Asian women, and Native American women.[7]

- A 20% drop in vaginal births after cesarean (VBAC) from 2000 to 2001 to 16.4%—access to VBAC is disappearing requiring many women who have cesarean scars to undergo surgery.[8]

- An induction rate of 20.5%—which has more than doubled since 1989 and continues to rise.[9]

- Many mothers traumatized by their treatment during birth, with as many as 30% exhibiting some signs of post-traumatic stress disorder[10] and 50% experiencing some aspect of postpartum depression (the highest such rate in the world).[1]

Moreover:

Of the eight most common surgical procedures in the U.S. four are obstetric in nature—episiotomy, repair of obstetric laceration, cesarean birth, artificial rupture of membranes. These are also the top four surgeries performed on women in the U.S.[12]

Obstetric procedures are the most common type of surgical procedures performed in the U.S. (6,209,000), slightly higher than cardiac procedures (5,939,000). Consider the following:

- obstetric procedures are only performed on women—more obstetric procedures are performed on women than the next two categories (cardiac and digestive) combined;

- there are over six million obstetric procedures, but just over four million births;

- these procedures are primarily performed on healthy women during a normal physiological process.

The problem has steadily gotten worse over the last two decades. All obstetric procedures combined have nearly doubled since 1980, while certain procedures, such as medical induction of labor, vacuum extraction, and manually assisted delivery increased more than ten-

fold in that time.[13] Each procedure carries with it risks to mothers and babies, and less invasive techniques exist for most of them. Furthermore, they are usually not medically necessary and are avoidable for the majority of women.

The Midwives Model of Care[14] and the evidence-based Mother-Friendly Childbirth Initiative[15] recognize birth as a normal, natural process and support the use of less invasive techniques, such as position changes, waiting, hydrotherapy, and perineal support, that carry fewer risks to mothers and babies and are usually more effective.

Research shows that midwives are the safest birth attendants for most women, with lower infant and maternal mortality rates and fewer invasive interventions such as episiotomies and surgical births (cesareans). In developed countries where midwives are the primary care providers for pregnant women, mortality and surgical birth rates are much lower than in the United States. However, legal, regulatory, and financial barriers to the practicing the Midwives Model of Care and Mother-Friendly care make it difficult for women to access either in the U.S.

REFERENCES

1. Martin, Joyce, et al., "Births Final Data for 2001," *National Vital Statistics Reports*, Vol. 51, No. 5, December 18, 2002, p. 1.

2. 1999 National Statistics, HCUPnet, Healthcare Cost and Utilization Project. Agency for Healthcare Research and Quality, Rockville, MD. http://www.ahrq.gov/data/hcup/hcupnet.htm.

3. *Child Health USA 2001*, Maternal Child Health Bureau, Health Resources and Services Administration, U.S. Department of Health and Human Services, p. 22, http://mchb.hrsa.gov/chusa02/main_pages/page_22.htm.

4. Hoyert, DL; et al., "Deaths: Final Data for 1999," *National Vital Statistics Report*, Vol. 49, No. 8, September 21, 2001, p. 11.

5. *State of the World's Mothers 2002*, Save the Children, http://www.savethechildren.org/mothers/sowm02/report/complete_index.pdf.

6. Hoyert, DL; et al., "Deaths: Final Data for 1999," *National Vital Statistics Report*, Vol. 49, No. 8, September 21, 2001, p. 89.

7. Martin, Joyce, et al., "Births Final Data for 2001," *National Vital Statistics Reports*, Vol. 51, No. 5, December 18, 2002, p. 16.

8. Ibid

9. Ibid, p. 15

10. Creedy DK, Shochet IM, Horsfall J. "Childbirth and the development of acute trauma symptoms: incidence and contributing factors." *Birth*, 2000 Jun; 27(2):104–11.

11. Wolf, Naomi, *Misconceptions: Truth, Lies, and the Unexpected on the Journey to Motherhood.* Doubleday, 2001, p. 216.

12. Kozak LJ, Hall MJ, Owings MF. *National Hospital Discharge Survey: 2000 Annual Summary with detailed diagnosis and procedure data.* National Center for Health Statistics. Vital Health Stat 13(153). 2002, p. 40, http://www.cdc.gov/nchs/data/series/sr_13/sr13_153.pdf.

13. Ibid, p. 46.

14. Developed in 1996 by Midwifery Task Force, www.midwiferytaskforce.org.

15. Developed in 1996 by the Coalition for Improving Maternity Services, www.mother-friendly.org.

"Ideals vs. Reality in U.S. Births"

from Citizens for Midwifery

	WHO Recommendations	**CIMS Suggestions**	**2004 U.S. Stats (4.1 million births)**
Birth Attendants	Midwives for normal pregnancy and birth	Access to professional midwifery care	Midwives 7.9% (325,000)
Place of Birth	Out-of-Hospital preferred	Where mother prefers	Hospitals 99.% (4.07 million)
Electronic Fetal Monitoring	Not routine	Not routine	No longer reported Last reported 85.%
Pain Relief Drugs in Labor	Not routine	Only for complications	80%*
Induction of Labor	10% or less	10% or less	21.2% (870,000)
Episiotomies (Vaginal Births)	Systematic use not justified	Goal of 5%	23.7%** (667,000)
Cesarean Rate	10–15%	10–15%	29.1% (1.19 million)
Breastfeeding After Birth	Immediately	WHO-UNICEF BFHI Guidelines	67%***

- *WHO Recommendations*–taken from a report on the *Appropriate Technology for Birth*, published by the World Health Organization in April, 1985.
- *CIMS Suggestions*–taken from *The Mother-Friendly Childbirth Initiative* from the Coalition for Improving Maternity Services (CIMS), 1996, www.motherfriendly.org. BFHI = Baby-Friendly Hospital Initiative.
- *2004 US Stats*–most taken from *Births: Final Data for 2004*, National Vital Statistics Report Vol. 55, No. 1, September 29, 2006 http://www.cdc.gov/nchs/data/nvsr/nvsr55/nvsr55_01.pdf.

No longer reported—In revising birth certificate reporting, NCHS no longer collects this information. Last reported rate (2003) is included here

Listening to Mothers Report, October 2002, p. 18
**"National Hospital Discharge Survey 2004: Advance Data," *Vital Health Statistics*, No. 371, May 5, 2006.
***Mothering Magazine*, No. 112, May/June 2002

"How Do Socioeconomic Factors Affect Disparities in Maternal Mortality?"

by Deborah Maine

Socioeconomic factors affect nearly every cause of death, but not always in the same ways. Understanding which components of socioeconomic development were responsible for the great declines in maternal mortality in the United States and Britain can help us design effective programs in developing countries. The literature shows that maternal mortality is most strongly influenced by women's access to medical care for complications of pregnancy. In addition to international disparities in maternal mortality, there are still great disparities among racial groups in the United States. Here, too, analysis of the factors at work may be helpful in tailoring interventions. (*JAMWA.* 2001;56:189–190)

Nearly every disease varies with socioeconomic status—among countries and among social groups within countries. But that does not mean that all causes of death are affected by the same factors. After all, socioeconomic status is composed of a variety of elements, including education, nutrition, income, social status, and access to medical care, that influence health and disease in different ways. Therefore, although infant and maternal mortality (MM) may both vary with socioeconomic status or stage of development, they may actually be affected by quite different forces. Examining historical patterns of mortality can help us identify which elements of socioeconomic status have the greatest influence on particular causes of death. This can, in turn, assist us in designing more effective programs to improve health.

Although maternal deaths are now very rare in developed countries, they are still everyday events in the developing world. More than half a million women die each year of complications of pregnancy and childbirth, 99% of them in developing countries. As Table 1 shows, MM ratios are estimated to be nearly 100 times higher in Africa than in North America. This is the greatest disparity between developed and developing countries of any commonly used public health indicator.

Clearly, MM shines a spotlight on the vast disparities in health between people in developing and developed countries. It also highlights some disparities in developed countries. For example, black women in the United States have had higher levels of MM than white women for as long as data have been available, and the gap widened during the 20th century.

One of the great truths of public health is that medical care is not the most important influence on the health status of populations. It was not an important factor in the steep decline in mortality in the 19th and early 20th centuries. Instead, improved living conditions in Europe and North America resulted in sustained and impressive declines in infant mortality long before medical technology to prevent or treat the major causes of death was developed. For example, there were more than 1200 deaths from measles among children in the United Kingdom in 1860. By 1940, the number of deaths had dropped to about 100, even though immunization was not introduced until decades later. Better food and

Area	Maternal Deaths, n	MM Ratios[†]
Africa	272 500	1006
Asia	217 000	276
Europe	2 200	28
North America	500	11
World	514 500	397

TABLE 1   Estimated Maternal Deaths and Maternal Mortality Ratios, Selected Regions and World, 1995*

*Data from Hill et al.
[†]Maternal deaths per 100 000 live births.

living conditions are presumed to have improved the ability of infants to survive infection.

In contrast, MM did not decline during this period. From 1840 (when the first MM statistics were available) to the mid-1930s, MM remained as high in Britain as it is today in many developing countries. This shows that nutrition, education, and general standard of living are not the major factors in MM. These factors had improved and are credited with causing the drastic declines in infectious diseases.

Then, after nearly a century of stagnation, MM declined so sharply that within 15 years it was no longer a major public health problem. This was largely because the technology to treat obstetric complications—including antibiotics (first sulfa drugs and then penicillin), banked blood, and safer surgical techniques—became available. In 1934, there were 441 maternal deaths per 100,000 births in England and Wales. By 1950, there were 87, and in 1960 there were only 39. Similar patterns are found in other European countries and in the United States, despite the great variety in patterns of care. For instance, in the United Kingdom, general practice physicians managed most deliveries, whereas in the Netherlands midwives played an important role, and the United States increasingly relied on obstetricians.

Not only was the decline in MM *not* the result of improvements in the general standard of living, but the usual relationship of mortality to social class was also reversed. For most causes, death is higher in disadvantaged groups. As Table 2 shows, in the early 1930s, the usual social class gradient was reversed in England and Wales, with the highest classes having the highest MM. In fact, this pattern persisted from at least the end of the 18th century through the early 20th century, although each time such statistics were published the reaction was usually "surprise bordering on disbelief."

The main explanation for this rare pattern is the practice of interventionist obstetrics among the physicians who delivered upper-class women. During the late 19th and early 20th centuries, for example, "the use of chloroform and forceps in ordinary domiciliary deliveries was often as high as 50% or even 70%." Consequently, at that time the death rate was higher among women delivered by physicians than among those delivered by midwives. As Table 2 shows, not only did the level of MM decline dramatically by the latter half of the 20th century, but the usual social class gradient was also restored.

Why spend so much time on the history of MM? Because much of it is relevant to present-day developing countries. Maternal deaths in developing countries are not caused by exotic conditions. They are caused by the same complications that were responsible for high levels of MM in now-developed countries. In fact, many women in industrialized countries still develop these complications, but very few die of them because they receive prompt, adequate treatment.

As Table 3 shows, hemorrhage, sepsis, and hypertensive disorders are still leading causes of MM in the United States. The major differences in causes between developed countries (represented here by the United States) and the world (composed mostly of developing countries) are in deaths from abortion, obstructed labor, and embolism. The availability of safe, legal abortion has virtually eliminated mortality from abortion complications. Unfortunately, in most developing countries abortion is either legally restricted or unavailable. There are almost no deaths from obstructed labor in the United States because almost all women deliver in medical facilities, where cesarean sections are readily available.

Thus, the literature strongly demonstrates that medical care—specifically, treatment of life-threatening

TABLE 2 Maternal Mortality by Social Class in England and Wales, 1930–1932 and 1979–1981*

Social Class	MMR, 1930–1932[†]	MMR, 1979–1981[‡]
1 & 2 (highest)	444	12
3	411	15
4 (or 4 & 5)	416	17
5	389	. . .
Worst/best ratio	1.14	1.42

*Data from Loudon and Turnbull et al.
[†]Maternal deaths per 100 000 births.
[‡]Maternal deaths per 100 000 legitimate, live births.

TABLE 3 Direct and Indirect Obstetric Deaths, by Cause: Global Estimates, 1993 and United States, 1987–1990*

Cause of Death	World 1993, %	United States 1987–1990, %
Hemorrhage	25	29
Embolism	[†]	20
Sepsis	15	13
Hypertensive disorders of pregnancy	12	18
Obstructed Labor	8	[†]
Unsafe abortion	13	[†]

*Data from WHO and Berg et al.
[†]Negligible.

complications—is the key to reducing MM in developing countries. Application of this knowledge varies, however. In many parts of the world, the first step is to make sure that care is available and accessible. Consider the example of cesarean section. Although this procedure is overused in some countries, it is necessary to save the lives not only of women with obstructed labor, but also of women with eclampsia and other complications. The World Health Organization and other agencies have estimated that 5% to 15% of deliveries should be done by cesarean section in order to preserve maternal and infant health.

In many countries in African and Asia, however, a sizeable proportion of government hospitals do not provide the full range of obstetric services. A study of 20 district hospitals in Bangladesh, for example, found that 6 of these hospitals had performed no cesarean sections at all during the previous year, even though each district had more than a million residents. Surveys have shown that the proportion of deliveries by cesarean section is well below the minimum in India (2.5%), Indonesia (4.3%), Morocco (2.0%), Nigeria (2.5%), and Pakistan (2.7%). The problem is especially serious in rural areas. For example, 5.7% of births among urban women in India in 1992-1993 were by cesarean section, compared to only 1.6% among women in rural areas, and MM ratios are much higher in rural areas.

In most countries, improving the availability of emergency obstetric care does not require building new hospitals or even increasing the ranks of health personnel. A substantial proportion of the need for emergency obstetric care could be met if existing facilities (such as district hospitals) functioned as they were meant to and if existing personnel were deployed more equitably. Furthermore, in some countries laws and regulations designed to "protect" women's health actually serve as barriers to health care. For example, in Morocco, general physicians are not permitted to perform surgery, even though many provincial hospitals do not have obstetricians. Similarly, in many countries midwives are not permitted to perform such critical functions as manual removal of retained placenta. For women who live far from functioning hospitals and experience postpartum hemorrhage, this can make the difference between life and death.

As noted earlier, racial disparities in MM are still a problem in the United States. As Table 4 shows, MM has been higher among nonwhite than white women in the United States since 1915 (the first year for which records exist), when the nonwhite/white MM ratio was 1.76. (This is higher than the gap between the lowest and highest classes in the United Kingdom, shown in

TABLE 4   Maternal Mortality Ratios in the United States, by Race, 1915–1990*

Year	Nonwhites[†]	Whites[†]	Nonwhite/ White Ratio
1915	1056.0	601.0	1.76
1930	1174.0	609.0	1.93
1945	455.0	172.0	2.65
1950	222.0	61.0	3.64
1990	26.7[‡]	6.5	4.11

*Data from USDHEW and Berg et al.
[†]Maternal deaths per 100 000 live births.
[‡]Data are for "black," not "nonwhite."

Table 2.) Moreover, as the 20th century progressed, the gap between races in the United States grew ever larger, until by 1990 the MM ratio was more than 4 times higher among black women than among white women.

The meaning of these data is not immediately clear. It might be that factors other than medical care are responsible for the racial disparity. For example, it might be due to a higher prevalence of risk factors (such as greater age or parity) among black women. However, a recent study found that these factors did not explain the racial difference. In fact, among women classified as high risk, black and white women had similar rates of death; it was among the low-risk women that the racial disparity was found. Furthermore, there was no major difference in leading causes of MM. Thus, health problems known to be more common in black women, such as heart disease, did not explain the difference. One can speculate that part of the racial disparity in the United States may be due to poorer quality of care for minorities, which has already been demonstrated for such conditions as congestive heart failure, pneumonia, and colorectal cancer.

Although MM generally reflects disparities in socioeconomic level, it does not automatically reflect women's status in the society, as the historical data from Britain (and the current low level of MM in Saudi Arabia) show. However, it does reflect women's access to treatment of obstetric complications. This, in turn, may provide us with insights into the values and priorities of a society. India, for example, has a vast medical system and a wealth of physicians, but large proportions of the population lack access to life-saving care for obstetric emergencies. And the fact that the racial disparity in MM in the United States not only persists, but has increased, is a national shame.

REFERENCES
A list of references is available in original source.

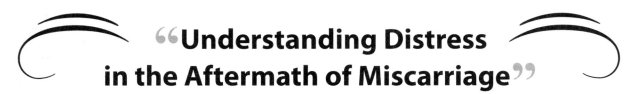

"Understanding Distress in the Aftermath of Miscarriage"

by Pamela A. Geller

Our culture typically associates pregnancy and childbirth with positive emotions and with motherhood, but this is not the case for all pregnancies or for all women. When a reproductive loss occurs, our society does not encourage women and their partners to discuss their experience, and in many cases even tends to minimize the loss.

Rates and Risk Factors

Miscarriage involves the spontaneous termination of an intrauterine pregnancy that results in fetal death. Although studies have varied widely in how they distinguish miscarriage from later reproductive loss, most studies define miscarriage as the unintended termination of pregnancy before 27 completed weeks of gestation.

Because many pregnancies end in miscarriage before the mother even knows she is pregnant, some estimates suggest that as many as 45 to 50 percent of all pregnancies end in miscarriage. Of clinically recognized pregnancies, however, 10 to 20 percent end in miscarriage. Risk appears to vary substantially by age; for example, rates are 9 percent for women age 20 to 24 years, but 75 percent for women older than 45. Stillbirth, defined as late fetal death with a fetus weighing more than 500 grams, has about a 1/1000 risk in singleton pregnancies and higher risk in multiple pregnancies.

Risk factors can be broadly classified as environmental (e.g., caffeine, nicotine and other drug use; toxins; electro-magnetic fields; stressful life events) or biological (e.g., genetic, including chromosomal abnormalities; endocrinologic; anatomic; immunologic; microbiologic).

Common Psychological Reactions

For many women, miscarriage constitutes an unanticipated, traumatic experience that can bring considerable physical pain and discomfort, and may even pose a serious threat to the life of the woman. Physiologically, miscarriage marks the end of a pregnancy, and psychologically, a myriad of reactions are possible, including sadness, distress, guilt, self-reproach, fear and even relief. Other typical responses can include loneliness; anger at oneself, family members, insensitive friends and often God; jealousy towards pregnant women or others with children; and physical sensations like tightness in the chest or hollowness in the stomach. When continued, these reactions can impact long-term adjustment and functioning. These include an intense "yearning" for the lost pregnancy and lost baby, and preoccupation with the loss.

Women who have miscarried may also be anxious about a number of issues, such as continued bleeding or discharge, possible underlying medical illness or genetic factors that may have contributed to the loss, and fears about their ability to carry a subsequent pregnancy to term. Anxiety symptoms may be even greater than depressive symptoms immediately post-miscarriage, and there may be an increased risk for posttraumatic stress disorder or a recurrent episode of obsessive-compulsive disorder.

Several issues make miscarriage a unique loss. First, it is usually untimely and unexpected; children are not expected to die before their parents. Miscarriage also is an "ambiguous loss" since it involves mourning what *would* have or *could* have been. Because the loss is early and the embryo has not fully developed, miscarriage is even less defined as a loss than is a stillbirth, neonatal or sudden infant death. Moreover, many social and legal definitions suggest that the fetus was never an actual human being. Regardless, it is still a baby in the mind of the parents.

Partner's Reaction

A severely neglected area of miscarriage research is that of the partner's reaction to the loss. To date, there had been little rigorous research addressing the impact on male partners, and no published research regarding the female partner's response in the case of lesbian couples. Initial uncontrolled studies suggest that although males may be affected by miscarriage, their depression and anxiety may be shorter-lasting than women's. In addition, they may have difficulty relating to their partner's intense emotional grief, their coping strategies may differ from those of women, and they may express their grief and distress somewhat differently. For example, men appear to cry less, want to talk less about the loss, express more anger, and attempt to cope by returning to work as soon as possible and using such maladaptive behaviors as substance use. Men who have seen an ultrasound scan of the living fetus may have greater difficulty coping and demonstrate greater despair compared to men who have not seen an ultrasound. Researchers hypothesize that men's coping difficulties are related to the demands of being the "comforter," compounded by feelings of inadequacy aroused by their inability to influence events while insufficiently attending to their own emotional response.

This emerging area of interest sorely needs systematic work that employs appropriate comparison groups and male as well as female partners of women who have miscarried, with greater numbers of lesbian couples making the decision to have children. In addition to addressing the female partner's responses to the loss itself (and how these responses may differ from those of male partners), researchers should also address other issues unique to lesbian couples (e.g., if the choice for one partner to conceive was made only after the other partner miscarried).

Societal Reactions

Society still sees miscarriage as an "unfortunate event," but one that is less tragic than the loss of a child. Women who have miscarried are often told that they can "try again," which suggests that the lost baby is interchangeable with another, something rarely expressed when an older child dies. Parents whose first child has died before birth are often not considered to be parents, making it more difficult to feel their grief is justified. In addition, this type of loss tends not to be socially legitimized or supported, as many people expect the grief to be mild and transient and do not understand that parents can grieve as intensely for a reproductive loss as for any other loss. For most parents, the relationship to the child begins long before birth, creating a host of expectations, hopes and feelings to grieve.

Since miscarriage involves a loss that often remains unknown to all but a woman's most intimate confidants and her health care providers, the grieving process may be compounded by limited social support and the challenge of managing feelings associated with the loss of a *potential* child. There are few memories and stories to share with others, so the parents are often isolated and may avoid social contact out of shame and others' discomfort. In addition, the mother may feel she has failed. Unlike other experiences that get easier to handle with

repetition, multiple miscarriages challenge coping resources to an even further degree.

Societal reactions may also differ by gender, with women's sense of self-identity more deeply affected than men's. Society pressures women, regardless of socioeconomic status, ethnic-racial status and religion, to view motherhood as our primary adult role. Violating these societal norms and expectations has both social and personal consequences. The stigma associated with childlessness involves social definitions of women as selfish, unfeminine, unnatural and inadequate—ideas that many women incorporate into their own self-concept.

Treatment Issues

Although supporters often struggle to find the "right thing to say," practically every empirical study has emphasized the *ability to listen over the ability to say something.* Speaking about loss aids in healing. To counteract the social negation of miscarriage, supporters should allow the parents to express their grief for what they lost individually, as a couple and as a family, regardless of the gestational age at loss. Because women may cope by socially isolating themselves, they need frequent reminders that someone is ready to listen and cares how they are feeling. Parents often require some validation and confirmation of the child's existence. They may need to remember and review their thoughts and feelings about the child from the very beginning of the pregnancy to make it seem real, and save mementoes or plan a farewell ritual to begin to feel some resolution. Additionally, since couples often attribute the miscarriage to something they have done, factual information about the probable cause of the miscarriage should be provided when possible.

Debate continues as to whether clinicians should advise women who have miscarried to try to conceive right away or to wait until their grief and depressive symptoms have resolved. Recent studies conclude that while women may be justifiably distressed or anxious during a subsequent pregnancy about the prospect of yet another loss, a subsequent pregnancy is in fact healing for many parents. Parents are encouraged to discuss their individual situation with their clinician and reach their own decision, particularly since a sense of choice and control is often a welcome relief in itself.

As a whole, little clinical attention has been paid to treating the grief and psychological distress associated with miscarriage, despite the fact that treatment in the early weeks after loss may help offset more serious psychological and psychiatric consequences. Since there is no systematic treatment protocol in place for women who have miscarried and their families, mental health referrals are varied and depend on the particular treating physician or hospital. This may be because health care providers generally have little understanding of the needs of these women and have limited training in grief counseling, along with time constraints and general discomfort with psychological issues. Compounding these issues is the reality that women who have miscarried often adopt a coping strategy of avoidance, further preventing them from receiving treatment.

Our national resource for information and support is SHARE: Pregnancy & Infant Loss Support Inc. (800-821-6819; www.nationalshareoffice.com).

REFERENCES
A list of references is available in the original source.

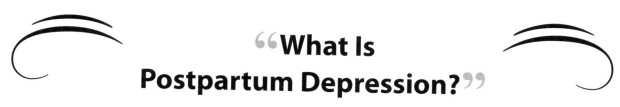

"What Is Postpartum Depression?"

by Leslie W. Tam

It's not what Andrea Yates, the Texas woman who drowned her five children, had. It appears that she was afflicted with postpartum psychosis, a much more severe postpartum illness. However, with the sensationalistic and often inaccurate media coverage that followed, it seems more important than ever to clarify what is meant by these often misunderstood disorders. The umbrella term "postpartum distress" or "PPD" actually refers to a range of postpartum mental disorders. These include the "baby blues," depression, anxiety and, in the worst cases, psychosis. Every woman who contemplates a pregnancy should be educated about the risks of these psychiatric complications and empowered to manage her particular situation with appropriate interventions.

Definitions

Most new mothers will experience the **"baby blues."** On the third or fourth day postpartum, 80 percent of women notice a brief period of mild weepiness, irritability and depressed mood. With the abrupt change in hormone levels once the baby and placenta are delivered, the baby blues are thought to be related to the biological changes taking place. Especially since they are so ubiquitous, the baby blues are considered a normal and self-limiting postpartum symptom, and their symptoms usually resolve within a week or two.

When the blues persist beyond two weeks or generalize to encompass sleep and appetite changes, frequent crying, disinterest in the infant or feelings of being overwhelmed, then the diagnosis is more likely to be major depression with postpartum onset. **Postpartum depression** occurs in 10 to 15 percent of new mothers and can actually have its onset at any time in the first postpartum year. Like the blues, postpartum depression is thought to be related to hormonal changes brought on by sleep deprivation, weaning and the resumption of the menstrual cycle. Prior or family history of depression also increases a woman's risk.

It is also common for **anxiety disorders**, such as panic disorder, generalized anxiety disorder or even obsessive-compulsive disorder (OCD), to present or recur in the postpartum period. Postpartum OCD is typically characterized by a mother's hypervigilance about possible harm to her baby, which then becomes a recurrent, unwanted thought or obsession. The mother may become compulsively protective of her infant to the extent that her functioning is impaired, or she may wish to avoid her baby or situations in which she fears she might do it harm.

The most serious and fortunately the most rare postpartum mental illness is **postpartum psychosis.** Unlike the other disorders, postpartum psychosis is thought to be primarily biologically based and related to hormonal changes in the immediate postpartum period.

Psychosis usually presents within a few day of giving birth, though there have been reports of later onsets. Women with underlying psychotic disorders are at heightened risk, but postpartum psychosis also can occur in women who seem to have no risk factors. The psychosis is most often an affective psychosis resembling acute mania. Affected women tend to have difficulty sleeping, are prone to agitation or hyperactivity, and intermittently experience delusions, hallucinations and paranoia.

Most concerning are psychotic thoughts that may include the wish to harm themselves or their infant. These symptoms wax and wane, making this disorder particularly difficult to diagnose. However, postpartum psychosis represents a medical emergency and usually requires hospitalization.

Risk Factors

Other factors that may play a role in the development of postpartum depressive or anxiety symptoms include an unexpected birth outcome, marital stress, lack of support and a troubled relationship between the new mother and her own mother. Mothers who have a traumatic or unsatisfying birthing experience also may blame themselves or feel that they have failed. Also, mothers who find themselves unable to breastfeed, for whatever reason, may experience disappointment or a sense of inadequacy.

The birth of a premature or severely compromised infant also can trigger symptoms; interestingly, however, the onset is usually after the baby's situation has been stabilized. It is as if the mother puts herself on hold to deal with the crisis of her severely ill newborn, and only when the crisis is over does she react to the psychological as well as biological stressors.

Marital or relationship stress can have a major role in the onset of postpartum symptoms in vulnerable women. The arrival of an infant tests a relationship in many ways. Fathers or partners can feel left out when an infant seems to monopolize the new mother's time and affections. Also, fathers or partners may have to take on more household responsibilities that the new mother may be unable to perform. Even in gay, lesbian or adoptive couples, this shift of responsibilities can breed resentment and foster discord.

By whatever means a woman becomes a parent, she will experience sleep deprivation, ambivalence and several other stressors that are part of the adjustment. New mothers require added support to meet the physical and emotional demands of parenthood; those who do not receive adequate support may be at risk for symptom development.

In my practice of reproductive psychiatry, I meet with couples before the baby arrives and help them consider the many types of assistance that may be needed: care for other children, house-cleaning, meal preparation, laundry, etc. In other cultures it is common for other women from the family, neighborhood or tribe to take over the new mother's responsibilities for the first 40 days or so after childbirth, freeing her to rest, recover and bond with her infant. Most western societies offer new mothers nothing of the sort!

What Postpartum Depression Isn't

In our society we operate under the assumption that new mothers can take care of their infants, continue to function in their previous roles and adjust in stride to all the changes that new motherhood brings. Many women I have treated sought help from their health care providers for what turned out to be postpartum depression but were told that their symptoms were a normal part of new motherhood, or that they would pass. Neither is true. Many women feel they are unable to live up to society's, their family's or their own expectations and so view themselves as having a character flaw or as just not trying hard enough. In reality, they are suffering from a postpartum illness that, when treated, resolves and allows them to return to their previous level of functioning. Attitudes and perceptions are extremely important in dealing with this population.

What Can Be Done?

In working with women with postpartum disorders, it has become clear to me that health care providers and others who advocate for greater awareness of postpartum mental health issues have a long way to go. The level of ignorance among providers about these disorders is astonishing. Several organizations work to educate the public and providers about these illnesses (see addenda). Education should also be a part of prenatal education. So many patients have told me they wish they had known that such illnesses were even a possibility.

We also need to empower women to make good decisions regarding their own health as well as that of their children. There are times, for instance, when it probably isn't advisable for a new mother to breastfeed. Even though advocates remind us that "breast is best," some women are too depressed, psychotic, fatigued or uncomfortable with their own bodies to breastfeed. Sometimes it is appropriate to treat pregnant or nursing mothers with medications, and yet many women are led to believe that no medications are safe. Yes, medication use can be risky for this group of women. However, it's best to weigh the risks and benefits to mother and baby of both the medication and the illness.

Despite the prevalence of postpartum disorders, there is no formal screening mechanism in the present standard of

U.S. health care. Very adequate screening questionnaires could be administered to new mothers at follow-up visits with obstetricians, at the pediatrician's office or in other systems that interface with them. It is encouraging to note that the U.S. House of Representatives passed a resolution (HR-163) to mandate screening for postpartum mental illness. However, it remains to be seen just how and when the screening will be implemented.

Recently, Rep. Bobby Rush (D-Illinois) introduced further legislation with the Melanie Stokes Postpartum Research and Care Act (HR-2380), which would appropriate more funding for postpartum research and treatment. The addendum lists a few organizations that provide further information about these disorders and that advocate for education and awareness.

As stated above, it is likely that Andrea Yates had a severe case of postpartum psychosis. In her confession, she stated that for weeks prior to the incident she believed that she was a terrible mother, that she had done irreparable harm to her children and that she should kill them to spare them further pain. These were clearly delusional thoughts. Fortunately, some of the media (see *Newsweek,* July 2, 2001) took the time to clarify the difference between depression and psychosis. Even so, I received several calls from depressed patients wondering if something like that might happen to them. All the more reason for the public and professionals to become informed about these serious and potentially dangerous disorders.

Selected References

Cox JL, Holden JM, Sagovsky R. "Detection of Postnatal Depression: Development of the 10 Item Edinburgh Postnatal Depression Scale." *British Journal of Psychiatry* 1987; 150: 782–86.

O'Hara M, Zekoski E. "Postpartum Depression: a Comprehensive Review." In R. Kumar and I. F. Brockington, Ed. *Motherhood and Mental Illness.* Wright, 1988; 17–63.

Miller LJ, ed., *Postpartum Mood Disorders*, American Psychiatric Press, 1999.

Sichel D and Driscoll JW, *Women's Moods: What Every Woman Must Know about Hormones, the Brain, and Emotional Health,*, William Morrow & Co., 1999.

Further Reading

This Isn't What I Expected, by Karen R. Kleiman, MSW and Valerie D. Raskin, MD, Bantam Books, 1994.

Mothering the New Mother, by Sally Placksin, Newmarket Press, 1994.

Postpartum Survival Guide, By Ann Dunneworld, PhD and Dian G. Sanford, PhD, New Harbinger Publications, 1994.

The Postpartum Husband, by Karen R. Kleiman, MSW, Xlibris Corporation, 2001.

Advocate Organizations

Postpartum Support Internationalat www.postpartum.net

Depression After Delivery, at: www.behavenet.com.

Formula for Profit
"How Marketing Breastmilk Substitutes Undermines the Health of Babies"

by Jennifer Coburn

Because of the strident societal and economic impact wielded by the formula industry, bottle-feeding has today become the social norm in the US. Fewer than half of all US babies are exclusively breastfed during their first day or two in the hospital. By the time they are six months old, only 19 percent of US babies receive any breastmilk, and only 2 percent of one year olds. Contrast this with the average age of weaning worldwide, which is 4.2 years. This country's societal hostility towards breastfeeding is such that many states have had to pass laws protecting a mother's right to breastfeed her child anywhere that she is otherwise permitted to be.

The very need for such legislation is a sad commentary on the lack of appreciation for the broad range of health, social, and environmental benefits of breastfeeding. Nevertheless, the slogan "breast is best" is no exaggeration. Breastmilk contains 400 nutrients that cannot be recreated in a laboratory, and several studies suggest that breastfeeding reduces the risk of sudden infant death syndrome. An absence of breastfeeding has been linked to an increased risk of hospitalization, childhood cancer, diarrheal diseases, lower respiratory illness, ear infections, bacterial infections, diabetes, infant botulism, Crohn's disease, ulcerative colitis, and even cavities. In *Milk, Money and Madness: The Culture and Politics of Breastfeeding,* Naomi Baumslag, MD, MPH, asserts that breastfed babies also have lower incidence of allergies, urinary tract infections, obesity, learning, behavioral and psychological problems, later-life heart disease, pneumonia, neonatal sepsis, and giardia infection.

Children are not the only ones who benefit from breastfeeding. Nursing mothers enjoy a reduced risk of premenopausal breast cancer, ovarian cancer, and osteoporosis. Breastfeeding is advantageous for people who are outside the mother-baby unit, when you consider healthier babies mean lower health insurance premiums for everyone, and lower absenteeism among working parents. The production of formula, bottles, plastic nipples, and formula cans, not to mention cleaning artificial feeding supplies—all create pollution and in some cases hazardous waste. Finally, breastmilk is also free and convenient, considerations that should give pause to families faced with an average yearly cost of $800 per baby if they choose to formula feed.

The economic implications of formula are certainly significant. The industry generates $5 to $6 billion in sales each year, and its executives reap huge profits—the CEO of Abbott Labs earns more than $4 million per year; his counterpart at Bristol-Myers Squibb (makers of Enfamil), nearly $13 million. Part of the reason the industry is so profitable is the fact that every dollar formula makers charge their retail distributions outlets costs them a mere 16 cents on production and delivery. Formula is, in short, big business—the result of a complex social marketing campaign that began half a century ago, one that has speciously managed to define artificial feeding as a convenient, liberating, and "modern" way of feeding one's infant.

Science Crushes Nature

"At the beginning of the 20th century, basically women breastfed, had a wet nurse or their babies died," says Mary Lofton, spokesperson for La Leche League International (LLLI). Insofar as artificial baby milk became available as a life-saving alternative to breastmilk, it was deemed a blessing. "The crucial social phenomenon," Lofton adds, "was the shift from home to hospital in childbirth. . . . Women were given anesthesia, babies were taken away, schedules were rigid, and all those interferences led to problems with breastfeeding."

Considering formula to be nutritionally equal to breastfeeding, doctors began recommending it to patients. Tangentially our society experienced a burgeoning captivation with science and technology, and became increasingly enamored with an efficiency-model of infant feeding and care. The advent of World War II encouraged women to work outside the home, which only furthered the reliance on artificial feeding. By the 1950s, infant formula gained the widespread endorsement of the pediatric community, and artificial feeding increasingly became seen as equal—if not superior—to nursing.

Marian Tompson, one of the founding mothers of LLLI, thinks the 1950s doctor acted out of ignorance. "I think anyone with half a brain would realize that human milk is species-specific," she says. "No one ever suggests that I feed my kittens with milk from the cocker spaniel next door." Nevertheless, with its decidedly scientific-sounding name, formula fit right into the landscape of an America mesmerized by the march of modernity, leisure, and ease. Measuring formula, sterilizing bottles, the modern mom became a domestic chemist. Bottle-feeding became a symbol of modern living, prosperity, and progress—indeed, healthful living! In contrast, breastfeeding took on the aspect of a primitive, retrograde thing to do.

The Role of the Medical Establishment

The campaign to normalize artificial feeding gains a great deal of its effectiveness from an unholy alliance between the pharmaceutical industry and the medical establishment. To promote artificial feeding, formula manufacturers spend millions of dollars securing exclusive distribution deals for formula samples, at a yearly average of $6,000 to $8,000 per doctor. They donate $1 million annually to the American Academy of Pediatrics in the form of a renewable grant that has already netted the AAP $8 million. The formula industry also contributed at least $3 million toward the building costs of the AAP headquarters.

The American College of Obstetrics and Gynecology received $548,000 from two of the four major formula makers in 1993. The American Medical Association television program is sponsored by the makers of Similac. Moreover, the American Dietetic Association, the National Association of Neonatal Nurses, and the Association of Women's Health, Obstetric and Neonatal Nurses all receive generous funding from the formula industry.

A 1994 study that was published in the *Journal of the American Medical Association* exposes the influence the formula industry wields over the medical establishment. "By giving physicians money," the authors found, "the [formula] companies are successful in influencing doctors to recommend their product."

Formula manufacturers play hardball to get hospital business. Take the example of Canada, where Mead Johnson secured an exclusive contract with Toronto's Women's College Hospital that pays the hospital $1 million the first year and $350,000 per subsequent year for a decade. Abbott Labs and Bristol-Myers Squibb got into a bidding war over the right to promote formula through Grace Hospital in Vancouver, Canada's largest birthing facility. Ross Labs offered to pay the Doctor's Hospital in Canada $1 million for a contract which would require that the hospital would give their product to all mothers in take home packages, supply breastfeeding mothers with Ross's instructions on nursing, and make sure mothers had "access" to Ross architectural services for nurseries.

Jack Newman, MD, author of *Dr. Jack Newman's Guide to Breastfeeding,* a book on the politics of formula use, characterizes the relationship between the pharmaceutical industry and medical establishment as bribery. From large donations to the "myriad of other little 'useful' items" such as pens, paper pads, measuring tape, growth charts, and coffee cups (all of which feature formula advertising), Newman considers these contributions wholly unethical.

Physical separation of hospital nurseries and maternity wards begin to erode the breastfeeding relationship right from the start. James McKenna, PhD, director of University of Notre Dame Mother-Infant Behavioral Sleep Laboratory, told me "Our studies of breastfeeding mother-baby pairs, where infants were about four months, reveal that proximity to mother, particularly the types of intimate contact that occur during bed-sharing that permit the infant to smell its mother's milk, doubles the amount of breastfeeding episodes, and triples the amount of nightly breastfeeding time."

Perhaps the most coveted payoff for formula makers, however, is the opportunity to exclusively distribute their products through hospital maternity wards. When a mother is released from a hospital or birthing center, she is often given a discharge gift basket that includes free formula. Research shows this tacit endorsement on the hospital's part is so effective in establishing brand loyalty that 93 percent of mothers who artificially feed continue using the brand of formula given to them by the hospital. Research suggest that exposure to formula advertising during pregnancy seriously undermines a future breastfeeding relationship.

Even more egregious than subjecting a mother to a barrage of formula advertising is veiling formula marketing as a form of health service, as the Nestle corporation has done. In past decades the company deployed sales staff, posing as "milk nurses," to promote artificial feeding to mothers in developing nations, compensating the sellers commensurate with the amount of artificial baby milk sold. To save money on the costly formula, mothers often diluted the mix. This on its own would have a deleterious, nutrition-depleting effect on the babies, but compounded with the lack of access to sterilized water, the use of formula in these countries led to many infant deaths. Formula use is still associated with the deaths of one and a half million children each year—both overseas and in the US.

Ross Laboratories' Mother's Survey

The formula industry's insistence on framing the debate on infant feeding even extends to their endeavor to collect and publish "national breastfeeding statistics." Barbara Heiser, executive director of the National Alliance for Breastfeeding Advocacy (NABA) says Ross Laboratories' role in tracking breastfeeding rates creates a conflict of interest. "We wouldn't ask the tobacco industry for statistics on lung cancer," she says. Daven Lee, a breastfeeding advocate and writer, says Ross is the only group that tracks national breastfeeding statistics—via a survey generated by their Marketing Department, and subsequently presented as unbiased research. "This way," Lee states, "Ross wins credibility and is cited as a resource in the media."

Clearly, Ross and other formula makers are competing not with each other, but with breastfeeding itself. In that light, breastfeeding mothers are caught in the crossfire. Heiser points out that mothers who purchase nursing pads often receive coupons for free formula. "Just recently a man was in renting a breast pump for his wife and he asked for two receipts because he could get a $10.00 coupon for formula with every breast pump rental receipt he sent in" to the formula makers, she remarks, an irony that lactation consultant and childbirth educator Linda Smith has also witnessed. "The breastfeeding mother gift packs companies give mothers," Smith says, "often contain breast pumps that are "uncomfortable and usually ineffective—along with bra pads and formula samples. These are very popular with mothers and nurses." And, for a new mom, sleep-deprived, and struggling to meet her baby's needs, tempting.

Indeed, an interesting inverted rationale exists whereby formula feeding is considered by some to be a pro-woman, even feminist practice. By aligning themselves with the feminist ideal of flexibility—including the freedom to return to work or to pursue personal interests—

the formula was originally embraced by the feminist movement. Marion Tompson says since then, however, "We've seen a total turnaround." In fact, she says, as far back as 1975 attorneys for the National Organization for Women (NOW) successfully fought to eliminate inquiries about a mother's breastfeeding status from the unemployment eligibility questionnaire. Prior to this, a nursing mother's commitment to finding employment was questioned and benefits could be denied.

More recently, women's groups have fought for public breastfeeding laws, unpaid time off to pump breastmilk, insurance coverage for lactation specialists, and the Family and Medical Leave Act, which allows a new mother to take a 12-week maternity leave without threat of losing her job. Not all of these measures were approved, but feminists signed on to every effort. So although formula makers are trying to link arms with the feminist movement, the courtship is arguably one-sided. In reality, it is extraordinarily paternalistic to withhold information from mothers about the profound inferiority of artificial feeding. Feminist ideals demand informed choice.

The WHO Code

The aggressive marketing of infant formula stands in direct conflict with the directives of the World Health Organization (WHO) and United Nations International Children's Education Fund (UNICEF), which jointly adopted an International Code of Marketing of Breastmilk Substitutes in 1981. The objective of the WHO Code is "to contribute to the provision of safe and adequate nutrition for infants, by the protection and promotion of breastfeeding and by the proper use of breastmilk substitutes, when these are necessary, on the basis of adequate information and through appropriate marketing and distribution." The code carries ten main provisions:

- No advertising of breastmilk substitutes
- No free samples of breastmilk substitutes to mothers
- No promotion of products through healthcare facilities
- No company-appointed "nurses" to "advise" mothers
- No gifts or personal samples to health workers
- No words or pictures idealizing artificial feeding, including pictures of infants, on the labels of the products
- Information to health workers should be scientific and factual
- All information on artificial feeding, including the labels, should explain the benefits of breastfeeding

and the costs and hazards associated with artificial feeding

- Unsuitable products, such as sweetened condensed milk, should not be promoted for babies
- All products should be of high quality and take into account the climatic and storage conditions of the country where they are used

Tompson, part of the group that drew up the guidelines in Switzerland, proposed that formula labels include health hazards of artificial feeding like the surgeon general's warning on cigarettes—a suggestion that the group, comprised of about 50 representatives of nongovernmental organizations (NGOs), as well as executives from the formula industry, rejected. Yet Tompson still thinks warning labels are a good idea. "Today when you see an ad on television for a drug, a soft voice lists all of the contraindications. . . . You don't hear that soft voice telling you all that can go wrong with formula," she adds. Nevertheless, the US' reluctance to sign onto the voluntary code—ten years after most other nations did—under-scores the fact that, however well intended, the WHO Code is as toothless as the infants it aims to benefit.

The Baby-Friendly Hospital Initiative

WHO and UNICEF have experienced greater breastfeeding promotion success with the Baby-Friendly Hospital Initiative (BFHI), established in 1991 to help hospitals and birthing centers create an environment that is conducive to breastfeeding. Resting on the foundation of the WHO Code and the Innocenti Declaration (a resolution prepared at an international breastfeeding conference for international policy makers in Innocenti, Italy, in 1990), the BFHI was drafted to encourage hospitals to educate mothers about the benefits of breastfeeding.

Although the ten criteria for baby-friendly status are easily attainable, the US lags behind: of 14,000 baby-friendly hospitals worldwide, only 23 are in the US, says Judy Lannon, project manager for the Baby-Friendly Hospital Initiative (BFHI). To earn this standing, a hospital "may not distribute gift packages to new mothers that contain formula" adds Lannon. The other requirements are that hospitals do the following:

- Have a written breastfeeding policy that is routinely communicated to all healthcare staff
- Train all healthcare staff in skills necessary to implement this policy
- Help mothers initiate breastfeeding within an hour of birth

- Show mothers how to breastfeed and how to maintain lactation, even if they should be separated from their infants
- Give newborn infants no food or drink other than breastmilk, unless medically indicated
- Practice "rooming in" by allowing mothers and infants to remain together 24 hours a day
- Encourage breastfeeding on demand
- Give no artificial teats, pacifiers, dummies, or soothers to breastfeeding infants
- Foster the establishment of breastfeeding support groups and refer mothers to them on discharge from the hospital or birthing center

Seventy-five US hospitals are currently holding "certificates of intent," meaning they are preparing to be reviewed for BFHI status in the near future. Lannon says that if a hospital fails to meet the criteria the first time, they are given recommendations and urged to reapply. There is no limit on how many times a hospital may apply, she adds.

In other nations, the BFHI has led to tremendous breastfeeding successes. In Chile, only 4 percent of infants were exclusively breastfed in 1985. By 1991, less than one year after the BFHI was launched, the rate had risen to 25 percent. Six years after Cuba adopted the BFHI, the rate of mothers who were breastfeeding at the time of hospital discharge jumped from 63 percent to 98 percent. In Iran, it took only five years for the rate of exclusively breastfeed infants to rise from 10 to 53 percent. China experienced comparable success: 6,300 hospitals reached baby-friendly status by 1996, along with regulations on the marketing of formula. A 1994 survey found that in just two years, breastfeeding rates increased from 10 percent to 48 percent for infants in urban areas; it rose from 29 percent to 68 percent in rural areas.

The Tobacco Connection

The formula industry's marketing tactics have been likened to big tobacco companies that give away free samples, and place their products in popular movies and television shows, while denying that their products are addictive. Likening formula marketing to tobacco marketing is an argument that gains credibility when one considers that 4,000 babies worldwide die every day because they are not breastfed. (According to the American Lung Association, 1,180 people die from smoking-related illnesses every day in the US.) Many Americans falsely believe that the alarming number of formula-related infant deaths is solely due to unsanitary water and overdilution in developing nations. But formula

feeding increases babies' health risks everywhere. In the US, four of every 1,000 infants born die because they are not breastfed. Healthcare savings would reach an estimated $2 to $4 billion annually if every child in the US were breastfed for as little as three months.

Smith says that there are some similarities in marketing formula and tobacco, but she's not sure the two are parallel. A significant difference, she believes, is that "there is a limited need for formula for some babies and mothers." In her work as a lactation consultant, Smith says she sees one case about every few years where "a loving and wonderful mother tries absolutely everything and she simply isn't able to breastfeed." Although formula does serve an important function for a small minority of children, it is clear that formula makers have every baby in their sights as they wage their aggressive marketing efforts. And the vast majority of mothers who experience insurmountable obstacles to breastfeeding have simply been failed by the medical establishment. Like prescription drugs, formula should be administered judiciously.

Formula Recalls

Artificial milk's health risks to young children are only compounded by the frequent occurrence of product recalls, of which there were 22 "significant" ones between 1982 and 1994. Seven of these were classified as Class I, potentially life threatening. Salmonella contamination, vitamin deficiencies, and bacterial contamination were among the most serious health risks, with the presence of glass particles from bottle chipping among the less serious, but not negligible, offenses.

In 1999, 120,000 cans of Mead Johnson's ProSobee formula were recalled for labeling errors after a parent called the company to inquire why the product smelled strange. It was discovered that cans labeled as infant formula contained, in fact, Vanilla Sustacal—an adult nutritional supplement that, if consumed by infants, could lead to what the Mead Johnson Corporation itself calls "severe medical problems." The formula in question was shipped to stores at least six months prior to the recall.

Nevertheless, Mead Johnson termed the recall an "extra precautionary" measure. Wouldn't extra precaution be to have caught the labeling error before the formula left the factory and spent half a year on supermarket shelves? We will never know how many mothers fed their babies the defective product, threw away the can, and later had no idea why their infants became ill.

Dr. Derrick Jelliffe, in a 1980 interview with the *Wall Street Journal,* characterizes the history of formula production as "a succession of errors." He adds, "Each stumble is dealt with and heralded as yet another breakthrough, leading to further imbalances and then more modifications."

The Food and Drug Administration (FDA) fact sheet on formula, titled the "Overview of Infant Formulas," maintains that "the composition of commercial formula is carefully controlled and the FDA requires that these products meet very strict standards." Further, the document boasts that the quality of formula is "ensured" by the Infant Formula Act, a law which gives the FDA authority to create and enforce formula production standards. This is a bold—and grossly inaccurate—statement about a product that has a track record of health-threatening production errors.

The Infant Formula Act was signed into federal law in 1980 after deficient formula hit the market and caused infant deaths, says Baumslag. Realizing that there were no guidelines to oversee formula production, Congress introduced this law and gave the FDA authority to set the standard for—and monitor—formula production.

But however well intended the Infant Formula Act may have been when introduced, it has not prevented significant health risks in formula production. In fact, in standardizing production methods, the IFA did not account for which ingredients were healthiest for infants. It simply considered which were most commonly used. This forced several smaller companies with alternative, perhaps healthier, ingredients out of the market. The legislation created an opportunity for major pharmaceutical companies to dominate formula sales.

How to Reverse the Trend

If doctors or parents ever had any questions about the cause and effect relationship between formula marketing and declining breastfeeding rates, they now can reference the first randomized, controlled study investigating the issue. Recently published by the *Journal of Obstetrics and Gynecology,* the "Office Prenatal Formula Advertising and Its Effects on Breastfeeding Patterns" concludes that prenatal exposure to formula advertising "significantly increased early termination of breastfeeding." Women who did not receive direct marketing materials from formula makers were more successful at maintaining the breastfeeding relationship.

The American Academy of Pediatrics policy on breastfeeding, which was revised in 1997, is "a huge step in the right direction," adds Smith. She says, "It shows that the AAP is now solidly on board with breastfeeding." The statement encourages doctors to learn more about human lactation and promote breastfeeding as the optimal source of nutrition for babies. It also made headlines by encouraging women to breastfeed for a minimum of one year. Smith adds that over the last five years she's also seen an emergence of lactation consultants in pediatric offices, another indication that the medical community is moving in the right direction. Still, this leaves the question of the economic ties between the medical establishment and formula makers.

The social marketing campaign launched by the formula industry has been a successful one, but this doesn't mean the trend is irreversible. The US can return to being a breastfeeding culture if healthcare providers, policy makers, and families make it a national priority. First, the medical establishment must financially disentangle itself from formula makers. The WHO Code must be enforced, and artificial baby milk must not be marketed through medical facilities. Second, birthing centers and hospitals should strive to meet the criteria of the BFHI and create a setting that is conducive to breastfeeding. Distribution deals and formula promotion in medical settings must cease because when mothers receive formula samples from trusted health providers, they assume artificial feeding offers health benefits, instead of considering the risks associated with infant formulas. The medical community has an ethical obligation not to violate their patients' trust or compromise their health for economic gain.

Finally, our entire culture must support breastfeeding. All workplaces should be equipped with lactation stations. Health insurance ought to provide coverage for lactation consulting. And no woman should ever be chided for breastfeeding in public or "too long." Then our culture will not just say breast is best. We'll act like it.

REFERENCES
A list of references is available in the original source.

Why the Precautionary Principle?

"A Meditation on Polyvinyl Chloride (PVC) and the Breasts of Mothers"

by Sandra Steingraber

Those of you who know me know that when I talk on these topics I usually speak out of two identities: biologist and cancer activist. My diagnosis with bladder cancer at age 20 makes more urgent my scientific research. Conversely, my Ph.D. in ecology informs my understanding of how and why I became a cancer patient in the first place: bladder cancer is considered a quintessential environmental disease. Links between environment and public health became the topic of my third book, *Living Downstream*, but since I have been given the task of speaking about the effect of toxic materials on future generations, I'm going to speak out of another one of my identities—that of a mother.

I'm a very new mother. I gave birth in September 1998 to my daughter and first child. So, I'm going to speak very intimately and in the present tense. You know it's a very powerful thing for a person with a cancer history to have a child. It's a very long commitment for those of us unaccustomed to looking far into the future. My daughter's name is Faith.

I'm also learning what all parents must learn, which is a new kind of love. It's a love that's more than an emotion or a feeling. It's a deep physical craving like hunger or thirst. It's the realization that you would lay down your life for this eight-pound person without a second thought. You would pick up arms for them. You would empty your bank account. It's love without boundaries and were this kind of love directed at another adult, it would be considered totally inappropriate. A kind of fatal attraction. Maybe, when directed at babies, we should call this "natal attraction."

I say this to remind us all what is at stake. If we would die or kill for our children, wouldn't we do anything within our power to keep toxics out of their food supply? Especially if we knew, in fact, there were alternatives to these toxics?

Of all human food, breast milk is now the most contaminated. Because it is one rung up on the food chain higher than the foods we adults eat, the trace amounts of toxic residues carried into mothers' bodies become even more concentrated in the milk their breasts produce. To be specific, it's about 10 to 100 times more contaminated with dioxins than the next highest level of stuff on the human food chain, which are animal-derived fats in dairy, meat, eggs, and fish. This is why a breast-fed infant receives its so-called "safe" lifetime limit of dioxin in the first six months of drinking breast milk. Study after study also shows that the concentration of carcinogens in human breast milk declines steadily as nursing continues. Thus the protective effect of breast feeding on the mother appears to be a direct result of downloading a lifelong burden of carcinogens from her breasts into the tiny body of her infant.

When it comes to the production, use, and disposal of PVC (polyvinyl chloride), the breasts of breast-feeding mothers are the tailpipe. Representatives from the vinyl industry emphasize how common a material PVC is, and they are correct. It is found in medical products, toys, food packaging, and vinyl siding. What they don't say is that sooner or later all of these products are tossed into the trash, and here in New England, we tend to shovel our trash into incinerators. Incinerators are de facto laboratories for dioxin manufacturer, and PVC is the main ingredient in this process. The dioxin created by the burning of PVC drifts from the stacks of these incinerators, attaches to dust particles in the atmosphere, and eventually sifts down to Earth as either dry deposition or in rain drops. This deposition then coats crops and other plants, which are eaten by cows, chickens and hogs. Or, alternatively, it's rained into rivers and lakes and insinuates itself into the flesh of fish. As a breast-feeding mother, I take these molecules into my body and distill them in my breast tissue. This is done through a process through which fat globules from throughout my whole body are mobilized and carried into the breast lobes, where, under the direction of a pituitary hormone called prolactin, they are made into human milk. Then, under the direction of another pituitary hormone called oxytocin, this milk springs from the grape-like lobes and flows down long tubules into the nipple, which is a kind of sieve, and into the back of the throat of the breast-feeding infant. My daughter.

So, this, then, is the connection. This milk, my milk, contains dioxins from old vinyl siding, discarded window blinds, junked toys, and used I.V. bags. Plastic parts of buildings that were burned down accidentally are also housed in my breasts. These are indisputable facts. They are facts that we scientists are not arguing about. What we do spend a lot of time debating is what exactly are the health effects on the generation of children that my daughter belongs to. We don't know with certainty because these kids have not reached the age at which a lot of diseases possibly linked to dioxin exposure would manifest themselves. Unlike mice and rats, we have long generational times. We do know with certainty that childhood cancers are on the rise, and indeed they are rising faster than adult cancers. We don't have any official explanation for that yet.

Let me tell you something else I've learned about breast feeding. It's an ecstatic experience. The same hormone (oxytocin) that allows milk to flow from the back of the chest wall into the nipple also controls female orgasm. This so-called let-down reflex makes the breast feel very warm and full and fizzy, as if it were a shaken-up Coke bottle. That's not unpleasant. Moreover, the mouths of infants—their gums, tongues, and palates—are perfectly designed to receive this milk. A newborn's mouth and a woman's nipple are like partners in a tango. The most expensive breast pump—and I have a $500 one—can only extract about half of the volume that a newborn baby can because such machines cannot possibly imitate the intimate and exquisite tonguing, sucking, and gumming motion that infants use to extract milk from the nipple, which is not unpleasant either.

Through this ecstatic dance, the breast-fed infant receives not just calories, but antibodies. Indeed the immune system is developed through the process of breast feeding, which is why breast-fed infants have fewer bouts of infectious diseases than bottle-fed babies. In fact, the milk produced in the first few days after birth is almost all immunological in function. This early milk is not white at all but clear and sticky and is called colostrum. Then, from colostrum you move to what's called transitional milk, which is very fatty and looks like liquid butter. Presumably then, transitional milk is even more contaminated than mature milk, which comes in at about two weeks post-partum. Interestingly, breast milk is so completely digested that the feces of breast-fed babies doesn't even smell bad. It has the odor of warm yogurt and the color of French mustard. By contrast, the excretions of babies fed on formula are notoriously unpleasant.

What is the price for the many benefits of breast milk? We don't yet know. However, one recent Dutch study found that schoolchildren who were breast fed as babies had three times the level of PCBs[*] in their blood as compared to children who had been exclusively formula fed. PCBs are probably carcinogens. Why should there be any price for breast feeding? It should be a zero-risk activity.

If there was ever a need to invoke the Precautionary Principle—the idea that we must protect human life from possible toxic danger well in advance of scientific proof about that danger—it is here, deep inside the chest walls of nursing mothers where capillaries carry fat globules into the milk-producing lobes of the mammary gland. Not only do we know little about the long-term health effects of dioxin and PCB exposure in newborns, we haven't even identified all the thousands of constituent elements in breast milk that these contaminants might act on. For example, in 1997 researchers described 130 different sugars unique to human milk. Called oligosaccharides, these sugars are not digested but function instead to protect the infant from infection by binding tightly to intestinal pathogens. Additionally, they appear to serve as a source of sialic acid, which is essential to brain development.

So, this is my conclusion. Breast feeding is a sacred act. It is a holy thing. To talk about breast feeding versus bottle feeding, to weigh the known risks of infectious diseases against the possible risks of childhood or adult cancers is an obscene argument. Those of us who are advocates for women and children and those of us who are parents of any kind need to become advocates for uncontaminated breast milk. A woman's body is the first environment. If there are toxic materials from PVC in the breasts of women, then it becomes our moral imperative to solve the problem. If alternatives to PVC exist, then it becomes morally imperative that we embrace the alternatives and make them a reality.

"The Mother's Milk Project"

from *Undivided Rights: Women of Color Organize for Reproductive Justice*

The Mother's Milk Project underlines the centrality of women's bodies and birthing in Native American culture. A woman's body is seen as the first environment and is not separable from the external environment.[1] With this understanding, reproductive rights struggles are part of struggles for sovereignty and land. Degrading the health of mothers and their children is organically connected to the degradation of Native lands. Protesting against General Motors for leaving behind a Superfund site[2] that has "tainted the land, water and ultimately the bodies of the Mohawk people, their babies included"[3] is thus a reproductive rights struggle. For Native American women, environmental justice and reproductive rights struggles intertwine in the body of each woman.

A community of about 8,000 Mohawk lives in Akwesasne—"land where the partridge drums."[4] This 25-square-mile reservation, also known as the St. Regis Mohawk Reservation, is located along the St. Lawrence River (Kariatarowaneneh, or "majestic river," in Mohawk) and the international border between northern New York and Canada. Akwesasne is well watered, thickly forested, and had some of the largest runs of sturgeon, walleyed pike, and bass in northeastern North America until the opening of the St. Lawrence Seaway in the late 1950s. At that time industries came to the region because of cheap power and easy access to both the Atlantic Ocean and the American heartland. Many corporations, like Reynolds Metals, General Motors, and Alcoa, came for the rich raw material resources. They stripped the land, operated manufacturing plants that used polychlorinated biphenyls (PCBs), dumped thousands of pounds of PCBs into the St. Lawrence, and poured toxic substances from their unfiltered smoke-stacks.[5] This industrial pollution has severely contaminated the land, air, and water and led to the discontinuation of a way of life for the Mohawk.

Akwesasne is also the home of Katsi Cook, a Mohawk woman and Native women's health activist. Katsi organized the Women's Health Dance Program and the Mother's Milk Project (MMP), two overlapping and related initiatives that promote Native sovereignty through Native women asserting control over the birthing process. Her projects are the focus of this chapter.

"I was born to a Mohawk woman from a reservation across the St. Lawrence River from Montreal, Kahawague, by the rapids,"[6] writes Katsi. Katsi describes growing up on the reservation as being "colonized"— her education in Christian schools undermining her connection to her own culture. As a young adult, Katsi began her personal process of decolonization as she rediscovered the customs and traditions of her people. A major turning point for Katsi was when, as a teenager, she attended her first traditional Women's Dance in Akwesasne. The structure and nature of the dance raised many questions for Katsi about women's roles and women's culture in her community. Most importantly, Katsi wanted to know why only women danced in this ritual. Katsi's first Women's Dance experience set her on a lifelong quest to realize who she was as a Native woman and to help other Native women make similar discoveries.

Katsi came to learn that Native women express their identity and connection to their culture through dance. Every aspect of the Long House women's dance she witnessed was invested with symbolic meaning. For example, in the shuffle, the dancers' feet never leave the ground, expressing the indivisible tie between women and Mother Earth. With their feet firmly on the ground, the women are reminded to live by the laws that govern this sacred relationship and of their responsibility to provide food, clothing, and shelter. Men do not participate in this particular dance but attend it to honor the women. In addition to being a tool for cultural education and social interaction, in Mohawk culture dance is recommended as a treatment for many ailments.[7] Thus, through traditional dance, women can heal themselves as well as find their identity and oneness with their culture and people. Katsi says, "Seeing traditional ways of thinking was a huge revolution for me as a colonized woman . . . [in] every part of my life."[8]

As a young woman, Katsi was familiar with the mainstream women's movement and some of its leading figures, among them Gloria Steinem and Betty Friedan.

She was intrigued by these feminists and their assertion of greater power and visibility for women; the issues raised by second wave feminists informed the questions she asked about the women's dances. However, in larger part, she did not find their gendered critiques of society pertinent to her life. The discrimination faced by her people as indigenous people was her primary concern.

Katsi was more deeply influenced by the Red Power Movement's commitment to self-determination and freedom from oppression than by the growing feminist movement.[9] In 1977, leaders of the Iroquois nation, including John Mohawk and Jeannie and Audrey Shenandoah, gathered to define for indigenous people of North America the meaning of sovereignty. Their definition included control over six key areas of life: land base, jurisprudence, education, psycho-religious life (including language restoration), and control over both production (the productive resources of the community) and reproduction. Katsi selected from the mainstream feminist movement what was useful to her and applied it in her efforts to address how Native women could simultaneously address issues of Native women's oppression and Native sovereignty.

Midwifery and Native Sovereignty: Rebirthing the Nation

As the daughter of a midwife, Katsi understood the role and tradition of the midwife as the key intersection of feminism and sovereignty and a space for critical activism that could affect both individuals and society. Committed to principles of Native sovereignty, Katsi believed that traditional midwives had an essential role to play in the rebirthing of the Nation. For Native Americans to control the destiny of their people, Native women had to be in charge of birth and death, "the most joyful and most terrifying moments in life . . . Without taking control over our lives, starting with the birthing process, we would simply be wards of the state."[10]

Thus, Katsi set forth to study midwifery in the Women's Health Training Program at the University of New Mexico and graduated in 1978 as a health specialist. She also attended a Planned Parenthood program that trained women specialists to run reproductive service clinics in underserved areas. As a fourth generation traditional *Kanienkehaka*[11] (midwife), Katsi incorporates traditions passed down through her lineage—especially from her grandmother, a noted Mohawk midwife—into her practice.

Mohawk midwifery, says Katsi, involves more than just helping women through labor. She speaks of the deep connection between childbirth and the land:

Everything we know in midwifery we learned from the corn. All our knowledge comes from the corn, and inside of each kernel of corn is many generations of knowledge. Part of my training as an aboriginal traditional Mohawk midwife was to raise fields of our original corn. The songs, the ceremonies that go with the growing of corn in the field also have to do with the gestation of the human baby, and so the corn plays a big part in the birth process also, and is also a good-quality protein when mixed with beans for the mother to eat.[12]

From her elders, Katsi learned that the mother is the first environment every human being experiences. A baby inside a woman's body sees through the mother's eyes and hears through the mother's ears:

At the time of the child's birth it is greeted by its family and is identified with the events that occur in the natural world at the time of its emergence from its mother's womb. At the breasts of women, the generations are nourished. From the bodies of women flows the relationship of those generations both to society and to the natural world. In this way the earth is our mother, grandma says. In this way, we as women are earth.[13]

According to the Mohawk, women need to be reawakened to the power that is inherent in the transformative birth process. Katsi talks about the excitement of seeing how a young woman working with her midwife can learn how to become self-determining. She explains that learning to make responsible decisions about their fertility enables women to make other important decisions in their lives and ultimately to become decision makers in their community.

Fundamentally, Katsi's work on birthing and women's health is also based on the belief that Native women must become whole again; as colonized women, they must find their cultural roots. For Katsi, these cultural roots include various Native traditions and conceptions of self and community. She believes that the relationship of trust and respect between a woman and her midwife empowers the woman to ask questions and obtain the information she needs to make real choices about her health and life. Furthermore, for a Native woman, making the right decisions for herself means that she also makes them for her people, because there is no strong separation between the individual and the society. People trust and respect women and the decisions that they must make, knowing that what is best for a woman is also best for her community. Thus, the concepts of society and self, when infused with honor and respect, are mutually reinforcing rather than dichotomous. Native women do not have to choose between Native sovereignty and self-determination; they are one and the same.

Working With Women of All Red Nations

After completing her training in New Mexico, Katsi followed the Mohawk tradition of practicing healing in other Native communities before returning to her own people.[14] In 1978, she went to the Dakotas, a center of American Indian Movement (AIM) activism, where she attended the founding meeting of Women of All Red Nations (WARN) in Rapid City. WARN women felt they could organize more effectively in a traditional sex-segregated social environment, which they saw as a political equivalent of traditional Native women's societies. WARN was committed to ensuring sovereign nation status for Native peoples and asserting control over their own affairs, without the interference of the US government. WARN believed that by embracing traditional culture, the ravages of colonialism could be remedied. As Phyllis Young, a co-founder of WARN, explains:

> What we're about is drawing on our traditions, regaining our strength as women in the ways handed down to us by our grandmothers and their grandmothers before them. Our creation of an Indian women's organization is not a criticism or division from our men . . . Only in this way can we organize ourselves as Indian women to meet our responsibilities, to be fully supportive of the men, to work in tandem with them as partners in a common struggle for the liberation of our people and our land . . . So, instead of dividing away from the men, what we are doing is building strength and unity in a traditional way.[15]

For WARN, struggles for Native sovereignty against the violation of treaty rights included opposition to sterilization abuse, the loss of children to extra-tribal adoption, the theft of Native lands, and the incarceration of Indians as political prisoners. WARN publicized the issue of sterilization abuse among Native women. While Katsi recognized the importance of sterilization abuse, she was also concerned about the issues underlying Native women's powerlessness.

Katsi saw that the lack of knowledge about their bodies led to a lack of control over their reproductive health. In New Mexico, she witnessed the banning of community-based and traditional Native American approaches to health and health care. The devaluation of Native approaches by white society caused Native communities to lose faith in their ability to take care of themselves.[16] For example, in the year that Katsi did her clinical training among the Navajo people she saw the terrible scars women bore from unnecessary cesarean sections that suited the convenience of the providers. She was dismayed to see how little women knew about their own health and, consequently, how powerless they were to challenge such practices. She became convinced that Native American activists had to go beyond taking the federal government to task for the abuses it perpetrated. In Katsi's view, for real change to occur, Native women needed to take responsibility for the birthing process. Community-controlled health care was essential if Native women were going to reassert political control over their lives

Reclaiming Health Through Culture

WARN members were impressed and inspired by Katsi's knowledge of midwifery and her commitment to the principles of Native sovereignty. They asked her to set up a clinic at the Red Schoolhouse in Minnesota to teach midwifery, investigate sterilization practices, and pioneer culturally appropriate health care, so that Native women would not be vulnerable to the abuses of inadequate and manipulative government health programs. Hence, the Women's Dance Health Program (DHP), initiated in 1979 as a project of the WARN Youth Program and based in Minneapolis/St. Paul, was dedicated to placing health care back in Native hands. Under Katsi's leadership, the program trained women to assist in birthing the traditional way. Once the women were trained, they became members of a Birthing Crew.

Native children, Katsi said, were "taught to be submissive, empty and have no identity."[17] The DHP worked with other regional organizations to implement healing practices for the sexual and mental health of children who had been educated in boarding schools. When Katsi left Minneapolis, the project was adopted by the Oneida of Wisconsin. Since 1980, other Native women dedicated to reproductive health care issues have focused their efforts on regaining knowledge of traditional practices and reclaiming traditional midwifery. Several Native American groups now work to promote reproductive health in their communities, providing culturally appropriate health education and services that give people knowledge so they can make their own choices about their health.

Organizing in Akwesasne

When Katsi returned to Akwesasne in 1980, the Native sovereignty movement was strong: 23 Iroquois leaders were under indictment for their political militancy, and a US military encampment had been set up at Akwesasne to contain the political situation. The Akwesasne

Freedom School, founded by Mohawk parents in 1979 to ensure the survival of their language and culture, demonstrated the commitment of the community to the principles of sovereignty. Akwesasne was also located in close proximity to a General Motors site that posed a serious environmental threat to the Mohawk. In this political context, Katsi introduced the DHP in Akwesasne.[18]

One of the first initiatives of the DHP was to train a Birthing Crew at Akwesasne. Crew members set out to "organize the families and the women to recover birth as the way to keep our people strong, to give our children a sense of community."[19] To build trust among community members, the crew offered prenatal classes and examinations, individual case counseling, and home births. Katsi reports:

> Birthing takes place primarily in our homes, often with children and relatives present. In this situation we find ourselves not building a long list of "clients" or "patients," but creating a web of family relationships which serves to further our goals in the natural course of community life.[20]

Providing midwifery services was the nucleus around which other Akwesasne community health programs grew. Katsi's programs at Akwesasne provide one-on-one woman-based health education—a goal of many other contemporary Native women's health programs. The DHP created a safe space that fosters trust between caregiver and patient—an essential part of providing Native women with the opportunity to make informed health decisions and, in doing so, realize their reproductive rights.[21]

A Ms. Foundation grant enabled the DHP to recruit more women to its well-trained Birthing Crew, to provide community health education, and to make resources on family health available to the community. As Katsi explains:

> Education is the most important work of the Women's Dance Health Project at Akwesasne. We now have available two basic kits for Birthing Crew use. One is an educational kit for midwifery skills and "patient education." This kit includes a pelvic model complete with fetus, cord, and placenta to demonstrate position, lie, and attitude of the fetus. It includes such items as the maternity center's birth atlas and disposable plastic speculums for demonstration of the pelvic exam—particularly useful for mothers who have never visualized a cervix . . . [The] videotapes, *1000 Births* and *Common Complications of Labor and Delivery*, are especially useful. Slides, charts, and information packets make up the remainder of the kit. It is in a portable trunk, and can be carried or loaned to workshops or conferences quite easily.

> The birthing kit includes all the equipment and supplies necessary for prenatal, birthing, and postpartum care. Because of the expense of critical items and the need for adaptability and versatility in rural areas (and in some cases even the deep woods!), the birthing kit has been put together with an eye towards portability and professional quality, and in keeping our birthing up to standards.[22]

Katsi served as project director for the DHP from 1983 to 1989. In 1989, Beverly Cook, a licensed nurse and former director of the Akwesasne emergency team, was hired on a part-time basis to serve as a liaison between the program and tribal organizations. Beverly facilitated a series of workshops and training sessions for the Birthing Crew and assisted with prenatal, birthing, and postpartum care. Other women, such as Priscilla Thompson and Niddie Thompson Cook from the Birthing Crew, trained for and also became involved in other aspects of the program.

Birthing Crew members included clan mothers who attended the home births of their relatives. Mothers brought their daughters and daughters-in-law for prenatal care or counseling. Teenagers who had taken the fertility awareness classes offered by the DHP were also involved in the program's activities. This high level of community engagement was an indicator of the need for health care and education. To develop this work further, group members organized conferences and training activities for health care providers in the region. A few doctors and practitioners also led trainings and workshops on the reservations. Dr. Nic Drouet and his wife Françoise, a French couple who visited Akwesasne, even supplied much-needed medical equipment to the Dance Health Program.

The Birthing Crew communicated with tribal programs and service organizations in the area to improve the quality of services they offered. They discussed their perspectives on Indian health issues with staff from the IHS. They reached out to other lay midwives and alternative birthing organizations in New York State through their participation in health conferences and networked with other Native women's groups and health projects. At the Awasis Atoskewin (working with children) conference in Regina, Saskatchewan, Katsi acquainted hospital staff and program directors with traditional Native values regarding maternal and infant health care. These conferences provided her with an opportunity to share this traditional knowledge with urban Iroquois women.

National and International Networking

In 1980, Katsi was invited to join the board of the National Women's Health Network (NWHN). She notes:

> It mattered a great deal to have respect and be given a seat at predominantly non-Native meetings—the NWHN was a wonderful time for me. [It] trained the community agent to see the bigger picture. Those women were wonderful. They invited me to speak at conferences about midwifery and helped me to work through our [Native American] pain.[23]

Through the NWHN, Katsi was introduced to both the national and the international women's health movements. For example, she learned about the work that Byllye Avery was doing on midwifery at the Birthing Center and became acquainted with important information and materials that enriched her own work. She feels this exposure to broader issues was invaluable: "I began to learn about community movements outside the tribe, which is very important as tribes have a different process."[24] She was also able to advocate on behalf of other Native women and to share her contacts and information. Katsi stayed on the network's board for only a year, as she was a young mother and found it hard to find the time to participate. However, in this short period, she made important friends, like Judy Norsigian and Norma Swenson from the Boston Women's Health Book Collective, who have remained allies over the years.

Katsi also speaks of the important role that Wilma Mankiller played in encouraging her and other Native women to speak out about their concerns. Mankiller's pioneering work on tribal development projects brought her national recognition. She was a member of the boards of many prestigious national social justice and women's organizations and used her position to amplify the voices and work of Native activists.[25] By the early 1980s, Katsi was often called upon as a spokesperson for Native American women in the women's health movement. During this time she also got involved in international campaigns, such as the Nestlé boycott.[26] Through this activism, she built an international network on birthing, midwifery, and Native women's health issues.

The Akwesasne Mother's Milk Project

Though much of Katsi's early work focused on midwifery, she was very interested in working with Native women on other issues related to their health. In the early 1980s, the community women with whom she interacted through her Birthing Crew work and the Nestlé boycott raised questions regarding the safety of breastfeeding. While the Nestlé boycott reinforced the health and cultural value of breastfeeding, corporate environmental devastation forced them to re-evaluate their decision in a scientific context. Mohawk women suspected that local industries were producing toxic chemicals that were released into the water, air, soil, and food chain, contaminating their breast milk and possibly causing birth defects. Katsi said:

> The fact is that women are the first environment [in which babies live] . . . We accumulate toxic chemicals like PCBs, DDT, Mirex, HCBs, etcetera, dumped into the waters by various industries. They are stored in our body fat and are excreted through breast milk. What that means is that through our own breast milk, our sacred natural links to our babies, [our babies] stand the chance of getting concentrated dosages [of these chemicals].[27]

Katsi and other women at Akwesasne were determined to understand the actual risks posed by this high level of pollution. In 1985, the Mother's Milk Project (MMP) was created to "understand and characterize how toxic contaminants have moved through the local food chain, including mother's milk."[28] Katsi approached scientists to investigate the toxicity of breast milk. The MMP also conducted its own community-based research that focused on analyzing organochlorines in mother's milk, fetal cord blood, and maternal and infant urine.

They invited scientists from the New York State Department of Health and the State University of New York School of Public Health to provide chemical analysis of breast milk samples. However, Katsi found that members of the MMP did not have the knowledge they needed to interpret the results that the scientists presented to them. To address the lack of scientific literacy among Mohawk women, the MMP trained about 125 Mohawk women to be health researchers and advocates. Since some of these women were also participants in the study, they became "researchers of their own reality."[29]

The MMP, together with members of the Tribes Environmental Office, conducted a bioaccumulative analysis of the entire food chain at Akwesasne, from fish to wildlife to breast milk. Katsi raised funds from General Motors, one of the contaminators, for this research project. The project studied new mothers each year for several years with a total of 50 new mothers participating in the study. The study documented a 200 percent greater concentration of PCBs in the breast milk of those women who consumed fish from the St. Lawrence River compared to the general population. This research showed how PCBs, fluorides, and hexachlorobenzene (HCB), all toxins dumped by local industries into the St. Lawrence River and into the air, made their way, through the food chain, into the bodies of local women, infants, and children. These toxins posed particular risks for women, since "PCBs mimic the reproductive hormone estrogen which is responsible for many of the physiological changes in a woman's body in puberty, menstruation, reproduction, and menopause."[30] Elevated levels of PCBs can trigger earlier puberty and menopause, each having a series of negative health impacts that are underresearched and not understood.

From Research to Action

The MMP published a newsletter, *First Environments*, to inform the community of the research process and its findings and issued advisories on prenatal and infant nutrition in a toxic environment to safeguard community health. When the studies indicated high levels, of contaminants in some community wells, the MMP alerted families and pregnant women to this danger and recommended actions they could take to ameliorate the problem. For example, they asserted that Native children are at greater risk from *not* being breastfed than from environmental contaminants, and worked to reestablish breastfeeding in the community by launching a breastfeeding promotion campaign. The MMP advised pregnant and nursing mothers to eliminate consumption of fish from contaminated waters, and to avoid excessive weight reduction during pregnancy and postpartum, since weight loss may mobilize the chemicals stored in fat tissues.[31]

As a result of these warnings and recommendations, Mohawk women stopped eating fish so they could protect their children from PCBs and still continue to breastfeed. However, Mohawk women were angered by the lifestyle changes they had to make to protect the health of their children. Katsi speaks for the local women when she states:

> Our traditional lifestyle has been completely disrupted, and we have been forced to protect our future generations. We feel anger at not being able to eat the fish. Although we are relieved that our responsible choices at the present protect our babies, this does not preclude the corporate responsibility of General Motors and other local industries to clean up the site.[32]

She explains the impact on Mohawk women's day-to-day activities" "We feel anger about not being able to . . . grow our gardens and practice our cultural ties to the earth. Our whole cycle of life has been affected."[33]

To strengthen community responses to issues of pollution, the MMP collaborates with the Akwesasne Task Force on the Environment (ATFE), which is made up of tribal and Mohawk council officials, the traditional Long House, and concerned members of the community. By sharing skills, research, contacts, and resources with the ATFE, the MMP has increased community awareness of the links between environmental degradation and health. The Mother's Milk Project has enhanced the self-esteem of Mohawk women and their families by giving them the information they need to fight critical environmental challenges. It has helped develop a network of environmental and health organizations that work to clean up the environment and compensate the victims.

The research gathered about breast milk also provided a great deal of information on other health issues of concern to Mohawk women. For example, the data indicated that the rate of induced abortion had increased considerably among Mohawk women. Katsi interpreted this as a result of more women being in the workforce and having greater access to health information, which enabled Mohawk women to exercise greater control over their fertility. The statistics also indicated a high level of thyroid disease in menopausal women. The MMP has been able to use such information to improve health awareness and education in Akwesasne. It continues to help with birthing, conducts on-site research, and provides environmental-health education.

The MMP collaborated with the Inuit of Canada and Alaska to protect aboriginal midwifery and share environmental health information. For example, when the Inuit of northern Ontario became aware of the presence of PCBs in the food chain, deposited on their land as a by-product of the American government's highway construction and in the operation of Distant Early Warning stations during the Cold War,[34] Inuit midwives shared the statistics on this subject with the Mother's Milk Project. Through its extensive networks in the Native community in the US and Canada, the MMP helped establish the Six Nations Birthing Center, which was funded by the Ministry of Health in Ontario. Commenting on their success, she states:

> In Ontario last year, 37 Mohawk and Seneca, Oneida, Onondaga, Tuscarora, and Cayuga babies were born into the hands of their own people, on their own land, using our traditions and culture, and taking back the responsibility of life. The door of life and the door of death are the same door, and when you lose the knowledge of how to be born, you lose the knowledge of how to die.[35]

The MMP worked with the Inuit of northern Quebec when they decided to restore the power of birth to their communities. Previously, they had a 20 percent cesarean rate. Under the government's evacuation policy, these women were flown out to cities in the south to have their babies alone, disrupting their families and depriving them of community support. Since 1985, they have had four practicing Inuit midwives and have reduced the cesarean rate in the village to 6 percent, with 95 percent of the births now conducted in their own language.[36]

Much of the work to promote aboriginal midwifery is done by Katsi herself. She initiated "Native Midwives," through which she works with aboriginal midwives across the United States and Canada, often serving as a trainer and a speaker at conferences, and developing educational and policy materials. She has also helped aboriginal women work with public health advocates to raise sufficient funds for research on traditional midwifery practices. Katsi has helped to establish aboriginal midwifery as a profession. She is currently working with the Aboriginal Nurses Association of Canada on a sexual and reproductive health issues guide for aboriginal communities.

The primary goal of the Mother's Milk Project is to create a society in which women are healthy. Holistic midwifery addresses all the factors that shape a mother and her baby's health and well-being: "whether it is [General Motors] contamination or the mental health of the mother, all must be cared for if the baby is to be healthy:"[37] MMP strengthens the social bonds of the community. As Katsi says: "One home birth will impact 30 people."[38] Katsi still hopes to see the development of a midwifery center in Akwesasne.

Linking Reproductive Health, Environmental Health, and Cultural Survival

Their work on reproductive health led MMP staff members to become environmental health activists. The contamination of their environment had both an immediate and long-term impact on the Mohawks' ability to practice their culture. For the Mohawk people, fish are a symbol of fertility and were traditionally fed to young women who wished to conceive healthy children. Mohawk mothers had to give up eating fish in order to protect their children and to continue breastfeeding. The absence of this excellent, low-cost protein has affected the ability of families to feed themselves. Thus, for Native American women, the right to a non-toxic environment is also a basic reproductive right.

The MMP also demonstrated that the reproductive health of the Native community is closely tied to issues of environmental contamination and cultural survival. Because Native people have close ties to and depend on their land for survival, Native women are distinctly aware of the connection between reproductive rights and environmental justice. The Mother's Milk Project continues to monitor the environment and press for a meaningful cleanup of the hazardous waste sites of local industries. They have been engaged in a lengthy battle with General Motors, Alcoa, General Electric, and Reynolds, some of the companies responsible for hazardous waste dumping in their area. The project's goal is to restore the environment so that people are able to eat fish and wildlife and resume traditional life-styles. As a result of these efforts, some financial settlements have been made on behalf of Native people.

The Mother's Milk Project is an example of how work on reproductive health can be made central to the life and cultural survival of communities. Katsi's life goal

> is to labor as an aboriginal midwife in the fields of social change of the Haudenosaunee and First Nations communities for the respect and empowerment of Onkwehon, . . . to restore the power of birth to the hands of women, and to work for the protection of the Seven Generations whose faces are yet coming towards us out of the mother earth.[39]

Contributions of the MMP

The Mohawk belief that a woman is the first environment makes the strong connection between women's health, the health of the entire community, and environmental justice. This holistic way of thinking is now gaining ground among medical and scientific professionals and is a significant conceptual contribution of the MMP and a model for activism that could be adopted by other communities.

The Dance Health Program and the MMP have helped restore competent, culturally appropriate midwifery services and women's health care to Mohawk women and their families. The revival of Native midwifery in Akwesasne has increased the support for it from health professionals and the Canadian government. There is a wider acknowledgment of the importance of midwifery in Native health care than there was in the past. Katsi's work has also had a significant impact on the Indian world. Today, Native reproductive health activists are aware that for Native women to control their reproductive health and future, midwifery is essential. By addressing health care in a holistic fashion, the Mohawk have created a template that other groups can use to build more comprehensive and culturally specific reproductive health programs. The MMP has also made the public more aware of the role of PCBs in the environment and led the Environmental Protection Agency (EPA) to initiate a health study at Akwesasne, a Superfund site.

Initially sparked by the "mothers' questions" in the 1980s, the MMP evolved into a remarkable model of community activism. Combining the knowledge and expertise of health research scientists, members of the community, and health care providers, the MMP initiated the first such study ever undertaken at a Superfund site. Mohawk women have been empowered by their participation in the research process. Not only has this participation deepened community understanding of environmental problems, it has also been a step towards greater health realization. By underlining the importance of Native women conducting their own research, Katsi has helped create opportunities for them in the fields of health sciences and education. There are now more than 20 Mohawk women involved in various aspects of research at Akwesasne, and several Native women, including one from Akwesasne, have pursued careers in science.

The partnership between the Mother's Milk Project and the Akwesasne Task Force on the Environment serves as a model in the Native American community for community control over research. The two groups have developed their own tribal Institutional Research Boards to ensure that their communities are made aware of, educated about, and involved in research. Researchers, including epidemiologists and physicians, who wish to study aspects of a community must first sign a contract which restricts them from entering the community without a member of the community accompanying them and stipulates that community members—not the researcher—own all the information obtained in the study. Anything that is published has to be approved by a community review board. Community members, rather than outsiders, are subcontracted by the researchers to conduct the work.[40]

The advocacy, research, and direct service programs of the MMP address many different community needs simultaneously. This is similar to the work of most of the other women of color groups we examined. The multi-issue agenda developed by the Mother's Milk Project serves as an important lesson for the mainstream reproductive rights movement: breaking away from single-issue politics empowers a movement to draw connections between several issues and in the process can galvanize new constituencies and new sources of funding to support reproductive rights and health.

Women's funds, notably the Ms. Foundation and the Ruth Mott Foundation, were of critical importance to the success of the work done at Akwesasne. Katsi's participation in the National Women's Health Network was also crucial, since it exposed her to the efforts of other women's groups. Her experience showed her how important it was to have Native American women in positions of influence in order to promote Native American concerns.

Instead of building one large organization to carry out all the projects her community needed, Katsi's work grew organically from the community and culture of which she is a part. As a leader, she empowered hundreds of Mohawk and other aboriginal women to develop important skills and to take political action for Native reproductive health.

NOTES
A list of endnotes is available in the original source.

WORKSHEET—CHAPTER 11

Childbirth and Lactation

1. Doris Haire's "The Cultural Warping of Childbirth" identified many common obstetrical practices from early pregnancy to postpartum that "served to warp and distort the childbearing experience in the U.S."

   a. List ten of the practices Haire identified.

   b. Choose two of these practices. For these two, discuss the known health benefits/risks of each; describe how this practice has changed or not since Haire wrote this article in 1972.
      In thinking about this question, it might be helpful to ask the woman or women you interview for question #2 about her/their experiences with these specific practices.

2. Interview two women who have given birth or one woman who has given birth at least twice. (If you have given birth, you are encouraged to answer these questions.) Ask the following questions about each pregnancy and birth.

    a. How was she treated in pregnancy by health providers and others? Was she healthy during the pregnancy? Did she have access to regular pre-natal care? During her pregnancy, did she have strong ideas about what she wanted her childbirth experience to be?

Birth 1	Birth 2

    b. For the birth event: Where was the birth? Who assisted in the delivery? What kind of birth was it (natural childbirth, some intervention, Ceasarean section)? Try to be specific about the interventions if there were any.

Birth 1	Birth 2

    c. Did the woman feel she had control in the process and did she have the childbirth experience she had hoped for?

Birth 1	Birth 2

3. For the two pregnancy and birth experiences described above, identify social and economic factors that you think influenced similarities and differences in the two experiences.

4. Many people think of childbirth experiences as one extreme (doctor assisted, with a great deal of medical intervention, birth in a hospital) or the other (non-doctor woman assisted, with no medical intervention, birth at home). However, it should be possible to negotiate all three factors: who assists; type of delivery, including interventions; location of the birth.

   Make up your own scenario of a birth plan, including the three factors above for a woman who does not want to have either of the extremes. Describe the advantages and disadvantages of each aspect of this plan as compared to the "extremes."

5. The introduction to this chapter emphasizes that increasing choices for women during childbirth must take into account that different women will benefit from different choices. Identify two examples of a "choice" in childbirth that some women might want, but that might not be desirable or appropriate for other women. Give a brief explanation if the explanation is not obvious.

6. The articles on breast feeding all emphasize the benefits of breast feeding. However, two articles also point out the risks of environmental toxins contaminating breast milk. List at least three benefits to the mother or baby of breast feeding. Suggest ways that a woman could work to reduce contamination of breast milk on a personal and a community level.

AGING, AGEISM, MID-LIFE *and* OLDER WOMEN'S HEALTH ISSUES

A core theme of this book is to remember that different women have different chances of being healthy and/or having access to health services appropriate to their needs. This chapter looks specifically at a few issues for mid-life and older women.

Ageing is certainly a woman's health issue because almost all people have more health concerns and call upon the health system more as they grow older. As women outnumber men in a ratio of 2:1 in the over-75 age group, health issues of aging are disproportionately women's health issues. Both because of women's roles and status in society and because of their longer life expectancy, women have very different experiences of aging and being old than men. Older women's incomes are on average 58 percent of the income of older men; women over 65 are almost twice as likely to have incomes below the poverty line as men over 65 (Ruth Sidel, "The Special Plight of Older Women" in *Women and Children Last*). Men are much more likely to be cared for by a loved one in their dying days; women are much more likely than men to spend their last days or years in nursing homes.

When young people suggest that the issues of aging are not relevant to their lives, it is very appropriate to point out that we are all, constantly, in the process of aging! Patsy Murphy's "Ageing" article brings this point home by looking at the issues of ageing from the vantage point of a 43-year old. Questions on the worksheet try to guide students of all ages to an awareness that ageing is a lifelong process and that taking care of our bodies in our younger years may be the best investment we can make to maximize on our old age. In the case of osteoporosis, young people who do weight-bearing exercise and eat a diet that promotes healthy bones literally build for their future; reaching age 35 with the strongest bones possible does more to prevent osteoporosis than most decisions made after 35. There is increasing evidence that the time between a woman's first period and her first pregnancy is the time when her body is most vulnerable to carcinogens. The decisions a woman makes in her teens and early twenties about exercise, fat consumption, alcohol use, and exposure to radiation, pesticides, or other environmental hazards (often not a choice at all) influence her chances of developing breast cancer later in life more than decisions she makes later. There is evidence that girls involved in athletics in high school and college have a decreased risk of breast cancer. Susan Love, breast-cancer specialist, concludes, "A theory has been very seriously put forth that I find delightful: put public health funding into high school athletics for girls—not a bad use of our resources. This would likely decrease breast cancer; also it strengthens bones and helps prevent heart disease." (*Dr. Susan Love's Breast Book*, 1995, p. 239). Rose Frisch's work has shown that women involved in college athletics not only have a significantly lower lifetime prevalence of breast cancer but also have a lower rate of uterine, ovarian, cervical, and vaginal cancers, and benign tumors of the breast and reproductive system than non-athletic peers. Very relevant to this chapter on ageing, Frisch emphasizes, "It's not too late to start exercising . . . Regular exercise has so many advantages that it is a lifestyle to adopt at any age" (Rose E. Frisch, *Female Fertility and the Body Fat Connection*, 2002, p. 120). The importance of *starting* health promotion at any age is most inspiringly described by Natalie Angier in *Women: An Intimate Geography*:

> Muscle is gracious. It does not hold grudges. Even an elderly woman who never learned
> to do cartwheels or bothered to join a fitness club in early adulthood can, in her oxidized

age, become a mighty virago. Her muscles will be there for her. Miriam Nelson, a physiologist at Tufts University, has taken women in their seventies, eighties, and nineties, women who couldn't leave their apartments or rise from their chairs, women in nursing homes, and she trained them twice a week with weights the way weightlifters in gyms train with weights—not timidly, not holding back for fear of their frailty or fear that they might, heavens, "bulk up," but with intensity, using as high a weight as the woman can manage. After only four months in the program, these women, these sedentary, often arthritic women with dowager's humps and hummingbird bones, grew astonishingly strong, were as though healed by a carnival preacher, tossing aside canes and walkers, getting down on their hands and knees to garden, canoe(ing), shovel(ing) snow . . . they doubled or trebled their strength. They became stronger than they had been in middle age. (pp. 319–320.)

In addition to the physical health issues related to the ageing process and being older, ageism is, of course, a mental health issue for older women. In "Women and Ageing: The Dreaded Old Woman Fights Back," Madge Sceriha identifies how sexism and society's lack of respect for older people come together in anophobia, the fear of old women. Although she describes this powerful social, economic, and political issue, as the title of her article suggests, she also emphasizes how older women are actively organizing and fighting against this oppression. Similarly, building on the theme that even women's movements have too often ignored the issues of older women, in "An Open Letter to the Women's Movement," Barbara Macdonald identifies ways we can all work against our own ageism.

To set the context for several articles that discuss a range of drugs offered to mid-life women, we first look at how the medicalization of menopause and mid-life issues has made people forget that this is a normal, healthy transitional time in women's lives. When we teach menopause workshops, we are surprised with how many women enroll primarily to find out *which* drugs to take. By the end of our workshops, many women are instead asking what convinced them that they needed to take *any* drugs for normal changes. In "Menopause's Milder Side," an anthropologist explores how women's experiences of menopause are vastly different in different parts of the world. She contrasts women's experiences in a number of Asian countries where few women notice "symptoms" associated with menopause with the U.S. where approximately two-thirds of women report hot flashes. She attributes the U.S. experience to the fact that "the medical vision of menopause has become the dominant way of understanding this midlife transition."

Major women's health news of this decade included the funding and implementation of the largest randomized, double-blind, perspective women's health study to ever be done (the Women's Health Initiative) and its significant findings that risks outweighed benefits for mid-life hormonal therapies.

"Hormone Replacement Therapy (HRT): Getting to the Heart of the Politics of Women's Health" can be viewed as an introduction to the response to the Women's Health Initiative findings and the medicalization of menopause and an analysis of how the HRT story represents wider recurring themes about women's health and the marketing of products. In the words of the National Women's Health Network, HRT was symbolic of "the triumph of marketing over science." Instead of letting the "dangers of HRT" news get framed as being about one particular product at one particular moment in time, it is important that women's health students identify the many ways that the HRT story is not unique. HRT is symbolic of a recurring pattern of untested, unneeded products being marketed to healthy women for pharmaceutical company-inspired "medical conditions." Both the media and the medical profession managed to present news of the dangers of HRT as shocking and totally unpredictable, but, in fact, no one should have been surprised to learn that HRT did not prevent heart disease, and that it presented health risks. Many researchers and activists had been saying this for over a decade. Since 1989, the National Women's Health Network (NWHN) had been publishing *Taking Hormones and Women's Health*, an accessible summary and critique of all the (mid-life) hormone studies. (This book started being published and distributed by Prima Publishers, as *The Truth About Hormone Replacement Therapy: How to Break Free from the Medical Myths of Menopause* in 2002.) This regularly updated publication continually warned that the benefits of hormones had not been proven and that the long-term risks were not fully understood. The NWHN played a key role in the early 1990s in advocating and lobbying for a large randomized trial [which eventually became the Women's Health Initiative, (WHI)] to study the risks and benefits of estrogen and HRT. As we now recognize the importance of this study, it is important to remember that the study almost didn't happen. "At various times, the trial is opposed by members of Congress who think it is too expensive, by epidemiologists who think the design is too complicated, and by leading gynecologists who think the heart disease benefit is so well proven that it is unethical to ask women to accept the possibility that they might get randomized to a placebo!" (*The Truth about HRT*, p.180). The importance of the WHI's findings on the dangers of both Hormone Replacement Therapy (HRT) and Estrogen Replacement Therapy (ERT) need to be a reminder of the importance of having large randomized trials for *all* products, especially for products marketed to healthy people.

In the years since the 2002 and 2004 headlines announcing the risks of HRT and ERT, the media has been full of stories focusing on a number of new products women can take to "replace" their "replacement" hormones. The obvious irony is that HRT has been widely used since the early 1980s but the crucial questions about its safety were only recently answered. The important thing to remember about new products is that they are *new*. (Recent changes in federal laws now require the Food and Drug Administration and pharmaceutical companies to work together to get new products to the market sooner, so long-term safety studies have not been done on most new products when they reach the market.)

Unless women start to demand safer, better-studied products, the National Women's Health Network asks the important question, "Who knows what is coming next? It is not hard to imagine that one of the new drugs people are taking today, believing that it makes them healthier, will be the HRT bombshell of tomorrow."

In their *The Women's Health Activist*, the National Women's Health Network tries to help women have scientifically accurate, personally empowering information for deciding which products to try from the smorgasbord offered to mid-life women—or whether to skip the smorgasbord until there are healthier, better studied choices. "When, How, and Which One? Navigating the Maze of Osteoporosis Drugs" and "A Bone to Pick with Bone Drugs" help women better understand osteoporosis, the range of products promoted to stop bone loss or strengthen bones, and that preventing falls is much more important than bone measurement screening. "Less Hormone Therapy, Less Breast Cancer" may be the most important little article you will ever read! Adriane Fugh-Berman reports on the stunning drop in breast cancer after the Women's Health Initiative results convinced many women to stop taking hormones and she concludes:

> at this point, many lines of evidence have proven that menopausal estrogen-progestin therapy *increases* breast cancer risk. Don't let anyone tell you otherwise.

In light of worries about HRT and other pharmaceutical products, many women are turning to "alternative medicine," "natural" hormones, and nutritional supplements. Because there is considerably less regulation of these products than of pharmaceutical drugs, it is extremely important that consumers make as informed decisions about these products as they do about FDA regulated medicines. Dr. Adriane Fugh-Berman's excellent *Alternative Medicine: What Works* (Odonian Press, 1996) and her chapter on alternatives to HRT in *The Truth about HRT* are recommended. Her critique of "bioidentical" or "natural" hormones is the topic of "Are Natural Hormones a Safe Alternative to Postmenopausal Hormone Drugs?" and we include her "Phytoestrogens: A New Alternative for Women?" as an example of the kinds of information women need to know in making decisions about whether to use plant products with estrogenic effects for menopausal concerns and disease prevention.

We remind readers that the National Women's Health Network's clear, succinct response to hormonal controversies, "Hormone Therapy: Six Steps Toward a Better Future," is the summary of the marketing chapter (Chapter 4.)

Ageing

by Patsy J. Murphy

I cried bitterly when I reached my twenty-third birthday because everyone else in my year in college was nineteen or thereabouts and I felt life passing me by. I dreaded thirty with a passion which in retrospect was idiotic—I had the happiest time of my life between thirty and thirty-five. I walked the beach at Dunquin on my fortieth birthday on a lovely June day and felt terrific, and when asked at forty-three to write on ageing I felt resentful—it's hip to be over forty in New York and ageing is something I wasn't thinking about anyway. Now I've been thinking about it for the last month and what I feel about ageing is GUILT. Lots of Guilt and mostly about the things that I haven't done that I thought I would have—I haven't written a book, made a movie, seen Vienna—I haven't, in short sorted out my life and it's time I did. . . . On the other hand, I've enjoyed myself, reared a daughter (almost), supported us both and today I am starting to sort out my life.

I believe that most of the time ageing isn't so dreadful. A friend of mine told me crisply that ageing is what other people notice about you—you don't monitor its progress. My daughter used to carefully count the lines on my forehead when I was thirty-three and I know they've increased and multiplied, but I remain unaware of it until I pass a shop window and see this Winnie-the-Pooh-shaped middle-aged woman and then I reel in horror at the vision that is me.

But the vision isn't as dreadful as the guilt, which has to do with things I've left undone. At my back I always hear time's winged chariot. I've run a questionnaire amongst some of my contemporaries, who are, as a French woman I know puts it, 'happy in their skin'—that is doing what they want to do and liking themselves. They don't mind ageing. I asked the cleverest woman I know how she felt about it and she said that 99 percent of the time she was totally unconscious of ageing—ageing was no bother. But the one percent was the awful, awful nostalgia about the past. I'll come back to the past later, but 99 percent is OK. The message for me is to do things that make me like myself and avoid the many, many things that make me hate myself—drinking too much, not making dental appointments. The message is the same for us all, sisters.

I asked a psychologist about guilt—it's normal he says, but it's useless: 'Take it out into the back garden and get rid of it,' he says. So, guilt apart, what does ageing mean? It means the body ain't what it used to be, but what the hell—the mind has more information and the body more experience. Ageing means that situations don't scare you as much as they did when you were young. I no longer feel terror when I walk into a room full of people. I no longer dread having to speak in public. I no longer think that someone else is going to sort out my life for me though I often wish that someone would.

For many women ageing brings freedom—a time to do things for themselves, by themselves, things that family responsibilities excluded for years. You don't have to be twenty to be knocked out by Venice, and the southern sun beams as benignly on your back at forty as at eighteen. A good book is still a good book. A glass of wine is still a glass of wine.

I've convinced myself that ageing has its compensations, but I'm still frightened of old age. I'm frightened of all the things that I presume everyone fears, being on my own, having no one to love, no one loving me, not being able to manage, the fear that the whole structure that one calls one's life, which I often feel I have small control over, will collapse around me and that I won't have the health or the energy to put it together again. Old age is not a subject one hears discussed. People on the radio and in books talk to the old, not about being old, but about their past, their part in the revolution, their girlhood, their village long ago. My fear of old age is the fear of death, which I have only experienced as the loss of other people, particularly the dreadful loss of my father. I couldn't bear his death—I hated to think of him in the cold ground. I still cannot face the idea of my own death.

I can face the more immediate horrors, though. I don't believe that the menopause is such a big deal or that it's going to make me feel useless. I imagine it must be quite a relief—no more periods—and it can hardly make me more evil-tempered than I can be now. So what is it that worries me? I'm back where I started. I'm back with my friend talking about the awful nostalgia. I'm there in my past looking at a photograph of us all sitting on a wall in Paris in 1958, skinny, happy, hopeful. . . . Or I'm back in a place of which I can say, like Edna O'Brien's green-eyed girl, 'I was happy here' and I feel my ghost, I see my former self, before motherhood, before mortgages, before security mattered. This is agony, the skewer in the heart and it has to be borne. Yeats felt it, Dylan Thomas, Simone de Beauvoir . . . we all feel it, bear it, hate it. Sometimes I want it back, my lovely lost past. Well, it's gone.

When I was young, I read a lot. I've continued to do so, and I will always do so, and if I'm blind I'll ask someone to read to me because books at any age are a passport to freedom. Once, in a very gloomy period of my existence, I kept sane by reading Simone de Beauvoir's series of autobiographies. I would mechanically get through my horrid day and then, clutching twenty cigarettes, get under the blanket and live a different life, a life that became more real than my own. Unhealthy, you may say, but it got me through a bad time in my life and I imagine that books will have to and will get me through more bad times. I don't have enough life left to read all that remains to be read. Apart from such old pleasures I've found new ones in middle age—gardening, listening to opera. The pleasures of the flesh? To be candid I haven't experienced them for some time but I don't think they have disimproved and I suppose everyone's life has lulls in sensuality.

Last week I saw David Shaw Smith's TV film on the life of Pauline Bewick, an artist whose work is a total celebration of womankind. In a very beautiful film, the thing that touched me most was her triumphant feeling about her future and her work now she's fifty. She looked to her future with such a shout of confidence. I would like to be like that, although I'm not.

Our friends are the most important source of pleasure. I still have the same friends that I had in my twenties, and the friendship of women is something that improves with time, because women share their sorrows, drink over them, laugh over them, grow close over them. I hope when we're old we'll be laughing more than crying.

My friends and I laughed a lot in our twenties, we got up late, looked out the window with a cup of coffee and a fag in hand and surveyed the long carefree day ahead. Then, as it was the sixties, we all got jobs we loved, and had love-lives and money and lots of crack. Then we got pregnant, and the hassles and stratagem and patchwork that are the lot of women who bring up children—especially on their own—followed. But we survived and we still enjoyed ourselves, frazzled, broke and unperceptibly ageing. We survived. What we lost with youth was freedom, the freedom, as one friend says wistfully, just to fling stuff into a rucksack and go. I was never one for rucksacks, but I know how she feels.

So I sit here at the typewriter aged forty-three and how I do feel? I think that I have not done all that I should with my life. There are moments when I feel panic-stricken and desolate: 'What if this or that happens?' 'What if it doesn't?' There are times when I trail home from work clutching the shopping and sink in front of the telly, immersed in *Hill Street Blues,* and scream silently to myself 'Is there a life out there in the world?' And yes, I know there is and I'm going out to tackle it one of these days. Perhaps I'll tackle it today. I'll put the photograph of our hopeful selves sitting on a wall in Paris in 1958 back in the album and I'll go out and confront this grey city and my life ahead.

Suggested Reading

Jane Barker and Rosie Graham, 'Change of Life?' *Spare Rib,* No. 51 (London: October 1976) pp. 41–3.

Colette, *Earthly Paradise: An Autobiography drawn from her lifetime writings,* Edited by Robert Phelps, (Harmondsworth: Penguin 1974).

Simone de Beauvoir, *All Said and Done* (Harmondsworth: Penguin 1977). *Old Age* (Harmondsworth: Penguin).

Barbara Macdonald with Cynthia Rich, *Look Me in the Eye: Old Women, Aging and Ageism* (London: The Women's Press 1984).

Adrienne Rich, *Of Woman Born. Motherhood as Experience and Institution* (London: Virago 1977).

Virginia Woolf, *A Room of One's Own* (Harmondsworth: Penguin 1963).

Women and Ageing
"The Dreaded Old Woman Fights Back"

by Madge Sceriha

Introduction

Ageism is one sociopolitical issue which has been conspicuously absent from the agenda of mainstream feminism over the years since its second wave surged some thirty years ago. For those feminists like myself who are presently facing the challenge of growing old, there is an immediacy to our concern that this omission be addressed. One compelling reason is that, while older women are increasingly evident in demographic data describing our ageing population, they are virtually *invisible* elsewhere in literature about women except as depressed, despairing, demented burdens.

Over the last decade, however, there has been a vocal and determined resistance movement gathering momentum among older women. To a large extent this represents a grassroots rebellion against the socially invalidating experience of older women's virtual invisibility within white, male-dominated western societies. Many within this movement have brought a feminist consciousness to the analysis of their experience and this has contributed to a more encompassing awareness of the effects of all forms of oppression on women throughout their lives. (Anike & Ariel 1987; Ford & Sinclair 1987; Job 1984; Rosenthal 1990; Scutt 1993; Walker 1985). Pioneers of second-wave feminism and public figures such as Germaine Greer (1991), Betty Friedan (1993) and Robin Morgan, the woman who coined the slogan 'the personal is political' and who is now editor-in-chief of *Ms Magazine,* have joined the ranks too and added strength to the movement.

It is still early days though, and inspiring women who are ageing to challenge the stereotype of the 'old woman' is no easy task. This chapter will highlight the insidiousness of ageism as it affects women: the 'links between the social devaluation of women and their own self deprecating beliefs' (Fook 1993, 15).

Anophobia

When I am an old woman I shall wear purple . . .'
(Jenny Joseph, cited in Martz 1991, 1)

These opening words from Jenny Joseph, in the now familiar poem 'Warning', sound as if they were written especially for feminists growing old. It certainly is a poem of protest against conventional role expectations for women and paints a picture of the old woman as defiant and outrageous. Yet such is the power of ageism that it is more than likely that the woman who emulates this poem's urgings would be ridiculed and her purpose in rebelling ignored or trivialised.

Most older women are not overtly rebellious. Instead they have learned to step out carefully amid the minefields of patriarchal capitalism and ever more so as they negotiate the added dangers of ageism. Were they to look more closely at ageism though, they would see that their experience of it is neither gender neutral nor new. In a different form, which Germaine Greer (1991, 2) has called 'anophobia', it has stalked them throughout their lives as women.

'Anophobia' means 'the irrational fear of old women'. This is the fear that has made being called an 'old woman' one of the most insulting things that can be said by one man about another man. This is the fear which, because it is internalized by women from an early age, complicates their own inevitable ageing experience. This is the fear that is in effect yet another way in which women are systematically oppressed in our white, male supremacist society. Anophobia is the fuel which feeds sexist ageism.

Anophobia is a most effective social control mechanism every time it silences the rage and pain of old women's existence as they struggle to survive against the constraints of economic, social and political marginalisation. It is effective too when it perpetuates divi-

---

siveness among women of different ages. Perhaps the worst outcome of all is its effectiveness in reinforcing fear and a sense of helplessness in women as ageing progresses and their capacity to serve others diminishes. For many, all that seems to be left for them is to passively serve out their time till death comes as a welcome release.

Serving and servicing others still characterises the work women do in the home and in the paid workforce and, although this 'women's work' has traditionally been devalued as low status in a male-defined model of work, it has provided many older women with a role identity over their lifetime. Where there is unquestioned commitment to this role, it can drain women physically and emotionally. An example of this is the work older women do in caring for a partner who is dying or who has some lingering illness requiring constant care. This work is all too easily taken for granted because most women in traditional marriages:

> . . . honour their commitment to selfless caregiving in line with religious beliefs as well as sex role expectations . . . [at the cost of] social isolation and problematic return to life outside family relations [when the caring role ends]. (Rosenthal 1990, 4)

The exploitation of women this represents is seldom if ever recognised on a societal basis nor is the work costed and thereby included as contributing to the economy. To have the courage to reject the caring role is not without its costs either, for the woman who fails to fulfil her role in selfless serving is all too often labelled selfish. This negative label is particularly effective as a means of social control when applied to women, especially those who are conditioned to put others' needs before their own.

The women's movement certainly has challenged structural inequalities with respect to work because such inequalities discount the value of what women do and consequently deny women as a social group access to economic power and independence. These structural inequalities have, however, not yet yielded to change fast enough or far enough for this to be reflected in major changes to women's identification with traditional roles. Ageing women therefore face an identity crisis when they contemplate a future in which they are increasingly likely to need the services of others rather than being the ones providing the services.

This identity crisis is exacerbated by the stereotypes which have been perpetuated under anophobic influence; stereotypes which infiltrate our awareness from an early age in fairy tales, legends, books, movies and television. Think about these all too familiar examples:

- the wicked witch with superhuman powers, sharp featured, hunched over her evil brew, cackling to herself or shrieking curses;
- this is not far removed from the feared and reviled matriarch who, with her razor-sharp tongue and control of the purse strings emasculates the males of the household and enslaves the females;
- in contrast there's the pathetic, useless, dried up, shabby shadow of a woman who is the ultimate form of female passivity and powerlessness, huddled in a lonely room waiting to die;
- then there's the old maid who, unfulfilled without a man and children in her life, is portrayed as an object of scorn or pity;
- for a good opportunity to ridicule think of Dame Edna Everage, an image created and exploited by a man which gives it just that extra impact;
- and of course there's Maggie in 'Mother and Son' whose image reminds us of our fears of becoming a burden, of losing our memories and doing outrageous things which shame our families and we're meant to laugh *at* her not *with* her;
- the best that is offered is the idealised grandmother image, but it is an image of a paragon of smiling, ever-available sacrifice whose own needs are always secondary to those of family and community.

Words too which are typically associated with old women are loaded with derision: 'dithering', 'dotty', 'doddering', 'little old lady', 'shrivelled shrew' and 'old bag' are telling examples. Woe betide her too if she's sexual because then she's grotesque or disgusting, especially if her partner is a younger man or, even more unspeakable, a woman.

Then there are the doom and gloom projections about the future sensationalised by the media which tell us that 'by the year 2021, 17% of our population will be over the age of 65' (Cross 1992, 13). We are warned that this will burden the young and strain the health services to say nothing of all the other services which will be clogged with these dependent, decrepit drains on the public purse. Let's face it though, the bulk of the older persons likely to be affected by such messages are women. It is women who are likely to spend most of our years supposedly 'past our prime' for it is suggested that 'women get pushed into the category of non-persons our society calls older people twenty years or so before men do.' (Cross 1992, 14). Because women also live longer on average than men, we are likely to experience the loss of status associated with ageing as a double burden—it starts earlier and lasts longer. Anophobia ensures also that we are likely to experience it more intensely.

This gender dimension has until recently been largely ignored in the literature on ageing as indeed has race and ethnicity. 'Very few Aboriginal people or Torres Strait Islanders survive to old age' we are reminded in a recent report. This report reminds us also of the 'growing numbers of migrants in the older population who are increasingly . . . from non-English speaking backgrounds,' (Davison, Kendig, Stephens & Merrill 1993, 16–17). These two facts can very easily be ignored when neither of the groups concerned has yet a voice (least of all a female voice) that commands attention in male-dominated, white, English-speaking Australian society.

The dominant societal voice is rather one that sounds out loudly and clearly that to be an old woman is the pits in the destiny stakes. Searching for an identity as an old woman is therefore fraught with anxiety when selfless sacrifice appears to be the only alternative to her more blatantly negative stereotypes. All too often we defend ourselves against this anxiety with denial, and fall back on the belief that age is a state of mind not a matter of chronological years. This belief is reflected in the observation that 'most people perceive themselves as essentially younger than they are' (Greer 1991, 272) and is exploited by advertisers every time they target older people and promote their products with images that evoke fantasies of passing for or emulating youth.

Every time we succumb to such propaganda we reinforce our own internalised anophobia. This is evident with regard to health and self-care products and procedures which are promoted through association with youthful attractiveness and youthful desirability. The success of sales of pills and potions from the health food stores, pins and tucks from cosmetic surgeons, the creams and dyes from the cosmetic houses, to say nothing of weight control regimes, is founded on unrealistic expectations for miracles of repair, restoration, reconstruction and, in terms of weight, reduction. What publicity there has been about the costs in economic terms, emotional anguish and often enough, the traumatising physical consequences of these examples of the pursuit of beauty has not had a marked impact on the thriving beauty industries which benefit from women's fear of growing old.

The Beginning of the End or the End of the Beginning

It hasn't been so easy though to deny the menopause which marks the end of women's reproductive years and, it is suggested, the end of her 'prime time' as well (Cross

1992, 14). Not so easy that is until the advent of the menopause industry. Working on the premise that menopause is an endocrine deficiency disease, the medical profession with quite a little help from the media has effectively promoted the idea that what women need to carry them through the 'dreaded change of life' is a steady dose of medicalisation in the form of hormone replacement therapy (HRT). It'll calm them down, keep them cool, and even allow them to have a bleed once a month if they want.

It's certainly a lot easier for the medical profession to prescribe pills than it is for them to deal with the social reality that this is likely to be a particularly stressful time in many women's lives. One such stressful social reality is the powerful influence of anophobia. Small wonder then that the 'quick fix' promise of HRT is so widely taken up when it is presented as providing the possibility 'of eliminating menopause and keeping all women both appetising and responsive to male demand from puberty to the grave [thereby] driving the dreaded old woman off the face of the earth forever' (Greer 1992, 2).

Women are certainly not expected to think about the fact that HRT is a very lucrative product for the drug companies if they can be assured of a population of consumers with some thirty years of consuming to do from menopause to death. We're not expected to think either about the costs to women (economic, emotional and physical) of a regime of HRT. Nor perhaps are we expected to remember that, before HRT, a woman at menopause who experienced symptoms which led her to seek out help was likely to be dismissed or trivialised, whereas now, as a potential consumer of HRT, the midlife woman is much sought after.

Nowhere is this more obvious than in the marketing of osteoporosis. In *The Menopause Industry* Sandra Coney cautions us to question the motives of that industry, in particular the pharmaceutical companies, that would have us believe that osteoporosis is a 'silent epidemic' with the potential to leave us all deformed past midlife. 'Osteoporosis sells things' she reminds us, like calcium supplements and HRT and its sales success is based on our fear of the little old lady who may turn out to be even 'littler' than our worst fears could imagine (Coney 1991, 105ff). Fear is the enemy as much as any potentially debilitating condition though, especially if we allow ourselves to be 'persuaded to feel anxious, fragile and prey to a host of unpleasant diseases [thereby] . . . worrying ourselves half to death,' (Coney 1991, 277).

We might otherwise recognise that osteoporosis could have as much to do with chronic dieting and overexercising and the tendency some women have to wear themselves out or starve themselves half to death because of an obsession with slenderness. It appears that there is advantage in the presence of a little padding as we grow older provided we also keep fit. Not only does carrying this weight benefit bone structure, it cushions any falls that could lead to fractures as well. It appears also that this padding is involved in the process of oestrogen production in our bodies after menopause. This process involves the conversion of androgens, which are produced by the ovaries and the adrenal glands, into a form of oestrogen called oestrone and this process takes place primarily in the fat of women's breasts and stomach (Coney 1991, 85, 149).

It is significant too that anophobic obsession with the idea that the young female is the yardstick of what is worthwhile and desirable in a woman is divisive and keeps women in competition with each other between and within age groupings. We must remember though that it is a particular image of the young female which is idealized. An image which, furthermore, is elusive because it is created by the media in collusion with advertisers who have no scruples about using the airbrush and computer technology to shape their models to their whim. Magazines, we are told,

> ignore older women or pretend they don't exist . . . [and] consciously or half consciously, must project the attitude that looking one's age is bad because $650 million of their ad revenue comes from people who would go out of business if visible age looked good. (Wolf 1990, 82–4)

That age is airbrushed off the faces of any older women who do happen to be featured 'has the same political echo that would resound if all positive images of blacks were routinely lightened, . . . that less is more' (Wolf 1990, 82–4).

Even within the covers of those magazines which target an older female population, the emphasis is on the message that 'it's all right to get older as long as you look as young as possible' (Gerike 1990, 42). Thus, although there are many articles featured in these magazines which take up social issues of concern to older women, they appear alongside a proliferation of advertisements in which the models are young, trim and trendy. For good measure there are the occasional accounts of celebrities like Elizabeth Taylor who at sixty still appear ever young and ravishing. It isn't surprising therefore that so many women find comfort and reassurance from being told that they've 'worn well' or they 'don't look their age' and who dread being judged as having 'let themselves go.'

There are limits to what is tolerated in the effort to pass as or emulate the young though, and this has been

very clearly demonstrated in the widespread controversy attendant on the news that two post-menopausal women have given birth after undergoing fertility treatment in an Italian clinic. Reports about the international uproar these events have caused focus on concerns for the future welfare of children of an elderly mother who might die or, for some other reason, not be able to care for her children (*Townsville Bulletin,* 31 December 1993). The double standard this represents is ignored, for males past 'their prime' who father a child are more than likely to get a pat on the back because what they've done shows that there's 'life in the old dog yet'.

Within the politics of reproduction, reproductive technology has emerged as a new frontier for the women's movement in its protracted struggle against patriarchal-capitalist power and control. 'Science and commercial enterprises (forms of institutional power) join forces with ideological forms of power (the control myth of woman as mother) in their attempt to control woman's procreative power' (Rowland 1988, 163–64). Reproductive technology stands alongside the medicalisation of childbirth and menopause, the radical invasive surgery of hysterectomy and the castration of women through oophorectomy as sociopolitical issues about which we need to develop a rigorous woman-honouring 'reproductive consciousness' (Rowland 1988, 165).

We certainly need such a consciousness to counteract complacency about the effects of the removal of a woman's uterus, cervix and ovaries when she is close to menopause. The removal of these organs is often justified on the basis of the argument that they are 'useless organs, sources of potential disease and decay' (Schumacher 1990, 58). Yet evidence is accumulating that, far from being useless, these organs have lifelong structural and functional significance for women's health and well-being other than that associated with reproduction. Not least of the functional aspects is the part these organs play in woman's sexual pleasure from arousal to orgasm. Women have been too easily persuaded to accept the 'take it all out' technique and then later, when they experience the very real sexual losses this entails, to accept that '[s]ex is all psychological' anyway (Schumacher 1990, 55).

Seldom though have we heard it suggested that we name the indiscriminate use of medical practices and procedures that experiment on, invade, mutilate and manipulate women's bodies for what they are—another form of sexual abuse (Schumacher 1990, 64). Seldom too do we reflect on the marked contrast there is in our attitudes to the prospect of hysterectomy as opposed to mastectomy. "Hysterectomy is trivialised where mastectomy is dramatised; the visible mutilation . . . is dreaded in the same irrational proportion as the internal mutilation is courted' (Greer 1992, 52). Prescriptive body image beliefs and the sexual objectification of women once again triumph when we fail to make such connections.

Women still trust the male-dominated medical profession to give them authoritative advice. Perhaps though we should remind ourselves of the absurdity of such authority about women's reproductive processes as it fuelled nineteenth-century arguments that women should not be admitted to universities. Then it was said that women's monthly bleeding would rob their brains 'of the constant and substantial flow of blood . . . required for intellectual activity' (Scutt 1993, 3). Keeping them out once menopause removed this impediment to participation was then left to other mechanisms of social control, not least of which was anophobic-driven sexist-ageism. Even today when menopause could be perceived as the beginning of another developmental stage in women's lives, prevailing medical authority favours a deficiency-disease diagnosis.

Medical authority is a form of institutionalised power which can influence our beliefs about ourselves. Where that authority influences us to believe the ageing woman's body is deficient and her once valued organs of reproduction are useless, it becomes another source of tacit legitimation for the continued medicalisation of women's lives and the social practices which devalue older women on the basis of their perceived biological inferiority. It is as if '[o]ur society has the idea that the value of women over 40 starts dropping rapidly and makes it a reality by turning the assumptions into facts' (Anike 1987, 26).

The Dreaded Old Women Unmasked

Devaluing is a form of social abuse which is 'so systematic that it . . . is considered normal by the society at large' (Dworkin 1988, 133). Its purpose is to marginalise and disempower and it is most successful when it generates feelings of revulsion and fear of the devalued group. Anophobia is such an abuse. Its obvious expression is in the pathological representation and negative stereotyping of women's ageing. It is much less obvious and therefore more difficult to confront when it takes the form of patronising tolerance. Worst of all though is when women start to feel that they are invisible, as this tends to silence them as well. It is not uncommon for women to remark that they really became aware of feeling old when they were ignored in shops and bumped into in the street as if they weren't there. Experiences of that sort soon erode self-esteem and self-confidence, especially if there were little of either at the outset.

The life expectancy of women in white Australian society has increased by some thirty years over this century and women outnumber men in all age groups after the age of 65 (Parliamentary Report 1992, 18–19). Women are the majority of the aged population and will be into the future and that population is projected to increase dramatically.

Alarmist reports in the media about the consequences of this demographic phenomenon refer to a '. . . "time-bomb" that threatens to blow the economy to pieces' (Parliamentary Report 1992, 52). It isn't difficult to see how the fear this has generated already in our society will attach to women in particular because they live longer. The double standard which persists in granting males as they age greater status and privilege than women accentuates this possibility. It is not that males are immune to ageist oppression but there is no male equivalent of anophobia nor is the image of unattractiveness, asexuality, passivity, dependency and incompetence associated with being old thrust upon them so early nor so destructively.

A 1992 Parliamentary Report observes,

Demographic change may expose inadequacies in economic and social institutions and practices, but the former is not in itself the problem . . . The debate over how best to run an economic system is not primarily an ageing discussion . . . the ageing of populations may have little to do with the outcome. (Parliamentary Report 1992, 68, 70)

We must therefore maintain a critical consciousness of how easily the aged (and most particularly women) could be scapegoated when politicians blame welfare spending for the country's economic crises. Our society would have more to fear if older women were to withdraw the unpaid caring work they do within family networks and as volunteers in the community which is a contribution they are likely to make as long as they are able. Research indicates that

older people are more likely to be providers than recipients of any kinds of support . . . [In addition it seems that more than 60% of the over 65 population have no limit on their functional ability and about 30% report only some minor restrictions to their activity. (Edgar 1991, 17)

There is a danger in focusing on 'use value' as a justification for older women's right to more visibility and respect though, especially where it is so closely linked to privatisation of service provision within the family structure. Such a view constrains women who want to 're-tire' from such role expectations and venture into other pursuits which interest them and negates those women who are frail or disabled. These issues are among the many which increasing numbers of older women are coming together to confront as part of an older women's movement which has the potential to become as politically significant as any of the radical movements which developed in the 1960s.

Accounts of this movement worldwide are proliferating. The Older Women's League (OWL) in America, The Older Feminist's Network and the Growing Older Disgracefully Collective in the United Kingdom, the Older Women's Network (OWN) in Australia and the Raging Grannies in Canada are examples of action groups that are inspiring older women to be who they are with courage, openness and a commitment to living more fully than they have ever before been allowed to think possible. These groups offer support and encouragement for women to explore their potential without imposing expectations for dramatic change. In such an environment it is more possible to become aware of internalised anophobia and all other forms of oppression which ageist prejudice exacerbates. They are not about establishing new stereotypes for old women for not all women have secret burning desires to abseil or bungee jump or even to join in direct social action. Not all women could, even if they wanted to, because of frailty, disability and/or economic constraints.

Many of these groups are encouraging women to write their own stories, to join in theatre workshops, to learn public speaking, to lead discussions, to learn self-defence, to be involved in environmental and peace issues and to link in with younger women's groups for events like International Women's Day and Reclaim the Night marches and rallies. Through involvement in such activities and action women can break down the barriers isolating them from each other within and between age groups, break the silence about their concerns and discover that the world of the young woman is no utopia nor is the world of the old woman necessarily a hell on earth.

That it is a hell on earth for too many is a fact that all women, both young and old, have a stake in addressing. We know that old women are likely to be victims of socio-economic violence (or what has been more euphemistically labelled the 'feminisation of poverty') because structural inequalities in our society continue to disproportionately disadvantage women throughout their lives. We know from the burgeoning literature on elder abuse that old women are often victims of emotional, physical and sexual violence just as their younger sisters are. We know that many feel isolated, lonely, hopeless and helpless because poverty, prejudice and powerlessness confine them to the margins of societal concerns. There is good reason, therefore, for all women to be actively anti-ageist and, in particular, anti-anophobic for it is an investment in their own future.

For references, see the original.

An Open Letter to the Women's Movement

by Barbara Macdonald

The following suggestions conclude a longer article entitled "An Open Letter to the Women's Movement" which deals with the widespread ageism in the women's community. The book from which this article is taken, *Look Me in the Eye*, is about women and ageing.

The following are a few suggestions to all of us for working on our ageism:

1. Don't expect that older women are there to serve you because you are younger—and *don't think the only alternative is for you to serve us.*

Reprinted with permission from *Look Me in the Eye* by Barbara Macdonald and Cynthia Rich, Spinsters/Aunt Lute Book Co., 1983. (Available from P.O. Box 410687, San Francisco, CA 94141).

2. Don't continue to say "the women's movement," . . . until all the invisible women are present—all races and cultures, and *all ages* of all races and cultures.

3. Don't believe you are complimenting an old woman by letting her know that you think she is "different from" (more fun, more gutsy, more interesting than) other older women. To accept the compliment, she has to join in your rejection of old women.

4. Don't point out to an old woman how strong she is, how she is more capable in certain situations than you are. Not only is this patronizing, but the implication is that you admire the way she does not show her age, and it follows that you do not admire the ways in which she does, or soon will, show her age.

5. If an old woman talks about arthritis or cataracts, don't think old women are constantly complaining. We are just trying to get a word in edgewise while you talk and write about abortions, contraception, premenstrual syndromes, toxic shock, or turkey basters.

6. Don't feel guilty. You will then avoid us because you are afraid we might become dependent and you know you can't meet our needs. Don't burden us with *your* idea of dependency and *your* idea of obligation.

7. By the year 2000, approximately one out of every four adults will be over 50. The marketplace is ready now to present a new public image of the aging American, just as it developed an image of American youth and the "youth movement" at a time when a larger section of the population was young. Don't trust the glossy images that are about to bombard you in the media. In order to sell products to a burgeoning population of older women, they will tell you that we are all white, comfortably middle class, and able to "pass" if we just use enough creams and hair dyes. Old women are the single poorest minority group in this country. Only ageism makes us feel a need to pass.

8. Don't think that an old woman has always been old. She is in the process of discovering what 70, 80, and 90 mean. As more and more old women talk and write about the reality of this process, in a world that negates us, we will all discover how revolutionary that is.

9. Don't assume that every old woman is not ageist. Don't assume that I'm not.

10. If you have insights you can bring to bear from your racial background or ethnic culture—bring them. We need to pool all of our resources to deal with this issue. But don't talk about your grandmother as the bearer of your culture—don't objectify her. Don't make her a museum piece or a woman whose value is that she has sacrificed and continues to sacrifice on your behalf. Tell us who she is now, a woman in process. Better yet, encourage *her* to tell us. I wish you luck in your beginning. We are all beginning.

"Menopause's Milder Side"

as answered by Margaret Lock

Questions for Dr. Margaret Lock, the well-known Canadian anthropologist on Japanese women, cultural nuances and the eastward creep of the western medical model.

Women's Health Activist: Your work studying women in Japan in 1983 and 1984 was some of the first to document that women's experiences of the physical effects of menopause are not the same everywhere. Among your most striking findings was that less than 20 percent of menopausal and post-menopausal Japanese women had experienced hot flashes, compared to about two-thirds of American women. How else is menopause different in Japan than in North America?

Margaret Lock: One of the most obvious differences involves the concept of menopause itself. In North America, we equate the end of menstruation with menopause; in fact, we've conflated the two. The word used in Japan, *konenki*, simply means a change in life. *Konenki* is much closer to the term once used in Europe, the climacteric, meaning a gradual change in midlife that can extend for a decade or more.

In my study, at least 25 percent of women I interviewed said they had no sign of *konenki*, yet they had finished menstruating at least a year before. Instead, they were more likely to mention a whole range of changes, including weakened eyesight, a bit of hearing loss, shoulder stiffness, headaches and lumbago [pain in the lower back].

One lesson to be learned from cross-cultural research is that unless you are sensitive to language nuances, your findings are not reliable. For instance, there is no Japanese word that means only a menopausal hot flash, although you can use three words that are close. A colleague of mine, a very good linguist, and I went to a lot of trouble to give Japanese women all three options for responding to questions about hot flashes. My impression when doing research in Japan was always that, if anything women were over-reporting, because they were trying so hard to be cooperative.

WHA: Your most recent trip to Japan was in 2003. Have things changed?

ML: Yes, things have changed because there's been an extensive effort on the part of Japanese gynecologists to medicalize menopause, with mixed success. There has been a massive amount of media coverage, with doctors appearing on television and publishing articles in popular magazines. I'm still in the process of analyzing these interviews, but my impression is that Japanese women are reporting more hot flashes than they did in the 80s, yet still many fewer than North American women reported at that time and presumably still are reporting.

I'm also finding, as I did in the earlier research, a very big difference in the severity and frequency of hot flashes. They're quite a bit milder in Japan than in North America, and for many women they simply don't happen at all. You would have to go a long way to meet a Japanese woman who needs to get up in the middle of the night to change her sheets. For the vast majority, hot flashes do not disrupt their daily activities much at all.

WHA: How are hot flashes treated in Japan?

ML: There are hormonal treatments, but most women don't want them; they're very concerned about the long-term side effects of medication and prefer to treat symptoms with herbals. Most Japanese gynecologists don't recommend lifetime usage [of hormone replacement therapy]; they start out recommending it for perhaps five years, then take women off it. Japanese women still do not routinely go to gynecologists, and family doctors usually don't do pelvic exams unless there's a problem. Japanese gynecologists want women to change their habits and come to see them regularly, but women are fairly resistant, it seems.

WHA: Where else is menopause treated differently than it is in North America, and is it always perceived in a negative light?

"Menopause's Milder Side," by Dr. Margaret Lock, originally published in the *Women's Health Activist*, March/April 2004, pp. 6–7, the newsletter of the National Women's Health Network (NWHN). It is reprinted with the permission of the author and the NWHN.

ML: Researchers have found consistently throughout Asia—in China, South Korea, India, Indonesia—that menopause is understood as a rather gradual midlife transition rather than simply as the end of menstruation. Low symptom reporting is also documented for many of these countries, and one group of researchers found no reporting of hot flashes among women in traditional Mayan society.

In rural India, this time seems to proffer increased status; women who are freed of the constraints of the modesty they had to have as younger, sexually active women can take greater part in the outside world. On the other hand, if you've had no children then it can be a terrible time because you have no one to look after you when you get old.

WHA: What do you think underlies the different perceptions and experiences of menopause around the world? Nutrition? Physical activity? Different attitudes toward aging women?

ML: Of course culture and attitudes contribute to differences and language does too, but I believe there's something biological going on as well. It could be to do with genetics; as we're learning from molecular genetics, even a small amount of genetic diversity can account for a significant difference in bodily experience. Or perhaps it's something to do with the destabilization of core body temperature when a woman has an FSH surge, and some women may be more vulnerable to this than others. Or, it could be to do with diet. The effect of soybeans is being checked out extensively in Japan, with mixed results.

It's also important to note that there is enormous concern about looking after one's health in Japan, particularly among women because they don't want to be a burden to someone else. Japanese women reported many fewer chronic problems than do North American women. They take herbal supplements, they're careful about dietary intake. On my last visit, I found that middle-aged women were reverting to traditional diets once their children had left the household and they no longer had to prepare western-style food for the younger generation. Japanese women also exercise a great deal, and most of them have never smoked or been big caffeine drinkers.

WHA: Some researchers have argued that women's cultures lead them to describe their experiences differently, but that their experiences are actually similar. How do you respond to the implication that women's biology is universal, and the physical effects of menopause must be universal too?

ML: I disagree with this line of argument very strongly. I spent hours and hours talking with Japanese women about menopause, and they have no inhibitions about discussing their bodily experiences. Japanese language and culture encourage one to pay close attention to the rhythms and changes of the body. I would also respond by pointing to epidemiological findings. It is undeniable that there are major differences in the incidence of common diseases in different parts of the world. This geographical variation is due in part to environment and diet, and also as a result of socioeconomic status, age, gender and so on. So why do we make the assumption that women's bones are the same everywhere; that physical changes at menopause are the same everywhere? As an anthropologist, I cannot accept that a woman who says she does not have hot flashes is wrong; one must take subjective reporting seriously and not assume that women are duped by their culture.

Obviously, women everywhere stop having their menstrual cycle around the age of 50, when estrogen levels drop. Something very predictable and biological is going on. However, we know that the way in which estrogen levels drop is not uniform: in some women the drop is rapid, in others it seems to go up and down in spikes, and yet other women experience a slow, steady decline. These differences are mediated by individual biology and by diet. Again, these differences may well be related to genetics. Everything we're learning tells us to pay attention to the fact that even a little bit of genetic variation can be significant in interesting and surprising ways.

I think there are two reasons why such differences in symptom reporting make people uncomfortable. One is the pressure of the medical world, which trains health care practitioners to think in terms of universal models. The other reason, particularly in the United States, I believe, is resistance to thinking about possible biological differences because they are so readily associated with race and racism.

WHA: In the U.S., attitudes toward menopause have evolved from considering it a time of "living decay" to a time when women hear they need screening tests, drugs and medical management to prevent diseases of aging. NWHN has been critical of both of these responses. What hopes do you have for women who will reach menopause in the future?

ML: I would like people to think more about the life-cycle as a whole rather than picking out menopause as one distinct and difficult period. So much of what happens as we grow older depends in large part on what we do when we're younger. With bone loss, clearly genetics puts some people at greater risk, but many people who have exercised and built up good strong bones when younger have enough bone mass for there not to be a problem later. It isn't just a matter of doing something when you're 48.

Secondly, as researchers such as Sonja McKinlay and Patricia Kaufert have shown, menopause isn't a particularly difficult time for the majority of women. Studies that make use of samples drawn from the population at large in North America show no statistical correlation between depression and the end of menstruation. This research also found that the majority of menopausal women do not suffer from troublesome hot flashes and that 40 percent never have hot flashes. These positive experiences need to be publicized much more.

The medical vision of menopause has become the dominant way of understanding this midlife transition. But a physician's viewpoint tends to be skewed as a result of seeing patients, many of whom are indeed suffering and need help. While being fully sympathetic with women who have a hard time at menopause and with those who are at high risk for osteoporosis, for example, this is not the whole story. For many women the end of menstruation is unremarkable, and becoming older isn't at all bad. I'm 68 next month, and I have to say a lot of marvelous things are happening at this stage of my life-cycle, including becoming a grandparent.

Hormone Replacement Therapy (HRT) "Getting to the Heart of the Politics of Women's Health?"

by Nancy Worcester[1]

In 2002, the National Institutes of Health announced that one arm of the largest hormone study ever to be done on healthy women was being stopped for safety reasons: the risks of hormone replacement therapy (HRT) outweighed the benefits. This paper explores how the HRT story can be used to politicize women and their health care providers about the recurring pattern of marketing untested products to healthy women. It also provides a history of the women's health movement's critique of the lack of scientific evidence that HRT was safe or effective, discusses the new Food and Drug Administration (FDA)-pharmaceutical industry partnerships that increase the medicalization of women's health, and shows that the HRT story is not unique. Emphasizing that the Women's Health Movement is as important as ever, this paper concludes with strategies for ensuring that the lessons learned from the HRT story are incorporated into practice and policy. Highlighted as well is the important role the National Women's Health Network (NWHN) played in the HRT story and its continuing crucial role in enhancing women's health.

Keywords: estrogen / Food and Drug Administration (FDA) / hormone replacement therapy (HRT) / National Women's Health Network (NWHN) / progestin / Women's Health Initiative (WHI) / Women's Health Movement

"The widespread popularity of hormone replacement therapy in the United States is a triumph of marketing over science and advertising over common sense." National Women's Health Network (2002, xii)

"Hormone Replacement Therapy (HRT): Getting to the Heart of the Politics of Women's Health?" by Nancy Worcester, *National Women's Studies Association Journal*, 16:3 (2004), pp. 56–69. © National Women's Studies Association Journal. Reprinted with permission of The Johns Hopkins University Press.

On July 9, 2002, the National Institutes of Health announced that the hormone replacement therapy (HRT), estrogen/progestin portion, of the largest hormone study to ever be done on healthy women was being stopped. Approximately three years before any results were expected, scientific investigators for the Women's Health Initiative (WHI) already had information they knew they had to share with the participants in the study and the public: the risks of estrogen plus progestin outweighed the benefits. Specifically, the study had shown that women taking HRT had a 26 percent increase in breast cancer, a 41 percent increase in strokes, and a 200 percent increase in the rates of blood clots in legs and lungs (National Women's Health Network [NWHN], 2002). Later analysis of the studies also showed that HRT does not improve "quality of life" issues or memory. The "good news" often highlighted by reporters who had sung the praises of HRT for years was that women taking HRT had 37 percent less colon cancer and 34 percent fewer hip fractures.

The Personal Is Political

Approximately six million women in the United States were taking HRT that day when headlines everywhere announced that, instead of preventing heart disease, this most important study had shown that hormone "replacement" therapy increased a healthy woman's risk of heart disease (Spake 2002). What were women to do with this news? What did women do with this news? One crucial question this paper asks is whether the HRT story was one where women saw that "the personal is political," or did six million women simply feel that "the personal is personal?" Instead of feeling a sense of outrage that once again women had been sold unsafe products, how many women felt alone and worried about their own individual, individualistic decision-making as they were bombarded with messages about how shocking this news was and new products they could try? Using this as a time for self-reflection within the Women's Health Movement, I challenge us to think about how we can use the HRT story to politicize women and their health care providers about "the triumph of marketing over science" in women's health. Instead of letting the HRT news get framed as being about one particular product at one particular moment in time, it is more important than ever that women's health activists, researchers, teachers, and policymakers identify that HRT is not a unique story. HRT is symbolic of the pattern of untested, unneeded products being marketed to healthy women for pharmaceutical-company inspired "medical conditions."

Responses to the July 2002 Announcement

"The post-study reality represents one of the biggest disconnects that has ever occurred in medicine." (Peter Wilson, Framingham Heart Study, quoted in Spake 2002, 42)

No one should have been surprised by the news that HRT did not prevent heart disease and that its long-term safety was questioned. Many researchers and activists have been saying this for over a decade. The Society for Menstrual Cycle Research conferences and publications have for many years brought together researchers, clinicians, and activists asking important questions about the medicalization of menopause and the safety of products marketed to midlife women. How many times has Cindy Pearson, Executive Director of the National Women's Health Network, asked an audience, "Does estrogen make women healthy or do healthy women take estrogen?" Since 1989, the NWHN has been publishing *Taking Hormones and Women's Health*, an accessible summary and critique of all the (midlife) hormone studies. This regularly updated publication continually warned that the benefits of hormones had not been proven and the long-term risks were not fully understood.

Arguing that every heart disease prevention drug used by men has been tested in a large randomized trial, the NWHN played a key role in the early 1990s in advocating and lobbying for a large randomized trial (which eventually became the Women's Health Initiative) to study the risks and benefits of estrogen (Estrogen "Replacement" Therapy [ERT]), and estrogen plus progestin (Hormone "Replacement" Therapy [HRT]) in healthy women. As we now recognize the importance of this study, it is important to remember that it almost did not happen: "At various times, the trial is opposed by members of Congress, who think it is too expensive, by epidemiologists, who think the design is too complicated, and by leading gynecologists, who think the heart disease benefit is so well proven that it is unethical to ask women to accept the possibility that they might be randomized to a placebo" (NWHN 2002, 180).

Published a few months before the July 2002 announcement, *The Truth About Hormone Replacement Therapy* contained the NWHN's version of a "center-page spread," a two-page fact sheet for women to give to their health practitioners in case "Your health care provider may still be under the 'impression' that HRT may somehow be good for your heart." This fact sheet reminded practitioners that both the safety and effectiveness (in relation to heart disease) of ERT and HRT have been questioned continually: in 1990, the FDA denied approval to Wyeth-Ayerst, manufacturer of Premarin, to market Premarin for heart disease prevention (neither ERT nor HRT were ever given FDA approval for heart disease); in 1998, the Heart and Estrogen/Progestin Replacement Study (HERS), the first randomized study to look at heart disease outcome, demonstrated that HRT did not help women who already had heart disease, and in March 2000, participants in the Women's Health Initiative study were sent letters letting them know that, in the earliest stages of the study, women on ERT and HRT were showing more heart attacks, blood clots, and strokes than women in the placebo group. (Interestingly, these were downplayed as "early findings," but some researchers felt they would be useful for keeping women motivated to stay in the study. In a climate where women and their physicians were constantly bombarded with "information" saying ERT and HRT prevented heart disease, it was challenging to find women who were willing to be a part of a study where they might be randomized to what they viewed as the "wrong" group.)

Precisely because the July 2002 Women's Health Initiative results were not surprising to any of us who had been evaluating the studies and critiquing the marketing of hormones, reaction to the announcement proved to be a useful barometer for measuring people's understanding of the politics of women's health. A great teaching project would be to have students assigned to read and contrast the actual results reported from the Women's Health Initiative (Writing Group for WHI 2002) and comment on how that information was covered in a wide range of popular media (Whatley, personal communication). While there were some delightful cartoons and refreshing commentaries that captured the real meaning of the HRT news story, I found the following reactions I encountered in the media, among students and colleagues, to be the most thought-provoking in exploring the challenges of building a more sophisticated consumer awareness of the recurring pattern of the marketing of unsafe and unneeded products to healthy women:

From a middle-aged woman doctor appearing on the evening news: In a great example of internalized sexism and ageism, this doctor appeared on July 9th news shows to discuss the WHI findings. She stated confidently that it was urgent that physicians have *something* to prescribe to mid-life women. She actually said that without some sort of

medication mid-life women were going to have all sorts of problems and their husbands would leave them! With absolutely no analysis of how menopause has been medicalized, here was a physician simply looking for one more product to prescribe for her patients.

From an undergraduate in a women's health course: In the spirit of this article, my teaching team was eager to use the HRT headline story as a teaching theme in the fall 2002 semester to demonstrate the ongoing problem of the medicalization of women's health. In October (only three months after the HRT study was stopped), an undergraduate criticized our dwelling on "old news," saying there was no reason to keep talking about the risks of HRT because people had known since July that it was dangerous so no one should be using it anymore. Despite our attempts to use HRT as one example among many unsafe products marketed to women, this undergraduate (who had enthusiastically chosen to take this Women's Studies women's health course) served as an example of someone who very much wanted as much information as possible for her own personal decision-making, but was not interested (yet!) in looking at the bigger picture of the politics of information.

From science graduate students applying to teach a women's health course: Asking applicants how they would handle the above HRT discussion situation (where an undergraduate fails to look beyond an individual issue to develop a broader analysis) proved to be a most useful interview question in selecting teaching assistants for my women's health course. Many feminist graduate students, particularly the social scientists, quickly realized they were being asked to describe how they would teach the politics of women's health and gave exciting answers. Interestingly, some more scientifically confident applicants totally missed the point of the question and immediately demonstrated how up to date they were on scientific issues by describing the Women's Health Initiative in much detail and saying that they would be able to share the scientific details of the study with students and that they would emphasize that the ERT part of the study continues and that there is still much potential for what will be learned about ERT.

From a male university colleague who works on communications: This colleague was intrigued with my quick "good-bye" the evening before the WHI results were to be announced. I had simply said to think of me as he listened to the next day's news and to remember that, "I told you so!" As someone who has read my work (as we are required to do for each other for annual peer reviews in a department where our research and teaching interests do not overlap), he had no trouble matching my good-bye comment to the HRT headlines. He was the person who most understood the significance of the HRT announcement: he immediately went on-line to watch the effect this would have on the stock market. In conversations since that day, it is obvious that he has developed a great appreciation for the politics of women's health by seeing the financial implications of that one announcement.

There is nothing scientific about my sample, but it certainly is thought-provoking. It is probably not a coincidence that the triumph of marketing over science or the triumph of wealth (of pharmaceutical companies) over (consumers') health was more apparent to someone who understands the stock market than to an undergraduate wanting information for personal decision-making, graduate students immersed in studying the details of health science, or a busy physician who has undoubtedly been greatly influenced by pharmaceutical industry-influenced "physician education."

Lessons from the Past Should Be Informing Present Debates

The HRT news was not just about one particular product at one particular moment in time. There is an incredible amount of money to be made any time a company can find a product to market to healthy women. Why are the companies that produce menstruation-related products willing to spend so much money on middle-school education resources or give so many free samples to girls starting their periods? Think of the money they can make if they hook someone into buying their particular brand for most of her reproductive years. My students love to calculate the amount of money an average woman spends in her lifetime on menstruation-related products.

Women of all ages should be aware that HRT is only the most recent addition to an ever-growing list of products sold to healthy women that turned out to be dangerous or lethal. Any consumer or clinician who will be involved in decision making about women's health products deserves to have, or has the responsibility to have, information on the recurring history of unsafe products hurting healthy women. The safety-monitoring committee of the Women's Health Initiative knew that it was important ethically to let participants know in March

2000 that early findings indicated some increased risks with hormones. Similarly, all consumers have the right to know much more about the risks they may be taking when they make the decision to use a product that has not been proven safe in large, long-term, double-blind, randomized studies.

Here are a couple examples of women's health history lessons that are important for safety-conscious consumers to know:

DES (Diethylstilbestrol)—This drug was widely used in the United States from 1941 to 1960. In the 1950s, 4 to 7 percent of all pregnant women took this drug. Although it was originally prescribed specifically for the treatment and prevention of miscarriage, both pregnant women and their clinicians liked the effect of the drug so it started to be used routinely in healthy women to promote healthy pregnancies. Two decades after the drug had become popular, it was discovered that some of the daughters who had been fetuses in pregnant women taking DES developed a very rare, potentially lethal, form of vaginal cancer when they were in their late teens or twenties. By the time the FDA withdrew DES from the market in 1971, approximately four million women had taken it. Today, *six decades* after this drug became available, researchers and consumers groups like DES Action are still trying to understand the long-term impact of this drug as it keeps unfolding in the daughters, sons, and grandchildren of women who took DES and in the women themselves. *The DES story should be the only one we need to remind us that we will never really know the long-term safety of a product until the long-term safety of that product has been proven* (Sloane 2002).

The Dalkon Shield—A crab-shaped intrauterine contraceptive device with a multi-filament tail became very popular in the 1970s due to a very aggressive marketing campaign where the manufacturer falsified safety studies and pregnancy prevention rates. The product was associated with a high rate of Pelvic Inflammatory Disease, a much-increased rate of infertility, and was blamed for causing at least fourteen deaths before it was withdrawn from the U.S. market in 1974. By that time the manufacturer had "dumped" many thousands of Dalkon Shields on unsuspecting consumers around the world where they might never hear of its dangers. Even in the United States, it was controversial as to whether it was safer to leave the device in place or risk damage to the uterus in having it removed. In speaking to executive officers of the company that marketed the Dalkon

Shield, Chief Judge Miles Lord of the U.S. District Court in Minnesota summarized the irresponsibility of selling women dangerous products:

> If one poor young man were by some act of his—without authority or consent—to inflict such damage upon one woman, he would be jailed for a good portion of the rest of his life. And yet your company, without warning to women, invaded their bodies by the millions and caused them injuries by the thousands. . . . Your company has, in fact, continued to allow women, tens of thousands of them, to wear a device—a deadly depth charge in their wombs, ready to explode at any time. The only conceivable reasons you have not recalled this product are that it would hurt your balance sheet and alert women who have already been harmed that you may be liable for their injuries. . . . This is corporate irresponsibility at its meanest. (Engelmeyer and Wagman 1985, 254–6)

Similarly, consumers need to know how certain menstrual products had to be removed from the market after their association with more than 100 toxic shock syndrome deaths (Riley 1986), how 1.2- to 2.4-million women were affected the day it was announced that the popular diet drug combination Fen-Phen was being removed from the market because of the deaths that it had caused and the fact that approximately 30 percent of people who had used the drug had heart valve abnormalities (Mundy 2001); that debates still continue about the long-term safety of Depo-Provera, oral contraceptives, and silicone breast implants; and that debates *should* be taking place about every new product (Sathyamala 2000; Sloane 2002; Zuckerman 1998; Worcester and Whatley 2000).

In 1986, Joan Rachlin wrote an excellent review of four books on the Dalkon Shield, Rely tampons, and toxic shock syndrome for *The Women's Review of Books*. She concluded:

> These books are important from both a historical and women's health perspective; they remind us that other substances, such as Depo-Provera, could well provide the material for the next set of books to be reviewed in these pages, if we don't learn well enough the lessons from the past. We have to exercise our rights and responsibilities as empowered consumers of health care services and products. We have to demand safe and effective pharmaceuticals, produced and marketed by honest and competent organizations and administered by caring and capable physicians. We can only, after all, really *rely* on ourselves; we need to be as informed and as involved as

possible if we are to navigate the medical-corporate complex. These books show us what the alternatives will continue to be. (Rachlin, 1986, 7–8)

Increased Medicalization of Women's Health

Nearly two decades later, now with the HRT story added to the DES, Dalkon Shield, Rely, and Fen-Phen stories, and the increasingly powerful partnership of the pharmaceutical industry, the FDA, the advertising industry, and industry-influenced medical education, Joan Rachlin's words are more important than ever. Consumer literacy and action related to demanding safe, effective products, marketed by ethical corporations, and administered by physicians who have accurate, science-based information is urgent. Important new trends in the 1990s in how drugs get to the market and how products can be marketed come together in a way that makes it more likely than ever that women will end up using products that are not necessary, are not effective, and may not be safe.

In the political climate of the late 1980s/early 1990s, there were major changes in the Food and Drug Administration's (FDA) relationship with the pharmaceutical industry, which affected the speed at which new drugs can get to the market. The FDA, the "watchdog" organization responsible for ensuring that only safe products are allowed on the market, was accused of being too cautious, so that it was said that it took too long for good drugs to be available to Americans. Primarily, conservatives in Congress and "friends of industry" pushed for a more industry-friendly FDA, but it is important to note that consumer activists, particularly AIDS activists, and later breast cancer activists, were also instrumental in demanding that promising drugs be made available to patients sooner. The contradictions in claiming this as a consumer victory are obvious and serve to highlight a consequence of the women's health movement's shift from broader, grassroots organizing for a more holistic, health-promoting approach to women's health to the more recent emphasis on specific disease-focused campaigns (Ruzek and Becker 1998.) There are extremely different ramifications of demanding speedy access to life (quality or quantity) enhancing drugs for terminally ill patients than of setting the safety standards for a drug that will be marketed to healthy woman to be consumed for many years. When drug companies started promoting ERT and HRT for heart disease and osteoporosis, they hoped to hook women into a product they would stay on for the rest of their lives; such products must be extremely safe.

The Prescription Drug User Fee Act (PDUFA) of 1992 requires that the FDA and pharmaceutical companies work together now in somewhat of a "partnership" so that "good" drugs get to the market sooner. PDUFA requires industry to pay a user fee to the FDA and in |exchange the FDA works with the company to help the process of drug approval go more quickly. Everyone acknowledges that there is a tension between ensuring the safety of products and speeding patient access to new drugs. There is certainly no doubt that more drugs are reaching the market faster as a result of PDUFA. While some media attention has focused on the number of drugs that have had to be withdrawn from the market (often with much public attention as in the Fen-Phen case) since the approval process has been speeded up, the FDA emphasizes that the *rate* of drug withdrawals has not changed significantly. (Approximately 2.8% of drugs are withdrawn *after* they have been on the market and problems emerge.) What matters to consumers wanting safe drugs is that the *number* of people impacted by taking drugs that later are recalled is much higher if the volume of drug approvals is higher, even if the *rate* of withdrawals is not increasing. Another major change for U.S. consumers is that approximately 80 percent of new drugs now go on the market in the United States before they are available elsewhere. In contrast, it used to be that most drugs were used and tested first in other countries so Americans had often heard about risks and undesirable side effects before new products reached the U.S. market (FDA 2002).

The important role of the FDA maintaining its role as our "watchdog" without too much influence from industry, is well documented and discussed in Philip J. Hilts' *Protecting America's Health: The FDA, Business, and One Hundred Years of Regulation*. In responding to New Right groups in Washington that continued to criticize the FDA as being too cautious so as to "filter out almost all harm," even after the PDUFA mandated the new FDA-industry collaborations and drug-approval processes had been speeded up, Hilts explained:

With the present FDA system (described as overcautious), drugs that are *reviewed and approved* kill about 100,000 people annually and seriously injure more than a million in the United States. The system has not filtered out all risk, apparently. No other cause of accidents approaches the level of injury attributed to pharmaceuticals. (A table of risk put together by Thomas Moore of George Washington University estimates the lifetime chance of being put in the hospital by accidents: severe injury by prescription drugs, 26 in 100; auto accident, 2 in 100; murder, 1 in 100; commercial air crash, 1 in 35,000.) And the vast majority of deaths occur not among people knowingly taking a risk, but among the innocent. We accept this high level of risk because we are seeking greater benefit—saving lives and preventing or minimizing illness. The FDA is not an overcautious agency by nature. (2003, 307–8)

In the weeks and months following the announcements about the risks of HRT, the media has been full of feature stories focusing on a number of new products that women could try to "replace" their "replacement hormones." The obvious irony is that HRT has been widely available since the early 1980s, but the important questions about its safety and effectiveness have only started to be answered. The important thing to remember about these new products is that they are *new:* some may prove to be wonder drugs, some may be less effective than promised, some may be dangerous. To have the kind of useful information we now have about HRT will require large, long-term randomized controlled studies.

In addition to its new influence on the FDA, the drug industry also has increasing influence on both consumers and health care providers. The drug industry speaks directly to women these days, coming into their minds and conversations through their televisions and radios, and in their magazines and newspapers. The industry-sponsored ads, industry-spokes-people, and industry-prepared ready-to-use health segments (which 100% of surveyed television news stations admit they use) not only powerfully influence the purchase of particular products, but also influence more broadly what women identify as health issues and fears, and what needs medication. Even before Merck had a product approved for osteoporosis (Fosamax was still going through FDA-approval processes at that stage), many women's magazines ran a two-page ad paid for by Merck. The very eye-catching image showed a young woman riding a bicycle, casting a large shadow of a wheelchair. The words, "The shadow of osteoporosis doesn't have to influence future independence" effectively sold women the fear of osteoporosis and the feeling that they should start taking *something* to prevent it. Advertising is so effective that many women enroll for menopause classes feeling they have to get more information on *which* medicine to take: inevitably they have been so influenced by the industry-promoted medicalization of menopause that they have forgotten there is a choice *not* to take *any* medication.

Television ads have been an especially powerful source of drug pushing since guidelines for direct-to-consumer ads were liberalized in 1997. By 1999, the pharmaceutical industry spent more than $1.8 billion on direct-to-consumer advertising. Because the ads often give misinformation, their power can be dangerous. The FDA does not pre-approve ads, so ads containing misinformation get pulled only after they have already been seen and it is too late to undo the message they gave. Although most consumers underestimate how much they personally are affected by advertising, studies consistently show that drug ads are incredibly influential in manipulating what consumers want. One-third of consumers have spoken to their health care providers about a product they saw advertised and 15 percent of consumers admit they might switch doctors if their doctor would not prescribe a medication they saw advertised and requested (NWHN 2002, 14).

The power of advertising may be the most detrimental to women's health when the advertising is geared toward her physician. In today's world where the FDA is pressured to get more drugs on to the market faster and where consumers are trained to ask for specific medications, the way-too-busy physicians, whose HMOs demand they see an almost impossible number of patients per hour, have ever-increasing responsibilities as the gatekeepers to the smorgasbord of medications available. Philip Hilts emphasizes the importance of this role in stating: "Drug approvals are in the hands of the FDA, but medicine is in the hands of doctors" (235). He identifies that the most common system failure in terms of the safety of medicine is in getting the appropriate knowledge to physicians:

> By the mid-1990s, the FDA, under pressure, was pinning its hopes on warning labels and doctors' care in prescribing. The burden of dangerous drugs thus shifted away from the agency. Good, but worrisome drugs are sent to market, and worries are often expressed on the label, rather than waiting for more data or proof of safety.
>
> That system may work if doctors read and heed the labels. Reviewers (at FDA) say the crafting of the label and related information is one of the chief satisfactions of the job—it amounts to giving the official word on what science knows about a drug. But as one reviewer said, "Doctors aren't often paying attention. We may put crucial information in a label and have it end up as a dead letter." Studies confirm it: the labels are largely unheeded and often completely unread. At the same time, pharmaceutical manufacturers effectively use the full arsenal of advertising and promotion to tout a drug's good qualities and downplay its problems. (2003, 234–5)

"Manufacturing Need, Manufacturing Knowledge" in *The Truth about Hormone Replacement Therapy* provides page after page of examples of how physicians' knowledge and prescribing practices are very carefully influenced by pharmaceutical companies. We all know about those mugs, pens, prescription pads, free lunches, and industry-supported conferences in Hawaii, but how many of us have thought about how much *our* physician's knowledge about *our* health is manipulated by the drug industry that has just managed—or not managed—to get a new product on the market? How many of the millions of women who have had prescriptions for ERT or HRT for the prevention of heart disease know that neither ERT nor HRT was ever given FDA approval for the prevention of heart disease? In one of the most important examples of the physicians' ultimate control of medicine, physicians have the right to prescribe a medication for a condition even if the FDA has never approved the medication for that condition, as long as the medication has had FDA approval for some condition. Because ERT and HRT have been approved for osteoporosis prevention, it is perfectly legal—and obviously was even considered "good medicine"—for a physician to prescribe it "off label" for heart disease. Keeping that in mind, it becomes even more obvious how influential a fast-talking drug rep, a slick PowerPoint presentation (designed and paid for by the drug company but actually delivered by a respected colleague), a study demonstrating the effectiveness of a particular drug (who reads the fine print to see that the drug company influenced the study design and funded the study; who knows how many industry-funded studies do not get published if they don't find the "right" answer?), or free samples of medications can be in helping that busy physician know what to prescribe. Drug companies know that money spent influencing physicians is money well spent. In 2001, they spent more than $16 billion on this line item. In other words, pharmaceutical companies pay $8,000–13,000 per year to influence *each* physician's drug prescribing practices (NWHN 2002, 3–18).

Using the HRT Story to Get to the Heart of the Politics of Women's Health

"Millions of healthy women were taking long-term hormone therapy for a preventative benefit not yet proven because medical practice was determined under the influence of industry rather than under the influence of (scientific) evidence" (Pearson 2003, 3). This was a statement made by the NWHN executive director, Cindy Pearson, at an October 24, 2003, National Institutes of Health meeting organized for the purpose of discussing the implications of the Women's Health Initiative.

Emphasizing the lessons that must be learned from the fact that "drug companies, professional societies, women's groups, policymakers, and government agencies had all been complicit in creating a 'climate of enthusiasm for hormone therapy' and allowing the needless suffering of tens of thousands of women," Pearson identified the following steps that must be taken:

- Get drug company money out of medical education.

- Give the FDA the authority to pre-approve direct-to-consumer advertisements for prescription medications.

- End industry payments to physicians for writing papers that appear in medical journals.

- Stop quoting medical experts in media reports on health without reporting on their financial relationship with industry.

- Clean up consumer groups' health education so that the all-too-common and dangerous influence of drug company money is replaced with healthy skepticism.

- Bar anyone with significant financial ties to industry from involvement in the development of professional guidelines. (2003, 3)

The role of the Women's Health Movement is as important as ever. We must

- Insist that large, long-term, randomized studies are done on all products that are marketed to healthy women. Science must triumph over marketing. Safety must be seen to be more important than money.

- Shift the emphasis to life-long health promoting practices. We must constantly ask whether the availability or overuse of drugs and other products distracts attention from looking at safer ways of taking care of women's health.

- Organize around the fact that consumer activism and consumer medical literacy are more important than ever so that common sense and health promotion triumph over marketing.

Note

1. While I take full responsibility for ideas expressed in this paper, I give much credit to the other members of the writing group of *The Truth About Hormone Replacement Therapy* (National Women's Health Network, 2002) and to the book for some of the ideas and information shared here.

REFERENCES
A list of references is available in original source.

When, How, and Which One?
"Navigating the Maze of Osteoporosis Drugs"

by Kristen Suthers

Osteoporosis (porous bone) is a disease that causes bones to become fragile and increases their risk of breaking. It is a real condition with serious effects on women's health and quality of life; at the same time, it's a condition that has become over-advertised and over-treated. What is osteoporosis? When should it be treated and which treatment is best? In recent years, the number of drugs available to address osteoporosis has grown exponentially, creating a dilemma for many women about the appropriate use of these medications. Specifically, women want to know when it is appropriate to take a drug for osteoporosis, and which treatments are safest and most effective.

"When, How, and Which One? Navigating the Maze of Osteoporosis Drugs," by Kristen Suthers, Ph.D., originally published in the *Women's Health Activist*, March/April 2006, pp. 1, 3, 5, the newsletter of the National Women's Health Network (NWHN). It is reprinted with the permission of the author and the NWHN.

While all women lose bone mass more quickly at the onset of menopause, all women don't develop osteoporosis. A woman is diagnosed with *osteoporosis* if her bone mineral density score is more than 2.5 standard deviations below the average for young adult Caucasian women. Bone density is measured either by X-ray equipment called a DEXA machine or by an ultrasound machine. The U.S. Preventive Services Task Force recommends that women over 65 be screened for osteoporosis; for women under 65, the decision to test depends on her risk for osteoporosis, her health, and her family history. It's important to know that the American College of Sports Medicine has stated that it's unclear whether these criteria are appropriate for women of color. Until standardized criteria for osteoporosis are available for non-Caucasian populations, health care practitioners will likely continue relying on the current diagnostic criteria.

Osteopenia identifies women with low bone mineral density who may be at-risk for osteoporosis; osteopenia is diagnosed when a woman's bone mineral density score is 1.0–2.5 standard deviations below the average. Although all women with osteoporosis once had osteopenia, not all women with osteopenia will develop osteoporosis. For this reason, and because it is unclear how much drugs benefit women at this stage, the World Health Organization recommends treating osteopenia only when other risk factors for fractures are apparent.

Hormones

The Food and Drug Administration (FDA) has approved estrogen and progestin treatment only to prevent, not to treat, osteoporosis. Both estrogen alone and combinations of estrogen and progestin reduce the risk of osteoporosis and bone fracture in women. As yet, no evidence indicates that doses lower than 0.625 mg are effective in preventing fractures. Taking these hormones, however, increase a woman's risk of breast cancer, heart attack, stroke, and pulmonary embolism. Therefore, estrogen and progestin should be the last choice for osteoporosis prevention and should be used only when other types of prevention are contraindicated. Further, there is insufficient scientific evidence to support using other types of non-traditional estrogens (i.e., 17 Beta-estradiol and 'bioidentical hormones') to prevent or treat osteoporosis.

Two other classes of medications have been approved only to treat women who already have osteoporosis: *teriparatide* and *calcitonin*. Teriparatide is a derivative of human parathyroid hormone (PTH), the primary regulator of calcium and phosphate metabolism in bones; 20 mg are injected daily to stimulate new bone formation and prevent vertebral and non-vertebral fractures in women with osteoporosis. Teriparatide (brand name: Forteo) is generally used only for women with severe osteoporosis, since side effects can include nausea, leg cramps, and dangerously high levels of calcium.

Calcitonin (not to be confused with calcium supplements) is a hormone that participates in calcium and phosphorus metabolism. While calcitonin prevents spinal fractures, it has not been shown to prevent hip, wrist, or other non-vertebral fractures. The hormone has been approved to treat women with osteoporosis, but the poor quality of the study evaluating calcitonin has made doctors reluctant to recommend it, and a review article in *The New England Journal of Medicine* stated that the use of calcitonin is generally not recommended. Women who do decide to take calcitonin must watch their intake of foods containing high calcium levels (e.g., milk, cheese), as excessive calcium in a woman's body may be dangerous. Calcitonin (brand names: Fortical or Miacalcin) can be administered as a nasal spray or as a skin injection; side effects may include nasal congestion and nausea.

Bisphosphonates

Bisphosphonates are non-hormonal drugs that reduce the risk of fracture without the problems associated with hormone therapy. The drugs include Alendronate (brand name: Fosamax), Risendronate (brand name: Actonel), and Ibandronate (brand name: Boniva). Bisphosphonates have been approved by the FDA to prevent bone loss and fractures in the entire skeleton. Side effects vary by type of bisphosphonate, but generally can include damage to the esophagus (esophagitis) and muscle pain. The initial 150 mg dose may also cause a one-time response of muscle pain, joint aches, and low-grade fever.

While bisphosphonates seem to have fewer risks than hormones, they have not been around very long and clinical trials have not explored the effects on women of taking bisphosphonates for more than 10 years. A woman who starts taking bisphosphonates at menopause is likely to have to continue on the drugs for several decades to benefit, since the risk of debilitating fractures becomes most significant after age 70. Bisphosphonates' effects in premenopausal women have also not yet been extensively studied. Long-term bisphosphonate use may also begin to suppress, rather than stimulate, new bone formation, which can lead to brittle bones. A woman who decides to take bisphosphonates should carefully weigh the risks and benefits in consultation with her health care provider.

The use of most bisphosphonates requires a woman to take a pill every day and then sit upright for 30–60 minutes to prevent esophageal damage. Since its approval, Boniva has been heavily marketed because it can be taken once a month, a great advantage over daily pills. Women need to understand, however, that Boniva is only approved to prevent vertebral fractures; not other types of breaks such as hip or wrist fractures. In January, 2006, the FDA approved intravenous Boniva, to be administered by a health care provider every three months. Despite Boniva's advantages, it has been available to the general population for a short time, which means there is only limited information on its effectiveness in preventing bone loss and fractures in the general public.

Selective Estrogen Receptor Modulators

Sometimes referred to as 'designer estrogens', the FDA has approved *Selective Estrogen Receptor Modulators* (SERM) for the treatment and prevention of osteoporosis. SERMs have different effects on estrogen receptors in different parts of the body, producing estrogenic effects in some sites, and acting like anti-estrogens in others. Raloxifene (brand name: Evista) seems to prevent osteoporosis without increasing the risk of cancers associated with other hormone treatments. But, raloxifene carries risks not found in non-hormonal drugs, including increased risk of blood clots, hot flashes, nausea, and leg cramps.

Large-scale, randomized, placebo-controlled trials over several years have indicated that raloxifene can prevent vertebral, but not non-vertebral fractures in postmenopausal women with osteoporosis. This is useful, as women who have multiple spinal fractures experience severe and debilitating pain, and difficulty with their daily activities. But the drug has not been shown to prevent non-vertebral fractures (such as hip or wrist fractures), and its efficacy has not been demonstrated in women without osteoporosis. It should be noted that raloxifene studies have not reported outcomes by race or ethnicity, since the studies lacked enough women of color to draw conclusive distinctions. Therefore, it is difficult to know how effective raloxifene is in preventing osteoporosis for women of color. While osteoporosis is more common among Caucasian and Asian women, the NWHN believes that these questions are important to all women regardless of ethnicity, and that any women's health study should include women of color.

In 2005, raloxifene's manufacturer, Eli Lilly, plead guilty to violating the Food, Drug, & Cosmetic Act and paid $36 million in fines for illegally promoting the drug to prevent and treat breast cancer and cardiovascular disease. The FDA has not approved raloxifene for these indications. This violation calls Eli Lilly's integrity into question. A woman who decides to take a drug to pre-

---

Risk factors you cannot change:
- **Gender** Osteoporosis is more common among, women because they have less bone tissue and lose bone faster than men due to changes that occur in menopause.
- **Age** The older you are, the greater your risk of osteoporosis as bones become thinner and weaker with age.
- **Body size** Small, thin-boned women are at greater risk.
- **Ethnicity** Caucasian and Asian women are at highest risk. African American and Hispanic women have lower, but significant, risk.
- **Family history** People whose parents have a history of fractures also seem to have reduced bone mass and may be at risk for fractures.

Risk factors you can change:
- **Sex hormones** Abnormal absence of menstrual periods, low estrogen levels, and low testosterone level in women can bring on osteoporosis.
- **Anorexia nervosa** The eating disorder increases the risk of osteoporosis.
- **Calcium and vitamin D intake** A lifetime diet low-in calcium and vitamin D makes you vulnerable to bone loss.
- **Medication use** Long-term use of glucocorticoids and some anticonvulsants can lead to loss of bone density and fractures.
- **Lifestyle** Inactive lifestyles or extended bed rest tends to weaken bones.
- **Smoking** Cigarettes are bad for bones as well as the heart and lungs.
- **Alcohol Intake** Excessive consumption increases the risk of bone loss and fractures.

Source: National Institutes of Health Osteoporosis and Related Bone Diseases Resource Center.

vent vertebral fractures should try bisphosphonates first; she should only consider raloxifene if she has osteoporosis and cannot tolerate bisphosphonates. There's no reason to try raloxifene first, because no other benefit has been definitively shown.

The Bottom Line

There are clear indications that the pharmaceutical industry is looking to expand its market for osteoporosis drugs; the latest efforts are targeting 'non-traditional' populations for osteopenia and osteoporosis screening, such as younger women and men. The NWHN believes many women under age 65 without critical risk factors are being inappropriately screened for osteopenia and osteoporosis; screening at this early age has not been shown to help prevent serious fractures unless there are significant risk factors present. We encourage women under age 65 to avoid bone density screening unless they are at an increased risk for osteoporosis based on multiple risk factors. (See box for more information on risk factors.)

There are a few other factors women need to consider when deciding whether to take osteoporosis drugs. The sequence of medications is important: some drugs cannot precede or follow others. In addition, the duration of treatment is critical in determining the effectiveness of prevention and treatment of osteoporosis: when a woman stops taking the drug, the preventive effects are lost. A woman shouldn't hesitate to ask her health care practitioner about the safety and efficacy of any osteoporosis medication, and inquire whether non-drug alternatives might be just as effective for her, based on her personal history and current health status.

For more information go to the National Institutes of Health Osteoporosis and Related Bone Diseases Resource Center's website: http://www.osteo.org/osteolinks.asp. The NWHN also has Fact Sheets on hormone therapy for osteoporosis and raloxifene at our website: www.nwhn.org.

"A Bone to Pick with Bone Drugs"

by Adriane Fugh-Berman

Worried about your bone density? Anti-osteoporosis drug makers hope you are. Osteoporosis is represented as a deadly disease, a silent killer affecting millions of women who go about their daily lives, unaware that their bones are dwindling to kindling. A 1995 book for consumers states. "If osteoporosis gets bad enough, a woman who has it could suffer a broken arm lifting a casserole out of the oven or reaching back to zip up her dress. She could break her foot stepping put of bed or a rib upon sneezing."[1]

The National Osteoporosis Foundation (NOF) says: "Osteoporosis is a major public health threat for an estimated 44 million Americans, or 55% of the people 50 years of age and older. In the U.S. 10 million individuals are estimated to already have the disease and almost 34 million more are estimated to have low bone mass, placing them at increased risk for osteoporosis."[2]

Seems to me that if more than half the population over 50 is so deficient in bone mass there should be a *lot* more people found in crumpled heaps by their ovens and beds.

NOF's website also says: "A hip fracture . . . can impair a person's ability to walk unassisted and may cause prolonged or permanent disability or even death." Another suspect statement. Breaking an arm doesn't kill people; why should breaking a hip? Associations between hip fracture, disability, and death are misleading because hip fracture is a marker for *frailty*. If you're frail and elderly (especially if you have other medical problems), being hospitalized for *any* major surgery, including to fix a hip fracture, can kill you.

The average age of hip fracture is 80. As one researcher put it, "High mortality, particularly in the first three months, is probably due to the combination of

"A Bone to Pick with Bone Drugs," by Adriane Fugh-Berman, M.D., originally published in the *Women's Health Activist*, March/April 2006, p. 11, the newsletter of the National Women's Health Network (NWHN). It is reprinted with the permission of the author and the NWHN.

trauma, major surgery in elderly people with concurrent medical problems, and a low physiological reserve."[3] One study of 2,448 patients admitted to the hospital with hip fracture found a high rate of post-operative complications. Patients with multiple medical problems before hospitalization did worse; about 10% died within a month, usually of chest infections or heart failure.[3] This doesn't mean that hip fractures were the culprit. In fact, researchers state, "Few of these deaths can be attributed to the hip fracture *per se*; most are due instead to chronic illnesses that led to both the fracture and to the patient's ultimate demise. Thus, whether prevention of hip fracture can extend life expectancy, and to what extent is unclear."[3]

Even if your bones look like Swiss cheese, avoiding falls is more important than building bone; falls cause more than 90% of hip fractures and 80% of other fractures. Preventing falls would prevent most fractures. Just increasing physical activity could cut falls by half. Fall risk factors include being older; having muscle weakness or limited mobility; being challenged by environmental hazards (e.g., throw rugs, slippery shoes); taking four or more medications or taking psychoactive drugs; having dementia, visual difficulties, or Parkinson's; and experiencing a stroke. Age is probably most important: women over 85 are nearly 8 times more likely to be hospitalized for hip fracture than women aged 65–74.

Nursing home residents contribute more than their fair share of broken bones and fall-related deaths to these statistics. Among older adults, the 5% who live in nursing homes suffer 20% of all fall-related deaths.[4] Up to three out of four nursing home residents fall annually, twice the rate of seniors living in the community. And, more than 1/3 of fall-related injuries in nursing homes occur to residents who weren't able to walk before the fall.[5]

Despite the scary scenarios perpetuated by drug makers, the absolute risk of hip fracture is low, especially in 50-year-olds. The risk that a 50-year-old woman will fracture her hip in the next 10 years is just 0.4%. The 10-year risk for a 60-year-old is 1.5%; at 70, the risk is 4.7%; and at 80, is 11%.[6] So, one 50-year-old of 250 will fracture her hip by age 60; at 70, one woman in 20 will fracture her hip in the next 10 years.

Osteoporosis is not a killer disease. It's not really a disease at all, but a structural abnormality. 'Osteopenia' is a term that's become popular recently as a way to expand market share for bone-building drugs. Let's see: osteopenia is a risk factor for osteoporosis: which is a risk factor for hip fracture; which is a risk factor for surgery, immobility and complications; which is a risk factor for death, but primarily in frail elderly nursing home residents (and not just the women)! A multimodal fall prevention and mitigation program—including eye exams, medication adjustments, strength training, environmental modifications, hip protectors and appropriate antiosteoporosis therapies—could have a real effect on decreasing fall-related disability and death. Scaring ambulatory, community-dwelling women into taking antiosteoporosis drugs benefits corporate coffers, not women's health.

REFERENCES

See: The Centers for Disease Control and Prevention. National Center for Injury Prevention and Control 'Falls and Hip Fractures Among Older Adults,' on-line: http://www.cdc.gov/ncipc/factsheets/falls.htm.: and Stevens, JA. Olson S. 'Reducing falls and resulting hip fractures among older adults.' *MMWR* 2000, 49 (RR-2):3–12.

1. Nachtigall L. Heilman J. *Estrogen. The facts can change your life! A complete guide to reversing the effects of menopause using hormone replacement therapy.* New York: HarperCollins, 1995.

2. National Osteoporosis Foundation, 'Fast Facts,' On-line: http://www.nof.org/osteoporosis/diseasefacts.htm.

3. Cummings SR. Melton L.J. 'Epidemiology and outcomes of osteoporotic fractures.' *Lancet* 2002;359:1761–67

4. Rubenstein LZ. 'Preventing falls in the nursing home.' *JAMA* 1997:278(7):595–6.

5. Thapa PB, Brockman KG, Gideon P, et al. 'Injurious falls in nonambulatory nursing home residents: a comparative study of circumstances, incidence and risk factors,' *Journal of the American Geriatrics Society* 1996:44:273–8.

6. van der Klift M, de Last CD, Pols HA. 'Assessment of fracture risk: who should be treated for osteoporosis?' *Best Pract Res Clin Rheumatol* 2005;19(6):937–5.

"Less Hormone Therapy, Less Breast Cancer"

by Adriane Fugh-Berman

The exodus from menopausal hormone therapy after the Women's Health Initiative (WHI) proved that the risks of this therapy outweighed its benefits has resulted in a stunning drop in breast cancer rates. A new study shows that, in 2003, the year after the estrogen-progestin arm of the WHI was stopped, breast cancer rates plummeted by seven percent.[1] It was expected that about 200,000 women would develop breast cancer in 2003, so about 14,000 fewer women were diagnosed with the disease than expected.

The decrease was most pronounced in women who were older than 50: women who were the prime target audience for hormone therapy. Breast cancer rates dropped 11 percent for women in their 50s and 60s—and 7 percent for women in their 70s. In contrast, breast cancer rates dropped only 1 percent for women in their 40s, who are less likely than older women to take hormones.

The effects of hormone therapy are linked more strongly to estrogen-receptor (ER)-positive tumors than to estrogen-receptor-negative tumors. The decrease in cancer rates was twice as high (8 percent versus 4 percent) in ER-positive tumors than it was in ER-negative tumors. Among women 50–69 years of age, the reduction in ER-positive tumors was three times higher than the reduction in ER-negative tumors (12 percent versus 4 percent). This study provides dramatic confirmation that combined hormone therapy increases the risk of developing breast cancer, particularly of developing ER-positive tumors.

Normally, one has to be cautious in interpreting cause and effect from associations. For example, birth rates that go up in a location in which the number of storks is also increasing doesn't prove that storks bring babies. The dramatic drop in breast cancer rates, however, is extremely unusual—especially without a change in other cancer rates. The decrease was seen in every cancer registry that reports data to the federal government. The fact that there were so many people using, and then abandoning, hormone therapy makes this into a sort of large-scale natural experiment.

The wide use of hormone therapy, of course, was due to marketing. Menopausal hormones were heavily promoted as a way to prevent disease during the 1990s. In fact, gynecologists were so convinced of its benefits that they ranked hormone use above smoking cessation as a positive means to prevent disease.[2] Fifty-eight million prescriptions for hormone therapy were written in 1995; between 1999 and 2002, 90 million prescriptions were written annually.[3] That means about a quarter of all women over 40 were taking hormones during this time.

Six months after the WHI found that menopausal hormones increased breast cancer rates and did not prevent cardiovascular disease, hormone prescriptions dropped by two-thirds. A year later, hormone prescriptions were down by 80 percent, compared to the number written before the WHI results were announced.[4] Other studies have also found that hormone use has dropped. The National Ambulatory Medical Care Survey and the National Hospital Ambulatory Medical Care Survey found that visits to physicians that resulted in hormone prescriptions being written decreased 43.6 percent from 2001 to 2003.[5]

Fluctuations in breast cancer rates appear to closely follow the use of hormones. While hormones were being most heavily promoted, breast cancer rates increased: between 1990 and 1998, the incidence increased 1.7 percent per year. Breast cancer incidence began to drift down gradually after that, declining about 1 percent a year. Then, in 2003, the rates suddenly plummeted 7 percent. This is an astoundingly large drop; cancer rates just don't change that fast without something major going on.

Hormone therapy is effective for hot flashes, and its short-term use may be worth the risks for some women with severe symptoms. But at this point, many lines of evidence have proven that menopausal estrogen-progestin therapy increases breast cancer risk. Don't let anyone tell you otherwise.

REFERENCES

1. Ravdin PM, Cronin KA, Howlander N et al. "A sharp decrease in breast cancer incidence in the United States in 2003." Data from MD Anderson, the National Cancer Institute, and Harbor UCLA Medical Center, presented at the San Antonio Breast Cancer Symposium, December 14, 2006.

2. Saver BG, Taylor TR, Woods NF et al. "Physician policies on the use of preventive hormone replacement therapy." *Am J Prev Med* 1997: 13(5):358–365.

3. Hersh AL, Stefanick ML, Stafford RS. "National use of postmenopausal hormone therapy: annual trends and response to recent evidence." *JAMA*, 2004 Jan 7; 291(1): 47–53.

4. Majumdar SR, Almasi EA, Stafford RS. "Promotion and prescribing of hormone therapy after report of harm by the Women's Health Initiative." *JAMA*. 2004 Oct 27; 292(16):1983–8.

5. Hing E, Brett KM. "Changes in U.S. prescribing patterns of menopausal hormone therapy, 2001–2003." *Obstet Gynecol*. 2006 Jul:108(1):33–40.

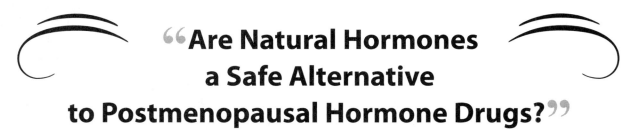

"Are Natural Hormones a Safe Alternative to Postmenopausal Hormone Drugs?"

by Maryann Napoll

When a landmark clinical trial reported in 2002 that the dangers of postmenopausal hormone drugs far outweighed the benefits, many more women turned to *bioidentical* or *natural* hormones. These products are widely portrayed in the media and on the Internet as safer than prescription hormone drugs like Prempro and Premarin for the relief of hot flashes and other menopausal symptoms. The idea that these products are safer or even natural is challenged in a paper by Adriane Fugh-Berman, MD, and Jenna Bythrow of the Complementary and Alternative Medicine Master's Program, Georgetown University School of Medicine.

Sold as topical creams and tablets over the Internet and in health food stores, bioidentical hormones are actually synthetic versions of female hormones, including estriol, estrone, estradiol, progesterone, testosterone, DHEA, thyroxine and cortisol. In their paper published recently in the *Journal of General Internal Medicine*, Fugh-Berman and Bythrow contend that *bioidentical* is a meaningless term coined by a business that knows what sells.

Compounding Pharmacies

Many of these products are prepared by compounding pharmacies that convert prescription and non-prescription drugs into different formulations. For example, converting a drug manufactured in tablet form to a syrup for people who have difficulty swallowing pills or a pet-sized dose of a drug meant for humans. In the case of bioidentical hormones, the pharmacies are reformulating the *standard prescription hormone drugs*, usually in weaker doses.

Because compounding pharmacies are not manufacturing facilities, they are not required by the FDA to prove safety or effectiveness. "Compounding pharmacies have their place," said Dr. Fugh-Berman in a telephone interview. "But [with bioidentical hormones] all these pharmacies are doing are buying hormones from Upjohn or some other drug company and following a recipe."

"Bioidentical hormones are chemically identical to hormones produced by the body," explained Dr. Fugh-Berman, but the term *bioidentical* is widely misunderstood. Most women surveyed at one compounding pharmacy either thought it meant "not man-made" or plant-derived; they no doubt got that impression from advertising and/or reading the product labels which often, for example, feature wild yams as the source of progesterone.

Bioidentical hormones are sometimes derived from starting materials of plants in a lab process, Dr. Fugh-Berman said, "but, you won't get progesterone from eating a yam. Plants have precursors in them, but not actual progesterone."

Because compounding pharmacies are unregulated, they can make unsubstantiated claims for their products. The most dangerous to Dr. Fugh-Berman are the claims that bioidentical hormones will prevent heart disease and breast cancer, as well as improve well-being—all of which have been discredited for standard hormone drugs in the landmark 2002 Women's Health Initiative trial.

Also, women with an intact uterus must protect it against estrogen-induced endometrial cancer with the addition of progesterone. Studies show that many bioidentical progesterone products contain much weaker doses of the standard progesterone prescription drugs, so they do not provide the level of needed protection.

For the many women who do not want to hear her message and will continue taking bioidentical hormones no matter what, Dr. Fugh-Berman has this advice, "Now we know that [the conventional prescription] hormones help only symptoms—hot flashes and vaginal dryness—they don't prevent disease," she said, referring to the results of the 2002 Women's Health Initiative trial. "So symptomatic women should take the lowest possible dose for the shortest period of time. Women without symptoms shouldn't use either bioidentical or conventional hormones for disease prevention. Bioidentical hormones should be assumed to have the same risks as conventional hormone drugs and should carry the same warning labels."

As for the standard claim that bioidentical hormones are natural, "Ironically, the estrogen in the best-selling hormone preparations Premarin, Prempro, and Premphase is derived from pregnant mare's urine, an inarguably natural source."

Phytoestrogens
"A New Alternative for Women?"

by Adriane Fugh-Berman

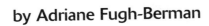
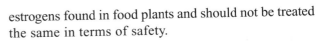

Phytoestrogens, or plant estrogens, are much weaker estrogens than our own bodies make. Phytoestrogens are only about 1/200th the strength of endogenous estrogens. There are two main kinds of phytoestrogens: lignans and isoflavones. Foods that contain lignans include oily seeds, especially flaxseed (also called linseed) and also cereal grains, beans, vegetables and fruits. Premenopausal women fed 10 grams a day of flaxseed powder multiplied their lignan excretion 3 to 285 fold. Isoflavones are less common, occurring mainly in soybeans, chickpeas, and other legumes (Knight). Some phytoestrogens are also found in black cohosh, clover and other medicinal herbs, but these are different than phyto-estrogens found in food plants and should not be treated the same in terms of safety.

Hot Flashes and Vaginal Dryness

Whole grains and beans (especially soybeans) are the most commonly eaten source of phytoestrogens. Asian women complain less of hot flashes than Western women do, and it may be that eating soy products serves as a type of hormone replacement therapy (Adlercreutz). There is evidence that supplementing with phytoestrogens can help hot flashes and vaginal dryness. A study of 145 Israeli women with menopausal symptoms found that the 78 women assigned to a phytoestrogen-rich diet had fewer hot flashes and less vaginal dryness than the

36 women in the control group who did not change their diet (Adlercreutz 1997). The study lasted twelve weeks and women in the treatment group substituted phytoestrogen-rich foods (including tofu, soy drink, miso, and flax seed) for approximately one fourth of their daily caloric intake (Brzezinski). Two studies have looked at whether supplementing the diet with phytoestrogens resulted in estrogenic changes in vaginal cells. One study found a positive result (Wilcox) and the other a negative result (Baird), but the study that did not find an effect used an unusual method of collecting vaginal cells that may have underestimated estrogenized cells (Knight).

Breast Cancer Prevention

What is the effect of phytoestrogens on breast cancer risk? Although there has not been a prospective study on this, studies of different populations show that groups that consume a lot of phytoestrogens have a lower rate of breast cancer. A recent case control study found that women with breast cancer excreted much lower amounts of phytoestrogens in their urine than women without breast cancer (Ingram).

However, this protective effect may be strongest in premenopausal women. Soybeans are quite high in phytoestrogens, and there is a high intake of soy products in some Asian countries, especially China, Japan, and Korea. A study of Chinese women in Singapore found that soy product intake seemed to protect premenopausal women, but not postmenopausal women, from breast cancer (Lee).

Different Effects in Premenopausal and Postmenopausal Women

The above result is not all that surprising because phytoestrogens may have opposite effects in premenopausal and postmenopausal women. Premenopausal women have nominally higher estrogen levels than postmenopausal women. In premenopausal women who eat a lot of plant estrogens, the weak plant estrogens perform some of the same functions as our own, stronger estrogens. Chemical messengers regulate estrogen in our bodies by determining when more or less estrogen is needed; when weak plant estrogens are meeting our estrogen needs, our own hormone factories take a break. So premenopausal women with normally high estrogen levels who eat plant estrogens everyday have a constantly lower rate of production of homegrown estrogens, and the total estrogen effect on their bodies (lower internal estrogen production plus weak plant estrogens) is lower. So in premenopausal women, the effect of a diet high in phytoestrogens is actually anti-estrogenic.

"Background" estrogen levels are already low in postmenopausal women, so eating phytoestrogens boosts the estrogen levels. So for postmenopausal women, phytoestrogens may have an estrogenic effect. This estrogenic effect may affect different organs differently. A high soy intake appears to protect against endometrial cancer in both premenopausal and postmenopausal women (Goodman).

Different Menopausal Experiences in Asian and Western Women

Some people theorize that hot flashes and other menopausal symptoms may be due less to low estrogen levels than to a sudden drop in estrogen levels. According to this theory, Asian women complain less of hot flashes and other menopause-related complaints because decades of eating soy products may have lowered estrogen levels sufficiently that the menopausal drop, especially cushioned by continued high intake of phytoestrogens, may be an easy hormonal descent. Westerners start at a higher estrogen level and fall to a lower level; we plummet over a hormonal cliff.

Other factors may be equally important, of course; it is difficult to determine the importance of the fact that Asians respect age while Westerners worship youth. The transition to menopause in the West might be very different if we looked forward to an honored place in society rather than discrimination and poverty.

If You Have Breast Cancer

Phytoestrogens in food have been consumed for thousands of years by Asian women, who have a lower risk of breast cancer than Western women at all ages, and the idea that these foods are dangerous is clearly absurd. For premenopausal women with breast cancer, phytoestrogen would be expected to lower circulating estrogen levels and thus be beneficial.

For postmenopausal women with breast cancer the situation is more complicated. Soybeans contain substances that are estrogenic and substances that are anticancer. It is not clear whether the estrogenic properties of soybeans could cause breast cancer to grow. In cultured breast cancer cells, both estradiol and a phytoestrogen stimulated cell growth, but when added together, little to no growth stimulation occurred. But in an immunocompromised mouse model, phytoestrogen implants caused estrogen receptor positive (but not estrogen receptor negative) breast cancer implants to grow (Helferich).

On the other hand, phytoestrogen supplementation in postmenopausal women markedly increased sex hormone binding globulin (SHBG) (Brzezinski). High levels of SHBG are associated with lower breast cancer risk.

The Network believes that supplementing one's diet with phytoestrogens makes sense for premenopausal women. Whether postmenopausal women with breast cancer should avoid supplementing with phytoestrogens is an open question. The Network believes that there is no need for postmenopausal women with breast cancer to actively avoid phytoestrogens, which are consumed in quantity in many countries with low breast cancer rates, and are found in many foods with high nutritive value. Whether or not to actively supplement a diet with phytoestrogens is a different story.

Some people argue that Asian women have lower breast cancer rates at all ages than Westerners, so phytoestrogen intake can't be harmful. But Asians consume high levels of phytoestrogens throughout their lifetime, and this may create a very different hormonal situation than a Western woman who has a low phytoestrogen intake premenopausally and then suddenly increases her phytoestrogen intake postmenopausally. It is theoretically possible that that scenario increases her lifetime exposure to estrogens. Also, other factors may contribute to a lower rate of breast cancer in Asian women, who generally consume a low-fat, high-fiber diet, and have different exposures to environmental factors. A case can be made for postmenopausal women with breast cancer to maximize or minimize phytoestrogen intake, but there is not adequate evidence to justify a strong recommendation either for supplementing or avoiding phytoestrogens.

Should breast cancer patients who are being treated with the hormonal drug tamoxifen supplement with phytoestrogens? These two substances have similar effects in terms of having some estrogenic and some antiestrogenic properties. There are no studies on what the effects are of combining the use of phytoestrogens and tamoxifen. The Network believes that once again, a case can be made either for supplementing or avoiding phytoestrogens, and that the most prudent decision may be to do neither.

Cardiovascular Disease

Soybeans also may have a beneficial effect on cardiovascular disease. A meta-analysis of 38 controlled clinical trials found that eating a lot of soy protein was associated with reduced cholesterol (9.3% less than controls), reduced LDL cholesterol (12.9%), reduced triglycerides (10.5%). HDL cholesterol was unaffected (Anderson).

Osteoporosis

The effect of phytoestrogens on bone has not been well studied, but there is reason to believe that there may be some effect on bone. Asians have a lower rate of osteoporotic bone fracture than Western women do, despite the fact that the bones of Asian women are thinner and their calcium intake is far lower than Western women. And genistein, the predominant isoflavone in soybeans, helps to maintain bone in rats that have had their ovaries removed (Knight).

If You Want to Supplement with Phytoestrogens

Soybean products are the most widely consumed source of isoflavones and also contain some lignan precursors. Chick peas (garbanzo beans), lima beans, other beans, and peas are also good sources of isoflavones.

In Asia, consumption of legumes (soybeans, lentils, other beans, and peas) provides 25–45 mg of total isoflavones a day, compared with Western countries, where less than 5 mg/day is eaten. In Japan, where soy consumption is very high, up to 200 mg/day of isoflavones are consumed (Knight).

Not all soy products are equal in terms of phytoestrogen content. Soy oil and soy sauce don't have measurable amounts of phytoestrogens in them.

Tofu (soy bean curd) comes in many different textures and is almost tasteless on its own; it easily takes on other flavors. "Silken" tofu is the softest and is best for blending; try making shakes with fruit juice or substituting it for oil in your favorite salad dressing recipe. Very firm tofu can be cut up and put into soups and curries or marinated and stir-fried with vegetables.

An added bonus for eating tofu is that many brands are made with calcium sulfate and can supply a significant amount of this important nutrient. According to the USDA, ¼ block (116 mg) of tofu made with calcium supplies 406 mg. of calcium, and ¼ block of firm tofu (81 gm) supplies 553 mg of calcium. Read the label to see if your brand of tofu is made with calcium.

You can increase your intake of lignans by eating more whole grains (especially rye) and eating flaxseed. Several breakfast cereals are made with flaxseed. It tastes nutty when toasted and can be sprinkled on hot or cold cereal, yogurt, etc.

Summary

The Network believes that phytoestrogens are safe and beneficial to the health of premenopausal women, and may alleviate menopausal symptoms in postmenopausal women, but that the safety of supplemental phytoestrogens in postmenopausal women with breast cancer has not been clearly established.

References are available from the office of the National Women's Health Network.

WORKSHEET—CHAPTER 12

Aging, Ageism, Mid-life and Older Women's Health Issues

1. Compare who you are physically, emotionally, and intellectually today to the person you were five years ago. Which of the changes are positive? Which changes are negative? How do you think the changes of the last five years are similar to and different than the changes you will go through in the next five years? How do the issues you have identified compare with those Pasty J. Murphy identifies in "Ageing?"

2. It is often hard to think about ageing when we are young. However, there are many lifestyle factors throughout our lives that can have an impact on the health we will experience when we get older. (Be sure to read the introduction to this chapter and the articles before completing these questions.)

   a. Examine your own health-related behaviors (nutrition, exercise, use of drugs, etc.) to see how these might affect risks for both osteoporosis and heart disease.

   b. What changes could you make now to decrease these risks? Be specific!

   c. Do you think the answers for question b will be different for a 20-year-old, a 40-year-old, and a 60-year-old?

   d. How could health policies and health education for young people be most appropriate for maximizing the possibility for a healthy old age?

3. Pretend you are a health educator designing a poster for mid-life (35 to 65 year old) women to encourage positive images and health promotion. Describe what your poster could look like.

4. Healthy mid-life women are a huge market. Observe how products and lifestyle issues are marketed to this group in magazines, in T.V. ads, and talk shows. What messages do women get about ageing? What information is given about specific products? Do you think women have the information they need to evaluate whether they "need" a product and whether it is safe?

5. Read the information on menopausal hormones and osteoporosis products in this chapter. (Or, do your own research on the latest scientific research on such products.) Compare what you know about the science of menopause, osteoporosis, hormones, and "alternatives" with what you see covered on these topics in the popular media, particularly ads aimed at mid-life women.

6. Interview two older women about the following issues, and summarize their answers.

a. Ask them their age and ask them to think about how one or two women's health issues have changed in their lifetimes. How do they think women's health issues are different for today's 20 to 30-year-old women than when they were that age?

Woman 1   Woman 2

b. Ask them to describe their attitudes and experiences of menopause and what they think influenced their attitudes and experiences? Were they surprised by the "news" that estrogen and HRT have serious health risks? How has that "news" and other information influenced their decisions about medication for menopause symptoms and for osteoporosis and heart disease prevention?

Woman 1   Woman 2

c. Ask them to identify key health issues in their lives today. How secure do they feel about being able to meet their health needs in the next five years and for the rest of their lives?

Woman 1   Woman 2

d. Compare the answers you heard from these two women. In comparing their answers, think about how differences or similarities in age, race, class, sexual identity, education, religion, or other issues may have impacted on the differences or similarities in their answers.

POLITICS *of* DISEASE, PREVENTION, *and the* ENVIRONMENT

The politics of disease can be seen in the decisions made by government agencies, pharmaceutical companies, and the healthcare industry regarding priorities in funding, research, services, and education. Another aspect of the politics of disease is how women interact as both consumers and practitioners with these systems to fight for the priorities we identify. The first section of this chapter focuses on breast cancer, which it is estimated that one out of seven women in the United States will develop. The excerpt, "Breast Cancer: Power vs. Prosthesis," from *The Cancer Journals* by Audre Lorde, an extraordinary writer who died of breast cancer, examines the complexities around Lorde's decision not to use a prosthesis after mastectomy. The reader is encouraged to think about ways this article illustrates a number of themes in this book. While some women feel the use of a breast prosthesis or implants will be an important part of their coping with or healing from breast cancer, other women will identify with Lorde in not wanting to hide the battle they are fighting or have won. Thus Lorde's "Power vs. Prosthesis" can be considered a critique of a medical system that too often assumes "one size fits all." Similarly, this important classic symbolizes body image issues where there is too narrow a definition of what women should look like and there is enormous pressure for women to "fit" this image, no matter how inappropriate it is for their health and well-being. (Also see Lorde's essays in Chapter 2: "Age, Race, Class, and Sex: Women Redefining Difference" and "There is No Hierarchy of Oppression.") The next article, by Stephanie Donne, provides an update on the ongoing debates and controversies about breast implants (silicone gel or saline) used for reconstruction after mastectomy. Questions are raised about both known and unknown health risks of these implants, including an effect crucial for women who have a breast cancer history to know: The implants interfere with the ability of mammograms to detect breast cancer.

We draw your attention to Rita Arditti and Tatiana Schreiber's "Breast Cancer: The Environmental Connection" because it so eloquently asks us to think about what it would mean to *prevent* breast cancer rather than merely detect it or treat it. The worksheet encourages students to compare what is known about the prevention, diagnosis, and treatment of cancers. Students are always surprised and disappointed with how little they can find about the prevention of cancers compared to what is known about detection and treatment. This certainly demonstrates the priorities and funding for cancer research and this reflects the pressure for researchers to be able to design quick-fix studies which will get measurable, statistically significant findings in the short time frame of most funding cycles. Contrast that to the reality of how cancer works. In the excellent *Dr. Susan Love's Breast Book*, Dr. Love suggests that breast cancer rates could be reduced by 25 percent by reducing the amount of fat in the diet and decreasing obesity in a population, but she quotes a researcher who has acknowledged "that the changes in the diet would probably have to start at age five, and would have a 20 year lag until an effect would even be seen, and (it would be) 80 years until the maximum effect would be realized. " (Love, 1995, p. 235.)

The short fact sheet on the rBGH campaign in Massachusetts gives one example of environmental activism that may help reduce the risk of cancers; it ties in well with the article on the Mother's Milk Project discussed in Chapter 11. As with many health issues, it is clear that *primary* prevention, which means preventing a disease before it starts to develop, may require a focus on the environment more than on the individual, and that we must pay attention to the Precautionary Principle (see Chapter 11). A crucial question about breast cancer, and about all other diseases, is how can we shift the medical interest and funding from detection and treatment to primary prevention? It is important that we *not* confuse prevention, detection, and treatment. For example, many people think of mammography as a form of prevention, but it is a form of *secondary* prevention, which translates as early detection of a disease that is already present.

Many women have been convinced to accept that mammography is always good and that early detection will save lives. Cynthia Pearson, in her article on mammography, presents a thoughtful, careful exploration of the complexities of mammography as a screening tool. This article is not intended to discourage women from having mammography. Instead, we hope this increases awareness of the limitations of mammography and the urgent need to shift action and research to breast cancer prevention. There is a whole pink-ribbon, mammography-promoting culture that has grown up around the inaccurate slogan, "early detection is your best prevention." Few know that this slogan and National Breast Cancer Awareness Month were conceived and promoted by Imperial Chemical Corporation, now Zeneca, the manufacturer of tamoxifen, an important drug in the treatment of breast cancer, and one of the world's largest producers and users of chlorinated products, which are believed to increase breast cancer. In spite of the powerful side effects (including increasing risk of endometrial cancer) of tamoxifen, it has moved from being successfully used for breast cancer *treatment* to being marketed to healthy women to supposedly prevent breast cancer.

The next group of articles in this chapter address different aspects of the politics of sexually transmitted infections (STIs). "The Gendered Epidemic: Women and the Risks and Burdens of HIV" presents a global, gendered analysis demonstrating why "a gender dimension needs to be a central part of all AIDS strategies . . . (and) that AIDS needs to be a part of all gender strategies." Whether we're looking at why women contract HIV more easily than men, how their expected caretaking roles mean AIDS epidemics fall disproportionally as an extra burden on women, or how violence against women relates to HIV, Peter Piot reminds us that:

> The impact of AIDS is gendered in its every aspect. Women's HIV vulnerability derives particularly from contexts in which they have little control over sex, whether as a consequence of the predominating power relations between men and women or as a function of the economic and life choices available to them.

The next article, "Scared to be Safe," follows up on the issue of women having "little control over sex" in relationship to prevention of disease transmission. Jiayan Chen, a young feminist intern at the National Women's Health Network, examines the question: "Why, if condoms are so effective in preventing HIV and pregnancy, don't more women use them?" The answer another intern gives is that "women simply don't command enough power in their relationships to insist on condoms." Using that answer as a springboard, the author raises important questions about gender relations, women's control of sexuality, and sexual health.

"With or Without the Dam Thing: The Lesbian Safer Sex Debates" is an all-too-rare and now classic article both because it specifically addresses lesbian sexual health and because it addresses disease (HIV) prevention in a sex-positive, explicit manner which looks at risks associated with specific activities. The material in this article will be useful, or at least thought-provoking, for anyone who is sexually active with a partner or partners.

Microbicides, substances that can kill a range of disease-causing agents, were mentioned in "Scared to be Safe" as possible alternatives for women to be able to have more control of their protection from STIs. Bindiya Patel's article focuses on the recent research and advocacy related to microbicide development. She points out that "microbicides are not going to be a magic bullet against HIV. It is important to note that while microbicides will help people reduce infection, they will never be as effective as condoms," adding that microbicides could be very important for couples who don't use condoms at all or consistently, and for women who may not have any control over when condoms are used.

The next two articles, by Adriane Fugh-Berman and Alicia M. Bell respectively, provide thoughtful critical analyses of the science and politics involved in the introduction of Gardisil, the first vaccine to prevent certain HPV infections, thereby *reducing* risk of cervical cancer. A vaccine that can prevent or reduce the risk of cancer would obviously receive a lot of attention and the HPV vaccine is complicated by the fact that it prevents cancer by preventing a sexually transmitted infection. In addition, this vaccine could be a gold mine for the pharmaceutical company that developed it. Refer back to "How Vaccine Policy Is Made: The Story of Merck and Gardisil" in Chapter 4 for more on the politics of marketing and public health policy involved.

Moving away from infectious diseases, the next articles look at conditions that affect many women and may be either ignored or overtreated. The title of the first of these, "Treat Incontinence Without Drugs or Surgery," sums up the main point of the article, as the author, Adriane Fugh-Berman, discusses safe and effective strategies to use before considering powerful drugs or invasive surgery. One of these safe alternatives is to do Kegel exercises, described in detail in the Worksheet for Chapter 9. The next article, on the very common condition of uterine fibroids, gives a clear explanation of what they are, what impact they may have on a woman's health, and how they can be treated. Doing nothing or having a hysterectomy, a very common form of often unnecessary surgery, used to be the only choices, but now there are other options available. "Live and Uncut" examines another frequently unnecessary surgery—removal of the ovaries (oophorectomy), which often accompanies hysterectomy even if the ovaries are completely healthy. The author concludes that "Most of these procedures, however, are done for no other reason than the surgeon is in the neighborhood."

Chronic Fatigue Immune Deficiency Syndrome (CFIDS, also known as Chronic Fatigue Syndrome or CFS) is a health issue that disproportionately affects women, and is often trivialized or assumed to be "all in her head." The next article, "David and Goliath," was written by a woman who had this disease, known in England as ME. She describes her battle to have a major study she did on the prevalence of ME in British schoolchildren taken seriously. This story parallels the battles many who live with CFIDS/ME fought to have the disease recognized as both real and serious, and this is a recurring story with many women's health issues. Similarly, the "Vagina Dialogues" describes a woman's extremely painful and stressful experiences with vulvodynia, a "chronic pain in the vulva . . . a little talked about problem affecting thousands of women, who are often led to believe it's all in their heads." Both articles emphasize the isolation and frustration of having a disease that is not taken seriously or is not talked about.

Endometriosis used to be one of those conditions that was not understood or talked about, but the Endometriosis Association (http://www.endometriosisassn.org) certainly changed that. The Endometriosis Association has long been one of the best examples of consumer activism and an organization built around giving voice to women who live with this disease. This group has been able to influence the health system by providing information about endometriosis, as learned from women who experience it, as well as providing support and information for women with endometriosis. "What Is Endometriosis?" explains what is known about this disease and what can be done about it. The next article, "Why Endometriosis Is an Environmental Issue," highlights the Endometriosis Association's increasingly visible role in drawing attention to the connections between environmental issues and endometriosis, and supporting research on identifying and reducing risks associated with endometriosis. Their environmental focus, as with work on contamination of breast milk and breast cancer prevention discussed previously, makes the important connection between health and the environment.

This chapter ends with a further discussion, by Emily Alexander, of the effects of environmental contamination on women's health. This article gives a very important reminder that it is easy to feel personally responsible for having made the "wrong" decision that may then have had a negative impact on health, when, in fact, an individual may not have many options. The author explains:

> In addition to empowering women with the best health information we have available, let's bring attention to the environments (social, political and physical) that increase the prevalence of toxic chemicals in our lives. Let's bring attention to the lack of access, support, education and job opportunities that influence the choices people can make about what they buy and how they treat their bodies.

This strong message about placing health in a broader context than individual responsibility is a fitting close to this book.

Breast Cancer
Power vs. Prosthesis

by Audre Lorde

On Labor Day, 1978, during my regular monthly self-examination, I discovered a lump in my right breast which later proved to be malignant. During my following hospitalization, my mastectomy and its aftermath, I passed through many stages of pain, despair, fury, sadness and growth. I moved through these stages, sometimes feeling as if I had no choice, other times recognizing that I could choose oblivion—or a passivity that is very close to oblivion—but did not want to. As I slowly began to feel more equal to processing and examining the different parts of this experience, I also began to feel that in the process of losing a breast I had become a more whole person.

After a mastectomy, for many women including myself, there is a feeling of wanting to go back, of not wanting to persevere through this experience to whatever enlightenment might be at the core of it. And it is this feeling, this nostalgia, which is encouraged by most of the post-surgical counselling for women with breast cancer. This regressive tie to the past is emphasized by the concentration upon breast cancer as a cosmetic problem, one which can be solved by a prosthetic pretence. The American Cancer Society's Reach for Recovery Program, while doing a valuable service in contacting women immediately after surgery and letting them know they are not alone, nonetheless encourages this false and dangerous nostalgia in the mistaken belief that women are too weak to deal directly and courageously with the realities of our lives.

The woman from Reach for Recovery who came to see me in the hospital, while quite admirable and even impressive in her own right, certainly did not speak to my experience nor my concerns. As a 44-year-old Black lesbian feminist, I knew there were very few role models around for me in this situation, but my primary concerns two days after mastectomy were hardly about what man I could capture in the future, whether or not my old boyfriend would still find me attractive enough, and even less about whether my two children would be embarrassed by me around their friends

My concerns were about my chances for survival, the effects of a possibly shortened life upon my work and my priorities. Could this cancer have been prevented, and what could I do in the future to prevent its recurrence? Would I be able to maintain the control over my life that I had always taken for granted? A lifetime of loving women had taught me that when women love each other, physical change does not alter that love. It did not occur to me that anyone who really loved me would love me any less because I had one breast instead of two, although it did occur to me to wonder if they would be able to love and deal with the new me.

In the critical and vulnerable period following surgery, self-examination and self-evaluation are positive steps. To imply to a woman that yes, she can be the "same" as before surgery, with the skillful application of a little puff of lambswool, and/or silicone gel, is to place an emphasis upon prosthesis which encourages her not to deal with herself as physically and emotionally real, even though altered and traumatized. This emphasis upon the cosmetic after surgery reinforces this society's stereotype of women, that we are only what we look or appear, so this is the only aspect of our existence we need to address. Any woman who has had a breast removed because of cancer knows she does not feel the same. But we are allowed no psychic time or space to examine what our true feelings are, to make them our own.

Ten days after having my breast removed, I went to my doctor's office to have the stitches taken out. This was my first journey out since coming home from the hospital, and I was truly looking forward to it. A friend had washed my hair for me and it was black and shining, with my new grey hairs glistening in the sun. Colour was starting to come back into my face and around my eyes, I wore the most opalescent of my moonstones, and a single floating bird dangling from my right ear in the name of grand asymmetry. With an African kentecloth tunic and new leather boots, I knew I looked fine, with that brave new-born security of a beautiful woman having come through a very hard time and being very glad to be alive.

The doctor's nurse, a charmingly bright and steady woman of about my own age who had always given me a feeling of quiet no-nonsense support on my other visits, called me into the examining room. On the way, she asked me how I was feeling.

"Pretty good," I said, half-expecting her to make some comment about how good I looked.

"You're not wearing a prosthesis," she said, a little anxiously, and not at all like a question.

"No," I said, thrown off my guard for a minute. "It really doesn't feel right," referring to the lambswool puff given to me by the Reach For Recovery volunteer in the hospital.

Usually supportive and understanding, the nurse now looked at me urgently and disapprovingly as she told me that even if it didn't look exactly right, it was "better than nothing," and that as soon as my stitches were out I could be fitted for a "real form."

"You will feel so much better with it on," she said. "And besides, we really like you to wear something, at least when you come in. Otherwise it's bad for the morale of the office."

I could hardly believe my ears! I was too outraged to speak then, but this was to be only the first such assault on my right to define and to claim my own body.

A woman who is attempting to come to terms with her changed landscape and changed timetable of life and with her own body and pain and beauty and strength, that woman is seen as a threat to the "morale" of a breast surgeon's office!

Yet when Moishe Dayan, the Prime Minister of Israel, stands up in front of parliament or on TV with an eye patch over his empty eye socket, nobody tells him to go get a glass eye, or that he is bad for the morale of the office. The world sees him as a warrior with an honourable wound, and a loss of a piece of himself which he has marked, and mourned, and moved beyond. And if you have trouble dealing with Moishe Dayan's empty eye-socket, everyone recognises that it is your problem to solve, not his.

Well, women with breast cancer are warriors, also. I have been to war, and still am. So has every woman who had had one or both breasts amputated because of the cancer that is becoming the primary physical scourge of our time. For me, my scars are an honorable reminder that I may be a casualty in the cosmic war against radiation, animal fat, air pollution, McDonald's hamburgers and Red Dye no. 2, but the fight is still going on, and I am still a part of it. I refuse to have my scars hidden or trivialised behind lambswool or silicone gel. I refuse to be reduced in my own eyes or in the eyes of others from warrior to mere victim, simply because it might render me a fraction more acceptable or less dangerous to the still complacent, those who believe if you cover up a problem it ceases to exist. I refuse to hide my body simply because it might make a woman-phobic world more comfortable.

Prosthesis offers the empty comfort of "nobody will know the difference." But it is that very difference which I wish to affirm, because I had lived it, and survived it, and wish to share that strength with other women. If we are to translate the silence surrounding breast cancer into language and action against this scourge, then the first step is that women with mastectomies must become visible to each other. For silence and invisibility go hand in hand with powerlessness. By accepting the mask or prosthesis, one-breasted women proclaim ourselves as insufficients dependent upon pretence.

In addition, we withhold that visibility and support from one another which is such an aid to perspective and self-acceptance.

As women, we cannot afford to look the other way, nor to consider the incidence of breast cancer as a private or secret personal problem. It is no secret that breast cancer is on the increase among women in America. According to the American Cancer Society's own statistics on breast cancer survival, of women stricken, only 50% are still alive after three years. This figure drops to 30% if you are poor, or Black, or in any other way part of the underside of this society. We cannot ignore these facts, nor their implications, nor their effect upon our lives, individually and collectively. Early detection and early treatment is crucial in the management of breast cancer if those sorry statistics of survival are to improve. But for the incidence of early detection and early treatment to increase, American women must become free enough from social stereotypes concerning their appearance to realize that losing a breast is infinitely preferable to losing one's life (or one's eyes, or one's hands . . .).

Although breast self-examination does not reduce the incidence of breast cancer, it does markedly reduce the rate of mortality, since most early tumours are found by women themselves. I discovered my own tumour upon a monthly breast exam, and so report most of the other women I know with a good prognosis for survival. With our alert awareness making such a difference in the survival rate for breast cancer, women need to face the possibility and the actuality of breast cancer as a reality rather than a myth, or retribution, or terror in the night, or a bad dream that will disappear if ignored. After surgery, there is a need for women to be aware of the possibility of bilateral recurrence, with vigilance rather than terror. This is not a spread of cancer, but a new occurrence in the other breast. Each woman must be aware that an honest acquaintanceship with and evaluation of her own body is the best tool of detection.

The greatest incidence of breast cancer in American women appears between the ages of 40 to 55. These are the very years when women are portrayed in the popular media as fading and desexualised figures. Contrary to the media picture, I find myself as a woman of insight ascending into my highest powers, my greatest psychic strengths, and my fullest satisfactions. I am freer of the constraints and fears and indecisions of my younger years, and survival throughout these years has taught me how to value my own beauty, and how to look closely into the beauty of others.

There is nothing wrong, *per se*, with the use of prostheses, if they can be chosen freely, for whatever reason, after a woman has had a chance to accept her new body. But usually prostheses serve a real function, to approximate the performance of a missing physical part. In other amputations and with other prosthetic devices, function is the main point of their existence. Artificial limbs perform specific tasks, allowing us to manipulate or to walk. Dentures allow us to chew our food. Only false breasts are designed for appearance only, as if the only real function of women's breasts were to appear in a certain shape and size and symmetry to onlookers, or to yield to external pressure. For no woman wearing a prosthesis can even for one moment believe it is her own breast, any more than a woman wearing falsies can.

Attitudes towards the necessity for prostheses after breast surgery are merely a reflection of those attitudes within our society towards women in general as objectified and depersonalised sexual conveniences. Women have been programmed to view our bodies only in terms of how they look and feel to others, rather than how they feel to ourselves, and how we wish to use them. As women, we fight this depersonalisation every day, this pressure towards the conversion of one's own self-image into a media expectation of what might satisfy male demand. The insistence upon breast prosthesis as "decent" rather than functional is an additional example of that wipe-out of self in which women are constantly encouraged to take part. I am personally affronted by the message that I am only acceptable if I look "right" or "normal," where those norms have nothing to do with my own perceptions of who I am. Where "normal" means the "right" colour, shape, size, or number of breasts, a woman's perception of her own body and the strengths that come from that perception are discouraged, trivialised, and ignored.

Every woman has a right to define her own desires, make her own choices. But prostheses are often chosen, not from desire, but in default. Some women complain it is too much effort to fight the concerted pressure exerted by the fashion industry. Being one-breasted does not mean being unfashionable; it means giving some time and energy to choosing or constructing the proper clothes. In some cases, it means making or remaking clothing or jewelry. The fact that the fashion needs of one-breasted women are not currently being met doesn't mean that the concerted pressure of our demands cannot change that.

Some women believe that a breast prosthesis is necessary to preserve correct posture and physical balance. But the weight of each breast is never the same to begin with, nor is the human body ever exactly the same on both sides. With a minimum of exercises to develop the habit of straight posture, the body can accommodate to one-breastedness quite easily, even when the breasts were quite heavy.

Women in public and private employment have reported the loss of jobs and promotions upon their return to work after a mastectomy, without regard to whether or not they wore prostheses. The social and economic discrimination practised against women who have breast cancer is not diminished by pretending that mastectomies do not exist. Where a woman's job is at risk because of her health history, employment discrimination cannot be fought with a sack of silicone gel, nor with the constant fear and anxiety to which such subterfuge gives rise. Suggesting prosthesis as a solution to employment discrimination is like saying that the way to fight prejudice is for Black people to pretend to be white. Employment discrimination against post-mastectomy women can only be fought in the open, with head-on attacks by strong and self-accepting women who refuse to be relegated to an inferior position, or to cower in a corner because they have one breast.

Within the framework of superficiality and pretence, the next logical step of a depersonalising and woman-devaluating culture is the advent of the atrocity euphemistically called "breast reconstruction." It should be noted that research being done on this potentially life-threatening practice represents time and research money spent—not on how to prevent the cancers that cost us our breasts and our lives—but rather upon how to pretend that our breasts are not gone, nor we as women at risk with our lives.

Any information about the prevention or treatment of breast cancer which might possibly threaten the vested interests of the American medical establishment is difficult to acquire in the country. Only through continuing scrutiny of various non-mainstream sources of information, such as alternative and women's presses, can a picture of new possibilities for prevention and treatment of breast cancer emerge.

The mortality for breast cancer treated by conventional therapies has not decreased in over 40 years (Rose Kushner, *Breast Cancer*, Harcourt, Brace & Jovanovitch, 1975, p. 161). Since the American medical establishment and the ACS are determined to suppress any cancer information not dependent upon western medical bias, whether this information is ultimately useful or not, we must pierce this silence ourselves and aggressively seek answers to these questions about new therapies. We must also heed the unavoidable evidence pointing towards the nutritional and environmental aspects of cancer prevention.

Cancer is not just another degenerative and unavoidable disease of the ageing process. It has distinct and identifiable causes, and these are mainly exposures to chemical or physical agents in the environment. In the medical literature, there is mounting evidence that breast cancer is a chronic systemic disease. Post-mastectomy women must be vigilantly aware that, contrary to the "lightning strikes" theory, we are the most likely of all women to develop cancer somewhere else in the body.

Every woman has a militant responsibility to involve herself actively with her own health. We owe ourselves the protection of all the information we can acquire about the treatment of cancer and its causes, as well as about the recent findings concerning immunology, nutrition, environment and stress. And we owe ourselves this information *before* we may have a reason to use it.

It was very important for me, after my mastectomy, to develop and encourage my own internal sense of power. At all times, it felt crucial to me that I make a conscious commitment to survival. It is physically important for me to be loving my life rather than to be mourning my breast. I believe it is this love of my life and myself, and the careful tending of that love which was done by women who love and support me, which has been largely responsible for my strong and healthy recovery from the effects of my mastectomy. But a clear distinction must be made between this affirmation of self and the superficial farce of "looking on the bright side of things."

Last week I read a letter from a doctor in a medical magazine which said that no truly happy person ever gets cancer. Despite my knowing better, and despite my having dealt with this blame-the-victim thinking for years, for a moment this letter hit my guilt button. Had I really been guilty of the crime of not being happy in this best of all possible infernos?

The idea that the cancer patient should be made to feel guilty about having had cancer, as if in some way it were all her fault for not having been in the right psychological frame of mind at all times to prevent cancer, is a monstrous distortion of the idea that we can use our psychic strengths to help heal ourselves. This guilt trip which many cancer patients have been led into (you see, it is a shameful thing because you could have prevented it if only you had been more . . .) is an extension of the blame-the-victim syndrome. It does nothing to encourage the mobilisation of our psychic defenses against the very real forms of death which surround us. It is easier to demand happiness than to clean up the environment. The acceptance of illusion and appearance as reality is another symptom of this same refusal to examine the realities of our lives. Let us seek "joy" rather than real food and clean air and a saner future on a liveable earth! As if happiness alone can protect us from the results of profit-madness.

Was I wrong to be working so hard against the oppressions afflicting women and Black people? Was I in error to be speaking out against our silent passivity and the cynicism of a mechanized and inhuman civilisation that is destroying our earth and those who live upon it? Was I really fighting the spread of radiation, racism, woman-slaughter, chemical invasion of our food, pollution of our environment, the abuse and psychic destruction of our young, merely to avoid dealing with my first and greatest responsibility—to be happy?

The only really happy people I have ever met are those of us who work against these deaths with all the energy of our living, recognising the deep and fundamental unhappiness with which we are surrounded, at the same time as we fight to keep from being submerged by it. The idea that happiness can insulate us against the results of our environmental madness is a rumour circulated by our enemies to destroy us. And what Woman of Colour in America over the age of 15 does not live with the knowledge that our daily lives are stitched with violence and with hatred, and to naively ignore that reality can mean destruction? We are equally destroyed by false happiness and false breasts, and the passive acceptance of false values which corrupt our lives and distort our experience.

The idea of having a breast removed was much more traumatic for me before my mastectomy than after the fact, but it certainly took time and the loving support of other women before I could once again look at and love my altered body with the warmth I had done before. But I did.

Right after surgery I had a sense that I would never be able to bear missing that great well of sexual pleasure that

I connected with my right breast. That sense has completely passed away, as I have come to realise that that well of feeling was within me. I alone own my feelings. I can never lose that feeling because I own it, because it comes out of myself. I can attach it anywhere I want to, because my feelings are a part of me, my sorrow and my joy.

I would never have chosen this path, but I am very glad to be who I am, here.

Breast Implants for Reconstruction
"A Closer Look"
by Stephanie Donne

Of the tens of thousands of American women each year who undergo mastectomies, approximately 75 percent go on to have one or both breasts surgically reconstructed, according to breastcancer.org. Roughly half of these women opt for surgery that rebuilds the breast using their own body tissue. Most of the rest decide on artificial implants.

The National Women's Health Network is extremely concerned about the safety of breast implants, and we believe that no implant should be approved without long-term data on safety and effectiveness. Yet despite a dearth of this data, breast implants are available in this country. Silicone gel-filled implants were first introduced in the 1960s and remain available through clinical trials for surgical reconstruction after mastectomy. In 2000, the Food and Drug Administration (FDA) also approved saline breast implants for reconstructive and augmentative use.

Silicone gel implants have not been available outside clinical trials since 1992, when the FDA banned them due to long-term safety concerns. In 2004, the FDA rejected Inamed's application to bring silicone gel implants back to the market, a decision NWHN supported.

Breast Implants Cause Known Health Problems

All women with silicone gel or saline implants can experience post-surgical complications, including pain, capsular contracture (hardening of the tissue that forms around the implant), infection, inflammation or irrita-

tion, breasts that are not the same size or shape, and breasts that look wrinkled.

These complications may require additional surgeries to remove or replace the implants. A study of Inamed's saline breast implants found that after three years, 21 percent of augmentation patients and 40 percent of reconstruction patients required additional surgeries. Inamed's study of its silicone gel implants showed that 20 percent of breast augmentation patients and 46 percent of breast reconstruction patients required additional surgeries within three years.

There are unanswered questions about systemic and long-term health problems associated with implants. A study by FDA scientists found a significant link between silicone gel implants and fibromyalgia, a disorder that causes pain and fatigue in the muscles, tendons and ligaments. A National Cancer Institute study found that women with silicone gel implants had increased risk of cancers of the brain, respiratory tract, cervix and vulva. It is not known if reconstruction patients are more likely to experience these problems than augmentation patients.

Silicone Gel Implants May Cause Unknown Health Problems

We still do not know enough about the long-term disease risk of women with implants. Women with silicone implants have reported a variety of autoimmune diseases, including scleroderma, rheumatoid arthritis and lupus. These diseases are rare and take many years to develop and be diagnosed, and all studies on silicone implants and autoimmune diseases have been short-term and have included small numbers of women. As a result, the connection between implants and long-term risk of these diseases remains unknown.

Researchers have suggested that if a woman is already more likely to develop an autoimmune disease for other reasons, her exposure to toxins in silicone gel may trigger the development of that disease.

Implants and Mammography

All breast implants interfere with accurate mammography readings and can be ruptured by breast compression during mammograms. Other potential adverse events, as identified in a recent study by FDA scientists, include delayed breast cancer detection, pain and soreness during and after the mammogram and, in the event of capsular contracture, inability to perform a mammogram. There are ways to minimize implants' interference with accurate mammography, but approximately 30 percent of the breast tissue will remain obscured in the image.

Breast Implants Break

Some implants break within the first few months of being implanted, and some last more than 15 years. But no implant lasts forever. At some point, all women with breast implants will require surgery to replace or remove their implants.

When saline implants rupture, the saline typically leaks out quickly and the implant deflates. Women are usually aware that their implant has ruptured because the breast changes in size or shape. When the saline leaks out of the implant, it is absorbed into the body. This in itself is usually harmless, but bacteria or fungus from inside the implant may also leak into the body.

Silicone gel implants are filled with a thick cohesive gel. When they rupture, women sometimes notice changes in the breast's size or shape, along with pain, swelling, numbness or tingling. But most silicone ruptures are known as silent ruptures and occur without any symptoms. The only way to accurately detect a silicone rupture is with MRI.

After a silicone rupture, silicone gel can remain within the capsule of scar tissue that forms around the implant, or it can leak outside the scar tissue and travel to distant points throughout the body. The long-term effects of silicone gel on the health of women have not been adequately researched. It is not known whether these effects may be different in women who have had cancer.

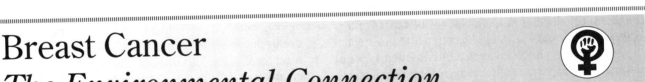

Breast Cancer
The Environmental Connection

by Rita Arditti and Tatiana Schreiber

Today in the United States, we live in the midst of a cancer epidemic. One out of every three people will get some form of cancer and one out of four will die from it. Cancer is currently the second leading cause of death; by the year 2000, it will likely have become the primary cause of death. It is now more than two decades since the National Cancer Act was signed, yet the treatments offered to cancer patients are the same as those offered 50 years ago: surgery, radiation, and chemotherapy (or slash, burn, and poison, as they are called bitterly by both patients and increasingly disappointed professionals). And in spite of sporadic optimistic pronouncements from the cancer establishment, survival rates for the three main cancer killers—lung, breast, and colo-rectal cancer—have remained virtually unchanged.

In the '60s and '70s, environmental activists and a few scientists emphasized that cancer was linked to environmental contamination, and their concerns began to have an impact on public understanding of the disease. In the '80s and '90s, however, with an increasingly conservative political climate and concerted efforts on the part of industry to play down the importance of chemicals as a cause of cancer, we are presented with a new image of cancer. Now it is portrayed as an individual problem that can only be overcome with the help of experts and, then, only if one has the money and know-how to recruit them for one's personal survival efforts. This emphasis on personal responsibility and lifestyle factors has reached absurd proportions. People with cancer are asked why they "brought this disease on themselves" and why they don't work harder at "getting well."

While people with cancer should be encouraged not to fall into victim roles and to do everything possible to strengthen their immune systems (our primary line of defense against cancer), it seems that the sociopolitical and economic dimensions of cancer have been pushed completely out of the picture. "Blaming the victim" is a convenient way to avoid looking at the larger environmental and social issues that form individual experiences. Here we want to talk about environmental links to cancer in general and to breast cancer in particular, the kinds of research that should be going on, why they're not happening, and the political strategies needed to turn things around.

Extensive evidence exists to indicate that cancer is an environmental disease. Even the most conservative scientists agree that approximately 80 percent of all cancers are in some way related to environmental factors. Support for this view relies on four lines of evidence: (1) dramatic differences in the incidences of cancer between communities—incidences of cancer among people of a given age in different parts of the world can vary by a factor of ten to a hundred; (2) changes in the incidence of cancer (either lower or higher rates) in groups that migrate to a new country; (3) changes in the incidence of particular types of cancer with the passage of time; and (4) the actual identification of the specific causes of certain cancers (such as the case of beta-naphthylamine, responsible for an epidemic of bladder cancer among dye workers employed at du Pont factories). Other well-known environmentally linked cancers are lung cancer, linked to asbestos, arsenic, chromium, bischloromethyl ether, mustard gas, ionizing radiation, nickel, polycyclic hydrocarbons in soot, tar, oil, and of course, smoking; endometrial cancer, linked to estrogen use; thyroid cancer, often the result of childhood irradiation; and liver cancer, linked to exposure to vinyl chloride.

The inescapable conclusion is that if cancer is largely environmental in origin, it is largely preventable.

Our Environment Is a Health Hazard

"Environment" as we use it here includes not only air, water, and soil, but also our diets, medical procedures, and living and working conditions. That means that the food we eat, the water we drink, the air we breathe, the radiation to which we are exposed, where we live,

what kind of work we do, and the stress that we suffer—these are responsible for at least 80 percent of all cancers. For instance, under current EPA regulations as many as 60 cancer-causing pesticides can legally be used to grow the most commonly eaten foods. Some of these foods are allowed to contain 20 or more carcinogens, making it impossible to measure how much of each substance a person actually consumes. As Rachel Carson wrote in *Silent Spring* in 1962, "This piling up of chemicals from many different sources creates a total exposure that cannot be measured. It is meaningless, therefore, to talk about the 'safety' of any specific amount of residues." In other words, our everyday food is an environmental hazard to our health.

Recently, a study on the trends in cancer mortality in industrialized countries has revealed that while stomach cancer has been steadily declining, brain and other central-nervous-system cancers, breast cancer, multiple myeloma, kidney cancer, non-Hodgkin's lymphoma, and melanoma have increased in persons aged 55 and older. Given this context, it is not extreme to suspect that breast cancer, which has reached epidemic proportions in the United States, may be linked to environmental ills. This year, estimates are that 180,000 women will develop breast cancer and 46,000 will die from it. In other words, in the coming year, nearly as many women will die from breast cancer as there were American lives lost in the entire Vietnam War. Cancer is the leading cause of death among women aged 35 to 54, with about a third of these deaths due to breast cancer. Breast cancer incidence data meet three of the four lines of reasoning linking it to the environment: (1) the incidence of breast cancer between communities can vary by a factor of seven; (2) the risk for breast cancer among populations that have migrated becomes that of their new residence within a generation, as is the case for Japanese women who have migrated to the United States; and (3) the incidence of breast cancer in the United States has swelled from one in twenty in 1940 to one in eight in the '90s.

A number of factors have been linked to breast cancer; a first blood relative with the disease, early onset of menstruation, late age at first full-term pregnancy, higher socioeconomic status, late menopause, being Jewish, etc. However, for the overwhelming majority (70 to 80 percent) of breast cancer patients, their illness is not clearly linked to any of these factors. Research suggests that the development of breast cancer probably depends on a complex interplay among environmental exposures, genetic predisposition to the disease, and hormonal activity.

Research on the actual identification of causal factors, however, is given low priority and proceeds at a snail's pace. We still don't know, for example, the effects of birth control pills and the hormone replacement therapy routinely offered to menopausal women. Hormonal treatments are fast becoming the method of choice for the treatment of infertility, while we know nothing about their long-range effects. And the standard addition of hormones in animal feed means that all women (and men) are exposed to hormone residues in meat. Since there is general consensus that estrogen somehow plays a role in the development of breast cancer, hormonal interventions (through food or drugs) are particularly worrisome.

A startling example of the lack of interest in the prevention of breast cancer is the saga of the proposed study on the supposed link between high-fat diets and breast cancer. The "Women's Health Trial," a fifteen-year study designed to provide conclusive data about the high fat-cancer link, was denied funding by the National Cancer Advisory Board despite having been revised to answer previous criticisms and despite feasibility studies indicating that a full-scale trial was worth launching. Fortunately, it now appears that the study will be part of the Women's Health Initiative, a $500-million effort that will look at women's health issues. This success story is a direct result of women's activism and pressures from women's health groups across the country.

But even if the high fat-breast cancer correlation is established, it is unlikely to fully explain how breast cancer develops. The breast is rich in adipose cells, and carcinogens that accumulate in these fat tissues may be responsible for inducing cancer rather than the fat itself or the fat alone. Environmental contamination of human breast milk with PCBs, PBBs and DDE (a metabolite of the pesticide DDT) is a widely acknowledged phenomenon. These fat-soluble substances are poorly metabolized and have a long half-life in human tissue. They may also interact with one another, creating an additive toxic effect, and they may carry what are called "incidental contaminants": compounds like dibenzofurans, dioxins, etc., each with its own toxic properties.

Among the established effects of these substances are: liver dysfunction, skin abnormalities, neurological and behavioral abnormalities, immunological aberrations, thyroid dysfunction, gastrointestinal disturbances, reproductive dysfunction, tumor growth, and enzyme induction. Serious concerns have been raised about the risks that this contamination entails for infants who are breast-fed. But what is outrageous in the discussion about human breast-milk poisoning is that little or no mention is made of the possible effects on the women themselves, particularly since it is known that most of these sub-

stances have *estrogenic* properties (that is, they behave like estrogen in the body). It is as if the women, whose breasts contain these carcinogens, do not exist. We witness the paradox of women being made invisible, even while their toxic breasts are put under the microscope.

The Pesticide Studies

Very recently, some scientists have at last begun to look at the chemical-breast cancer connection. In 1990, two Israeli scientists from Hebrew University's Hadassah School of Medicine, Elihu Richter and Jerry Westin, reported a surprising statistic. They found that Israel was the only country among 28 countries surveyed that registered a real drop in breast cancer mortality in the decade 1976 to 1986. This happened in the face of a worsening of all known risk factors, such as fat intake and age at first pregnancy. As Westin noted, "All and all, we expected a rise in breast cancer mortality of approximately 20 percent overall, and what we found was that there was an 8 percent drop, and in the youngest age group, the drop was 34 percent, as opposed to an expected 20 percent rise, so, if we put those two together, we are talking about a difference of about 50 percent, which is enormous."

Westin and Richter could not account for the drop solely in terms of demographic changes or improved medical intervention. Instead, they suspected it might have been related to a 1978 ban on three carcinogenic pesticides (benzene hexachloride, lindane, and DDT) that heavily contaminated milk and milk products in Israel. Prior to 1978, Westin said, "at least one of them [the three pesticides] was found in the milk here at a rate 100 times greater than it was in the U.S. in the same period, and in the worst case, nearly a thousand times greater." This observation led Westin and Richter to hypothesize that there might be a connection between the decrease in exposure following the ban and the decrease in breast cancer mortality. They believed the pesticides could have promoted enzymes that in turn increased the virulence of breast cancer in women. When the pesticides were removed from the diet, Westin and Richter speculated, there was a situation of much less virulent cancer and the mortality from breast cancer fell.

Westin and Richter are convinced that there is a critical need to increase awareness about environmental conditions and cancer. Health care clinicians, for example, could play an important role in the detection of potential exposures to toxic chemicals that might be missed in large studies. This is a refreshing view since it encourages individual physicians to ask questions about work environments, living quarters, and diet, the answers to which could provide important clues about the cancer-environment connection.

In the United States, only one study we know of has directly measured chemical residues in women who have breast cancer compared to those who do not. Dr. Mary Wolff, a chemist at New York's Mount Sinai School of Medicine, recently conducted a pilot study with Dr. Frank Falck (then at Hartford Hospital in Hartford, Connecticut) that was published in *The Archives of Environmental Health*. In this case-controlled study, Falck and Wolff found that several chemical residues from pesticides and PCBs were elevated in cases of malignant disease as compared to nonmalignant cases.

The study involved 25 women with breast cancer and the same number of women who had biopsies but did not have breast cancer. The results showed differences significant enough to interest the National Institute for Environmental Health Sciences, which will fund a larger study to look at the level of DDT and its metabolites in the blood samples of 15,000 women attending a breast cancer screening clinic in New York. A recent report just released by Greenpeace, entitled "Breast Cancer and the Environment: The Chlorine Connection," provides further evidence linking industrial chemicals to breast cancer.

In the United States, levels of pesticide residues in adipose tissue have been decreasing since the 1970s (following the banning of DDT and decreased use of other carcinogenic pesticides) while the breast cancer rate continues to rise. This observation would seem to contradict the pesticide hypothesis. However, it is important to remember that the chemicals could act differently at different exposure levels, they are unlikely to act alone, and the time of exposure may be important. For example, if a child is exposed during early adolescence, when breast tissue is growing rapidly, the result may be different than exposure later in life.

Radiation and Mammography

Another area that demands urgent investigation is the role of radiation in the development of breast cancer. It is widely accepted that ionizing radiation at high doses causes breast cancer, but low doses are generally regarded as safe. Questions remain, however, regarding the shape of the dose-response curve, the length of the latency period, and the importance of age at time of exposure. These questions are of great importance to women because of the emphasis on mammography for early detection. There is evidence that mammography screening reduces death from breast cancer in women aged 50 or older. However, Dr. Rosalie Bertell (director of the International Institute of Concern for Public Health, author of *No Immediate Danger: Prognosis for a Radioactive World* [1985] and well-known critic of the nuclear establishment) raises serious questions about mammography screening. In a paper entitled "Comments on Ontario Mammography Program," Bertell criticized a breast cancer screening program planned by the Ontario Health Minister in 1989. Bertell argued that the program, which would potentially screen 300,000 women, was a plan to "reduce breast cancer death by increasing breast cancer incidence."

Bertell's critique of mammography suggests that the majority of cancers that would have occurred in the group could have been detected by other means. A recent Canadian mammography study on 90,000 women looked at cancer rates between 1980 and 1988. Preliminary results show that for women aged 40 to 49, mammograms have no benefits and may indeed harm them: 44 deaths were found in the group that received mammograms and 29 in the control group. The study also suggests that for women aged 50 to 69, many of the benefits attributed to mammography in earlier studies "may have been provided by the manual breast exams that accompanied the procedure and not by the mammography," as Bertell noted in her paper. Not surprisingly, the study has been mired in controversy. As study director Dr. Anthony Miller remarked, "I've come up with an answer that people are not prepared to accept."

According to Bertell, the present breast cancer epidemic is a direct result of "above ground weapons testing" done in Nevada between 1951 and 1963, when 200 nuclear bombs were set off and the fallout dispersed across the country. Because the latency period for breast cancer peaks at about 40 years, this is an entirely reasonable hypothesis.

Other studies have looked at the effect of "low-level" radiation on cancer development. A study investigating the incidence of leukemia in southeastern Massachusetts found a positive association with radiation released from the Pilgrim nuclear power plant. (The study was limited to cases first diagnosed between 1978 and 1986.) In adult cases diagnosed before 1984, the risk of leukemia was almost four times higher for individuals with the greatest potential for exposure to the emissions of the plant. Other types of cancer take a greater number of years to develop, and there is no reason to assume that excessive radiation emission was limited to the 1978-to-1986 time frame. In other words, as follow-up studies continue, other cancers (including breast cancer) may also show higher rates.

The Surveillance Theory

Current theory supports the concept that cancerous mutations are a common phenomenon in the body of normal individuals and that the immune system intervenes before mutated cells can multiply. Known as the "surveillance" theory of cancer, the basic premise is that cancer can develop when the immune system fails to eliminate mutant cells. Carcinogenic mutations can be induced by radiation or chemicals, for instance, and if immunological competence is reduced at a critical time, the mutated cells can thrive and grow.

Given the apparent importance of the immune system in protecting us from cancer, we ought to be concerned not only with eliminating carcinogens in our environment but also with making certain that our immune systems are not under attack. Recent evidence that ultraviolet radiation depresses the immune system is therefore particularly ominous. At a hearing on "Global Change Research: Ozone Depletion and Its Impacts," held in November 1991 by the Senate Committee on Commerce, Science, and Transportation, a panel of scientists reported that ozone depletion is even more serious than previously thought. According to the data, the ozone layer over the United States is thinning at a rate of 3 to 5 percent per decade, resulting in increased ultraviolet radiation that "will reduce the quantity and quality of crops, increase skin cancer, *suppress the immune system,* and disrupt marine ecosystems" [our emphasis]. (The report also states that a 10 percent decrease in ozone will lead to approximately 1.7 million additional cases of cataracts world-wide per year and at least 250,000 additional cases of skin cancer.) As the writers make chillingly clear, since this is happening literally over our heads, there is no place for us to run.

In addition, dioxin (an extremely toxic substance that has been building up steadily in the environment since the growth of the chlorinated-chemical industry following World War II) can produce alterations that disrupt the immune system. "Free radicals" created by exposure to low-level radiation can cause immune system abnormalities. In other words, our basic mechanisms of defense against cancer are being weakened by the chemical soup in which we are immersed.

It follows that an intelligent and long-range cancer-prevention strategy would make a clean environment its number one priority. Prevention, however, is given low priority in our national cancer agenda. In 1992, out of an almost $2 billion National Cancer Institute (NCI) budget, $132.7 million was spent on breast cancer research but only about 15 percent of that was for preventive research. Moreover, research on the cellular mechanism of cancer development, toward which much of the "prevention" effort goes, does not easily get translated into actual prevention strategies.

In his 1989 exposé of the cancer establishment, *The Cancer Industry,* Ralph Moss writes that until the late '60s, the cancer establishment presented the view that "cancer is . . . widely believed to consist of a hereditable,

and therefore genetic," problem. That line of thinking is still with us but with added emphasis on the personal responsibility we each have for our cancers (smoking and diet) and little or no acknowledgement of the larger environmental context. In a chapter appropriately titled "Preventing Prevention," Moss provides an inkling of why this is so.

The close ties between industry and two of the most influential groups determining our national cancer agenda—the National Cancer Advisory Board and the President's Cancer Panel—are revealing. The chair of the President's Cancer Panel throughout most of the '80s, for example, was Armand Hammer, head of Occidental International Corporation. Among its subsidiaries is Hooker Chemical Company, implicated in the environmental disaster in Love Canal. In addition, Moss, formerly assistant director of public affairs at Memorial Sloan-Kettering Cancer Center (MSKCC), outlines the structure and affiliations of that institution's leadership. MSKCC is the world's largest private cancer center, and the picture that emerges borders on the surreal: in 1988, 32.7 percent of its board of overseers were tied to the oil, chemical and automobile industries; 34.6 percent were professional investors (bankers, stockbrokers, venture capitalists). Board members included top officials of drug companies—Squibb, Bristol-Myers, Merck—and influential members of the media—CBS, the *New York Times,* Warner's Communications, and *Reader's Digest*—as well as leaders of the $55-billion cigarette industry.

Moss's research leaves little doubt about the allegiances of the cancer establishment. Actual cancer prevention would require a massive reorganization of industry, hardly in the interest of the industrial and financial elites. Instead of preventing the generation of chemical and toxic waste, the strategy adopted by industry and government has been one of "management." But as Barry Commoner, director of the Center for the Biology of Natural Systems at Queens College in Brooklyn, New York, put it rather succinctly, "The best way to stop toxic chemicals from entering the environment is to not produce them."

Instead, the latest "prevention" strategy for breast cancer moves in a completely different direction. A trial has been approved that will test the effect of a breast cancer drug (an antiestrogen, tamoxifen) in a healthy population, with the hope that it will have a preventive effect. The trial will involve 16,000 women considered at high risk for breast cancer and will be divided into a control group and a tamoxifen group. The National Women's Health Network (a national public-interest organization dedicated solely to women and health) is unequivocal in its criticism of the trial. Adriane Fugh-Berman, a member of the Network board, wrote in its September/October 1991 newsletter, "In our view the trial is premature in its assumptions, weak in its hypothesis, questionable in its ethics and misguided in its public health ramifications." The criticisms center on the fact that tamoxifen causes liver cancer in rats and liver changes in all species tested and that a number of endometrial cancers have been reported among tamoxifen users. Fugh-Berman points out that approving the testing of a potent, hormonal drug in healthy women and calling that "prevention" sets a dangerous precedent. This drug-oriented trial symbolizes, in a nutshell, the paradoxes of short-sighted cancer-prevention strategies: more drugs are used to counteract the effect of previous exposures to drugs, chemicals or other carcinogenic agents. It is a vicious circle and one that will not be easily broken.

Cancer, Poverty, Politics

Though it is often said that affluent women are at higher risk for breast cancer, this disease is actually on the rise (both incidence and mortality) among African-American women, hardly an "affluent" population overall. The African-American Breast Cancer Alliance of Minnesota, organized in October 1990, has noted this steady increase and the limited efforts that have been made to reach African Americans with information and prevention strategies. People of color often live in the most polluted areas of this country, where factories, incinerators, garbage, and toxic waste are part of the landscape. Native American nations are particularly targeted by waste-management companies that try to take advantage of the fact that "because of the sovereign relationship many reservations have with the federal government, they are not bound by the same environmental laws as the states around them."

Poverty and pollution go hand in hand. The 1988 Greenpeace report *Mortality and Toxics Along the Mississippi River* showed that the "total mortality rates and cancer mortality rates in the counties along the Mississippi River were significantly higher than in the rest of the nation's counties" and that "the areas of the river in which public health statistics are most troubling have populations which are disproportionately poor and black." These are also the areas that have the greatest number of toxic discharges. Louisiana has the dubious distinction of being the state with the most reported toxic releases—741.2 million pounds a year. Cancer rates in the Louisiana section of the "Chemical Corridor" (the highly industrialized stretch of river between Baton Rouge and New Orleans) are among the highest in the nation. Use of the Mississippi River as a drinking-water source has been linked to higher than average rates of cancer in Louisiana. The rates of cancer of the colon, bladder, kidney, rectum, and lung all exceed national averages. Louisiana Attorney General William J. Guste, Jr., has criticized state officials who claimed that people of color and the poor *naturally* have higher cancer rates. You can't "point out race and poverty as cancer factors," said Guste, "without asking if poor people or blacks . . . reside in less desirable areas more heavily impacted by industrial emissions."

It follows that African-American women, living in the most contaminated areas of this country, would indeed be showing a disproportionate increase in breast cancer incidence. However, widespread epidemiological studies to chart such a correlation have not been undertaken. For instance, given the evidence implicating pesticides in the development of breast cancer, studies of migrant (and other) farm workers who have been exposed to such chemicals would seem imperative.

Women's groups around the country have started organizing to fight the breast cancer epidemic. A National Breast Cancer Coalition was founded in 1991. Its agenda is threefold: to increase the funding for research, to organize, and to educate. All of the recently organized groups consider prevention a priority, and one of their tasks will undoubtedly entail defining what effective prevention really means. In Massachusetts, the Women's Community Cancer Project, which defines itself as a "grassroots organization created to facilitate changes in the current medical, social, and political approaches to cancer, particularly as they affect women," has developed a Women's Cancer Agenda to be presented to the federal government and the NCI. Several demands of the agenda address prevention and identification of the causes of cancer. The group has received endorsements of its agenda from over 50 organizations and individuals working in the areas of environmental health, women's rights, and health care reform and is continuing to gather support. This effort will provide a networking and organizing tool, bringing together different constituencies in an all-out effort to stop the cancer epidemic.

Cancer *is* and needs to be seen as a political issue. The women's health movement of the '70s made that strikingly clear and gave us a road map to the politics of women's health. In the '80s, AIDS activists have shown the power of direct action to influence research priorities and treatment deliveries. In the '90s, an effective cancer-prevention strategy demands that we challenge the present industrial practices of the corporate world, based solely on economic gains for the already powerful, and that we insist on an end to the toxic discharges that the government sanctions under the guise of "protecting our security." According to Lenny Siegel, research director of the Military Toxic Network, the Pentagon has produced more toxic waste in recent years—between 400,000 tons and 500,000 tons annually—than the five largest multinational chemical companies combined.

Indeed, if we want to stop not only breast cancer but all cancers, we need to think in global terms and to build a movement that will link together groups that previously worked at a respectful distance. At a worldwide level, the Women's World Congress for a Healthy Planet (attended by over 1500 women from 92 countries from many different backgrounds and perspectives) presented a position paper, Agenda 21, at the 1992 United Nations Earth Summit conference in Brazil. The paper articulates a women's position on the environment and sustainable development that stresses pollution prevention, economic justice, and an end to conflict resolution through war and weapons production, probably the greatest force in destroying the environment.

On February 4, 1992, a group of 65 scientists released a statement at a press conference in Washington, D.C., entitled "Losing the 'War against Cancer'—Need for Public Policy Reforms," which calls for an amendment to the National Cancer Act that would "re-orient the mission and priorities of the NCI to cancer causes and prevention." The seeds of this movement have been sown. It is now our challenge to nourish this movement with grassroots research, with demonstrations, and with demands that our society as a whole take responsibility for the environmental contamination that is killing us.

Author's note: Many thanks to the women of the Women's Community Cancer Project in Cambridge, Massachusetts, for their help and support. A longer version of this article with complete footnotes and references appeared in the Resist newsletter (May/June 1992).

"rBGH Campaign in Massachusetts"

by Rita Arditti

What Is rBGH?

rBGH is a genetically modified hormone that is injected into dairy cows to increase milk production 5–15%. Monsanto created this synthetic hormone, sold under the name Posilac, using the cow gene from Bovine Growth Hormone (a hormone naturally produced by the pituitary gland of cows) and DNA from a bacteria, *Escherichia coli*. It is estimated that about 35% of dairy cows in the U.S. receive the drug.

Harm to Cows and to the Quality of Milk

The increased milk production comes at a high cost. The warning label given to farmers lists 20 adverse effects: 79% increase in mastitis (a contagious bacterial infection leading to painful inflammation of the udder); weight loss; aberrations of the reproductive system; alterations in the quality of milk. Mastitis leads to an increase of pus in the milk. Also the milk contains increased residues of the antibiotics used to treat the mastitis

Harm to Humans

Antibiotics Antibiotics in our milk and other dairy products can lead to antibiotic-resistant bacteria in our bodies making it harder to fight infection.

Increased Cancer Risk rBGH increases milk production through the stimulation of another hormone, called insulin-like growth factor-1 (IGF-1). IGF-1 is a naturally occurring potent growth hormone and cell-death inhibitor that has been implicated in breast, colon, prostate, lung, and other cancers as well as abnormal cell growth. IGF-1 is chemically identical in humans and cows. This means that when we drink milk from rBGH cows we are adding the IGF-1 from that milk to our own IGF-1 levels.

Labeling   Millions of people in the USA are unknowingly consuming rBGH dairy products. After pressure from Monsanto the FDA ruled that dairy produced from rBGH treated cows does not require a label. Monsanto has sued some of the companies that voluntarily labeled their milk rBGH-free.

Countries Banning rBGH   The 25 nations of the European Union, as well as Canada, Australia, New Zealand, and Japan have banned the used of rBGH. The United Nations food safety organization, Codex Alimentarium, has declined three times to declare the drug safe.

What We Can Do

Put pressure on schools, supermarkets, hospitals, coffee-shops, restaurants, etc, to use only rBGH-free dairy products. Buy organic products or products labeled "rBGH-free."

In truth, the story of what has happened with rBGH during the last 15 years speaks of the incredible power of the Monsanto Corporation and the dairy lobby to intimidate, silence its critics, and continue its relentless pursuit of profit while putting our health and lives at risk.

rBGH Web Resources

- *Food and Water Watch: Dairy* (http://www.foodandwaterwatch.org/food/dairy) Information on this site includes a *rBGH Fact Sheet*, a *list* of dairy companies nationwide that do not use rBGH, and the latest on a *campaign* to convince Starbucks to switch to rBGH-free milk.
- *Position Statement on rGBH* (.pdf) (http://www.noharm.org/details.cfm?ID=1104&type=document) The position statement of *Health Care Without Harm*, an international organization working to make the health care sector safer for patients, workers, public health and the environment.
- *Campaign for Safe Food* (http://www.oregonpsr.org/programs/campaignSafeFood.html) Information on the Oregon chapter of Physicians for Social Responsibility's campaign to boost the production of non-genetically altered foods.
- *rBGH & rBST Information* (http://www.organicconsumers.org/rbghlink.cfm) News and articles about the use of rBGH from the Organic Consumers Association.
- *Center for Food Safety* (http://www.centerforfoodsafety.org/rbgh2.cfm) This site examines the issue of rBGH within a wider critique of genetic engineering. Includes a *list of experts* on genetic engineering and information on the history of rBGH and the FDA.
- *Environmental Research Foundation* (http://www.rachel.org/bulletin/index.cfm?St=2) The organization's newsletter, "Rachel's News," documents the research and controversy surrounding rBGH from 1994–2003. To read the articles, type "rBGH" in the search box on this page.

Screening Mammograms
"When Fighting for Coverage and Quality Isn't Enough"

by Cynthia Pearson

Sometimes the work of women's health activists is easy. We find out that a new procedure or service can help improve women's health, we advocate for all women to have access to it, we do everything we can to ensure that it is provided in a high quality way, and then we celebrate the gains made. Sometimes it's more complicated, though, and the case of mammography screening for breast cancer is a painful example of a complicated women's health issue.

Mammography was originally studied as a screening tool in the 1960s. The first trial seemed to show screening saved lives: asymptomatic women were screened every year or two; smaller cancers were found than in similar, but unscreened women; these cancers were treated promptly; and fewer women died of breast cancer. This trial was followed by a large demonstration study that showed the average radiologists outside a highly structured clinical trial could identify small breast cancers. Based on these promising results, it appeared that mammography screening should be made available to all women at-risk of developing breast cancer.

In the aftermath of this early research, NWHN advocated strongly for mammography access. In the late 1980s, we lobbied Congress for Medicare coverage of screening mammograms. At that time, Medicare didn't cover any screening tests, and its managers were reluctant to expand the program's scope. In fact, I still remember testifying before Congress in favor of Medicare coverage of screening mammograms—and being opposed by a government accountant who said that it would be "too expensive" to pay the health care costs for all the women who would live many years longer if their breast cancer was cured after being found on a screening mammogram! Thankfully, Congress expanded Medicare's coverage even after the accountant's dire warning.

After Medicare began to cover screening mammograms, private insurance companies followed suit, and programs aimed at reaching women without insurance began. With access expanding, NWHN next turned its advocacy efforts to quality—and found we had work to do. Provision of screening mammography wasn't regulated back then, and the quality of machines used varied greatly, as did the training and experience of technicians and radiologists. Many women received very high-quality services, but not everyone did. And, as we pointed out, a bad mammogram is worse than no mammogram at all. The Network created a guide to the important elements of high-quality mammography, and many NWHN members volunteered to check out facilities in their hometowns. When members found inconsistent quality, we took this information to Congress and sought federal regulations. Other women's and cancer advocacy groups joined in this effort and, in the early 1990s, the Mammography Quality Standards Act was passed. We were especially proud that the Act gave women the right to get their own copy of their mammograms.

But, just when we thought we'd accomplished our work, the original premise of mammography (that screening saves women's lives) came into question. In 1992, NWHN began analyzing the benefit women really got from mammography screening. And, it turned out, the benefit wasn't as big as originally thought, nor did it apply equally to women of all ages. NWHN dove into this work, not because we thought we were exposing a sham—we'd promoted screening mammography, after all—but because our members want to know if researchers had doubts about the effectiveness of any treatment. NWHN members have told us that they don't want overly optimistic information or simplistic messages that are better at motivating than educating.

"Screening Mammograms: When Fighting for Coverage and Quality Isn't Enough," by Cynthia Pearson, originally published in the *Women's Health Activist*, January/February 2007, pp. 1 & 3, the newsletter of the National Women's Health Network (NWHN). It is reprinted with the permission of the author and the NWHN.

What we discovered in the 1990s was disheartening. In the aftermath of mammography screening's first trial, several other trials were undertaken, without impressive results. Screening's life-saving benefit was not found in all trials. It certainly wasn't found in the one trial designed to show the benefit of beginning mammography at age 40. NWHN went public with this information, and in 1993, issued a position paper recommending against screening mammography for pre-menopausal women—a very controversial position. The breast cancer advocacy movement was just getting started back then, and many organizations had a hard time accepting the idea that screening mammography might not really be very effective.

We also found that many people were shocked at the very idea that screening could, in fact, be harmful. Here's why: screening leads diagnosis, which leads to treatment. There is no treatment without risks. Treatment is often worth the risk when a condition is causing symptoms or is dangerous. But early cancer found through screening, when no symptoms are present, doesn't always progress to life-threatening, advanced cancer. We wanted to be sure that treating everyone found to have early cancer would actually help save women's lives. It was these considerations that led NWHN to tell women we believe that breast cancer screening should not be recommended for pre-menopausal women until it's been well-proven to do more good than harm.

Times have changed but, unfortunately, the complicated nature of mammography screening hasn't. The same seven screening mammography trials still generate controversy, just as they did in the early '90s. But the emergence of several wonderful breast cancer advocacy organizations that do their own independent analysis of science and clinical trials now makes it much easier for women to find excellent information on this complicated subject. The Network stopped doing our own analysis of the issue a few years ago, when we realized that other organizations can follow and analyze breast cancer screening reports as well as, and often more quickly than, NWHN.

The Myth of the Baseline Mammogram

While many things about screening mammograms are uncertain, there's at least one thing that is certain: baseline mammograms shouldn't be recommended as a routine part of health care for women. There is complete agreement about this, even among organizations that disagree on almost every other aspect of mammography.

But, despite this agreement that baseline mammograms aren't necessary and shouldn't be recommended, many women tell us that their practitioners start recommending baseline mammograms at age 35. Why is this? In part, it's because the American Cancer Society (ACS) spent over a decade promoting baseline mammograms as an essential part of screening for breast cancer. The ACS recommendation had no scientific evidence to support it—there are absolutely no studies showing any benefit of a baseline mammogram in women under 40—but the ACS recommendations reached and influenced the majority of U.S. physicians, nurse practitioners, and physician assistants.

The ACS received steady criticism of its recommendation in favor of baseline mammograms and finally withdrew it in 1992. The ACS did not, however, promote this change and the message still hasn't gotten out to well-meaning practitioners who continue to tell women in their 30s that its time for their baseline mammogram.

For more information about the history of the mammography debate, see: Sharon Batt, *Patient No More: The Politics of Breast Cancer*, Charlottetown, PE: Gynergy Books, 1994. Barron Lerner, MD., *The Breast Cancer Wars: Hope, Fear and the Pursuit of a Cure in Twentieth-Century America*, New York: Oxford University Press, 2001.

REFERENCE

"Chronological History of ACS Recommendations on Early Detection of Cancer." On-line at: http://www.cancer.org/docroot/PED/content/PED_2_3X_Chronological_History_of_ACS_Recommendations_on_Early_Detection_of_Cancer.asp?sitearea=PED.

A Gendered Epidemic
"Women and the Risks and Burdens of HIV"

by Peter Piot

The world has known about acquired immune deficiency syndrome (AIDS) for 20 years, and during that time, the severity of the epidemic has continued to surpass even the most pessimistic predictions. Despite the devastation that human immunodeficiency virus (HIV) has already caused, it is now clear that we are still in the early stages of the epidemic. As the epidemic has progressed, it has also become clear that it is fueled by the forces of inequality, social exclusion, and economic vulnerability.

This progression is most evident in the increasing impact of HIV on women. Where the HIV epidemic has been established longest and spread furthest, women represent an increasing proportion of those infected. Today, women make up just less than half the global total of nearly 34 million adults living with HIV, 55% of the 24 million adults living with HIV in sub-Saharan Africa, and 30% of total adult infections in the rest of the world.[1]

The largest gender difference is at younger ages: Average infection rates among teenage girls in sub-Saharan Africa are more than 5 times higher than those among teenage boys and in some countries of the region as much as 16 times higher. Women in their early 20s in sub-Saharan Africa are infected on average at 3 times the rate of men their age.[1]

The disproportionately high rates of infection among girls and young women is accounted for in large part by age mixing: younger women with older male sex partners. Not only are older male partners more likely to be infected than age-equivalent partners would be, but the relative immature genital tracts in younger women make them more susceptible to infection.

Women have come to comprise the majority of the HIV-infected population in sub-Saharan Africa because the rate of women's infection peaks at a younger age than men's, younger age groups are a large proportion of the population, and those infected at younger ages tend to survive longer. Elsewhere in the world, rates of HIV infection among women are continuing to rise. Parts of the Caribbean are characterized by longstanding epidemics and similar age mixing to that found in sub-Saharan Africa, with similar consequences. In parts of Central America, where heterosexual transmission of HIV predominates and is exacerbated by economic and race-based disparities, the epidemic is becoming generalized across populations, and women are increasingly affected. Antenatal testing has found HIV prevalence of 3% to 7% in several of Caribbean littoral countries.[1]

Women are an increasing proportion of the epidemic in many high-income countries. Over time, the epidemic follows patterns of social disadvantage, so that in many cases, the women who have been most affected are those from disadvantaged or minority ethnic populations.

The rapidly growing epidemic in Eastern Europe, where transmission through injection drug use predominates, is also rapidly spreading to the sex partners of injection drug users. The epidemic in Asia is affecting women who are particularly vulnerable, such as sex workers, and those whose lives do not fit conventional notions of "risk." For example, 93% of 400 female attendees at a sexually transmitted diseases clinic in Pune, India, were married, and 91% had never had sex with anyone but their husbands, yet 14% were infected with HIV.[2]

The burden of HIV/AIDS on women continues to increase. Women bear a disproportionate burden of HIV-related care. The growing number of AIDS orphans—at least 13 million worldwide, mainly in Africa—have, in many communities, already exceeded the capacity of extended families to cope. Women in some African villages are helping child-headed households to cope, by ensuring that the house door is locked at the end of the day, for example.[1]

The HIV/Aids epidemic is driven by the interlocking dynamics of risk, vulnerability, and impact. The immediate risks of HIV exposure through sex or injection drug use are structured by underlying forces of HIV-related vulnerability—the extent to which individuals have the capacity to control their risks. Women's HIV vulnerability derives in particular from contexts in which they have little control over sex, whether as a consequence of the predominating power relations between men and women or as a function of the economic and life choices available to them.

In turn, the impact of the epidemic itself creates additional HIV-related vulnerabilities. Populations suffering the stresses of a substantial AIDS toll have weakened resources to resist further spread of the epidemic. Women and girls from families whose productive capacities have been weakened by AIDS may have to resort to risky sex for their livelihoods. And planning for the future becomes a more distant goal in the face of current devastation.

Breaking the vicious cycle of HIV risk, vulnerability, and impact requires a systematic, sustained, and multi-sectoral AIDS response. Addressing the social and economic circumstances of women and girls is key to the effectiveness of a sustained AIDS response, as are strategies that address relations between men and women.

For some time, UNAIDS, together with many other governmental and non-governmental agencies, has argued that a gender dimension needs to be a central part of all AIDS strategies. It is now time to add that AIDS needs to be a part of all gender strategies.

AIDS constitutes a global development crisis. In the worst-affected countries, AIDS is turning life expectancy back by decades, cutting economic production by 1% to 2% a year, and putting development goals out of reach. Elsewhere, it has the potential to cause similar damage, unless sustained intervention holds the epidemic in check.

The precise form of effective, society-wide AIDS responses will differ in different settings, but there are a number of conditions of success that are both universally applicable and that will bring rapid results.

Women's organizations and women-led civil society responses are vital building blocks of the AIDS response, demonstrated repeatedly in contexts as diverse as the care, support, and prevention services of The AIDS Support Organization in Uganda and the empowerment of female sex workers in Sonagachi in Calcutta. Increasingly important are organizations that provide a direct voice for HIV-positive women.

Voluntary counseling and testing is the entry point for HIV care. Its effectiveness in preventing the spread of HIV is greatly enhanced where it addresses both men and women, and, especially, couples.

Preventing HIV transmission from mother to infant has become technically feasible and relatively inexpensive, yet more than one million infants are born with HIV annually, because their mothers do not have access to antenatal or postnatal care, HIV testing, antiretroviral therapy, or safe alternatives to breastfeeding. Extending the reach of care to prevent transmission from mother to child should also be the platform for extending HIV care

to women as the necessary infrastructure for HIV testing and care is made more widely accessible.

Keeping girls in school addresses HIV risk, vulnerability, and impact. As epidemics mature, HIV prevalence has been found to be associated with lower levels of education. The most effective school-based interventions simultaneously address both the skills children need and their social context. Tanzania, for example, is extending successful approaches that combine life-skills education, peer involvement, school-based AIDS committees (including parents), and guardian schemes to protect girls from sexual harassment.

Micro-finance initiatives, mainly involving women, are increasingly addressing AIDS by countering the social exclusion that makes some women particularly vulnerable. Micro-finance institutions have community education infrastructures that provide a venue for HIV-related community education. Micro-finance can be integrated into community coping mechanisms, as for example in the Uganda Women's Effort to Save Orphans, where micro-finance assists the caretakers of AIDS orphans.

The impact of AIDS is gendered in its every aspect: in conflict and emergency situations where rape is used as a weapon and in situations of extreme privation where sex is one of the only commodities; in the application of inheritance law where AIDS widows can lose their capacity to maintain family livelihood; in prevention commodities where female condoms, having proven acceptable, now need to become accessible; and in research where public subsidy is needed to accelerate the development of an effective microbicide, which would place a major HIV-prevention tool under women's control.

The recent UN General Assembly Special Session on AIDS saw nations sign on to a comprehensive set of AIDS targets, including a commitment to the participation of women in national AIDS strategies, reducing HIV prevalence in young people by 25%, a 20% reduction in transmission to infants by 2005 and a 50% reduction by 2010, as well as commitments to strengthened responses in relation to care, vulnerability, and conflict.

These commitments set a new benchmark of accountability for national and global AIDS responses. They will remain unachievable until and unless responding to AIDS becomes a central plank in worldwide efforts to empower women and, correspondingly, that gender becomes a central consideration across the totality of AIDS responses.

REFERENCES

1. *Report on the Global HIV/AIDS Epidemic*. Geneva: UNAIDS;2000. UNAIDS/00.13EO

2. Gangakhedkar RR, Bentley ME, Divekar AD, et al. Spread of HIV infection in married monogamous women in India. *JAMA*. 1997; 278:2090–2092.

"Scared to Be Safe"

by Jiayan Chen

It was one of those topics that rarely makes its way into daily conversation. The three other NWHN interns and I had just finished watching a video on microbicides—female-controlled contraceptives that are being developed as a way to provide women with protection against HIV and other sexually transmitted infections (STIs)—when we found ourselves in a discussion about contraceptive use. We wondered why, if condoms are so effective in preventing HIV and pregnancy, don't more women use them?

The question was finally answered when someone mustered up the courage to speak the hard truth: many women simply don't command enough power in their relationships to insist on condoms. In situations where cooperation from both partners (and particularly from the man) is required to use a specific method, we Network interns agreed that women may encounter obstacles, rather than encouragement, when they try to protect themselves. As a student who lives in a sorority with 60 other women, I can attest that condom use and safe sex are rarely discussed. That so many intelligent, sexually autonomous, and independent women still consider condoms taboo can't be dismissed as an isolated phenomenon.

The issue of mutual cooperation highlights a rather unsettling situation: despite the fact that condoms are the only form of contraception that protects against STIs and transmission of HIV, they aren't widely used as a primary means of protection. Consider these statistics from 2002.[1]

- Oral contraception (which doesn't protect against STIs) was the most commonly used contraception, used by 30.6% of women aged 15–44, and 53% of teens aged 15–19.

- Eighteen percent of women aged 15–44 rely on condoms as their primary form of contraception, down from 20% in 1995.

- Among teenage women aged 15–19 who use contraception, 45% use condoms either alone (19%) or with another method (25%).

What these facts reveal is that—although latex condoms are the only well-proven option for preventing both pregnancy and STIs (including HIV), are available over-the-counter, are inexpensive, and are relatively easy to use—a small percentage of sexually active women relies on condoms as their primary means of protection. (Preliminary research shows that diaphragms offer some protection against infection, but more work on this is needed.) This is particularly problematic for young women, who are have the highest rates of Chlamydia and Gonorrhea infection in the U.S., and who make up a growing proportion of new HIV infections. Condom use is more likely among teens and women in their 20s, but the rates could be much higher. Seven percent of sexually active teens don't use any form of contraception, and 21 percent of women don't use any form of contraception the first time they have sex.[1] Consequently, women are still potentially exposing themselves to pregnancy and STIs even if they use condoms more often than not.

Although the benefits of condom use are obvious, social norms that govern dating and sex are not as evolved and accommodating to women's need for protection as might be hoped. Male motivation for having a condom is unquestioned—when the back pocket of his jeans display a condom package's slight, round protrusion, a man escapes without ridicule or censure. Consider, on the other hand, a young woman who keeps condoms in her purse, or dares to bring condoms with her when she goes out for the evening. The typical reaction includes lots of questions: Is she expecting to have sex tonight? Does she know *who* she'll have sex with, or is she bringing a condom "just in case"? The sad fact is that women—far more than men—are expected to explain themselves when they chose condoms.

While it's true that women have come a long way in advancing our status, too often we are still beleaguered by out-dated notions of "appropriate" female identity and sexuality. In relationships where the man has the upper hand, women are discouraged to place "excessive"

"Young Feminists: Scared to Be Safe," by Jiayan Chen, originally published in the *Women's Health Activist*, March/April 2006, pp. 8–9, the newsletter of the National Women's Health Network (NWHN). It is reprinted with the permission of the author and the NWHN.

burden on her partner, and expecting him to use a condom easily belongs in this category. Women are anxious about asking their partners to use condoms because many men complain they decrease pleasure; women also may not want to foster an aura of mistrust that may arise from the request. It is worth mentioning that many young women avoid condoms for the same reason as their male counterparts, citing a loss of sensation or interruption of spontaneity. Ironically, young women who are less likely to be in long-term, monogamous relationships are the ones who really should be more concerned about practicing safe sex. Embarrassing stigmas about female sexuality hamper women from being empowered to be prepared and ready to protect themselves.

The problem persists even in long-term, intimate relationships, where an unequal distribution of power can still occur. I can recall conversations with my female friends who've said. "If he doesn't bring out the condom before sex, we usually don't use one." Typically, in these situations, condoms weren't used because the woman was too embarrassed or too afraid to ask; if she initiates the subject, it becomes her issue and something her partner must now address and is, thus, inconvenienced by.

The idea that women, like men, have sexual needs, desires, and concerns must replace the prevailing notion that only men can direct how sexuality is experienced. Only then can sexual relationships become an arena in which both partners are comfortable expressing their concerns about protection. One way we can achieve this is to expand sexuality education, and to focus educational efforts on younger men and women who are just beginning to experience and understand their sexuality. Condom use is on the rise for first-time sexual intercourse, which shows that safer sexuality education is effective and can help people protect themselves.

In addition to sexuality education, women need forms of protection that don't require male cooperation. Expanding the variety of woman-controlled contraceptives and barrier methods is essential to increasing women's control over their sexuality, particularly in preventing STIs. In some countries, female condoms are much more widely used than in the U.S., and we need to do more to make them more embraced in this country, as well. Microbicides are another promising development that offer a new way for women to protect themselves from STIs and HIV—but the lack of both funding for research and overall public awareness threaten the method's timely introduction into the public market. While we wait, we must establish a more encouraging environment in which outdated and stereotypical notions of gender are removed from efforts to promote safer sex and contraception.

REFERENCES

1. Mosher. W., Martinez, G., Chandra. A. et. al. 'Use of Contraception and Use of Family Planning Services in the United States: 1982–2002.' Advance Data 2004:(350): 1–46. See http://www.agi-usa.org/pubs/fb_contr_use.html.

With or Without the Dam Thing
The Lesbian Safer Sex Debate

by Carol Camlin

I have a rare lesbian safer sex poster on my office wall that shows two young white women embracing, naked and wet, in a steamy public bath. One woman sits on a tiled ledge with her legs spread, hair tossed in her face, smiling blissfully. The other is on her knees, leaning into her lover's open thighs, her head arched back. The text, in lavender, reads: "Wet your appetite for safer sex."

As a lesbian HIV/AIDS educator at the AIDS Action Committee of Massachusetts, I pay keen attention to the few safer sex messages and images produced for lesbians by national and international HIV/AIDS service organizations. For one thing, this environment brimming with gay male erotic safer sex posters would make any healthy lesbian long for a few pictures of nude women.

I also pay attention to keep abreast of the raging debate about lesbian sexual transmission of HIV—the so-called dam debate—among those who advocate either for or against the use of dental dams for oral sex (dental dams are small latex squares available at your local dental supply store: just masquerade as a dentist and ask for the 100-pak).

The lesbian safer-sex poster on my wall is different from gay male posters in one significant way. The scene evokes the eroticism of wetness, and seems to encourage comfort with bodily fluids. Wetness is sexy but, in the context of HIV, has come to seem dangerous. Although the poster would probably be a turn-on for most lesbians, I would imagine that The Terrence Higgins Trust (THT), the British AIDS service organization that produced the poster, has taken some flak for this one. The poster introduces the idea that there is such a thing as lesbian safer sex, without directly advocating the use of dental dams.

Carrying this message one step further, at the VIII International Conference on AIDS in July, THT unveiled a poster that directly advocates that lesbians *not* use dental dams. "Very low risk in oral sex," it advised, "so ditch those dental dams. Don't bother with gloves unless it turns you on." The poster immediately unleashed a storm of protest. Dozens of ACT UP members (most of them men) zapped the THT display booth, chanting "Shame!," spray painting it and modifying the poster with messages like "This poster is killing lesbians."

The intense controversy surrounding woman to woman sexual transmission of HIV is largely due to the fact that a very little HIV-prevention education information is geared to lesbians, despite our involvement in all aspects of the epidemic.

How many lesbians either harbor exaggerated fears of HIV or assume they're at no risk of HIV infection (or any other sexually transmitted disease)? How many lesbians are tacitly restricting their sexual practices, and so their sexual pleasure, out of fear of the unknown? How many HIV-positive lesbians know what they can safely do with their HIV-negative girlfriends? How many HIV- negative lesbians worry about how to have sex with their HIV-positive girlfriends without putting them at risk of an immune-threatening infection? Why this dearth of information?

In her July 1992 *Herizons* article, "Damned If You Do, Damned If You Don't," Lesli Gaynor of the AIDS Committee of Toronto argues: "The exclusion of lesbians and lesbian sexuality from AIDS education is not only a reflection of homophobia within mainstream education, but also a sign of the systematic sexism that exists within the gay community."

Lesbians need and deserve to get the facts abut AIDS, but the rare attempts to define safer sex for lesbians have focused almost exclusively on the use of dental dams. As a result, many lesbians have a vague idea that they should be using these devices, yet as Nancy Solomon notes in her Spring 1992 *Out/Look* article, "Risky business", very few women do—including lesbian safe sex educators who issue public pronouncements about dental dams.

Given the lack of availability of dental dams and their sexual unattractiveness, is it any surprise that we're not using them? I've heard the "damn dams" described as "about as sexy as a pair of rubber pants for the diaper wearing set" in Jenifer Firestone's "Memoirs of a Safe Sex Slut" (in *Bad Attitude*) and cunnilingus with a dam described as "chewing on a rubber tire."

Most lesbian health educators acknowledge that the three-inch-by-three-inch dental dams are small and difficult to use. How do you know when your spit ends and her fluids begin, unless you're really alert? Some educators advocate plastic wrap as an option for oral sex, because it's convenient, and it's larger. "Also," as one plastic-wrap aficionado puts it, "you can see through it, and that's nice."

Still others question barrier use in the first place. Louise Rice, a lesbian health educator and nurse at the AIDS Action Committee observes in her August 1992 *Sojourner* article, "Rethinking Dental Dams": "Barrier protection against HIV in vaginal fluids has no proven efficacy. Dental dams provide false security for an activity (going down) that already carries a relatively low risk."

Instead of broadening the topic of lesbian safer sex, the dam debate has sometimes obscured a deeper and more detailed discussion about the range of behaviors and activities which put lesbians at highest risk for infection with HIV and other STDs. After all, cunnilingus is not *all* we do. Do we focus on the use of dental dams because that's all we know how to talk about? Do we avoid discussion about the behaviors which put us at highest risk because of deep-seated taboos within the lesbian community?

Most HIV-positive lesbians became infected by sharing injection drug needles, or having sex with men without a condom. Several studies have shown that at least one-third of lesbians in the 20 to 35 year-old age group have slept with men, even after coming out. Simply having a lesbian identity does not make you "immune" to HIV: Our community must come to terms with the facts that lesbians sometimes use IV drugs and sometimes have sex with men.

Although these two risk factors are primarily responsible for the incidence of HIV among lesbians, it is possible for HIV to be transmitted sexually from woman to woman. Even those who aren't lesbian latex zealots agree that we are not "God's Chosen People." Lesbian sexual transmission of HIV is very rare—but just how rare, exactly how it happens, and how to prevent it are all points of debate. The information available to lesbians about what constitutes safer sex for lesbians is ambiguous and diverse in opinion.

AIDS service organizations offer advice to lesbians ranging from "stock up on latex condoms or dams" to AIDS Committee of Toronto's provocative suggestion "a little more sex, a little more leather, a little more lace, a little LESS LATEX." Somewhere in the middle of this, a growing number of lesbian health educators argue that, well into the second decade of this epidemic, enough is known about HIV transmission to suggest that HIV prevention education for lesbians need not include the "dental dams at all times under all circumstances" message. What exactly are the HIV transmission risks with woman to woman sex?

Let's review the facts. For someone to get infected, HIV not only has to get OUT of one person, via an infected body fluid, it also has to get INTO another person's bloodstream, via the mucous membranes or a break in the skin.

How the Virus Leaves the Body The highest concentration of HIV can be found in blood, and the next highest in semen. In vaginal fluid and pre-seminal fluid (or pre-cum, the fluid that men emit before ejaculation), the concentration is much lower. In some fluids such as tears or saliva, the concentration of HIV is so low or non-existent that there's no risk of infection.

The Chance of Infection via Oral Contact with Vaginal Fluid Is Very Low, and It Depends on the Presence of Blood Products However, several factors can increase the likelihood of the presence of HIV: menstrual blood, vaginal infections (such as yeast) and sexually transmitted diseases (such as herpes and chlamydia) can elevate levels of HIV in vaginal fluid, because all would contain white blood cells which harbor HIV. In later stages of HIV disease all bodily fluids contain higher concentrations of HIV. Also, the pH, or level of acidity, of the vaginal fluid can influence whether HIV is present. The pH of vaginal fluid is normally low, or acidic, and "inhospitable" to HIV (the pH of semen, on the other hand, is higher, or alkaline—and therefore more "hospitable" to HIV). Vaginal fluid is more alkaline during menstruation and ovulation.

How the Virus Enters the Body You can become infected with HIV if someone else's infected body fluid enters your bloodstream via breaks in the skin or via mucous membranes. Mucous membranes line the rectum, vagina and mouth (and in men also the urethra and glans—the tip of the penis); they're also found in the inside of your nose and eyelids. Some mucous membranes are thick and strong, and others are thin, and easier for the virus to pass through. The rectum is the most vulnerable because the walls of the rectum are very thin and there are tiny blood vessels at its surface which are easily ruptured during anal intercourse. The walls of the vagina are tougher and thicker, therefore less vulnerable to fissures and tears (with well-lubricated penetration and trimmed fingernails). The mucous membranes in the mouth are thicker than either the rectum or the vagina. It's therefore difficult for HIV to enter the bloodstream through your mouth. Moreover, saliva has a neutralizing effect on HIV, making it harmless when present in a low concentration, such as in vaginal fluid.

Reducing Your Risks "Lesbians do everything from nibbling on each other's ears to fisting—and in between there are a lot of things that are safe and some things that aren't," notes Amelie Zurn, Director of Lesbian Services at the Whitman-Walker Clinic in D.C. "The point is, risk is relative . . . for some people, any risk at all is unacceptable. For other people, more risk is okay."

The key to safer sex is communication: defining your limits and talking to your partner about what you want. To assess your risks and decide what to do, communicate with your partner.

Get to Know Your Vagina "Vaginal fluids have not been studied enough," Louise Rice acknowledges, "but women are capable of doing the studying. Getting to know your vagina, your discharges and smells, and those of a partner, can alert you to changes and potential infections. Unrecognized and untreated infections are a concern for all women, not just those with HIV. When HIV is present, an infection can quickly become disabling."

Get to Know Your Mouth Remember, even if you go down on a woman and she is menstruating or has a vaginal infection, the virus still has to find its way into your bloodstream. You may want to use a barrier under those circumstances—but if you don't there are ways to make oral sex even safer than it is, without having to use a barrier.

If you have a cold sore, or bleeding gums, or a cut on your tongue, "wait until you've healed so that you don't have to waste time and needless worry," Lesli Gaynor of Toronto advises. "If you have a contagious mouth condition like herpes, it's only courteous to consider the other person's health."

Gaynor offers an additional tip for safe licking: "Don't brush [or floss] your teeth before oral sex—use mouthwash to get that just-brushed fresh feeling." If your partner is HIV-positive, you may want to use mouthwash as a matter of course, to protect her from germs in your mouth.

You also may want to go down on your partner BEFORE you penetrate her with your hand or a sex toy. This will reduce the chance of there being blood present in the vaginal fluid.

Gaynor also suggests, "Take a closer look at what you're about to eat. If there are sores or areas of concern, don't panic but avoid contact. Kiss the surrounding areas lovingly."

Rimming Oral contact with the anus isn't a risk for HIV transmission unless the rectum contains blood (such as following "rough" anal penetration, and even then bleeding may not necessarily occur). But, you could contract another kind of infection via rimming, such as hepatitis A or amoebas. It's a good idea to use a barrier for rimming.

Fingerfucking or Using a Dildo HIV can be transmitted if menstrual or other blood of an HIV-positive woman gets into the vagina or anus of her partner. The safest option is to use your own toy. Wash thoroughly after each use with soap and water. If you share toys, use a condom and put on a new condom (with plenty of water-based lubricant) before you share. Or, wash thoroughly before sharing.

Remember, **intact skin is a good barrier against HIV infection.** If you have open cuts on your fingers and she's menstruating or has a vaginal infection, use latex or vinyl gloves or finger cots when penetrating her. A message to all you "Lee-Press On" femmes: trim those finger nails if you're planning to fuck her! The lesbian fashion of trimmed, smooth fingernails is in place for good reason: you don't want to cut or tear the lining of the vagina.

If you or your partner is HIV-positive, latex or vinyl gloves serve the function of not exposing an HIV-positive woman to bacteria and other germs under the fingernails, and reducing the risk of a cut in your or her vagina which could allow the germs to pass through to the bloodstream.

Fisting This can result in fissures or tears in the vaginal (or rectal) lining, which can result in both the presence of blood and access to the bloodstream. Fisting is an activity which can place both partners at risk, since tears may occur on the skin of the person doing the fist-

ing. Use latex or vinyl gloves with plenty of water-based lubricant when fisting, and if you plan to go down on her, either do so before you penetrate her or use a barrier.

Piercing, Cutting and Other S/M Activities Let the above principles of HIV transmission, and common sense be your guide in assessing risks and taking precautions with S/M activities. Invest in your own favorite equipment: latex or rubber toys, leather goods or metal equipment. The surest and safest guide is to not share equipment at all. If, however, it's not possible for you to supply your own, every precaution should be taken by you and your partner to make sure that equipment is properly cleaned prior to any sexual scene: (1) wash your equipment thoroughly, (2) soak it for several hours in a solution of one-part bleach to ten-parts water, and (3) rinse it thoroughly several times to be sure that all the bleach has been removed. These guidelines are adapted from the brochure "AIDS-Safe S/M," distributed by the AIDS Action Committee of Mass. For further information about S/M safety, see Pat Califia's *The Lesbian S/M Safety Manual: Basic Health and Safety for Woman-to-Woman S/M* Denver: Lace Publications, 1988.

Do I think cunnilingus is an effective way of spreading HIV? No . . . and the reason is that cunnilingus is not an effective way of spreading things which are much more infectious, like hepatitis B, which has 100,000 times more viral particles per cubic milliliter of blood than HIV. There has never been a single reported case of woman-to-woman transmission of hepatitis B via oral sex. In addition, given the number of lesbians infected with HIV, we would be seeing many, many cases of women getting infected via oral sex with other women—and we aren't

When HIV/AIDS educators talk to gay men about oral sex, most say, "Oral sex is very low risk. You can make it safer by not taking his come into your mouth. To be absolutely safe, you can use a condom." Very few gay men use condoms for oral sex, yet studies have shown that only about two dozen gay men worldwide, of the millions infected with HIV, have become infected via oral sex—and in those cases, almost all the men had taken ejaculate in the mouth, there were usually severe dental or gum problems, and often a high number of sexual partners (in the hundreds).

Dental dam advocates argue that data on lesbian transmission is fragmentary, since the Centers for Disease Control (CDC) doesn't include woman-to-woman transmission among the risk factors they normally track. Any well-informed AIDS activist knows that the CDC AIDS surveillance system is faulty, because it is based on the identity rather than the behavior of the person with AIDS. The sexual orientation of a person with AIDS does not explain how they became infected. The category "male homosexual/bisexual" doesn't tell us, for example, whether a man had insertive or receptive anal sex. The "heterosexual" category doesn't differentiate between those who became infected via anal or vaginal intercourse.

Although the right questions are not asked, the surveillance data is based on a hierarchy of transmission grounded in medical research and the real experience of people who've become infected with HIV. Sharing injection drug needles will put you in the "IV Drug User" category whether you are a gay or straight woman. Having unprotected intercourse with a man will put you in the "Heterosexual" category even though you identify as a lesbian. Both of those behaviors are much more likely to have caused your infection with HIV than going down on your girlfriend, because HIV is transmitted very efficiently and easily via blood to blood or semen to blood contact. To know the scope of the epidemic in the lesbian community at large, we need among other things a national seroprevalence survey of self-identified lesbians.

Most lesbian health educators acknowledge that although lesbians with HIV haven't been studied well, several lesbian health studies do exist. In studies of hundreds of lesbians with AIDS, only four cases of woman-to-woman transmission of HIV via sex have been reported in the medical literature. In the first case, both partners reported oral, anal and a vaginal contact with blood during sex (*Annals of Internal Medicine,* vol. 105, no. 6). The second case involved a woman whose female partner, an injection drug user, was in the late stages of HIV disease (*Annals of Internal Medicine,* vol. 111, no. 11). In the final two cases the HIV-positive lesbians' sexual partners were HIV-negative, and they reported no IV drug use or sex with men (*The Lancet,* 7/87 and *AIDS Research,* vol. 1, 84). The problem with these last three cases is that it is not reported exactly how the women became infected. There are several other anecdotal, word-of-mouth reports of sexual transmission of HIV between women. We may never know the full story with those cases, but we need only return to what we know about HIV transmission to be able to assess risks and make decisions about what we want to do sexually.

HIV prevention education for gay men is usually very sex-positive. Why do we reserve all of our sexual conservatism for lesbians, by passing out dams and gloves and issuing blanket statements to lesbians such as "oral sex on a woman is risky" and "putting your fingers inside her can be risky"? Most HIV/AIDS educators

wouldn't dream of telling a heterosexual man to wear a glove when putting his fingers in his girlfriend's vagina.

Many lesbian educators and activists are feeling that lesbians already have so much stacked against our sexual pleasure and freedom: internalized homophobia, racism and sexual abuse drain our self-esteem and sexual power; sexism and the puritan tradition subtly pervade how we think about sexuality and our bodies; our parents inculcated sexual shame in most of us, and that shame and guilt is only multiplied when we realize that we are queer.

Coming out can be an explosion of that shame into delight and power—and yet well-publicized phenomena such as "Lesbian Bed Death" and the general perception hat lesbians do it less than everybody else ("Bullshit!" some of us say; "Well quantity and quality are two separate things," other of us say) are signs that these various forms of oppression have taken their toll on our community.

The implicit question asked by many lesbian educators is: Do we want to be a part of what's keeping lesbians from getting it on and enjoying themselves, by exacerbating fears and encouraging lesbians to restrict themselves sexually? Absolutely not. We do need to continue to get the information out about what's risky and what's not.

"Every day, women make decisions about the risk of different activities," Louise Rice noted, "Most of these activities (smoking or driving a car, for example) carry a far greater risk than cunnilingus. Thousands of lesbians' lives could be saved if we were to devote half the attention to mammograms and breast self-awareness that has been focused on dental dams."

Having put out all of this provocative information, I'd like to suggest that we turn our political focus outward and turn our activism towards improving the lives of ALL women with AIDS—not just lesbians with AIDS. In the United States, women with AIDS make up only 4 percent of all clinical trials, although women make up 13 percent of all people with AIDS (and that's an underestimate of about 28 percent). Fourteen million women still don't have access to health insurance. The CDC case definition of AIDS still doesn't include life-threatening gynecological manifestations of AIDS. The number-one HIV transmission risk for women is IV-drug use: We need to make clean needles available and drug treatment accessible. All of these issues are lesbian health issues. And we can achieve victories on many of these fronts if we ACT UP louder and in greater numbers. Meantime, let's talk about sex—and have as much as we want.

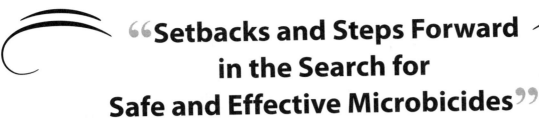 

"Setbacks and Steps Forward in the Search for Safe and Effective Microbicides"

by Bindiya Gillenwater Patel

Worldwide, women are disproportionately impacted by the HIV AIDS epidemic. More women are newly infected with HIV than men, primarily through having sex with men who are HIV-positive.[1] In the U.S., more than 250,000 women are living with HIV/AIDS, and the disease is the number one cause of death among African American women aged 25–34.[1,2] And, internationally, around half of the 38.6 million people living with HIV are women.[3] For this reason, advocates around the world have long voiced the need for an HIV prevention method that women can control.

Microbicides—products that are designed to be used in a gel, tablet, or vaginal ring to help prevent HIV/AIDS—could provide exactly that. Due to advocates' work around the world, and the recent attention on microbicides at the 2006 International AIDS Conference in Toronto, millions of people have heard about microbicides. The challenge the field now faces is to find the correct balance between building enthusiasm and political support for microbicides, while avoiding raising unrealistic expectations in the media or in our outreach work.

Microbicides are not going to be a magic bullet against HIV. It is important to note that, while microbicides will help people reduce risk of infection, they will never be as effective as condoms. We still need to improve people's access to the interventions that we know work now: making sure that male and female condoms are available and affordable (for more on this, see: www.prevention now.net, as well as http://www.populationaction.org/resources/publications/condomscount/index.htm); ensuring that pregnant women get access to services that prevent maternal transmission to their babies (www.pedaids.org); and promoting appropriate male circumcision programs (http://www.global-campaign.org/malecircumcision.htm).

Nonetheless, microbicides have the potential to be an important way for women and couples to reduce their risk of infection. The hope is that couples will be able to use microbicides more consistently than they currently do condoms. We need to encourage people to continue to use condoms if they possibly can, and suggest additional use of microbicides for back-up protection and added pleasure.

Timing for Microbicide Availability

Although microbicides do not yet exist, ten products are currently being tested in clinical trials, and anticipation is building: results from the first microbicide effectiveness trials could be available in 2008. Then it will take at least one or two years for the products to be reviewed and approved. Thus, while a microbicide could be ready for introduction by 2010, it's likely only to happen in a few countries, most likely through smaller scale, introductory programs. If the products currently in effectiveness trials do not prove effective, the timeline will be longer. There are several second-generation leads already in human testing, and we need to ensure that the entire pipeline of products advances.

In January, 2007, however, the search for an effective microbicide faced a major setback when the trials of one potential product were stopped due to safety concerns. Shortly thereafter, in March 2007, the U.S. House of Representatives and Senate both introduced legislation to provide a much-needed boost to the microbicides field. We'll discuss both of these developments below.

Cellulose Sulfate Trials Close Due to Safety Concerns

In order to fully understand the recent microbicide trial closures, a bit of background information on clinical

"Setbacks and Steps Forward in the Search for Safe and Effective Microbicides," by Bindiya Gillenwater Patel, MPA, originally published in the *Women's Health Activist*, May/June 2007, pp. 1, 3, 7, the newsletter of the National Women's Health Network (NWHN). It is reprinted with the permission of the author and the NWHN.

Women and HIV

Women are at higher risk of HIV infection than men partly because of biology, partly because of economics, and partly because of culture. Women are more vulnerable to HIV because they are exposed to more virus for a longer period of time during sexual intercourse.[4] Young girls are especially at risk because their reproductive tracts are not fully mature and are more vulnerable to infection.

Economically, women often have less access than men to education, job opportunities, property, or credit, which makes them financially dependent on their partners.[5] As a result, women often cannot afford to leave relationships that put them at risk of HIV and other STIs, to refuse sex, or demand condoms. Culture also plays a role. Here and abroad, women are expected to be faithful but men are not, and their male partner's infidelity is one of the greatest HIV risks women face. In addition, gender-based violence is a big factor in women's risk.[6]

The current prevention methods (abstinence, fidelity, and condom use) often require active acceptance, participation, consent and cooperation by both partners. But women don't always have control over when and how they have sex. While we are making important progress on delivering treatment, we still need to do everything we can to give people more prevention options—especially those that they themselves can control. Microbicides provide an alternative for women who ask, "I just can't make him use a condom; isn't there something else I can do to protect myself?" Once microbicides become available, we'll be able to tell her that, while the new products aren't as effective as condoms, they're much better than nothing. And, as we all know, a lot of women are getting infected because "nothing" is all they have.

trials is useful. Before any new drug is available to consumers, it goes through a rigorous series of clinical tests in people. The first two levels of these safety tests, called Phase I and Phase 2 trials, look for evidence that the product could be harmful. If a product gets through Phase 1 and 2 safety trials without evidence that it might cause harm, it can then move to Phase 3 effectiveness trials, which compares the new product to a standard product or a placebo. The microbicide gel cellulose sulfate (CS) went through II Phase 1 and 2 trials, without results to indicate that it was harmful. CS proceeded to Phase 3 trials, in which one group of women used the experimental gel (CS), while a second group used a placebo gel without the active ingredient.

Extensive measures are taken to help all microbicide trial participants understand that they should not count on the gel for protection from HIV, that half would receive the placebo gel, and that they have the right to withdraw from the trial at any time. All participants receive monthly HIV prevention counseling, free condoms, and prompt diagnosis and treatment for any sexually transmitted infections. Finally, an independent Data Safety Monitoring Board (DSMB) exists for each microbicide trial. The DSMB is composed of individuals with expertise in statistics, medicine, clinical trials,

and community issues; it serves to protect participant safety and recommends whether a particular trial should continue.

Cellulose sulfate was one of four microbicides in Phase 3 effectiveness trials for HIV/STI prevention (the other three are BufferGel, Carraguard, and PRO2000). CONRAD was conducting. Phase 3 trials to assess CS' effectiveness in Benin, India, South Africa, and Uganda. A similiar trial, sponsored by Family Health International (FHI), was also underway in Nigeria. Both sponsors are U.S.-based nonprofit research groups dedicated to advancing health in developing countries. In January, at the recommendation of their respective DSMBs, both groups discontinued their CS trials after CONRAD's DSMB found evidence suggesting that the microbicide might be contributing to an increased risk of HIV infection. (In other words, more HIV infections occurred in women using the experimental gel than among women using the placebo.) Although review of the data from the Nigerian trial found no evidence of increased risk, FHI felt that the only responsible course of action was to halt its study also. Interim results of the other three ongoing Phase 3 trials have been reviewed by their respective DSMBs, which have found no evidence of similar safety concerns.

Once their trials closed, the FHI and CONRAD investigators quickly shifted their efforts to notifying the trial participants, collecting any unused gels, and ensuring that participants received appropriate follow-up care—including counseling, HIV testing, and medical referrals, if needed. In response to demands from advocates, many trial sponsors now develop written agreements before trials begin. In this case, both trial sponsors had prepared written agreements in advance with local providers to assure that any women infected while enrolled in the trial would get ongoing care and treatment.

In the days following the closure of the CS trial, women from around the world voiced a strong demand for information about what went wrong with these trials and support for continuing the search for a safe, effective microbicide. Women still don't have the tools they need to protect themselves from HIV. The Global Campaign for Microbicides and the African Microbicide Advocacy Group are continuing to answer advocates' questions; facilitate dialogue and debate; and develop and advocacy agenda that prioritizes participants' rights, enhances scientific transparency, and encourages deep scientific reflection. (Learn more about this work at: www.global-campaign.org/cellulose-sulfate.htm).

Demonstrating Public Demand in the U.S.—The Microbicide Development Act

In the wake of the CS trials' closure, advocates, researchers and legislators are working together to ensure sufficient public funding for the continued search for a safe and effective microbicides. Since the pharmaceutical industry has not yet invested significantly in this field, microbicide research depends on governmental and philanthropic investment. Yet, right now, barely three percent of the U.S. budget for HIV/AIDS research is spent on developing microbicides.

To mark International Women's Day on March 8, 2007, a bipartisan group of senators and representatives introduced the Microbicide Development Act (MDA) of 2007. Sponsors include Sen. Barack Obama (D-IL). Sen. Olympia Snowe (R-ME), Rep. Jan Schakowsky (D-IL), and Rep. Christopher Shays (R-CT). The Act calls for improved coordination and expanded resources for microbicide research and development activities at the National Institutes of Health, the Center for Disease Control, and the U.S. Agency for International Development. NWHN members can play a pivotal role by contacting your legislators to support the MDA. A petition, sample letter, and advocacy email system are at: http://www.global-campaign.org/legislativeadvocacy.htm. If you call your Congress members, give them this simple message: "I am calling to ask Representative/Senator _____ to sponsor the H.R.1420/S.823 Microbicide Development Act. This bill can really make a difference in addressing the AIDS pandemic by supporting the development of important HIV prevention options that women can control."

The real heroines and heroes are the women who enroll in these trials. Over two years, on average, trial participants each attend 29 study visits—including monthly visits for HIV and pregnancy tests—and go through II pelvic exams. Without their participation and commitment, it would be impossible to discover an effective microbicide. This month, take a moment to write or call your legislators to honor their commitment and move one step closer to getting a new prevention tool into women's hands.

REFERENCES

1. The Centers for Disease Control and Prevention (CDC), "Cases of HIV Infection and AIDS In the United States and Dependent Areas, 2005," *HIV/AIDS Surveillance Report* 2007; 17:11–12. 36–37.

2. Kaiser Family Foundation, *Women and HIV/AIDS in the United States, HIV/AIDS Policy Fact Sheet*, Menlo Park, CA: Kaiser Family Foundation, December 2006. p. I.

3. Joint United Nation Programme on HIV/AIDS (UNAIDS), *Report on the Global AIDS Epidemic: 2006.* Geneva: World Health Organization, 2006. pp. 8, 45–46.

4. European Study Group on Heterosexual Transmission of HIV. "Comparison of female to male and male to female transmission of HIV in 563 stable couples," *British Medical Journal* 1992; 304:809–813.

5. UNAIDS. Economic Security for Women Fights AIDS. Global Coalition on Women and *AIDS Report, Issue #3*, Geneva. Switzerland: UNAIDS, 2005.

6. Garcia-Moreno, C. and C. Watts, "Violence against women: its importance for HIV/AIDS," *AIDS* 2000; 14(Suppl 3): S253–S265.

"Cervical Cancer Vaccines in Context"

by Adriane Fugh-Berman

In Washington D.C., in the 1970s, I volunteered at a Latino health fair that offered various health screenings, including Pap smears to look for precancerous cells. When the results came back, about one of four of the Paps was abnormal. An abnormal Pap doesn't equal a diagnosis of cervical cancer, but follow-up colposcopy (examination of the cervix with a lighted microscope) is necessary, and some women should have further procedures as well. Colposcopy is a specialized procedure, usually done by gynecologists, and we couldn't identify qualified physicians who were willing to perform this procedure without charge, so we couldn't provide this follow-up. I don't know what happened to the women whose abnormal Paps were identified during the health fair; without adequate follow-up, some may have developed cervical cancer by now.

Paps are crucial to preventing deaths . . . but only if women can get them, and if they're followed up by appropriate diagnostics and treatment. Worldwide, cervical cancer rates are much higher in other countries than in the U.S.; more than 80% of cases occur in underserved, resource-poor communities. In parts of Africa, Central and South America, and Micronesia, there are more than 50 cases of cervical cancer per 100,000 women.

In the U.S., there are 6.6 cases of cervical cancer for every 100,000 White women, and 10.5 cases for every 100,000 African American women. Since the Pap smear was introduced in 1949. U.S. cervical cancer incidence and mortality have dropped by three-quarters, although rates are higher in the rural South and some cities, including D.C. (The combined Pap/human papilloma virus test that's now common was invented in the 1990s.) Today, about half of the U.S. women diagnosed with cervical cancer had never been screened by a Pap test prior to their diagnosis.

There are hundreds of types of human papilloma virus (HPV), some of which cause genital warts (especially HPV types 6 and 11), and others of which cause cervical cancer (especially HPV types 16 and 18). Infection with HPV, including with the cancer-associated types, is *extremely* common: about 15% of the population's infected with some form of HPV. Yet, most women with HPV, including those with types 16 and 18, never develop either cervical cancer or abnormal cells. In fact, in most people, HPV cures itself. About 70% of women test negative for the virus a year after their diagnosis and about 90% test negative after two years.

Only about 10% of women who are infected with HPV stay infected; it is these women with persistent infections who are at the highest risk for HPV to progress to cervical cancer. In the U.S., even presistent HPV rarely causes cervical cancer, as regular screening catches precancerous changes and available treatment of precancerous changes prevents cancer. In the U.S., in 2006, an estimated 9,710 cases of invasive cervical cancer occurred, and about 3,700 women died from it. Worldwide, however, cervical cancer is the 2nd most common cancer death among women, causing about 288,000 deaths annually. In June 2006, the Food and Drug Administration (FDA) approved Gardasil, a vaccine against HPV types 6, 11, 16 and 18 Gardasil is the first vaccine against cervical cancer to be approved, although a second vaccine will reach the market soon. The development of a cervical cancer vaccine is a public health breakthrough with the potential to save many lives worldwide. It won't end cervical cancer, however, although it will reduce the need for Pap smears over time. This is because some cervical cancers are caused by viral strains not covered by the vaccine, and we don't know yet how long protection lasts for the covered strains (we do know that it's still going strong at five years), so booster shots may be required.

The vaccine only works well if it is administered before a woman is exposed to HPV. Merck (Gardasil's manufacturer) just curtailed its efforts to lobby state legislatures to require vaccination of schoolgirls, as part of which it donated an undisclosed sum to Women in Government, an advocacy group of women state lawmakers. Bills have been introduced, or are being drafted, in about 20 states to require HPV vaccination for schoolgirls.

There's been a public backlash against the idea of this mandatory vaccination. I support the backlash, but I also support the use of HPV vaccines. HPV vaccines are expected to reduce deaths from cervical cancer, and to reduce the risk of precancerous changes, which are not trivial. Treatment of precancerous conditions involves cutting, burning, or freezing part of the cervix, and can cause complications that affect childbearing. Reducing the number of these procedures will benefit women's health.

There should be a public outcry against mandatory HPV vaccine laws not because the vaccines are experimental (they are well-tested) or because they are dangerous (they aren't). The currently proposed laws should be opposed because public health policy should never be orchestrated by corporations. The debate over mandatory HPV vaccination is an important one, but the debaters should be restricted to those who will not turn a profit from the decisions.

Although the HPV vaccine's touted as the first vaccine against cancer, the hepatitis B virus (which can be transmitted sexually) increases the risk of liver cancer, and hepatitis vaccines are available. And in terms of sexually transmitted infections, hepatitis and HIV together cause many more deaths than HPV, Condoms, of course, are still the best protection against all sexually transmitted infections, including HPV. But these are not mutually exclusive strategies. We need public health education about condoms, cervical cancer screening—and cervical cancer vaccines.

See: The Centers for Disease Control and Prevention (CDC). "Human papillomavirus; HPV information for clinicians." Atlanta: CDC. Nov. 2006. Online: http://cdc.gov; and Saslow D, Castle PE, Cox JT et al. "American Cancer Society Guidelines for human papillomavirus (HPV) vaccine use to prevent cervical cancer and its precursors." *Cancer J Clin* 2007; 57:7–28. Online. http://caonline.amcancersoc.org/cgi./content/full/57/1/7.

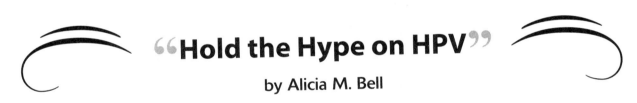

"Hold the Hype on HPV"

by Alicia M. Bell

A week before my 27th birthday, I've been thinking beyond my usual self-assessments and musings on the number of candles on my birthday cake. I can't stop wondering where women my age see themselves in the context of the ongoing, frenzied debate over Gardasil, the only FDA-approved vaccine for the human papillomavirus (HPV). In addition to its marketing campaign, Merck, Gardasil's manufacturer, aggressively pushed for legislation to require mandatory vaccination of school-aged girls. In the wake of the resulting major public outcry, Merck abandoned this tactic, but its political faux pas further complicated the murky issues surrounding HPV's link to cervical cancer. (See the March 2007 issue of the *Women's Health Activist* for Adriane Fugh-Berman's column on the campaign.)

The HPV discussion currently focuses largely on young, school-aged girls—because Merck's controversial push for mandatory, vaccination in this population caused a general knee-jerk, parental freakout. Many parents are probably uncomfortable with the HPV vaccine because it makes them think of their children one day having sex, which they almost certainly will (an issue they don't have to consider with other childhood vaccinations!) Eventually, the dust will settle and public health authorities will promote a stronger, more cohesive and (I hope) less biased public message on the HPV vaccine. But, in the meantime, where does this leave women who are past the age of school vaccinations? Women over 18, like me, must decide whether to get vaccinated on our own.

Gardasil has been approved for use in females between the ages of 9 and 26, so there are many young adult women who will have to deal with pressure to get the

"Young Feminists: Hold the Hype on HPV," by Alicia M. Bell, originally published in the *Women's Health Activist*, May/June 2007, pp. 8–9, the newsletter of the National Women's Health Network (NWHN). It is reprinted with the permission of the author and the NWHN.

vaccine. Doctors are allowed to prescribe a therapy for any purpose in any population after its approval by the Food and Drug Administration (FDA), so it's possible that doctors will advise women over 26 to receive the vaccination. It is also possible that women over 26 may demand vaccination because, "Hey, it can't hurt." One's level of sexual activity is, however, the important determinant in whether to get vaccinated. The HPV vaccine makes the most sense for women who have never had sex or had very few sex partners. Although Gardasil isn't approved for use in men, men are most often the carriers who infect their female partners. If the vaccine is shown to be effective in men, then vaccinating males might be good for women, too. Currently, there are lots of questions about the choices that can be made to prevent cervical cancer—questions that are unlikely to be answered in the politically charged climate.

I first heard about HPV several years ago while in college, where I learned that it is sexually transmitted, that people may not have symptoms when infected, and that it causes the majority of cervical cancers. At least 80 percent of women will have had an HPV infection by the time they are 50.[1] At first, I was angry. You always hear about HIV, gonorrhea, syphilis, and herpes—so why hadn't I heard about this virus before? Then I saw a television episode of "Law and Order: Special Victims' Unit", in which a woman who had been sexually assaulted was diagnosed with HPV. The fictional detectives wanted to find the young woman quickly so that she could get treated for the infection immediately, since HPV can cause cancer. Although this was just a TV show, I wondered about this: was HPV an emergency? What treatment could the woman get? I thought there was no treatment for HPV!

I learned about treating HPV firsthand some time later. Over a year ago, a doctor nonchalantly informed me that I had genital warts caused by HPV, and that I could treat them with a cream or she could burn the warts off. It really bothered me that she acted like it was no big deal, and I was a bit taken aback because I worried that my chances of getting cervical cancer later in life had automatically increased with the HPV infection. My next emotional reaction was guilt that I had been sexually irresponsible. I wondered if I should tell my past partners that I had HPV. I worried about how long I had been infected. I felt really confused; was HPV something I should stay up nights worrying about, or was it as normal a part of women's life as yeast infections?

It turns out that HPV is quite common—so common that a gynecologist told me women could think of it as *normal flora*. HPV infection often goes unrecognized

because there may be no symptoms, but it can be diagnosed through an abnormal Pap test or from the presence of genital warts. The genital warts caused by certain types of HPV (including types 6 and 11) can be removed with gels, creams, cryotherapy (literally burning them off), or surgery, but there is no cure for HPV.[2] Luckily, this is generally not a problem because the infection almost always goes away on its own: 90 percent of women with cervical HPV infection have no detectable virus within two years.[1] Additionally, the types of HPV that cause genital warts are not the same types that can lead to cervical cancer. Therefore, HPV is only a cancer risk for women who have persistent infection with high-risk HPV, such as types 16 and 18.[2]

After I learned that HPV is very common, that most people clear the virus, and that genital warts are not caused by the type of HPV associated with cervical cancer, I was no longer worried. Condom use dramatically reduces the risk for HPV infection, but it is not fully protective; HPV can be transmitted through skin that isn't covered by a condom (such as the vulva, scrotum, or perianal region).[2] Wow—I wish I had known this *before* the doctor told me that I had HPV.

Considering all this, should sexually active young women run out and get the HPV vaccine? Maybe not. The vaccine is not very effective in those who have already been exposed to one of the types of HPV it targets.[3] If you have never had sex (or had very few sex partners), you may benefit from the vaccine. If you have had multiple sex partners, you are unlikely to benefit from the vaccine because your level of sexual activity is a more important determinant than age for getting HPV. Also, HPV exposure usually occurs within the first few years after a person becomes sexually active—that's why it's recommended that women get the vaccine before having sex (or very soon thereafter). Nearly one-quarter of U.S. teens have had sex by age 15, and 70 percent have had sex by the time they are 18—that's why vaccination at a much younger age is the most effective public health intervention.[3]

A general sense of dread surrounds HPV and cervical cancer, and I think most women are relieved there is a vaccine. But I worry that the public is getting an oversimplified view of HPV and its relation to cervical cancer. From a public health perspective, it makes sense to vaccinate all girls before they've had sex. But for women who have had sex, the number of sexual partners—not age—should be the most important factor in the decision to get vaccinated. I fear that many women will be subjected to unnecessary vaccinations, or stop seeking regular cervical cancer screening. It is possible that confusion surrounding the vaccine could lead to a misuse of resources and could become a barrier to achieving the best possible health outcomes for women.

Cervical cancer screening through regular Pap tests is still crucial, especially since the currently available HPV vaccine does not protect against all types of high-risk HPV strains. The Pap test has truly been the first line of defense against developing cervical cancer and U.S. screening programs have greatly reduced deaths from cervical cancer in this country. The single most important factor associated with developing invasive cervical cancer is never (or rarely) getting screened.[4] The American Cancer Society estimates that in 2007, 11,150 women will develop invasive cervical cancer in the U.S. and 3,670 will die.[1] Even in the U.S., most of the women who die of cervical cancer never had regular Pap tests.[1]

The World Health Organization (WHO) estimates that there are 250,000 annual cervical cancer deaths worldwide, making it the second most common cause of female cancer deaths.[3] The vast majority of these deaths are in countries where women do not have access to regular screening, and the HPV vaccine has amazing potential to save many lives in these countries. Despite the hype now surrounding HPV, regular Pap tests and condom use are still key to reducing risk for genital HPV infection and the HPV-associated problems of genital warts and cervical cancer—even if you do decide to get the HPV vaccine.

References are available from editor@nwhn.org, or online.

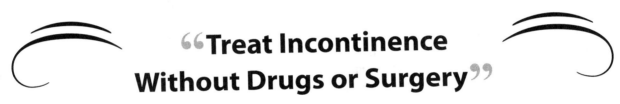

"Treat Incontinence Without Drugs or Surgery"

by Adriane Fugh-Berman

My cousin's child, at about age 4, didn't make it to the bathroom in time, and burst into tears of embarrassment because she had piddled on the floor. "It's just an accident, nothing to worry about," I said, soothingly, "You know, even *grown-ups* have accidents." She was so astonished that she stopped crying, mid-sob.

Adults don't talk about it much, but incontinence is common, especially among women. There are two sorts of urinary incontinence. "Stress incontinence", the loss of urine during coughing, laughing, sneezing, or exercise; "urge incontinence" is a sudden urge to urinate immediately followed by involuntary urine loss.

The most effective, safest, and cost-effective therapies for treating urinary incontinence are pelvic floor muscle (PFM) exercises and a kind of behavioral therapy called "bladder retraining." PFM exercises are what my generation called Kegel exercises. Named for U.S. physician A.H. Kegel, the exercises involve strengthening the muscles located in and near the vagina that keep us continent. While Kegeling was promoted to my gen-

eration as a sex improvement technique, it may be even more important for preventing and treating incontinence.

To do PFM (or Kegel) exercises, tighten the vaginal muscles as though you were stopping urine flow, and then tighten the muscles of the anus as though you were trying to stop a bowel movement. For both exercises, pull upwards and inwards, hold for a count of three, then relax. Do a set of 5–10 several times daily and try to work up to holding the positions for 10 seconds. Alternate sets of long slow contractions with sets of fast flicks. Try not to involve the abdomenal or buttock muscles.

If you have trouble identifying the muscles to tighten, insert 1–2 fingers into your vagina and try to squeeze your fingers with your vaginal muscles. Or, try to stop your urine flow midstream (don't do this on a regular basis, as it creates turbulence in the bladder, which is bad for you—but it's okay to do it while learning the technique). PFM exercises can be done anywhere; while watching TV, commuting, or in meetings, in elevators—the possibilities are endless.

"Treat Incontinence Without Drugs or Surgery," by Adriane Fugh-Berman, M.D., originally published in the *Women's Health Activist*, March/April 2005, p. 15, the newsletter of the National Women's Health Network (NWHN). It is reprinted with the permission of the author and the NWHN.

Some people find PFM exercises difficult to learn leading to the invention of vaginal weightlifting aids. Vaginal cones, which are sold through catalogs are weighted plastic, tampon-like devices that are placed into the vagina, and fall out if the pelvic muscles are inadequately contracted. The weights are graduated so that after successfully learning to hold in lighter weights a woman moves on to heavier ones.

If these measures don't work, biofeedback—preferably with bladder retraining—should be the next step. The biofeedback technique teaches people how to control their muscle tone (or other bodily processes) by using audio or visual signals. For incontinence one tries to contract the PFM muscles while relaxing the abdominal muscles (which may seem impossible to do simultaneously at first). Several techniques can be used, including one where a small device placed into the vagina translates information about muscle tone through beeps or visual images. By learning to control these signals, women can learn which muscles to contract. The machines are unnecessary once the technique is mastered.

Behavioral training sessions help people learn alternatives to bolting desperately for the bathroom when they experience the urge to urinate. Behavioral training involves learning "urge strategies", which involve sitting down, relaxing, contracting their pelvic muscles repeatedly, then proceeding to the toilet at a normal pace once the feeling of urgency subsides.

Many randomized controlled trials have demonstrated the effectiveness of these therapies in diverse populations, including homebound elders, women who have just given birth, and female soldiers with exercise-induced incontinence.

Physicians often prescribe drugs (like oxybutynin and tolterodine) but biofeedback-assisted behavioral therapy is just as effective. Incontinence drugs relax muscle cells in the urinary tract, but also slow motility in the gut, so constipation can be a problem. Other side effects include dry mouth and eyes, headaches, abnormal vision, and urinary retention. Various surgeries have also become popular; while it can be effective, surgery should be a *last* resort. For urinary incontinence, biofeedback and behavioral therapies should always be tried first.

Your doctor may not know about PFM exercises and biofeedback, but now you do. Tell your friends! For more information or a referral to a biofeedback therapist in your area, contact:

Biofeedback Certification Institute of America:
10200 West 44th Ave, #310, Wheat Ridge, CO 80033, 303.420.2902 Website: www.bcia.org

Association for Applied Psychophysiology and Biofeedback:
10200 West 44th Ave, #304, Wheat Ridge, CO 80033, 303.422.8436 Website: www.aapb.org

REFERENCES
References for this article are available from email editor@nwhn.org.

Women and Fibroids
"Making the Best Decisions"

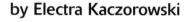

by Electra Kaczorowski

Uterine Fibroids are extremely common, but not a very well-understood women's health topic. When a woman is told that she has fibroids, her first question is usually "What do I do?" While this is a perfectly reasonable question, finding the answers often leads her to embark on a confusing journey in which she is likely to receive misleading information about treatment options. Often, the woman becomes more anxious than she was before. The truth is that fibroids, while sometimes painful, are almost never a cause for worry. In the vast majority of cases, women can take the time needed to consider all of their options and find the treatment plan (if one is even necessary) that works best for them.

Fibroids (medically known as *uterine leiomyomas*) are benign lumps of muscle and tissue that grow in and around the uterus. *Submucosal* fibroids grow underneath the uterine lining; *intramural* fibroids grow between the muscles of the uterus; and *subserosal* fibroids are formed on the outside of the uterus. Fibroids are extremely common, potentially affecting three-quarters of all women of reproductive age.[1] While fibroids have no known cause, African American women are three to five times more likely to develop them than are women of other racial and ethnic backgrounds.

Common Symptoms of Fibroids

The two main symptoms from which women usually seek relief are heavy bleeding and abdominal pain. Other possible symptoms of fibroids include anemia, a constant urge to urinate, constipation, pelvic pressure (a "full" feeling in the lower abdomen), pain during intercourse, and lower back pain. While many women with fibroids have healthy and uneventful pregnancies, fibroids can contribute to reproductive problems such as early onset of labor, miscarriage, or difficulty conceiving.

Most women with fibroids have no symptoms and remain unaware of the condition until a gynecologist makes an identification during a routine pelvic exam. These women often find that fibroids do not affect their quality of life or physical health in any way. For other women, some of the symptoms of fibroids can significantly reduce their quality of life. These women often need to search for the best solution to their fibroid-related problems. Like many women's health issues, there is no magic bullet for fibroids, and no "one size fits all" treatment.

The Power of Language

Before delving into treatment options, it is worth exploring the intimidating (and often insensitive) language used to describe fibroids. Fibroids are, technically, tumors. But, telling a woman that she has a tumor in her uterus sounds misleadingly alarming, and is unlikely to alleviate her fears—even when a provider emphasizes that the tumor is benign. Instead, women should receive a proper explanation of fibroids, so that they understand what they are beyond just knowing that they are "tumors."

A woman with fibroids may be told that her uterus' size is comparable to that of a pregnant woman's uterus at a certain stage of pregnancy. A fibroid's size is also often compared to different types of fruit, such as plums, oranges, or grapefruits. When a woman hears that her uterus is carrying the weight of a five-month fetus—or contains a grapefruit-sized tumor—her anxiety is bound to increase, causing thoughtful decision-making to become more difficult.

Using different words or ways to describe fibroids will not stop a woman's bleeding or banish her pain, but it can impact the way she feels about the situation, and influence how she addresses fibroid-related symptoms. Most importantly, avoiding unnecessarily frightening terms normalizes the situation. This may help the woman feel more in control of her health care which, in turn, increases the likelihood that she will make the best decision for herself from among her various options.

Watchful Waiting

The first thing many women with fibroids consider is whether they need to take any action at a given time. The term "watchful waiting" describes an approach in which a woman tracks any symptoms and has regular pelvic exams to monitor her fibroids. This approach is ideal for asymptomatic women, as well as for women who can use pain management or other non-medical techniques to manage their symptoms. Women who are approaching menopause may also want to consider watchful waiting, as many fibroids shrink after the menopausal transition. Watchful waiting is an important option that, while not for everyone, should not be overlooked.

Heavy bleeding during menstruation (*menorrhagia*) can be intimidating, but it is fairly common among women with fibroids, and often needs no treatment. Many women who are near menopause experience an increase in blood flow that goes away after a month or two. Women are often able to manage this bleeding on their own without medical intervention. Interestingly, a Scottish study found that women who present with menstrual complaints tend to be diagnosed with menorrhagia or dysfunctional uterine bleeding—even if they did not report their bleeding as problematic. These diagnoses may, in turn, lead to inappropriate treatment, including hysterectomy.[2]

If a woman's menstrual bleeding is unmanageable and does not decrease on its own, however, a health care provider should be consulted to rule out endometrial cancer. For women who feel that their fibroids require medical intervention, there are several options, described below.

Treating Fibroids: Non-Surgical and Surgical Methods

Often, discomfort from fibroids can be eased with pain medications such as aspirin or ibuprofen, or with drugs called GnRH agonists which decrease the body's production of estrogen, often shrinking the fibroids. Some women find that lifestyle changes, such as increasing exercise, discontinuing hormone use, and/or avoiding caffeine and alcohol help fibroid-related symptoms. Commonly, however, fibroids are treated with the following interventions, described in order from the least to the most invasive:

Uterine Artery Embolization

Uterine Artery Embolization (UAE), also sometimes called Uterine Fibroid Embolization, is a relatively new procedure introduced in the U.S. in 1997. UAE is designed to shrink fibroids by cutting off their blood supply. During UAE, a woman is put under conscious sedation and an incision is made in her groin. Using a catheter, small particles of polyvinyl alcohol (a type of plastic) are injected into the uterine arteries which provide blood to the uterus. The particles are then guided by the bloodstream and positioned next to the fibroids, thereby inhibiting the fibroids' blood supply.

This procedure is the least invasive surgical procedure, but is not 100 percent effective, and some fibroid growth is still possible after UAE. While pregnancy after UAE is possible, there is a higher incidence of miscarriage and placenta problems in these pregnancies. For this reason, UAE is not recommended for women who want to preserve their fertility. Due to the lack of long-term data, UAE is not yet considered a standard of care, but interest in the procedure is rapidly growing.

Myomectomy

Myomectomy is a process by which the fibroids are surgically removed in small pieces and the uterus is left in place while the woman is under general anesthesia. It can be performed through a vaginal or abdominal incision, depending on the size and location of the fibroids.

Although the uterus is left intact, some women need additional surgeries to repair the uterine walls after the initial surgery. In addition, 20 percent of women who have had myomectomy find that their fibroids grow back after the surgery.[3] Myomectomy is not performed very frequently in the United States, although it is more common in other countries, such as France. The procedure is recommended for women who want to become pregnant at a later date.

Hysterectomy

Hysterectomy is the surgical removal of the uterus. This procedure is performed while the woman is under general anesthesia, through either a vaginal or abdominal incision. It may or may not include the removal of the cervix, fallopian tubes, or ovaries. Hysterectomy is the

procedure most often mentioned to women after they learn they have fibroids. In reality, however, a hysterectomy is the *last* option a woman should consider. Although hysterectomy is the only sure way to completely remove fibroids, it is major surgery that comes with its own host of risks and considerations, including surgical complications, increased risk of heart attack, changes in sexual desire and function, and depression.

The majority of hysterectomies performed in this country are elective and the National Women's Health Network believes that most hysterectomies are medically unnecessary.[4] Further, fibroids are the leading reason for which women are told they should have a hysterectomy.[5] Women should explore other options before choosing to have a hysterectomy, although they may need to seek several opinions before finding a health care provider who is willing to discuss alternatives to the procedure.

How to Decide

The experiences of women with fibroids vary greatly, and it is really up to each woman to reflect on which of her symptoms needs addressing, and how she wants to do so. It is important to keep in mind that not all fibroids require surgery. Health care providers should be careful not to unnecessarily alarm women about having fibroids. Women, for their part, should feel actively involved in the process of monitoring and treating their fibroids. Once this occurs, much unnecessary over-treatment of fibroids can be avoided.

For more information about fibroids, visit our website at http://www.nwhn.org/content/index.php?pid=134.

REFERENCES

1. National Institute of Child Health and Human Development (NICHD), National Insitutes of Health, Department of Health and Human Services. *Uterine Fibroids.* Washington, DC: NICHD. 2005.

2. Warner, P, Critchley H, Lumsden M, et al. "Referral for Menstrual Problems: Cross Sectional Survey of Symptoms, Reasons for Referral, and Management." *BMJ* 2001; 323:24–28.

3. Skilling, Johanna. *Fibroids: The Complete Guide to Taking Charge of Your Physical, Emotional, and Sexual Well-Being.* New York: Marlow and Company. 2000.

4. Boston Women's Health Book Collective, *Our Bodies, Ourselves.* New York: Touchstone. 2005. p. 637.

5. U.S. Department of Health and Human Services (HHS). "Hysterectomy; Frequently Asked Questions." Washington, DC: HHS, 2006. Posted on the National Women's Health Information Center Website: http://www.4woman .gov/FAQ/hysterectomy.htm; accessed October 6, 2006.

Live and Uncut
"Unnecessary Castration on the Rise"

by Adriane Fugh-Berman

It's bad enough that most hysterectomies are unnecessary, but castrating women at the same time is unconscionable. There are 600,000 hysterectomies performed in the U.S. every year, 90% of which are performed for benign reasons: usually fibroids or endometriosis, which often need no treatment or, if they cause symptoms, can be treated in other ways than through surgery. *Oophorectomy* (removal of the ovaries) is commonly done during hysterectomy even when there is nothing wrong with the ovaries. A study presented in a poster session at the American College of Obstetrician-Gynecologists' 2005 meeting indicated that the practice of removing the ovaries along with the uterus rose from 45% to 64% between 1979 and 2001 for women over the age of 50.[1] For women under 50, the proportion of those castrated nearly doubled in the same period, from 26% to 46%.

Prophylactic oophorectomy, the medical term for removal of perfectly healthy ovaries, is promoted under the guise of improving health. The standard line is that removing the ovaries removes the risk of ovarian cancer. Well, sure, removing the kidneys reduces the chance of kidney cancer, too, but no one's promoting that as good preventive medicine. The cavalier attitude towards ovaries in menopausal women may be partly due to doctors' mistaken belief that ovaries drop dead at menopause, their useless corpses just waiting to develop cancer. In fact, ovaries remain functional after menopause and are a vital source of several hormones, including estrogen and testosterone. Ovaries continue to produce hormones even when women are in their 80s.[2,3,4] And, ovarian cancer is *very* uncommon. The chances that a woman 50–80 years old will die of ovarian cancer in the next five years is less than two tenths of one percent.[5] There is *no* evidence that removing ovaries from healthy women decreases death rates from ovarian cancer or anything else. Oophorectomies should be done to treat ovarian cancer, and are not an unreasonable choice to reduce the risk of ovarian or breast cancer in women at high familial risk for developing these diseases. But, they should *not* be performed in women with an average risk for an uncommon disease.

Just because a specialty is devoted to women doesn't mean that it respects them. In fact, gynecology could be said to have been founded on misogyny. Gynecology arose in the latter half of the 19th century, during a time when women's sexuality was thought to make them mad. Gynecology was founded amidst claims that women were deteriorating, and that doctors could help them. Physicians believed that masturbation, orgasm, the use of contraception, and abortion were all symptoms of mental illness and, starting in the 1860s, surgical treatment of psychiatric disorders became common.

Because women's organs were thought to cause insanity, the obvious cure was to remove them. For example, after the Civil War, removal of the clitoris was popular. (Clitoridectomy was invented in England in 1858 by Isaac Baker-Brown, but British medicine had the sense to censure the procedure; the practice died with the inventor in England, but lived on in the U.S. until the early 20th century). Robert Battey invented the removal of normal ovaries in 1872 as a way to induce menopause and reduce chronic gynecologic conditions. The operation became popular among gynecologists who performed the procedure for, among other indications: 'troublesomeness, eating like a ploughman, masturbation, attempted suicide, erotic tendencies, persecution mania, simple "cussedness", and dysmenorrhea [menstrual cramps].[6] Oophorectomy for psychological reasons flourished until about 1910. Hysterectomies also were performed during this time for psychological reasons.

One can't help wondering whether these surgeries were a backlash to the growing rebellion of women against their restrictive societal roles. The first women's rights convention was held in 1848. Mary Livermore, a

"Live and Uncut: Unnecessary Castration on the Rise," by Adrian Fugh-Berman, M.D., originally published in the *Women's Health Activist*, January/February 2006, p. 11, the newsletter of the National Women's Health Network (NWHN). It is reprinted with the permission of the author and the NWHN.

women's suffrage worker in the late 19th century, denounced the "unclean army of gynecologists who seem desirous to convince women that they possess but one set of organs—and that these are always diseased."[7]

Well, some things have changed and some things haven't. Hysterectomies and oophorectomies aren't done for psychiatric reasons anymore—but most are not performed for medical reasons either. A few oophorectomies are done to treat or prevent ovarian or breast cancer. Most of these procedures, however, are done for no other reason than that the surgeon was in the neighborhood.

REFERENCES

1. Barrows LJ. 'Prophylactic castration at the time of hysterectomy in the United States 1979–2001.' Poster presentation, American College of Obstetrician-Gynecologists, 2005.

2. Davison SL, Bell R, Donath S et al. 'Androgen levels in adult females: changes with age, menopause, and oophorectomy.' *J Clin Endocrinol Metab*. 2005; 90(7):3847–53.

3. Sowers MF, Beebe JL, McConnell D et al. 'Testosterone concentrations in women aged 25–50 years; associations with lifestyle, body composition, and ovarian status.' *Am J Epidemiol*. 2001; 153(3):256–64.

4. Hughes CL Jr, Wall LL, Creasman WT. 'Reproductive hormone levels in gynecologic oncology patients undergoing surgical castration after spontaneous menopause.' *Gynecol Oncol*. 1991;40(1):42–5.

5. SEER data. Quoted in Parker WH, Broder MS, Liu Z et al. 'Ovarian conservation at the time of hysterectomy for benign disease.' *Obstet Gynecol*. 2005;106(2):219–26.

6. Barker-Benfield, quoted in Ehrenreich B and English D. *For Her Own Good: 150 Years of the Experts' Advice to Women*. New York: Anchor Books. 1989. p. 124.

7. *For Her Own Good: 150 Years of the Experts' Advice to Women*. New York: Anchor Books. 1989. p. 115.

"Davida and Goliath"

by Jane Colby

"**H**ow dare they. How *dare* they?!" I stared in disbelief at the most recent issue of the *British Medical Journal* (*BMJ*). Not one, but three articles in the prestigious periodical had publicly trashed my research. The entire medical establishment of England seemed ranged against me.

They were attempting to discredit my five-year project. The one that had studied a third of a million school pupils; a properly peer-reviewed study that had been conducted with a famous microbiologist and published in a reputable U.S. medical journal; research that when I first went public with it, took top spot on the national newspapers and TV news networks.

You don't believe it? Believe it.

Steeling myself, I sat down to flip through the pages of Britain's top medical journal. The articles on us included one by a leading pediatrician alleging research bias, and an end-piece questioning *my* personal integrity and motivation.

"Oh yeah? Right, guys. We'll see about that."

This had to be put right, and now. Sure, I thought about my reputation, but mostly I thought, *If I don't fight back, who will take the kids seriously? Who will help them if I don't?* It'd be a daunting task to take on the medical establishment. *Can I do it?* I wondered. I had to think about it—for all of one minute.

If I could survive the same horrendous illness the children had, including the years of pain and disability, and if I could survive that harrowing two-day media frenzy of last May, when I first released the research results, I sure as hell could sort this.

What was their problem? Didn't they want to know the truth?

Schools Hit by ME Plague, ran the front-page headline of Britain's leading newspaper last spring. With that, the country's top medics were caught with their pants down. That was what hurt. They should have known. They, themselves, should have done the study and fronted the cameras—not me. They didn't take it kindly, hearing it from a writer and one-time school principal. Especially when they had been denying there was any problem at all. Now, smarting, they chose to attack instead of acknowledge the truth about this disabling disease.

You're asking, What is this illness? What was all the fuss about?

I'll tell you what. We'd discovered that ME (Myalgic Encephalomyelitis), also known as Chronic Fatigue Syndrome (CFS), was much more prevalent than previously known. Our research proved that over half the country's kids on long-term sick leave had it. And yes, it is a physical illness, not an emotional one. Brain scans and other tests have proven that. Chronic Fatigue Syndrome? It may have been given a pathetic name, and some outdated doctors may still refuse to recognize it, but ME/CFS is a devastating disease.

I know firsthand.

ME/CFS can be triggered by a number of things. I got it after contracting a viral illness related to polio. Then for twelve years I was in constant pain and bedridden, slowly moving from a wheelchair to a walking aid. I gave up my career as a school principal to concentrate on getting well. As I got stronger, I retrained myself as a journalist and, with a consultant microbiologist, spent half a decade investigating 333,000 schoolchildren. In the end, our study showed ME/CFS was the single biggest cause of long-term sick leave in British schools, bigger than cancer and leukemia combined. No other illness came close. In short, we'd found a cluster pattern, a plague, in our schools. And yes, it exists in the United States, and in South Africa, Europe, Australia, Japan, wherever. Thousands upon thousands of kids have it. Most of them aren't listened to or believed when they say they are too exhausted to move, too brain fogged to think clearly, or in too much body pain to go to school.

But we listened. That was why we did the study. That was why I now couldn't ignore the attacks. No one would take our work seriously if the *BMJ* said it was flawed. So I set out to make them admit it wasn't. I began a campaign to get Goliath, Britain's medical establishment, to acknowledge the health crisis at hand.

First we sent a strongly worded complaint stating they had published incorrect information. We backed up our claim with data proving the accuracy of our research. Then we threatened "further action" if a published correction and apology were not given. I followed up with resolute and persistent phone calls.

It took six months, but finally, once again, I was staring in disbelief at the prestigious *BMJ*. This time it was what I *wanted* to see. My tenacity had paid off: *Journal Was Wrong to Criticize Study in Schoolchildren*, ran their headline.

With that apology, our research was affirmed, thereby helping the country realize the critical role ME/CFS played in our children's health. In addition, I, as co-researcher, was recognized; I was made a member of the UK Chief Medical Officer's Working Group, as well as Children's Officer for a noted national charity. But the icing on the cake came the day the esteemed pediatrician who had originally attacked me in the *BMJ* now publicly introduced me.

"We know," he said, "that ME/CFS is responsible for more long-term sickness absence in schoolchildren than any other disease. One of the authors of the paper is sitting here beside me."

I smiled and got ready to speak.

For additional information on Chronic Fatigue Syndrome, contact:

The CFIDS Association of America
P.O. Box 220398
Charlotte, NC 28222-0398
Toll-free Info Line: (800) 442-3437
Resource Line: (704) 365-2343
Fax: (704) 365-9755
E-mail: info@cfids.org.
Website: www.cfids.org

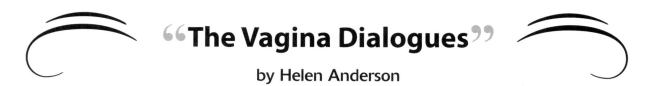

"The Vagina Dialogues"

by Helen Anderson

Our bodies are beautiful. Our bodies are to be celebrated. Having grown up in the 90s as a self-identified feminist, I've heard and repeated all of the current feminist discourse on women's bodies and sexuality. In high school, I volunteered as a safe-sex peer educator for four years. Later, as a graduate student, I was co-director of my university's production of *The Vagina Monologues*, a production whose aim was to encourage women to feel good about having a vagina and to feel good talking about it. There was only one problem. I hated my vagina. I wished it would disappear. And because I hated my vagina, I hated sex.

For as long as I can remember, any kind of sexual penetration has been incredibly painful for me. At 16, during my first visit with a gynecologist, I mentioned to her that sex—other than clitoral stimulation—was really painful. She told me that it was because I was so young and that my body would get used to it. In the meantime, I was advised to just use more lubrication.

Well okay, so this is normal, I thought. I will just have to wait it out. So I waited. And waited. Two years later, I figured I had waited long enough and I went to see another doctor. By this time, sexual relations with my long-term partner had dwindled to nearly nothing and our relationship was beginning to suffer. I began to develop really distorted views about sex. Because sex (specifically intercourse) was so painful for me, it seemed to me that if my partner wanted to have sex, he must want to cause me pain. I began to think that my partner was some kind of sadist.

Another doctor I went to see told me to stop all sexual activity and then slowly reintroduce physical intimacy at a pace I was comfortable with. This approach didn't address the physical pain I was having.

Inevitably, my relationship of four-and-a-half years failed. I began to avoid physical intimacy of any kind; and then I began to avoid my partner completely. I also thought that perhaps the problem was my sexual partner (he was my only sexual partner up to that point).

Shortly after our breakup, I became involved in another relationship. Sex with my new partner was fantastic and I finally felt a connection between my body and my mind that I knew I was supposed to have. When I reached orgasm during intercourse, I cried because I hadn't thought it was possible. For four months we enjoyed an amazing physical relationship. However, this eventually led to a series of urinary tract and yeast infections, which, despite treatment, kept coming back. Then I began to experience the symptoms of infection, even though my test results were negative. I spent almost every moment in class trying to ignore the pain and the urge to urinate frequently.

When I started grad school, the pain and irritation became unbearable. It affected every aspect of my life. I couldn't sit down without experiencing pain and discomfort. I stopped training for the triathlon I had dreamed of finishing, because running, swimming and biking became impossible. I began to gain weight and started to feel poorly about my body. My studies suffered as well, because I couldn't get my mind off of the pain.

But what was I supposed to do? Emailing my profs, "Please excuse Helen from class because her vagina hurts" just wouldn't cut it. Meanwhile, my doctor at school insisted that nothing was physically wrong with me and implied that it was a mental condition. She continued to pump me full of antibiotics to deal with non-existent urinary tract infections. She also gave me a prescription for a heavy painkiller, which didn't help the symptoms, but kept me in a drug-induced stupor while I tried to continue my studies.

After ending up in a hospital emergency room one night begging for relief, I received two pills that were supposed to treat the symptoms of urinary tract infections and I was told to make a doctor's appointment the next day. I told my doctor I couldn't deal with the pain any more and she offered to try to get me an emergency appointment with a urologist. This emergency would involve a two-month wait.

Eventually, I found a urologist in Toronto and made an appointment to have a procedure that would test for interstitial cystitis, an oversensitivity of the bladder. I made the three-hour trip home from school, and the excruciatingly painful test revealed that I did not have interstitial cystitis. The doctor told me I was fine.

I felt so defeated. I wasn't fine, but I felt like there was nothing I could do. I found my way into a gynecologist's office in Toronto. I had seen 13 doctors since the beginning of this journey, and this time someone finally knew what was wrong with me. I had a form of vulvodynia called vestibulitis. Vulvodynia, as explained in *The Vulvodynia Survival Guide* by Howard I. Glazer and Gae Rodke (New Harbinger Publications, 2002), is characterized by "chronic vulvar itching, burning and pain that causes physical, sexual and psychological distress," while vestibulitis is the occurrence of this pain in the vulval vestibule.

I was ecstatic to have a name to describe what was wrong with me and relieved to know it wasn't just in my head. However, my elation faded fast when I discovered that there is no known cause of vestibulitis nor a cure. Some doctors speculate that vestibulitis may be triggered by a yeast or urinary tract infection. Glazer and Rodke speculate that vestibulitis results from chronic inflammation, which can lead to a greater production of nerve fibres and therefore greater sensitivity. Different methods are used to treat symptoms, and the different approaches have varying success rates in each case.

My first treatment was an anti-fungal cream applied to the affected area twice a day. The symptoms got worse. I then tried a prescription used for people with overactive bladders, which didn't help either. A low-dose antidepressant was prescribed to alter the transmission of pain impulses. Still no relief. I tried an anti-yeast diet, which didn't work. I am now trying a low-oxalate diet. Oxalates, according to Glazer and Rodke, are natural by-products secreted in urine which can form crystals that resemble broken glass under a microscope. The crystals may be irritants that can contribute to vulvodynia. Other approaches I have yet to try include acupuncture, anticonvulsants, estrogen therapy and surgery.

Although I haven't found a treatment that can cure my symptoms, I have discovered a few ways to minimize them and to prevent flare-ups. I wear boxer shorts or 100 percent cotton underwear (or no underwear). I wear skirts. I use fragrance-free natural soap and gentle laundry detergent. I wear natural, unbleached menstrual pads or reusable cotton pads. I use glycerine-free lubricant; I always urinate after intercourse as well as wash the genital area (a spray bottle in the bathroom is great for this). I am also shopping for a good sex therapist to help me deal with the emotional symptoms that have resulted from this condition.

The hardest part of dealing with vulvodynia has been the loss of a connection with my body and my mind. I began to hate my body, to see it as a traitor. It just wasn't co-operating with me. I just wanted sex to disappear. I was torn as a feminist. Even within feminist circles, I found it difficult to talk about something being wrong with my vagina. In the words of ani difranco, I felt as though "my cunt is built like a wound that won't heal."

Trying to connect with my body and my sexuality has been difficult, but I am working on it. I have started yoga classes and now work out, which makes me feel stronger and more in tune with my physical being. I eat things that are good for me. I read everything I can find on the subject of vulvodynia.

Although my health problems are yet to be solved, I am doing a good job of resolving the emotional problems that can follow from chronic vaginal pain. I am now confident that I will discover solutions that will allow me to enjoy pain-free living that includes pain-free sexuality.

RESOURCES

National Vulvadynia Association www.nva.org

Vulval Pain Society www.vul-pain.dircon.co.uk

Vulval Pain Foundation www.vulvarpainfoundation.org

The Hassle Free Clinic www.hasslefreeclinic.org/VulvarVestibulitis.html

For Women Only: A Revolutionary Guide to Reclaiming Your Sex Life by Jennifer and Laura Berman (Henry Holt and Co., 2001)

The Vulvodynia Survival Guide: How to Overcome Painful Vaginal Symptoms and Enjoy an Active Lifestyle, by Howard I. Glazer and Gae Rodke (New Harbinger. 2002)

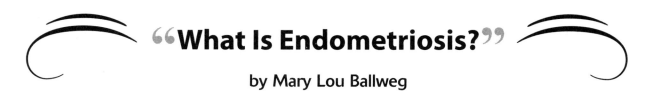

"What Is Endometriosis?"

by Mary Lou Ballweg

Endometriosis is a puzzling hormonal and immune disease affecting girls and women from as young as eight to post menopause. The name comes from the word endometrium, which is the tissue that lines the inside of the uterus and builds up and sheds each month in the menstrual cycle. In "endo," as this disease is called for short, tissue like the endometrium is found outside the uterus in other areas of the body. In these locations outside the uterus, the endometrial tissue develops into what are called "nodules," "tumors," "lesions," "implants," or "growths." These growths can cause pain, infertility, and other problems.

The most common locations of endometrial growths are in the abdomen—involving the ovaries, fallopian tubes, ligaments supporting the uterus, area between the vagina and the rectum, outer surface of the uterus, and lining of the pelvic cavity. Sometimes the growths are also found in abdominal surgery scars, on the intestines, in the rectum, or on the bladder, vagina, cervix, and vulva (external genitals). Endometrial growths have also been found outside the abdomen, but these are uncommon.

It is possible, though relatively rare, for endo lesions to become cancerous. In addition, recent research has indicated women and girls with endo and their families are at greater risk for cancer, particularly ovarian and breast cancer, as well as melanoma, non-Hodgkin's lymphoma, brain, and thyroid cancers. They and their families are also at risk for certain autoimmune diseases, such as multiple sclerosis and rheumatoid arthritis, in which the immune system attacks the body's own tissues. Because of these risks and the life-disrupting nature of endo in many cases, women and girls are encouraged not to ignore symptoms.

Like the lining of the uterus, endometrial growths usually respond to the hormones of the menstrual cycle. They build up tissue each month and break down. The result is internal bleeding, degeneration of the blood and tissue shed from the growths, inflammation of the sur-

rounding areas, and formation of scar tissue (adhesions). Other complications can be rupture of cysts (which can spread endo to new areas), intestinal bleeding or obstruction (if the growths are in or near the intestines), interference with bladder function (if the growths are on or in the bladder), and other problems. Symptoms seem to worsen with time, though cycles of remission and recurrence are the pattern in some cases.

Symptoms

The most common symptoms of endo are pain before and during periods (usually worse than "normal" menstrual cramps), pain during or after sexual activity, fatigue, infertility, and heavy bleeding. Other symptoms may include painful bowel movements with periods, lower back pain with periods, and diarrhea and/or constipation and other intestinal upset with periods. Many women with endo also experience a range of immune disorders, including allergies, asthma, eczema, and certain autoimmune diseases. Infertility affects about 30-40% of women with endo and is a common result with progression of the disease.

The amount of pain is not necessarily related to the extent or size of the growths. Tiny growths (called "petechial") have been found to be more active in producing prostaglandins, which may explain the significant symptoms that often seem to occur with small implants. Prostaglandins are substances produced throughout the body, involved in numerous functions, and thought to cause many of the symptoms of endo.

Theories About the Cause of Endometriosis

The cause of endo is not known with certainty, but a number of theories have been advanced. One theory is the retrograde menstruation or transtubal migration theory. According to this theory, during menstruation some of the menstrual tissue backs up through the fallopian tubes, implants in the abdomen, and grows. Research

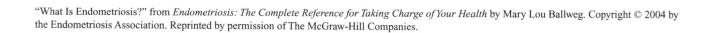

shows most, if not all, women experience some menstrual tissue backup, so experts believe that an immune system problem and/or hormonal problem allows this tissue to take root and grow in women who develop endo. Another theory suggests that the endometrial tissue is distributed from the uterus to other parts of the body through the lymph or blood. A genetic theory suggests that certain families may have predisposing factors for the disease. Research spearheaded by the Association since 1992 has shown that environmental toxins such as dioxin and PCBs, which act like hormones in the body and damage the immune system, can cause endometriosis.

Another theory suggests that remnants of tissue from when the woman was an embryo may later develop into endo or that some adult tissues retain the ability they had in the embryo stage to transform into reproductive tissue under certain circumstances. Surgical transplantation has also been cited as a cause in cases where endo is found in abdominal surgery scars. However, endo has also been found in such scars when direct accidental implantation seems unlikely.

Diagnosis

Diagnosis of endo is generally considered uncertain until proven by laparoscopy. Laparoscopy is a surgical procedure done under anesthesia. The patient's abdomen is distended with carbon dioxide gas to make the organs easier to see, and a laparoscope (a tube with a light in it) is inserted into a tiny incision in the abdomen. By moving the laparoscope around the abdomen, the surgeon can check the condition of the abdominal organs and see the endometrial implants, if the surgeon is careful and thorough.

A doctor can sometimes feel endometrial implants during a pelvic examination, and symptoms will often indicate endo, but it is not good practice to treat this disease without confirmation of the diagnosis. (Ovarian cancer, for instance, sometimes has the same symptoms.) A laparoscopy also indicates the locations, extent, and size of the growths and may help the doctor and patient make better-informed long-range decisions about treatment and pregnancy.

Treatment

Treatment for endo has varied over the years, but no sure cure has yet been found. Hysterectomy and removal of the ovaries has been considered a "definitive" cure, but research by the Association and others has found such a high rate of continuation/recurrence that women need to be aware of steps they can take to protect themselves.

(Please see The Endometriosis Sourcebook and the chapter on menopause and endo in Endometriosis: The Complete Reference for Taking Charge of Your Health for more information.) Painkillers are usually prescribed for the pain of endo. Treatment with hormones aims to stop ovulation for as long as possible and can sometimes force the disease into remission during the time of treatment and sometimes for months or years afterward. Hormonal treatments include oral contraceptives, progesterone drugs, a testosterone derivative (danazol), and GnRH drugs (gonadotropin-releasing hormone drugs). New drugs are being tested. With all hormonal treatments, side effects are a problem for some women.

Because pregnancy often causes a temporary remission of symptoms and because it is believed that infertility is more likely the longer the disease is present, women with endo are often advised not to postpone pregnancy. However, there are numerous problems with the "prescription" of pregnancy to treat endo. The woman might not yet have made a decision about childbearing, certainly one of the most important decisions in life. She might not have critical elements in place to allow for childbearing and child rearing (partner, financial means, etc.). She may already be infertile.

Other factors may also make the pregnancy decision and experience harder. Women with endo may have higher rates of tubal pregnancy and miscarriage, and one study has found they have more difficult pregnancies and labors. Research also shows there are family links in endo, increasing the risk of endometriosis and related health problems in the children of women with the disease.

Conservative surgery, either major or through the laparoscope, involving removal or destruction of the growths, is also done and can relieve symptoms and allow pregnancy to occur in some cases. As with other treatments, however, recurrences are common. Surgery through the laparoscope (called operative laparoscopy) has rapidly replaced major open abdominal surgery. In operative laparoscopy, surgery is carried out through the laparoscope using laser, electrosurgical equipment, or small surgical instruments. Radical surgery, involving hysterectomy (removal of the uterus) and removal of all growths and the ovaries (to prevent further hormonal stimulation), may become necessary in cases of long-standing, troublesome disease.

Menopause also is believed to end the activity of mild or moderate endo, although little research has been done in postmenopausal women. Even after radical surgery or menopause, however, a severe case can be reactivated by estrogen replacement therapy or continued hormone production. Some authorities suggest no estrogen be given for a short time after hysterectomy and removal of the ovaries for endo.

Many complementary treatments, including nutritional approaches, immunotherapy, traditional Chinese medicine, allergy management techniques, and others, are being used by women with endo. A survey of 4,000 women with endo found some of these treatments to be the most successful of all the treatments they had tried. See our books for more information.

Learning About Endometriosis

Endo is without question one of the most puzzling diseases affecting women and girls. More is being learned about it as time goes on, and this knowledge is dispelling some of the assumptions of the past. One of these past assumptions was that nonwhite women did not generally get endo. This has now been shown to be untrue. Often nonwhite women were not getting the kind of medical care to have endo diagnosed.

Another myth about endo is that very young women do not get it—an idea that probably arose because formerly teenagers and younger women endured menstrual pain (often one of the early symptoms) in silence and did not get diagnosed until the disease progressed to unbearable proportions. It was also believed in the past that endo more often affected well-educated women. Now we know that this notion developed because well-educated women were those getting better medical care and were more often persistent enough to obtain explanations for their symptoms.

Another assumption sometimes made about endo is that it is not a serious disease because it is not a killer like cancer, for instance. However, anyone who has talked with many women with endo about their actual experiences with the disease soon learns otherwise. While some women's lives are relatively unaffected by it, too many others have suffered severe pain, emotional stress, have at times been unable to work or carry on normal activities, and have experienced financial and relationship problems because of the disease. Perhaps someday soon we will understand this perplexing disease and end all the myths, pain, and frustration that go with it!

How the Endometriosis Association Can Help

The Endometriosis Association is a self-help organization of women and families with endo, doctors and scientists, and others interested in exchanging information about the disease, offering mutual support and help to those affected by endo, educating the public and medical community about the disease, and promoting research related to endo. Those affected by the disease help each

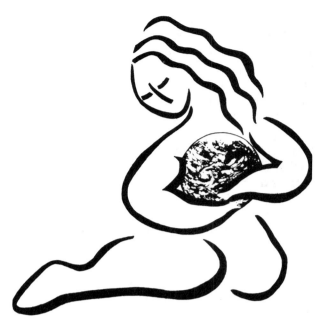

From *Building Parnerships That Work: Grassroots, Science, and Social Change, The Endometriosis Association Story.* Reprinted by permission from Endometriosis Association, Inc., international headquarters, Milwaukee, Wisconsin.

other by ending the feeling of being alone, sharing with others who understand what one is going through, counteracting the lack of information and the misinformation about endo, and learning from each other.

The Association is an international organization with headquarters in Milwaukee, Wisconsin (USA), members in numerous countries, and chapters and activities worldwide. Elected officers guide the Association, with help and suggestions from an advisory board of medical professionals and others. The Association, founded in Milwaukee in 1980 by Mary Lou Ballweg and Carolyn Keith, was the first group in the world dedicated to helping women with endo.

The Support Program provides a wide range of services to help girls, women, and their families. These services include support groups, counseling/crisis call help, assistance finding knowledgeable doctors, a prescription drug savings plan, networking, and other help. At the local group level, meetings and activities are planned according to each group's wishes. Usually some meetings are planned to allow informal sharing of information and support. Other meetings offer speakers and presentations on various aspects of the disease. Group activities also may include fund-raising and outreach into the community to teach about endo.

The Education Program provides a wide range of literature, books, CDs, DVDs, and other educational items to help individuals and the public learn about the disease. Members of the Association receive a popular newsletter covering the latest treatment and research news, as well as Association activities. The Association also provides ongoing help to the media and medical community to aid in the dissemination of accurate information about endometriosis.

The Association's Research/Translational Medicine Program includes maintaining the world's largest database on the disease, major research partnerships with Vanderbilt University School of Medicine, and the U.S. National Institutes of Health, and funding of promising research worldwide. The Association also serves as a clearinghouse for information on the disease and conducts programs to alert healthcare providers about the latest research and clinical findings on endo.

Mary Lou Ballweg is president and executive director of the Endometriosis Association, an organization she cofounded in 1980. Besides founding and leading the Association, she has overseen the publication of the Association's three books and its educational videotapes, an extensive body of literature on the disease, and the development of two million-dollar-plus educational awareness campaigns, four public-service announcement campaigns, and many other outreach efforts. She is editor of the Association's bimonthly newsletter and has produced numerous articles and chapters for journals, magazines, newsletters, and medical textbooks.

Together with Karen Lamb, Ph.D., she established the world's first research registry for endo. She was responsible for a major breakthroughh in research linking dioxin to endo, helped develop groundbreaking work on cancer and endo, and has collaborated with the National Institutes of Health on research on autoimmune diseases and endo. She was instrumental in estabishing Association research programs at Dartmouth Medical School and Vanderbilt University of Medicine.

Prior to founding the Endometriosis Association, Ballweg was a communications consultant with her own national business producing film and audiovisual materials and training programs on affirmative action and race/cultural/gender understanding in the corporate and social environments. Earlier she was a scriptwriter-director at a film and public relations company and managing editor of a monthly magazine. She was also one of the founders of a women's community health clinic and has been recognized in numerous Who's Who listings, including *Who's Who in the World*, *International Who's Who in Medicine*, and *The World Who's Who of Women*.

Endometriosis Association
8585 N. 76th Place, Milwaukee, WI 53223
www.EndometriosisAssn.org

"Why Endometriosis Is an Environmental Issue"

by Lynn Castrodale

The following information applies to you whether you are female or male, a construction worker, a homemaker, a factory worker, an accountant, a lawyer, a nurse, a librarian, a scientist, or a pastor. It applies to moms, dads, grandmothers, teenagers, students, and retirees. It applies to people on all continents, even people in the Arctic regions. If you live on Planet Earth,

you may want to know the following because it affects your life and is worthy of your attention.

There is a struggle going on—a struggle between sustainability and the degradation of our environment. Toxic chemicals are building up in our bodies and the environment. These chemicals are causing terrible harm and disease. The good news is that we have the choice to fight for sustainability and against persistent toxic chemicals in order to protect ourselves and future generations.

The purpose of this chapter is to describe the "big picture" of health risks from toxic chemicals in the environment. Scientific research has established the link between endometriosis and environmental toxins. This article will explain how our health and the environment are inseparable, how persistent toxic chemicals are related to endo and other diseases, and how to empower yourself to take action.

The Real Definition of Environment

The spirit of the old saying "You are what you eat" should no longer be restricted to food. Perhaps the more contemporary way to state it is, "You are the environment, and the environment is you." The word *environment* does not just mean the forests, lakes, and oceans; it includes our cities, our backyards, our homes, and our bodies. From the air we breathe to the clothes we wear and the furniture we sit on—all are part of the environment.

Our bodies reflect the state of the environment around us. Our health and the health of our world are intertwined. When the planet and its environment are diseased with toxic chemicals, our individual bodies become diseased and sick. When we eat contaminated food or live in a toxic building, we are polluting our most important environment, ourselves. We require clean air, water, and food to keep ourselves and our families healthy.

J. P. Myers, Ph.D., coauthor of *Our Stolen Future*, a powerful book about endocrine-disrupting chemicals, made the following statement in a presentation to the United Nations Commission on the Status of Women: "Throughout human evolution we have always had a refuge from our mistakes. Early on, if we depleted the game in one valley we moved to the next. As we polluted one river course, there was always another . . . and if the pollution wiped out one clan or one township, well, in the grand scheme of things, there were always other people somewhere else. No pollutants affected everyone. This is now changed irrevocably and fundamentally. There is no next valley waiting to be filled. There is no watershed completely lacking of pollutants. None."

The waste that we produce today will be in tomorrow's water, air, and soil. Toxic chemicals that are created in factories and incinerators end up in our food and drinking water. Toxins that we unknowingly breathe or ingest must be processed by our bodies and can overload our systems. No one is immune to our toxic environment, and our immune systems pay dearly.

It is worth mentioning that many people have the notion that "environmentalists" are confrontational extremists who hug trees. But if you care about your home and the town you live in, you could be considered an envi-

ronmentalist. Planting a garden, trimming dead branches off a tree, recycling aluminum cans, giving your old clothes to the Salvation Army—these are all examples of caring about the world you live in. If you care about yourself and your surroundings, then it is important to take positive actions to protect and nurture them. If we acknowledge that we all play a part in caring for our health and our environment, then we can each accept the awesome responsibility of protecting our health and planet from threats like toxic chemicals.

Our Bodies Are Absorbing Harmful Chemicals

Of the thousands of manufactured chemicals in our world (experts estimate there are over 88,000), very few have been tested for health effects on adults, even fewer for health effects on children. Every baby born on the planet today has "persistent toxic chemicals" in his or her body. One thing that makes these chemicals so dangerous to human health is that they accumulate in our bodies (starting before birth and continuing throughout life) and resist breakdown. These persistent toxic chemicals are among the most threatening to human life and our natural environment.

Using state-of-the-art blood testing, researchers find that all of us, no matter where or how we live, have a minimum of 200 detectable manufactured chemicals in our blood.[1] And although some are worse for our health than others, we really do not know how these chemicals will affect us today or twenty years from now. We do not know which ones interact with each other to cause potentially larger effects than they do individually. Human beings, at present, lack the scientific ability and resources to test them together to uncover their synergistic chemical reactions. Yet these chemicals continue to intermingle in our bodies.

This is especially frightening for the parents of children of this era, as exposures to toxic chemicals can affect a child's development. "A growing body of evidence is raising concerns that exposure to toxic chemicals may harm children and developing babies far more than adults," according to Bill Moyers's report "Trade Secrets" on PBS.[2] Infants and children breathe more rapidly and inhale more pollutants per pound of body weight than do adults. They also eat more food and drink more water, milk, and juice per unit of body weight than most adults.[3] Until recently, safety testing and regulation of environmental substances has not been taking this difference into account. The U.S. Environmental Protection Agency (EPA) first began taking children's biological differences into account in 1996. Before then, it was assumed that children were just miniature adults, an assumption that is scientifically invalid.[4]

How the Environment Fits into the Endometriosis Puzzle

It has been established that endo is a disease related to environmental toxins. In fact, it is one of the first diseases (outside of cancers) to be linked to persistent organic pollutants like dioxin in humans. Since 1992, research findings have been showing that dioxins and polychlorinated biphenyls (PCBs) can cause the development of endo. This has shifted the previous perception of endo from an unexplained gyn disease to a disease that is most likely triggered or worsened by the environment in which we live. In addition, it may be possible that endo is just one part of a larger disease family resulting from exposure to these chemicals.

Scientific evidence implicates dioxins, PCBs, and many other chemicals in disrupting the immune and endocrine (hormonal) systems. We already know that endo is a disease of the immune and endocrine systems. Now an important study shows that the prevalence of other hormonal or immune disorders is higher in women with endo than in the general female population. These diseases include hypothyroidism, fibromyalgia, chronic fatigue immune dysfunction syndrome (CFIDS), rheumatoid arthritis, lupus, Sjögren's syndrome, and multiple sclerosis.[5]

Moving beyond endo to view the big picture of diseases plaguing our society today, it is important to know that dioxin and other environmental toxins have also been linked to childhood cancers (at least preliminarily), attention deficit disorder, reproductive cancers, Parkinson's disease, chronic fatigue immune dysfunction syndrome (CFIDS), diabetes, and asthma. As we watch scientific evidence link more and more diseases to environmental toxins, we have to ask ourselves if this is why health issues are escalating out of control in our society. It is too early to know for sure which diseases are linked to which toxins or how the diseases themselves are related, but it is never too early to educate ourselves on the key toxins.

Dioxins and PCBs

Dioxins are a class of seventy-five chemicals with similar properties that are known to be the most toxic chemicals ever produced. Dioxins are the by-products of industrial processes that involve chlorine or the burning or incineration of chlorinated material with organic matter. The most toxic form of dioxin is 2,3,7,8-tetrachlorodibenzo-p-dioxin (TCDD), a known carcinogen. This was the type of dioxin fed to rhesus monkeys in the groundbreaking study that first linked dioxin to endo. Monkeys that ingested TCDD in amounts as small as five parts per trillion developed the disease.[6]

According to the U.S. EPA, the average American adult has enough dioxin in his or her body today to cause adverse health effects. Some have even more. For example, people living near a vinyl plant in Louisiana were found to have an average combined dioxin level of 68 parts per trillion. Four people tested showed levels of 150 parts per trillion, and several girls in the area developed endo as teenagers.[7]

The top three sources of dioxin are municipal waste incineration, backyard burn barrels (individuals burning their trash in their yards), and medical waste incineration.[8] Other sources include chemical and vinyl (PVC, or polyvinyl chloride plastic) manufacturing, metal smelting, and pulp and paper bleaching. Dioxin emissions from smokestacks and discharge pipes travel long distances in the atmosphere via air currents. After the dioxin falls to the ground, it is often consumed by livestock that graze on the dioxin-contaminated crops or soil. Dioxin is fat soluble and accumulates in the tissues of the animals. The higher an animal is on the food chain, the more dioxin it will accumulate. Therefore, animal products that we eat, such as beef, dairy, chicken, pork, fish, and eggs, are regularly contaminated with dioxin. The EPA estimates that over 95 percent of human exposure to dioxin is through our food. People who live near incinerators or manufacturing plants, such as the vinyl plant in Louisiana mentioned previously, are unfortunately exposed to additional dioxin through air, soil, and possibly water.

Certain types of PCBs behave similarly to dioxin in the environment and our bodies. PCBs are a group of nonflammable chemicals that were used as insulation and/or coolants in electrical transformers, as well as lubricants, hydraulic fluids, cutting oils, liquid seals, and in carbonless paper. In the United States, they were widely used between 1929 and 1977. Because PCBs are incredibly persistent chemicals, it can take 20 to 160 years for them to completely break down. Unfortunately, companies that manufactured PCBs for industrial use dumped millions of pounds of these toxins directly into rivers and lakes before the U.S. government banned them. They are now found in the body fat of almost every living creature on our planet and are especially concentrated in fish from polluted waterways.

Endocrine-Disrupting Chemicals

Certain types of dioxins and PCBs, in addition to many other types of chemicals, are known to be endocrine disruptors. The endocrine system is a complex system of glands (such as the thyroid, pituitary gland, and ovaries) and hormones that regulate activities such as reproduction in human beings and animals. Hormones are biochemical messengers secreted by endocrine glands into

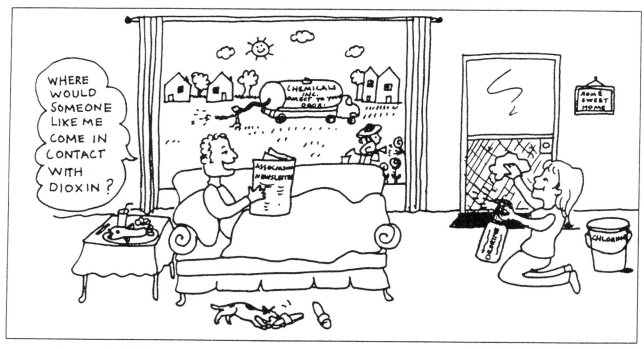

Cartoon reprinted with permission from *Endometriosis: The Complete Reference for Taking Charge of Your Health*, New York: McGraw-Hill, 2003.

the bloodstream to control and direct the function of specific organs. Nearly all animals, including mammals, fish, amphibians, reptiles, birds, and invertebrates, have endocrine systems.

"Endocrine disruptors" are substances that mimic hormones, fooling the body into overresponding, responding at inappropriate times, or blocking the effects of a natural hormone. Endocrine disruptors "may directly stimulate or inhibit the endocrine system, causing overproduction or underproduction" of the body's hormones.[9] They can mimic estrogen, block progesterone, or affect testosterone levels. Many chemicals are known endocrine disruptors, and more are being discovered every year. Many of them are in pesticides, detergents, cosmetics, and the plastics used to package food. Through the air we breathe, the water and food we consume, and the substances that touch our skin, our bodies are regularly exposed to endocrine-disrupting chemicals.

Endocrine disruptors can have negative effects on the female reproductive system, including increased risk of breast cancer, early puberty, altered menstruation, decreased fertility, increased miscarriages, and early menopause.[10] For males, it has been found that exposure in the womb to a compound present in common plastics causes abnormality in the adult male prostate.[11] A group of common chemicals called phthalates can "damage the developing testes [testicles] of animal offspring and cause malformations of the penis and other parts of the reproductive tract."[12]

Endocrine disruptors and other persistent chemicals do not necessarily cause health effects overnight. There is often a long time lag between exposure and the health problem, which adds to our confusion about cause and effect. Exposure in the womb may not manifest in health problems until the child becomes an adult.

Toxicity of a chemical may not be scientifically proven until years after it is spread throughout the environment (and our bodies). Take the scientific history of lead poisoning, for example. In 1975 it was considered harmless for a tenth of a liter of human blood to contain thirty-nine micrograms of lead. Today we know that thirty-nine micrograms can cause severe brain damage in children. Many scientists believe that *any* amount of lead can damage the central nervous system and reduce IQ. However, the lead industry still hires scientists to dispute these conclusions.[13] Fortunately, society has been made aware of the danger of lead exposure. This is not yet the case for dioxin and many endocrine-disrupting chemicals.

Protecting Health or Profits?

While people generally have had faith in governments and corporations to protect us from harm and injustice, today it is clear these institutions are not living up to that expectation. One example close to the hearts of women with endo, given the link between dioxin and endo, is the EPA's report on the sources and health effects of dioxin commonly referred to as the Dioxin Reassess-

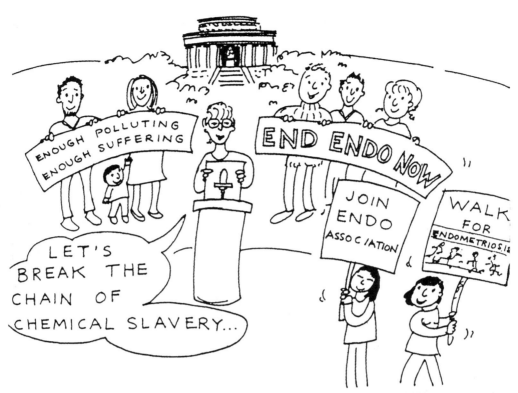

Cartoon reprinted with permission from *Endometriosis: The Complete Reference for Taking Charge of Your Health*, New York: McGraw-Hill, 2003.

ment. The following history shows how long people have been waiting for the U.S. government to complete a key report meant to protect human health.

In 1977 animal studies first indicated that dioxin causes cancer. In 1985 the U.S. EPA published the first Dioxin Risk Assessment, which was a scientific review of the health effects of dioxin. This assessment prompted the establishment of an "acceptable" daily dose of dioxin of 0.006 picogram (a picogram is one trillionth of a gram) per kilogram of body weight per day. (The assumption regarding "acceptable daily doses" is that small amounts of chemicals are safe as long as they do not exceed a certain daily amount. The same dose is set for all people, regardless of whether they are sick or healthy, young or old.)

In the late 1980s, dioxin-producing industries claimed that the established daily dose was too low and that higher levels, like those set in some other countries at that time, were more appropriate. These industries requested that the EPA do a reassessment of the 1985 Dioxin Risk Assessment, expecting an increase in the acceptable dose. By 1990 the chlorine industry had succeeded in persuading the EPA to undertake a formal reassessment of dioxin, and in 1994 the EPA released the first Draft Reassessment. This document revealed that our environment is full of dioxin, dioxin has accumu-

lated in our bodies, and any additional exposure is too much. Findings included the following:

- The data strengthen the conclusion that dioxin causes cancer in people. The EPA found that dioxin is the most important cancer-causing chemical for the general population and that the average adult has a risk factor of 1 in 100 of getting cancer from dioxin exposure. EPA's "acceptable" risk level for cancer is 1 in 1 million.

- Noncancer health problems may have even more impact on public health than the cancer-causing effects of dioxin because they are passed down from generation to generation. (In addition to being carcinogenic, there is evidence of dioxin's immunotoxicity, developmental toxicity, reproductive toxicity, and endocrine disruption.) Endometriosis is just one example of a noncancer health problem.

- Suppression of the immune system and other health effects of dioxin were found to occur "at or near levels to which people in the general population are exposed."[14]

Realizing that the eventual release of the final Dioxin Reassessment would eliminate any doubt about the danger of dioxin and may precipitate federal regulations to reduce dioxin production and exposure, the dioxin-producing industries have campaigned to stop the final report from being issued. They have succeeded in blocking its release for over seven years. (At the time of this writing, the final report has still not been issued.) Meanwhile, the evidence regarding the serious health problems associated with dioxin exposure continues to accumulate, while the U.S. government still has not taken action to protect the public's health.[15]

Currently, the profits of industry and a "business as usual" attitude appear to come before the health of living beings. Just like the tobacco industry, chemical industries are paying experts to downplay the toxicity of chemicals and confuse the issues. Vinyl, or polyvinyl chloride (PVC) plastic, is known to create dioxin throughout its life cycle—during the manufacturing process and when burned or incinerated. In addition, many more toxic chemicals, including lead, cadmium, and phthalates, are added to raw PVC to stabilize or plasticize it for use in a wide range of consumer products.[16, 17] According to a comprehensive public television documentary by highly regarded journalist Bill Moyers, the industry has been aware of many toxic health effects from vinyl production but has worked to keep them secret from the public and government agencies.[18, 19]

Precautionary Principle

While powerful corporations and others with vested interests spend money to defend their harmful chemicals and shroud the emerging science in a veil of uncertainty, we are all taking part in uncontrolled scientific experiments that risk our fundamental rights to healthy lives. The current system of regulating chemicals forces the public to "prove harm" *after* the chemicals are on the market and in the environment. By the time scientists are able to prove harm, it is too late—harm has already occurred in those exposed. Once released into the environment, damaging chemicals are impossible to recall.

The current reactive, rather than proactive, system of monitoring chemical health effects has several inadequacies:[20]

- Millions of people have to become sick before regulators can begin to prove harm.

- The current system fails to take into account the cumulative effects of thousands of small, supposedly safe exposures to that chemical.

- There is no way to account for the fact that all living creatures are subject to *multiple* exposures of many different environmental contaminants.

- The "prove harm" regulatory system bases its determinations on what current science alone can prove—often industry-sponsored science—omitting many essential human values such as personal philosophies, religion, and other values (such as not feeding babies contaminated milk or formula). Currently, the right to pollute outweighs the right to be born without toxins in your body.

Taking proactive, precautionary actions when developing potentially toxic chemicals is one solution to this problem. The 1998 Wingspread Statement on the Precautionary Principle was drawn up by top scientists and experts in this field, who discussed their concerns and defined the Precautionary Principle. Key components of the principle include "upholding the basic right of each individual and future generations to a healthy, life-sustaining environment" and "placing responsibility on originators of potentially dangerous activities to thoroughly study and minimize risks." When there is credible evidence that a substance will cause harm to public health or the environment, policy changes should be made, even if the magnitude of the harm in not fully proven.[21]

This brings us to the discussion of "environmental justice" and how it relates to endometriosis. Just as the past and present neglect toward women in diagnosing and treating endo is sometimes a result of inequality issues between women and men in our society, environmental injustice springs from inequality among races, socioeconomic groups, and developing and developed nations. Waste incinerators are often strategically placed in poorer communities, pesticides that are banned in the United States are exported to developing countries, and "company towns" housing toxic industries exploit and poison the workers and their families who are too poor or dependent on the jobs to move away. Their rights are ignored in the name of profit, "progress," and economic growth.

Historically, the environmental justice movement has been made up of many important groups, especially human rights leaders, community-based activists, and labor unions. Peter Montague, editor of *Rachel's Environmental and Health Weekly News*, believes that there is a new, powerful group of "people whose health has been affected by multiple chemical sensitivities, birth defects, breast cancer, endometriosis, lymphoma, diabetes, chronic fatigue, veterans affected by Agent Orange and Gulf War Syndrome, and many others"[22] now becoming part of the environmental justice movement.

Things You Can Do Every Day to Help Yourself and the Environment

- You can improve the environment and your health through your purchasing practices. Everyday items such as detergent, toilet paper, and toothbrushes with "greener" ingredients or materials are available. Support companies that make environmentally safe and healthy products by buying their products. Find these products at ecomall.com and other websites, as well as at your local natural or health food stores.
- Certain plastics (especially PVC) can leach toxic chemicals into food. Be especially careful to avoid letting plastic wrap touch food, and do not cook in plastic containers. Glass, ceramic, and stainless steel are preferable materials in most cases.
- Choose cosmetics, shampoos, and personal care products without harsh chemicals and phthalates. For more information on phthalates in cosmetics, visit nottoopretty.com.
- Request the use of PVC-free products for medical procedures involving IV bags, including laparoscopies. See noharm.org or aaa.dk/pvc for information on alternatives to PVC medical devices.
- Avoid chlorine and chlorine-based products (such as PVC plastic) because they can create and possibly contain dioxin. Replace chlorine-bleached materials such as paper, tampons, and coffee filters with unbleached or non-chlorine-bleached alternatives.
- Contact manufacturers to ask what materials are used in their products. Tell them they should disclose materials and ingredients on the package. If it is made with PVC (polyvinyl chloride plastic, or vinyl, marked with the number 3 inside the recycle symbol), ask for PVC-free alternatives. See greenpeaceusa.org for more information.
- Dioxin and many persistent toxins build up in meats and other animal products, particularly in the fatty portions. To minimize PCB and dioxin consumption, eat lowfat meats and dairy products, preferably certified organic ones. Cut nonorganic meats and dairy products out of your diet whenever possible (or altogether).
- Fish are the main sources of PCBs in food, especially fish caught in contaminated lakes or rivers. Avoid eating contaminated fish and game (such as ducks). Call your local health department to find out about any fishing advisories, and obey them. Remember to peel vegetables and fruit, because PCBs and pesticides concentrate in the lipid, or fatty, layer of their skins.
- Avoid pesticides and herbicides, indoors and out, because they are toxic to adults, children, and pets. Try organic pest control, integrated pest management, and home remedies (for example, jalapeño pepper bug spray to repel ants). For more information, see beyondpesticides.org or panna.org.
- If you like to garden, consider growing your own organic food.
- Recycling is an important way of improving our environment. Plastics marked with numbers 1 (PETE) and 2 (HDPE) are the most commonly recycled. PVC (numbered 3) is not recycled, even if they pick it up at your curb, and can contaminate batches of other plastics. This is another good reason to avoid PVC. Plastics marked 6 (PS) and 7 are often not recyclable, either.
- Avoid plastics that leach suspected endocrine disruptors. These include plastics numbered 3 (PVC), 6 (PS), and 7 (PC or "other").
- Avoid using electrical devices and appliances, including old fluorescent lighting fixtures, TVs, and refrigerators, that were made before 1979. These items may leak small amounts of PCBs into the air when they get hot during operation.
- PCBs can be rapidly absorbed through the skin. Do not disturb or handle dirt near hazardous waste sites or in areas where there was a transformer fire. Prevent or limit skin contact with the shore soil and water in contaminated areas.
- For gifts and holidays, consider buying environmentally friendly products and services for your family members and friends.
- Raise your children, nieces and nephews, and/or grandchildren to respect the environment and other people. Many educational books and videos deal with the subject of the environment. Your actions are usually the best teacher. For more information on children's environmental health, visit iceh.org and partnersforchildren.org.
- Be aware that some product marketers are trying to "greenwash" the public by using slogans such as "all natural." Reading labels and ingredient lists is more trustworthy than reading just the marketing slogans. (Be aware that some products have undisclosed chemical ingredients.)

Creating Change and Healing

Future generations depend on those living today to leave them with a safe and healthy environment. How do we, as people whose health has been compromised by environmental toxins, create change for ourselves and for future generations? The key is to become empowered advocates for our health and the health of others. Women and girls with endo can empower themselves and go from being victims to being part of the solution.

Victims don't heal anything, just as caterpillars don't fly. The caterpillar must go through a process of transformation before it emerges as a weightless butterfly. For a woman with a disease who feels incapable or insignificant, becoming empowered can truly be a metamorphosis. A period of fear, anger, and feelings of being overwhelmed may be a necessary stage of this transformation, much like the cocoon stage for the caterpillar. Emerging from the cocoon as an advocate for yourself and the environment, you can help your situation (and that of many others) immensely.

If you are learning to be assertive with your healthcare providers—partnering with them instead of expecting them to "fix" you, for example—then you are halfway there. You may no longer accept the inequalities of our current world, and you fight for your rights, whether they are women's rights, minority rights, healthcare rights, or something else. Take the same approach to the environment, and watch the empowered person you have become accomplish substantial and significant change. Remember, every small action that you take to help the environment counts.

If the human mind can produce new technology that is dangerous and destructive, it can also use its ingenuity to create technology, products, and inventions that are safe and empowering. Use your own creative talents, whether as architect, investor, consumer, scientist, cook, parent, or nurse to create healthy, environmentally friendly contributions to our world. Using your creativity toward this goal will help heal the planet, not to mention your own health.

The most important victory we can influence with our actions is a "climate of opinion" change. This battle is not fought in the complicated political and regulatory arena only. "Climate of opinion" is a concept illustrating that social acceptability of inequalities can change.[23] At one time in history (only one hundred years ago), it was understood and accepted that women were not allowed to vote. The suffrage movement succeeded in securing this right for women. Today, our society would not consider going back in time and revoking a woman's right to vote. It is unthinkable. The civil rights movement is another example. We will not go backward and segregate the races again—that would be absurd.

ALIVE/TO TESTIFY
Wanna Wright

I's got to reach out to keep 'em alive
din you can teach 'em to testify
'bout de air an de waters
dat's killin us daughtus.

So pleas don't dis me caus my ribbon's pink
I wears it to make my sistas think
(more soft)
bout breakin' down barriers, bout choosin life
(more oft)
bout early detection—maybe even da knife.

We got problems you don't know
we sheddin layers, we tryin to grow
to trust—to believe—to claim our power
to save lives lost hour after hour

we hafta save lives one at a time
we's got to catch up—we's behind
so save us a place, we's on our way
gettin stronga ev'ry day by day.

we makin it known, makin it unda'stood
soon no toxins/Dioxins allowed in da Hood
but first we got to stay alive—
Then we will stand—(with you) to testify.

"Alive/To Testify," by Wanna Wright, as appeared in *Endometriosis: The Complete Reference for Taking Charge of Your Health*. Reprinted by permission of the author.

The issue of toxic chemicals will be another example someday. When all of us speak out and educate others about the unacceptable health hazards of persistent toxic chemicals, public opinion will change. The new climate of opinion will evolve on this vital issue, just as it has evolved with others. The health and rights of humans and all other forms of life will finally outweigh the rights of toxic polluters. They will be held accountable, and destructive products, such as PVC plastic, will be completely replaced with alternatives that have been proven safe for our health and the environment. It is only a matter of time until we free ourselves from the hold that these toxic chemicals have over our lives, and we will be able to look back and know that we helped make it happen.

The right to live freely in a clean environment is a part of our collective civil rights movement affecting all races, ages, sexes, and nationalities. The fact that these toxins spread around the globe makes this a *worldwide* issue. Cumulative actions by people around the planet can force the cleanup of contaminated areas, the replacement of toxic chemicals with safer alternatives, and the phaseout of persistent toxic chemicals altogether. Together we make a difference!

Join with Others to Make a Difference!

A number of wonderful organizations sponsor worthy efforts. Consider joining in!

- Get involved in an environmental campaign through the Endometriosis Association (visit EndometriosisAssn.org or call 414-355-2200) or a local environmental group.
- Support the Center for Health, Environment and Justice (CHEJ), and get involved when you can. For more details about their campaigns, go to chej.org.

- Become a member of the Collaborative on Health and the Environment (CHE). CHE is a network of health-affected groups and patients, physicians, scientists, environmental health advocates, concerned citizens, and funders interested in working together to improve environmental health. For more information, visit cheforhealth.org.
- For updated information on endocrine-disrupting chemicals, visit ourstolenfuture.org.
- Get a free subscription to *Rachel's Environmental and Health Weekly News*. Go to rachel.org for more details.
- Support organized boycotts against foods or products that are proven to be unsafe.
- Support legislation that will increase research on environmental health issues, such as endocrine disruption.
- If you live in the United States, find out what companies are polluting your area by going to scorecard.org and entering your zip code.

Environmental Health Education and Awareness

 ## "Avoiding the Personal Responsibility Trap"

by Emily Alexander

At a recent women's health conference, I attended a panel on the health impact of environmental contaminants and chemicals on women, and specifically on reproductive health. In addition to dangerous pollutants and pesticides that can affect health, synthetic chemicals found in common plastics and many cosmetic products can act as endocrine disruptors and interfere with our bodies' hormones. Despite growing concerns, of the thousands of chemicals registered for use in the United States, only 10 percent have been tested for their possible effects on human health.[1]

So far, there are data to suggest a link between select contaminants and an increased risk for endometriosis, fertility problems, and adverse effects on early fetal development.[1] For instance, phthalates, a plasticizer found in some personal care products, may negatively affect the fetus' reproductive organs. Additionally, traces of mercury, a known reproductive toxin, have been found in some mascara products.[2] While the

"Young Feminists: Environmental Health Education and Awareness: Avoiding the Personal Responsibility Trap," by Emily Alexander, originally published in the *Women's Health Activist*, November/December 2007, pp. 8–9, the newsletter of the National Women's Health Network (NWHN). It is reprinted with the permission of the author and the NWHN.

conference panel presented multiple ways that our bodies absorb harmful contaminants, the audience immediately responded to the specific warnings against chemicals in body products and common plastics. But instead of voicing outrage that such commonly available and widely used products contain potentially harmful toxins, advocates and health care providers focused on how their individual choices could protect them, and their patients, from chemical exposure.

My favorite part of being an advocate is finding effective ways to synthesize complicated health concepts into effective education and policy opportunities. To this end, we are increasing health research and developing more and more guidelines and advice about what women should or shouldn't do to their bodies. While past guidelines have focused on personal behaviors during pregnancy, with the addition of last year's preconception care guidelines from the CDC, women now have 10 recommendations that emphasize the importance of personal responsibility and behavior throughout their reproductive years. Yet women are simultaneously losing health care access and coverage while being trapped in physical and social environments that do not foster and support healthfulness.

Advocacy surrounding the potential dangers of cosmetic products is particularly complicated. Change depends on advocates' ability to raise awareness about the dangers of chemicals whose names are so complex that it is nearly impossible to recognize them on ingredient labels. Making matters worse, many of the chemicals of concern are not included on ingredient labels at all.[3] In this context, it is hard to find a way to empower women with the most current and accurate health information without feeding the cultural discourse that already, shamelessly judges women's relationships with their bodies and reproductive health. To succeed, we must move beyond individual behavior to broader, systemic change. An integral part of meeting this challenge will be our work to demand that policymakers and industry better regulate chemicals, workplace conditions, and the environments in which people live.

During my childhood, my family ran a natural foods grocery store before this trend became part of mainstream culture. The recent increased attention to environmental contaminants' impact on fertility and women's health reminds me of the work my family did with food to educate our consumers to use their purchasing power to influence food markets and culture.

My experience at my family's grocery store led me to work in health policy. While I appreciate the benefits of an approach that promotes individual empowerment, behavior change and advocacy, I also worry about its

tremendous pitfalls. Instead of putting the burden on consumers to avoid harmful chemicals, I believe that the federal government should take responsibility and adopt policies to decrease the contaminants in our lives.

Environmental women's health education and advocacy provides an opportunity to direct the focus away from personal responsibility and consumer behaviors and toward the need for better regulation. The U.S. barely regulates either the presence of chemicals in our products or the industries that increase pollution in our communities. Cosmetics, for example, have no real safety standards. Further enforcement of existing laws on these products is desperately needed; yet, to date, the U.S. has only banned five chemicals from cosmetics.[4] The regulatory structure in this country only addresses acute reactions to chemicals, and unfortunately, there are no defined safety standards to which manufacturers must adhere.[4] Growing concerns about these chemicals arise from the question of how consistent exposure to small amounts of toxins impacts our health. Advocacy groups have gathered together information about possible toxins present in personal care products; the Environmental Working Group has produced "Skin Deep" a comprehensive database of ingredients found in thousands of products (see: www.cosmeticsdatabase.com).

Partly because of the inability of the federal government to regulate the cosmetics industry, in 2005, California passed the Safe Cosmetics Act—the first law to specifically address the chemicals found in personal care products. The law stipulates that corporations must notify the State if their products contain chemicals that have been linked to either cancer or adverse reproductive health effects.[5] Still, notification is not the same as regulation. The federal government should better regulate the products allowed to be on the market. With loopholes in federal law, apart from a handful of ingredients, corporations can put products on the market without an FDA review.

Further, consumer choices and personal behaviors related to health are not only shaped by information and choice, but also by access, the availability of resources, and other social determinants. We should use every possible opportunity to highlight lack of access and bring attention to the government's inadequacy in providing health coverage and support services to those in need.

In addition to empowering women with the best health information we have available, let's bring attention to the environments (social, political, and physical) that increase the prevalence of toxic chemicals in our lives. Let's bring attention to the lack of access, support, education and job opportunities that influence the choices people can make about what they buy and how they treat their bodies. With this lens, we have a better chance of making lasting change at the policy level on topics that include, but go beyond, environmental health. These changes will help increase freedoms and therefore improve personal behaviors, leading to better health for everybody. For more information, see the Environmental Working Group (www.ewg.org): The Campaign for Safe Cosmetics (www.safecosmetics.org); and Women's Voices for the Earth (www.womenandenvironment.org).

REFERENCES

1. Women's Health & the Environment, *What We Know: New Science Linking our Health and the Environment*, Bolinas, CA: Women's Health & the Environment, April, 2007. On-line: http://wwww.womenshealhandenvironment.org/toolkit.

2. The Campaign for Safe Cosmetics, *Unmasked: 10 Ugly Truths Behind the Myth of Cosmetic Safety*, The Campaign for Safe Cosmetics. Retrieved September 29, 2007 from: http://www.safecosmetics.org/action/materials.cfm.

3. Houlihan J., Brody C., Schwan B. *Not Too Pretty: Phthalates, Beauty Products & the FDA*. Washington, DC: Environmental Working Group, July 2002.

4. Women's Health & the Environment. *What We Can Do Community Efforts to Protect Our Health*. Bolinas, CA: Women's Health & the Environment, April 2007. On-line: http://www.womenandtheenvironment.org/toolkit.

5. The Campaign for Safe Cosmetics, "Governor Signs Safe Cosmetics Bill," The Campaign for Safe Cosmetics, October, 2005. Retrieved August 31, 2007 from http://www.safecosmetics.org/newsroom/press.cfm?pressReleaseID=13.

WORKSHEET—CHAPTER 13

Politics of Disease, Prevention, and the Environment

1. Fill in the chart below, showing what is available in terms of prevention, detection, and treatment for each of the three cancers listed.

Cancer	Prevention	Detection	Treatment
Breast			
Cervical			
Endometrial			

2. Think about what you learned from doing question # 1. Was it easier to find some information than other information? What do you think this represents in terms of the priority given to prevention, detection, and treatment of cancers?

3. Why do you think it is dangerous for there to be confusion about primary prevention vs. detection for cancers? How could health education and health policies emphasize prevention?

4. Several articles point out the silence around certain diseases. The authors of the articles on CFIDS/ME and on vulvodynia discuss how isolated and unsupported they felt; the Endometriosis Association is an example of an organization which has brought women together throughout the world to talk about their condition and

support each other. Identify the roles that self-help support groups could have for women. Pick a specific disease or condition around which you might organize a support group. Describe how you might find other people to join the group and imagine the topics the group might discuss. Identify advantages and disadvantages of doing this in person or through the internet.

5. Drawing on issues raised in this chapter and in Chapter 1's "How To Tell Your Doctor a Thing or Two," design a poster or leaflet for college women on how they can reduce the risk of STI infections.

6. One of the most rapidly growing groups of people infected with HIV is that of adolescents, many of whom become infected through heterosexual intercourse.

   a. If you were to design an educational program for highschool students to help prevent transmission of HIV, what specific information would you want to include?

   b. What obstacles might there be to presenting this information in the public schools? Discuss how you might present an argument for inclusion of the prevention program.

   c. Discuss any ideas you might have for overcoming adolescents' belief in their own invulnerability ("It can't happen to me.") when teaching about HIV/AIDS.

   d. "With or Without the Dam Thing" addresses HIV-prevention in a sex-positive, explicit manner, addressing risks associated with specific sexual activities. Can you imagine using ideas from this article to design information for heterosexual, gay, or lesbian teens?

7. "Women's HIV vulnerability derives particularly from contexts in which they have little control over sex, whether as a consequence of the predominating power relations between men and women or as a function of the economic and life choices available to them." Discuss how this statement specifically about HIV, in "The Gendered Epidemic" article, could be expanded to talk about women's vulnerability to other sexually transmitted infections and unwanted pregnancies.

Chapter 1: Women and the Health Care System

Gynecological Exam

Feminist Women's Health Center: Gynecological Self-Exam
www.fwhc.org/health/selfcare.htm

MS Magazine: What to Ask Your Gynecologist!
www.msmagazine.com/aug00/stds.asp

Women's Health Specialists of California
(An organization providing information on the gynecological exam and women's reproductive health issues.)
www.womenshealthspecialists.org/

Your First Gynecologist Visit
Scarleteen: Sex Ed for the Real World
www.scarleteen.com/article/pink/your_first_gynecologist_visit

Female Anatomy

National Institutes of Health–Female Anatomy
http://0-www.nlm.nih.gov.catalog.llu.edu/medlineplus/ency/imagepages/1112.htm

University of Ohio Medical School–Female Pelvic Anatomy
www.oucom.ohiou.edu/dbms-witmer/Downloads/OConnor%20pelvis.pdf

American Medical Association: Atlas of the Body
www.ama-assn.org/ama/pub/category/7140.html

Scarleteen's Sexual Anatomy Tour
www.scarleteen.com/body/female_anatomy.html

Women's Health Resources

Center for Women's Health
University of Wisconsin Medical School
www.womenshealth.wisc.edu/

Feminist Women's Health Center
(FWHC is a nonprofit organization that promotes and provides resources for women to choose and receive reproductive health care.)
www.fwhc.org/welcome.htm

Health Facts
(Provides consumers accurate, science-based information to make medical decisions.)
www.medicalconsumers.org

The Guttmacher Institute
(An organization that uses scientific evidence for promoting sexual and reproductive health, policy analysis and public education.)
http://guttmacher.org

Go Ask Alice
(An interactive health question and internet resource run by Columbia University's Health Services.)
www.goaskalice.columbia.edu/

National Women's Health Network
(Provides information from a network of organizations and individuals committed to giving women more of a voice in the healthcare system.)
www.womenshealthnetwork.org/

National Women's Health Resource Center
(A nonprofit organization that provides up-to-date health information based upon the latest advances in medical research and practice.)
www.healthywomen.org/

Office of Women's Health
U.S. Department of Health & Human Services
(Provides information and resources on 100+ women's health topics, including health services and preventative care.)
www.4women.gov/

Office of Women's Health
U.S. Food and Drug Administration
(The OWH provides information to help women navigate the healthcare system. The website also has information on food and product safety specific to women's health needs.)
www.fda.gov/womens/

Our Bodies Ourselves
Boston Women's Health Book Collective
(OBOS provides history of the Women's Health Movement, and information of women's health issues.)
www.ourbodiesourselves.org/

PNHP: Physicians for a National Health Program
www.pnhp.org

Raising Women's Voices (for the health care we need)
www.raisingwomensvoices.net/

U.S. Dept. of Health & Human Services, Source for Women's Health Information
www.Womenshealth.gov/

Women's Health
Centers for Disease Control and Preventions
(Health information and resources from the CDC for women at every stage of life.)
www.cdc.gov/Women/

Women's Health Initiative
U.S. Dept. of Health and Human Services
National Institutes of Health
(Established in 1991 the WHI studies the most common causes of morbidity and mortality in post-menopausal women.)
www.nhlbi.nih.gov/whi/

Women's Health: Take Time to Care Grassroots Campaign
Food and Drug Administration of Women's Health
(An FDA campaign providing women with knowledge to use medicines wisely.)
www.fda.gov/womens/taketimetocare/progsumm.html

Resources for the Un/Underinsured
Covering Kids and Families
(A national program working to enroll children and adults in low-cost or free health care coverage programs.)
www.coveringkidsandfamilies.org/

HRSA: Health Resources and Services Administration
U.S. Department of Health and Human Services
(A network of federally funded health care centers that provide affordable care to those without health insurance.)
http://findahealthcenter.hrsa.gov/

FreeClinic
(Currently under construction this website will provide information on free health care facilities and services nationwide.)
www.freeclinic.net

Free/Low-Cost Meds
NeedyMeds.com
(A non-profit helping people who cannot afford medicine or healthcare costs.)
www.needymeds.com

Rx Assist: Patient Assistance Program Center
(A directory of patient assistance programs run by pharmaceutical companies to provide free medications to people who cannot afford to buy their medicine.)
www.rxassist.org/

Chapter 2: Inequalities and Health
Note: For LGBTQ Health Resources please see Chapter 9: Sexuality.
For Economic Health Resources please see Chapter 1: Women and the Health Care System.

Disabilities
Adaptive Sports Association
(The ASA helps to enrich and transform the lives of people with disabilities through sports.)
www.asadurango.org

CROWD: Center for Research on Women with Disabilities
www.bcm.edu/crowd/

DisabilityResourcex.org: Women with Disabilities
(Provides resources and links for disabled women of different backgrounds.)
www.disabilityresources.org/WOMEN.html

Disabled Women on the Web
www.disabilityhistory.org/dwa/

ILI: Independent Living Institute
www.independentliving.org/

Women with Disabilities Education Program
(This organization educates patients in self-management and trains health professionals.)
www.womenwithdisabilities.org

World Enable
http://www.worldenable.net

Immigrant Women's Health
Citizens and Immigrants for Equal Justice
http://ciej.org

Immigration Equality
http://lgirtf.org

National Immigration Forum
http://immigrationforum.org

National Network of Immigrant and Refugee Rights
http://nnirr.org

Health Disparities and Minority Health Resources

AMSA: American Medical School Association
(On health disparities)
www.amsa.org

Center to Reduce Cancer Health Disparities
http://crchd.nci.nih.gov/

Center for Research on Minority Health
University of Texas MD Anderson Center
(The CRMH works to provide resources for reducing the prevalence of cancer in ethnic minority and medically underserved populations.)
http://www.mdanderson.org/departments/CRMH/

The Health Center Program: Special Populations
Health Resources and Services Administration
U.S. Department of Health and Human Services
http://bphc.hrsa.gov/about/specialpopulations.htm

Institute of Women and Ethnic Studies
http://iwes.org

Minority Women's Health
The National Women's Health Information Center
U.S. Department of Health and Human Services,
Office on Women's Health
(A resource for minority with links for African American, Latina, API, and Native American women.)
www.4woman.gov/minority/

Minority Health
National Institutes of Health
(A health information resource with links for minority and women's health issues.)
http://health.nih.gov/search.asp/26

National Women's Alliance
http://nwaforchange.org

The Office of Minority Health
U.S. Department of Health & Human Services
(This website provides statistics, and information on funding, cultural competency, many health topics, and resources for specific minority groups.)
www.omhrc.gov/

Afghan Women

Afghan Women's Association International
http://awai.org

African American Women

African American Women Evolving
http://aaweonline.org

Black Radical Congress
(The BRC promotes dialogue and activism to promote progressive political, social and cultural movements, and too renew the Black radical movement.)
http://blackradicalcongress.org/

Black Women's Health Imperative
(An organization dedicated to eliminating the health disparities that exist for Black women.)
www.blackwomenshealth.org

Center for Black Women's Wellness
(A non-profit organization that provides low-cost services to empower black women, and their families, toward physical, mental and economic wellness.)
www.cbww.org/

Asian and Pacific Islander American Women

AANCART: Asian American Network for Cancer Awareness, Research and Training
(A cancer awareness and training partnership between the National Cancer Institute and the University of California, Davis focused on the APT community.)
www.aancart.org/

APIAHF: Asian and Pacific Islander American Health Forum
(Health and political organizing resources for the API community.)
www.apiahf.org

NAWHO: National Asian Women's Health Organization
(A non-profit organization providing resources for Asian women and their families to achieve health equity.)
www.nawho.org/

Latinas

Latino Commission on AIDS
(A non-profit that uses programs and grassroots organizing to fight the spread of HIV/AIDS in the Latino community.)
www.latinoaids.org/

National Alliance for Hispanic Health
(An resource for Latino community health, with specific information and links to programs on women's health issues.)
www.hispanichealth.org/

National Latina Health Network
(A non-profit organization that addresses critical health concerns affecting Latinas and their families.)
www.nlhn.net/

National Latina Institute for Reproductive Health
(An organization committed to changing policy and mobilizing communities to provide Latinas with reproductive healthcare.)
www.latinainstitute.org/

Native American Women

IHS: Indian Health Service on Women's Health
(Federal government healthcare resources and information for American Indians and Alaska Native women.)
www.ihs.gov/MedicalPrograms/MCH/W/index.cfm

Indigenous Women's Network
http://indigenouswomen.org

Indigenous Women's Reproductive Rights and Pro-choice Page
http://nativeshop.prg/pro-choice.html

National Indian Women's Health Resource Center
(A non-profit organization founded to assist American Indian and Alaska Native women to achieve health while staying committed to their roots and communities.)
www.niwhrc.org/

Native Shop: Native American Women's Health Education Resource Center
(A resource for Native women for health issues, education, land and water rights, and economic development.)
www.nativeshop.org/

Cultural Awareness

Georgetown University National Center for Cultural Competence
http://www11.georgetown.edu/research/gucchd/nccc/

Diversity Rx
http://www.diversityrx.org/

ThinkCulturalHealth
https://cccm.thinkculturalhealth.org/

Transgender Resources
Note: For a complete list of transgender resources please see Chapter3: Sex, Gender, Roles, and Health.

Transgender Warrior
(Leslie Feinberg's web site with resources, support and activist opportunities to help the transgendered community.)
http://transgenderwarrior.org/

Chapter 3: Sex, Gender Roles, and Health

Note: For environmental health and women's occupational health please see Chapter 13: The Politics of Disease, Prevention, and the Environment.

Female Genital Cutting

RAINBO-Research, Action and Information Network for the Bodily Integrity of Women
www.rainbo.org/

Gender Roles and Health

AL Fatiha
(A foundation with resources for LGBTIQ Muslims, those exploring their sexual orientation or gender identity, and their allies, families and friends.)
http://al-fatiha.org/

AlterHeros
http://alterheros.com

American Boyz
http://amboyz.org

American Institute of Bisexuality
www.bisexual.org/

Center for Health and Gender Equality
http://genderhealth.org

GLAD: Gay & Lesbian Advocates & Defenders
http://glad.org/

glaad: Gay & Lesbian Alliance Against Defamation
http://glaad.org/

Gay & Lesbian Medical Association
www.glma.org/

Gay, Lesbian, Straight Education Network
www.glsen.org/

Human Rights Campaign
(A civil rights organization working for gay, lesbian, bisexual and transgender equality.)
www.hrc.org

National Association of Lesbian, Gay, Bisexual, and Transgender Community Centers (NAKGBTCC)
www.lgbtcenters.org/

NCLR: National Center for Lesbian Rights
(An organization dedicated to the advancement of civil and legal rights of LGBT individuals through litigation, policy advocacy, and public education.)
www.nclrights.org/

National Gay and Lesbian Task Force
www.thetaskforce.org/

National Latina/o Lesbian, Gay, Bisexual, and
Transgender Organization
http://iglhrc.org

National Youth Advocacy Coalition
http://nyacyouth.org

PFLAG: Parents and Friends of Lesbians and Gays
www.pflag.org

Sexual Minority Youth Assistance League
http://smyal-dc.org

Youth Gender Project
http://youthgenderproject.org

Women's Initiatives for Gender Justice
http://iccwomen.org

Intersex

Bodies Like Ours: Intersex Information and Peer
Support
www.bodieslikeours.org/forums/

Intersex Initiative
http://intersexinitiative.org

Intersex Society of North America
http://isna.org

Transgender Resources

National Center for Transgender Equality
www.nctequality.org/

NTAC: National Transgender Advocacy Coalition
www.ntac.org

National Transgender Law Institute
   (Legal affairs activist site with updates on changed
in state or federal law, and databases on employer
transgender policies.)
www.transgenderlaw.org

IFGE: International Federation for Gender Education
   (The leading Trans oriented web site.)
www.ifge.org

IGLHRC: International Gay and Lesbian Human
Rights Commission
www.iglhrc.org/site/iglhrc/

PFLAG Transgender Network:
   (Support organization for transgender individuals,
their families and friends)
http://www.pflag.org/TNET.tnet.0.html

Transgender Warrior
   (Leslie Feinberg's web site with resources, support
and activist opportunities to help the transgendered
community.)
http://transgenderwarrior.org/

Chapter 4:   Medicalization, Marketing, and the Politics of Information

American Medical Student Association: Concise
& Evidence-Based Sources of Pharmaceutical
Information
http://www.amsa.org/hp/cleansources.cfm

Center for Drug Evaluation and Research
www.fda.gov/cder/

Center for Medical Consumers
www.medicalconsumers.org

Cochrane Collaboration: Evidence-Based Healthcare
Databases
www.cochrane.org/

De-Fib: Demanding Evidence, Forgoing Industry Bias
www.de-fib.org/index.html

Feminist Internet Gateway: Health
Feminist Majority Foundation
*http://www.feminist.org/gateway/feministgateway
-results.asp?category1=health*

HealthRatings.org
www.healthratings.org

Healthy Skepticism: Countering Misleading Drug
Promotion
www.healthyskepticism.org/

AdWatch by Healthy Skepticism
   (Critical view on current drug advertisements.)
http://www.healthyskepticism.org/adwatch.php

The James Lind Library
   (For fair tests of treatments in health care.)
www.jameslindlibrary.org/

Journal of the American Medical Women's
Association
www.jamwa.org

The National Institute for Health and Clinical Excellence (UK)
www.nice.org.uk/

National Research Center for Women and Families
www.center4research.org/womenhlth1.html

New York Online Access to Health
www.hoah-health.org/

No Free Lunch "Just Say No to Drug Reps".
http://nofreelunch.org/

PharmedOut
www.pharmedout.org/

The Prescription Project: Advancing Medical Practice and Policy
www.prescriptionproject.org/

Pushing Prescriptions: How the drug industry sells its agenda at your expense
http://projects.publicintegrity.org/rx/

Society for Women's Health Research
www.womenshealthresearch.org

Where Women Have No Doctor
www.hesperian.org/index.php

Women's Health
Agency for Healthcare Research and Quality
U.S. Department of Health and Human Services
www.ahrq.gov/research/womenix.htm

Women's Health Matters
www.womenshealthmatters.ca/index.cfm

Women's Health Resource Site
http://userpages.umbc.edu/~korenman/wmst/links.html

Chapter 5:   Menstruation

Note: For contraception/birth-control please see Chapter 10: Reproductive Justice, Fertility, and Infertility.

For the marketing resources about women's health please see Chapter 4: Medicalization, Marketing, and the Politics of Information.

Female Adolescence

Getting Your Period
Girlshealth.gov
U.S. Department of Health and Human Services
www.girlshealth.gov/body/period/index.cfm

GirlsInc.
www.girlsinc.org/

Planned Parenthood: Teen Health
www.plannedparenthood.org/health-topics/teens-4315.htm

Puberty: Adolescent Female
www.healthsystem.virginia.edu/uvahealth/peds_growth/paf.cfm

Puberty, Periods, and Girls
www.avert.org/puberty2.htm

Your First Pelvic Exam
Center for Young Women's Health
Children's Hospital Boston
www.youngwomenshealth.org/pelvicinfo.html

Menstruation

The Centre for Menstrual Cycle and Ovulation Research
www.cemcor.ubc.ca/

Feminist Women's Health Center (on menstruation)
www.fwhc.org/health/moon.htm

Menstruation
MedlinePlus
National Institutes of Health
www.nlm.nih.gov/medlineplus/menstruation.html

Menstruation and the Menstrual Cycle
WomensHealth.gov
U.S. Department of Health & Human Services
www.womenshealth.gov/faq/menstru.htm#a

Menstruation Resource Center
Association of Reproductive Health Professionals
www.arhp.org/healthcareproviders/resources/menstruationresources/index.cfm

Museum of Menstruation & Women's Health
www.mum.org

The Red Web Foundation: Creating Lifelong Menstrual Health Through Community & Education
www.theredweb.org/

Society for Menstrual Cycle Research
http://menstruationresearch.org/

SPOT: The Tampon Health Website
www.spotsite.org/

Alternative Menstrual Products

Guide to Alternative Menstrual Products
www.youngwomenshealth.org/alternative_menstrual.html

Introduction to Menstrual Product Alternatives
www.oasisdesign.net/health/moon/new.htm

Non-Chlorine Bleached Cotton Pads and Tampons

Natracare
www.natracare.com

Pandora
www.pandorapads.com

Seventh Generation
*www.seventhgeneration.com/Organic-Cotton
-Tampons*

Washable Cloth Pads

GladRags
www.gladrags.com

Lunapads
www.lunapads.com

Natural Sponges

Sea Pearls
www.seapearls.co.uk/buyonline.php

GladRags
www.gladrags.com/category/sea-sponge-tampons

Menstrual Cups

The Keeper (latex)
www.keeper.com

The Diva Cup (hypoallergenic silicone)
www.divacup.com

The Instead Softcup
www.softcup.com

PMS: Premenstrual Syndrome and PMDD: Premenstrual Dysphoric Disorder

National Association for Premenstrual Syndrome
(U.K)
www.pms.org.uk/

Premenstrual Syndrome
The Federal Governement Source for Women's Health
Information
U.S. Department of Health and Human Services
*www.womenshealth.gov/faq/pms.htm?PHPSESSID
=232c4dfb919991006d4b188f044075d6*

Premenstrual Syndrome
MedlinePlus
National Institutes of Health
*www.nlm.nih.gov/medlineplus/
premenstrualsyndrome.html*

Premenstrual Syndrome
Women's Health, MayoClinic.com
*www.mayoclinic.com/health/premenstrual
-syndrome/DS00134*

PreMenstrual Dysphoric Disorder: A Severe Form
of PMS
Ask a Women's Health Specialist
MayoClinic.com
www.mayoclinic.com/health/pmdd/AN01372

The Marketing of Premenstrual Syndrome and Premenstrual Dysphoric Disorder

Note: For more on marketing and health see Chapter 4: Medicalization, Marketing, and the Politics of Information.

Direct to Consumer Advertising
Navigating the Health Care System
Our Bodies Ourselves Resource Center
*www.ourbodiesourselves.org/book/companion.asp
?compID=69&id=30*

Misleading Ads and How They Hurt Us
Direct to Consumer Advertising
Navigating the Health Care System
Our Bodies Ourselves Resource Center
*www.ourbodiesourselves.org/book/companion.asp
?id=30&compID=69&page=4*

Prime Time Pushers
Mother Jones Magazine
*www.motherjones.com/news/feature/2001/03/
drug.html*

Selling Sickness: The Pharmaceutical Industry and
Disease Mongering
British Medical Journal
www.bmj.com/cgi/content/full/324/7342/886

Making the Female Cycle a Disease: The Pharmaceutical Industry Markets More than Comfort
Women's Health
*http://womenshealth.suite101.com/article.cfm/
making_the_female_cycle_a_disease*

Sarafem: Treatment of PMDD
Warner Chilcott Pharmaceutical Company
(Remarketing of Prozac as a treatment for PMDD.
This website is included to show how PMS and
PMDD are medicalized and treated. This website is
not included to provide accurate scientific information
for women.)
www.pmdd.com/

There is Help for PMDD Suffers
Lilly Pharmaceuticals
   (This website is included to show how after PMDD becomes a medicalized condition Lilly Pharmaceutical Company can treat it. This website is not included to provide information on a 'cure' for PMS of PMDD.)
www.lilly.com/products/health_women/pmdd/index.html

Chapter 6:   Mental Health
Women's Mental Health
Adult Survivors of Childhood Sexual Assault
RAINN: Rape, Abuse & Incest National Network
www.rainn.org/get-information/effects-of-sexual-assault/adult-survivors-of-childhood-sexual-abuse

Emotional Health
Center for Young Women's Health
www.youngwomenshealth.org/emotional_menu.html

Depression in Wisconsin Women
Report of the Task Force on Women and Depression in Wisconsin
www.ltgov.state.wi.us

National Empowerment Center
   (Practical information for recovering from mental illness.)
www.power2.org/

National Center for Posttraumatic Stress Disorder
www.ncptsd.va.gov/ncmain/index.jsp

PsychCentral
   (Information about mental health and medications.)
http://psychcentral.com/

Resources on Depression in Mothers
www.granitescientific.com/depressionfrontpage.htm

SSRI Antidepressants: Their Place in Women's Lives
Women and Health Protection (Canada)
www.whp-apsf.ca/en/documents/ssri.html

Gender and Women's Mental Health
World Health Organization
www.who.int/mental_health/prevention/genderwomen/en/

Women and Mental Health
National Institute of Mental Health
www.nimh.nih.gov/health/topics/women-and-mental-health/index.shtml

Women and Mental Health
World Health Organization
www.who.int/mediacentre/factsheets/fs248/en/index.html

Women's Mental Health
The National Women's Health Information Center
U.S. Department of Health and Human Services
www.4woman.gov/mh/

Depression in Wisconsin Women
Report of the Task Force on Women and Depression in Wisconsin
www.ltgov.state.wi.us

Co-dependency
Co-Dependency
Mental Health America
www.nmha.org/go/codependency

Information about Codependency
www.faqs.org/health/topics/80/Codependency.html

Chapter 7:   Violence Against Women
Domestic Violence/Rape
The Alabama Coalition Against Domestic Violence
www.acadv.org/

American Institute on Domestic Violence, Inc.
www.aidv-usa.com/

Battered Women's Justice Project
www.bwjp.prg/menu.htm

Chicago Metropolitan Battered Women's Network
www.batteredwomensnetwork.org

Coalition Against Violence Network
www.cavnet.org/

Communities Against Rape and Abuse
http://cara-seattle.org

Domestic Abuse Intervention Project
www.duluth-model.org/

Domestic Violence Survival Kit
www.dvguide.com/content.html

Family Violence Prevention Fund
http://endabuse.org

Incite! Women of Color Against Violence
http://incite-national.org

Institute on Domestic Violence in the African American Community
www.dvinstitute.org/

Jane Doe, Inc.
http://janedoe.org

Legal Defense and Education Fund
National Organization of Women
http://nowldef.org

Minnesota Center Against Violence and Abuse
www.mincava.umn.edu/

National Coalition Against Domestic Violence
http://ncadv.org

National Domestic Violence Hotline
1-800-799-SAFE
www.ndvh.org/

National Network to End Domestic Violence
www.nnedv.org/

The Network/La Red
http://thenetworklared.org

Rape, Abuse & Incest National Network (RAINN)
   (Hotline for survivors of sexual assault" 800-656-HOPE)
www.rain.org

Silent Witness National Initiative
www.silentwitness.net/

Survivor Project
http://survivorproject.org

U.S. Department of Justice, Office on Violence Against Women
www.ojp.usdoj.gov/vawo/

Women's Rural Advocacy Programs
www.letswrap.com/

Domestic Violence and Teens

Breaking the Cycle: Domestic Violence and Teens
Genderal Federation of Women's clubs
www.gfwc.org/content_1239.cfm

Bursting the Bubble
   (Information for teenagers about abuse, domestic violence, family violence.)
www.burstingthebubble.com

Dating Violence
Alabama Coalition Against Domestic Violence
www.acadv.org/dating.html

South East Centre Against Sexual Assault:
Information for Teenagers
www.secasa.com.au/index.php/survivors/52

Teens and Dating Violence
National Domestic Violence Hotline
1-800-799-SAFE
www.ndvh.org/help/teen-help.html

Teens and Dating Violence
University of Minnesota Extension
www.extension.umn.edu/info-u/families/BE912.html

Teens and Domestic Violence
Chicago Metropolitan Battered Women's Network
www.batteredwomensnetwork.org/id71.html

When Love Hurts: A Guide on Love, Respect and Abuse in Relationships
www.dvirc.org.au/whenlove/

Chapter 8:   Food, Body Image, and Body Modification
Body Positive & Feminist Media

Bitch Magazine
   (A feminist response to pop-culture.)
http://bitchmagazine.org/

Feminist Media Project
www.feministmediaproject.com/

Feminist Majority Foundation
   (Feminist links and resources.)
www.feminist.org/gateway/

Girls, Women and Media Project
www.mediaandwomen.org/

Guerilla Girls
http://guerillagirls.com

MS Magazine
www.msmagazine.com/

Women's E News
http://womensenews.org

Body Image, Body Projects and Disordered Eating

About Face
   (An organization that provides resources for girls to resist harmful media messages that affect self-esteem and body image.)
www.about-face.org

Adios Barbie
www.adiosbarbie.com

Celebrate Your Body: Transforming Negative Body Image
www.bodycelebration.com/

EDC: Eating Disorders Coalition
www.eatingdisorderscoalition.org/

EDREFERRAL.COM
Eating Disorder Referral and Information Center
www.edreferral.com/body_image.htm

Girls Incorporated
www.girlsinc.org

Jean Kilbourne
www.jeankilbourne.com

Largesse: The Network for Size Esteem
www.eskimo.com/~largesse/

National Eating Disorders Association
www.nationaleatingdisorders.org

Size Wise: Your World, Your Size
www.sizewise.com/

Nutrition
Arbor Nutrition Guide
www.arborcom.com

Dietary Guidelines for Americans
U.S. Department of Health & Human Services
www.health.gov/dietaryguidelines/

The Food Allergy Network
www.foodallergy.org

National Association of Nutrition Professionals
www.certifiednutritionist.com

Cosmetics and Health
Warning on Cosmetic Safety
Center for Food Safety and Applied Nutrition
U.S. Food and Drug Administration
www.cfsan.fda.gov/~dms/cos-prd.html

Obesity
The Obesity Society
www.Obesity.org

Chapter 9:   Sexuality
Note: For Disability Resources please see Chapter 2: Inequalities and Health.

For Resources on Women and Aging please see Chapter 12: Aging, Mid-Life and Older Women's Issues.

Sexuality
AASECT: American Association of Sex Educators, Counselors, and Therapists
www.aasect.org

The Birds & Bees Project
   (This website provides information for making informed decisions about sexual and reproductive health, emotional well-being, and lifetime goals.)
http://birdsandbees.org/

Coalition for Positive Sexuality
   (A grassroots direct-action group dedicated to providing young adults information needed to both talk and make decisions about sex, sexuality and reproductive control.)
www.positive.org/Home/index.html

PPFA: Planned Parenthood Federation of America
   (Provides resources under 'health topics' for relationships, sexuality, sexual orientation & gender, and STIs).
www.plannedparenthood.org/health-topics/health -topics-11.htm

Sex, Etc.
   (A leader in teen-to-teen sexuality education.)
www.sexetc.org/

The Sexual Health Network
http://sexualhealth.com/

Scarleteen: Sex Ed for the Real World
www.scarleteen.com

SIECUS: Sexuality Information and Education Council of the United States
www.siecus.org

SEXoutLOUD
   (A resource for sex positive education and activism.)
www.sexoutloud.com/

The Working Group on a New View of Women's Sexual Problems
www.fsd-alert.org

Safe Sex & STIs
National Center for HIV, STD and TB Prevention
Division of Sexually Transmitted Diseases
Centers for Disease Control and Prevention
www.cdc.gov/std

HIV InSite: Safer Sex Methods
(Up-to-date information on HIV/AIDS and other STI treatment, prevention and policy from UC, San Francisco.)
http://hivinsite.ucsf.edu/

International Herpes Alliance
www.herpesalliance.org

Medicine.net
(Sexually transmitted infections in women: Causes, symptoms, diagnosis and treatment.)
www.medicinenet.com/sexually_transmitted _diseases_stds_in_women/article.htm

Sexually Transmitted Diseases: Overview
U.S. Department of Health and Human Services Office on Women's Health
www.womenshealth.gov/faq/stdsgen.htm

The STD World of Resource Network
www.sworn.org/main.html

LBTQ Resources
Lesbian STD
www.lesbianstd.com

Mautner Project: The National Lesbian Health Organization
(An organization centered on improving the health care system for lesbians, bisexual, and transgender women.)
www.mautnerproject.org/

The National Coalition for LGBT Health
www.lgbthealth.net/

Youth Support
Effective Sex Education
Advocates for Youth
www.advocatesforyouth.org

National Youth Advocacy Coalition
www.nyacyouth.org/

LYRIC: Lavender Youth Recreation and Information Center
www.lyric.org

TransKids Purple Rainbow Foundation
www.transkidspurplerainbow.org/

Teen Voices
www.teenvoices.com

Youth TIES: Youth Trans & Intersex Education Services
http://youthgenderproject.org

Trans-Specific Resources
Philadelphia Trans-Health Conference
www.trans-health.org/

Trans-Health Online Magazine
http://trans-health.com

Chapter 10: Reproductive Justice, Fertility, and Infertility
Abortion/Reproductive Rights
AAP: Abortion Access Project
www.abortionaccess.org

AGI: Alan Guttmacher Institute
www.agi-usa.org/sections/abortion.html

California Abortion and Reproductive Rights Action League
http://choice.org

The Center for Reproductive Rights
www.reproductiverights.org

Choice USA
www.choiceusa.org

EXHALE
http://4exhale.org

Ipas USA
www.ipas.com

Law Students for Choice
http://ms4c.org

Medical Students for Choice
http://ms4c.org

NARAL Pro-Choice America
www.naral.org

The National Abortion Federation
www.prochoice.org

National Family Planning & Reproductive Health Association
http://nfprha.org

National Network of Abortion Funds
www.nnaf.org

Physicians for Reproductive Choice & Health
http://prch.org

Pro-Choice Public Education Project
http://protectchoice.org

The Religious Coalition for Reproductive Choice
www.rcrc.org

Contraception

Public Citizen Page on Oral Contraceptive Safety
www.notmypill.org

Cervical Barrier Advancement Society
(An organization that promotes cervical barrier methods for preventing pregnancy and that provides information on microbicides, and preventing STI and HIV infection in women.)
www.cervicalbarriers.org

CONRAD Program
Eastern Virginia Medical School
www.CONRAD.org

Feminist Women's Health Center
www.fwhc.org/birth-control/index.htm

The Fertility Awarness Network
www.FertAware.com

Justisse Healthworks for Women
(Fertility education, natural birth control & holistic reproductive health.)
www.justisse.ca/

National EC Hotline
888-NOT-2-LATE
www.rhtp.org/ec/ec_hotline.htm
www.not-2-late.com

PPFA: Planned Parenthood Federation of America
www.ppfa.org/bc

Infertility and Reproductive Technology

American Fertility Association
www.theafa.org

American Society for Reproductive Medicine
www.asrm.org

Council for Responsible Genetics
www.gene-watch.org

Infertility Network
www.infertilitynetwork.org

Internation Council on Infertility Information Discrimination
www.inciid.org

Reproductive Health Technologies Project
http://rhtp.org

RESOLVE, Inc.
www.resolve.org/

Overpopulation

Pop/Dev: The Population and Development Program, Hampshire College
(This program promotes reproductive rights, economic justice, and social equality for women. It challenges the traditional views of over-population and immigration as primary causes of environmental degradation, political instability and poverty.)
http://popdev.hampshire.edu/home

Reproductive Justice/Freedom

APIAHF: Asian and Pacific Islander American Health Forum
(Health and political organizing resources for the API community.)
www.apiahf.org

CLPP: Civil Liberties and Public Policy
(A program dedicated to educating, training and inspiring new reproductive justice activists.)
http://clpp.hampshire.edu/

Indigenous Women's Reproductive Rights and Pro-choice Page
http://nativeshop.prg/pro-choice.html

National Indian Women's Health Resource Center
(A non-profit organization founded to assist American Indian and Alaska Native women to achieve health while staying committed to their roots and communities.)
www.niwhrc.org/

National Latina Institute for Reproductive Health
(An organization committed to changing policy and mobilizing communities to provide Latinas with reproductive healthcare.)
www.latinainstitute.org/

Reproductive Freedom Task Force
http://refuseandresist.org/repro/idx.php

Sistersong Women of Color Reproductive Health Collective
www.sistersong.net/index.html

Chapter 11:   Childbirth and Lactation
Loss of Pregnancy

Hygeia Foundation, Inc., and Institute for Perinatal Loss and Bereavement
www.hygeia.org

SHARE Pregnancy Loss and Infant Support, Inc.
www.nationalshareoffice.com

The MISS Foundation
www.missfoundation.org

Wisconsin Stillbirth Service Program
www.wisc.edu/wissp

Parenting Resources

Childfree Resources
www.fred.net/turtle/kids/resources

National Adoption Information Clearinghouse
http://naic.acf.hhs.gov/

National Guardianship Association, Inc.
www.guardianship.org

ParentsPlace.com
www.parentsplace.com

Postpartum Depression Support Page
www.ppdsupportpage.com

Pregnancy Resources and Choices in Childbirth

Association of Labor Assistants and Childbirth
Educators
www.alace.org

Childbirth.org
www.childbirth.org

Citizens for Midwifery
www.cfmidwifery.org

Doulas of North America
www.dona.org

International Cesarean Awareness Network
www.ican-online.org

International Childbirth Education Association
www.icea.org

Lamaze Institute for Normal Birth
http://normalbirth.lamaze.org/instotute/

Maternity Center Association
www.maternitywise.org

Midwifery Today
www.midwiferytoday.com

Mothering
www.mothering.com

National Association of Childbearing Centers
www.birthcenters.org

Lactation

Breastfeeding
Office on Women's Health
U,S. Department of Health and Human Services
800-994-WOMAN
www.4woman.gov/owh/breastfeeding.htm

La Leche League USA
www.lllusa.org

International Lactation Consultants' Association
www.ilca.org

Blue Vinyl
(A video made by Judith Helfand in 2002 documenting the presence of PVC in breast milk and the effects of PVC on environmental health.)
www.bluevinyl.org

Chapter 12:   Aging, Ageism, Mid-Life and Older Women's Issues
Aging for Women

Eldercare Locator
www.wldercare.gov

Gray Panthers
www.graypanthers.org

National Family Caregivers Association
www.thefamilycaregiver.org

National Hispanic Council on Aging
www.nhcoa.org

National Program on Women and Aging
http://iasp.brandeis.edu/womenandaging/

National Program on Women and Aging–Research
http://iasp.brandeis.edu/womenandaging/research.htm

OWL: Older Women's League
The Voice of Midlife and Older Women
www.owl-national.org

Senior Action in a Gay Environment
www.sageusa.org

Women's Health, Aging A-Z
Centers for Disease Control and Prevention
www.cdc.gov/women/az/aging.htm

Alzheimer's Disease

Alzheimer's Association
www.alz.org/index.asp

Alzheimer's Disease Education & Referral Center
National Institute on Aging
National Institutes of Health
www.nia.nih.gov/Alzheimers/

Contraception
Contraception after 40
Women's Health Watch
Queensland Wide Inc.
www.womhealth.org.au/factsheets/contraception _after_40.htm

Menopause
Menopause Expert
   (Information, articles and resources for menopause.)
www.menopauseexpert.com/

Menopause Resource Center
Association of Reproductive Health Professionals
www.arhp.org/healthcareproviders/resources/ hrtresources/index.cfm?ID=290

North American Menopause Society
www.menopause.org/

Menopause
Planned Parenthood
www.plannedparenthood.org/health-topics/womens -health/menopause-4807.htm

Menopause and Heart Disease
The Canadian Women's Health Network
www.cwhn.ca/resources/faq/menoHeartDis.html

The Menopause Experience
Project Aware
www.project-aware.org/Experience/experience.shtml

Women's Health: Working Toward a Better Understanding of Menopause
Study of Women's Health Across the Nation
http://mediwire.skyscape.com/main/Default.aspx ?P=Content&ArticleID=138161

Hormone Replacement Therapy
A Marketing Breakthrough
MEDIAWATCH
   (Information on use of hormone replacement therapy in Australia where law prohibits drug companies advertising directly to the public.)
www.abc.net.au/mediawatch/transcripts/s1390967.htm

Hormone Replacement Therapy Side Effects
www.hormone-replacement-therapy-side-effects.com/

WHI: Women's Health Initiative
   (A 15 year NIH study on the common causes of health problems for postmenopausal women.)
www.nhlbi.nih.gov/whi/index.html

WHI: Menopausal Hormone Therapy Information
National Institutes of Health
www.nih.gov/PHTindex.htm

WHI: Facts About Postmenopausal Hormone Therapy
National Institutes of Health
www.nhlbi.nih.gov/health/women/pht_facts.htm

WHI: Questions and Answers about the Women's Health Initiative Estrogen-Plus-Progestin Study—
National Institutes of Health
www.nhlbi.nih.gov/health/women/q_a.htm

WHI: The Estrogen-Alone Study of the Women's Health Initiative
www.nhlbi.nih.gov/whi/index.html#estrogen

WHI: The Estrogen-Plus Progestin Study
www.nhlbi.nih.gov/whi/estro_pro.htm

WHI: Oral Contraceptives and Cardiovascular Disease
www.nhlbi.nih.gov/new/press/04-12-15.htm

WHI: Postmenopausal Hormone Therapy
National Institutes of Health
www.nhlbi.nih.gov/health/women/index.htm

Hormone Replacement Therapy Alternatives
Alternatives to Hormone Replacement Therapy/ Phytoestrogens
Women's Health Queensland Wide Inc.
www.womhealth.org.au/factsheets/alternativestoHRT .htm

Bone Health and Phytoestrogens
Menopause and Osteoporosis
   (all see "Osteoporosis" below)
National Insititues of Health
Department of Health and Human Services
www.niams.nih.gov/Health_Info/Bone/Osteoporosis/ Menopause/bone_phyto.asp

Marketing Menopause
Women's Desk
National Radio Project
http://radioproject.org/archive/1999/9908.html

Menopause Resource Center
Association of Reproductive Health Professionals
www.arhp.org/healthcareproviders/resources/ hrtresources/index.cfm

National Center for Complementary and Alternative Medicine
http://nccam.nih.gov/

"Natural" Hormones: Are They a Safe Alternative
Health and Sexuality
Association of Reproductive Health Professionals
*www.arhp.org/healthcareproviders/onlinepublications/
healthandsexuality/hormonetherapy/naturalhormones
.cfm*

Natural Hormone Education and Research Library
Virginia Hopkins Health Watch
The Science of Alternative Medicine
www.virginiahopkinstestkits.com/library.html

Phytoestrogens and Breast Cancer
   Program on Breast Cancer and Environmental Risk
Factors
Cornell University
*http://envirocancer.cornell.edu/FactSheet/Diet/fs1
.phyto.cfm*

Women and Osteoporosis
National Osteoporosis Foundation
www.nof.org/

Osteoporosis
The National Women's Health Information Center
U.S. Department of Health and Human Services
www.4woman.gov/faq/osteopor.htm

Osteoporosis and Bone Physiology
http://courses.washington.edu/bonephys/

Osteoporosis in Postmenopausal Women: Diagnosis
and Monitoring
Agency for Healthcare Research and Quality
U.S. Department of Health &Human Services
www.ahrq.gov/clinic/epcsums/osteosum.htm

Chapter 13:   Politics of Disease, Prevention, and the Environment
Arthritis
The Arthritis Foundation
www.arthritis.org

Chronic Fatigue Syndrome
CFIDS Association of America, Inc.
www.cfids.org

Endometriosis
Endometriosis Organization
www.endometriosis.org/

Endometriosis
U.S. Dept. of Health & Human Services
www.4woman.gov/faq/endomet.htm

The Endometriosis Association
www.endometriosisassn.org/

National Institutes of Health–Endometriosis
www.nlm.nih.gov/medlineplus/endometriosis.html

Fibroids
Fibroids
U.S. Dept. of Health & Human Services
www.4woman.gov/FAQ/fibroids.htm

Information on Fibroids
www.fibroids.net

Fibromyalgia
Fibromyalgia Network
www.fmnetnews.com/

Graves' Disease
EndocrineWeb
www.endocrineweb.com/hyper4.html

Heart Disease, Heart Attack, Hypertension, and Stroke
American Heart Association
www.americanheart.org

American Stroke Association
www.strokeassociation.org

Canadian Cardiovascular Society
www.ccs.ca

Hysterectomy and Oophrectomy
Hysterectomy Educational Resources and Services
www.hersfoundation.com/facts.html

Mayo Clinic: Use of Prophylactic Oophorectomy for
Breast Cancer Prevention
   (Provides information on oophorectomy vs. mastectomy for breast cancer prevention.)
www.mayoclinic.com/health/breast-cancer/WO00095

Incontinence
Urinary Incontinence in Women
National Kidney and Urologic Diseases Information
Clearinghouse
National Institutes of Health
*http://kidney.niddk.nih.gov/kudiseases/pubs/uiwomen/
index.htm*

Lupus
Lupus Foundation of America
www.lupus.org/

Microbicides
Alliance for Microbicide Development
www.microbicide.org/

Global Campaign for Microbicides
www.global-campaign.org/

International Partnership for Microbicides
www.ipm-microbicides.org/

Microbicides
World Health Organization
http://www.who.int/hiv/topics/microbicides/microbicides/en/

PCOS
Polycystic Ovarian Syndrome Association
www.psossupport.org

Scleroderma
American College of Rheumatology
www.rheumatology.org/public/factsheets/scler.asp

Sjögren's Syndrome
Sjögren's Syndrome Foundation
www.sjogrens.org

Urinary Track Infections/Disorders and Interstitial Cystitis
Interstitial Cystitis Association
www.ichelp.com

Women and Cancer
Breast Cancer Action
www.bcaction.org/index.html

Dr. Susan Love Research Foundation
  (Provides health information on menopause, hormone replacement therapy and breast cancer).
www.susanlove.md.com

NCCC: National Cervical Cancer Coalition/National HPV Cancer Coalition
  (A grass-roots, nonprofit organization providing women information and resources about cervical cancer and HPV disease.)
www.nccc-online.org/

MAMM: Women, Cancer and Community
  (A magazine providing women with breast and reproductive cancer the latest information on cancer diagnosis, treatment and support.)
www.mamm.com/

National Alliance of Breast Cancer Organizations
  (A non-profit resource providing information and education on breast cancer from over 400 members nationwide.)
www.naboc.org

Silicone and Saline Breast Implant Information for Mastectomy and Breast Reconstruction
www.breastimplantinfo.org/recon_hp.html

Women's Cancer Network
www.wcn.org/

Women's Cancer Information Center
www.womenscancercenter.com/

Women's Cancers Home Page
National Cancer Institute
National Institutes of Health
www.cancer.gov/cancertopics/types/womenscancers

Women's Cancer Research Institute
Cedars-Sinai Women's Cancer Research Institute
www.csmc.edu/7199.html

Women and HIV/AIDS
AVERT.org
www.avert.org/womenstata.htm

AIDS Action
http://aidsaction.org

The Body: The Complete HIV/AIDS Resource
www.thebody.com/index/whatis/women.html

Community HIV/AIDS Mobilization Project
http://champnetwork.org

Fact Sheet on Women and AIDS
Centers for Disease Control and Prevention
www.cdc.gov/hiv/topics/women/resources/factsheets/women.htm

Global AIDS Alliance
http://globalaidsalliance.org

The Global Coalition on Women and AIDS
http://womenandaids.unaids.org/

HIV Infection in Women
U.S. National Institutes of Health
www.niaid.nih.gov/factsheets/womenhiv.htm

HIV Positive: Women and Children
www.hivpositive.com/f-Women/WoChildMenu.html

National AIDS fund
http://aidsfund.org

National AIDS Hotline
Centers for Disease Control and Prevention
www.ashastd.org/nah/index.html

National Center for HIV, Viral Hepatitis, STD, and TB Prevention
Divisions of HIV/AIDS Prevention
www.cdc.gov/hiv

Project Inform
www.projinf.org

UNIFEM—Gender & HIV/AIDS
United Nations Development Fund for Women
www.genderandaids.org

Women & HIV/AIDS
U.S. Dept. of Health & Human Services
www.womenshealth.gov/hiv/

Women's Occupational Health/ Environmental Health

Association of Occupational and Environmental Clinics
www.aoec.org

Center For Health, Environment and Justice
www.chej.org

Women's Environment and Development Organization
www.wedo.org

Committee on Women, Population, and the Environment
http://cwpe.org

COSH: National Council for Occupational Safety and Health
www.coshnetwork.org

Chemical Exposure and Multiple Chemical Sensitivity

Rachel's Environment and Health News, Environmental Research Foundation
www.rachel.org

DES Action
www.desaction.org

Vulvodynia

National Vulvodynia Association
www.nva.org